Textbook of Clinical Pediatrics

Abdelaziz Y. Elzouki

Harb A. Harfi, Hisham M. Nazer, F. Bruder Stapleton, William Oh and Richard J. Whitley (Editors)

Textbook of Clinical Pediatrics

Second Edition

Volume 5

With 990 Figures and 812 Tables

Springer

Editors
Abdelaziz Y. Elzouki
Professor of Pediatrics
Faculty of Medicine
Umm Al-Qura University
Makkah
Saudi Arabia

Harb A. Harfi
Director
National Center of Allergy,
Asthma & Immunology (NCAAI)
Riyadh
Saudi Arabia

Hisham M. Nazer
Consultant Pediatric Gastroenterology & Hepatology
Islamic Hospital
Amman
Jordan

F. Bruder Stapleton
Professor and Chair Department of Pediatrics
Seattle Children's Hospital University of Washington
School of Medicine
Seattle, WA
USA

William Oh
Professor of Pediatrics
Alpert Medical School of Brown University
Woman and Infants Hospital
Providence, RI
USA

Richard J. Whitley
Professor of Pediatrics
University of Alabama
Birmingham, AL
USA

ISBN 978-3-642-02201-2 e-ISBN 978-3-642-02202-9
ISBN (print + eReference) 978-3-642-02203-6
DOI 10.1007/978-3-642-02201-2
Springer Heidelberg Dordrecht London New York

Library of Congress Control Number: 2011931523

First Edition Lippincott Williams & Wilkins 2001

Printed on acid-free paper

Springer is part of Springer Science+Business Media (www.springer.com)

Preface to the Second Edition

I am pleased to present the second edition of the *Textbook of Clinical Pediatrics.* The first edition of this textbook (published in 2001) proved to be both a scientific and a clinical success. Scholarly reviews recommended the book as a primary textbook for residents and medical students and an excellent resource for practicing pediatricians as well as other pediatric health care providers.

The primary goal of the editor of any clinically oriented textbook is to make sure that the text is comprehensive, with updated knowledge, and draws together best practices in practical clinical management. This can be achieved only by utilizing the expertise of those colleagues who have special knowledge and talent in the discipline of pediatrics as a whole and in its various sub-specialties. It is with great pleasure that I welcome along with Harb Harfi and Hisham Nazer, the new co-editors—Dr. Bruder Stapleton (University of Washington School of Medicine), Dr. William Oh (Brown University School of Medicine) and Dr. Richard Whitley (University of Alabama School of Medicine) who have brought in their deep knowledge and practical expertise to harness the best available knowledge in pediatrics. All of us together are also delighted to welcome our very eminent panel of outstanding leaders who performed the role of editing various topical sections on pediatric sub-specialties strengthening them with their specialized knowledge, authority, and experience. The second edition includes an expanded team of 17 new section editors who contribute to a wider coverage and scope of this new edition. We are pleased to welcome our 389 expert contributors from leading medical schools and medical centers around the world who contributed chapters.

This second edition constitutes a major revision, update, and reorganization of the textbook based on systematic reviews of advances in pediatric science and clinical application while retaining the reader- and practitioner-friendly features of the first edition. It is designed to cover contemporary pediatrics totally in logical sequence and with maximum authority. All pediatric sub-specialties are covered and discussed. The textbook's size and number of illustrations have been increased significantly. The scope of this text is wider than most other textbooks of pediatrics—this is deliberate and reflects the growth of knowledge in the field as well as the changing trends in medical practice and education. The contents have therefore been redeveloped to serve as a substantial and comprehensive pediatric text, balanced scientifically and clinically to be a problem- and evidence-based global reference for clinicians.

To this end, many fields have been extensively rewritten, including—genetic disorders, neonatology, infectious diseases, blood diseases, endocrine disorders, cardiology, pediatric oncology, developmental, learning and behavioral disorders, allergic disorders, primary immunodeficiency disorders, respiratory disorders, neurology, kidney and urinary tract disorders, disturbances in acid-base and electrolyte disorders, critical care, rheumatology, pediatric orthopedics, and disorders of the skin. Three new sections have been added on pediatric surgery (intended to help practitioners to benefit from the knowledge and clinical management experience of medically important pediatric surgery problems through the eyes of expert pediatric surgeons), on adolescent medicine (an important new area of knowledge related to the practice of pediatrics), and on drug dosing in pediatrics (providing important reference information to busy practitioners on dosage and value).

A total of 155 new chapters have been added including—principles of genetic testing, treatment of genetic disorders, surfactant replacement therapy, ECMO, neonatal neurology, common procedures in neonatology, ethics and decision making in neonatology, autism spectrum disorders, children in disaster, nutritional modulation of intestinal gene expression, animal and human bites, infection associated with medical devices, Chlamydial infections, Listeria monocytoenes, Mycoplasma infection, Actinomycosis, influenza, 2009 H1N1, rotaviruses and noro-and caliciviruses, innate immune defect, immune dysregulation, cutaneous disorders of neonate, pediatric surgical dermatology, skin barrier management and topical treatment in pediatric dermatology, pain amplification syndromes, autoinflammatory diseases, post-infectious arthritis and related conditions, probiotics in gastrointestinal disorders, capsule endoscopy in childhood, intestinal transplantation in children, mitochondrial hepatopathies and Reye's syndrome, pulmonary complications of the immunocompromised patients, cardiovascular genetics, sudden cardiac death and pre-participation sports screening, secondary cardiac morbidities, noninvasive cardiovascular imaging, interventional cardiology, cardiomyopathies and heart transplantation, acute respiratory failure, mechanical ventilation, and infections in PICU.

In addition there are chapters on the management of snake bites and spider bites, clinical disorders associated with altered potassium metabolism, care of the child refusing blood products, thrombosis, sleep and its disorders in childhood, stroke in children, headache and head pain, pediatric neurorehabilitation and many others.

The textbook places special emphasis on the clinical aspects of various practical pediatric problems. Actual prototype case histories, intended to reinforce the basic principles in clinical management, are presented in sections where it contributes to an enhanced understanding of the subject, such as genetic disorders, inborn errors of metabolism and immunology.

Sections also have been enriched with chapters on clinical scenarios that form the basis for discussion of the relevant clinical problem and are commonly encountered by practitioners and residents, such as anemia, child with recurrent infections, failure to thrive, cough, chest pain, abdominal pain, diarrhea, vomiting, abdominal masses, limping child, heart murmur, metabolic acidosis, metabolic alkalosis, proteinuria, hematuria, and enlarged lymph nodes. These chapters provide an overview of the background for these clinical problems as well as an approach for managing the problem.

Wherever possible, the textbook has based its contents on the best available evidence. The level of evidence preferred is the systematic review of randomized control trials. It is the editors' earnest hope that these efforts provide for a significant enhancement of the management and care for sick children around the world.

On a personal note, I would also like to add for those interested, a short history of the development of this work. It was several years ago in Benghazi (Libya), my home town, where I thought to edit a textbook that would cover new ground clinically and yet be of global relevance. Dr. Hassan Majeed was the first person who accepted the idea and gave his guidance and support. Dr. Ahmad Teebi contributed to the first edition as section editor for genetic disorders. Both were inspiring teachers with unique clinical competence (Majeed syndrome, Teebi syndrome). It is sad that both these giants of clinical pediatrics passed away in 2010. Majeed and Teebi will not be forgotten and will be missed by all who were inspired by them to work with children.

The editors and I also thank the staff at Springer who did a great job to ensure the best major reference work possible. Particularly, Sandra Fabiani, Anil Chandy, and Sunali Mull from Springer's major reference work division as well as Marion Kraemer and Sverre Klempe from the Clinical Medicine editorial division.

For this new edition, I also appreciate and acknowledge the support of the Faculty of Medicine, Umm Al-Qura University.

The editors and I like to dedicate this textbook to our contributors and section editors. It is their book and it is their work that has given our textbook its strength and authority.

September 2011

Abdelaziz Y. Elzouki
Makkah, Saudi Arabia

Preface to the First Edition

It is with great pleasure, that we launch the first edition of the *Textbook of Clinical Pediatrics.* The textbook went through several stages of ideas, development, design, writing, revision, editing and extensive critical review by authorities in their field before it was submitted for publication. All the above stages demanded a great amount of effort. The aim was to produce a textbook that has both a global appeal and interest and would help practicing pediatricians, pediatric residents and family practitioners to manage sick children in a practical way, but on a sound scientific basis. The textbook is also intended to help pediatricians in training who are preparing for board or membership examinations and to function as a desk reference with updated information for practicing physicians and pediatricians. Our aim was also to develop a textbook that covers in some detail prevalent childhood diseases. In doing so, we are privileged to acknowledge the contribution of over 100 distinguished pediatricians and scientists from 34 well-known medical schools, major hospitals and health centers from five continents. Therefore, this textbook is enriched with international experience in childhood health care.

Almost all pediatric subspecialties are well covered in this textbook, including blood diseases, neoplastic disorders, infectious diseases, respiratory disorders, allergic disorders, immunodeficiency disorders, inborn metabolic disorders, rheumatic disorders, cardiovascular disorders, diseases of the kidney and urinary tract, nutritional disorders, neonatology, endocrinology, oral and craniofacial disorders, gastrointestinal and liver disorders, neurological disorders, skin diseases, orthopedic, otolaryngology, ophthalmological disorders, pediatric poisoning, critical care, burns, acid base and electrolytes disturbance. The textbook puts special emphasis on the clinical aspects of various practical pediatric problems. Prototype actual case histories, to enforce the basic principles in clinical management, are presented in sections where we think it will make the subject more understandable, such as in inborn errors of metabolism and immunology. Some sections also have been enriched with a chapter on a clinical scenario that forms the basis for discussion of relevant clinical problems. For example, in the hematology section, there is a chapter on approach to a child with anemia; in the kidney and urinary tract disorders section there is a chapter on clinical approach to a child with urinary tract obstruction; in the section on malignant and neoplastic disorders, there is a chapter on clinical approach to a child with abdominal mass, and lymph node enlargement; in the immunology section, there is a chapter on approach to a child with recurrent infection; and in the genetic section, there is a chapter on approach to the child with dyamorphic features.

We would like to dedicate this textbook to all those who contributed to it either directly, such as our contributors, section leaders and supportive staff, or indirectly by being supportive and patient during the preparation, writing and editing of this text, including our families and colleagues. Special appreciation is due to the staff of Lippincott Williams & Wilkins who took a keen interest and labored to ensure the best book possible. We particularly thank Ellen DiFrancesco and James D. Ryan, Vice President of Lippincott Williams & Wilkins.

We wish to give a special mention and acknowledgment to King Khalid Foundation, Saudi Arabia for their generous contribution and support.

Abdelaziz Y. Elzouki
Harb A. Harfi
Hisham M. Nazer

Editor

Abdelaziz Y. Elzouki
Professor of Pediatrics
Faculty of Medicine
Umm Al-Qura University
Makkah
Saudi Arabia

Co-Editors

Harb A. Harfi
Director
National Center of Allergy,
Asthma & Immunology (NCAAI)
Riyadh
Saudi Arabia

Hisham M. Nazer
Consultant Pediatric Gastroenterology & Hepatology
Islamic Hospital
Amman
Jordan

F. Bruder Stapleton
Professor and Chair Department of Pediatrics
Seattle Children's Hospital University of Washington
School of Medicine
Seattle, WA
USA

William Oh
Professor of Pediatrics
Alpert Medical School of Brown University
Woman and Infants Hospital
Providence, RI
USA

Richard J. Whitley
Professor of Pediatrics
University of Alabama
Birmingham, AL
USA

Section Editors

Abdul-Rahman M. Abu-Taleb
Department of Pediatrics
King Saud Bin Abdulaziz University for Health Sciences – National Guard Health Affairs
Western Region
Jeddah
Saudi Arabia
Section: Critical Care

Mohamed O. Abuzeid
Department of Otolaryngology Head and Neck Surgery
King Faisal Specialist Hospital and Research Centre
Riyadh
Saudi Arabia
Section: Pediatric Otolaryngology

Khaled Al Haidari
Scientific Board of Pharmacy
Saudi Commission for Health Specialties
Riyadh
Saudi Arabia
Section: Pediatric Poisoning

Selwa A. F. Al-Hazzaa
Department of Ophthalmology
King Faisal Specialist Hospital and Research Centre
Riyadh
Saudi Arabia
Section: Pediatric Ophthalmology

Nada S. Al-Qadheeb
Division of Pharmacy Services
King Faisal Specialist Hospital and Research Centre
Riyadh
Saudi Arabia
Section: Pediatric Poisoning

Peter N. Cox
Department of Critical Care Medicine
Hospital for Sick Children
Toronto, ON
Canada
Section: Critical Care

J. Burton Douglass
Cumberland Gap Orthodontics, Inc.
Harrogate, TN
USA
Section: Oral and Craniofacial Disorders

Craig P. Eberson
Division of Pediatric Orthopedics
Alpert Medical School of Brown University
Providence, RI
USA
Section: Pediatric Orthopedics

Generoso G. Gascon
RHCI for Children
Forestdale, MA
USA
Section: Neurology

Gabriel G. Haddad
Divisions of Respiratory Medicine and Neurosciences
Department of Pediatrics
University of California San Diego
Rady Children's Hospital San Diego
San Diego, CA
USA
Section: Respiratory Disorders

Harb A. Harfi
Director
National Center of Allergy, Asthma & Immunology (NCAAI)
Riyadh
Saudi Arabia
Sections: Allergic Disorders
Primary Immunodeficiency Disorders

Fuad K. Hashem
Department of Surgery
King Faisel Specialist Hospital and Research Center
Riyadh
Saudi Arabia
Section: Pediatric Burns

Pamela High
Developmental, Learning and Behavioral Disorders
The Warren Alpert Medical School of Brown University
Providence, RI
USA
Section: Developmental, Learning and Behavioral Disorders

Khalid Hussain
The London Centre for Paediatric Endocrinology and Metabolism
Hospital for Children NHS Trust
London
UK
Section: Endocrine Disorders

Martin Keszler
Department of Pediatrics
Women and Infants Hospital,
Warren Alpert Medical School
Brown University
Providence, RI
USA
Section: Neonatology

Bruce R. Korf
Department of Genetics
University of Alabama
Birmingham, AL
USA
Section: Genetic Disorders

Mark B. Lewin
Heart Center
Seattle Children's Hospital
Seattle, WA
USA
Section: Cardiology

Alberto Martini
Department of Pediatrics
University of Genoa
Pediatria II e Reumatologia Istituto G. Gaslini
Genoa
Italy
Section: Rheumatology

Hisham M. Nazer
Consultant Pediatric Gastroenterology & Hepatology
Islamic Hospital
Amman
Jordon
Sections: Gastrointestinal and Liver Disorders
Pediatric Nutrition

Stacy Nicholson
Department of Pediatrics
Division of Pediatric Hematology/Oncology
Oregon Health & Science University
Portland, OR
USA
Section: Pediatric Oncology

Pinar T. Ozand
Department of Pediatrics and Department of Biological and Medical Research
King Faisal Specialist Hospital and Research Centre
Riyadh
Saudi Arabia
Section: Inborn Errors of Metabolism

Kristine A. Parbuoni
Department of Pharmacy Services
University of Maryland Medical Center
Baltimore, MD
USA
Section: Drug Dosing in Pediatrics

Michael Recht
Division of Pediatric Hematology-Oncology
Oregon Health and Science University
Portland, OR
USA
Section: Blood Diseases

Zbigniew Ruszczak
Division of Dermatology
Department of Medicine
Institute of Medicine
Sheikh Khalifa Medical City
Abu Dhabi
UAE
Section: Disorders of the Skin

F. Bruder Stapleton
Department of Pediatrics
Seattle Children's Hospital University of
Washington School of Medicine
Seattle, WA
USA
Sections: Disturbances in Acid - base and Electrolytes Disorders
Kidney and Urinary Tract Disorders

Thomas F. Tracy
Department of Surgery
Alpert Medical School Brown University
Providence, RI
USA
Section: Pediatric Surgery

Leslie R. Walker
Division of Adolescent Medicine
Department of Pediatrics
Children's Hospital and Regional Medical Center
University of Washington
Seattle, WA
USA
Section: Adolescent Medicine

Richard J. Whitley
Professor of Pediatrics
University of Alabama
Birmingham, AL
USA
Section: Infectious Diseases

Yvette E. Yatchmink
Pediatric Developmental Behavioral Health
Providence, RI
USA
Section: Developmental, Learning and Behavioral Disorders

List of Contributors

Shaden Abdel Hadi
Division of Dermatology
Institute of Medicine
Sheikh Khalifa Medical City
Abu Dhabi
UAE

Ruba A. Abdelhadi
Department of Pediatrics and Communicable
Diseases, Pediatric Gastroenterology
University of Michigan Medical School
C. S. Mott Children's Hospital
Ann Arbor, MI
USA

Asaad M. A. Abdullah Assiri
Head Division, Paediatric Gastroenterology, Hepatology
& Nutrition
King Khalid University Hospital
King Saud University
Riyadh
Saudi Arabia

Anisha Abraham
Department of Pediatrics, Adolescent Medicine
Georgetown University School of Medicine
Washington, DC
USA

Kabir M. Abubakar
Division of Neonatology
Georgetown University Children's Medical Center
Washington, DC
USA

Abdul-Rahman M. Abu-Taleb
Department of Pediatrics
King Saud Bin Abdulaziz University for Health Sciences –
National Guard Health Affairs
Western Region
Jeddah
Saudi Arabia

Mohamed O. Abuzeid
Department of Otolaryngology Head and Neck Surgery
King Faisal Specialist Hospital and Research Centre
Riyadh
Saudi Arabia

William P. Adelman
Walter Reed Army Medical Center and National
Naval Medical Center
Uniformed Services University of the Health Sciences
Bethesda, MD
USA

Adetunji Adeyokunnu
Department of Pediatrics
King Fahad National Guard Hospital
Riyadh
Saudi Arabia

H. Hesham A-Kader
Division of Gastroenterology, Hepatology and Nutrition
College of Medicine
University of Arizona
Tucson, AZ
USA
and
Department of Pediatrics
College of Medicine
University of Arizona
Tucson, AZ
USA

Kathryn Akong
University of California, San Diego
Rady Children's Hospital of San Diego
San Diego, CA
USA

Tekin Akpolat
Department of Nephrology
Ondokuz Mayis University
School of Medicine
Samsun
Turkey

Sulaiman Al Alola
Department of Pediatrics
King Fahad National Guard Hospital
Riyadh
Saudi Arabia

Roaa Al Gain
Pharmacy Division
King Faisal Specialist Hospital & Research Centre
Riyadh
Saudi Arabia

M. M. Al Qattan
Department of Surgery
King Saud University
Riyadh
Saudi Arabia

Manal Alasnag
Pediatric Intensive Care Unit/King Fahd Armed Forces Hospital
Jeddah, KSA
Saudi Arabia

Zaina H. Albalawi
Department of Internal Medicine
University of Alberta
Edmonton, AB
Canada

Assunta Albanese
Paediatric Endocrine Unit
St George's Hospital
London
UK

J. Elaine-Marie Albert
Division of Pediatric Critical Care Medicine
Seattle Children's Hospital
University of Washington School of Medicine
(J.E.A. and H.E.J.)
Seattle, WA
USA

Youssef A. Al-Eissa
Department of Pediatrics
College of Medicine
King Saud bin Abdulaziz
University for Health Sciences
Riyadh
Saudi Arabia

Mohammed Al-Essa
Department of Biological and Medical Research
King Faisal Specialist Hospital and Research Centre
Riyadh
Saudi Arabia

Khaled M. Al-Haidari
Scientific Board of Pharmacy
Saudi Commission for Health Specialties
Riyadh
Saudi Arabia

Sami Al-Hajjar
Department of Pediatrics
King Faisal Specialist Hospital & Research Centre
Riyadh
Saudi Arabia
and
Department of Pathology and Laboratories
King Faisal Specialist Hospital & Research Center
Riyadh
Saudi Arabia

Selwa A. F. Al-Hazzaa
Department of Ophthalmology
King Faisal Specialist Hospital and Research Centre
Riyadh
Saudi Arabia

Rana AlMaghrabi
Department of Pediatrics
King Faisal Specialist Hospital & Research Centre
Riyadh
Saudi Arabia

Fadheela Al-Mahroos
College of Medicine and Medical Sciences
Arabian Gulf University
Manama
Bahrain

Saleh Al-Muhsen
Pediatric Allergy and Immunology
Department of Pediatrics
King Faisal Specialist Hospital and Research Centre
Riyadh
Saudi Arabia

Mohammad Almutawa
Medical School Division of Internal Medicine
Kuwait University
Aljabria
Kuwait

Abdallah Al-Nasser
King Fahad National Centre for Children's Cancer
King Faisal Specialist Hospital & Research Centre
Riyadh
Saudi Arabia

Nada S. Al-Qadheeb
Division of Pharmacy Services
King Faisal Specialist Hospital and Research Centre
Riyadh
Saudi Arabia

Soud A. Al-Rasheed
Pediatrics
King Saud bin Abdulaziz
University for Health Sciences
Riyadh
Saudi Arabia

Mohammad Al-Shaalan
Department of Pediatrics
King Soud bin Abdulaziz
University for Health Sciences
Riyadh
Saudi Arabia

Jeffrey Alten
Division of Pediatric Critical Care
University of Alabama at Birmingham
Birmingham, AL
USA

Asa'd Al-Toonsi
Department of Pediatrics
King Faisal Specialist Hospital and Research Centre
Riyadh
Saudi Arabia
and
Saudi Board Program
Maternity Children Hospital
Makkah
Saudi Arabia

Mercedes C. Amado
Section of Allergy, Asthma & Immunology
The Children's Mercy Hospitals & Clinics
University of Missouri-Kansas
City School of Medicine
Kansas City, MO
USA

Kyle Anderson
Dermatology and Plastic Surgery Institute
Cleveland Clinic
Cleveland, OH
USA

Kathleen Angkustsiri
Department of Pediatrics
UC Davis Children's Hospital and UC Davis MIND Institute
Sacramento, CA
USA

Ronen Arnon
Department of Pediatrics
Mount Sinai Kravis Children's Hospital
Mount Sinai School of Medicine
New York, NY
USA

Stephen Ashwal
Department of Pediatrics
Loma Linda University School of Medicine
Loma Linda, CA
USA

Farahnak Assadi
Professor of Pediatrics, Director, Section of Nephrology
Rush Children's Hospital
Rush University Medical Center
Chicago, Illinois
USA

Tadej Avčin
Department of Allergology, Rheumatology and Clinical Immunology
University Children's Hospital Ljubljana
University Medical Center
Ljubljana
Slovenia

Yasser Awaad
King Fahad Medical City
Riyadh
Saudi Arabia

Kenneth S. Azarow
Children's Hospital Omaha
University of Nebraska
Omaha, NE
USA

Sakra S. Balhareth
Pharmacy Services Division
King Faisal Specialist Hospital and Research Center
Riyadh
Saudi Arabia

Mark Ballow
Division of Pediatric Allergy and Immunology
Department of Pediatrics
Women and Children's Hospital of Buffalo
Buffalo, NY
USA

Robert S. Baltimore
Department of Pediatrics
Yale University School of Medicine
Associate Hospital Epidemiologist
For Pediatrics Yale-New Haven Hospital
New Haven, CT
USA

Hany Banoub
Queen Mary's Hospital for Children
Epsom & St. Helier University Hospitals NHS Trust
Carshalton, Surrey
UK

Dinesh Banur
Queen Mary's Hospital for Children,
Epsom St Helier University NHS Trust
Carshalton, Surrey
UK

Keith J. Barrington
Department of Pediatrics
University of Montreal
Sainte-Justine Hospital
Montreal, Quebec
Canada

Cristina Basso
Cardiovascular Pathology
Department of Medical-Diagnostic Sciences
University of Padua
Padua
Italy

Asim Belgaumi
King Fahad National Centre for Children's Cancer
King Faisal Specialist Hospital & Research Centre
Riyadh
Saudi Arabia

Alexandre Belot
Unit of Pediatric Nephrology and Rheumatology
Femme Mère Enfant Hospital, Lyon 1 University
Lyon
France

Fabrizio de Benedetti
Direzione Scientifica
IRCCS Ospedale Pediatrico Bambino Gesù
Rome
Italy

Henry Berman
Adolescent Medicine
Seattle Children's Hospital, M/S: W-7831
Seattle, WA
USA

Jorge A. Bezerra
Pediatric Liver Care Center and Division of Pediatric Gastroenterology, Hepatology, and Nutrition of Cincinnati Children's Hospital Medical Center and the Department of Pediatrics
University of Cincinnati
Cincinnati, OH
USA

Ibrahim Bin-Hussain
Department of Pediatrics
King Faisal Specialist Hospital & Research Centre
Riyadh
Saudi Arabia

Michael S. Blaiss
College of Medicine
University of Tennessee Health Science Center
Germantown, TN
USA

Gregory Blaschke
Department of Pediatrics
Oregon Health & Science University
Portland, OR
USA

Joseph M. Bliss
Department of Pediatrics
Women & Infants Hospital of Rhode Island
The Warren Alpert Medical School of Brown University
Providence, RI
USA

Suresh B. Boppana
Department of Pediatrics
University of Alabama School of Medicine
Birmingham, AL
USA

Lynn Boshkov
Medicine & Pediatrics
Oregon Health & Science University
Portland, OR
USA

Mahmoud Bozo
Pediatric Gastroenterology and Nutrition
Damascus Hospital
Damascus
Syria

Heather Bradeen
Department of Pediatrics
University of Vermont
Burlington, VT
USA

Brian R. Branchford
The Children's Hospital Denver
Center for Cancer and Blood Disorders
Aurora, CO
USA

David J. Breland
Adolescent Medicine
Seattle Children's Hospital M/S: W-7831
University of Washington
Seattle, WA
USA

Cora Collette Breuner
Division of Adolescent Medicine
Department of Pediatrics
Orthopedics and Sports Medicine
Seattle Children's Hospital, M/S: W-7831
Seattle, WA
USA

Nicola A. Bridges
Chelsea and Westminster Hospital
NHS Foundation Trust
London
UK

Vivian Brown
Walgreens
Sequim, WA
USA

William D. Brown
Department of Clinical Neuroscience
Brown University
Seekonk, MA
USA

Khalid K. Bshesh
Cardiovascular Department
Pediatric Intensive Care Unit/King Faisal Specialist
Hospital and Research Center
Jeddah, KSA
Saudi Arabia

Rubén Burgos-Vargas
Department of Rheumatology
Hospital General de México Universidad Nacional
Autónoma de México
México, DF
Mexico

Tyler Burpee
Division of Gastroenterology, Hepatology and Nutrition
Seattle Children's Hospital
Seattle, WA
USA

Gale R. Burstein
Department of Pediatrics
Division of Adolescent Medicine
State University of New York at Buffalo School of Medicine and Biomedical Sciences
Buffalo, NY
USA

Karen Buysse
Center for Medical Genetics
Ghent University Hospital
Ghent
Belgium

William J. Cashore
Department of Pediatrics
Women & Infants Hospital of Rhode Island
Providence, RI
USA

Bill H. Chang
Pediatric Hematology & Oncology
Doernbecher Children's Hospital
Oregon Health & Science University
Portland, OR
USA

Eugenia Chang
St. Luke's Mountain States Tumor and Medical Research Institute
Boise, ID
USA
and
Department of Pediatrics
University of Utah
SLC, UT
USA

Margaret A. Chen
PreventionGenetics
Marshfield, WI
USA

Ravi Chetan
Endocrinology & Diabetes
Southend University Hospital
London
UK

Robert L. Chevalier
Department of Pediatrics
School of Medicine
University of Virginia Health System
Charlottesville, VA
USA

Edward Chien
Division of Maternal-Fetal Medicine
Department of Obstetrics and Gynecology
Women and Infants' Hospital of Brown University
Providence, RI
USA

Tanuja Chitnis
Partners Pediatric Multiple Sclerosis Center
Department of Pediatric Neurology
Massachusetts General Hospital for Children
Boston, MA
USA

Sonny K. F. Chong
Queen Mary's Hospital for Children
Epsom & St. Helier University Hospitals NHS Trust
Carshalton, Surrey
UK
and
St. George's Hospital Medical School
London
UK

Nadine F. Choueiter
Division of Pediatrics
University of Washington
Seattle, WA
USA

Thomas H. Chun
Departments of Emergency Medicine and Pediatrics
Department of Pediatric Emergency Medicine
The Alpert Medical School of Brown University
Providence, RI
USA

Terrence U. H. Chun
Heart Center
University of Washington School of Medicine
Seattle Children's Hospital
Seattle, WA
USA

Christina E. Ciaccio
Section of Allergy, Asthma & Immunology
The Children's Mercy Hospitals & Clinics
University of Missouri-Kansas City School of Medicine
Kansas City, MO
USA

Rachel Clingenpeel
Child Protection Program
Department of Pediatrics
Warren Alpert Medical School of Brown University
Providence, RI
USA

Pierre Cochat
Centre de référence des maladies rénales rares &
Inserm U820
Hospices Civils de Lyon & Université de Lyon
Lyon
France
and
Service de pédiatrie
Hôpital Femme Mère Enfant
Bron cedex
France

Gordon Cohen
Heart Center
Seattle Children's Hospital
Seattle, WA
USA

Jeffrey A. Conwell
Division of Pediatric Cardiology, Heart Center
University of Washington School of Medicine
Seattle Children's Hospital
Seattle, WA
USA

Rosanna Coppo
Nephrology, Dialysis and Transplantation Unit
Regina Margherita University Children's Hospital
Turin
Italy

Domenico Corrado
Division of Cardiology
Department of Cardiac, Thoracic and Vascular Sciences
University of Padua Medical School
Padova
Italy

Paula Costanzo
Division of Respiratory Medicine
Rady Children's Hospital of San Diego
San Diego, CA
USA

Robert A. Cowles
Morgan Stanley Children's Hospital of
NewYork-Presbyterian
Columbia University Medical Center
New York, NY
USA

Peter N. Cox
Department of Critical Care Medicine
Hospital for Sick Children
Toronto, ON
Canada

Mara G. Coyle
Department of Pediatrics
Alpert Medical School of Brown University
Providence, RI
USA
and
Department of Pediatrics
Brown Medical School Women & Infants Hospital
Providence, RI
USA

T. Coyne-Beasley
Division of General Pediatrics and Adolescent Medicine
University of North Carolina
Chapel Hill, NC
USA

Amanda W. Dale-Shall
Department of Pediatrics
Division of Nephrology and Hypertension
Levine Children's Hospital at Carolinas Medical Center
Charlotte, NC
USA

Peter Davis
The Royal Women's Hospital
Melborne, VIC
Australia

Meghan Delaney
Puget Sound Blood Center
Seattle, WA
USA

Thomas G. DeLoughery
Division of Hematology/Medical Oncology
Department of Medicine and Division of
Laboratory Medicine
Department of Pathology, Hematology L586
Oregon Health Sciences University
Portland, OR
USA

Penelope H. Dennehy
Division of Pediatric Infectious Diseases
Department of Pediatrics
Hasbro Children's Hospital
The Alpert Medical School of Brown University
Providence, RI
USA

Meena P. Desai
Sir Hurkisondas Nurrotumdas Hospital &
Research Centre
Mumbai
India

Maria Descartes
Department of Genetics
University of Alabama
Birmingham, AL
USA

Shireesha Dhanireddy
Division of Allergy & Infectious Diseases
University of Washington
Seattle, WA
USA

Alicia Dixon Docter
Department of Family and Child Nursing
Seattle Children's Hospital M/S: W-3726
University of Washington
Seattle, WA
USA

William K. Dolen
Department of Pediatrics
Division of Allergy-Immunology and Rheumatology
Medical College of Georgia at the Georgia Health
Sciences University
Augusta, GA
USA

Tavey Dorofaeff
Royal Children's Hospital
Herston, Brisbane
Australia

Ami Doshi
Division of Hospital Medicine
Department of Pediatrics
University of California San Diego
Rady Children's Hospital
San Diego, CA
USA

J. Burton Douglass
Cumberland Gap Orthodontics, Inc.
Harrogate, TN
USA

Craig P. Eberson
Department of Orthopaedics
Warren Alpert School of Medicine Brown University
Providence, RI
USA

Burhan Edrees
Umm Al-Qura University
Makkah
Saudi Arabia

Jochen H. H. Ehrich
Department of Pediatric Kidney, Liver and
Metabolic Diseases
Children's Hospital
Hannover Medical School
Hannover
Germany

Mohammad El Baba
Division of Pediatric Gastroenterology
Wayne State University School of Medicine
Children's Hospital of Michigan
Detroit, MI
USA

Mohamed A. El Guindi
Hepatology, and Nutrition, National Liver Institute
Menoufiya University
Cairo
Egypt

Mohammad I. El Mouzan
Department of Pediatrics (gastroenterology)
College of Medicine & King Khaled University Hospital
King Saud University
Riyadh
Saudi Arabia

Hassan El Solh
King Fahad National Centre for Children's Cancer
King Faisal Specialist Hospital & Research Centre
Riyadh
Saudi Arabia

Mohammed El-Bali
Department of Medical Parasitology
Umm Al-Qura University
Makkah
Saudi Arabia

Afif El-Khuffash
Department of Neonatology
Hospital for Sick Children
Toronto, ON
Canada

Mortada El-Shabrawi
Department of Pediatrics
Cairo University
Mohandesseen, Cairo
Egypt

Abdelaziz Y. Elzouki
Faculty of Medicine
Umm Al-Qura University
Makkah
Saudi Arabia

Ilgi O. Ertem
Department of Pediatrics
Developmental-Behavioral Pediatrics Unit
Ankara University School of Medicine
Ankara
Turkey

Yolanda Evans
Adolescent Medicine, General Pediatrics
Seattle Children's Hospital, M/S: W-7831
Seattle, WA
USA

Melanie D. Everitt
Division of Pediatric Cardiology
University of Utah
Salt Lake City, UT
USA

Paul D. Fadale
Warren Alpert Medical School of Brown University/
Rhode Island Hospital
Providence, RI
USA

Leonard G. Feld
Department of Pediatrics
Levine Children's Hospital at Carolinas Medical Center
Charlotte, NC
USA

Heidi M. Feldman
Department of Pediatrics
Stanford University School of Medicine
Palo Alto, CA
USA
and
Department of Pediatrics
Stanford University School of Medicine
Stanford, CA
USA

Philip R. Fischer
Department of Pediatric and Adolescent Medicine
Mayo Clinic
Rochester, MN
USA

Peter G. Fitzgibbons
Department of Orthopedics
Warren Alpert Medical School of Brown University
Providence, RI
USA

Thomas A. Fleisher
Department of Laboratory Medicine
NIH Clinical Center
National Institutes of Health
Bethesda, MD
USA

Veronica H. Flood
Department of Pediatrics
Medical College of Wisconsin
Milwaukee, WI
USA

Joseph T. Flynn
Division of Nephrology
Seattle Children's Hospital
Seattle, Washington, DC
USA

John W. Foreman
Department of Pediatrics
Duke University Medical Center
Durham, NC
USA

John R. Fowler
Department of Orthopaedics
Temple University Hospital
Philadelphia, PA
USA

Doris Franke
Department of Pediatric Kidney, Liver and Metabolic Diseases
Children's Hospital
Hannover Medical School
Hannover
Germany

Aaron Friedman
Medical School Dean's Office
University of Minnesota
Minneapolis, MN
USA

John N. Gaitanis
Division of Biology and Medicine
The Warren Alpert School of Medicine at Brown University
Hasbro Children's Hospital
Providence, RI
USA

Christopher Gasbarre
Dermatology and Plastic Surgery Institute, Cleveland Clinic
Cleveland, OH
USA

Generoso G. Gascon
RHCI for Children
Forestdale, MA
USA

Marco Gattorno
UO Pediatria II (2nd Division of Pediatrics)
G. Gaslini Scientific Institute for Children
Genoa
Italy

Nicole Gebran
Department of Pharmacy Services
Tawam Hospital
Al Ain, Abu Dhabi
UAE

Fayez K. Ghishan
Department of Pediatrics
Steele Children's Research Center
University of Arizona
Tucson, AZ
USA
and
Department of Pediatrics
College of Medicine University of Arizona
Tucson, AZ
USA

Ann Giesel
Pediatrics, Adolescent Medicine
Seattle Children's Hospital M/S: W-7831
Seattle, WA
USA

Mark A. Gilger
Pediatric Gastroenterology, Hepatology & Nutrition,
Baylor College of Medicine
Texas Children's Hospital
Houston, TX
USA

Mary Margaret Gleason
Tulane University School of Medicine
New Orleans, LA
USA

Jason Glover
Pediatric Hematology & Oncology
Doernbecher Children's Hospital, Oregon Health & Science University
Portland, OR
USA

Neil A. Goldenberg
Department of Hematology
The Children's Hospital-Denver and University of Colorado Hemophila and Thrombosis Center
Aurora, CO
USA

Allan M. Goldstein
Department of Pediatric Surgery
Massachusetts General Hospital
Harvard Medical School
Boston, MA
USA

Harald P. M. Gollnick
Department of Dermatology & Venereology
Otto-von-Guericke University
Magdeburg
Germany

Marah Gotcsik
Department of Pediatrics
University of Washington
Seattle, WA
USA

Phillip W. Graham
Behavioral Health and Criminal Justice Division
RTI International
NC
USA

Daniel Greenberg
Oregon Health Sciences University
Portland, OR
USA

Elke Griesmaier
Department of Pediatrics IV, Neonatology, Neuropaediatrics and Metabolic Diseases
Medical University Innsbruck
Innsbruck
Austria

Erica R. Gross
Division of Pediatric Surgery
Morgan Stanley Children's Hospital
New York-Presbyterian
Columbia University
New York, NY
USA

Linda S. Grossman
Baltimore County Department of Health
Baltimore, MD
USA

James T. Guille
Division of Pediatrics Orthopaedics
Brandywine Orthopaedics
Pottstown, PA
USA

Michelle Gurvitz
Department of Cardiology/BACH
Children's Hospital Boston
Boston, MA
USA

Robin H. Gurwitch
National Center for School Crisis and Bereavement
Division of Developmental and Behavioral Pediatrics
Cincinnati Children's Hospital Medical Center
Cincinnati, OH
USA

Generoso Gutierrez-Gascón
Pediatric Neurology Unit
Department of Neurology
Massachusetts General Hospital
Boston, MA
USA

Raúl Gutiérrez-Suárez
Department of Rheumatology
Hospital General de México
México DF
México

Gabriel G. Haddad
Divisions of Respiratory Medicine and Neurosciences
Department of Pediatrics
University of California San Diego
Rady Children's Hospital San Diego
San Diego, CA
USA

Issam M. Halabi
Department of Pediatrics
University of Illinois
College of Medicine
Peoria, IL
USA

Kristina M. Haley
Pediatric Hematology/Oncology
Oregon Health & Science University
Portland, OR
USA

Margaret R. Hammerschlag
Division of Infectious Diseases
Department of Pediatrics
State University of New York Downstate Medical Center
Brooklyn, NY
USA

Abdel-Hai Hammo
Department of Pediatrics
Tufts University Brockton Hospital
Brockton, MA
USA

Eckart Haneke
Dermatology Practice
Dermaticum
Freiburg
Germany
and
Department of Dermatology
University of Berne
Inselspital
Switzerland
and
Centro de Dermatología
Inst CUF
Porto
Portugal
and
Department of Dermatology
Acad Hosp, University of Ghent
Belgium

Coral D. Hanevold
Division of Pediatric Nephrology
University of Washington School of Medicine Seattle
Children's Hospital
Seattle, WA
USA

Robin L. Hansen
Department of Pediatrics
UC Davis Children's Hospital and UC Davis MIND
Institute
Sacramento, CA
USA

Bruce G. Hardy
Division of Pediatric Cardiology
University of Washington School of Medicine
Seattle, WA
USA

Harb A. Harfi
National Center of Allergy, Asthma
and Immunology (NCAAI)
Riyadh
Saudi Arabia

Fuad Hashem
Department of Surgery
King Faisel Specialist Hospital and Research Center
Riyadh
Saudi Arabia

Fetouh Hassanin
Misr International University
Cairo
Egypt

Kirsten Hawkins
Department of Pediatrics, Adolescent Medicine
Georgetown University School of Medicine
Washington, DC
USA

Elise M. Herro
Division of Dermatology
University of California
San Diego - Rady Children's Hospital
San Diego, CA
USA

Geoffrey Heyer
Division of Child Neurology
Ohio State College of Medicine
Columbus, OH
USA

Rosemary D. Higgins
Pregnancy and Perinatology Branch, Center for Developmental Biology and Perinatal Medicine
Eunice Kennedy Shriver National Institute of Child Health and Human Development, National Institutes of Health
Bethesda, MD
USA

Pamela High
Developmental and Behavioral Pediatrics
The Warren Alpert Medical School of Brown University
Providence, RI
USA

Omar M. Hijazi
Division of Pediatric Cardiac ICU
Department of Cardiac Sciences
King Abdul Aziz Cardiac Center
King Abdul Aziz Medical City
King Fahad National Guard Hospital
Riyadh
Saudi Arabia

Yamini Jagannath Howe
Developmental and Behavioral Pediatrics
The Warren Alpert Medical School of Brown University
Providence, RI
USA

Peter F. Hoyer
Department of Pediatric Nephrology
University Children's Hospital
Essen
Germany

Taosheng Huang
Department of Pediatrics
University of California
Irvine, CA
USA

Michael J. Hulstyn
Warren Alpert Medical School of Brown University/
Rhode Island Hospital
Providence, RI
USA

Khalid Hussain
The London Centre for Paediatric Endocrinology and Metabolism
Great Ormond Street Hospital for Children NHS Trust
London
UK
and
Developmental Endocrinology Research Group
Molecular Genetics Unit
Institute of Child Health
University College London
London
UK

Jeffrey W. Hutchinson
Department of Adolescent Medicine
National Naval Medical Center and Walter Reed Army Medical Center
Uniformed Services University
Bethesda, MD
USA

Donna Huynh
University of Maryland School of Pharmacy
Baltimore, MD
USA

Lisa F. Imundo
Department of Pediatrics
Columbia University Medical Center
New York, NY
USA

Natascia Di Iorgi
Department of Pediatrics, IRCCS
Giannina Gaslini - University of Genova
Genova
Italy

Michael B. Ishitani
Division of Pediatric Surgery
Mayo Clinic and Foundation
Rochester, MN
USA

Sharon E. Jacob
Department of Dermatology and Cutaneous Surgery
University of California
San Diego - Rady Children's Hospital
San Diego, CA
USA

Richard F. Jacobs
Department of Pediatrics
University of Arkansas for Medical Sciences College of Medicine
Little Rock, AR
USA

Chela James
The London Centre for Paediatric Endocrinology and Metabolism
Great Ormond Street Hospital for Children NHS Trust
WC1N 3JH and the Institute of Child Health University College
London
UK

Annie Janvier
Department of Pediatrics and Clinical Ethics
Sainte-Justine Hospital
University of Montreal
Montreal, Quebec
Canada

Howard E. Jeffries
Division of Pediatric Critical Care Medicine
Seattle Children's Hospital
University of Washington School of Medicine
(J.E.A. and H.E.J.)
Seattle, WA
USA

Troy A. Johnston
Heart Center
University of Washington/Seattle Children's Hospital
Seattle, WA
USA

Deborah P. Jones
University of Tennessee Health Science Center
Children's Foundation Research Center at Le Bonheur Children's Medical Center
Memphis, TN
USA

Suliman Al Jumaah
Department of Pediatrics, MBC 58
King Faisal Specialist Hospital and Research Centre
Riyadh
Saudi Arabia

Tara Karamlou
Heart Center
Seattle Children's Hospital
Seattle, WA
USA

Clifford E. Kashtan
Department of Pediatrics
Division of Pediatric Nephrology
University of Minnesota Medical School
Minneapolis, MN
USA

Laura Kastner
Department of Psychiatry & Behavioral Sciences
School of Medicine
University of Washington
Seattle, WA
USA

Julia A. Katarincic
Department of Orthopedic Surgery
Warren Alpert Medical School Brown University
Providence, RI
USA

Jeremy Katcher
Kirkwood, MO
USA

Elizabeth M. Keating
Mayo Medical School
Mayo Clinic
Rochester, MN
USA

Steven Keiles
Ambry Genetics
Aliso Viejo, CA
USA

Matthias Keller
Department of Pediatrics I, Neonatology and Pediatric Neurology
University Hospital Essen
Essen
Germany

Mariska S. Kemna
Division of Cardiology
Department of Pediatrics
Seattle Children's Hospital
University of Washington
Seattle, WA
USA

Sean E. Kennedy
Department of Nephrology
Sydney Children's Hospital & School of Women's & Children's Health University of New South Wales
Sydney, NSW
Australia

Martin Keszler
Department of Pediatrics
Women and Infants Hospital of Rhode Island
The Warren Alpert Medical School of Brown University
Brown University
Providence, RI
USA

Melissa Ketunuti
Division of Infectious Diseases
Department of Pediatrics
The Children's Hospital of Philadelphia
University of Pennsylvania
Philadelphia, PA
USA

Najwa Khuri-Bulos
Pediatric Infectious Diseases
Jordan University Hospital
Amman
Jordan

David W. Kimberlin
Division of Pediatric Infectious Diseases
Sergio Stagno Endowed Chair in Pediatric Infectious Diseases
The University of Alabama at Birmingham
Birmingham, AL
USA

Shyla Kishore
Paediatric Gastroenterology
St. George's Hospital NHS Health Care Trust
London
UK

Aziz Koleilat
Department of Pediatrics
Makassed University General Hospital
Beirut
Lebanon

Isabelle Koné-Paut
Department of Pediatrics and Pediatric Rheumatology
National Reference Center for
Auto-Inflammatory Disorders
Bicêtre University Hospital
Le Kremlin Bicêtre
France

Bruce R. Korf
Department of Genetics
University of Alabama
Birmingham, AL
USA

Michael P. Koster
Hasbro Children's Hospital
Alpert Medical School of Brown University
Providence, RI
USA

Sanjeev Kothare
Division of Sleep Medicine
Harvard Medical School
Boston, MA
USA

Martin A. Koyle
Division of Pediatric Urology
The Hospital for Sick Children
Toronto, ON
USA

James Krebs
Experiential Education
University of New England
College of Pharmacy
Portland, ME
USA

Douglas W. Kress
Children's Hospital of Pittsburgh
University of Pittsburgh 11279 Perry Highway
Wexford, PA
USA

Vibha Krishnamurthy
Ummeed Child Development Center
Mumbai, Maharashtra
India

Karthik Krishnan
Department of Pediatrics
Division of Allergy-Immunology and Rheumatology
Medical College of Georgia at the Georgia Health Sciences University
Augusta, GA
USA

Matthew P. Kronman
Division of Infectious Diseases
Department of Pediatrics
Seattle Children's Hospital
University of Washington
Seattle, WA
USA

Arlet G. Kurkchubasche
Department of Surgery
Alpert Medical School of Brown University
Providence, RI
USA
and
Hasbro Children's Hospital
Providence, RI
USA

Peter Kurre
Department of Pediatrics
Oregon Health and Science University
Portland, OR
USA

John D. Lantos
Children's Mercy Bioethics Center
Children's Mercy Hospital
Kansas City, MO
USA

Bianca Lattanzi
Dipartimento di Scienze Pediatriche G. De Toni
Istituto di Ricovero e Cura a Carattere Scientifico G. Gaslini
Genoa
Italy

Yuk M. Law
Division of Cardiology
Department of Pediatrics
Seattle Children's Hospital
University of Washington
Seattle, WA
USA

Mark C. Lee
Pediatric Orthopaedic Surgery
University of Connecticut
Connecticut Children's Medical Center
Hartford, CT
USA

Ting-Wen An Lee
Division of Pediatric Endocrinology
Children's Hospital at Montefiore
Albert Einstein College of Medicine
Bronx, NY
USA

Mark B. Lewin
Heart Center
Seattle Children's Hospital
Seattle, WA
USA

Meerana Lim
Division of Respiratory Medicine
University of California, San Diego
Rady Children's Hospital of San Diego
San Diego, CA
USA

Susan J. Lindemulder
Department of Pediatrics
Oregon Health and Science University
Portland, OR
USA

Jonathan Lipton
Department of Neurology
Center for Pediatric Sleep Disorders
Children's Hospital Boston
Boston, MA
USA

Warren Lo
Division of Child Neurology
Ohio State College of Medicine
Columbus, OH
USA

Sara A. Lohser
Department of Dermatology
Institute of Dermatology and Plastic Surgery
Cleveland Clinic Foundation
Cleveland, OH
USA

Rebecca Loret de Mola
Department of Pediatrics
Division of Hematology/Oncology
Oregon Health and Science University
Portland, OR
USA

Edward J. Lose
Department of Genetics
University of Alabama
Birmingham, AL
USA

Michael Loubser
Infinity Health Clinic
Dubai
UAE

Francois I. Luks
Division of Pediatric Surgery
Hasbro Children's Hospital
Providence, RI
USA
and
Division of Pediatric Surgery
Alpert Medical School of Brown University and
Hasbro Children's Hospital
Providence, RI
USA

John B. Lynch
University of Washington School of Medicine
Seattle, WA
USA

Andrew James Lyon
Simpson Centre for Reproductive Health
Royal Infirmary of Edinburgh
Edinburgh, Midlothian
UK

Michelle M. Macias
Medical University of South Carolina
Charleston, SC
USA

Benjamin Mackowiak
University of Washington Medical Center
Seattle, WA
USA

Kenneth J. Mack
Division of Child and Adolescent Neurology
Mayo Clinic
Rochester, MN
USA

Mohamad Maghnie
Department of Pediatrics
IRCCS Giannina Gaslini, Gaslini
University of Genova
Genova
Italy

Anthony E. Magit
Rady Children's Hospital of San Diego
San Diego, CA
USA

Pierre Quartier dit Maire
Hematology and Rheumatology Unit
Universite Paris-Descartes and Pediatric Immunology
Necker-Enfants Malades Hospital
Paris
France

Suman Malempati
Department of Pediatrics
Division of Pediatric Hematology/Oncology
Oregon Health & Science University
Portland, OR
USA

Daniel P. Mallon
Department of Pediatrics
University Washington School of Medicine
Seattle, WA
USA

Ahmad A. Mallouh
Jordan Hospital
Amman
Jordan

Trond Markestad
Department of Pediatrics
Institute of Clinical Medicine
Haukeland University Hospital
University of Bergen
Bergen
Norway

Carol Marquez
Department of Radiation Medicine
Oregon Health and Science University
Portland, OR
USA

Alberto Martini
Department of Pediatrics
University of Genoa
Pediatria II e Reumatologia
Istituto G. Gaslini
Genoa
Italy

Michael J. Mason
Department of Education and Human Services
366 Villanova University
Villanova, PA
USA

Christine A. Matarese
Division of Child and Adolescent Neurology
Mayo Clinic
Rochester, MN
USA

Abdulrahman M. Al Mazrou
Section of Pediatric Infectious Diseases
Department of Pediatrics
King Saud University and King Fahad Medical City
Riyadh
Saudi Arabia

Evelina Mazzolari
Department of Pediatrics
University of Brescia
Brescia
Italy

Elizabeth McCauley
Department of Psychiatry & Behavioral Sciences
Division of Child Psychiatry
University of Washington/Seattle Children's Hospital
Seattle, WA
USA

Kenneth L. McClain
Department of Pediatrics
Texas Children's Cancer Center and Hematology Service
Baylor College of Medicine
Houston, TX
USA

Jonathan A. McCullers
Department of Infectious Diseases
St. Jude Children's Research Hospital
Memphis, TN
USA

Patrick J. McNamara
Department of Neonatology
Hospital for Sick Children
Toronto, ON
Canada

Robyn Mehlenbeck
Department of Psychology
George Mason University
Fairfax, VA
USA

Hector Mendez-Figueroa
Division of Maternal-Fetal Medicine
Department of Obstetrics and Gynecology
Women and Infants' Hospital of Brown University
Providence, RI
USA

David J. Michelson
LLU Division of Child Neurology
Loma Linda University School of Medicine
Loma Linda, CA
USA

Giorgina Mieli-Vergani
Paediatric Liver, GI and Nutrition Centre
King's College London School of Medicine at King's College Hospital
London
UK

Federico Migliore
Division of Cardiology
Department of Cardiac, Thoracic and Vascular Sciences
University of Padua Medical School
Padova
Italy

Michelle A. Miller
Pediatric Physical Medicine and Rehabilitation
The Ohio State University Medical School/Nationwide Children's Hospital
Columbus, OH
USA

Tamir Miloh
Department of Pediatrics
Mount Sinai School of Medicine New York University
New York, NY
USA

Mohamad Miqdady
Pediatric Institute
Sheikh Khalifa Medical City/Managed by Cleveland Clinic
Abu Dhabi
UAE

Neena Modi
Section of Neonatal Medicine
Department of Medicine
Imperial College London
Chelsea & Westminster campus
London
UK

Hadi Mohseni-Bod
Department of Critical Care Medicine
University of Toronto
Hospital for Sick Children
Toronto
Canada

Keith O. Monchik
Department of Orthopedic Surgery
Warren Alpert Medical School of Brown University/
Rhode Island Hospital
Providence, RI
USA

John Moore
Section of Cardiology
Department of Pediatrics
University of California San Diego School of Medicine
Rady Children's Hospital
San Diego, CA
USA

Jill A. Morgan
University of Maryland School of Pharmacy
Baltimore, MD
USA

Colin J. Morley
Department of Neonatal Medicines
Royal Women's Hospital
Carlton, VIC
Australia

Amir Mostofi
Hand and Upper Extremity Surgery
Risser Orthopaedic Group
Pasadena, CA
USA

Manuel Moya
Pediatric Department
University M. Hernández/Hospital Universitario S.Juan
San Juan, Alicante
Spain

Maka Mshvildadze
Chachava Scientific-Research Institute of Perinatal Medicine Obstetrics and Gynecology
Tbilisi, GA
USA

Mary K. Mulcahey
Department of Orthopedic Surgery
Warren Alpert Medical School of Brown University/
Rhode Island Hospital
Providence, RI
USA

Christopher S. Muratore
Department of Surgery
Division of Pediatric Surgery
Rhode Island Hospital/Hasbro Children's Hospital
Providence, RI
USA

Mahmoud M. Mustafa
Jimmy Everest Cancer Center
Children's Hospital of Oklahoma
Oklahoma City, OK
USA

Radhika Muzumdar
Division of Pediatric Endocrinology
Children's Hospital at Montefiore
Albert Einstein College of Medicine
Bronx, NY
USA

Arti Nanda
Pediatric Dermatology
As'ad Al-Hamad Dermatology Center
Salmiya
Kuwait

Jack H. Nassau
Division of Child and Adolescent Psychiatry
The Warren Alpert Medical School of Brown University
Providence, RI
USA

David Nathalang
Division of Pediatric Critical Care
University of Arizona
Tucson, AZ
USA

Simona Nativ
Department of Pediatrics
Columbia University Medical Center
Children's Hospital of New York
New York, NY
USA

Kellie J. Nazemi
Department of Pediatrics
Division of Hematology/Oncology
Oregon Health and Science University
Portland, OR
USA

Dena Nazer
Department of Pediatrics
Wayne State University
Children's Hospital of Michigan
Detroit, MI
USA

Lama H. Nazer
Department of Pharmacy
King Hussein Cancer Center
Amman
Jordan

Hisham M. Nazer
Pediatric Gastroenterology, Hepatology and Clinical Nutrition
University of Jordan
Islamic Hospital
Amman
Jordan

Deepika Nehra
Department of Surgery
Massachusetts General Hospital
Harvard Medical School
Boston, MA
USA

Eneida R. Nemecek
Department of Pediatrics
Oregon Health and Science University
Portland, OR
USA

Josef Neu
Division of Neonatology
University of Florida
Gainesville, FL
USA

Patrick Niaudet
Service de Nephrologie Pediatrique
Hôpital Necker-Enfants Malades
Université Paris-Descartes
Paris
France

H. Stacy Nicholson
Department of Pediatrics
Division of Pediatric Hematology/Oncology
Oregon Health & Science University
Portland, OR
USA

Cory Noel
Seattle Children's Hospital
Seattle, WA
USA

Luigi D. Notarangelo
Division of Immunology
Children's Hospital Harvard Medical School
Boston, MA
USA

Cyrus Nozad
Cordova, TN
USA

William Oh
Department of Pediatrics
Warren Alpert Medical School of Brown University
Women and Infants Hospital
Providence, RI
USA

Aaron K. Olson
Heart Center
Seattle Children's Hospital
University of Washington
Seattle, WA
USA

Jordan S. Orange
Department of Pediatrics
The Children's Hospital of Philadelphia University of Pennsylvania School of Medicine
Philadelphia, PA
USA

Fatih Ozaltin
Department of Pediatric Nephrology and Rheumatology
Hacettepe University
Ankara
Turkey

Pinar T. Ozand
Department of Genetics
King Faisal Specialist Hospital
Riyadh
Saudi Arabia
and
Department of Pediatrics and Department of Biological and Medical Research
King Faisal Specialist Hospital and Research Centre
Riyadh
Saudi Arabia

Seza Ozen
Department of Pediatric Nephrology and Rheumatology
Hacettepe University
Ankara
Turkey

M. Jason Palmer
The Hand Center
Greenville, SC
USA

Vincent J. Palusci
Frances L. Loeb Child Protection and Development Center Bellevue Hospital Center
New York University School of Medicine
New York, NY
USA

Lars Pape
Department of Pediatric Kidney, Liver and Metabolic Diseases
Children's Hospital
Hannover Medical School
Hannover
Germany

Kristine A. Parbuoni
Department of Pharmacy Services
University of Maryland Medical Center
Baltimore, MD
USA

Sung Min Park
Division of Respiratory Medicine
Rady Children's Hospital of San Diego
San Diego, CA
USA

Bradley Peterson
Division of Pediatric Critical Care
Rady Children's Hospital of San Diego
San Diego, CA
USA

Juan Piantino
Department of Pediatrics
University of Chicago Medical Center
Chicago, IL
USA

Richard Plavka
Department of Obstetrics and Gynecology
Division of Neonatology
Charles University
Prague
Czech Republic

Nina Poliak
Department of Pediatrics
The Children's Hospital of Philadelphia University of Pennsylvania School of Medicine
Philadelphia, PA
USA

Jennifer K. Poon
Medical University of South Carolina
Charleston, SC
USA

Jay M. Portnoy
Section of Allergy, Asthma & Immunology
The Children's Mercy Hospitals & Clinics
University of Missouri-Kansas City School of Medicine
Kansas City, MO
USA

Priya Prabhakaran
Division of Pediatric Critical Care
University of Alabama at Birmingham
Birmingham, AL
USA

Rowena C. Punzalan
Department of Pediatrics
Medical College of Wisconsin
Milwaukee, WI
USA
and
Blood Center of Wisconsin
Milwaukee, WI
USA

Jose Bernardo Quintos
Department of Pediatrics
The Warren Alpert Medical School of Brown University
Providence, RI
USA

Tonse N. K. Raju
Eunice Kennedy Shriver National Institute of Child Health and Human Development
Bethesda, MD
USA

Jayashree Ramasethu
Division of Neonatology
Georgetown University Hospital
Washington, DC
USA

Soud Al Rasheed
King Saud bin Abdulaziz University for Health Sciences
Riyadh
Saudi Arabia

Angelo Ravelli
Istituto di Ricovero e Cura a Carattere Scientifico G. Gaslini
Genoa
Italy
and
Dipartimento di Scienze Pediatriche G. De Toni
Università degli Studi di Genova
Genoa
Italy

Mohamed Rawashdeh
Department of Pediatric Gastroenterology & Nutrition, The Medical School
Jordan University of Science & Technology
Irbid
Jordan

Jamal Raza
National Institute of Child Health
Karachi
Pakistan

Michael Recht
Division of Pediatric Hematology-Oncology
Oregon Health and Science University
Portland, OR
USA

Lesley Rees
Department of Nephrology
Great Ormond Street Hospital for Children NHS Trust
London
UK

Gabriela M. Repetto
Centro de Genética Humana
Department of Pediatrics and Unidad de Gestión
Clínica del Niño
Facultad de Medicina
Clínica Alemana-Universidad del Desarrollo
Clínica Alemana and Hospital Padre Hurtado
Lo Barnechea, Santiago
Chile

Jorge D. Reyes
Department of Surgery
University of Washington School of Medicine
Seattle, WA
USA

Nameeta P. Richard
Pediatric Hematology/Oncology
Oregon Health & Science University
Portland, OR
USA

Steve E. Roach
Division of Child Neurology
Ohio State College of Medicine
Columbus, OH
USA

Stephen S. Roberts
Department of Pediatrics
Uniformed Services University of the Health Sciences
Bethesda, MD
USA

C. Anita Robinson
Department of Pediatrics and Adolescent Medicine
Albert Einstein Medical Center
Philadelphia, PA
USA

Andrew R. Rosenberg
Department of Nephrology
Sydney Children's Hospital & School of Women's & Children's Health University of New South Wales
Sydney, NSW
Australia

Carlos D. Rose
Pediatric Rheumatology
DuPont Children's Hospital and Thomas Jefferson University
Wilmington, DE
USA

Shannon A. Ross
Department of Pediatrics
University of Alabama School of Medicine
Birmingham, AL
USA

Nicolino Ruperto
IRCCS G. Gaslini
Università di Genova
Pediatria II – Reumatologia – PRINTO
EULAR Centre of Excellence in Rheumatology
2008-2013
Genoa
Italy

Zbigniew Ruszczak
Division of Dermatology
Department of Medicine
Institute of Medicine
Sheikh Khalifa Medical City
Abu Dhabi
UAE

Julie Ryu
Department of Pediatrics
Division of Respiratory Medicine
University of California San Diego and
Rady Children's Hospital of San Diego
La Jolla, CA
USA

Camille Sabella
Center for Pediatric Infectious Diseases
Children's Hospital
Cleveland Clinic Foundation
Cleveland, OH
USA

Paul Saenger
Division of Pediatric Endocrinology
Children's Hospital at Montefiore
Albert Einstein College of Medicine
Bronx, NY
USA

Brian Safier
Division of Pediatric Allergy and Immunology,
Department of Pediatrics
Women and Children's Hospital of Buffalo
Buffalo, NY
USA

Mustafa A. M. Salih
Division of Pediatric Neurology
Department of Pediatrics
College of Medicine and King Khalid University Hospital
King Saud University
Riyadh
Saudi Arabia

Maria A. Salinas
Department of Pediatrics
Stanford University School of Medicine
Stanford, CA
USA

Hugh A. Sampson
Department of Pediatrics
Jaffe Food Allergy Institute
The Mount Sinai Medical Center
New York
USA

Ian R. Sanderson
Centre for Digestive Diseases
Blizard Institute
Barts and The London School of Medicine and Dentistry
Queen Mary
University of London
London
UK

Sami A. Sanjad
Department of Pediatrics and Adolescent Medicine
American University of Beirut
Beirut
Lebanon

Fernando Santos
Facultad de Medicinia
Hospital Universitario Central de Asturias
University of Oviedo
Oviedo, Asturias
Spain

Jonathan R. Schiller
Department of Orthopaedics
Warren Alpert Medical School Brown University
Providence, RI
USA

David J. Schonfeld
National Center for School Crisis and Bereavement
Division of Developmental and Behavioral Pediatrics
Cincinnati Children's Hospital Medical Center
Cincinnati, OH
USA

Amy H. Schultz
Heart Center
Seattle Children's Hospital
Seattle, WA
USA

Andrea Secco
Department of Pediatrics, IRCCS
Giannina Gaslini - University of Genova
Genova
Italy

Senthil Senniappan
The London Centre for Paediatric Endocrinology and Metabolism
Great Ormond Street Hospital for Children NHS Trust
WC1N 3JH and the Institute of Child Health
University College London
London
UK

Stephen P. Seslar
Heart Center
Seattle Children's Hospital
Seattle, WA
USA

Taraneh Shafii
Department of Pediatrics
Division of Adolescent Medicine
University of Washington School of Medicine
Seattle, WA
USA
and
Public Health-Seattle & King County
Seattle, WA
USA

Nalini S. Shah
Seth G. S. Medical College
K. E. M. Hospital
Parel, Mumbai
India

Jumana Shammout
Franklin Lakes, NJ
USA

Stephanya Shear
Pediatric Urology
Seattle Children's Hospital
Seattle, WA
USA

Samir Shehab
Department of Pediatrics
Doernbecher Children's Hospital
Oregon Health and Science University
Portland, OR
USA

Masako Shimamura
Department of Pediatrics
University of Alabama School of Medicine
Birmingham, AL
USA

Salah Shohieb
Faculty of Medicine
Tanta University
Tanta
Egypt

Janelle Shumate
Wake Teen Medical Services
Raleigh, NC
USA

Namita Singh
Division of Gastroenterology, Hepatology and Nutrition
Seattle Children's Hospital
Seattle, WA
USA

Justin Skripak
Department of Pediatrics
The Mount Sinai Medical Center
New York
USA

Rania Slika
Department of Pharmacy Services
Tawam Hospital
Al Ain, Abu Dhabi
UAE

Brian D. Soriano
Heart Center
Seattle Children's Hospital
Seattle, WA
USA

Mark A. Sperling
Department of Pediatrics
Division of Endocrinology
University of Pittsburgh School of Medicine
Children's Hospital of Pittsburgh
Pittsburgh, PA
USA

F. Bruder Stapleton
Department of Pediatrics
Seattle Children's Hospital University of Washington
School of Medicine
Seattle, WA
USA

Laurel Steinmetz
Seattle Children's Hospital
University of Washington School of Medicine
Seattle, WA
USA

Bonnie E. Stephens
The Warren Alpert Medical School of Brown University
Providence, RI
USA
and
Department of Pediatrics
Women and Infants Hospital
Providence, RI
USA

Karen Stout
Heart Center
Seattle Children's Hospital
University of Washington
Seattle, WA
USA

Stephanie H. Stovall
Department of Pediatrics
University of Arkansas for Medical Sciences College of Medicine
Little Rock, AR
USA

Erin R. Stucky
Division of Hospital Medicine
Department of Pediatrics
University of California San Diego
Rady Children's Hospital San Diego
San Diego, CA
USA

S. H. Subramony
Department of Neurology
McKnight Brain Institute
University of Florida
College of Medicine
Gainesville, FL
USA

Fredrick J. Suchy
The Children's Hospital Research Institute
The Children's Hospital
Department of Pediatrics
Child Health Research University of Colorado School of Medicine
Aurora, CO
USA
and
Department of Pediatrics
Mount Sinai School of Medicine New York University
New York, NY
USA

Gaafar I. Suliman
Dr. Gaafar Ibnauf Children's Specialized Hospital
Khartoum
Sudan

Andrea P. Summer
Department of Pediatrics
Medical University of South Carolina
Charleston
USA

Manika Suryadevara
Department of Peidatrics
Upstate Medical University
Syracuse, NY
USA

Jordan M. Symons
Department of Pediatrics
University of Washington School of Medicine
Seattle, WA
USA

Brian G. Tang
Department of Pediatrics
Stanford University School of Medicine
Stanford, CA
USA

Lloyd Y. Tani
Division of Pediatric Cardiology
University of Utah
Salt Lake City, UT
USA

J. Channing Tassone
Children's Hospital of Wisconsin
Milwaukee, WI
USA

James S. Taylor
Department of Dermatology
Institute of Dermatology and Plastic Surgery
Cleveland, OH
USA

AbdulWahab M. A. Telmesani
Department of Pediatrics
College of Medicine
Umm Al-Qura University
Makkah
Saudi Arabia

Rajan K. Thakkar
Department of Surgery
Alpert Medical School of Brown University and Rhode Island Hospital
Providence, RI
USA

Gaetano Thiene
Cardiovascular Pathology
Department of Medical-Diagnostic Sciences
University of Padua
Padua
Italy

Kenneth J. Tomecki
Department of Dermatology
Institute of Dermatology and Plastic Surgery
Cleveland Clinic Foundation
Cleveland, OH
USA

Jeffrey A. Towbin
Department of Pediatrics
Divisions of Pediatric Cardiology and Genetics
Cincinnati Children's Hospital Medical Center and University of Cincinnati College of Medicine
Cincinnati, OH
USA

Thomas F. Tracy
Department of Surgery
Alpert Medical School Brown University
Providence, RI
USA

Tu-Anh Tran
Department of Pediatrics and Pediatric Rheumatology
National Reference Center for Auto-Inflammatory Disorders
Bicêtre University Hospital
Le Kremlin Bicêtre
France

Richard S. Trompeter
Great Ormond Street Hospital for Children NHS Trust
London
UK

Daniel S. Tsze
Department of Pediatrics
Division of Pediatric Emergency Medicine
Columbia University College of Physicians and Surgeons
New York, NY
USA

Christer Ullbro
Department of Dentistry
King Faisal Specialist Hospital and Research Center
Riyadh
Saudi Arabia

Anton H. van Kaam
Department of Neonatology
Emma Children's Hospital
Academic Medical Center
Amsterdam
The Netherlands

Marcia Wenner VanVleet
Department of Pediatrics
The Warren Alpert Medical School of Brown University
Providence, RI
USA
and
Women and Infants Hospital
Providence, RI
USA

Roshni Vara
Department of Inherited Metabolic Disease
Evelina Children's Hospital
St Thomas' Hospital
London
UK

Louise Elaine Vaz
Department of Pediatrics
Virgina Mason Medical Center
Sand Point Pediatrics
Seattle, WA
USA

Maximo Vento
Neonatal Research Unit
Division of Neonatology
University Hospital Materno-Infantil La Fe
Valencia
Spain

Joris Robert Vermeesch
Center for Human Genetics
Catholic University of Leuven
Leuven
Belgium

Margaret MacMillan Vernon
Heart Center
Seattle Children's Hospital
Seattle, WA
USA

Bernadette Vitola
Children's Hospital of Wisconsin
Milwaukee, WI
USA

Betty R. Vohr
The Warren Alpert Medical School of Brown University
Providence, RI
USA
and
Department of Pediatrics
Women and Infants Hospital
Providence, RI
USA

Leslie R. Walker
Division of Adolescent Medicine
Department of Pediatrics
Children's Hospital and Regional Medical Center
University of Washington
Seattle, WA
USA

John A. Walker-Smith
University Department of Pediatric Gastroenterology
Royal Free Hospital
London
UK

Bradley A. Warady
Pediatric Nephrology
Children's Mercy Hospital
Kansas City, MO
USA

Garry L. Warne
Department of Endocrinology and Diabetes
Royal Children's Hospital
Melbourne
Australia

Sandra L. Watkins
Department of Pediatrics
University of Washington Seattle Children's Hospital
Seattle, WA
USA

Elizabeth W. Weber
Orthopedic Surgery
Connecticut Children's Medical Center
Hartford, CT
USA

Lucy R. Wedderburn
Rheumatology Unit
Institute of Child Health
University College London (UCL)
London
UK
and
Great Ormond Street Hospital
London
UK

Lynn M. Wegner
Division of Developmental-Behavioral Pediatrics
University of North Carolina
Chapel Hill, NC
USA

Leonard Weiner
5410 University Hospital
Upstate Medical University
Syracuse, NY
USA

Eric Werner
Division of Pediatric Hematology/Oncology
Children's Specialty Group
Eastern Virginia School of Medicine
Children's Hospital of The King's Daughters
Norfolk, VA
USA

Richard J. Whitley
Department of Pediatrics
The University of Alabama at Birmingham
Birmingham, AL
USA

Matthew S. Wilder
Division of Pediatric Critical Care
Department of Pediatrics
University of California
San Diego
Rady Children's Hospital
San Diego, CA
USA

Joseph I. Wolfsdorf
Department of Medicine (Division of Endocrinology)
Children's Hospital Boston
Boston, MA
USA

Trisha E. Wong
Puget Sound Blood Center
Seattle, WA
USA
and
Pediatric Hematology/Oncology
Seattle Children's Hospital
Seattle, WA
USA

Carine H. Wouters
Pediatric Rheumatology
Leuven University Hospital
Leuven
Belgium

Hassan M. Yaish
Department of Pediatrics
Primary Children Hospital
University of Utah
Salt Lake City, UT
USA

Hui-Kim Yap
Department of Pediatrics
Yong Loo Lin School of Medicine
National University of Singapore
Singapore

Ilya Yemets
Cardiac Surgery
The Children's Cardiac Center
Kyiv
Ukraine

Rae S. M. Yeung
Department of Pediatrics, Immunology and Medical Science
University of Toronto
The Hospital for Sick Children
Toronto, ON
Canada

Karyn Yonekawa
Nephrology A-7931
Seattle Children's Hospital
Seattle, WA
USA

Christopher Young
Division of Neonatology
University of Florida
Gainesville, FL
USA

Delphine Yung
Division of Pediatric Cardiology
University of Washington
School of Medicine, Seattle Children's Hospital
Seattle, WA
USA

Alessandro Zorzi
Division of Cardiology
Department of Cardiac, Thoracic and Vascular Sciences
University of Padua Medical School
Padova
Italy

Francesco Zulian
Pediatric Rheumatology Unit
Department of Pediatrics
University of Padova
Padua
Italy

Table of Contents

Volume 2

Volume 3

Volume 4

Volume 5

Volume 6

300 Congenital Nephrotic Syndrome

Patrick Niaudet

Congenital nephrotic syndrome is present at birth or appears during the first 3 months of life. Onset of nephrotic syndrome between 3 months and 1 year defines infantile nephrotic syndrome. Most cases have a genetic basis (➲ *Table 300.1*) and a poor outcome. The diagnosis of the disease responsible for the nephrotic syndrome is based on clinical, biological, histological, and genetic studies.

Congenital Nephrotic Syndrome of the Finnish Type (CNF)

This type of congenital nephrotic syndrome initially described by Hallman et al. is more frequent in Finland with an incidence of 1.2 per 10,000 births. It has also been reported in various ethnic groups around the world.

Genetics

The disease is inherited as an autosomal recessive trait. The gene was mapped to chromosome 19q13.1 in 17 Finnish families and other families around the world, and no genetic heterogeneity has been reported. The gene, called *NPHS1*, has a 26 kb size and contains 29 exons. It encodes for a 1,241-residue transmembrane protein of the immunoglobulin superfamily of cell adhesion molecules named "nephrin." Many different mutations of *NPHS1* have been reported. In Finnish patients, the two most common mutations, Fin-major and Fin-minor account for 90% of all patients, as homozygous mutations or compound heterozygous mutations. Fin-major mutation is a two base pair deletion in exon 2 that causes a frameshift and a translation stop in the same exon. Fin-minor is a nonsense mutation in exon 26.

The same gene is responsible for the disease in non-Finnish patients with CNF. The mutation-carrying chromosomes descend from different ancestors without evidence of a founder effect. Beside the two "Finnish mutations," more than 50 other mutations have been detected mainly outside Finland. The mutations including deletions, insertions, nonsense, missense, and splicing mutations are scattered along the entire gene. Interestingly, eight out of nine patients with an atypically mild disease (of which five were in remission) were homozygous for R1160X, a mutation also associated with the classical form suggesting the presence of genetic or other modifying events.

By immunoelectron microscopy, it has been shown that nephrin is specifically located at the slit diaphragm between the podocyte foot processes. Two decades ago, electron microscopic observations revealed a zipper-like structure at the slit diaphragm, with a width between 20 and 50 nm. It has been hypothesized that nephrin molecules extending between two opposite foot processes may interact with each other in the slit diaphragm through homophilic interactions. Since nephrin mutations are associated with massive proteinuria, it can be concluded that this protein is crucial for the maintenance of the glomerular filtration size-selective barrier.

Pathology

The kidneys are enlarged in the initial stages of the disease. Light microscopic examination early in the course of the disease show mild mesangial hypercellularity and increased mesangial matrix in the glomeruli. Irregular microcystic dilatation of proximal tubules is the most striking feature, although this change is not specific. No immune deposits are detected by immunofluorescence studies. Later in the course, interstitial fibrosis, lymphocytic and plasma cell infiltration, tubular atrophy, and periglomerular fibrosis develop in parallel with glomerular sclerosis.

Clinical Features

Massive proteinuria occurs in utero and the symptoms at birth are related to the protein deficiency. Most infants are born prematurely (35–38 weeks), with a low birth weight for gestational age. The placenta is enlarged, being more

Abdelaziz Y. Elzouki (ed.), *Textbook of Clinical Pediatrics*, DOI 10.1007/978-3-642-02202-9_300,

Table 300.1
Genetic forms of congenital and infantile nephrotic syndrome

Disease	Locus	Transmission	Gene	Protein
Finnish type NS	19q13.1	AR	*NPHS1*	Nephrin
SRNS	1q25-31	AR	*NPHS2*	Podocine
SRNS or DMS	10q23	AR	*NPHS3*	Phospholipase C ε 1
Denys–Drash syndrome or isolated DMS	11p13	AD	*WT1*	WT1 protein
Galloway syndrome	?	AR	?	
Pierson syndrome	3p21	AR	*LAMB2*	Laminine beta 2
Nail–patella syndrome	9q34.1	AD	*LMX1B*	Transcription factor
Mitochondrial cytopathies	mtADN	Maternal	mtADN	Respiratory chain protein

than 25% of the total birth weight. Fetal distress is frequent. The cranial sutures are widely separated due to delayed ossification. Infants often have a small nose and low ears. Flexion deformities of the hips, knees, and elbows are frequent.

Edema is present at birth or appears during the first week of life. The nephrotic syndrome is severe with marked ascites. The proteinuria is highly selective early in the course of the disease and hematuria is uncommon. The urinary protein losses are accompanied by profound hypoalbuminemia and severe hypogammaglobulinemia. As a result, nutritional status and statural growth are poor, and affected infants are highly susceptible to bacterial infections (peritonitis, respiratory infections) and to thromboembolic complications due to the severity of the nephrotic syndrome. Hypothyroidism due to urinary losses of thyroxine-binding protein is also common. Cholesterol and triglycerides are markedly elevated. The blood urea and creatinine concentrations are initially normal.

Renal ultrasonography shows enlarged hyperechogenic kidneys without the normal corticomedullary differentiation.

End-stage renal failure usually occurs between 3 and 8 years of age. However, some *NPHS1* mutations are associated with end-stage renal failure occurring much later in life.

Prenatal Diagnosis

CNF can be diagnosed prenatally as it becomes manifest during early fetal life, beginning at the gestation age of 15–16 weeks. Fetal proteinuria leads to a more than tenfold increase in the amniotic fluid alpha-fetoprotein (AFP) concentration. A parallel, but less important increase in the maternal plasma AFP level is observed. However, positive results may occur in heterozygous carriers leading to false diagnosis.

Genetic linkage and haplotype analyses may diminish the risk of false positive results in informative families. The four major haplotypes, which cover 90% of the CNF alleles in Finland, have been identified, resulting in a test with up to 95% accuracy. When the mutation responsible for the disease has been identified in a child, antenatal diagnosis may be proposed for a sibling following trophoblast biopsy.

Treatment

The nephrotic syndrome in CNF is always resistant to corticosteroids and immunosuppressive drugs. Furthermore, these drugs may be harmful due to the already high susceptibility to infection.

Standard conservative treatment includes daily or every other day albumin infusion, gamma globulin replacement, nutrition with a high-protein, low-salt diet, vitamin and thyroxine substitution, and prevention of infections and thrombotic complications. The diet is often provided by tube feeding. The rate of intercurrent complications remains high and growth and development are usually retarded. Some patients may require bilateral nephrectomy to prevent continued massive protein losses before the development of renal failure.

A possible medical alternative to nephrectomy is the combination of an angiotensin converting enzyme inhibitor and indomethacin therapy, which in some children lead to a decrease in protein excretion and improvement in nutritional status and growth.

If nephrectomy is performed, dialysis is provided until the patient reaches a weight of 8–9 kg. At this stage, renal transplantation can be considered. Nephrotic syndrome can develop after transplantation. This occurred in 13 of 51 allografts (25%), but only in children with the Fin-major/Fin-major genotype, which is associated with the absence of nephrin in the native kidneys. Anti-nephrin antibodies were observed in most affected patients. Plasma exchanges and oral cyclophosphamide may induce a remission.

Idiopathic Nephrotic Syndrome and *NPHS2* Mutations

Idiopathic nephrosis rarely occurs at birth, more commonly presenting during the first year of life. All the morphological variants of idiopathic nephrotic syndrome seen in older children can occur at this time including minimal change disease, diffuse mesangial proliferation, and focal and segmental glomerular sclerosis.

Steroid-responsiveness with a favorable course can be seen. However, most affected infants are resistant to therapy and many progress to end-stage renal disease. *NPHS2* mutations have been detected in some of these cases. *NPHS2* encodes an integral membrane protein, podocin, which is found exclusively in glomerular podocytes. Some patients with congenital nephrotic syndrome were found to lack *NPHS1* mutations. In two of five such patients, Koziell et al. found homozygous *NPHS2* mutations. Schulteiss et al. found homozygous or compound heterozygous *NPHS2* gene mutations in 11 out of 27 (41%) patients with CNS. Two additional cases had similar findings in terms of mutations in *NPHS2*, but not NPHS1, were also reported in a study of 13 unrelated patients from Japan.

In addition, some patients have both *NPHS1* and *NPHS2* mutations, resulting in a triallelic abnormality (homozygous mutations in one gene and a heterozygous mutation in the other). These findings demonstrate the genetic heterogeneity of congenital nephrotic syndrome and the absence of genotype/phenotype correlations.

Diffuse Mesangial Sclerosis

Diffuse mesangial sclerosis is the second cause of early nephrotic syndrome progressing to end-stage renal failure. It is seen exclusively in young children. Homozygous truncating mutations of the *PLCE1* gene, which encodes phospholipase C epsilon, was reported in eight children out of 12 children from six families with isolated diffuse mesangial sclerosis. Other patients have a Pierson syndrome, a Denys–Drash syndrome or an isolated form of diffuse mesangial sclerosis.

Clinical Features

Nephrotic syndrome may be present at birth or even detected in utero on the finding of elevated maternal alpha-fetoprotein serum level. The antenatal discovery of large hyperechogenic kidneys mimicking polycystic kidneys may be the first symptom of the disease. Most often, the patients are normal at birth and have a normal birth weight. Nephrotic syndrome develops progressively during the first or the first 2 years of life after a period of increasing proteinuria. Renal insufficiency may be present from the onset of renal symptoms. Various types of extrarenal signs have been reported in a few patients: nystagmus, nystagmus with mental retardation, cataract, mental retardation with microcephaly and myocarditis, severe myopia with cardiac arrhythmia, muscular dystrophy and dysmorphic features of the face.

Pathology

The glomerular lesions are characterized in the early stages by a fibrillar increase in mesangial matrix without mesangial cell proliferation. The capillary walls are lined by hypertrophied podocytes. The fully developed lesion consists of the combination of thickening of the glomerular basement membranes and massive enlargement of mesangial areas, leading to reduction of the capillary lumens. The mesangial sclerosis contracts the glomerular tuft into a sclerotic mass within a dilated urinary space (➊ *Fig. 300.1*). There is usually a corticomedullary

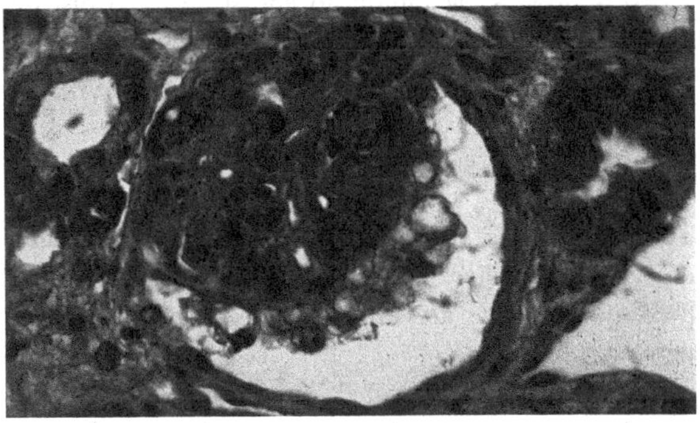

Figure 300.1

gradient of involvement, with the deepest glomeruli being less affected. Tubules are severely damaged, especially in the deeper cortex where they are markedly dilated and often contain hyaline casts.

Electron microscopy reveals hypertrophic mesangial cells surrounded by an abundant mesangial matrix, which often contains collagen fibrils. The podocytes are hypertrophied and contain many vacuoles. There is also irregular effacement of foot processes with focal detachment of the epithelial cell from the glomerular basement membrane.

Immunofluorescence shows mesangial deposits of IgM, C3, and C1q in the least affected glomeruli, while deposits of IgM and C3 outline the periphery of the sclerosed glomeruli. These deposits are probably nonspecific, occurring in areas of previous injury.

Therapy

Nephrotic syndrome secondary to diffuse mesangial sclerosis is always resistant to corticosteroids and immunosuppressive drugs. The nephrotic syndrome is usually less severe than in the CNF. Treatment is supportive and consists of maintenance of electrolyte and water balance and adequate nutrition, prevention and treatment of infectious complications, and management of renal failure. Bilateral nephrectomy is considered at the time of transplantation because of the theoretical risk of developing a Wilms' tumor. It is mandatory if a *WT1* mutation has been identified. Recurrent disease does not develop in the transplant.

Denys–Drash Syndrome

Denys–Drash syndrome (DDS) is characterized by the triad of severe glomerulopathy with diffuse mesangial sclerosis progressing rapidly to end-stage renal disease, male pseudohermaphroditism, and Wilms' tumor.

Genetics

The Denys–Drash syndrome is usually sporadic, and heterozygous germline mutations in the Wilms' tumor predisposing gene are observed in nearly all affected patients.

The *WT1* gene, located on chromosome 11p13, encodes a transcription factor presumed to regulate the expression of a series of target genes through DNA binding. It plays a critical role in kidney and gonad development and, when mutated, in the occurrence of kidney tumor and glomerular nephropathies. The target genes potentially regulated, most often negatively, by *WT1* include genes which code for transcription factors as well as for growth factors or their receptors.

WT1 is strongly expressed during embryofoetal life. In the mature kidney, *WT1* expression persists only in podocytes and epithelial cells of the Bowman's capsule. Disruption of *WT1* gene in mice results in the absence of both kidneys and gonads suggesting a crucial role of *WT1* in the development of the genitourinary tract. *WT1* play a major role in the induction of the ureteric bud, the mesenchymal to epithelial differentiation, the progression of nephrogenesis, and the maintenance of podocyte function.

More than 60 germline mutations have been reported in patients presenting with complete or incomplete DDS. They are de novo mutations, most of them missense mutations located within exons 8 or 9 encoding zinc fingers 2 and 3, respectively. The most common *WT1* lesion is a missense 1180 C to T transition converting the arginine located at the top of the third zinc finger (ZF3) to tryptophan (R394W). These *WT1* mutations change the structural organization of the respective zinc fingers and, consequently, result in loss or alteration of their DNA binding ability as confirmed by in vitro experiments. DDS mutations appear to act in a dominant negative fashion. *WT1* gene mutations, identical to those observed in DDS, have been reported in a few patients with isolated diffuse mesangial sclerosis.

Clinical Features

The nephropathy is usually discovered after several months of life, sometimes at birth. Proteinuria is accompanied by nephrotic syndrome. There is no hematuria. Blood pressure is often elevated. Progression to ESRD before the age of 4 years is the rule. Some patients progress rapidly within a few weeks to end-stage renal failure. There is no recurrence of the original disease after renal transplantation. Diffuse mesangial sclerosis is a constant feature of the Denys–Drash syndrome. It is associated with the two other components of the triad in the complete form, but with only one of the two in the incomplete forms. Wilms' tumor may be the first clinical manifestation of the syndrome. Thus, careful renal ultrasonography should be performed, looking for nephroblastoma, in any patient found to have diffuse mesangial sclerosis. The tumor may be unilateral or bilateral. Male pseudohermaphroditism, characterized by ambiguous genitalia or female phenotype with dysgenetic testis or streak gonads, is observed in all 46 XY patients. In contrast, 46 XX children appear to have a normal female phenotype.

Pierson Syndrome

Pierson syndrome is an autosomal recessive syndrome with congenital nephrotic syndrome with diffuse mesangial sclerosis and ocular malformations (microcoria, abnormal lens with cataracts, and retinal abnormalities). This disorder is due to mutations in the *LAMB2* gene, which encodes laminin beta 2. Laminin beta 2 is abundantly expressed in the glomerular basement membrane where it plays a role in anchoring and in the development of podocyte foot processes. *LAMB2* knockout mice exhibit congenital nephrotic syndrome in association with anomalies of the retina and neuromuscular junction. *LAMB2* mutations have also been found in patients with congenital nephrotic syndrome and either no or less severe ocular abnormalities.

Galloway Syndrome

The Galloway syndrome is characterized by microcephaly, mental retardation, hiatus hernia, and the nephrotic syndrome of early onset with a mean age at discovery of 3 months. It appears to be transmitted as an autosomal recessive trait. The nephrotic syndrome is usually severe, resistant to steroid therapy, and progresses to end-stage renal failure. Renal biopsy reveals minimal changes or focal and segmental glomerulosclerosis. The underlying defect is not known.

Congenital Nephrotic Syndrome Secondary to Infections

Congenital syphilis can cause membranous nephropathy. Histological examination often shows a mixed pattern with membranous nephropathy and mesangial proliferation. Penicillin treatment leads to the resolution of the syphilis and the renal abnormalities.

The nephrotic syndrome may be induced by congenital toxoplasmosis. Proteinuria may be present at birth or may develop during the first 3 months, in association with ocular or neurologic symptoms. Histological examination often shows mesangial proliferation with or without focal glomerulosclerosis. Treatment of toxoplasmosis or steroid therapy usually leads to remission of the proteinuria.

Congenital or infantile nephrotic syndrome has been reported in association with cytomegalovirus, rubeola virus, human immunodeficiency virus, and mercury intoxication.

Other Causes of Congenital Nephrotic Syndrome

Congenital nephrotic syndrome has been reported in association with type I carbohydrate-deficient glycoprotein syndrome in a neonate with neurologic abnormalities and diffuse mesangial sclerosis. It has also been reported in association with infantile sialic acid storage disease and more recently in association with mitochondrial respiratory chain deficiency.

Antenatal nephrotic syndrome due to membranous nephropathy has been reported in infants whose mothers have mutations in the metallomembrane endopeptidase gene, which encodes the podocyte protein neutral endopeptidase (NEP). During pregnancy, the absence of NEP protein induces an alloimmunisation against NEP presented by fetal cells, resulting in a fetal podocyte injury which may lead to chronic renal failure.

References

Boute N, Gribouval O, Roselli S et al (2000) NPHS2, encoding the glomerular protein podocin, is mutated in autosomal recessive steroid-resistant nephrotic syndrome. Nat Genet 24:349–354

Bredrup C, Matejas V, Barrow M et al (2008) Ophthalmological aspects of Pierson syndrome. Am J Ophthalmol 146:602–611

Debiec H, Nauta J, Coulet F et al (2004) Role of truncating mutations in MME gene in fetomaternal alloimmunisation and antenatal glomerulopathies. Lancet 364:1252–1259

Denys P, Malvaux P, Van Den Berghe H et al (1967) Association of an anatomo-pathological syndrome of male pseudohermaphroditism, Wilms' tumor, parenchymatous nephropathy and XX/XY mosaicism. Arch Fr Pédiatr 24:729–739

Drash A, Sherman F, Hartmann WH et al (1970) A syndrome of pseudohermaphroditism, Wilms' tumor, hypertension, and degenerative renal disease. J Pediatr 76:585–593

Galloway WH, Mowat AP (1968) Congenital microcephaly with hiatus hernia and nephrotic syndrome in two sibs. J Med Genet 5:319–321

Goldenberg A, Ngoc LH, Thouret MC et al (2005) Respiratory chain deficiency presenting as congenital nephrotic syndrome. Pediatr Nephrol 20:465–469

Habib R (1993) Nephrotic syndrome in the 1st year of life. Pediatr Nephrol 7:347–353

Habib R, Loirat C, Gubler MC et al (1985) The nephropathy associated with male pseudohermaphroditism and Wilms' tumor (Drash syndrome): a distinctive glomerular lesion – report of 10 cases. Clin Nephrol 24:269–278

Hallman N, Norio R, Rapola J (1973) Congenital nephrotic syndrome. Nephron 11:101–110

Hata D, Miyazaki M, Seto S et al (2005) Nephrotic syndrome and aberrant expression of laminin isoforms in glomerular basement membranes for an infant with Herlitz junctional epidermolysis bullosa. Pediatrics 116:e601–e607

Hinkes B, Wiggins RC, Gbadegesin R et al (2006) Positional cloning uncovers mutations in PLCE1 responsible for a nephrotic syndrome variant that may be reversible. Nat Genet 38:1397–1405

Hinkes BG, Mucha B, Vlangos CN et al (2007) Nephrotic syndrome in the first year of life: two thirds of cases are caused by mutations in 4 genes (NPHS1, NPHS2, WT1, and LAMB2). Pediatrics 119:e907–e919

Holmberg C, Antikainen M, Ronnholm K et al (1995) Management of congenital nephrotic syndrome of the Finnish type. Pediatr Nephrol 9:87–93

Holmberg C, Laine J, Ronnholm K et al (1996) Congenital nephrotic syndrome. Kidney Int Suppl 53:S51–S56

Huttunen NP, Rapola J, Vilska J et al (1980) Renal pathology in congenital nephrotic syndrome of Finnish type: a quantitative light microscopic study on 50 patients. Int J Pediatr Nephrol 1:10–16

Jeanpierre C, Beroud C, Niaudet P et al (1998a) Software and database for the analysis of mutations in the human WT1 gene. Nucleic Acids Res 26:271–274

Jeanpierre C, Denamur E, Henry I et al (1998b) Identification of constitutional WT1 mutations, in patients with isolated diffuse mesangial sclerosis, and analysis of genotype/phenotype correlations by use of a computerized mutation database. Am J Hum Genet 62:824–833

Kestila M, Mannikko M, Holmberg C et al (1994) Congenital nephrotic syndrome of the Finnish type maps to the long arm of chromosome 19. Am J Hum Genet 54:757–764

Koziell A, Grech V, Hussain S et al (2002) Genotype/phenotype correlations of NPHS1 and NPHS2 mutations in nephrotic syndrome advocate a functional inter-relationship in glomerular filtration. Hum Mol Genet 11:379–388

Lenkkeri U, Mannikko M, McCready P et al (1999) Structure of the gene for congenital nephrotic syndrome of the Finnish type (NPHS1) and characterization of mutations. Am J Hum Genet 64:51–61

Losito A, Bucciarelli E, Massi-Benedetti F et al (1979) Membranous glomerulonephritis in congenital syphilis. Clin Nephrol 12:32–37

Montini G, Malaventura C, Salviati L (2008) Early coenzyme Q10 supplementation in primary coenzyme Q10 deficiency. N Engl J Med 358:2849–2850

Niaudet P (2004) Genetic forms of nephrotic syndrome. Pediatr Nephrol 19:1313–1318

Niaudet P (2007) Utility of genetic screening in children with nephrotic syndrome presenting during the first year of life. Nat Clin Pract Nephrol 3:472–473

Patrakka J, Martin P, Salonen R et al (2002a) Proteinuria and prenatal diagnosis of congenital nephrosis in fetal carriers of nephrin gene mutations. Lancet 359:1575–1577

Patrakka J, Ruotsalainen V, Reponen P et al (2002b) Recurrence of nephrotic syndrome in kidney grafts of patients with congenital nephrotic syndrome of the Finnish type: role of nephrin. Transplantation 73:394–403

Pelletier J, Bruening W, Kashtan CE et al (1991) Germline mutations in the Wilms' tumor suppressor gene are associated with abnormal urogenital development in Denys–Drash syndrome. Cell 67:437–447

Sako M, Nakanishi K, Obana M et al (2005) Analysis of NPHS1, NPHS2, ACTN4, and WT1 in Japanese patients with congenital nephrotic syndrome. Kidney Int 67:1248–1255

Salviati L, Sacconi S, Murer L et al (2005) Infantile encephalomyopathy and nephropathy with CoQ10 deficiency: a CoQ10-responsive condition. Neurology 65:606–608

Schultheiss M, Ruf RG, Mucha BE et al (2004) No evidence for genotype/phenotype correlation in NPHS1 and NPHS2 mutations. Pediatr Nephrol 19:1340–1348

Shahin B, Papadopoulou ZL, Jenis EH (1974) Congenital nephrotic syndrome associated with congenital toxoplasmosis. J Pediatr 85:366–370

VanDeVoorde R, Witte D, Kogan J et al (2006) Pierson syndrome: a novel cause of congenital nephrotic syndrome. Pediatrics 118: e501–e505

Zenker M, Tralau T, Lennert T et al (2004a) Congenital nephrosis, mesangial sclerosis, and distinct eye abnormalities with microcoria: an autosomal recessive syndrome. Am J Med Genet A 130:138–145

Zenker M, Aigner T, Wendler O et al (2004b) Human laminin beta2 deficiency causes congenital nephrosis with mesangial sclerosis and distinct eye abnormalities. Hum Mol Genet 13:2625–2632

301 Nephrotic Syndrome in Children

Patrick Niaudet

Nephrotic syndrome is defined by a proteinuria higher than 50 mg/kgBW/day and hypoalbuminemia <30 g/l. A nephrotic syndrome is always secondary to a glomerular disease.

Different mechanisms have been described in the nephrotic syndrome: circulating nonimmune factors in idiopathic nephrotic syndrome, circulating immune factors in several types of glomerulonephritis, mutations in podocyte, or slit diaphragm proteins in inherited forms of nephrotic syndrome.

Proteinuria in glomerular disease is due to increased filtration of macromolecules (such as albumin) across the glomerular capillary wall. The latter consists of three components: the fenestrated endothelial cell, the glomerular basement membrane (GBM), and the epithelial cell foot processes. The pores between the foot processes are closed by a thin membrane called the slit diaphragm. The filtration of macromolecules across the glomerular capillary wall is normally restricted by charge-selectivity and size-selectivity. The GBM have a net negative charge which creates a barrier to the filtration of anions such as albumin. In comparison, circulating IgG is predominantly neutral or cationic and its filtration is not limited by charge.

In minimal change disease, the most common cause of nephrotic syndrome in children, there is a loss of anionic charge without structural damage by light microscopy. However, electron microscopy demonstrates epithelial foot processes effacement. In glomerular diseases other than idiopathic nephrotic syndrome, structural injury seen by light microscopy results in an increase in the number of large pores in the GBM. This structural damage allows movement of normally restricted proteins of varying sizes (including large neutral proteins, such as IgG) across the filtration barrier.

Clinical Features

The nephrotic syndrome is responsible for edema which increases gradually and becomes detectable when fluid retention exceeds 3–5% of body weight. It is often initially apparent around the eyes and misdiagnosed as an allergy. Edema is gravity dependent. During the day, periorbital edema decreases while it localizes to the lower extremities. In the reclining position, it localizes to the back. It is white, soft, and pitting. Edema of the scotum and penis or labiae may also be observed. Anasarca may develop. The abdomen may bulge with umbilical or inguinal hernias. When ascitis build up rapidly, the child complains of abdominal pain and malaise. Abdominal pain may also result from severe hypovolemia, peritonitis, pancreatitis, thrombosis, or steroid-induced gastritis. Blood pressure is often normal, but may be elevated depending on the underlying disease. Shock is not unusual after sudden fall of plasma albumin as observed in idiopathic nephrotic syndrome.

The nephrotic syndrome may be discovered during routine urine analysis or during the evaluation of a patient with hematuria. It may also be revealed by a complication such as peritonitis, deep vein or arterial thrombosis, or pulmonary embolism.

Laboratory Findings

Urine Analysis

Nephrotic range proteinuria is defined as urinary protein excretion greater than 50 mg/kg/day or 40 mg/m^2/h. It is higher at onset and decreases as plasma albumin concentration falls. In young children, it may be difficult to obtain a 24-h urine collection, and urinary protein to creatinine ratio or albumin to creatinine ratio in untimed urine specimens is useful. For these two indices, the nephrotic range is 200–400 mg/mmol. The selectivity of proteinuria may be appreciated by polyacrylamide gel electrophoresis or by the evaluation of the Cameron index that is the ratio of IgG to transferrin clearances. A favorable index would be below 0.05 and 0.10; a poor index is above 0.15 or 0.20. Proteinuria is most often highly selective, consisting of albumin and lower-molecular-weight proteins in case of minimal change disease whereas a poor Cameron index is often associated with more severe histologic lesions. However, there is a considerable overlap in results, and the test has limited value.

The urine sediment often contains fat bodies. Hyaline casts are also usually found in patients with massive

Abdelaziz Y. Elzouki (ed.), *Textbook of Clinical Pediatrics*, DOI 10.1007/978-3-642-02202-9_301,

proteinuria, but granular casts are not present unless there is associated acute renal failure and acute tubular necrosis. Urinary sodium is low, 1–2 mmol/day, resulting in sodium retention and edema

Blood

Plasma protein levels are markedly reduced, less than 50 g/l, due to hypoalbuminemia. Plasma albumin level is lower than 30 g/l and may be less than 10 g/l. Electrophoresis shows a typical pattern with low albumin, increased α2-globulins, and, to a lesser extent, β-globulins, whereas the level of γ-globulins depends on the cause of the nephrotic syndrome. For example, IgG levels are markedly reduced in minimal change disease and elevated in systemic lupus erythematosus. Lipid abnormalities include high levels of cholesterol, triglyceride, and lipoproteins. The result is that prolonged nephrotic syndrome contributes to the development of atherosclerosis and possibly to theprogression of renal damage. Total cholesterol and low-density lipoprotein cholesterol are elevated, whereas high-density lipoprotein cholesterol remains unchanged or low, particularly high-density lipoprotein 2, leading to an increased low-density lipoprotein to high-density lipoprotein cholesterol ratio. Patients with severe hypoalbuminemia have increased triglycerides and very-low-density lipoprotein. Apoproteins and apolipoproteins B, CII, and CIII are also elevated. The levels of lipoprotein (a) are elevated in nephrotic patients.

Serum sodium is often reduced due in part to hyperlipemia and in part to the dilution from renal retention of water due to hypovolemia and inappropriate antidiuretic hormone secretion. Hyperkalemia may be observed in cases of renal insufficiency. Hypocalcemia is related to hypoalbuminemia, and the level of ionized calcium is usually normal.

Hemoglobin levels and hematocrit are increased in patients with plasma volume contraction. Thrombocytosis is common and may reach 5×10^8/l or 10^9/l. Fibrinogen and factors V, VII, VIII, and X are increased, whereas antithrombin III, the heparin cofactor, and factors XI and XII are decreased. These abnormalities contribute to a hypercoagulable state.

Complications

Acute renal failure: Some patients with idiopathic nephrotic syndrome have a reduction of the glomerular filtration rate (GFR) attributed to hypovolemia, with complete return to normal after remission. A reduced GFR may be found despite normal effective plasma flow. This reduction is transitory, with a rapid return to normal after remission.

Renal failure may be secondary to bilateral renal vein thrombosis that can be diagnosed by sonography. Acute renal failure has also been reported with interstitial nephritis. Skin rash and eosinophilia are suggestive of this diagnosis, which is often associated with furosemide or other medication

Acute renal failure is usually reversible, often with intravenous albumin and high-dose furosemide-induced diuresis.

Renal failure may be related to severe histologic lesions in patients with primary or secondary glomerulonephritis.

Infections: Bacterial infections are frequent in nephrotic children. Sepsis may occur at the onset of the disease. The most common infection is peritonitis, often with *S. pneumoniae.* Other organisms may be responsible: *Escherichia coli, Streptococcus bovis, Haemophilus influenzae,* and other Gram-negative organisms. Apart from peritonitis, children may develop meningitis, pneumonitis, or cellulitis. Viral infections may be observed in patients receiving corticosteroids or immunosuppressive agents. Varicella is often observed in young children and may be life threatening if acyclovir therapy is not promptly initiated.

Thrombosis: Nephrotic patients are at risk of developing thromboembolic complications. Several factors contribute to this increased risk of thrombosis: a hypercoagulable state, hypovolemia, immobilization, and infection. The incidence of thromboembolic complications in nephrotic children is reported to be approximately 3%. However, this percentage may underestimate the true incidence. In one series, systematic evaluation by ventilation-perfusion scans showed defects consistent with pulmonary embolism in 28% of all patients with steroid-dependent minimal change disease. Pulmonary embolism should be suspected in cases with pulmonary or cardiovascular symptoms and may be confirmed by angiography or angioscintigraphy. Renal vein thrombosis should be suspected in patients with nephrotic syndrome who develop sudden macroscopic hematuria or acute renal failure. In such cases, Doppler ultrasonography shows an increase in kidney size and the absence of blood flow in the renal vein. Thrombosis may also affect the arteries (e.g., pulmonary arteries) or other deep veins (cerebral veins).

Hypovolemia: Hypovolemia is common and typically observed at onset of idiopathic nephrotic syndrome or early during a relapse. Sepsis, diarrhea, or diuretics may precipitate hypovolemia. Hypovolemic children often have abdominal pain, low blood pressure, and cold extremities. Hemoconcentration with a raised hematocrit accompanies hypovolemia.

Symptomatic Treatment

Diet: Diet includes a protein intake of 130–140% of the normal daily allowance according to statural age. Salt restriction is necessary for the prevention and treatment of edema. A very-low-salt diet is necessary in case of edema. Fluid restriction is recommended for moderate to severe hyponatremia (plasma sodium concentration <125 mmol/l). A reduction of saturated fat is advisable. Carbohydrates are given preferentially as starch or dextrin-maltose, avoiding sucrose, which increases lipid disturbances.

Hypovolemia: Hypovolemia, a consequence of rapid loss of serum albumin may be aggravated by diuretics. When symptomatic, this complication requires emergency treatment by rapid infusion of plasma (20 ml/kg) or albumin 20% (1 g/kg) administrated with monitoring of heart rate, respiratory rate, and blood pressure.

Diuretics: Diuretics should only be used in cases of severe edema, after hypovolemia has been corrected. Patients with anasarca may be treated with furosemide (1–2 mg/kg) or, if necessary, furosemide and salt-poor albumin (1 g/kg infused over 4 h) to increase the rate of diuretic delivery to the kidney. This approach is immediately effective, but not long lasting. Moreover, respiratory distress with congestive heart failure has been observed in some patients. Spironolactone (5–10 mg/kg) may be prescribed, provided serum creatinine is normal. Amiloride may also be used in combination with furosemide. Diuretics may induce intravascular volume depletion with a risk of thromboemboli and of acute renal failure. Refractory edema with serous effusions may require drainage of ascites and/or pleural effusions. Head-out immersion has been reported to be helpful in these cases.

Thromboemboli: Patients with severe hypoalbuminemia are at risk for thromboembolic complications. Prevention includes mobilization, avoiding hemoconcentration and treating early sepsis or volume depletion. Prophylactic warfarin may be given to patients with a plasma albumin concentration below 20 g/l, a fibrinogen level >6 g/l, or an antithrombin III level <70% of normal. Patients at risk may be treated with low-dose aspirin and dipyridamole, although no controlled trials have been performed to demonstrate their efficacy for preventing thrombosis.

Heparin is given initially if thrombosis occurs, alone or with thrombolytic agents. The heparin dose necessary to obtain a therapeutic effect is often greater than normally, due to decreased antithrombin III levels.

Antihypertensive drugs: Hypertension is treated, using a β-blocker or a calcium channel blocker during acute episodes. In cases of permanent hypertension, an angiotensin converting enzyme inhibitor or an inhibitor of angiotensin II receptor is preferred.

Infections and immunizations: Prophylaxis of *S pneumoniæ* with oral penicillin is often prescribed to children during initial corticosteroid treatment. Vaccination with the conjugated pneumococcal vaccine (7vPCV) is recommended. In cases of peritonitis, antibiotics against both *S pneumoniæ* and Gram-negative organisms are started after peritoneal fluid sampling. Varicella is a serious disease in patients receiving immunosuppressive treatment or daily corticosteroids. Varicella immunity status should therefore be assessed. In case of exposure, early prevention by acyclovir must be instituted. Immunization with the varicella vaccine is effective and safe in children on low-dose alternate day steroid therapy.

Reduction of proteinuria: There is evidence that proteinuria per se is toxic for the tubules and can favor the progression of renal fibrosis. Therefore, reduction of proteinuria should be a goal in patients with persistent proteinuria. The best results are obtained with ACE inhibitors and AT1 receptor antagonists, alone or in combination. Several studies have demonstrated the renoprotective effects of ACE inhibitors in proteinuric patients, suggesting that this strategy is appropriate in patients with prolonged nephrotic syndrome.

Causes of Nephrotic Syndrome in Children

Idiopathic Nephrotic Syndrome

It is the main cause of nephrotic syndrome in children (INS) representing more than 90% of cases before age 10 years and 50% after 10 years. INS is defined by the association of a nephrotic syndrome with minimal glomerular changes (➋ *Fig 301.1*) or nonspecific histological lesions such as focal and segmental glomerular sclerosis or diffuse mesangial proliferation. Most often, no immunoglobulin or complement deposit is seen on immunofluorescent examination. However, IgM deposits may be observed and the clinical significance of such deposits is controversial. Electron microscopy shows an effacement of the podocyte foot processes.

Most patients with minimal change lesions respond to corticosteroids with complete remission. Conversely,

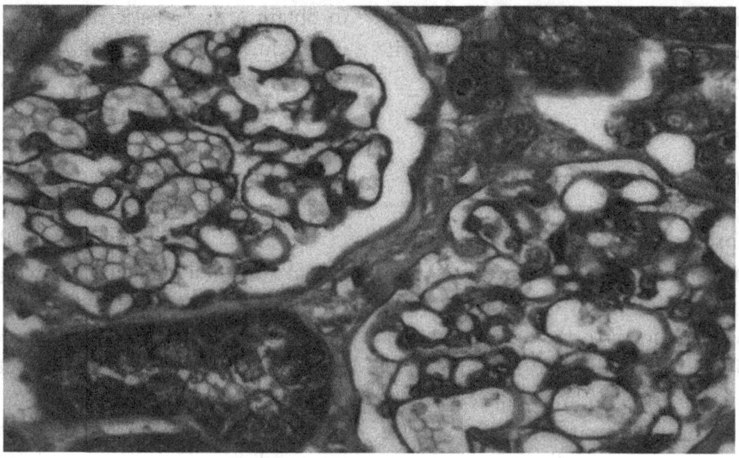

Figure 301.1

patients in whom the renal biopsy shows FSGS or diffuse mesangial proliferation often do not respond to corticosteroids. This is the reason why several authors believe that minimal change disease is a distinct entity, and FSGS, diffuse mesangial proliferation, and IgM nephropathy are also distinct entities. However, serial renal biopsies show that some patients with minimal changes on initial biopsy may later develop FSGS. Furthermore, some patients with FSGS respond to corticosteroids and have a favorable long-term outcome. Experience has shown that response to steroid therapy carries a greater prognostic weight than the histological features on initial biopsy. Therefore, two types of INS are described according to the response to corticosteroids; steroid sensitive INS in which proteinuria rapidly resolves and steroid-resistant INS in which proteinuria persists despite corticosteroids.

Initial Treatment

Steroid therapy is started when the diagnosis of INS is most likely in a child older than 1 year and younger than 11 years of age, without hypertension, gross hematuria or extra-renal symptoms, and normal complement levels. In some cases, the treatment is started after a renal biopsy has been performed. Prednisone remains the reference drug. Prednisolone has the advantage of being soluble in water, making treatment easier in young children. The ISKDC regimen consists of prednisone, 60 mg/m^2/day with a maximum of 80 mg/day, in divided doses for 4 weeks followed by 40 mg/m^2 on alternate days for 4 weeks. A response occurs in most cases within 10–15 days. Approximately 90% of responders enter in remission within 4 weeks after starting steroids, whereas less than 10% go into remission after 2–4 more weeks of a daily regimen or three to four pulses of methylprednisolone (1 g/1.73 m^2). This latter regimen seems to be associated with fewer side effects than prolongation of daily high-dose steroids.

The number of children with frequent relapses is decreased with a longer course of prednisone. A longer duration is more important than the cumulative dose of prednisone in reducing the risk of relapse. This relative risk decreases by 0.133 (13%) for every additional month of treatment up to 7 months.

Steroid-responsive INS

In the majority of children, INS is steroid responsive. Approximately 30% of them have only one attack and are definitively cured after a single course of steroids. Ten to 20% of patients experience relapses several months after stopping treatment and most of them are cured after three to four relapses which respond to a standard course of steroids. The remaining 50–60% relapse as soon as steroid therapy is stopped or when the dosage is decreased. These steroid-dependent patients often raise difficult therapeutic problems. As long as the nephrotic syndrome responds to therapy, there is very little risk of progression to chronic renal failure.

Treatment of Relapses

Fifty to sixty percent of children experience relapses as soon as steroid therapy is stopped or when dosage is decreased. Steroid-dependent patients may be treated with repeated courses of prednisone. Another option consists of treating relapses with daily prednisone, 40–60 mg/m^2, until proteinuria has disappeared for 4–5 days. Thereafter, prednisone is switched to alternate days and the dosage is tapered to 15–20 mg/m^2 every other day, according to the steroid threshold. Treatment is then continued for 12–18 months. This regimen is associated with less steroid side effects as the cumulative dosage is lower. The risk of relapse during upper respiratory tract infections is decreased when steroid therapy is given daily for 5–7 days rather than on alternate days.

Alternative Treatments

An alternative treatment is indicated in children who develop severe side effects of steroid therapy such as statural growth impairment, in children at risk of toxicity (diabetes or during puberty), in children with severe relapses accompanied by thrombotic complications or severe hypovolemia, and in those with poor compliance.

Levamisole at a dose of 2.5 mg/kg every other day reduces the risk of relapse in steroid-dependent patients. However, the beneficial effect of levamisole is not sustained after stopping treatment. Side effects occasionally include neutropenia, agranulocytosis, vomiting, cutaneous rash, vasculitis, and neurological symptoms including insomnia, hyperactivity, and seizure.

Alkylating agents such as cyclophosphamide and chlorambucil can induce long-lasting remissions in patients who are frequent relapsers or steroid dependent. Data from the literature show a remission rate of 67–93% at 1 year and 36–66% at 5 years following a course of cyclophosphamide. The therapeutic effect is related to the duration of treatment. The response to cyclophosphamide is also related to the pattern of response to steroids. The duration of remission is higher in frequent relapsers as compared to steroid-dependent patients. Cyclophosphamide is given at a dose of 2 mg/kg/day (cumulative dose 168 mg) to patients with steroid dependency who have evidence of steroid toxicity.

Remissions may also be obtained with chlorambucil. The recommended dosage is 0.2 mg/kgBW for 2 months.

Side effects of alkylating agents limit their use. Bone marrow toxicity requires regular blood cell counts. The treatment should also be discontinued in case of infection. The risks of varicella should be explained to the parents in order to rapidly start acyclovir treatment. Alopecia and hemorrhagic cystitis rarely occurs with the dosage used in these patients. Gonadal toxicity is well established and the risk is greater in boys than in girls. The gonadal toxicity threshold is between 200 and 300 mg/kgBW for cyclophosphamide and 8–10 mg/kgBW for chlorambucil.

Mycophenolate mofetil (MMF) treatment has a beneficial effect in children with steroid-dependent INS and allows to decrease or stop steroid therapy in 40–75% of children. However, relapses are nearly constant after cessation of treatment. Doses of 450–600 mg/m^2 day in two divided doses are usually given. Side effects including gastrointestinal disturbances (abdominal pain, diarrhea) and hematologic abnormalities are rare. Many authors now recommend the use of MMF rather than alkylating agents in children with steroid-dependent INS who suffer from side effects of steroid therapy.

Cyclosporine is effective in inducing or maintaining remission in 85% of patients with frequently relapsing or steroid-dependent NS, thereby allowing withdrawal of prednisone. The dose should preferably not exceed 5 mg/kg/day in two oral doses. Most patients relapse within the few months following cessation of treatment. Thus, cyclosporine may have to be administered for long periods of time, exposing patients to its potential nephrotoxicity. As a result, the plasma creatinine concentration should be monitored regularly. Serial renal biopsies after 18 months of therapy can demonstrate histologic lesions of nephrotoxicity without clinical evidence of renal function impairment. Other side effects include hypertension, hyperkalemia, hypertrichosis, gum hypertrophy, and hypomagnesemia.

Rituximab has been reported to be effective in patients with severe steroid-dependent nephrotic syndrome. In a multicenter series, 22 children with severe steroid-dependent nephrotic syndrome or steroid-resistant but cyclosporin-sensitive INS were treated with two to four infusions of rituximab. Rituximab was effective in all patients when administered during a proteinuria-free period in association with other immunosuppressive agents. Remission was induced in three of the seven proteinuric patients. One or more immunosuppressive treatments could be withdrawn in 19 patients (85%), with no relapse. When relapses occurred, they were always associated with an increase in CD19 cell count. Adverse effects were observed in 45% of cases, but most of them were mild and transient.

Steroid-resistant INS

It represents 10% of cases of INS and is a heterogeneous entity as different diseases are included under the same denomination.

During the recent years, there have been several reports on the molecular basis of familial cases of FSGS.

Mutations in several genes such as NPHS2, NPHS1, or WT1 may be responsible for steroid-resistant nephrotic syndrome with FSGS (➋ Table 301.1). Podocin mutations are found in more than 40% of autosomal recessive steroid-resistant INS and 10–20% cases of sporadic steroid-resistant INS. Because immunosuppressive therapy has not been shown to be effective in treating children with SRNS due to NPHS2, NPHS1, or WTI mutations, identifying these patients can avoid unnecessary exposure to these medications and their side effects. Thus, screening for such mutations should be performed in those with a familial history of SRNS and children with steroid-resistant disease

The optimal approach to the treatment of steroid-resistant INS not due to a genetic defect is uncertain. A treatment with cyclosporine and prednisone may be given provided the glomerular filtration rate is normal. There is evidence that tacrolimus is effective in a significant proportion of patients with steroid-resistant INS. A course of methylprednisolone pulses with alkylating agents may be another option. There is no evidence that mycophenolate mofetil is beneficial to these patients.

The long-term prognosis of steroid-resistant INS is dominated by the risk of progression to end-stage renal failure. Renal survival rate in Caucasian children is approximately 50% at 10 years. Progression to ESRF has been reported to be more frequent and more rapid in patients with African or Hispanic descent when compared to Whites.

About 30% of patients with steroid-resistant INS who progress to renal insufficiency present a recurrence of proteinuria after renal transplantation. Several risk factors for recurrence have been identified: onset of disease after 6 years of age, a rapid progression to renal failure, diffuse mesangial proliferation on initial renal biopsy, and a recurrence on a first graft.

Primary Glomerulonephritis

Membranous glomerulonephritis (MGN) is characterized by a diffuse thickening of the capillary walls due to immune deposits on the epithelial side of the GBM. By immunofluorescence, these deposits are granular and peripheral. They are stained mainly with anti-IgG serum. Patients with MGN develop proteinuria which may be asymptomatic and responsible for a nephrotic syndrome. Microscopic hematuria is frequent. Hypertension and renal insufficiency are exceptional early in the course of the disease. The prognosis is often good with a disappearance of proteinuria within a few months or years. Less than 10% of cases progress to renal failure. MGN may be secondary to systemic lupus erythematosus, an infection (hepatitis B, congenital syphilis), or to the administration of drugs such as penicillamin or gold salts. The treatment depends on the underlying disease and the severity of the clinical manifestations.

Membranoproliferative glomerulonephritis (MPGN) is characterized by mesangial hypercellularity, an increase of mesangial matrix, and a thickening of the capillary walls secondary to subendothelial extension of the mesangium. MPGN have been subdivided in three types according to morphological features. Type I MPGN, with subendothelial deposits, the most frequent, is associated with classical complement pathway activation. Type II MPGN or dense deposit disease is associated with an alternate complement pathway activation and intramembranous dense deposits and represent 10–20%

Table 301.1
Genetic forms of nephrotic syndrome with FSGS

Disease	Locus	Transmission	Gene	Protein
SRNS + FSGS	1q25–31	AR	*NPHS2*	Podocine
SRNS + FSGS or DMS	10q23	AR	*NPHS3*	Phospholipase C ε 1
CNS ou SRNS	19q13.1	AR	*NPHS1*	Nephrin
Susceptibility to FSGS	2q34–36	AR	*CD2AP*	CD2 associated protein
SRNS + FSGS	9q13	AD	*ACTN4*	α-Actinine
SRNS + FSGS	11q	AD	*TRPC6*	Calcium channel
Schimke syndrome	6p12	AR	*SMARCAL1*	Regulator of chromatin
Frasier syndrome	11p13	AD	*WT1*	WT1 protein
Mitochondrial cytopathies	mtADN	Maternal	mtADN	Respiratory chain protein

of cases. Type III MPGN, observed in less than 5% of cases, is characterized by subenthothelial and subepithelial deposits and by complex alterations of the GBM. More than 50% of patients have a low concentration of C3 due to the activation of the C3 convertase by autoantibodies, called nephritic factors (NeF). The C3NeF of the amplification loop is an IgG autoantibody which reacts with activated factor B of the C3 convertase and is observed in dense deposit disease with or without partial lipodystrophy. The C3NeF of the terminal pathway is observed in type III MPGN and also in some patients with Type I MPGN. Patients may present with acute nephritic syndrome, asymptomatic proteinuria, or nephrotic syndrome. Hematuria, macroscopic or microscopic, is most often present. MPGN may occur in patients with HBV or HCV infection. In the long term, more than 50% of patients progress to renal failure. Some children with MPGN respond to steroid therapy.

IgA nephropathy (Berger disease) is a frequent glomerular disease which affects boys more often than girls. The age at discovery is variable, but more often between 7 and 13 years. Macroscopic hematuria is the presenting symptom in 75% of cases. Recurrent episodes of macroscopic hematuria occur often within 2 days following an episode of upper respiratory tract infection. In other children, the disease is discovered at routine urine analysis because of microscopic hematuria and proteinuria. Blood pressure is usually normal. Serum IgA levels are increased in 50% of cases. Renal biopsy shows moderate histological lesions with mesangial deposits and mesangial hypercellularity, and less frequently segmental and focal glomerulonephritis (*Fig 301.2*) or endo-extracapillary glomerulonephritis. Mesangial deposits stains mainly for IgA, and less for IgG and C3. The presence of permanent proteinuria with or without nephrotic syndrome is a factor of poor prognosis with a possible progression to renal failure which occurs in 10% of cases after 10–15 years.

Anti-GBM nephritis is rare in children. It may be isolated or present with pulmonary hemorrhage (Goodpasture syndrome). Renal symptoms consist of hematuria, proteinuria with nephrotic syndrome, and renal failure. The diagnosis is confirmed by the presence of circulating IgG antibodies to the GBM by ELISA assay or by indirect immunofluorescence on normal kidney. Renal biopsy shows crescentis glomerulonephritis with linear deposits of IgG along the GBM by immunofluorescence. A prompt diagnosis is mandatory as only an early treatment with steroids, cyclophosphamide, and plasma exchanges may prevent the progression to end-stage renal failure.

Renal vasculitis the most frequent type of glomerulonepritis is microscopic polyangiitis involving glomerular capillaries. ANCA are present in most cases and are directed against myeloperoxydase (P-ANCA). In children, Wegener's granulomatosis is rare. Upper-respiratory symptoms are frequent and ANCA are directed against proteinase 3 (C-ANCA). Renal biopsy shows

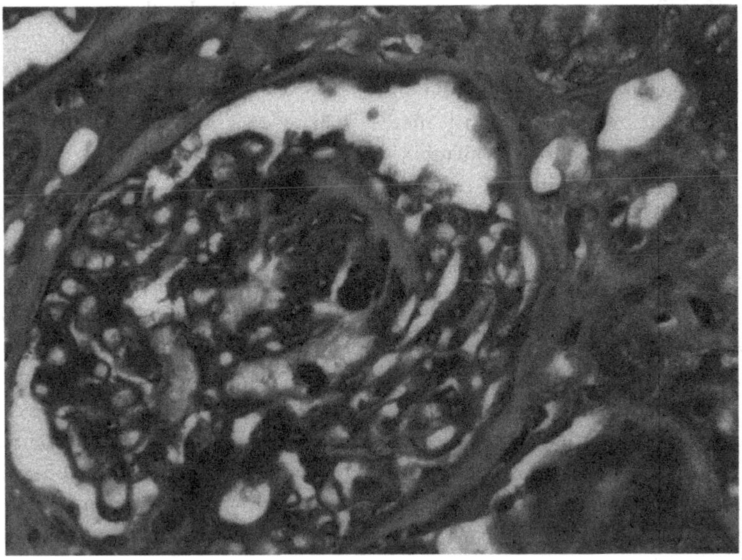

Figure 301.2

necrotizing glomerulonephritis with extracapillary proliferation without immune deposits. Corticosteroids and cyclophosphamide have greatly improved the prognosis.

Secondary Glomerulonephritis

Acute post-infectious glomerulonephritis occurs most often 10–20 days after a streptococcal infection. The child presents with an acute nephritic syndrome including hematuria, proteinuria, hypertension, and renal failure. Some patients develop nephrotic syndrome. Complement abnormalities include low CH50 and low C3. Renal biopsy, when performed, shows proliferative glomerulonephritis with infiltrating neutrophils and subepithelial humps. In severe cases, cellular crescents develop. C3 deposits are present in the mesangium and along the capillary walls. Most patients recover normal renal function within 3 weeks with supportive therapy. Steroid-pulse therapy is proposed to patients with rapidly progressive glomerulonephritis and extensive crescent formation.

Schönlein-Henoch purpura (SHP) nephritis is observed in 30–50% of children with SHP and manifests most often during the first 3 months. Hematuria, almost constant, may be accompanied by proteinuria and nephrotic syndrome. Renal biopsy shows IgA deposits and variable mesangial and extracapillary cell proliferation. Patients with nephrotic syndrome often have severe histological lesions with crescentic glomerulonephritis and a risk of progression to end-stage renal failure. In such cases, steroid therapy may be proposed.

Systemic lupus erythematosus renal disease is frequent in children with SLE. Nephrotic syndrome is observed in patients with more severe renal involvement, often in association with acute renal failure. Renal biopsy may show diffuse proliferative glomerulonephritis or membranous nephropathy with immunoglobulin and complement deposits. The presence of anti-DNA antibodies is highly suggestive of SLE and low C3 concentration is suggestive of an active disease.

Bacterial infections infective endocarditis may be associated with glomerulonephritis. The clinical manifestations are similar to those observed in acute glomerulonephritis. Nephrotic syndrome is unusual. Nephrotic syndrome is more frequent in shunt nephritis secondary to infected ventriculoatrial shunt. C3 and C4 levels are reduced in both conditions, and renal biopsy may show a pattern of membranoproliferative glomerulonephritis or acute post-streptococcal glomerulonephritis.

Other Causes

Amyloidosis

In children, amyloidosis is most often secondary to chronic inflammatory diseases (chronic juvenile arthritis, Crohn disease), to prolonged infections (tuberculosis, osteomyelitis, bronchestasis), to cystic fibrosis or familial Mediterranean fever. Amyloid deposits are present in the mesangium, the capillary walls, and the tubular basement membranes. In case of glomerular deposits, patients often present with proteinuria and nephrotic syndrome. The treatment of the cause, if possible, may prevent the progression to renal failure.

Alport Syndrome

Alport syndrome is an inherited renal disorder characterized by a progressive hematuric nephritis with ultrastructural changes of the glomerular basal membrane and sensorineural hearing loss. Mutations in the *COL4A5* gene are responsible for the more frequent X-linked form of the disease. All affected males progress to renal failure, whereas in most female patients, the course is considered to be benign. Mutations in the *COL4A3* or *COL4A4* genes are responsible for an autosomal recessive form of the disease observed in approximately 15% of patients. The disease is as severe in male as in female. The presence of massive proteinuria with nephrotic syndrome is suggestive of a poor prognosis and is associated with a progression to ESRD.

Nail–Patella Syndrome

The nail–patella syndrome or osteo-onychodysplasia is an autosomal dominant disorder characterized by hypoplastic or absent patella, dystrophic fingernails and toenails, and dysplasia of elbows and iliac horns. Renal symptoms are present in approximately 50% of patients. The most frequent symptoms are proteinuria, sometimes with a nephrotic syndrome, and hematuria. End-stage renal disease develops in approximately 30% of cases. The abnormal gene, located at the distal end of the long arm of chromosome 9, encodes a transcription factor of the LIM-homeodomain type named *LMX1B*, which plays an important role for limb development in vertebrates.

Hemolytic Uremic Syndrome

Hemolytic and uremic syndrome is characterized by the association of hemolytic anemia, thrombopenia, and renal disease secondary to thrombotic microangiopathy. The typical form is the most frequent in children occurring after an episode of diarrhea caused by *Escherichia coli.* Other germs may be responsible for HUS such as *Shigella dysenteriae* or *Streptococcus pneumoniae.* Children present with acute renal failure which is reversible in most cases. Atypical HUS is less frequent but of poorer prognosis. The patients may develop nephrotic syndrome and renal failure. Atypical HUS may be associated with mutations in the genes for complement proteins including C3, factors H, B, and I, and CD46. It is estimated that approximately 50 percent of cases of atypical HUS result from mutations in these genes. Atypical HUS may also be associated with von Willebrand factor-cleaving protease deficiency, congenital intracellular defects of vitamine B12 metabolism, or may be of unknown origin. Familial forms are frequent.

Sickle Cell Disease

Proteinuria with nephrotic syndrome and sometimes renal failure may develop in patients with sickle cell disease. Renal biopsy shows glomerular enlargement and focal and segmental glomerular sclerosis and less often a picture of membranoproliferative glomerulonephritis with IgG and C3 deposits.

Renal Hypoplasia and or Dysplasia

Children with renal hypoplasia or renal dysplasia usually do not have signs of glomerular involvement. The occurrence of proteinuria is often related to lesions of focal and segmental glomerular sclerosis secondary to severe nephron reduction and is observed in association to chronic renal failure.

References

Afzal K, Bagga A, Menon S et al (2007) Treatment with mycophenolate mofetil and prednisolone for steroid-dependent nephrotic syndrome. Pediatr Nephrol 22:2059–2065

Agarwal N, Phadke KD, Garg I et al (2003) Acute renal failure in children with idiopathic nephrotic syndrome. Pediatr Nephrol 18:1289–1292

Appenzeller S, Zeller CB, Annichino-Bizzachi JM et al (2005) Cerebral venous thrombosis: influence of risk factors and imaging findings on prognosis. Clin Neurol Neurosurg 107:371–378

Baldwin DS (1997) Poststreptococcal glomerulonephritis. Am J Med 62:1–11

Barletta GM, Smoyer WE, Bunchman TE et al (2003) Use of mycophenolate mofetil in steroid-dependent and -resistant nephrotic syndrome. Pediatr Nephrol 18:833–837

Boyer O, Moulder JK, Grandin L et al (2008) Short- and long-term efficacy of levamisole as adjunctive therapy in childhood nephrotic syndrome. Pediatr Nephrol 23:575–580

Cakar N, Yalcinkaya F, Ozkaya N et al (2001) Familial Mediterranean fever (FMF)-associated amyloidosis in childhood. Clinical features, course and outcome. Clin Exp Rheumatol 19:S63–S67

Cansick JC, Lennon R, Cummins CL et al (2004) Prognosis, treatment and outcome of childhood mesangiocapillary (membranoproliferative) glomerulonephritis. Nephrol Dial Transplant 19:2769–2777

de Groot K, Jayne D (2005) What is new in the therapy of ANCA-associated vasculitides? Take home messages from the 12th workshop on ANCA and systemic vasculitides. Clin Nephrol 64:480–484

Drash A, Sherman F, Hartmann W et al (1970) A syndrome of pseudohermaphroditism, Wilms' tumor, hypertension and degenerative renal disease. J Pediatr 76:585–593

Emre S, Bilge I, Sirin A et al (2001) Lupus nephritis in children: prognostic significance of clinicopathological findings. Nephron 87:118–126

Flynn JT, Smoyer WE, Bunchman TE, Kershaw DB, Sedman AB (2001) Treatment of Henoch–Schonlein Purpura glomerulonephritis in children with high-dose corticosteroids plus oral cyclophosphamide. Am J Nephrol 21:128–133

Furth SL, Arbus GS, Hogg R et al (2003) Varicella vaccination in children with nephrotic syndrome: a report of the Southwest Pediatric Nephrology Study Group. J Pediatr 142:145–148

Galloway WH, Movat AP (1968) Congenital microcephaly with hiatus hernia and nephrotic syndrome in two sibs. J Med Genet 5:319–321

Gansevoort RT, Sluiter WJ, Hemmelder MH et al (1995) Antiproteinuric effect of blood-pressure lowering agents: a meta-analysis of comparative trials. Nephrol Dial Transplant 10:1963–1974

Guigonis V, Dallocchio A, Baudouin V et al (2008) Rituximab treatment for severe steroid- or cyclosporine-dependent nephrotic syndrome: a multicentric series of 22 cases. Pediatr Nephrol 23:1269–1279

Hodson EM, Craig JC, Willis NS (2005) Evidence-based management of steroid-sensitive nephrotic syndrome. Pediatr Nephrol 20: 1523–1530

Hofstra JM, Deegens JK, Steenbergen EJ et al (2007) Rituximab: effective treatment for severe steroid-dependent minimal change nephrotic syndrome? Nephrol Dial Transplant 22:2100–2102

Hogg RJ, Fitzgibbons L, Bruick J et al (2006) Mycophenolate mofetil in children with frequently relapsing nephrotic syndrome: a report from the Southwest Pediatric Nephrology Study Group. Clin J Am Soc Nephrol 1:1173–1178

Homlberg C, Laine J, Ronnholm K et al (1996) Congenital nephrotic syndrome. Kidney Int 53:S51–S56

Hoyer P, Gonda S, Barthels M et al (1986) Thromboembolic complications in children with nephritic syndrome: risk and incidence. Acta Paediatr Scand 75:804–810

Jafar TH, Stark PC, Schmid CH et al (2001) Proteinuria is a modifiable risk factorfor the progressionof non-diabetic renal disease. Kidney Int 60:1131–1140

Kashtan CE (1998) Alport syndrome and thin glomerular basement membrane disease. J Am Soc Nephrol 9:1736–1750

Kasiske B, Lakatua JD, Ma JZ et al (1998) Hyperlipidemia in patients with chronic renal disease. Am J Kidney Dis 32:S142–S156

Kovacevic L, Reid CJ, Rigden SP (2003) Management of congenital nephrotic syndrome. Pediatr Nephrol 18:426–430

Llach F (1985) Hypercoagulability, renal vein thrombosis, and other thrombotic complications of nephrotic syndrome. Kidney Int 28:429–439

Makker SP (2003) Treatment of membranous nephropathy in children. Semin Nephrol 23:379–385

Makker SP, Kher KK (1989) IgA nephropathy in children. Semin Nephrol 9:112–115

Martin Hernandez E (2000) Acyclovir prophylaxis of varicella in children with nephrotic syndrome. Pediatr Nephrol 15:326–327

Mehta KP, Ali U, Kutty M, Kolhatkar U (1986) Immunoregulatory treatment for minimal change nephrotic syndrome. Arch Dis Child 61:153–158

Meyrier A, Niaudet P (2005) Minimal changes and focal-segmental glomerulosclerosis. In: Davison AM, Cameron JS, Grünfeld JP, Ponticelli C, Ritz E, Winearls CG, von Ypersele C (eds) Oxford textbook of clinical nephrology, 3rd edn. Oxford University Press, Oxford, pp 439–467

Niaudet P (2004) Genetic forms of nephrotic syndrome. Pediatr Nephrol 19:1313–1318

Niaudet P, Boyer O (2009) Idiopathic nephritic syndrome in children: clinical aspects. In: Avner ED, Harmon WE, Niaudet P, Yoshikawa N (eds) Pediatric nephrology, 6th edn. Springer, Berlin, Heidelberg, pp 667–702

Niaudet P, Habib R (1998) Methylprednisolone pulse therapy in the treatment of severe forms of Schonlein-Henoch purpura nephritis. Pediatr Nephrol 12:238–243

Niaudet P, The French Society of Pediatric Nephrology (1994) Treatment of childhood steroid resistant idiopathic nephrosis with a combinaison of cyclosporine and prednisone. J Pediatr 125:981–985

Niaudet P, Drachman R, Gagnadoux MF, Broyer M (1984) Treatment of idiopathic nephrotic syndrome with levamisole. Acta Paediatr Scand 73:637–641

Perfumo F, Martini A (2005) Lupus nephritis in children. Lupus 14:83–88

Rai Mittal B, Singh S, Bhattacharya A, Prasad V, Singh B (2005) Lung scintigraphy in the diagnosis and follow-up of pulmonary thromboembolism in children with nephrotic syndrome. Clin Imaging 29:313–316

Samuelson O, Mulec H, Knight-Gibson C (1997) Lipoprotein abnormalities are associated with increased rate of progression of human chronic renal insufficiency. Nephrol Dial Transplant 12: 1908–1915

Tune BM, Mendoza SA (1997) Treatment of idiopathic nephrotic syndrome: regimens and outcomes in children and adults. J Am Soc Nephrol 8:824–832

Wasserstein AG (1997) Membranous glomerulonephritis. J Am Soc Nephrol 8:664–674

Weber S, Gribouval O, Esquivel EL et al (2004) NPHS2 mutation analysis shows heterogeneity of steroid-resistant nephrotic syndrome and low post-transplant recurrence. Kidney Int 66:571–579

West CD (1986) Childhood membranoproliferative glomerulonephritis: An approach to management. Kidney Int 29:1077–1093

Zenker M, Tralau T, Lennert T et al (2004) Congenital nephrosis, mesangial sclerosis, and distinct eye abnormalities with microcoria: an autosomal recessive syndrome. Am J Med Genet 130:138–145

302 Juvenile Nephronophthisis

Abdelaziz Y. Elzouki · Laurel Steinmetz

Renal cysts are derived from tubular epithelium that proliferates abnormally to generate the wall delineating the cyst; fully developed renal cysts are, in fact, tumor masses that are filled with liquid rather than with cells. Cysts may occur in cortex, medulla, or both regions. Hereditary renal cystic disorders are a diverse group of clinical categories having in common only the presence of cystic structures in renal parenchyma. The following two chapters focus on the major hereditary renal cystic diseases that have clinical importance in the pediatric population, including juvenile nephronophthisis (NPH), medullary cystic kidney disease (MCD), autosomal recessive polycystic kidney disease (ARPKD), and autosomal dominant polycystic kidney disease (ADPKD).

Juvenile Nephronophthisis

Juvenile NPH is responsible for 10–20% of chronic renal failure in children and is the most common genetic cause of end-stage renal disease in children. The onset of NPH is insidious, and the condition is usually not clinically diagnosed until the patient is in advanced renal failure. MCD is clinically and histologically indistinguishable from NPH; nevertheless, the two forms can be distinguished on the basis of inheritance and evolution – NPH is an autosomal recessive disorder while MCD is autosomal dominant disorder, in NPH end-stage renal failure is encountered during early adolescence while it occurs after fourth decade of life in MCD.

Epidemiology

NPH affects girls and boys equally.The incidence is approximately 0.13 for 10,000 live births in Finland, whereas in Canada, it is 1 per 50,000 live births and in United States 9 per 8.3 million. The disorder has been reported worldwide.

Genetics

These disorders include juvenile nephronophthisis, Senior-Loken syndrome, Joubert syndrome, Meckel-Gruber syndrome, and medullary cystic kidney disease. While renal imaging and histology are similar, there is a diverse phenotypic range in both renal disease progression and extrarenal manifestations. Several different gene mutations have been implicated in this heterogeneous group of disorders. Amongst those are NPHP1-9 and AHI1 in nephronophthisis (➋ *Table 302.1*) and MCDK1-2 in MCDK. NPHP1 was the first gene mutation identified and the most prevalent. NPHP1 homozygous deletion is present in 20–40% of nephronophthisis cases. The other mutations are much less common accounting for less than 2% of the cases individually. While most of these mutations have been associated with retinitis pigmentosa, NPHP5 and 6 are often associated with more severe retinal disease such as Leber's congenital amaurosis.

Etiology

Through recognition of these genes and others implicated in cystic kidney diseases, a new unifying theory of renal cystogenesis has emerged. This theory states that proteins implicated in renal cyst development are expressed in the centrosome, basal body, or primary cilia. Cilia are hair-like structures found on almost every type of vertebrate cell explaining the extrarenal involvement associated with these disorders. The proteins involved in ciliary function are highly conserved amongst organisms and many of the gene products implicated in renal cystic disease interact with each other in the ciliary complex. These findings support reclassification of many cystic kidney diseases as ciliopathies. Several potential mechanisms for renal cyst development in nephronophthisis exist. They include: (1) the mechanosensory mechanism whereby ciliary bending defects lead to changes in calcium influx altering cell

Abdelaziz Y. Elzouki (ed.), *Textbook of Clinical Pediatrics*, DOI 10.1007/978-3-642-02202-9_302,

Table 302.1

Genetic heterogeneity and overlap of nephronophthisis (NPH), Senior–Loken, Joubert, and Meckel-Gruber syndromes

Locus	Chromosome	Gene[a]	Clinical manifestations
NPHP1/SLSN1	2q13	*NPHP1* (nephrocystin-1)	Juvenile nph (mild JBTS, mild RP, Cogan)
NPHP2	9q31	*NPHP2/INVS* (Inversin)	Infantile nph (RP, liver fibrosis, HT)
NPHP3/SLSN3	3q22	*NPHP3* (nephrocystin-3)	Juvenile nph (liver fibrosis, RP)
NPHP4/SLSN4	1p36	*NPHP4* (nephrocystin-4 or nephroretinin)	Juvenile nph (Cogan, RP)
NPHP5/SLSN5	3q21	*NPHP5/IQCB1*	Juvenile nph + severe RP
NPHP6/SLSN6/JBTS5/MKS4	12q21	*NPHP6/CEP290*	Juvenile nph + JBTS + severe RP, isolated RP, (MKS)
NPHP7	16p	*NPHP7/GLIS2*	Juvenile nph
NPHP8/JBTS7/MKS5	16q	*NPHP8/RPGRIP1L*	Juvenile nph + JBTS (MKS)
NPHP9	17q11	*NPHP9/NEK8*	Juvenile and infantile nph

Reproduced from Salomon R, Saunier S, Niaudet P (2009) Nephronophthisis. Pediatr Nephrol 24(12):2333–2344, Table 1

JBTS Joubert syndrome type B, *RP* retinitis pigmentosa, *MKS* Meckel-Gruber syndrome, *HT* arterial hypertension

[a]The name of the protein is indicated when it is not the same as the gene

signaling pathways, (2) defective membrane and centrosome proteins lead to disruption of normal cell–cell and cell–matrix signaling, (3) improper planar polarity of tubules due to dysregulation of the WNT pathway, (4) abnormal apoptosis of normal renal cells leading to proliferation of cystic lesions at the expense of normal kidney tissue which is unique to nephronophthisis compared to the polycystic kidney diseases with enlarged kidneys.

Pathology

The disease is characterized by the presence of cysts in the medulla and corticomedullary junction. The size of the cysts ranges from less than 0.5 mm to 2 cm in diameter. The characteristic pathologic feature in renal biopsy is the presence of chronic tubulointerstitial inflammation and fibrosis (➲ *Fig. 302.1*).

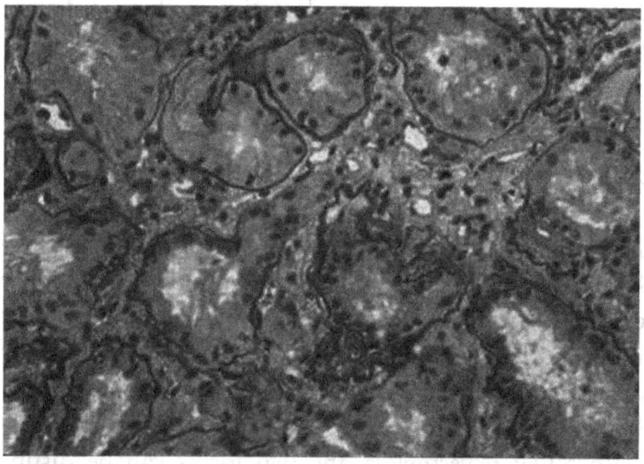

Figure 302.1
Renal histology of nephronophthisis showing diffuse interstitial fibrosis and various tubular changes (Reproduced from Salomon R, Saunier S, Niaudet P (2009) Nephronophthisis. Pediatr Nephrol 24(12):2333–2344, fig. 1)

Clinical Features

Usually the child presents with clinical and laboratory findings of chronic renal failure at the age of 10–12 years. Other characteristic clinical features include history of polyuria and polydipsia, history of salt craving, failure to thrive, normal blood pressure, parental consanguinity, and the presence of retinal abnormalities. Urinalysis is unremarkable, but urinary concentrating ability is impaired.

Extrarenal manifestations (➲ *Table 302.2*):

1. A retinopathy known as a tapetoretinal degeneration also known as retinitis pigmentosa (➲ *Fig. 302.2*) (Senior-Loken syndrome), seen in 18% of cases.

Table 302.2
Extrarenal manifestations in nephronophthisis

Ocular
Isolated oculomotor apraxia (Cogan syndrome)
Retinitis pigmentosa (Senior-Løken syndrome)
Coloboma
Nystagmus (Joubert syndrome)
Ptosis (Joubert syndrome)
Neurological
Mental retardation (Joubert syndrome or isolated)
Cerebellar ataxia with vermis hypoplasia (Joubert syndrome)
Hypopituitarism (RHYNS syndrome)
Liver
Elevation of hepatic enzymes
Fibrosis, biliary duct proliferation (Boichis syndrome)
Skeletal
Phalangeal cone-shaped epiphyses (Saldino-Mainzer or cono-renal syndrome)
Short ribs (Jeune or asphyxiating thoracic dystrophy syndrome)
Postaxial polydactyly
Skeletal dysplasia (Sensenbrenner syndrome or cranioectodermal dysplasia)
Other:
Situs inversus
Cardiac malformations
Bronchitis[a]
Sterility[a]
Hyperlipemia[a]
Ectodermal dysplasia (Sensenbrenner syndrome)

Reproduced from Salomon R, Saunier S, Niaudet P (2009) Nephronophthisis. Pediatr Nephrol 24(12):2333–2344, Table 2
[a]Personal data

Retinitis pigmentosa(RP) has been observed in association with mutations in most NPHP genes (except NPHP7), but whereas RP is always present and severe in patients with NPHP 5 and NPHP 6 mutations, the symptoms are in general mild in patients with mutations in the other NPHP genes.

2. Leber congenital amaurosis. In the early-onset form, affected children are blind from birth, have specific electroretinogram findings, and develop retinitis pigmentosa. In the late-onset type, blindness occurs later in childhood. Other eye abnormalities include coloboma, cataracts, amblyopia, and nystagmus.
3. Neurologic associations such as cerebellar ataxia, developmental delay (Joubert syndrome) JS is autosomal recessive neurological disorders can be associated with NPH and is characterized by complex cerebellar and brain stem malformation the so called "molar tooth sign" observed by MRI (➋ *Fig. 302.3*).

   Other neurological associations with NPH include recurrent seizures and mental retardation.
4. Congenital hepatic fibrosis.
5. Skeletal abnormalities, including cone-shaped epiphyses in the hand phalanges, metaphyscal chondrodysplasia of the femoral necks (Saldino-Mainzen syndrome), and Jeune asphyxiating thoracic dysplasia.
6. Other syndromes that feature NPH are described in ➋ *Table 302.3*.

Diagnosis

Medullary cysts, although regarded as the hallmark of this condition, are seldom seen in percutaneous renal biopsy specimens, even though medullary tissue may be present, presumably because of their uneven distribution. Ultrasonography has been used, but there are many other medical causes of chronic renal failure that show parenchymal heperechogenicity and loss of corticomedullary differentiation echogenic, and cysts may be too small to be detected by ultrasonography. Computerized tomography (CT) scan has been underutilized as a diagnostic tool in this disease entity. The recommended technique for CT scan examinations is contrast-enhanced 1- to 2-mm sections throughout the kidneys. Lesions are usually shown as multiple cysts, typically located at the medulla and corticomedullary region (➋ *Fig. 302.4*). The thin 1- to 2-mm sections recommendation is based on the fact that the size of the cysts ranges from less than 0.5 mm to 2 cm in diameter.

The detection of homozygous mutations by polymerase chain reaction (PCR) amplification permit fast and accurate diagnostic evidence. When a deletion has been demonstrated in one child, it should be sought in siblings to determine those who are affected.

Management

Usually the patient presented with clinical features of chronic renal failure. The immediate and long-term

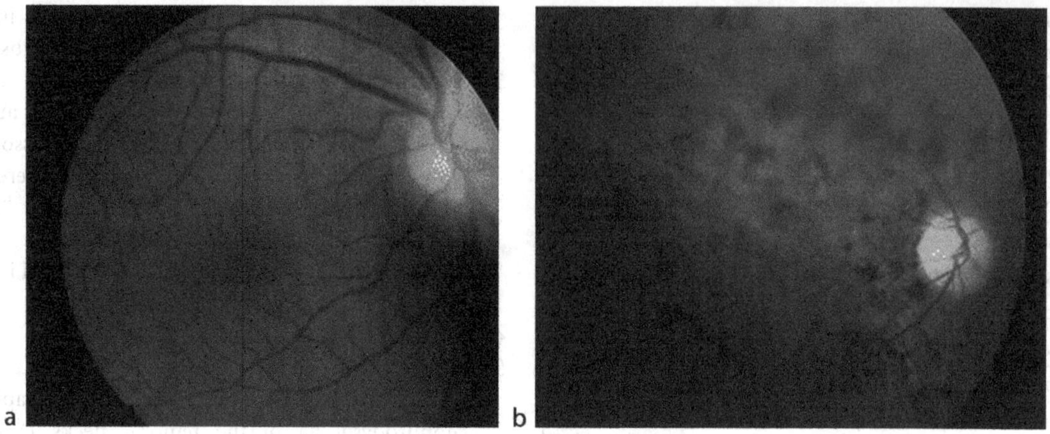

◘ Figure 302.2
Retinitis pigmentosa ophthalmoscopic examinations of a control subject (a) and an affected individual (b) showing typical retinitis pigmentosa fundus characterized by very thin retinal vessels, retinal pigment epithelium atrophy, abnormal pigmentary migrations, and pallor of the optic disk (Reproduced from Salomon R, Saunier S, Niaudet P (2009) Nephronophthisis. Pediatr Nephrol 24(12):2333–2344, fig. 2)

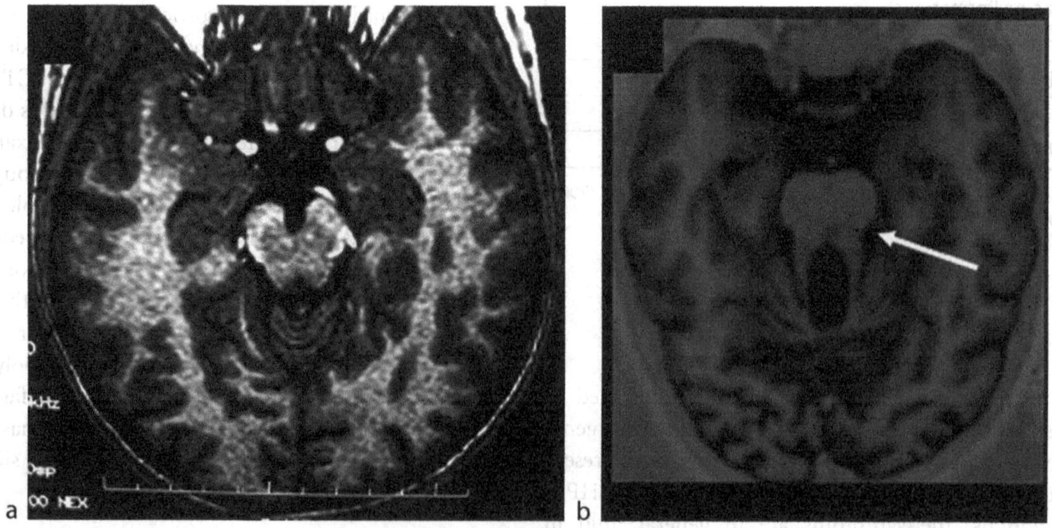

◘ Figure 302.3
Molar tooth sign on brain magnetic resonance imaging (MRI) axial image at the level of superior cerebellar peduncles of a control subject (a) and an affected individual (b) showing abnormally increased depth of the interpeduncular fossa, narrowing of the midbrain tegmentum, and thickening of the superior cerebellar peduncles, all of which contribute to the radiologic feature known as the molar tooth sign (*white arrow*) (Reproduced from Salomon R, Saunier S, Niaudet P (2009) Nephronophthisis. Pediatr Nephrol 24(12):2333–2344, fig. 3)

Table 302.3
Syndromes featuring nephronophthisis or associated with mutations of NPHP genes

Senior-Løken
Cogan
Joubert (type B)
Meckel-Gruber
Saldino-Mainzer (cono-renal syndrome)
Sensenbrenner (cranioectodermal dysplasia)
Ellis van Creveld (ectodermal dysplasia)
Jeune (asphyxiating thoracic dystrophy syndrome)
RHYNS (retinitis pigmentosa, hypopituitarism, and skeletal dysplasia)
Alstrom (retinal dystrophy, hearing impairment, obesity, type two diabetes mellitus)
Arima-Dekaban
Boichis

Reproduced from Salomon R, Saunier S, Niaudet P (2009) Nephronophthisis. Pediatr Nephrol 24(12):2333–2344, Table 3

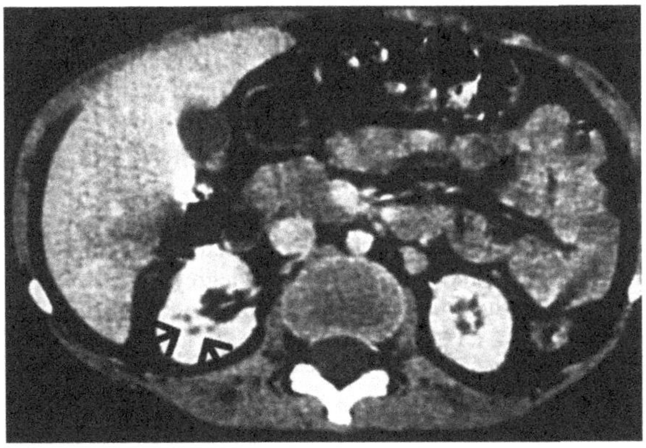

Figure 302.4
Contrast-enhanced computerized tomography cut through kidneys in a child with a diagnosis of juvenile nephronophthisis. Note the multiple small medullary and corticmedullary cysts in both kidneys (*arrows*) (Reproduced from chap. 108, first edition, fig.1)

management is as for children with chronic renal failure (see Chap. 313, "Chronic Renal Failure"), which includes correction of metabolic acidosis and electrolyte imbalance, treatment of osteodystrophy, nutritional support, and dialysis or kidney transplant.

Infantile Nephronophthisis

A chronic autosomal recessive tubulointerstitial nephritis with cortical microcysts progressing to end-stage renal disease before 2 years of age, severe hypertension is common. Ultrasonography usually shows moderately enlarged kidneys.

References

Delous M, Baala L, Solomon R et al (2007) The ciliary gene RPGRIPIL is mutated in cerebello-oculo-renal syndrome (Joubert syndrome type B) and Meckel syndrome. Nat Genet 39:875–889

Donaldson MD, Warner AA, Trompter RS et al (1985) Familial juvenile nephronophthisis, Jeune syndrome and associated disorders. Arch Dis Child 60:426–434

Elzouki A, Mirza K (1994) Juvenile nephronophthisis clinical quiz. Pediatr Nephrol 8:825–826

Elzouki AY, Al-Suhibani H, Mirza K et al (1996) Thin-section computed tomography scans detect medullary cysts in patients believed to have juvenile nephronophthisis. Am J Kidney Dis 27:216–219

Gangadoux MF, Bacri JL, Broyer M, Habib R (1998) Infantile chronic tubulo-interstitial nephritis with cortical microcysts: variant of nephronothisis or new disease entity? Pediatr Nephrol 3:50–55

Gusmano R, Ghiggeri GM, Caridi G (1998) Nephronophthisis-medullary cystic disease: clinical and genetic aspects. J Nephrol 11:224–228

Hildebrant F, Zhou W (2007) Nephronophthisis-associated ciliopathies. J Am Soc Nephrol 18:1855–1871

Konrad M, Saunier S, Heidet L et al (1996) Large homozygous deletions of the 2q13 region are a major cause of juvenile nephronophthisis. Hum Mol Genet 5:367–371

Salomon R, Saunier S, Niaudet P (2009) Nephronophthisis. Pediatr Nephrol 24(12):2333–2344

Scolari F, Puzzer D, Amoroso A et al (1999) Identification of a new locus for medullary cystic disease, on chromosome 16p12. Am J Hum Genet 64:1655–1660

Steele BT, Lirenman DS, Beattie CW (1980) Nephronophthisis. Am J Med 68:531–538

303 Autosomal Dominant Polycystic Kidney Disease/Autosomal Recessive Polycystic Kidney Disease

Abdelaziz Y. Elzouki · Laurel Steinmetz

Autosomal Dominant Polycystic Kidney Disease

ADPKD, the most prevalent hereditary renal cystic disorder, affects approximately 1:400 to 1:1,000 persons in the United States and is the fourth leading cause of chronic renal failure throughout the world. ADPKD is rarely diagnosed in infancy and childhood. Most reported cases present at birth with an abdominal mass or are found through screening members of families with ADPKD.

Genetics

ADPKD is inherited in an autosomal dominant fashion with full penetrance. A family history of ADPKD is elicited in approximately 60% of affected persons. A lack of family history is probably related to the variability of expression of the disease. ADPKD is a genetically heterogeneous disease with multiple different mutations in two genes, PKD1 and PKD2. PKD1 mutations tend to lead to end-stage renal disease at a younger age than mutations in PKD2. However, no specific mutations have been correlated with disease phenotype. PKD1 is a large gene on chromosome 16p13.3 and its mutations account for 85% of cases. PKD2 is a smaller gene on 4q21–23 and accounts for 14% of cases.

Only 5–10% of mutations are sporadic.

Preliminary evidence indicates that a third genotype, PKD3, has been identified in 1% of patients, but no genomic locus has been assigned.

Etiology

Cystogenesis in ADPKD is related to defects in polycystins, proteins, which localize to the cell membrane and cilia. Specifically defects in polycystin 1, coded for by PKD1, and polycystin 2, coded for by PKD2 contribute to cyst development. Polycystin 1 is expressed in heart, brain, bone, and muscle while polycystin 2 is expressed in reproductive organs, vascular smooth muscle, kidney, heart, and small intestine. Evidence suggests that these two proteins form a complex in the primary cilia contributing to its mechanosensory ability and that disruption of this ability contributes to cystogenesis. Polycystin 1 is also involved in cell–cell signaling, mechanosensory machinery, intracellular signaling including cell cycle regulation and proliferation, fluid production, and cell polarity. Polycystin 2 is responsible for intracellular calcium influx thought to alter gene expression. Evidence suggests that cystogenesis in ADPKD requires a two hit hypothesis where a patient inherits one mutation and then later develops a second somatic mutation leading to cyst development. The two hit hypothesis would explain why the cyst pattern in ADPKD is focal. This theory may also explain why cysts form at different times even amongst individuals who inherit the same genetic mutations.

Pathology

Renal architecture is distorted by multiple cysts whose number and size increase with increasing age. Cysts may be seen in liver and pancreas. Approximately 10% of patients develop berry aneurysms of the cerebral circulation, and hepatic fibrosis occurs occasionally.

Clinical Features

There are four ways in which ADPKD presents in childhood: (1) prenatal or neonatal presentation, which resembles the clinical presentation of ARPKD (i.e., bilateral renal mass, hypertension, respiratory distress, and renal insufficiency; (2) evaluation of asymptomatic siblings of families with ADPKD; (3) symptomatic children with a family history of ADPKD; and (4) symptomatic patients

Abdelaziz Y. Elzouki (ed.), *Textbook of Clinical Pediatrics*, DOI 10.1007/978-3-642-02202-9_303,

with no family history of polycystic kidney disease (PKD) for whom a parent is found to have PKD as a result of the evaluation of the parents. Usually these symptomatic children present with gross hematuria or hypertension and renal cysts on ultrasonography.

Extrarenal complications include cardiac valve abnormalities, cerebral berry aneurysms, hepatic, pancreatic, and spleen cysts.

Many studies in adults have been shown that patients with mutations in the PKD2 gene have a better prognosis than do PKD1 patients: In a study on genotype–phenotype correlation in children with ADPKD, PKD1 children had more and larger renal cysts, larger kidneys, and higher ambulatory blood pressure than PKD2 children. Prenatal finding of renal cysts or postnatal enlarged kidneys were observed only in patients with mutations in PKD1 gene.

Diagnosis

The renal ultrasonography of a neonate with ADPKD demonstrates large kidneys with hyperechoic parenchyma and no differentiation between cortex and medulla. It is possible to diagnose ADPKD prenatally with the use of DNA obtained from amniocentesis or chorionic villus sampling by the gene linkage techniques, but clinicians do not think this late-onset disease warrants interruption of pregnancy. In older children the renal ultrasonography demonstrates the cyst (➲ *Fig. 303.1*). The sensitivity of CT scan is greater than that of ultrasonography (➲ *Fig. 303.2*). In adult patients younger than 30 years of age, the presence of two cysts, either unilateral or bilateral, is sufficient to make the diagnosis. In patients 30–59 years old, at least two cysts in each kidney are essential for the diagnosis. DNA linkage analysis testing is useful in determining the disease status of relatives with normal kidneys who wish to be considered as potential donors for living kidney transplantation.

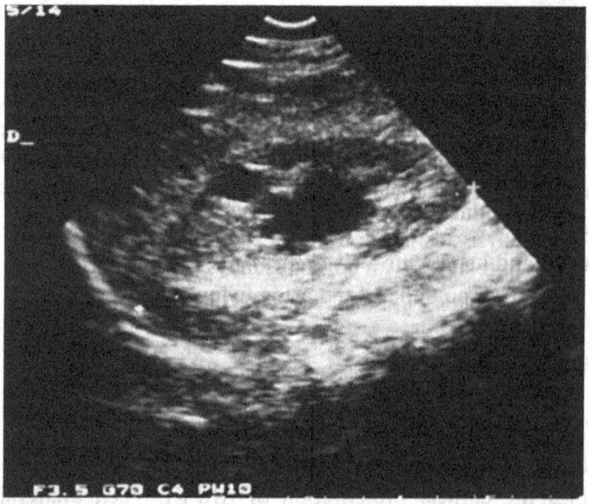

Figure 303.1
Renal ultrasonography in a child with a diagnosis of ADPKD. Note the large cyst (Reproduced from chap. 108, first edition, fig. 2)

Treatment

Early disease detection has traditionally led to problem with insurability and later employment but has offered these individuals little benefit if any in term of treatment option. New potential targets for therapies stemming from animal and bench research have been surfaced these include:

1. Clinical trials to explore the role of inhibition of renin-angiotensin-aldosterone system(RAAS), utilizing combination therapy ACEI and ARB in treatment of hypertensive individuals with ADPKD.
2. Agents that inhibit cell growth and proliferation utilizing an inhibitor of the mammalian target of rapamycin mTOR, treatment studies are now underway in adults with ADPKD to determine if Sirolimus that is widely used in transplant recipients is effective in slowing the progression of the disease.
3. Vasopressin V2 receptor antagonists are also demonstrating potential therapeutic benefits in APKD.

Although the translation of these new potential targets for therapies into meaningful safe remedies in human will

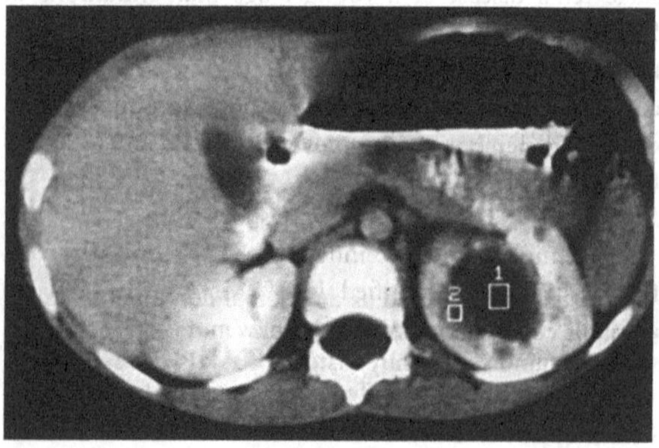

Figure 303.2
Contrast-enhanced computerized tomography scan demonstrates large cyst in left kidney in a child with a diagnosis of ADPKD (Reproduced from chap. 108, first edition, fig. 3)

take time and scrutiny, it is likely that children with ADPKD will benefit from those outstanding scientific contributions in near future.

Autosomal Recessive Polycystic Kidney Disease

ARPKD has previously been referred to as "infantile polycystic kidney disease"; however, the disease can present at any age, from the prenatal period through adolescence, and in a few patients ARPKD is not recognized until adulthood.

The pathologic findings of the disease include varying degrees of cystic dilation of the distal tubules and collecting ducts throughout the cortex and medulla, varying degrees of biliary dysgenesis, and hepatic fibrosis.

Epidemiology

The reported prevalence varies from 1:600 to 1:55,000 live births. Gene frequency is in a range from 1:40 to 1:100.

Genetics

This disease is inherited in an autosomal recessive pattern. Mutations have been found in the PKHD1 gene on chromosome 6p21. This gene is large and multiple different types of mutations have been found. Variability in age of onset is related to different expression of mutation and modifier genes. Patients with two truncating mutations will die in the perinatal period. Missense mutations tend to cause less severe phenotypes. PKHD1 encodes the protein fibrocystin, also known as polyductin.

Etiology

Fibrocystin is thought to contribute to normal ciliary development. However, its precise function has not been elucidated. Studies suggest that it complexes with polycystin 1 and 2 and plays a role in intracellular calcium signaling. It also may contribute to normal tubule morphogenesis. In addition, cyclic AMP and epidermal growth factor receptor also play a role in cystogenesis in ARPKD models.

Clinical Presentation

Prenatally the findings of oligohydramnios, bilateral enlarged kidneys that are diffusely echogenic, and the absence of fluid in the fetal bladder are consistent with a diagnosis of ARPKD. Elevation of α-fetoprotein levels in maternal serum and amniotic fluid may complement the prenatal ultrasonographic diagnosis.

The newborn usually presents with bilateral massively enlarged kidneys and respiratory distress, which is a complication of pulmonary hypoplasia or pneumothorax. Severely affected neonates may demonstrate the Potter phenotype (i.e., deep-set eyes, flat beaked nose, micrognathia, low-set ears, and joint deformities). Later in infancy and childhood, those who survive the neonatal period will develop the sequelae of renal insufficiency (i.e., failure to thrive, anemia, and renal osteodystrophy). The majority of patients have a concentrating defect with polyuria and polydipsia. Hyponatremia and metabolic acidosis have been described.

Hypertension occurs in nearly all patients with ARPKD. It was reported that all affected infants who had blood pressure measurements at 3 months of age were hypertensive. The degree of hypertension has been noted to be most severe in the first year of life and may be responsible for early death in many of these patients.

Extrarenal manifestations include:

Liver Disease. The liver disease in ARPKD is primarly manifest by two major types of pathophysiology biliary disease and portal hypertension.There is considerable variability in the severity of liver disease in ARPKD.

The complications of hepatic fibrosis and portal hypertension are seen more frequently in older children. These complications include hepatosplenomegaly, bleeding esophageal varices, and hypersplenism sequelae (i.e., anemia, thrombocytopenia, and leukopenia).

The most common manifestations of biliary disease are sepsis/cholangitis and or complication of cholelithiasis.

Standard liver biochemical testing is typically normal in children with ARPKD with liver disease and thus may not necessary be useful as screening tools.

A combination of physical examination (finding of splenomegly) and CBC (finding of cytopenia) and abdominal ultrasonography is a reliable method for screening for evidence of portal hypertension.

Intracranial Aneurysm. The incidence of intracranial aneurysm is well-known extrarenal manifestation of ADPKD, the incidence is about 10%; there are reported cases of intracranial aneurysm in patients with ARPKD (➋ *Fig. 303.3*).

Diagnostic Imaging

The abdominal ultrasound usually shows enlarged kidneys with hyperechoic parenchyma and no differentiation

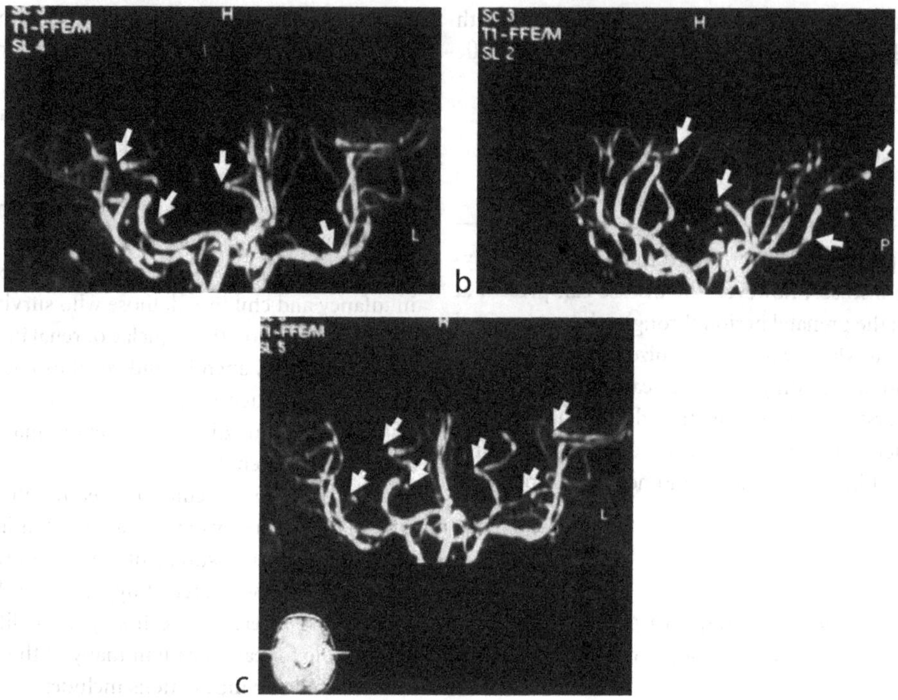

■ **Figure 303.3**

Magnetic resonance of brain angiography of multiple intracranial aneurysms in the branches of middle and posterior cerebral arteries (Reproduced from Lilova MI, Petkov DL (2001) Intracranial aneurysm in a child with Autosomal Recessive Polycystic Kidney Disease. Pediatr Nephrol 16:1030–1032)

between cortex and medulla (➋ *Fig. 303.4*). The liver is usually normal in size and less echogenic than the kidney; dilated intrahepatic biliary ducts may be demonstrated. The presence of portal hypertension on Doppler ultrasonography indirectly indicates the presence of hepatic fibrosis. The intravenous pyelogram usually shows the classic findings of enlarged kidneys, and delayed nephrogram with medullary streaking (accumulation of contrast in dilated medullary collecting ducts). The intravenous pyelogram is not essential for diagnosis and certainly not recommended.

Magnetic Resonance (MR) cholangiography is more sensitive test for identifying biliary ectasia, recommended the MR cholangiography be performed at least once in children with ARPKD.

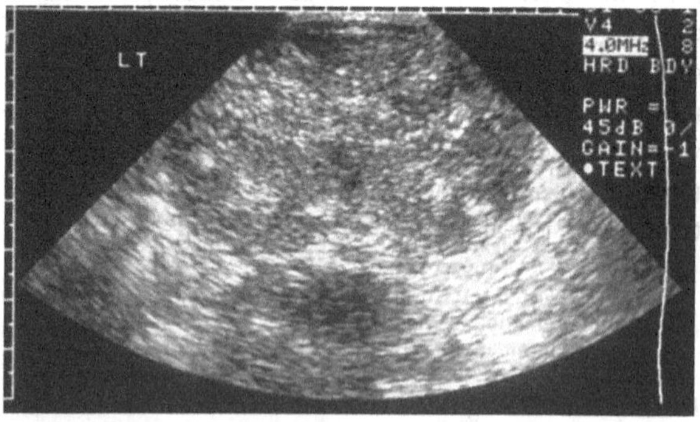

■ **Figure 303.4**

Renal ultrasonography in a child with a diagnosis of ARPKD. Note enlarged kidney with hyperechoic parenchyma and no differentiation between cortex and medulla (Reproduced from chap. 108, first edition, Fig. 4)

Management

Hypertension can be treated with calcium-channel blockers, β blockers, angiotensin-converting enzyme inhibitors, and vasodilators. Hypertension may require multiple antihypertensive agents for effective control.

Supplemental bicarbonate therapy is needed for those with metabolic acidosis. The same treatment as that used for chronic renal failure (see ➋ Chap. 313, "Chronic Kidney Disease"), as well as dialysis and/or transplant, are indicated when children with ARPKD reach end-stage renal disease. For hepatic involvement, close monitoring for the complications of portal hypertension and hypersplenism is necessary. Surgical intervention with portocaval and splenorenal shunts may be needed. Appropriate antimicrobial therapy should be given to those patients with a suspected diagnosis of cholangitis.

Caroli Syndrome

Caroli syndrome is characterized by the presence of autosomal recessive polycystic kidney disease, congenital hepatic fibrosis, and nonobstructive dilation of the intrahepatic bile ducts. On hepatic ultrasonography, there are saccular dilated bile ducts containing intraluminal protrusions and crossbridges, and contrast-enhanced CT scan reveals liver cysts with a "central dot sign" (➋ *Fig. 303.5*).

How to Differentiate Between ADPKD and ARPKD

Distinguishing between ADPKD and ARPKD based on clinical findings may be unreliable. Both ADPKD and ARPKD produce renal masses and hypertension in childhood. Ultrasonography may show enlarged hyperechoic kidneys in both entities; conversely, macroscopic cysts may be detected in older patients with ARPKD. The use of liver biopsy has been proposed as a means of distinguishing between ADPKD and ARPKD. The diagnosis of ARPKD cannot be supported in the presence of a normal liver. The presence of hepatic fibrosis, however, does not exclude a diagnosis of ADPKD. Congenital hepatic fibrosis has occurred in association with ADPKD. The single most useful investigation in the evaluation of a child with early onset of cystic renal disease is ultrasound of the parents and/or genetic analysis, the detection of homozygous mutations by polymerase chain reaction (PCR) amplification permit fast and accurate diagnosis evidence.

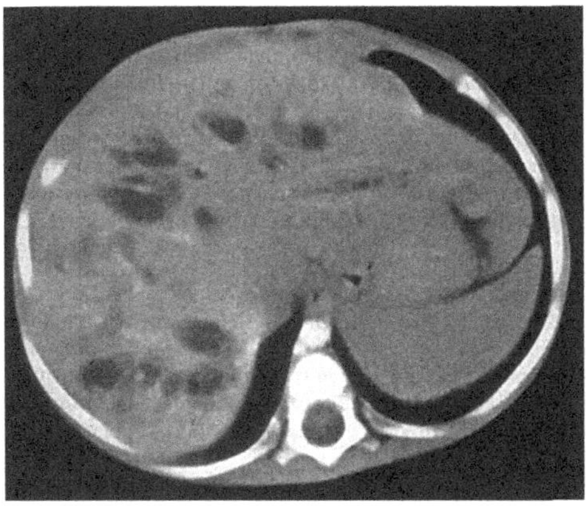

Figure 303.5
Computerized tomography scan demonstrates liver cysts with a "central dot sign" in a child with a diagnosis of Caroli syndrome (Reproduced from chap. 108, first edition, Fig. 5)

References

Alvarez V, Málaga S, Navarro M et al (2000) Analysis of chromosome 6p in Spanish families with recessive polycystic kidney disease. Pediatr Nephrol 14:205–207

Bergmann C, Senderek J, Windelen E et al (2005) Clinical consequences of PKHD1 mutations in 164 patients with autosomal-recessive polycystic kidney disease (ARPKD). Kidney Int 67:829–848

Cole BR (1990) Autosomal recessive polycystic kidney disease. In: Gardner KD Jr, Bernstein J (eds) The cystic kidney. Kluwer, Boston, pp 327–350

Daoust MC, Reynolds DM, Bichet DG, Somolo S (1995) Evidence for a third genetic locus for autosomal dominant polycstic kidney disease. Genomics 25:733–736

European Polycystic Kidney Disease Consortium (1994) The polycystic kidney disease 1 gene encodes a 14 Kb transcript and lies within a duplicated region on chromosome 16. Cell 77:1–20

Fencl F, Janda J, Blahova K et al (2009) Genotype-phenotype correlation in children with autosomal dominant polycystic kidney disease. Pediatr Nephrol 24:983–989

Gabow PA (1990) Autosomal dominant polycystic kidney disease. In: Gardner KD Jr, Bernstein J (eds) The cystic kidney. Kluwer, Boston, pp 295–326

Guay-Woodford LM, Desmond RA (2003) Autosomal recessive polycystic kidney disease: the clinical experience in North America. Pediatrics 111(5 Pt 1):1072–1080

Harris PC, Torres VE (2009) Polycystic kidney disease. Annu Rev Med 60:321–337

Igarashi P, Somlo S (2002) Genetics and pathogenesis of polycystic kidney disease. J Am Soc Nephrol 13(9):2384–2398

Jung G, Benz-Bohm G, Kugel H et al (1999) MR cholangiography in children with autosomal recessive polycystic kidney disease. Pediatr Radiol 29:463–466

Kaplan BS, Fay J, Shah V et al (1989) Autosomal recessive polycystic kidney disease. Pediatr Nephrol 3:43–49

Kimberling WJ, Kumar S, Gabaw PA et al (1993) Autosomal dominant polycystic kidney disease: localization of the second gene to chromosome 4q13–923. Genomics 18:467–472

Lilova MI, Petkov DL (2001) Intracranial aneurysm in a child with autosomal recessive polycystic kidney disease. Pediatr Nephrol 16:1030–1032

Martinez JR, Grantham JJ (1995) Polycystic kidney disease etiology, pathogenesis and treatment. Dis Mon 41:693–765

Menezes LF, Onuchic LF (2006) Molecular and cellular pathogenesis of autosomal recessive polycystic kidney disease. Braz J Med Biol Res 39(12):1537–1548

Murcia NS, Woychik RP, Avner ED (1998) The molecular biology of polycystic kidney disease. Pediatr Nephrol 12:721–726
Ogborn MR (1994) Polycystic kidney disease-a truly paediatric problem. Pediatr Nephrol 8:762–767
Parfrey PS, Bear JC, Morgan J et al (1990) The diagnosis and prognosis of autosomal dominant polcystic kidney disease. N Engl J Med 323:1085–1090
Peters DJM, Sandkuijl LA (1992) Genetic heterogenicity of polycstic kidney disease in Europe. Contrib Nephrol 97:128–139
Rick GM, Johnson AM, Strain JD et al (1993) Characteristics of very early onset autosomal dominant polycystic kidney disease. J Am Soc Nephrol 3:1863–1870
Rizk D, Chapman A (2008) Treatment of autosomal dominant polycystic kidney disease (ADPKD): the new horizon for children with ADPKD. Pediatr Nephrol 23:1029–1036
Saunders AJ, Denton E, Stephens S et al (1999) Cystic kidney disease presenting in infancy. Clin Radiol 54:370–376
Shaikewitz ST, Chapman A (1993) Autosomal recessive polycystic kidney disease: issues regarding the variability of clinical presentation. J Am Soc Nephrol 3:1858–1862
Shneider BL, Magid MS (2005) Liver disease in autosomal recessive polycystic kidney disease. Pediatr Transplant 9:634–639
Slovis TL, Bernstein J, Gruskin A (1993) Hyperechoic kidneys in the newborn and young infant. Peditar Nephrol 7:294–302
Torres V, Harris P (2009) Autosomal dominant polycystic kidney disease: the last 3 years. Kidney Int 76:149–168
Zerras K, Mucher G, Bachner L et al (1994) Mapping of the gene for autosomal recessive polycystic kidney disease (ARPKD) to chromosome 6P21. Nat Genet 7:429–432

304 Proximal Renal Tubular Disorders

Sami A. Sanjad

Definition and Classification

Diseases affecting the renal tubules occur due to structural or functional abnormalities in the different segments of the nephron. From a quantitative point of view the proximal tubular cells perform a remarkable job in reabsorbing the filtered plasma and its accompanying solutes. The distal tubules continue that process but are more involved in fine tuning operations, acidification of the urine, and diluting or concentrating it as necessary. In diseases of the proximal tubules, variable qualitative and quantitative degrees of aminoaciduria may be present with or without bicarbonaturia, glucosuria, uricosuria, or phosphaturia. Any combination of abnormal solute excretion is theoretically conceivable and may be found in different syndromes of proximal tubular dysfunction.

Etiology: General

Disorders of proximal tubular function may be secondary to congenital or hereditary diseases or due to acquired defects. The hereditary or congenital defects are much more prevalent and may be due to: (a) absent or defective Na-solute cotransport system in the proximal tubular cells, as seen in cystinuria, Hartnup disease, renal glucosuria, vitamin D resistant rickets, and proximal renal tubular acidosis; (b) altered gene affecting more than one transport system – adult Fanconi syndrome; (c) mutant genes resulting in endogenous tubulotoxic substances accumulated from extra renal metabolic pathways (cystinosis, galactosemia, tyrosinemia, hereditary fructose intolerance, Wilson's disease); (d) abnormal solute transport due to structural changes associated with congenital renal and urinary tract malformations (cystic diseases, nephronophthisis, and hydronephrosis).

Acquired defects of proximal tubular function are usually drug induced or related to intrinsic renal diseases (see below). This chapter covers three major disease entities associated with proximal tubular dysfunction: (1) Fanconi syndrome, (2) proximal renal tubular acidosis, and (3) disorders of phosphate transport.

Fanconi Syndrome

Also known by many other eponyms (Lignac-Fanconi, de Toni-Debré-Fanconi syndrome), the Fanconi syndrome represents a heterogeneous group of disorders which may be hereditary or acquired with a common denominator being abnormalities in the transport of multiple solutes by the proximal tubular cells. Solutes normally reabsorbed by the proximal tubules are lost in the urine in variable proportions. These include glucose, amino acids, phosphate, bicarbonate, uric acid, and low-molecular-weight proteins and cations. Most cases of Fanconi syndrome in children are secondary to inherited metabolic diseases associated with specific enzyme defects, or due to transport abnormalities across the tubular cells. Acquired Fanconi syndrome is usually due to tubulotoxic effect of several drugs and toxins or due to intrinsic renal diseases with a significant tubulointerstitial component (➲ *Table 304.1*). When no identifiable cause is found, the Fanconi is known as primary or idiopathic and may be familial or occur sporadically.

Clinical Findings

The clinical manifestations of the Fanconi syndrome and the onset of symptoms vary with the underlying etiology. Most patients with inherited disorders present in the first year of life with failure to thrive, frequently with anorexia and vomiting. Polyuria and polydipsia with bouts of fever and dehydration may also be present. Rickets is invariably seen at some stage of the disease and may be the presenting manifestation in some children.

Pathogenesis

The pathogenesis of the Fanconi syndrome is incompletely understood and probably varies with the underlying

Abdelaziz Y. Elzouki (ed.), *Textbook of Clinical Pediatrics*, DOI 10.1007/978-3-642-02202-9_304,

Table 304.1
Etiology of the Fanconi syndrome

Hereditary causes	Acquired causes
Cystinosis	Drugs and Toxins
Glycogen storage disease	Ifosfamide
Tyrosinemia type I	Heavy metals
Galactosemia	Glue sniffing
Hereditary fructose intolerance	Gentamicin
Lowe's syndrome	Outdated tetracycline
Mitochondrial cytopathies	
Metachromatic leukodystrophy	Disorders of Protein
Glutathione synthetase deficiency	Metabolism
	Light chain proteinuria
	Amyloidosis
	Nephrotic syndrome
	Multiple myeloma
	Other
	Renal transplantation

etiology. It is quite possible that a dysfunction of the basolateral membrane Na-K-ATPase pump, brought about by an endogenous or exogenous toxin, would result in impaired energy production for solute reabsorption by the proximal tubule. This has been observed in several clinical and experimental disorders associated with the Fanconi syndrome.

Diagnosis

The diagnosis of the Fanconi syndrome is easily made when the above constellation of findings are seen in association with euglycemic glucosuria and mild proteinuria on routine urinalysis. Proteinuria is primarily tubular in origin and is characterized by low-molecular-weight proteins, usually less than 30,000 Da. They include lysozyme and beta$_2$-microglobulin but also a small amount of filtered albumin that escapes reabsorption by the proximal tubule. Serum analysis reveals hyperchloremic metabolic acidosis, normal urea and creatinine levels (unless severe dehydration is present), hypophosphatemia, hypokalemia, hypouricemia, and hyponatremia. This low plasma solute concentration is a reflection of their losses in the urine as a result of decreased reabsorption by the proximal tubular cells. Urine amino acid analysis reveals generalized, nonspecific aminoaciduria. Once the diagnosis of Fanconi syndrome has been reached on clinical grounds, every effort should be made to obtain an etiologic diagnosis.

Etiology of Specific Forms of the Fanconi Syndrome

Hereditary Causes of the Fanconi Syndrome

Cystinosis

Cystinosis is cited in the western literature as the most common cause of the Fanconi syndrome with an incidence of 1:200,000 live births. It is not to be confused with cystinuria which (a) does not cause the Fanconi syndrome; (b) is predominantly associated with increased urinary excretion of cystine, ornithine, lysine, and arginine; and (c) is frequently associated with cystine urolithiasis.

Cystinosis is an autosomal recessive lysosomal storage disease characterized by the accumulation of cystine in several organs including the kidney, liver, gut, spleen, bone marrow, lymphatic system, leukocytes, cornea, thyroid, and other organs. The biochemical defect is unknown but a defective transport of cystine across the lysosomal membrane appears to be the most likely cause. Three forms of cystinosis are recognized: (1) infantile or nephropathic form being the most common, (2) adolescent or late form, and (3) adult or benign ocular cystinosis.

Clinical Findings in Cystinosis

The clinical and laboratory manifestations of nephropathic cystinosis are those of the Fanconi syndrome described above and they usually become apparent in early infancy. Polyuria and polydipsia are particularly common early manifestations. Some patients may present with severe hypokalemia and alkalosis mimicking Bartter's syndrome. Growth failure is severe and associated with hypophosphatemic rickets and hyperchloremic acidosis. Although glomerular filtration rate is normal in the early phases of the disease, progressive deterioration is the rule. By the end of the first decade most children with nephropathic cystinosis will develop end stage renal disease necessitating dialysis and renal transplantation.

The extra renal manifestations of cystinosis are secondary to the accumulation of cystine crystals in different organs. Thus, corneal deposition is responsible for photophobia, excessive tearing, and blepharospasm. Hypothyroidism, characterized by high TSH levels, is a frequent occurrence, particularly in older children, but clinical hypothyroidism is uncommon. Muscular weakness and hypotonia secondary to hypokalemia and carnitine deficiency are commonly observed. Testicular deposition of cystine crystals may explain the incomplete pubertal development frequently seen in males with cystinosis. This is associated with reduced plasma levels of testosterone but normal pituitary function. The central nervous system, initially thought to be spared in cystinosis, is now a well-known site of involvement in older patients with the disease. Symptoms vary from difficulty in walking to dysphagia, speech difficulty, and dementia. Cranial nerve involvement and pyramidal tract signs may also be seen. Retinopathy develops in a few patients and may be progressive and lead to blindness.

Adolescent and adult type cystinosis are less frequent. The clinical manifestations are insidious and the Fanconi syndrome is usually milder, occurring after the age of 8 years in the adolescent form. In the adult form of cystinosis, also known as ocular cystinosis, there is no renal involvement, but patients may complain of photophobia due to cystine deposition in the cornea.

Diagnosis

Cystinosis may be diagnosed by slit lamp examination of the cornea where cystine crystals may be seen. Bone marrow, liver or kidney biopsy may also reveal cystine crystals. Unequivocal diagnosis is made by demonstrating increased cystine content in leukocytes or rectal mucosa from affected individuals. The leukocyte cystine content is 5–15 nmol of ½ cystine/mg protein in the infantile form and less than 0.2 in normal individuals. Prenatal diagnosis is now possible by measuring amniotic fluid or cultured fibroblasts for cystine content. Molecular genetic studies have shown mapping of the cystinosis gene to chromosome 17p13. The *CTNS* gene encodes a 367-amino acid protein called cystinosin which is widely expressed in many organs, particularly pancreas, kidney and muscle. All patients with cystinosis tested have had mutations in the CTNS gene with no evidence thus far of genetic heterogeneity.

Glycogen Storage Disease (GSD)

The proximal tubular dysfunction associated with GSD is referred to as Fanconi-Bickel syndrome (GSD type 11) and was first described in 1949. Patients present typically in early infancy with failure to thrive, hypotonia, hepatomegaly, and rickets. Hyperchloremic acidosis with bicarbonate wasting is usually severe. The kidneys are usually enlarged and are loaded with glycogen. Many patients develop hypoglycemia with prolonged fasting and show impaired galactose utilization. One of the most striking abnormalities that characterizes this syndrome is the massive glucosuria, which may reach 100 g/m^2/day in some patients.

GSD appears to be relatively common in certain parts of the world. In Saudi Arabia it was diagnosed in more than one half of the cases of Fanconi syndrome (15 of 29) referred to a tertiary care center. In our experience many of these patients have a decreased or absent activity of the enzyme phosphorylase b kinase (pbk) involving liver and kidney. This was documented on liver homogenates from several patients with GSD and Fanconi syndrome who also had renal glycogen storage documented by histochemical assay. It has been subsequently shown, however, that mutations in the facilitative glucose transporter GLUT2 are causative of this syndrome and the low pbk activity detected in our patients is probably a secondary phenomenon that contributes to the deposition of glycogen in response to the intracellular glucose retention caused by GLUT2 deficiency.

Proximal tubular dysfunction has been described in a few patients with GSD type 1 (von Gierke's disease) but these are usually mild and not associated with a complete Fanconi syndrome. A more prevalent and serious finding in these patients who now are living longer than before is focal glomerulosclerosis with proteinuria and at times progressive renal failure.

Tyrosinemia Type I

Also known as hepatorenal tyrosinemia, this autosomal recessive disorder is characterized clinically by early onset of nodular hepatic cirrhosis, failure to thrive, and Fanconi syndrome. Rickets may be severe and crippling in untreated patients (➋ *Figs. 304.1* and ➋ *304.2*). Abdominal ultrasonography reveals hepatosplenomegaly and enlarged kidneys which, combined with the biochemical findings of the Fanconi syndrome, should arouse suspicion of tyrosinemia. A presumptive diagnosis of tyrosinemia is made when the urinary excretion of succinyl acetone (SA) is elevated. Delta aminolevulenic acid (DALA) is also excreted in large amounts in the urine of patients with tyrosinemia. The metabolic defect is related to deficiency of the enzyme fumaryl acetoacetate hydrolase (FAH) which leads to accumulation of toxic precursors including SA and DALA. The FAH gene has been cloned recently and mapped to chromosome 15 (15q23–q25). Several missense mutations have been described with no evidence of phenotype genotype correlation with different clinical manifestations sometimes observed

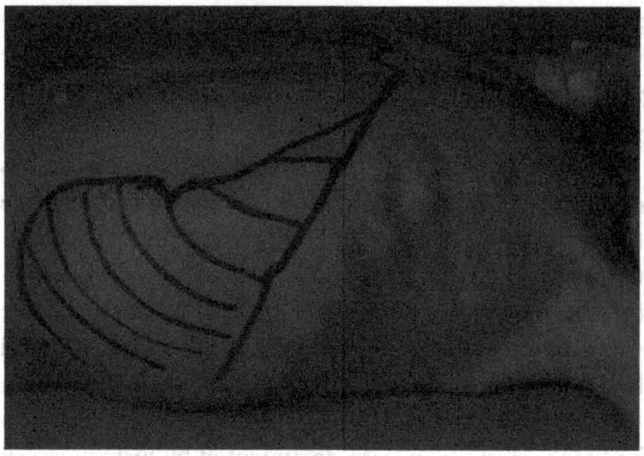

Figure 304.1
Massive splenomegaly and rachitic rosary in a 7-year-old male with tyrosinemia type 1

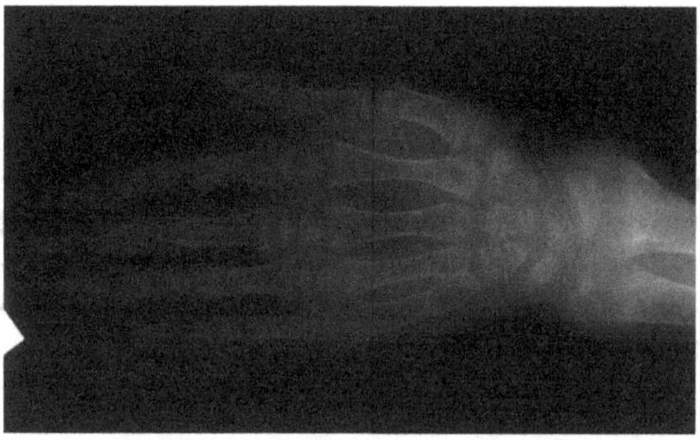

Figure 304.2
Severe rachitic changes in a patient with hepatorenal tyrosinemia

within the same family. This phenomenon may due to mutation reversion which has been described in patients with tyrosinemia.

Galactosemia

Galactosemia may result from many inherited enzyme deficiencies. Only that associated with Gal-1-PO_4 uridyl transferase deficiency results in the Fanconi's syndrome, which is incomplete, in that glucosuria is absent and phosphaturia is seldom severe to result in hypophosphatemia. Renal tubular acidosis is probably of the proximal type and associated with bicarbonaturia. Galactosemia and galactosuria are invariably seen. The diagnosis should be suspected in any infant with a history of failure to thrive, jaundice, hepatomegaly with or without cataracts, and non-glucose reducing substance in the urine. Definitive diagnosis is made by determining red blood cell Gal-1-PO_4 uridyl transferase activity. The molecular diagnosis of galactosemia has been identified recently by mutations in the GALT gene located on chromosome 9p13. The most common of these is a missense mutation of *Q188R* (replacement of glutamine-188 by arginine) but several other mutations have been identified as well.

Hereditary Fructose Intolerance

Hereditary fructose intolerance is an autosomal recessive inborn error of fructose metabolism caused by deficiency of fructose-1-phosphate (F1-PO_4) aldolase B activity in the liver, renal cortex, and small intestine. Several mutations in the human aldolase *B* gene have been identified, the most common being the A149P mutation in exon 5 located on chromosome 9_q 21.3_q 22.2. The clinical manifestations that develop following fructose ingestion are acute in nature and consist of nausea, vomiting, and diarrhea. Liver failure may develop within days. An acute Fanconi syndrome with *hyperuricemia*, hyperlactic acidemia, and hypermagnesemia develops within 30–60 min of ingestion of a large amount of fructose. In extreme cases, seizures, lethargy, and coma may develop. Ingestion of small amounts of fructose is not associated with symptoms.

The renal tubular abnormalities as well as the other manifestations of the disease are probably secondary to accumulation of F-1-PO_4 with depletion of inorganic phosphate, thus limiting ATP regeneration. This may lead to reduced transport of multiple solutes across the proximal tubular epithelial cell characteristic of the Fanconi's syndrome. Fructose withdrawal promptly reverses the acute changes and the renal tubular dysfunction. In patients with chronic fructose ingestion, however, liver damage may be irreversible.

Lowe's Syndrome (Oculocerebrorenal Syndrome)

Lowe's syndrome is an X-linked recessive disease characterized by congenital cataracts, glaucoma, developmental and growth retardation, hypotonia, and a renal Fanconi syndrome. The gene locus (OCRL) has been mapped to X 25–26 by linkage analysis. More specifically the gene product is a 105 kD protein localized to the Golgi complex.

The Fanconi syndrome is usually mild or incomplete but it may be quite severe in some cases. In many patients glomerular insufficiency develops later in childhood in spite of adequate symptomatic treatment for the tubular abnormalities. Dialysis and transplantation are usually not prescribed because of the moderate to severe mental retardation seen in most patients with Lowe's syndrome.

Dent's Disease

This is a rare X-linked disorder characterized by hypercalciuria, hyperphosphaturia, low-molecular-weight proteinuria, and aminoaciduria, and an incomplete Fanconi syndrome. If untreated, many patients develop nephrolithiasis and renal failure. In addition, one third of the patients develop rickets or osteomalacia. The gene has been localized to chromosome Xp11.22 and has been identified as a chloride channel gene *CLCN5*. There are actually four diseases associated with mutations in this gene: Dent disease, X-linked recessive nephrolithiasis (XRN), X-linked recessive hypophosphatemic rickets (XLRH), and idiopathic low-molecular-weight proteinuria of Japanese children (ILMWP). All share many similarities as described above but patients with Dent disease and XLRH develop rickets while the others do not. Renal failure is only seen in patients with Dent disease and XRN. Female carriers are asymptomatic but frequently have low-molecular-weight proteinuria.

Wilson's Disease

Wilson's disease is an autosomal recessive disease primarily affecting the liver and brain where marked amounts of copper are deposited. It is caused by mutations in the *ATP7B* gene located on chromosome 13 (13q14.3) and is expressed primarily in the liver, kidney, and placenta. The gene codes for a P-type (cation transport enzyme) ATPase that transports copper into bile and incorporates it into ceruloplasmin. Mutations can be detected in 90% of patients and most of these are homozygous.

The classical triad of hepatic cirrhosis, Kayser-Fleischer rings in the cornea, and neurological symptoms are pathognomonic findings. Renal involvement appears later with more advanced liver disease but it may precede hepatic failure. It is characterized by tubular dysfunction as seen in other cases of the Fanconi syndrome, but glucosuria is infrequent.

Other Hereditary Causes of the Fanconi Syndrome

The Fanconi syndrome has been described in association with several other rare inborn errors of metabolism including mitochondrial cytopathies, metachromatic leukodystrophy, pyruvate carboxylase deficiency (Leigh's syndrome), and glutathione synthetase deficiency. ➲ *Table 304.2* outlines some of the inherited disorders of proximal tubular function with and without the Fanconi syndrome. It includes some of the salient clinical findings, enzymatic defects, and inheritance pattern.

Acquired Disorders Causing the Fanconi Syndrome

These are primarily disorders associated with heavy metal exposure (lead, mercury, platinum), drug induced lesions as with ifosfamide, outdated tetracycline, aminoglycosides, toluene inhalation, and with abnormalities in protein metabolism as in amyloidosis, Sjögren's syndrome, and the nephrotic syndrome. The development of Fanconi syndrome in a child with nephrosis is an ominous sign indicating tubulointerstitial nephropathy, usually in association with focal segmental glomerulosclerosis. The Fanconi syndrome may also be acquired following renal transplantation where the mechanism is probably immune mediated.

Of all the drugs causally related to the Fanconi syndrome, ifosfamide is probably the most predictable since tubular dysfunction occurs in a relatively high percentage of treated patients. Ifosfamide is a cyclophosphamide analog used to treat several solid tumors. The Fanconi syndrome develops acutely during treatment and is usually heralded by glucosuria and hypophosphatemia. Both proximal and distal RTA may be observed in addition to aminoaciduria and uricosuria. Hypokalemia may be severe and beta$_2$-microglobulinuria is quite pronounced. The tubular toxicity is thought to be due to chloracetaldehyde, one of the metabolites of ifosfamide. Glomerular toxicity and reduced GFR may also occur with ifosfamide toxicity. Hemorrhagic cystitis occurs with much less frequency than with cyclophosphamide.

General Treatment of the Fanconi Syndrome

Metabolic Acidosis and Electrolyte Abnormalities

Patients with Fanconi syndrome frequently require large doses of bicarbonate or citrate to replace the ongoing losses

Table 304.2
Inherited disorders of proximal tubular function

Disorder	Clinical findings	Biochemical defect	Urine abnormalities	Inheritance, gene locus, mutations
Fanconi syndrome Cystinosis	Progressive renal failure; cystine storage in multiple organs	Defective cystine transport across lysosomal membrane	Usual for FS	AR 17p13, D17S1584, CTNS
GSD 11 Fanconi-Bickel syndrome	Hepatomegaly Nephromegaly Hypoglycemia	Phosphorylase b kinase deficiency in some patients due to massive glycogen accumulation secondary to impaired glucose transport	Massive glucosuria	AR 3q26.1–26.3 Mutations in *GLUT2*
Tyrosinemia	Nodular cirrhosis Portal hypertension Liver failure, hepatosplenomegaly nephromegaly	Fumaryl acetoacetate hydrolase deficiency	SA, DALA	AR 15q23–q25
Galactosemia	Jaundice Hepatosplenomegaly Cataracts Mental retardation	Gal-I-PO_4 uridyl transferase deficiency	Galactose No glucosuria	AR *GALT* gene on 9p13 Mutation of *Q188R*
Hereditary fructose intolerance	Hypoglycemia, seizures, jaundice, hyperuricemia, ↑Mg	F-I-PO_4 aldolase B deficiency	Fructose	AR chromosome 9q213–q22.2 *A149P* mutations
Lowe's syndrome	Mental retardation, cataracts, glaucoma	Abnormal inositol PO_4 metabolism	Usual for FS	XLR Xq25–26 OCRL-1 is 105 kD protein located in Golgi complex
Other P.T. disorders Proximal RTA with osteopetrosis	Growth failure Mental retardation Cranial nerve abnormalities Fractures	↓T_{HCO3} CAII deficiency	Bicarbonaturia Bicarbonaturia	AD, AR 8q22 – several mutations – intron 2
HVDRR	Rickets, hypophosphatemia	↓TRP Impaired calcitriol synthesis	Phosphaturia	XLD, AD *Hyp* gene Xp22.1 *PHEX, FGF23*
Cystinuria	None, urolithiasis, renal failure from obstructive uropathy	Defective transport of cystine and dibasic amino acids in proximal tubules and intestine	Cystine, ornithine, lysine, arginine	Chromosome 2p Mutations in *SLC3A1* gene

AD autosomal dominant, *AR* autosomal recessive, *XLD* X-linked dominant, *XLR* X-linked recessive, *SA* succinyl acetone, *DALA* delta aminolevulenic acid, *FS* Fanconi syndrome, *TRP* tubular reabsorption of phosphate, *CA* carbonic anhydrase, T_{HCO3} tubular reabsorption, bicarbonate

through the urine. If the fractional excretion of bicarbonate is very high the alkali requirement is proportionately larger. Some patients require 10–20 mEq/kg/day in four or more divided doses. If higher doses are needed, the large amount of sodium may lead to ECV expansion and further bicarbonate wasting. In such cases, salt and water should be restricted and a thiazide diuretic (2 mg/kg/day hydrochlorothiazide) administered to produce a mild ECV contraction and enhance bicarbonate reabsorption. Potassium supplements are frequently needed to replace renal potassium wasting and treat hypokalemia. Potassium citrate or lactate is ideally suited for treatment because they will also help in correcting metabolic acidosis. Calcium and magnesium supplements may be needed in patients with hypocalcemia and renal magnesium wasting. A prostaglandin synthetase inhibitor such as Indomethacin

(1–3 mg/kg/day) may be useful in reducing the urinary sodium, potassium, and water losses that are frequently seen in many patients with the Fanconi syndrome. Their use is contraindicated in the face of deterioration of renal function as seen in later stages of nephropathic cystinosis.

Hypophosphatemia and Bone Disease

While hypophosphatemia plays a major role in the bone disease in Fanconi syndrome, other factors including reduced calcitriol synthesis, chronic acidosis, and hypercalciuria are also important. Vitamin D therapy in the form calcitriol or one-alpha hydroxy-D3 is frequently needed to correct rickets. Doses vary from 0.25 to 3.0 μg/day. Phosphate supplements are always needed in high and frequent doses, depending on the severity of the phosphaturia. Most patients require 1–2 g/day in four divided doses. With adequate phosphate supplementation it is possible to promote bone healing with smaller doses of vitamin D.

Specific Treatment of the Fanconi Syndrome

Cystinosis

The use of the aminothiols cysteamine or phosphocysteamine has shown promising results in depleting cystine from the lysosome of affected cells. This is accomplished by an intralysosomal reaction between cystine and cysteamine to form a cysteine-cysteamine disulfide that exits the cell via a lysine carrier system. Treatment should be started as soon as the diagnosis of cystinosis is confirmed. The starting dose is 10 mg/kg/day in four divided doses. This is raised progressively to 60 mg/kg/day and titrated against leukocyte cystine content. Cysteamine treatment has been associated with improvement in the Fanconi syndrome and possible delay in the onset of renal failure. If and when renal failure develops, dialysis and transplantation offer the only hope for prolonged survival. The results of renal transplantation in patients with cystinosis are more successful than renal transplantation performed for other chronic renal diseases. This may be due to reduced immune responsiveness induced by intracellular cystine accumulation. The Fanconi syndrome does not recur but interstitial and mesangial accumulation of cystine has been reported.

Tyrosinemia Type 1

Until recently the only effective therapy for tyrosinemia type 1 was liver transplantation, preferably prior to the development of severe liver failure and hepatocellular carcinoma, known complications of nodular cirrhosis. An experimental drug that underwent clinical trials over the past 10 years or so appears to have stood the test of time and has shown promising results for patients with tyrosinemia type 1. The drug, 2-nitro-trifluoromethylbenzoyl-1, 3-cyclohexanedione (NTBC), inhibits 4-OH-phenylpyruvate dioxygenase, the second enzyme in the degradation pathway of tyrosine which is two steps proximal to the enzyme defect in tyrosinemia. The drug was recently approved for commercial use as an orphan drug and marketed as Nitisinone. Studies with NTBC therapy show an impressive reduction in the plasma level and the urinary excretion of SA and DALA and alpha-fetoprotein levels with a marked reduction in hepatosplenomegaly. Tubular dysfunction also improves significantly with NTBC treatment.

Other

In some cases of the Fanconi syndrome where the underlying cause is known, withdrawing the offending agent will reverse the tubular dysfunction. This is true for galactose in galactosemia and fructose in hereditary fructose intolerance. A diet low in tyrosine and methionine in patients with tyrosinemia results in moderate improvement in the Fanconi syndrome associated with the disease. Cornstarch therapy for GSD may cause regression of hepatomegaly but has no effect on the tubular dysfunction. Chelating agents such as Penicillamine-D and Zinc therapy for Wilson's disease are associated with significant reduction in serum copper levels as well as clinical improvement.

Prognosis in Fanconi Syndrome

Prognosis depends on the underlying etiology of the Fanconi syndrome. For patients with cystinosis, the most common cause of the syndrome, long term treatment with cysteamine improves long term patient outcome, but even in patients who have undergone successful renal transplantation a significant number of extra renal abnormalities persisted or worsened over time. These included hypothyroidism, pulmonary insufficiency, myopathy, diabetes mellitus, and others. One third of the transplanted patients died at a mean age of 28 years or 16 years post transplant. In tyrosinemia, long term outcome has improved appreciably with early institution of Nitisinone therapy (see above) which should be started prior to development of nodular cirrhosis.

Proximal Renal Tubular Acidosis (Type II, PRTA)

Definition

Defective bicarbonate reclamation by the proximal tubule is referred to as proximal RTA. It is usually seen in association with other proximal tubular transport defects as part of the Fanconi syndrome, but it may also be observed less commonly as an isolated condition where it is referred to as primary proximal RTA.

Etiology/Pathophysiology

The basic defect in PRTA is impaired renal bicarbonate reabsorption by the proximal tubules. Hypothetically, any of the mechanisms responsible for the reclamation of bicarbonate from the proximal tubular cells could be implicated in the etiology of PRTA. For a better understanding of PRTA a brief review of the mechanisms involved in bicarbonate reabsorption is in order (*Fig. 304.3*).

In the proximal tubular cells, a specific electroneutral Na^+–H_+ exchanger (NHE-3) at the luminal basement membrane, together with basolateral transport of bicarbonate by an electrogenic Na^+-HCO_3^- cotransporter (NBC-1), accounts for the reabsorption of 85% of the filtered bicarbonate back to the plasma. The remaining 15% of the filtered bicarbonate is reabsorbed in the more distal segments of the tubule, primarily by the thick ascending limb of Henle's loop (TALH). *NHE-3* is the main isoform of the NHE family responsible for the Na^+ exchange with H^+. It is localized exclusively in the apical cells of the proximal tubules and the cells of the TALH. The human *NHE-3* gene (*SLC9A3*) maps to chromosome 5p15.3.

Filtered bicarbonate combines with hydrogen (exchanged for sodium) to form carbonic acid (H_2CO_3) which is rapidly dehydrated to CO_2 and water, a process catalyzed by luminal carbonic anhydrase (CA IV) in the brush border of the proximal tubular cell. Luminal CO_2 diffuses freely into the cell and is rehydrated by cellular carbonic anhydrase (CA II) to form carbonic acid, which dissociates into H^+ and HCO_3^-. Both CA IV and CA II are maximally stimulated in chronic metabolic acidosis. The regenerated bicarbonate is returned to the blood via the NBC-1 to maintain normal bicarbonate levels. About one third of the hydrogen secreted and exchanged for sodium is derived from an electrogenic H-ATPase pump in the luminal basement membrane. PRTA (type 2 RTA) could occur if any of the forces involved in bicarbonate reabsorption, singly, or in combination became defective.

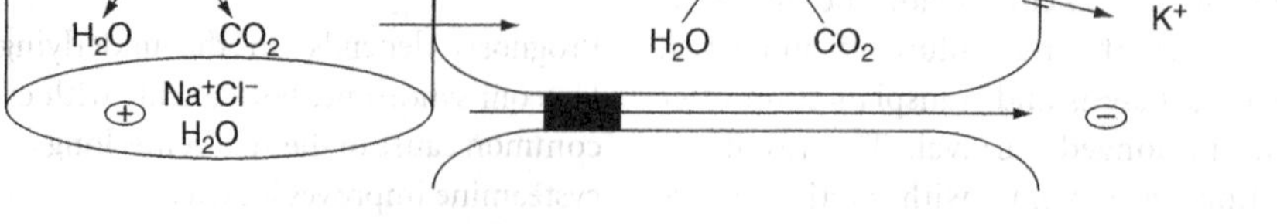

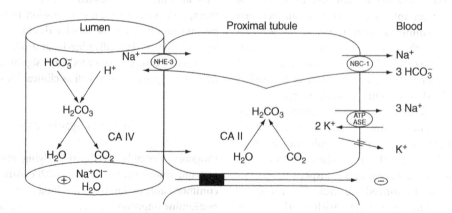

Figure 304.3
Bicarbonate reabsorption in proximal tubular cell. About two third of H^+ secreted is counter-transported with Na (NHE-3) and one third by a H^+-ATPase pump in the luminal membrane. HCO_3^- transport at the basolateral membrane is via a 1 Na^++3HCO_3 cotransporter (NBC-1). Cellular carbonic anhydrase II (CA II) and membrane-bound carbonic anhydrase IV (CA IV) are necessary for HCO_3^- reabsorption

These might be secondary to mutations in NHE3, NBC-1, carbonic anhydrase II or IV, or the H-ATPase pump. An abnormality in the Na-K-ATPase pump causes impaired reabsorption of all solutes ordinarily cotransported with sodium and results in the Fanconi syndrome. Bicarbonate reabsorption in the proximal tubule is a high capacity, low gradient process that bears an inverse proportion to changes in extracellular fluid volume. Other factors influencing HCO_3^- reabsorption include intraluminal flow rate, tubular and peritubular HCO_3-concentration, parathyroid hormone, pCO_2, chloride and potassium concentrations.

Incomplete bicarbonate reabsorption results in a large excretion of the filtered load of bicarbonate causing a fall in the plasma bicarbonate level. This excess bicarbonate will flood the distal tubules and impair urinary acidification. The urine pH will be alkaline and remain so until plasma bicarbonate falls below the renal threshold, after which it becomes bicarbonate free and properly acidified by the intact distal secretion of hydrogen ion. During acidemia in untreated patients, the urine pH is always less than 5.5.

PRTA in Association with the Fanconi Syndrome

The hereditary forms of the renal Fanconi syndrome are usually secondary to autosomal recessive metabolic diseases, the most common being cystinosis, tyrosinemia type 1, and glycogen storage disease (below). Renal bicarbonate wasting in the Fanconi syndrome occurs as part of a generalized proximal tubular transport defect. This is the result of a dysfunctional basolateral Na-K ATPase pump which is the driving source of energy for solute reabsorption. Glycogen storage disease appears to be a relatively common cause of the Fanconi syndrome in the Middle East, particularly in Saudi Arabia. This form of GSD, known as the Fanconi-Bickel syndrome, is due to mutations in the glucose transporter gene GLUT2. Other disease entities associated with the Fanconi syndrome and PRTA are listed in ➋ *Table 304.1*.

Isolated PRTA

This is a rare disease entity. The clinical features of isolated PRTA are those of failure to thrive and vomiting usually detected in early infancy, but the disease may not be diagnosed until early childhood. Unlike patients with the Fanconi syndrome, rickets, hypercalciuria are not features of this disease but hypokalemia has been observed in some patients. Most reported cases have been (a) sporadic, (b) autosomal dominant, and (c) autosomal recessive with ocular abnormalities.

Sporadic PRTA

Most cases of sporadic PRTA occur in early infancy and may be explained on an immature NHE3 or NBC1 transporter systems. Patients with this condition require therapy with alkalinizing agents but the majority outgrows the disease with time.

Autosomal Dominant PRTA

This variant of PRTA must be extremely rare and was reported once in a Costa Rican family about 30 years ago. All affected members had moderately severe hyperchloremic acidosis associated with growth retardation. Family pedigree in these patients was compatible with an autosomal dominant pattern of inheritance. Molecular studies have not been performed but the gene encoding the NHE3 appears to be a good candidate. Studies in knockout mice lacking the gene encoding NHE3 (*SLC9A3*) reveal significant reduction in proximal tubular reabsorption of bicarbonate but with only a mild degree of metabolic acidosis.

Autosomal Recessive PRTA

This entity was first described about 30 years ago by Donckerwolcke et al. This is another rare disorder which is invariably associated with ocular abnormalities including glaucoma, cataracts, and band keratopathy and, at times, physical and mental retardation, basal ganglia calcification, and enamel defects. The metabolic abnormalities reveal a fairly severe hyperchloremic, hypokalemic metabolic acidosis. The few patients described with this disease have been mostly from Europe and Japan. At the molecular level, several inactivating mutations in the gene encoding NBC-1 (*SLC4A4*) have been identified. These include nonsense mutations R298S, R510H, and a stop codon Q29X. The ocular abnormalities can be explained by the fact that the *NBC1* gene is expressed in several ocular tissues.

PRTA with Osteopetrosis

A unique syndrome of PRTA associated with osteopetrosis, cerebral calcification, and carbonic anhydrase II deficiency has been reported in several families from the Arab world. The syndrome is inherited as an autosomal recessive trait and is characterized clinically by failure to thrive, recurrent fractures, mental retardation in the majority of patients, and cranial nerve abnormalities. Over two third of the cases have been from Middle Eastern and North African countries where genetic heterogeneity is suggested by a more severe variant of the disease. In addition to the PRTA, a distal acidification defect has been suggested in many of these patients. The gene locus has been mapped to chromosome 8q22. Several mutations have been identified in patients with carbonic anhydrase II deficiency, but the most common is the Arabic one, which is a splice junction mutation in intron 2. More recently, mutations in the gene OC16, encoding the a3 subunit of the osteoclast V H^+-ATPase, have been shown to cause infantile malignant osteopetrosis.

Acquired PRTA

Drugs inhibiting carbonic anhydrase such as acetazolamide will cause a reduction in bicarbonate reabsorption in the proximal tubular cell (➜ *Fig. 304.3*) resulting in a mild form of PRTA. More recently, Topiramate, a drug initially approved as an antiepileptic agent, is being increasingly used in the treatment of several neurologic and metabolic disorders. The drug also inhibits renal carbonic anhydrase activity, resulting in a proximal acidification defect similar to that observed with acetazolamide. The drug also causes hypocitraturia, hypercalciuria, and increased urine pH, all conducive to increased risk for kidney stone disease.

Diagnosis of PRTA

The diagnosis of PRTA should be considered in any infant (male > female) with failure to thrive and unexplained hyperchloremic acidosis. A urinary pH below 5.5 is strong evidence against distal RTA. If urinary pH falls in the equivocal zone (5.5–6.0) an acute acid load test with ammonium chloride should clarify the issue. This test is not necessary, and could be hazardous, if moderate to severe acidosis is present to begin with. The urine pH in PRTA is variable and depends on the plasma bicarbonate concentration. The diagnosis is confirmed by demonstrating a fractional excretion of bicarbonate (FE_{HCO3}) in excess of 15%. FE_{HCO3} is calculated during intravenous bicarbonate infusion or oral bicarbonate therapy by simultaneous measurement of urine and plasma bicarbonate and levels after ensuring an adequate rise in plasma bicarbonate:

$$FE_{HCO3} = \frac{U_{HCO3} \times P_{Cr}}{U_{Cr} \times P_{HCO3}}$$

where U and P represent urine and plasma concentration of bicarbonate (HCO_3) and creatinine (Cr) respectively.

Treatment of Proximal RTA

Treatment of PRTA usually requires large and frequent doses of sodium bicarbonate or citrate (5–20 mEq/kg/day). Potassium supplements may be necessary especially with large doses of bicarbonate, as this will aggravate potassium wasting by the kidney. In patients requiring large doses of alkali therapy, a thiazide diuretic may be used to reduce ECV expansion and enhance bicarbonate reabsorption by the proximal tubules.

Prognosis of PRTA

The prognosis of PRTA depends on the underlying etiology. If associated with the Fanconi syndrome, as the majority of cases are, the outcome will vary with the specific etiology of the Fanconi syndrome and its response to therapy (see above).

Disorder of Renal Phosphate Transport

Several disease entities have been described in association with hypophosphatemia, some are heredofamilial and some are acquired.

Heredofamilial Hypophosphatemia

Several terms have been used to describe this entity: vitamin D resistant rickets, X-linked hypophosphatemic rickets, primary hypophosphatemic rickets, familial hypophosphatemia, and phosphate diabetes. The disease represents the most common form of rachitic bone disease in North America, Western Europe, and in industrialized countries where nutritional rickets is no longer a significant problem.

Heredofamilial hypophosphatemia is transmitted as an X-linked dominant (XLH) or autosomal dominant trait (ADHR) with the former being much more prevalent (1 in 20,000). A rare autosomal recessive variant (ARHR) was also described recently.

XLH

In XLH, affected males (hemizygotes) will always manifest the disease, whereas females (heterozygotes) have a milder form of hypophosphatemia with mild bowing of the legs.

Etiology, Genetics, and Pathogenesis

The mutant gene of XLH has been mapped recently to the short arm of the X chromosome (Xp 22). One third of cases occur sporadically and may represent new mutations. Two murine homologues, *Hyp* and *Gy*, have helped significantly in detecting the mechanisms for renal phosphate wasting in XLH. The gene responsible for XLH was identified recently by positional cloning and designated *PHEX* (*PH*osphate regulating gene with homology to *E*ndopeptidases on the *X* chromosome). Several inactivating mutations in this gene have been identified in patients with XLH and in the murine models as well. It is thought that under normal circumstances, *PHEX* is involved in the inactivation of a phosphaturic hormone or the activation of a phosphate conserving hormone. Therefore loss *of PHEX* function is associated with either an excess of this phosphaturic hormone or a deficiency in the phosphate conserving hormone. In either case, renal other Na/P cotransporter would be down regulated and phosphaturia would ensue. However, endogenous *PHEX* substrates have not yet been identified. Recently it has been shown that *FGF23* gene expression is increased in Hyp mouse bone and Hyp osteoblast cultures, suggesting that *PHEX* normally inhibits FGF23 expression. Thus, an inactivating PHEX mutation results in abnormal regulation of FGF23 and possibly other molecules, resulting in the phenotype of XLH.

Clinical Findings

Children with XLH present at the onset of walking or later when weight bearing will lead to the classical bone deformities and growth failure. Genu varum occurs more frequently than genu valgum. Coxa vara is common, leading to the typical waddling and unsteady gait. Craniotabes and rachitic rosary, commonly seen with vitamin D deficiency rickets, are seldom observed with XLH. Tooth eruption may be delayed, but unlike in hypocalcemic forms of rickets, the enamel is normal. Sensorineural deafness appears to be relatively common. Radiologically, the findings are those of rickets with loss of provisional zone of calcification, widening of the epiphyseal plate, and coarse trabecular pattern. These changes are more pronounced in the lower extremities. Long bones are short and thickened, resulting in short and stubby appearance.

Pathophysiology

The pathophysiology of bone disease in XLH remains a controversial issue. It is possible that the primary genetic defect (*PHEX* mutations) causes (a) decreased renal tubular transport of phosphate leading to phosphaturia and hypophosphatemia (b) defective renal 1-alpha hydroxylase activity leading to inappropriately low levels of 1,25 $(OH)_2D_3$ relative to the low serum phosphate. This latter defect could be acquired since calcitonin stimulation of 1-alpha hydroxylase is normal in patients with HVDRR. This combination (a and b) is synergistic in causing the bone disease characteristic of XLH. The inadequate levels of 1, 25 $(OH)_2$ D_3 will also lead to reduced calcium and phosphate absorption from the gut, further contributing to the pathogenesis of the disease. Although PTH levels in XLH are usually normal, increased proximal tubular sensitivity to PTH may contribute to the renal phosphate wasting.

Diagnosis

The clinical manifestations described above are usually suggestive of the diagnosis. This is confirmed Biochemically where XLH is characterized by variable degrees of hypophosphatemia with normal serum calcium, elevated alkaline phosphatase and normal or slightly elevated PTH levels. The urinary findings reveal evidence of hyperphosphaturia with urinary phosphate excretion exceeding 20 mg/kg/day. Tubular reabsorption of phosphate (TRP) is derived by simultaneous measurement of urine and plasma phosphate and creatinine and calculated by the formula:

$$TRP = 1 - \frac{U_p \times P_{Cr}}{U_{Cr} \times P_p}$$

where U_p and U_{Cr} indicate urine phosphate and creatinine concentrations, respectively, and P_{Cr} and P_p represent plasma creatinine and phosphate concentrations. Normally, TRP ranges between 0.80 and 0.90. In patients with XLH, TRP is frequently below 0.50 (0.40–0.70). The test should be done while the patient is receiving adequate phosphate supplements for a few days.

ADHR

Patients with ADHR have similar clinical findings as those with XLH but differ in their mode of inheritance. The *ADHR* gene locus was mapped to chromosome 12p13.3. The gene responsible for ADHR has been found by positional cloning to be a fibroblast growth factor, *FGF23.* It has been subsequently shown that infusion of FGF23 in experimental animals results in phosphaturia and hypophosphatemia. At the renal proximal tubule brush border, FGF23 infusion rapidly decreases expression of Na/P cotransporter. Parathyroid hormone (PTH) also directly decreases Na/P cotransporter at the renal proximal tubule brush border *via* a cAMP/protein kinase A–mediated pathway, but infusion of FGF23 in thyroparathyroidectomized rats causes hypophosphatemia suggesting that the action of FGF23 on renal phosphate reabsorption is independent of PTH and may be complementary.

Treatment and Prognosis of XLH and ADHR

Since rickets in XLH and ADHR is primarily due to hypophosphatemia the goal of therapy is directed at raising plasma phosphate to normal levels. Phosphate supplements, in large and frequent doses, were recommended in the past to compensate for the ongoing urinary losses. Large doses of phosphate are usually associated with gastrointestinal complaints (vomiting and diarrhea) which may be a limiting factor in the treatment. Another drawback of raising plasma phosphate is the simultaneous lowering of the plasma ionized calcium which will lead to secondary hyperparathyroidism that can further aggravate the bone disease and increase the phosphaturia. For these reasons the addition of calcitriol to the therapeutic regimen offers the following advantages: (1) less phosphate will be needed and less gastrointestinal complications; (2) calcium and, to a lesser degree, phosphate absorption from the gut are enhanced leading to bone healing and improved linear growth; and (3) low incidence of hyperparathyroidism. The recommended dose for oral phosphate supplement is 1–2 g/day in four to five divided doses. Calcitriol in a dose of 0.25–1.0 μg/day is usually sufficient but some patients may require higher doses. Lower limb deformities appear to correct better if treatment is started before the age of 6 years, but final adult height remains significantly lower than the expected mean for age. Many patients require unilateral or bilateral corrective osteotomies for severe and persistent rachitic changes in the lower extremities. Some patients may benefit from growth hormone therapy.

Recent data suggest that adjunctive therapy with thiazide diuretics in combination with salt restriction will enhance proximal tubular reabsorption of phosphate. We have tried this combination in 6 patients with XLH but were not encouraged with the results, but thiazides may be effective in reducing the hypercalciuria and nephrocalcinosis associated with vitamin D therapy.

Other Hypophosphatemic Syndromes

Hypophosphatemic rickets or osteomalacia may be seen with chronic intake of phosphate binding gels.

Oncogenic hypophosphatemia with osteomalacia also known as tumor induced osteomalacia (TIO) has been reported with certain tumors of mesenchymal origin, usually sclerosing hemangiomas. Patients with TIO may present with fatigue, bone pain, fractures, and proximal muscle weakness. Children develop rickets and lower extremity deformities similar to those in ADHR and XLH. Many of these tumors are small and may be difficult to locate. Multiple imaging techniques including, magnetic resonance imaging, and positron emission tomography may be required to localize the tumor, which when found and removed reverses the phosphate, vitamin D, and bone abnormalities. The vast majority of these tumors are benign. Tumors that cause TIO usually overexpress FGF23, a known phosphaturic substance. Pathologic samples of patients with TIO have detected FGF23 in more than 80% of specimens tested.

The syndromes of hereditary hypophosphatemia with hypercalciuria must be differentiated from HLH and ADHR. Two forms are recognized. One is a rare autosomal recessive with phosphaturia and hypophosphatemia but appropriately elevated calcitriol levels. Hypercalciuria is probably due to increased intestinal absorption of calcium. Phosphate supplement without vitamin D reverses the rickets and osteomalacia. The other form is known as Dent's disease and is associated with X-linked nephrolithiasis and hypophosphatemic rickets. Hypercalciuria, uricosuria, and renal potassium wasting with progression to chronic renal failure is frequently observed.

Hyperphosphatemic Syndromes

Disorders associated with hypoparathyroidism, whether congenital or acquired are associated with hyperphosphatemia and hypocalcemia. The various conditions associated with these abnormalities are discussed in the section of endocrinology. A new syndrome of congenital hypoparathyroidism, dysmorphic features, severe growth failure, and mental retardation was reported recently in Arabian infants with normal cardiovascular systems and normal cellular immunity. Their dysmorphic features are quite distinctive from those of DiGeorge's syndrome and consist of deep-set eyes, microcephaly, thin lips, beaked nose tip, external ear anomalies, depressed nasal bridge, micrognathia, and other minor anomalies. The mode of inheritance of this syndrome is autosomal recessive as suggested by the very high rate of consanguinity (11 of 12 patients), equal occurrence in both sexes, and familial incidence. Molecular studies have recently identified the genetic basis of this disease. Mutations in the tubulin-specific chaperone, *TBCE*, have been found consistently in these patients. Treatment with pharmacologic doses of vitamin D and calcium supplements improves their biochemical abnormalities but growth retardation shows no response.

References

ADHR Consortium (2000) Autosomal dominant hypophosphatemic rickets is associated with mutations in *FGF23*. Nat Genet 26:345–348

Alper SL (2006) Molecular physiology of SLC4 anion exchangers. Exp Physiol 91:153–161

Aronson PS (1983) Mechanisms of active H^+ secretion in the proximal tubule. Am J Physiol 245:F647–F659

Baum M (1993) Cellular basis of the Fanconi syndrome. Hosp Pract 28:137–142

Brenes LG, Brenes JM, Hernandez MM (1997) Familial proximal renal tubular acidosis. A distinct clinical entity. Am J Med 63:244–252

Brooks CC, Tolan DR (1993) Association of the widespread *A149P* hereditary fructose intolerance mutation with newly identified sequence polymorphisms in the aldolase B gene. Am J Hum Genet 52:835–840

Burwinkel B, Sanjad SA, Al-Sabban E, Al-Abbad A, Kilimann MW (1999) A mutation in *GLUT2*, not in phosphorylase kinase subunits, in hepatorenal glycogenosis with Fanconi syndrome and low phosphorylase kinase activity. Hum Genet Sep 105(3):240–243

Demers SI, Russo P, Lettre F, Tanguay RM (2003) Frequent mutation reversal inversely correlates with clinical severity in a genetic liver disease, hereditary tyrosinemia. Hum Pathol 3:1313–1320

Donckerwolcke RA, Van Stekelenburg GJ, Tiddens HA (1970) A case of bicarbonate-losing renal tubular acidosis with defective carbonic anhydrase activity. Arch Dis Child 45:769–773

Econs MJ, Rowe PS, Francis F et al (1994) Fine structure mapping of the human X-linked hypophosphatemic rickets gene locus. J Clin Endocrinol Metab 79:1351–1354

Foreman JW, Roth KS (1989) Fanconi syndrome – then and now. Nephron 51:301–306

Fukumoto S, Yamashita T (2002) Fibroblast growth factor-23 is the phosphaturic factor in tumor-induced osteomalacia and may be phosphatonin. Curr Opin Nephrol Hypertens 11:385–389

Gahl WA, Thoene JG, Schneider JA (2002) Cystinosis. N Engl J Med 347:111–121

Halperin ML, Kamel S, Ethier JH, Magner PO (1989) What is the underlying defect in patients with isolated, proximal renal tubular acidosis? Am J Nephrol 9:265–268

Hu PY, Roth DE, Skaggs LA et al (1992) A splice junction mutation in intron 2 of the carbonic anhydrase II gene of osteopetrosis patients from Arabic countries. Hum Mut 1(4):288–292

HYP Consortium (1995) A gene (PEX) with homologies to endopeptidases is mutated in patients with X-linked hypophosphatemic rickets. Nat Genet 11:130–136

Igarashi T, Sekine T, Inatomi J, Seki G (2002) Unraveling the molecular pathogenesis of isolated proximal renal tubular acidosis. J Am Soc Nephrol 13:2171–2177

Imel EA, Econs MJ (2005) Fibroblast growth factor 23: roles in health and disease. J Am Soc Nephrol 16:2565–2575

Kalatzis V, Nevo N, Cherqui S et al (2004) Molecular pathogenesis of cystinosis: Effect of CTNS mutations on the transport activity and subcellular localization of cystinosin. Hum Mol Genet 13: 1361–1371

Kornak U, Schulz A, Fiedrich W et al (2000) Mutations in the a3 subunit of the vacuolar H^+-ATPase cause infantile malignant osteopetrosis. Hum Mol Genet 9(13):2059–2063

Latta K, Hisano S, Chan JCM (1993) Therapeutics of X-linked hypophosphatemic rickets. Pediatr Nephrol 7:744–748

Lindstedt S, Holme E, Lock EA (1992) Treatment of hereditary tyrosinemia type I by inhibition of 4-hydroxyphenyl pyruvate dioxygenase. Lancet 340:813–817

Manz F, Bickel H, Brodehl J et al (1987) Fanconi-Bickel syndrome. Pediatr Nephrol 1:509–518

Markello TC, Bernardini IM, Gahl WA (1993) Improved renal function in children with cystinosis treated with cysteamine. N Engl J Med 328:1157–1162

Ng WG, Xu YK, Kaufman FR et al (1994) Biochemical and molecular studies of 132 patients with galactosemia. Hum Genet 94:359–363

Olivos-Glander IM, Janne PA, Nussbaum RL (1995) The oculocerebrorenal syndrome gene product is a 105 kD protein localized to the Golgi complex. Am J Hum Genet 57(4):817–823

Parvari R, Hershkovitz E, Grossman N et al (2002) Mutations of *TBCE* cause hypoparathyroidism-retardation-dysmorphism and autosomal recessive Kenny-Caffey syndrome. Nat Genet 32:448–452

Phaneuf D, Labelle Y, Berube D et al (1991) Cloning and expression of the cDNA encoding human fumaryl acetoacetate hydrolase, the enzyme deficient in hereditary tyrosinemia. Assignment of the gene to chromosome 15. Am J Hum Genet 48:525–535

Sanjad SA (1997) Hereditary and acquired renal tubular disorders: the Saudi experience. Saudi J Kidney Dis Transplant 8:247–259

Sanjad SA (2003) Renal tubular acidosis in the Arab world. Saudi J Kidney Dis Transplant 14:305–315

Sanjad SA, Sakati NA, Abu-Osba YK et al (1991) A new syndrome of congenital hypoparathyroidism, severe growth failure, and dysmorphic features. Arch Dis Child 66:193–196

Sanjad SA, Kaddoura RE, Nazer HM et al (1993) Fanconi's syndrome with hepatorenal glycogenosis associated with phosphorylase b kinase deficiency. Am J Dis Child 147:957–959

Santer R, Schneppenheim R, Dombrowski A et al (1997) Mutations in *GLUT2*, the gene for the liver-type glucose transporter in patients with Fanconi-Bickel syndrome. Nat Genet 17:324–326

Seikaly MG, Browne RH, Baum M (1994) The effect of phosphate supplementation on linear growth in children with X-linked hypophosphatemia. Pediatrics 94:478–481

Skinner R, Pearson AD, Price L et al (1990) Nephrotoxicity after ifosfamide. Arch Dis Child 65(7):732–738

Tenenhouse HS, Murer H (2003) Disorders of renal tubular phosphate transport. J Am Soc Nephrol 14:240–247

The Cystinosis Collaborative Research Group (1995) Linkage of the gene for cystinosis to markers on the short arm of chromosome 17. Nat Genet 10:246–248

Tieder M, Modai D, Samuel R et al (1985) Hereditary hypophosphatemic rickets with hypercalciuria. N Engl J Med 312:611–617

Town M et al (1998) A novel gene encoding an integral membrane protein is mutated in nephropathic cystinosis. Nat Genet 18:319–324

Wang T, Yang D-L, Abbiati T et al (1999) Mechanism of proximal bicarbonate absorption in NHE-3 deficient mice. Am J Physiol 277: F298–F302

Welch B, Graybeal D et al (2006) Biochemical and stone-risk profiles with topiramate treatment. Am J Kidney Dis 48:555–563

Winsnes A, Monn E, Stokke O, Feyling T (1979) Congenital persistent proximal type renal tubular acidosis in two brothers. Acta Paediatr Scand 68:861–868

305 Disorders of Distal Tubular Transport of Sodium and Potassium

Sami A. Sanjad · John W. Foreman

Under normal circumstances, the urinary excretion of sodium matches the dietary intake such that a zero external balance is maintained. The factors that control sodium balance have been briefly alluded to in the section on renal function. A detailed account of the different factors modulating sodium balance are beyond the scope of this chapter, but suffice it to say that after the first year of life, the kidney is able to reduce urinary excretion of sodium to negligible values if the need arises (low-salt diet, ECV contraction).

Disorders Associated with Isolated Renal Salt Wasting

Etiology

Solute Diuresis Associated with Nephron Hyperfiltration

This is typically seen in patients with chronic renal failure, particularly those with a significant tubulointerstitial component. Renal salt wasting is usually mild but occasionally can be severe enough to cause ECV contraction, hypotension, and further deterioration of renal function. The diagnosis is made from the history and physical examination and tests of renal function which reveal increasing azotemia, hyponatremia, hyperkalemia, and metabolic acidosis. Urinary sodium is usually in excess of 60–120 meq/L in spite of ECV contraction.

Impaired Tubular Sodium Transport

Both congenital and acquired defects in sodium transport along different segments of the nephron may be associated with variable degrees of renal salt wasting.

Acute and chronic interstitial nephritis – Various segments of the nephron may be involved in abnormalities of sodium transport. Many renal diseases with a prominent tubulointerstitial involvement may be associated with renal salt wasting. These include obstructive uropathies, nephrocalcinosis, analgesic nephropathy, allergic interstitial nephritis, amyloidosis, and others.

Medullary cystic disease/Juvenile nephronophthisis – Renal salt wasting may be a prominent feature in children and adolescents with this disease.

Drugs – Several drugs known to cause interstitial nephritis may cause some degree of salt wasting. Prominent among these are *cis*-platinum and Amphotericin B.

Renal tubular acidosis – Patients with both proximal and distal RTA exhibit variable degree of salt wasting. In proximal RTA, this occurs only with sodium bicarbonate treatment when plasma bicarbonate exceeds the renal tubular threshold. In distal RTA, a mild degree of renal salt wasting occurs at all levels of plasma bicarbonate, and fractional excretion of sodium is usually between 2% and 5% (normal <1%).

Transient Pathophysiologic States Associated with Renal Salt Wasting

Transient renal salt wasting may be seen during the recovery phase of acute tubular necrosis. In children recovering from acute post streptococcal glomerulonephritis, a mild degree of salt wasting may occur for a few months following recovery, but this is of no clinical significance. Massive renal salt wasting may occur in the early post renal transplant period, and to a lesser degree following relief of urinary tract obstruction. Diuretics, by definition, interfere with sodium reabsorption at different sites of the nephron and thus will cause reversible renal salt wasting.

Conditions Associated with Deficient Mineralocorticoid Activity

These are typically observed in patients with Addison's disease, isolated hypoaldosteronism, and pseudohypoaldosteronism type 1. Congenital adrenal hyperplasia,

Abdelaziz Y. Elzouki (ed.), *Textbook of Clinical Pediatrics*, DOI 10.1007/978-3-642-02202-9_305,

due to 21-α-hydroxylase deficiency is one of the most common extra renal causes of renal salt wasting. This entity is discussed separately in the section on endocrinology.

Treatment

Treatment of isolated renal salt wasting states will depend on the underlying mechanism and the severity of the renal sodium losses, its effect on renal function, blood pressure, serum sodium, potassium, and acid–base balance (see below). Liberalizing salt intake, parenterally, or orally if tolerated, will usually reverse these abnormalities. If concomitant metabolic acidosis is present, sodium bicarbonate or citrate should be used in addition to sodium chloride.

Disorders Associated with Renal Salt Wasting and Hypokalemia

Bartter's Syndrome

Since Bartter and colleagues' original description of two patients with severe hypokalemic metabolic alkalosis and hyperaldosteronism in 1962, there have been several series and case reports describing a similar clinical presentation.

Clinical Manifestations

Older patients with Bartter's syndrome present typically with hypokalemia, fatigue, muscle weakness and cramps, neuromuscular irritability, polyuria, and polydipsia. The hypokalemia is usually moderate to severe and is secondary to renal potassium wasting, with urinary potassium concentrations frequently exceeding 40 meq/L. Serum bicarbonate values usually exceed 30 meq/L and are accompanied by arterial pH values that are often above 7.50. This metabolic alkalosis is chloride resistant as urine chloride levels exceed 20 meq/L with resultant hypochloremia.

Many other abnormalities have been described in patients with Bartter's syndrome. Urine concentrating ability is impaired, presumably from the long-standing hypokalemia. Hyperplasia of the juxtagomerular cells is common but this is not pathognomonic of Bartter's syndrome as originally thought because it may be seen in other conditions associated with extracellular volume contraction and hyperreninemia, such as Addison's disease, laxative or diuretic abuse. Hyperplasia of renal medullary interstitial cells, the probable source of the increased prostaglandin secretion typically observed in this syndrome, has also been described. In children, growth retardation is common and may be the presenting complaint. Mild mental retardation and facial dysmorphism has also been noted in some patients. A more severe and common variant of Bartter's syndrome is seen in the neonate or early infancy and is referred to as antenatal Bartter's syndrome. These babies have a history of maternal polyhydramnios and are usually born prematurely and small for gestational age. Hypercalciuria is invariably present in association with nephrocalcinosis. Prostaglandin E2 is markedly elevated and has led to the name hyperprostaglandin E2 syndrome. These infants have been reported to respond especially well to cyclooxygenase inhibitors.

Etiology and Pathogenesis

The past 12 years have witnessed major developments in the fields of molecular and cell biology that have led to our understanding of the pathogenesis of Bartter's syndrome. Until the mid-1990s, the pathogenesis of this syndrome remained elusive and pathophysiologic constructs of the syndrome were circular making the initiating event difficult to define.

Because the biochemical and physiologic changes in Bartter syndrome are similar to those seen in patients receiving loop diuretics, the Bumetanide-sensitive Na–K-2Cl cotransporter, *NKCC2*, was sought as a candidate gene due to its role in Cl and Na reabsorption in the TALH segment. This transporter is the site of action for loop diuretics where they inhibit sodium, potassium, and chloride reabsorption. Thus, chronic administration of loop diuretics will result in hypokalemia, metabolic alkalosis, hyperreninemia, hyperaldosteronism, chloride wasting, hypercalciuria, and hyperprostaglandinism which are findings typically observed in patients with Bartter's syndrome (➔ *Fig. 305.1*). Also, physiologic studies with hypotonic saline or water diuresis had clearly demonstrated impaired sodium chloride reabsorption in the thick ascending limb of Henle's loop in the majority of patients studied.

The etiology of Bartter's syndrome has been characterized recently at the molecular level. Simon and associates demonstrated linkage of Bartter's syndrome to the renal Na–K-2Cl cotransporter gene *NKCC2* and identified several inactivating mutations for this gene that cosegregate with the disease – Bartter's type 1. Genetic heterogeneity was demonstrated subsequently by the

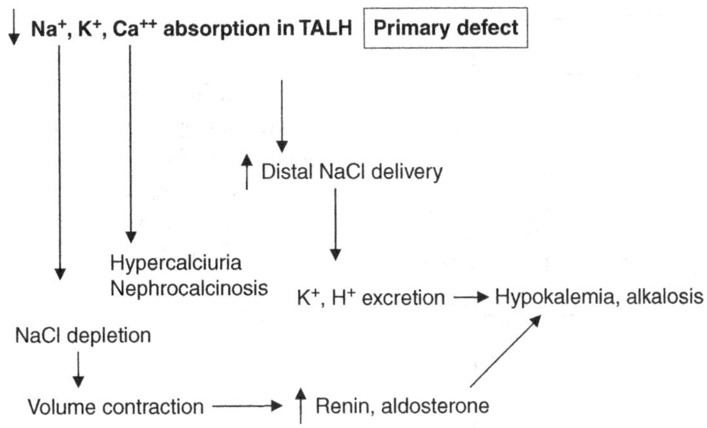

Figure 305.1
Pathophysiology of Bartter's syndrome

Table 305.1
Hereditary renal hypokalemic alkalosis

Disorder	Bartter's 1	Bartter's 2	Bartter's 3	Bartter's 4	Bartter's 5	Gitelman's
Inheritance	AR	AR	AR	AR	AD	AR
Gene/Locus	*SLC12A1*/15q15-21	*KCNJ1*/11q24	*CLCNKB*/1p36	*BSND*/1p31	*CASR*/3q21	*SLC12A3*/16q13
Protein	NKCC2	ROMK	ClCN-Kb	Barttin	CaR	NCCT
Polyuria, dehydration, polyhydramnios	Yes	Yes	Variable	Yes Deafness	Hypocalcemia, convulsions	Rare
Nephrocalcinosis hypercalciuria	Yes	Yes	Rare	Yes	Yes	Hypocalciuria
Antenatal Variant	Yes	Yes	Very rare	Yes	No	No

same group of investigators who identified mutations in two additional genes that act as regulators of the Na–K-2Cl cotransporter. The first is ROMK, an ATP-sensitive K channel, which recycles reabsorbed K back to the tubular lumen to allow sustained cotransport activity – Bartter's type 2. The second is a chloride channel gene *CLCNKB* which is important in Cl absorption across the basolateral membrane to the peritubular blood – Bartter's type 3. A fourth genotype of Bartter's syndrome was identified by positional cloning in ten families with the usual abnormalities but in association with sensorineural deafness. The gene encodes a protein called Barttin, a beta subunit of the *CLCNKB,* which is also expressed in the potassium-secreting epithelial cells of the inner ear. Thus, inactivating mutations of the gene impair function of the chloride channel, causing Bartter's syndrome and sensorineural deafness – Bartter's type 4. All these variants of Bartter's syndrome are inherited by autosomal recessive genes and disease prevalence is more common in communities with high rate of consanguineous marriages. Lastly, a fifth variant of Bartter's syndrome was discovered in association with another rare syndrome of autosomal dominant hypocalcemia. The mutated gene is the Calcium Sensor Receptor, *CASR,* which is also expressed in the TALH. When maximally activated due to gain of function mutations, this results in decreased sodium and chloride reabsorption primarily due to inhibition of the ROMK channel. With the advent of the molecular identification of the various types of Bartter's syndrome, it is now possible to develop phenotype–genotype correlations, although considerable overlap remains. *Table 305.1* and *Fig. 305.2* summarize the various phenotypes and genotypes of Bartter's syndrome.

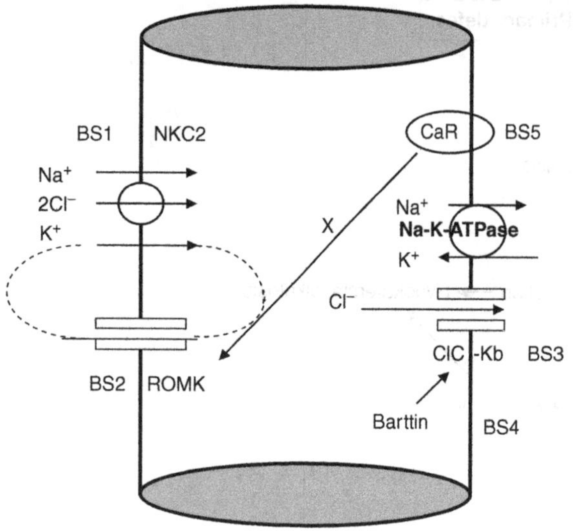

Figure 305.2
The main transport proteins and ion channels in the TALH. Mutations in the NKCC2, ROMK, CLC-KB, Barttin, and CaR cause Bartter's syndrome (BS) types 1, 2, 3, 4, 5, respectively

Table 305.2
Hypokalemic, metabolic alkalosis in children

Non-hypertensive	Hypertensive
Pyloric stenosis	Renal artery stenosis
Gastric suction	Primary aldosteronism
Cystic Fibrosis	Cortisol synthesis enzyme defects
Diuretics – laxatives	11-Beta-hydroxylase
Chloride deficient formula	17-Alpha-hydroxylase
Bartter's syndrome	Cortisol degradation enzyme defect
Gitelman's syndrome	11-Beta-cortisol dehydrogenase
Neonatal Bartter's – hyperprostaglandin E syndrome	Glucocorticoid remediable hypertension
	Liddle's syndrome
Congenital chloride diarrhea	Licorice abuse

Differential Diagnosis

The differential diagnosis of Bartter's syndrome and other forms of hypokalemic, metabolic alkalosis in children is shown in ➋ *Table 305.2.*

Gitelman's Syndrome

In 1966, Gitelman and Welt described a familial disorder characterized by hypokalemia, metabolic alkalosis, and hypomagnesemia. Most patients presented in late childhood, or as young adults, frequently with tetany. Compared to Bartter's syndrome, they have less pronounced hypokalemia, hyperreninemia, and hyperaldosteronism. Hypocalciuria and hypomagnesemia are other distinguishing features and they usually have normal stature. Genetic studies of patients with Gitelman's syndrome have identified several inactivating mutations in the thiazide-sensitive Na–Cl cotransporter (NCCT) in the early distal tubule. Impaired function of this transporter would increase sodium delivery to the more distal portions of the nephron leading to increased potassium and hydrogen ion secretion. The cause of the increased magnesium excretion seen in this syndrome is unclear, but it may also be seen in patients receiving thiazides chronically. ➋ *Table 305.3* shows some of the salient features that differentiate Bartter's from Gitelman's syndromes.

Treatment and Prognosis

The major goal in treating Bartter's syndrome is to normalize the serum potassium. However, this is usually difficult to achieve and patients require large doses of supplemental KCl. "Potassium sparing" agents, such as amiloride, spironolactone, and triamterene, are helpful but many of these patients remain hypokalemic in spite of large doses of KCl and potassium sparing drugs. Nonsteroidal anti-inflammatory drugs (NSAIDS) are somewhat useful in correcting the hypokalemia and volume contraction, presumably by inhibiting prostaglandin synthesis and their effect on blocking the tubuloglomerular feedback caused by decreased chloride reabsorption. Prostaglandin inhibitors also reduce the hypercalciuria and are reported to be especially useful in "neonatal Bartter's" or hyperprostaglandin E2 syndrome. In many patients, these agents are useful initially, but not on a long-term basis. Angiotensin converting enzyme inhibitors have been shown to improve the hypokalemia, but many patients cannot tolerate their hypotensive effects. In spite of the severe and long-standing potassium depletion, cardiac arrhythmias are infrequent and these patients tolerate general anesthesia relatively well. In Gitelman's syndrome, magnesium supplementation is especially important, in addition to potassium. In contrast to Bartter's syndrome patients,

Table 305.3
Differentiation between Bartter's and Gitelman's syndromes

	Bartter's syndrome	Gitelman's syndrome
Age of presentation	Early (may be neonatal)	Anytime – often as adults
Presenting complaint	Polyuria, polydipsia, FTT	Tetany
Inheritance	Autosomal recessive or sporadic	Autosomal recessive
Maximal urine concentration	Decreased	Usually normal
Serum magnesium	Normal	Low
Urinary calcium	>4 mg/kg/day	Low or normal
Defect	Mutations in cotransporter NKCC2, ROMK, CLCNKB/A Channels, Barttin, CaSR	Mutations in thiazide-sensitive NaCl transporter in renal distal tubule

Gitelman's syndrome patients require relatively modest doses of KCl to correct the potassium defect and NSAIDS are not required.

Disorders Associated with Renal Salt Wasting and Hyperkalemia

Autosomal Recessive Pseudohypoaldosteronism Type 1 (AR PHA1)

This is a rare autosomal recessive disorder characterized by life-threatening dehydration in neonatal life and early infancy secondary to severe renal salt wasting, hypotension, hyponatremia, and hyperkalemic metabolic acidosis. There is also marked elevation of plasma renin activity and aldosterone levels. Genetic analysis of affected offspring showed linkage to chromosomes 12p13 and 16p13 which contain genes encoding different subunits of the sodium epithelial channel, ENaC. Several inactivating homozygous mutations in the three subunits (α-, β-, and γ-ENaC) of this gene have been identified. These mutations are associated with persistent and longer open probability of the channels leading to renal salt wasting from the distal collecting tubules and a secondary defect in hydrogen and potassium ion secretion with resultant hyperkalemia and metabolic acidosis (*Figs. 305.3* and *305.5*). Since the ENaC is also expressed in the respiratory epithelial cells, from the nose to the terminal bronchioles and alveoli, patients with the PHA1 frequently present with increased airway secretions and lower respiratory infections.

The differential diagnosis of PHA1 includes (1) salt wasting congenital adrenal hyperplasia with mineralocorticoid deficiency, (2) isolated hypoaldosteronism (very rare), and (3) autosomal dominant PHA1.

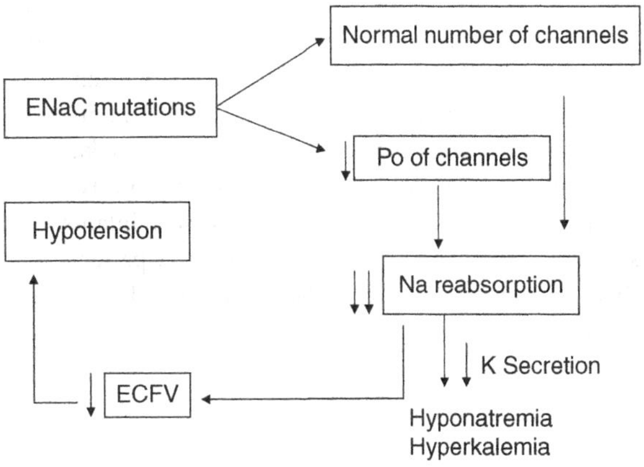

Figure 305.3
Pathophysiology of AR pseudohypoaldosteronism type 1. *ENaC* sodium epithelial channel, *Po* open probability

Autosomal Dominant Pseudohypoaldosteronism Type 1 (AD PHA1)

This entity has a similar but, usually, a less severe clinical presentation than the recessive type. Heterozygous mutations in the gene (*NR3C2*) encoding the mineralocorticoid receptor are found in 75% of reported families as well as in some sporadic cases. In many patients, the symptoms related to renal salt wasting remit with time.

Treatment of PHA1

In order to keep up with high urinary losses of sodium, a high salt intake is an essential aspect of the management of patients with PHA1 with some requiring as much as 20–30 mmol of sodium/kg/day. In addition, most infants and children will require K-binding resins to prevent hyperkalemia which may be lethal at times.

Disorders with Renal Salt Retention and Hypokalemia

Liddle's Syndrome

Liddle and colleagues described a family with hypokalemia and hypertension in which the clinical manifestations resembled primary aldosteronism, but the serum and urine aldosterone levels were suppressed. It was also noted that an inhibitor of the aldosterone receptor was not effective in treating hypertension, but triamterene, which inhibits potassium secretion through a mechanism other than aldosterone receptor blockade, was effective. Several kindreds have been described to date and this syndrome is inherited as an autosomal dominant disorder. The signal feature, besides hypertension, is hypokalemia, occurring in 50% of patients. Hypertension typically begins in adolescence, but has been noted in infants. The severity of the hypertension varies between patients, but there is an excess of cerebral hemorrhage and premature death in most kindreds.

Pathogenesis

Linkage analysis of the original kindred showed complete linkage of the disease to the beta subunit of the amiloride-sensitive epithelial sodium channel (β-ENaC). This sodium channel resides on the luminal membrane of the renal cortical collecting duct and plays an important role in sodium reabsorption in this nephron segment. It has been subsequently shown that activating, gain of function, mutations in both β and γ subunits of the ENaC are causative of Liddle's syndrome presumably, the defective subunit increases the number of open channels and maintains the distal nephron in a sodium avid state, even when the patients are salt repleted and aldosterone is inhibited. The avid sodium reabsorption maintains a lumen negative electrical gradient, which enhances potassium and hydrogen ion excretion. This leads to hypokalemia, volume expansion, hypertension, and metabolic alkalosis (➋ *Figs. 305.4* and ➋ *305.5*).

Diagnosis

The diagnosis of Liddle's syndrome should be suspected in patients with hypertension and hypokalemia. The finding

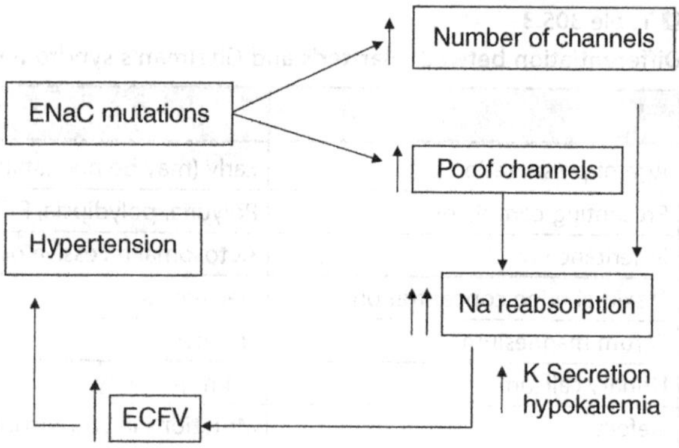

Figure 305.4
Pathophysiology of Liddle' Syndrome. *ENaC* sodium epithelial channel, *Po* open probability

of suppressed aldosterone levels confirms this suspicion, especially if there is a strong family history of hypertension. A urine aldosterone to potassium ratio of <60 (ng/mmol) appears to be the most sensitive measure of aldosterone suppression. Patients with Liddle's syndrome usually have high TTKG values (greater than 9–10) which fall to low levels following treatment with sodium channel blockers (see below).

Differential Diagnosis

Other causes of hypokalemic hypertension include renal artery stenosis, renin secreting tumor, primary hyperaldosteronism, and glucocorticoid remediable aldosteronism (GRA). All of these can be distinguished from Liddle's syndrome by the presence of hyperaldosteronism. Enzymatic deficiencies that lead to hypokalemic hypertension include 11-beta-hydroxylase and 17-alpha-hydroxylase in the cortisol and aldosterone biosynthetic pathway. Deficiency of 11-beta-hydroxylase is characterized by virilization and deficiency of 17-alpha-hydroxylase with hypergonadotropic hypogonadism. Both are also associated with decreased cortisol levels that stimulate corticotropin release. This stimulates steroid formation proximal to the block, including deoxycorticosterone that has mineralocortoid effects through the aldosterone receptor. These patients have low cortisol levels and abnormal levels of steroid metabolites in their urine. They respond to spironolactone, unlike patients with Liddle's syndrome. The enzyme, 11-beta-hydroxysteroid dehydrogenase, protects the aldosterone receptor from interacting with cortisol by converting it to cortisone. Patients with 11-beta-hydroxysterone dehydrogenase deficiency have low levels of aldosterone and abnormal levels

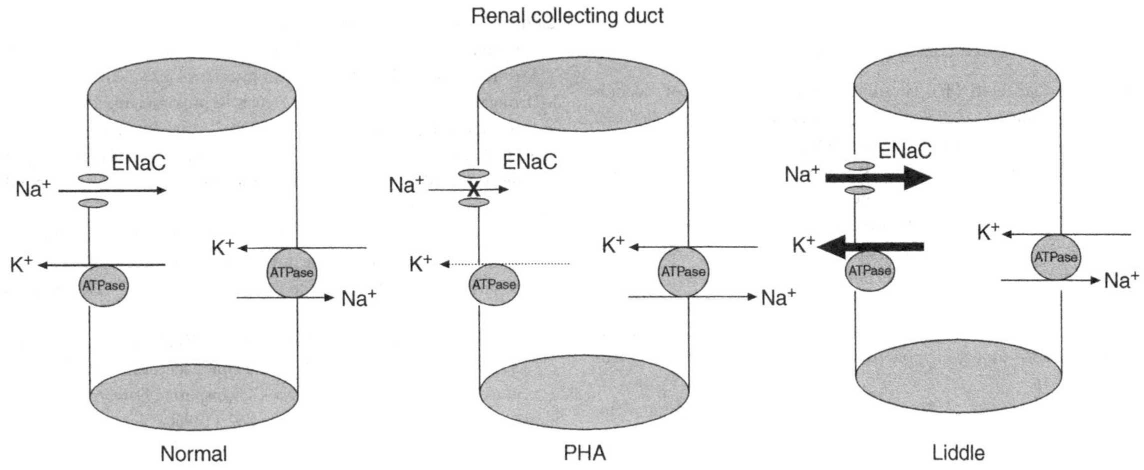

Figure 305.5
Pathophysiology of Pseudohypoaldosteronism type 1 and Liddle's syndrome

of cortisol to cortisone metabolites in their urine. Glycyrrhetinic acid found in licorice inhibits this enzyme mimicking 11-beta-hydroxysterone dehydrogenase deficiency. GRA results from an abnormal gene that consists of the ACTH responsive portion of the gene coding 11-beta-hydroxylase to aldosterone synthetase gene. This gene fusion mutation confers ACTH regulation to aldosterone synthesis, leading to excess aldosterone. All these enzyme defects demonstrate a reduction in blood pressure with physiologic doses of dexamethasone.

Treatment

The first aspect of Liddle's syndrome treatment is to block the open sodium channel with the potassium sparing diuretics, amiloride or triamterene. Spironolactone, acting through the aldosterone receptor is not useful. However, sodium restriction may still be necessary in some patients to reduce the volume expansion and maintain blood pressure control. In spite of maximal doses of amiloride and sodium restriction, some patients will require additional antihypertensive agents.

Disorders with Salt Retention and Hyperkalemia

Pseudohypoaldosteronism Type 2 (Gordon Syndrome)

In 1970, Gordon and associates described a 10-year-old girl with hypertension, severe hyperkalemia, acidosis, suppressed renin and aldosterone activity, and normal GFR. At least 40 patients with similar findings have been reported since then. Many of these have been members of the same family and an autosomal dominant inheritance has been suggested, but a clear-cut mode of transmission has not been determined in most cases. The syndrome is very rare and has been reported in both children and adults, and represents the prototype of pseudohypoaldosteronism type II. Hyperkalemia may be quite severe and is associated with hyperchloremic acidosis, moderate to severe hypertension, and ECV expansion, with secondary suppression of renin, aldosterone, and prostaglandins. These findings are diametrically opposite to those of Bartter's and Gitelman's syndromes. The proximate cause of this rather unique salt-sensitive syndrome of hypertension and hyperkalemic acidosis has been found recently to be due to activating, gain of function, mutations in the novel genes *WNK1* and *WNK4* both of which enhance the activity of the thiazide-sensitive NaCl cotransporter, NCC, in the distal collecting tubule. In addition, these mutated genes have an inhibitory effect on the potassium channel ROMK thus leading to avid sodium chloride reabsorption and potassium retention.

Treatment

Treatment consists of moderate salt restriction alone, or in combination with furosemide or thiazides. This completely reverses the hyperkalemic acidosis, restores renin, aldosterone, and prostaglandins, and normalizes blood pressure. In some patients with refractory hyperkalemia, cation exchange resins may be necessary.

References

Bertinelli A, Bianchetti MG, Girardin E et al (1992) Use of calcium excretion values to distinguish two forms of primary renal alkalosis: Bartter and Gitelman syndromes. J Pediatr 120:38–43

Birkenhager R, Otto E, Schurmann MJ, Vollmer M et al (2001) Mutation of BSND causes Bartter syndrome with sensorineural deafness and kidney failure. Nat Genet 29:310–314

Brochard K, Boyer O, Blanchard A et al (2009) Phenotype-genotype in antenatal and neonatal variants of Bartter's syndrome. Nephrol Dial Transplant 24:1455–1464

Cao L, Joshi P, Sumoza D (2002) Renal salt-wasting syndrome in a patient with cisplatin-induced hyponatremia: case report. Am J Clin Oncol 25:344–346

Chesney RW, Rogers SE (1976) Salt losing nephropathy in prune-belly syndrome. Reversal following unilateral nephrectomy. Am J Dis Child 130:778–779

Clive JM (1995) Bartter's syndrome: the unsolved puzzle. Am J Dis Child 25:813–823

Coleman AJ, Arias M, Carter NW et al (1966) The mechanism of salt wastage in chronic renal disease. J Clin Invest 45:1116–1125

Gitelman HJ, Graham JB, Welt LG (1966) A familial disorder characterized by hypokalemia and hypomagnesemia. Trans Assoc Am Physicians 79:221–235

Gordon RD (1986) The syndrome of hypertension and hyperkalemia with normal GFR. A unique pathophysiological mechanism for hypertension? Clin Exp Pharma Physiol 13(4):329–333

Gordon JA, Stokes JB III (1994) Understanding and treating Bartter's syndrome. Hosp Pract 29(5):103–110

Gordon RD, Geddes RA, Pawsey CJK et al (1970) Hypertension and severe hyperkalemia associated with suppression of renin and aldosterone and completely reversed by dietary sodium restriction. Aust Ann Med 19:287–294

Liddle GW, Bledsoe T, Coppage WS Jr (1963) A familial renal disorder simulating primary hyperaldosteronism but with negligible aldosterone secretion. Trans Assoc Am Physicians 76:199–213

McDougal WS, Wright FS (1972) Defect in proximal and distal sodium transport in post-obstructive diuresis. Kidney Int 2:304–317

Sanjad SA, Keenan BS, Hill LL (1983) Renal hypoprostaglandism, hypertension, and type IV renal tubular acidosis reversed by furosemide. Ann Int Med 99(5):624–627

Sebastian A, McSherry E, Morris RC Jr (1976) Impaired renal conservation of sodium and chloride during sustained correction of systemic acidosis in patients with type I classic renal tubular acidosis. J Clin Invest 58:454–469

Simon DB, Nelson-Williams C, Bia MJ et al (1996a) Gitelman's variant of Bartter's syndrome; inherited hypokalemic alkalosis, is caused by mutations in the thiazide-sensitive Na–Cl transporter. Nat Genet 12:24–30

Simon DB, Karet FE, Hamdan JM et al (1996b) Bartter's syndrome, hypokalemic alkalosis with hypercalciuria, is caused by mutations in the Na–K-2Cl cotransporter *NKCC2*. Nat Genet 13:183–188

Simon DB, Karet FE, Rodriguez-Soriano J et al (1996c) Genetic heterogeneity of Bartter's syndrome revealed by mutations in the K^+ channel, ROMK. Nat Genet 14:152–156

Simon DB, Bindra RS, Mansfield TA et al (1997) Mutations in the chloride channel gene, CLCNKB, cause Bartter's syndrome type III. Nat Genet 17:171–178

Stein JH (1985) The pathogenetic spectrum of Bartter's syndrome. Kidney Int 28:85–93

Uribarri J, Oh MS, Carroll HJ (1983) Salt-losing nephropathies. Am J Nephrol 3:193–198

Watanabe S, Fukumoto S, Chang H et al (2002) Association between activating mutations of calcium-sensor receptor and Bartter's syndrome. Lancet 360:692–694

Wilson FH, Disse-Nicodeme S, Choate KA et al (2001) Human hypertension caused by mutations in WNK kinases. Science 293:1107–1112

306 Distal Renal Tubular Acidosis (TYPE I, DRTA)

Sami A. Sanjad

Introduction

The kidney plays a major role in acid–base homeostasis. This is accomplished by two essential mechanisms, both involving the exchange of filtered sodium from the tubular lumen with secreted hydrogen from the tubular cells. The first mechanism is quantitatively more important and occurs primarily in the proximal tubule. It accounts for the reabsorption or reclamation of 85–90% of the filtered bicarbonate back to peritubular capillaries, thus maintaining the concentration of bicarbonate in the plasma fairly constant. This process is catalyzed both by: (a) luminal carbonic anhydrase IV, which causes the dehydration of carbonic acid; and (b) cellular carbonic anhydrase II, which rehydrates the absorbed CO_2 to form carbonic acid. The latter dissociates into H^+ and HCO_3. This regenerated bicarbonate is returned to the blood and maintains normal bicarbonate levels (➋ Fig. 288.2, ➋ Chap. 288, "Overview of Renal Function").

The second mechanism also involves the exchange of luminal sodium for cellular hydrogen ions secreted in the distal tubule. The hydrogen ions combine with filtered buffers (mainly phosphate) and are excreted in the final urine as titratable acid. As this is not enough to excrete all the daily acid load, a new buffer, NH_3, derived from the deamination of glutamine in the tubular cells, diffuses passively into the lumen and combines with hydrogen ion, also secreted from the tubular cells. The resulting NH_4^+ ion is "trapped" (does not diffuse back into the cell) and is excreted in the final urine (➋ Fig. 288.3, ➋ Chap. 288, "Overview of Renal Function"). Net acid excretion (NAE) is the term used to express the sum of TA and NH_4^+ minus any HCO_3 (negligible) that may be excreted. The steady state net acid excretion is equal to hydrogen ion generated from endogenous and exogenous (diet) sources. This is also equal to the net addition of bicarbonate by the kidneys to the body fluids (40–60 meq/m^2/day).

Definition

DRTA is a rare renal tubulopathy characterized by persistent hyperchloremic (normal anion gap) metabolic acidosis due to impaired secretion of hydrogen ion from the distal collecting duct cells to the tubular lumen resulting in relatively high urine pH in the face of systemic acidosis. Although frequently considered in the differential diagnosis of infants and children with failure to thrive, it is seldom detected as the cause.

Pathophysiology of DRTA

Until recently, all patients with DRTA were thought to have a single underlying pathogenetic mechanism: an inability of the distal nephron to generate and maintain steep pH gradients between peritubular blood and urine. The implication was that the distal tubular cells were capable of proton secretion but, because of a leaky membrane, hydrogen ions back diffused to the circulation leaving behind a relatively alkaline urine. This was referred to as gradient defect RTA. The prototype of such a defect in acidification is seen in patients treated with Amphotericin B.

Three types of cells in the distal nephron contribute to acid–base homeostasis: (1) the alpha-intercalated cells, which contain a luminal H^+-ATPase pump and an H^+–K^+-ATPase pump; (2) the principal cells, which have an indirect but important effect in urine acidification (see below, ➋ Voltage-dependent DRTA); and (3) the beta intercalated cells, which have a limited role in acidification but may be involved in bicarbonate secretion in vegetarians ingesting an alkaline ash diet. With this background, it is now possible to characterize DRTA from a mechanistic point of view (➋ *Fig. 306.1*).

The alpha-intercalated cell of the distal collecting ducts plays a pivotal role in the fine regulation of acid–base balance by the human kidney. This is accomplished by the H^+-ATPase pump at the luminal membrane, which

Abdelaziz Y. Elzouki (ed.), *Textbook of Clinical Pediatrics*, DOI 10.1007/978-3-642-02202-9_306,

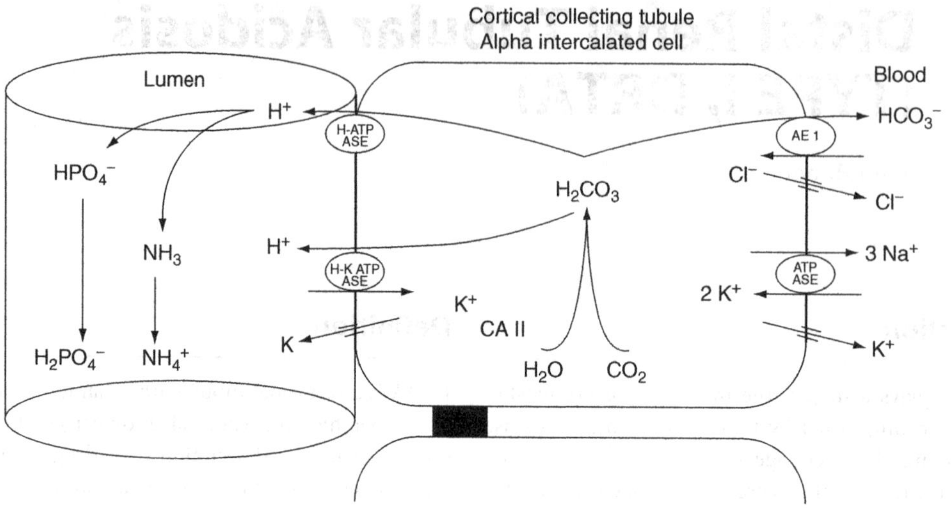

Fig. 306.1
Excretion of fixed acids in the distal nephron. Hydrogen secretion by the alpha-intercalated cells takes place via the H^+-ATPase pump in the luminal basement membrane. About 40% of the secreted hydrogen ions combine with filtered phosphate to form titratable acid. Most of the remaining hydrogen secreted combines with NH_3 to form NH_4^+, but a small amount remains as free hydrogen ions and regulates urinary pH. Bicarbonate reclamation occurs by Cl^-/HCO_3^- exchanger AE1 at the basolateral membrane

secretes H^+, and by the HCO_3^-/Cl^- (AE1) exchanger at the basolateral membrane, which is responsible for bicarbonate regeneration. Failure of either mechanism underlies the cellular and molecular etiology of distal RTA. Several mutations in the genes responsible for these transport systems have been identified recently, revolutionizing our understanding of the molecular basis of DRTA. Both hereditary and acquired forms are recognized in patients with DRTA, but this chapter will deal primarily with the hereditary forms of DRTA that prevail in infants and children.

Etiology of DRTA

Hereditary DRTA

The past 10 years have witnessed major advances in molecular biology that have allowed for a better understanding and classification of the hereditary forms of DRTA at the cellular and subcellular level. In infants and children, the autosomal recessive forms of RTA are more prevalent, whereas in adults the less severe, dominant forms are more common.

Autosomal Dominant Distal RTA

Randall and Targgart were the first to report RTA with nephrocalcinosis and osteomalacia in successive generations suggesting an autosomal dominant transmission. Subsequent reports confirmed this mode of transmission in several families. Clinical manifestations and the degree of acidosis in reported patients have been milder and therefore detected much later in life than in those with autosomal recessive distal RTA.

Chaabani and colleagues reported on large kindred with RTA with evidence of autosomal dominant transmission. As in previously reported cases, metabolic acidosis was well tolerated and often asymptomatic. Only 3 of 28 patients, with both parents affected, developed hypercalciuria, nephrocalcinosis, and growth retardation.

More recently, molecular studies in several kindreds with autosomal dominant RTA have consistently revealed mutations in the *SLC4A1* gene encoding the Cl^-/HCO_3^- exchanger AE1. These have been mostly missense mutations in codon Arg 589 suggesting an important role for this residue in the normal acidification process. It has been shown that these mutations in the *AE1* gene are not associated with loss of function of the Cl^-/HCO_3^- exchanger and that they probably affect the acidification process by targeting of *AE1* from the basolateral to the luminal membrane of the alpha-intercalated cell. Mutations in the erythrocyte isoform of the *AE1* are associated with hemolytic anemias due to ovalocytosis or spherocytosis, but seldom with RTA.

Autosomal Recessive DRTA

This entity appears to be relatively common in Middle Eastern countries. Karet et al. have elucidated the mechanisms responsible for the acidification defect in patients with recessive distal RTA. Molecular studies involving genome-wide linkage analysis in a cohort of several, mostly consanguineous, kindreds with distal RTA localized two genes: one on chromosome 2p13 associated with sensory-neural deafness (SND) and another on chromosome 7q33–34 associated with normal hearing. Both genes encode kidney-specific subunits of the proton pump of the alpha-intercalated cell. The majority of patients in both groups were of Arab or Turkish descent. Patients with distal RTA and SND were found to have several mutations in the gene encoding the B-1 subunit of the H^+-ATPase, *ATP6V1B1*, which is localized on chromosome 2p. Most of these mutations were found to disrupt the structure or alter the production of the normal B-1 subunit protein. It was also demonstrated that *ATP6V1B1* messenger RNA was expressed in the fetal and adult cochlea as well as the endolymphatic sac, findings that may explain the SND in these patients.

In patients with distal RTA and normal hearing, linkage analysis led to a defective gene on chromosome 7. This gene (*ATP6V0A4*) encodes a newly identified kidney-specific a4 isoform of the H^+-ATPase pump subunit. The clinical and biochemical manifestations are indistinguishable from patients with RTA with SND. Long-term follow-up, however, has revealed that many patients in this group develop mild hearing loss in later life. Stover and colleagues have recently demonstrated that the *ATP6V0A4* gene is also expressed within the human cochlea, again providing an explanation for the hearing defect. Recent reports from the Far East have identified different mutations in the AE1 in association with autosomal recessive distal RTA with or without ovalocytosis. This appears to be confined to Thailand and has not been documented in Caucasians.

Mixed RTA (Type 3)

Renal tubular acidosis combining features of both proximal and distal acidification defects may be observed in infants and children as a transient defect (previously known as type 3 RTA) and could be related to immaturity of one or more of the several transport systems described above. A syndrome of mixed RTA associated with osteopetrosis, cerebral calcification, and carbonic anhydrase II (CA II) deficiency has been reported in several families from the Arab world (➋ Chap. 304, "Proximal Renal Tubular Disorders"). The syndrome is inherited as an autosomal recessive trait and is characterized clinically by failure to thrive, recurrent fractures, mental retardation, and cranial nerve abnormalities. Over 70% of the cases have been from Middle Eastern and North African countries where genetic heterogeneity is suggested by a more severe variant of the disease. More than 70 cases have been documented in the literature, with more than half from Saudi Arabia. A recent study by Fathallah and colleagues documents evidence for a founder effect in 24 patients with osteopetrosis and CAII deficiency from 14 Tunisian families. A filiation study led to the tracing of a gene to a common Arabic tribe that settled in the Maghreb in the tenth century. The gene locus for CAII has been mapped to chromosome 8q2 with several mutations identified, the most common being the Arabic one, which is a splice junction mutation in intron 2. More recently, mutations in the gene *OC16*, encoding the a3 subunit of the osteoclast V-H^+-ATPase, have been shown to cause infantile malignant osteopetrosis.

Clinical Findings in DRTA

In infants and children the clinical manifestations of proximal and DRTA are similar, namely, growth failure, vomiting, and recurrent bouts of dehydration. Hypokalemia occurs in about 30% of patients with DRTA. Muscle weakness, sometimes progressing to skeletal or respiratory muscle paralysis may occur if hypokalemia is severe. Potassium depletion will also cause impaired urinary concentration resulting in polyuria and polydipsia with a tendency for extracellular fluid volume contraction and secondary hyperaldosteronism, which will further aggravate renal potassium wasting. Rickets or osteomalacia are frequently observed in untreated DRTA. Hypocitraturia, together with the alkaline urine, and hypercalciuria in patients with DRTA play an important role in the pathogenesis of nephrocalcinosis, which is found in more than two thirds of the cases (➋ *Fig. 306.2*). Nephrocalcinosis is seldom observed in patients with PRTA. The sequelae of impaired hydrogen ion secretion by the distal tubule are illustrated in ➋ *Fig. 306.3*

Differential Diagnosis of DRTA

➋ *Table 306.1* lists the different clinical entities considered in the differential diagnosis of DRTA. In infants the hereditary forms should be suspected in the face of a positive family history and consanguineous parents. The acquired forms of DRTA may be seen at any age and should be considered in patients with tubulointerstitial renal diseases such as chronic pyelonephritis, obstructive uropathies, and post-renal transplantation.

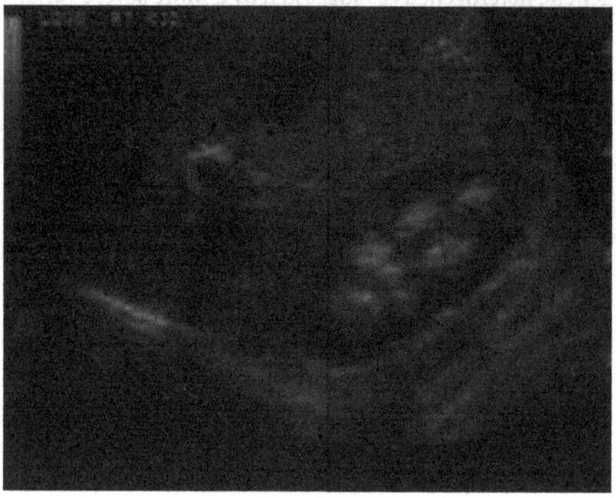

Fig. 306.2
Medullary nephrocalcinosis in an infant with dRTA

Hyperkalemic DRTA (Type 4)

The hereditary forms of hyperkalemic RTA are extremely rare and are usually seen in association with pseudohypoaldosteronism of which two types are recognized (see Chap. 305, "Disorders of Distal Tubular Transport of Sodium and Potassium").

Type I Pseudohypoaldosteronism

Clinically, these patients present in early infancy with renal salt wasting, hypovolemia, hyperchloremic acidosis, and hyperkalemia. Plasma and urinary aldosterone are elevated. Two modes of inheritance are recognized. The autosomal dominant is relatively mild and the defect is restricted to the kidneys. It is caused by heterozygous mutations in the mineralocorticoid receptor gene. The autosomal recessive form is much more serious and associated with severe renal salt wasting and potentially lethal hyperkalemia. The disease has been characterized recently at the molecular level and found to be due to loss of

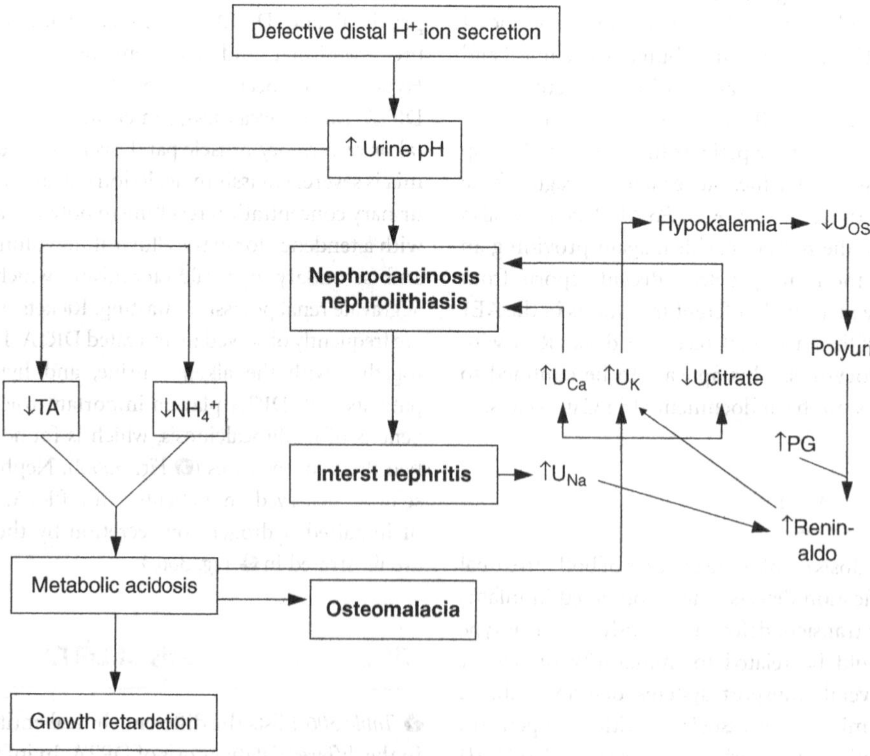

Fig. 306.3
The sequelae of impaired distal H^+ ion secretion by the distal collecting ducts

Table 306.1
Some diseases associated with DRTA

(A) Primary
Hereditary-permanent
1. Autosomal dominant: mutations in *SLC4A1* gene encoding the Cl-/HCO3- exchanger AE1.
2. Autosomal Recessive: Mutations in V-H-ATPase
(a) B1 subunit on chromosome 2p13 with SND
(b) a-4 subunit on chromosome 7q33-34 no or late onset SND
Sporadic-transient
(B) Secondary to associated diseases
1. Renal diseases
(a) Chronic pyelonephritis (b) Obstructive uropathy (c) Interstitial nephritis (d) Renal transplantation
2. Genetic diseases
(a) Sickle-cell anemia – nephropathy (b) Hereditary elliptocytosis (c) Ehlers–Danlos syndrome (d) Associated with sensory-neural deafness
3. Auto-immune diseases
(a) Systemic lupus erythematosus (b) Thyroiditis (c) Sjögren's syndrome
4. Associated with nephrocalcinosis
(a) Hyperparathyroidism (b) Hypercalciuria (c) Medullary sponge kidney
5. Drug induced
(a) Amphotericin B (b) Lithium

function mutations in the alpha, beta, and gamma subunits of the sodium epithelial channel, ENaC. In addition to the kidney, the salivary glands, the gastrointestinal and pulmonary systems may be also affected.

Type II Pseudohypoaldosteronism

This is a rare autosomal dominant disease with few case reports having appeared in the literature since the original description by Gordon and associates (see Chap. 305, "Disorders of Distal Tubular Transport of Sodium and Potassium"). It is characterized by hyperkalemic acidosis, hypertension secondary to plasma volume expansion, and suppression of renin and aldosterone. The proximate cause has been discovered recently to be secondary to gain of function mutations in the WNK1 and WNK4 kinases, which may enhance transcellular and paracellular chloride conductance as well as decreasing potassium efflux by inhibition of the potassium channel ROMK.

Voltage-Dependent RTA

Electronegativity of the distal luminal fluid is maintained by the principal cell that is involved in sodium absorption and potassium secretion. A lumen negative voltage due to reduced sodium reabsorption will indirectly impair hydrogen secretion by the alpha-intercalated cells and potassium secretion by the principal cells. Loss of sodium uptake into the cells of the distal nephron reduces the transepithelial potential for potassium and proton secretion, explaining the hyperkalemia and metabolic acidosis. The urinary pH is greater than 5.5, but will be appropriately acidic if the defect in sodium reabsorption is reversible. Voltage-dependent RTA may be observed in children with severe ECV contraction in which distal sodium delivery is significantly reduced. It may also be seen with urinary obstruction, sickle-cell disease, and lupus nephritis and as a side effect of several drugs, such as amiloride, triamterene, lithium, and trimethoprim.

Combined Voltage and Secretory Defects

Such a combined defect might explain the distal RTA observed in clinical states associated with reduced nephron mass and aldosterone deficiency or resistance. Patients with type IV RTA fall into this category and may be classified under various syndromes of hypoaldosteronism. In this subtype there is substantial reduction in renin production usually associated with chronic interstitial nephropathy. As a result, renin-dependent aldosterone secretion falls leading to low circulating levels with subsequent hyperkalemia and hyperchloremic acidosis. The condition is usually seen in adult patients with mild azotemia due to diabetic nephropathy, gout, chronic pyelonephritis, and interstitial nephropathy. It may also be seen in children with hydronephrosis and as a side effect of several drugs including nonsteroidal anti-inflammatory drugs, heparin and spironolactone.

Aldosterone Deficiency

This may occur with glucocorticoid deficiency as in adrenogenital syndrome and Addison's disease or as an isolated defect due to reduced aldosterone biosynthesis. Salt wasting is usually severe and hyperkalemia may be life threatening.

Infantile Type IV RTA (Partial Aldosterone Resistance)

This represents a relatively common type of hyperkalemic RTA in infants and young children. In this condition there seems to be partial resistance to the action of aldosterone with hydrogen and potassium retention, but normal sodium reabsorption and therefore no renal salt wasting. The clinical presentation is like that of other types of RTA, with failure to thrive and vomiting. There is no sex predilection and familial occurrence has been reported. This condition tends to be self-limited and most patients will no longer require alkali therapy by the age of 5 years. It is quite possible, therefore, that the condition represents a maturational defect in distal tubular physiology that may be related to the mineralocorticoid receptor gene or the sodium epithelial channel. A transient post-receptor defect remains a possibility. Some of the clinical findings and differential diagnosis of hyperkalemic RTA are outlined in ➲ *Table 306.2.*

Other Types of DRTA

Rate-Dependent DRTA

This is a rather mild defect in acidification also involving the alpha-intercalated cells of the collecting ducts and is due to a decreased number of H^+-ATPase pumps or their rate of operation. Patients with rate-dependent RTA are able to lower urine pH when properly challenged but have a reduced maximal rate of hydrogen ion excretion. Rate-dependent RTA is typically seen in patients with mild renal transplant rejection and in some cases of interstitial nephritis.

Incomplete DRTA

This entity is rare in children and is defined as an inability of the distal nephron to acidify the urine maximally with an exogenous acid load in the absence of systemic acidemia. It is often discovered in patients being investigated for nephrolithiasis and nephrocalcinosis. Incomplete RTA may also be seen in some patients with familial renal magnesium wasting and hypercalciuria.

With any of the above defects, excretion of titratable acid and ammonium (net acid excretion) will be reduced resulting in positive hydrogen ion balance. In patients with type IV hyperkalemic RTA, urinary pH is appropriately acidic and titratable acid is usually normal, but ammoniagenesis and ammonium transport are suppressed

Table 306.2
Hyperkalemic distal RTA (Type IV RTA)

	PRA	ALDO	BP	URINE Na
Hypoaldosteronism				
1.0 Mineralocorticoid deficiency	↑	↓	↓	↑
Hyporeninemic hypoaldosteronism	↓	↓	N↑	–
Renal disease – diabetes, gout, interstitial nephritis Drugs				
NSAIDS, cyclosporin, trimethoprim	↓	↓	↑	↓
ACE inhibitors	↑	↓	↓	↑
Pseudohypoaldosteronism				
PHA1 AR	↑	↑	↓	↑
PHA 1 AD	↑N	↑N	N	N
PHA 2 (Gordon's syndrome)	↓	↓	↑	↓

PRA plasma renin activity, *ALDO* aldosterone, *NSAIDS* nonsteroidal anti-inflammatory drugs, *PHA* 1,2 pseudohypoaldosteronism types 1 and 2, *AD* autosomal dominant, *AR* autosomal recessive by the high serum potassium resulting in decreased ammonium and net acid excretion. A mild degree of renal bicarbonate wasting may be seen in patients with distal RTA. Moderate bicarbonaturia (up to 15% of the filtered load) is commonly seen in infants with a secretory defect but tends to improve with time.

The clinical and laboratory findings that help distinguish the different types of RTA, including PRTA, appear in *Table 306.3.*

Diagnostic Evaluation of Patients with DRTA

1. Determine serum anion gap: $Na-[Cl+HCO_3]=$ $12-16$ mmol/L. In the absence of diarrhea or carbonic anhydrase inhibitors, a normal anion gap acidosis establishes the presence of RTA.
2. Measure capillary pH and pCO_2 and serum potassium to establish the severity of acidemia and the degree of respiratory compensation and diagnose hypo- or hyperkalemia.
3. Urine pH on a freshly voided specimen. If less than 5.5 and serum potassium is normal or low in the presence of acidemia, proximal RTA is the most likely diagnosis. This is confirmed if urine anion gap is negative (see below).
4. Assess glomerular function by blood urea and creatinine levels, creatinine clearance, and radionuclide scan if indicated. These are usually normal.
5. Assess global tubular function by measuring urine osmolality, glucose, amino acids, phosphate, uric acid, sodium, potassium, calcium, and magnesium to rule out Fanconi syndrome.
6. Radiologic evaluation to rule out nephrocalcinosis and rickets.
7. Determine urine anion gap (U_{AG}) by subtracting urine chloride from the sum of urine sodium and potassium concentrations: $U_{AG}=[U_{Na}+U_K]-U_{Cl}$. A negative value indicates that there is another unmeasured cation, ammonium (NH_4^+), signifying a normal distal acidification and ruling out distal RTA. A positive U_{AG} with a normal or low serum potassium and urine pH of >5.5 is highly suggestive of a secretory or gradient defect RTA. This can be substantiated by simultaneous determination of urine and blood pCO_2 (U-B pCO_2) during bicarbonate loading or following carbonic

Table 306.3
Clinical and laboratory findings in RTA

		Distal RTA		
		Type I		Type IV
	Proximal RTA (Type II)	Secretory or gradient defect	Voltage defect	Hypoaldosteronism Pseudohypoaldosteronism
Age	Infancy, childhood	Infancy	Any age	Any age
Sex	M>F	F>M	M>F	M>F
Nephrocalcinosis	Rare	Common	Rare	Unknown
Rickets osteomalacia	Common (with Fanconi syndrome)	Occurs	Rare	No
Urine pH (during acidosis)	<5.5	>5.5	>5.5	<5.5
NAE	N	↓	↓	↓
Serum K^+	N,↓	Usually ↓	↑	↑
Urine Ca	N,↑	↑	N↑	N↑
Urine citrate	N	↓	↓	N
Urine AG	Neg	Pos	Pos	Pos
IV_{HCO3^-}				
U-BpCO_2	>20 mmHg	<20 mmHg	<20 mmHg	>20 mmHg
FE_{HCO3}	>15%	3–15%	<5%	5%–15%
Alkali requirement (mg/kg/day)	5–20	2–14	2–3	2–3

NAE net acid excretion=(NH_4^+ titratable acid), *Urine AG* urine anion gap, *U-BpCO$_2$* simultaneous measurements of pCO_2 in urine and blood during intravenous bicarbonate infusion and urine alkalization (U pH>7.5), *FE_{HCO3}* fractional excretion of HCO_3 – or percentage of filtered load of bicarbonate excreted in the urine anhydrase inhibition and urine alkalinization. If distal hydrogen ion secretion is intact, hydrogen will combine with bicarbonate to form H_2CO_3. Due to the absence of luminal carbonic anhydrase IV in the distal tubule, H_2CO_3 will be dehydrated slowly to CO_2, and will raise tubular urine pCO_2 levels (Fig. 306.4 and Table 306.3).

Because of the impermeant nature of the uroepithelial membranes, this rise in pCO_2 will be reflected in the final urine. With normal distal hydrogen ion secretion, urine pCO_2 values rise above 70 or 80 mmHg and the U-B pCO_2 is greater than 20 mmHg. If the U_{AG} is positive (low NH_4^+) in the presence of hyperkalemic RTA, a urine pH above 5.5 is indicative of a voltage-dependent RTA. If urine pH is below 5.5, the diagnosis of hypoaldosteronism or any of the syndromes of pseudohypoaldosteronism should be considered.

8. Ammonium Chloride Load: (100 meq/m^2 po)/Furosemide-Fludrocortsone. This test of urine acidification should be used only in equivocal or borderline cases of suspected RTA when plasma bicarbonate is above 16–17 mmol/L and the urine pH is greater than 5.5. A normal test will result in lowering of the urine pH to less than 5.5 (usually less than 5.0) and yield a net acid excretion in excess of 40 μeq/min/m^2. Many patients tolerate NH_4Cl ingestion poorly because of gastric irritation and develop nausea and vomiting.

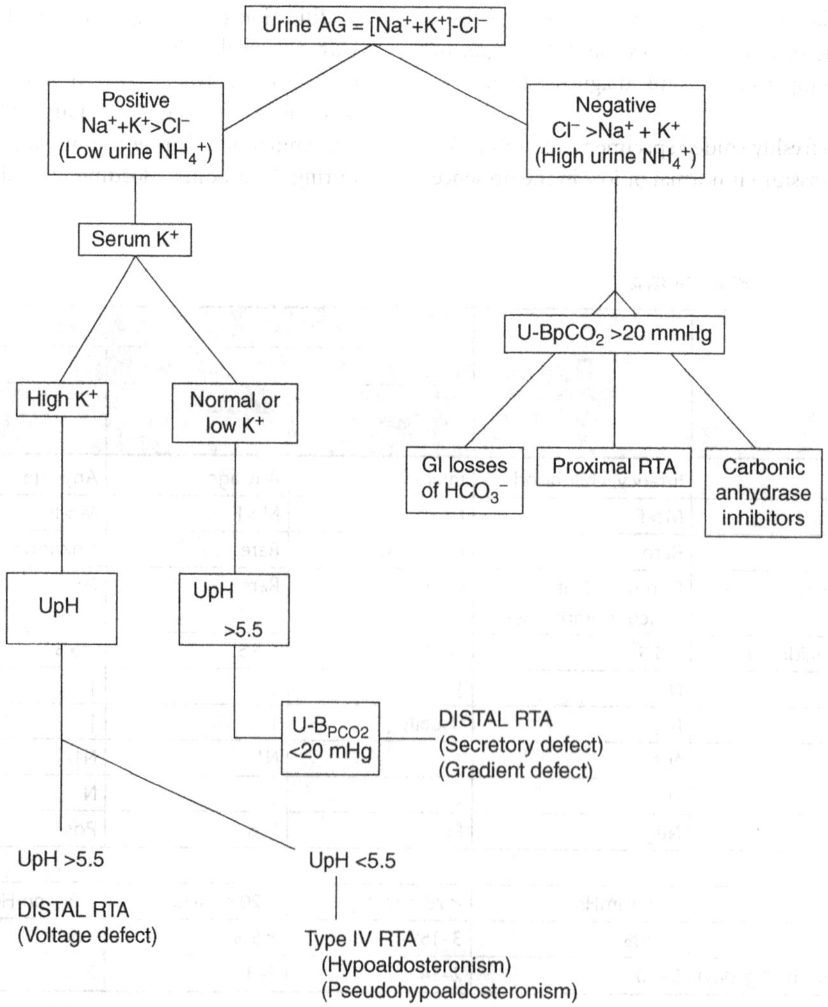

Fig. 306.4
Urine anion gap in the differential diagnosis of RTA (Modified from Lash and Arruda (1993)

An alternative way to test the capacity for distal acidification is to administer furosemide and mineralocorticoid fludrocortisone simultaneously. The combination of both, increased distal Na^+ delivery and mineralocorticoid effect, will stimulate distal H^+ secretion by both increasing the luminal electronegativity and having a direct stimulatory on H^+ secretion.

Treatment and Prognosis of DRTA

The treatment of distal RTA consists of adequate alkali replacement to normalize plasma bicarbonate. Infants with the classical variety require 2–3 meq/kg/daily in three divided doses. This corresponds to the endogenous acid production. Those with renal bicarbonate wasting may require higher doses of alkali (3–14 meq/kg/day) in four or more divided doses depending on the extent of their urinary losses. For patients with moderate or severe hypokalemic RTA, potassium citrate alone or in combination with sodium citrate (Polycitra) is the treatment of choice. One milliliter of Polycitra yields 2 meq of bicarbonate, 1 meq of sodium, and 1 meq of potassium. With correction of acidosis a "catch-up" growth is seen within a few months and normal stature is eventually attained. Correction of acidosis also corrects the hypocitraturia and prevents nephrocalcinosis and deterioration in renal function, if treatment is instituted before the age of 3 years. Partial correction of metabolic acidosis with inadequate alkali replacement will not prevent the development of nephrocalcinosis and possible chronic renal failure. The sensorineural deafness associated with autosomal recessive DRTA does not improve with treatment, even if initiated early in the course of the disease.

In the secondary forms of distal RTA, the therapy will depend on the underlying disease. Most patients will require 2–3 meq/kg/day of sodium bicarbonate in divided doses. In patients with severe rachitic bone disease a short course of vitamin D will accelerate the healing process.

In patients with hyperkalemic RTA, treatment is tailored to the underlying disease process. In voltage-dependent hyperkalemic RTA, a high sodium and low potassium intake with or without a thiazide or loop diuretic will lower serum potassium and raise bicarbonate to normal levels, but alkali therapy may be required in some patients. For patients with the various syndromes of hypoaldosteronism, and pseudoaldosteronism, treatment will consist of adequate salt intake to replace urinary losses and a mineralocorticoid supplement if necessary (Florinef .05–0.1 mg/day). In patients with hyporeninemic hypoaldosteronism, the use of Furosemide 1–2 meq/kg/day may be sufficient to correct the hyperkalemia and acidosis, but alkali therapy may also be necessary in some patients.

References

Albright F, Burnett CH, Parson W, Reifenstein EC, Roos A (1946) Osteomalacia and late rickets. Medicine 25:399–479

Arruda JAL, Cowell G (1994) Distal Renal tubular acidosis: molecular and clinical aspects. Hosp Pract 29:75–88

Awad M, Al-Ashwal AA, Sakati NA et al (2002) Long-term follow up on carbonic anhydrase deficiency syndrome. Saudi Med J 23:25–29

Batlle DC, Arruda JAL, Kurtzman NA (1981) Hyperkalemic distal renal tubular acidosis associated with obstructive uropathy. N Engl J Med 304:373–380

Batlle DC, Hizon M, Cohen E et al (1988) The use of the urine anion gap in the diagnosis of hyperchloremic metabolic acidosis. N Engl J Med 318:594–599

Butler A, Wilson J, Farber S (1936) Dehydration and acidosis with calcification at the renal tubules. J Pediatr 8:489

Chaabani H, Hadj-Khlil A, Ben-Dhia N, Braham H (1994) The primary hereditary form of distal renal tubular acidosis: clinical and genetic studies in 60-member kindred. Clin Genet 45:194–199

Cohen EP, Bastani B, Cohen MR et al (1992) Absence of H^+-ATPase in cortical collecting tubules of a patient with Sjögren's syndrome and distal renal tubular acidosis. J Am Soc Nephrol 3:264–271

Dafnis E, Spohn M, Lonis B et al (1992) Vanadate causes hypokalemic distal renal tubular acidosis. Am J Physiol 262:F449

Fathallah DM, Bejaoui M, Lepaslie D et al (1997) Carbonic anhydrase II deficiency in Maghrebian patients: evidence for founder effect and genomic recombination at the CA II locus. Hum Genet 99:634–637

Fuster D, Zhang J, Xie X, Moe O (2008) The vacuolar-ATPase B1 subunit in distal tubular acidosis: Novel mutations and mechanisms for dysfunction. Kidney Int 73:1151–1158

Geller DS, Rodriguez-Soriano J, Vallo Boado A et al (1998) Mutations in the mineralocorticoid receptor gene cause autosomal dominant pseudohypoaldosteronism type 1. Nat Genet 19:279–281

Ghishan FK, Knobel SM, Summer M (1995) Molecular cloning, sequencing, chromosomal localization, and tissue distribution of the human Na^+/H^+ exchanger (SLC9A2). Genomics 30:25–30

Hamed IA, Crerwinskiaw CB, Kaufmann C, Altmiller DH (1979) Familial absorptive hypercalciuria and renal tubular acidosis. Am J Med 67:385–391

Hu PY, Roth DE, Skaggs LA et al (1992) A splice junction mutation in intron 2 of the carbonic anhydrase II gene of osteopetrosis patients from Arabic countries. Hum Mut 1(4):288–292

Igarashi T, Inatomi J, Sekine T et al (1999) Mutations in *SLC4A4* cause permanent proximal renal tubular acidosis with ocular abnormalities. Nat Genet 23:264–266

Ismail EA, Saad A, Sabry MA (1997) Nephrocalcinosis and urolithiasis in carbonic anhydrase II deficiency syndrome. Eur J Pediatr 156: 957–962

Jentsch TJ, Keller SK, Koch M, Wiederholt M (1984) Evidence for coupled transport of bicarbonate and sodium in cultured bovine corneal endothelial cells. J Membr Biol 81:189–204

Kaitwatchrai C, Vasuvatakul S, Yenchitsomanus P et al (1999) Distal renal tubular acidosis and high urine carbon dioxide tension in a patient with Southeast Asia ovalocytosis. Am J Kidney Dis 33:1147–1152

Karet FE (2000) Inherited renal tubular acidosis. Adv Nephrol 30:147–161

Karet FE, Gainza FJ, Gyory AZ (1998) Mutations in the chloride-bicarbonate gene exchanger AE1 cause autosomal dominant but not autosomal recessive distal renal tubular acidosis. Proc Natl Acad Sci USA 95(11):6337–6342

Karet FE, Finberg KE, Nelson RD et al (1999a) Mutations in the gene encoding the B1 subunit of H^+-ATPase cause renal tubular acidosis with sensorineural deafness. Nat Genet 21:84–90

Karet FE, Finberg KE, Nayir A et al (1999b) Localization of a gene for autosomal recessive distal renal tubular acidosis with normal hearing to 7q33-34. Am J Hum Genet 65:1656–1665

Kornak U, Schulz A, Fiedrich W et al (2000) Mutations in the a3 subunit of the vacuolar H^+ATPase cause infantile malignant osteopetrosis. Hum Mol Genet 9(13):2059–2063

Lash JP, Arruda JAL (1993) Laboratory evaluation of renal tubular acidosis. Clin Lab Med 13:117–129

Lightwood R (1935) Calcium infarction of the kidneys in infants. Arch Dis Child 10:205–206

Nash MA, Torrado AD, Greifer I, Spitzer A, Edelmann CM Jr (1972) Renal tubular acidosis in infants and children. J Pediatr 80:738–748

Ocal G, Berberoglu M, Adiyaman P et al (2001) Osteopetrosis, renal tubular acidosis without urinary concentration abnormality, cerebral calcification and severe mental retardation in three Turkish brothers. J Pediatr Endocrinol Metab 14:1671–1677

Pines KL, Mudge GH (1951) Renal tubular acidosis with osteomalacia. Am J Med 11:302–311

Quilty JA, Li J, Reithmeier RA (2002) Impaired trafficking of distal renal tubular acidosis mutants on the human kidney anion exchanger kAE1. Am J Physiol Ren Physiol 282(5):F810–820

Randall RE, Targgart WH (1961) Familial renal tubular acidosis. Ann Intern Med 54:1108–1116

Richard P, Wrong OM (1972) Dominant inheritance in a family with familial renal tubular acidosis. Lancet II:998–999

Rodriguez Soriano J (2000) New insights into the pathogenesis of renal tubular acidosis-from functional to molecular studies. Pediatr Nephrol 14:1121–1136

Sanjad SA (1997) Hereditary and acquired renal tubular disorders. Saudi J Kidney Dis Transplant 8(3):247–259

Sanjad SA, Mansour FM, Hernandez RH, Hill LL (1982) Severe hypertension, hyperkalemia, and renal tubular acidosis responding to dietary sodium restriction. Pediatrics 69(3):317–324

Seedat YK (1963) Some observations of renal tubular acidosis-a family study. S Afr Med J 38:606–610

Smith AN, Skaug J, Choate KA et al (2000) Mutations in *ATP6N1B* encoding a new kidney vacuolar proton pump 116-kD subunit, cause recessive renal tubular acidosis with preserved hearing. Nat Genet 26:71–75

Stover EH, Borthwick KJ, Bavalia C (2002) Novel *ATP6B1* and *ATP6N1B* mutations in autosomal recessive renal tubular acidosis, with new evidence for mild hearing loss. J Med Genet 39:796–803

Tanphaichitr VS, Sumboonnanonda A, Ideguchi H et al (1998) Novel AE1 mutations in recessive distal renal tubular acidosis. Loss of function is rescued by glycophorin A. J Clin Invest 102:2173–2179

Vassuvattakul S, Yenchitsomanus PT, Vachuanichsanong P et al (1999) Autosomal recessive distal renal tubular acidosis associated with Southeast Asian ovalocytosis. Kidney Int 56:1674–1682

Walsh S, Shirley D, Wrong O, Unwin R (2007) Urinary acidification assessed by simultaneous furosemide and fludrocortisone treatment: an alternative to ammonium chloride. Kidney Int 71:1310–1316

Zelikovic I (1995) Renal tubular acidosis. Pediatr Ann 24:48–54

307 Nephrogenic Diabetes Insipidus

Deborah P. Jones

Definition/Classification

Diabetes insipidus (DI, *insipidis*, from Greek, "to pass through" and Latin, "without taste") is a disorder characterized by inability of the kidney to concentrate urine. It is complicated by polyuria, polydipsia, and increased risk for hypertonic dehydration. DI may result from defects in the central nervous system, which impair production/release of antidiuretic hormone (ADH, also known as vasopressin), a condition known as central DI, or from inability of the kidney to respond to ADH, known as nephrogenic DI (NDI). In central DI, because the kidney's response to ADH is preserved, ADH is used as therapy.

Etiology

Proper concentration of urine requires a hypertonic renal medulla (the result of normal function of the ascending limb of the loop of Henle) and normal function of the collecting duct, which controls water excretion. In the collecting duct, ADH increases luminal permeability to water by its action on the membrane abundance of apical water channels (aquaporin 2 channels, AQP2). Activation of the vasopressin 2 receptor (V2R) stimulates an intracellular signaling cascade, which stimulates the recruitment of previously synthesized water channels contained in endocytic vesicles to be inserted into the luminal membrane thus allowing the passive movement of water into the cell; water exits via other aquaporin channels (type 3 and 4) found on the basolateral membrane of the collecting duct cell.

Pathogenesis

In childhood, NDI is most often the result of congenital disease resulting from mutations of the transport systems required for active water reabsorption in response to vasopressin. (➋ *Fig. 307.1*) Genetic mutations of the vasopressin receptor are responsible for 90% of affected individuals with NDI, and mutations of the aquaporin 2 channel account for 10%. The X-linked form of NDI resulting from mutations in the AVPR2 gene, located on the X chromosome, explains the male predominance of this disorder. The incidence of X-linked NDI in the province of Quebec, Canada is estimated at 8.8/million live male births. In Nova Scotia, another Canadian province, the incidence is much higher (58/million male births) due to a founder effect from those who arrived to the region on the Ship Hopewell. Although most affected individuals are able to translate the V2R protein, it is not properly folded and thus not translocated to its proper location on the basolateral membrane; thus, absence of receptor or abnormal receptor interrupts the G-protein coupled cellular response following V2R activation.

Autosomal dominant and recessive modes of inheritance result from mutations of the AQP2 gene located on chromosome 12. Affected individuals with this form of NDI also appear to have intracellular trafficking abnormalities, which lead to retention of the protein within the endoplasmic reticulum instead of endosomes ready for recruitment to the apical membrane. The lack of apical AQP2 on the apical membrane prevents normal water movement in response to a normal vasopressin-induced intracellular signaling cascade. To date, there are no clinical characteristics that allow distinction between the two major underlying genetic forms of NDI. In addition, some individuals with clinical NDI have not been found to have either of these known defects in collecting duct water transport.

Case

A 2-year-old WM was referred by his pediatrician for polyuria and polydipsia. His mother reports that he drinks 200–300 oz of water each day. He wakes up every night to drink water and requires numerous diaper changes during the night due to a large urinary volume. When deprived of fluids, his lips become red and dry; he has been seen drinking water from the garden hose, gutter downspout drain, toilet, and pet bowl. He was the 8 lb product of an uneventful pregnancy. He was nursed until the age of

Abdelaziz Y. Elzouki (ed.), *Textbook of Clinical Pediatrics*, DOI 10.1007/978-3-642-02202-9_307,

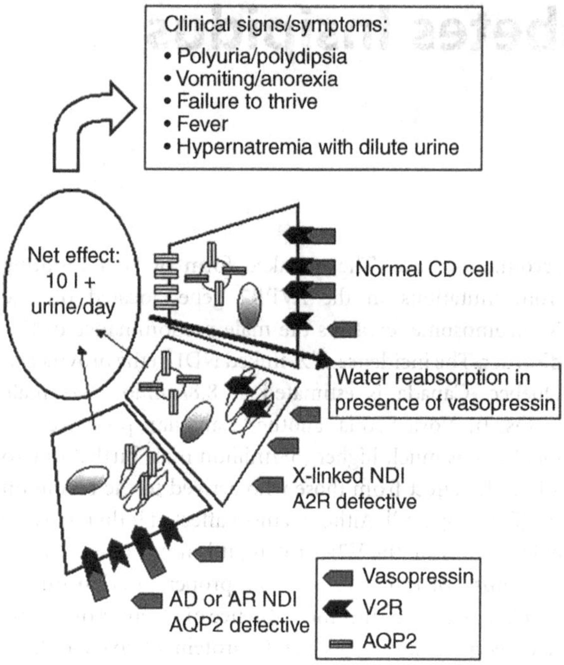

Figure 307.1
Cellular events involved in the vasopressin-induced water reabsorption in the normal collecting duct cell and in those resulting from mutations of either the V2R or AQ2 gene are represented. Common clinical symptoms/signs that accompany the underlying defect in water transport (reabsorption) are listed

6 months. Mother was often told that she was feeding him too much as he nursed constantly and also had vomiting during early infancy. Past medical history is without serious illness or hospitalization. Developmental milestones have been met. Family history is negative for kidney disease, specifically conditions with polyuria. Physical exam reveals an active and well-appearing boy who is drinking water directly from the exam room faucet. Weight was at the 50th and height at the 10th percentile.

Clinical Manifestations

The clinical presentation of NDI can be nonspecific particularly in infancy. The most common symptoms and signs at presentation are vomiting/anorexia (72%), failure to thrive (52%), fever (41%), constipation (34%), polydipsia (14%), and psychomotor retardation (3%). In a recent case series of genetically confirmed cases (30 males) the median age at diagnosis was 9 months, and mean age was 25 months. More than half were diagnosed by 12 months of age, and 87% were diagnosed by 18 months. Serum sodium is often increased, along with signs of dehydration and inappropriately dilute urine is found. Interestingly, family history was present in 25% of cases and six previous infant deaths were discovered to have likely been the result of undiagnosed NDI among families of identified cases. Given the nonspecific symptoms and often the lack of family history, diagnosis of NDI may be delayed. Previous case series indicated that up to 80% of affected individuals had signs of mental retardation. This is suspected to have been the result of repeated episodes of dehydration, fever, etc. With the trend toward earlier diagnosis in the past 2 decades, the prevalence of psychomotor retardation in children with NDI appears to be decreasing. Infants who receive mother's milk, which has a lower solute load, may also be somewhat protected. In the experience of this author, parents often give impressive histories describing extraordinary water craving: i.e., drinking from the outdoor waterspout, from the dog's bowl, and from the toilet. In, addition, infants with NDI often prefer water to milk or food in contrast to otherwise healthy children.

Case, continued: Laboratory evaluation sent at referral included a sodium level of 140 mmol/L, creatinine 0.5 mg/dL, urine specific gravity 1.005, and urine osmolality was 72 mOsm/kg. He underwent an abbreviated water deprivation test. At 4 h, the plasma osmolality was 309 mOsm/kg, sodium 149 mmol/L, and urine osmolality was 118 mOsm/kg. An ADH level was drawn and he was given DDAVP 1.5 mg/m^2 by subcutaneous injection; the highest urine osmolality obtained was 141 mOsm/kg, and at 1 h post ADH, the test concluded. His plasma ADH level was high – 38.1 pg/mL.

Differential Diagnosis

Polyuria, which is the clinical manifestation of inability to concentrate urine, may result from disorders other than DI. These disorders include other congenital renal tubular disorders such as Bartter/Gitelman syndrome and Fanconi syndrome. In contrast to NDI, these conditions are characterized by abnormalities in electrolyte handling, which are accompanied by hypokalemic metabolic alkalosis with or without hypomagnesemia (Bartter/Gitelman syndrome) and by hypokalemic, hypophosphatemic acidosis often with rickets (Fanconi syndrome). In addition, primary polydipsic syndromes may also cause polyuria. Acquired forms of NDI include lithium intoxication, hypercalcemia, protein malnutrition, sickle cell nephropathy, hypokalemia, juvenile nephronopthisis, and obstructive uropathy.

Diagnosis is dependent upon demonstration of inappropriately dilute urine in the setting of hyperosmolar plasma. In the case of individuals who present with hypernatremia and hyperosmolality, water deprivation is not required. In such a clinical setting, documentation of a urine osmolality of less than 300 mOsm (should be >800 in a normal child) is sufficient to indicate a significant concentrating defect. Administration of vasopressin is followed by measurement of urinary osmolality; individuals with central DI are able to increase the urine osmolality by at least 200 mOsm. Those with NDI show no significant increase in urine osmolality after vasopressin. In some cases in which the primary complaint is polydipsia and polyuria in the presence of normal serum sodium and plasma osmolality a short water deprivation test may be performed under close supervision. It is advised that this test be performed by those experienced in its procedure and interpretation. Measurement of plasma vasopressin may also be helpful in differentiating central from nephrogenic DI, as levels are lower than normal in central DI and elevated in NDI. Although NDI is much more common among males, females may be affected. The mutation may be expressed in females depending upon which X chromosome becomes inactivated in early embryogenesis. Therefore, the presence of clinical symptoms and signs suggestive of a concentrating defect in a female does not eliminate the possibility of NDI.

Given that 10 L of urine may be required to be excreted by the urinary tract, urologic complications of NDI are not uncommon. These complications include severe hydronephrosis, renal pelvic dilation, transient ureteral dilation, acute urinary retention, urinary infection, and nocturnal enuresis. Therefore, interval renal ultrasounds are recommended in the management of these patients. Growth may also be abnormal particularly in the first year of life. This aspect may be related to the feeding intolerance and the need to consume large volumes of water rather than food.

Case, continued: Imaging of the kidneys and bladder by ultrasound was normal. He was started on hydrochlorothiazide and amiloride. His mother reported a marked decrease in urine volume and increased appetite after initiation of treatment. A de novo mutation in the patient's vasopressin receptor gene was confirmed; his mother was not a carrier. Renal imaging studies at 5 years of age were still normal. At last follow-up, at 5 years of age, his height was at the 50th and weight at the 75th percentile. He continues to have polyuria and polydipsia, which is manageable during the day. Nighttime urine volume continues to be challenging.

Treatment

Treatment starts with access to water at all times. For infants, this may require creative methods. The mother of one of the author's patients fashioned a nipple attached to a large water bottle, which traveled wherever the child went – in stroller or bed. Dietary therapy is aimed at reduction of renal solute load. Previously prescribed low-protein diets are no longer recommended as they result in protein malnutrition. Low dietary salt is still recommended. Drug therapy most often initiates with thiazide diuretics (HCTZ 3 mg/kg/day, divided BID) in combination with the potassium sparing diuretic amiloride (0.3 mg/kg/day) and/or potassium supplementation. Although administration of diuretics to patients with polyuria seems counter intuitive, the thiazide diuretic hydrochlorothiazide reduces urine volume. This effect was initially attributed to increased proximal tubular water and solute reabsorption; however, recent studies indicate that thiazide diuretics increase water permeablility in the inner medullary collecting duct. In addition, hypokalemia should be avoided due to its potential contribution to abnormal urinary concentration. Nonsteroidal anti-inflammatory drugs such as indomethacin (2–3 mg/kg/day, divided BID) have also proven useful for NDI. These agents increase proximal tubular fluid and solute reabsorption; they seem to be tolerated fairly well. Unfortunately, they may be accompanied by gastrointestinal and renal toxicity. Although reduced by as much as 70% below baseline values with pharmacologic therapy, urine volumes and water intake are still excessive: one case series reported that despite therapy with HCTZ/amiloride, oral intake ranged from 125 mL/kg/day to 250 mL/kg/day and urine output from 3 mL/kg/h to 10 mL/kg/h. Most children continue to awaken at night to drink water and continue to demonstrate nocturnal enuresis despite optimal drug therapy. An algorithm for evaluating a child with polyuria is found in ➲ *Fig. 307.2.*

Although rare, the diagnosis of NDI should be considered in any child with polyuria and polydipsia, and in the setting of hypertonic dehydration in which dilute urine is found. Molecular characterization of the results of genetic mutations in the V2R and AQP2 have allowed a much better understanding of the underlying defects commonly found in children with NDI. Drug therapy is available which appears to be well tolerated and to support near normal growth. Unfortunately, most affected children

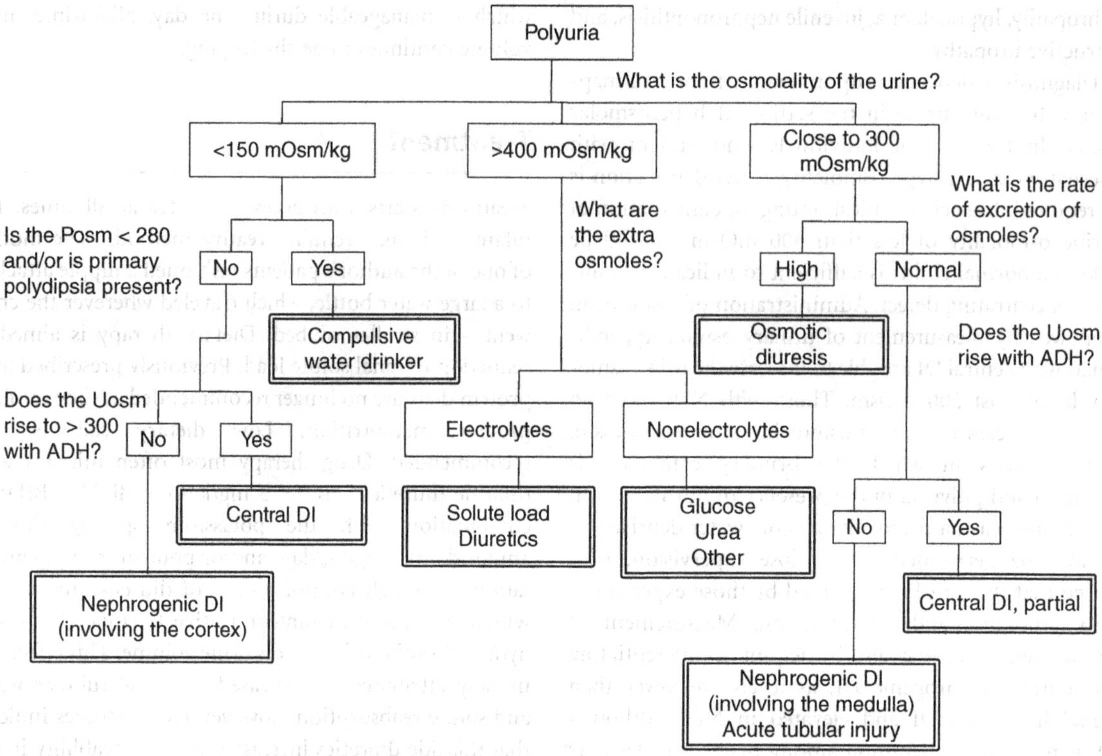

Figure 307.2
An algorithm for evaluating a child with polyuria

continue to display some symptoms and signs of excessive urinary volume.

Treatment: Future Development

Given that both V2R and AQP2 mutations have been associated with protein trafficking abnormalities, the potential for specific drug therapies aimed at escorting the miss-targeted proteins to their appropriate location on the basolateral or apical membrane of the collecting duct may eventually be available.

References

Bichet DG, Oksche A, Rosenthal W (1997) Congenital nephrogenic diabetes insipidus. J Am Soc Nephrol 8:1951–1958

Fujuwara TM, Bichet DG (2005) Molecular biology of hereditary diabetes insipidus. J Am Soc Nephrol 16:2836–2846

Halperin ML, Kamel KS, Narins RS (1992) Use of urine electrolytes and osmolality: bringing physiology to the bedside. In: Narins RG, Stein JH (eds) Diagnostic Techniques in Renal Disease. Churchill Livingstone, New York, NY, pp 1–46

Kirchlechner V, Koller DY, Seidl R, Waldhauser F (1999) Treatment of nephrogenic diabetes insipidus with hydrochlorothiazide and amiloride. Arch Dis Child 80:548–552

Knoers N, Monnens LAH (1992) Nephrogenic diabetes insipidus: clinical symptoms, pathogenesis, genetics and treatment. Pediatr Nephrol 6:476–482

Liffing J (2004) Paradoxical anti-diuretic effect of thiazides in Diabetes Indipidus: another piece of the puzzle. J Am Soc Nephrol 15:2948–2950

Sands JM, Bichet DG (2006) Nephrogenic diabetes insipidus. Ann Intern Med 144:186–194

Van Lieburg AF, Knoers NVAM, Monnens LAH (1999) Clinical presentation and follow-up of 30 patients with congenital nephrogenic diabetes insipidus. J Am Soc Nephrol 10:1958–1964

308 Urinary Stone Disease

Burhan Edrees · Soud Al Rasheed

Overview

Definition

Nephrolithiasis is the formation of stones in the kidney, while urolithiasis is stone in the urinary system. The existence of nephrolithiasis was known to Hippocrates, who described the symptoms of renal colic: "An acute pain is felt in the kidney, the loins, the flank and the testis of the affected side; the patient passes urine frequently; gradually the urine is suppressed. With the urine, sand is passed."

Nephrocalcinosis, when there is generalized increase in Calcium content of the kidney, which can be microscopic or macroscopic when you can see abnormal renal tissue using radiologic evaluation.

Epidemiology

Geographical Distribution

The incidence of urolithiasis in a given population is dependent on the geographic area, racial distribution, and socioeconomic status of the community.

Changes in socioeconomic conditions over time, and the subsequent changes in dietary habits, have affected not only the incidence but also the site and chemical composition of calculi.

In different series of patients of all ages with renal stone, prevalence in children ranges from 2 to 2.7%, can go up to 17% in some countries like Turkey, where urolithiasis is considered to be endemic. In the pediatric population, recent studies have shown that the annual incidence in children may be increasing in the West. In a series from Iceland, the annual incidence of kidney stones was 5.6 and 6.3 per 100,000 children under 18 and 16 years of age. The overall probability that an individual will form stones varies in different parts of the world. In view of adult literatures, the risk of developing urolithiasis in adults appears to be higher in the western hemisphere (5–9% in Europe, 12% in Canada, 13–15% in the USA) than in the eastern hemisphere (1–5%), although the highest risks have been reported in some Asian countries such as Saudi Arabia (20.1%). In Europe, it is reported that the occurrence of urolithias in the nineteenth century population was quite similar to that of the twentieth century in Asia. The rate of hospital admissions due to renal stone disease varies widely in different geographic regions, from 0.001 to 0.1% in the USA to 7% in Asia. This rate is one tenth of that seen in the adult population. Boys show a mild preponderance for stone disease, with a male to female ratio of 1.4:1 to 2.1:1, with more preponderance in white children in USA, and with African American and Asian children only rarely affected.

Renoureteral calculosis featuring mainly calcium oxalate and phosphate is currently more frequent in economically developed countries, whereas vesical calculosis (urinary bladder stone) is fairly widespread in Asia, with calculi composed of ammonium urate and calcium oxalate.

Stone composition has changed substantially over the past decades, with a progressive increase in frequency of calcium oxalate and calcium phosphate stones. Recent epidemiology studies from different continents and countries report that calcium oxalate accounts for 60–90% of stones in children, followed by calcium phosphate (10–20%), struvite (1–14%), uric acid (5–10%), cystine (1–5%), and mixed or miscellaneous (4%). Hypercalciuria is recognized worldwide as the most frequent underlying factor in calcium oxalate stones, although, in some countries of the eastern hemisphere, hypocitraturia has been reported as the leading cause. Other less frequent metabolic risk factors are hyperuricosuria and hyperoxaluria. However, increased urinary oxalate excretion might be underestimated and might even be a more prevalent risk factor than hypercalciuria for stone disease in some populations. Struvite or infection-related stones, which were very common in children until the last century, are rarely seen today in industrialized countries, possibly due to improved management of both pediatric obstructive uropathy and urinary tract infections. Bladder stones based on malnutrition during the first years of life are currently a frequent finding in various areas of Turkey,

Abdelaziz Y. Elzouki (ed.), *Textbook of Clinical Pediatrics*, DOI 10.1007/978-3-642-02202-9_308,

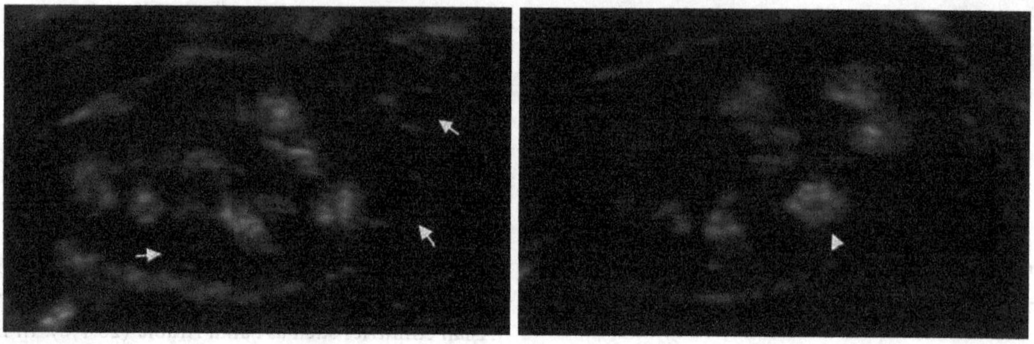

Figure 308.1
Renal ultrasound showing hypoechoic areas consistent with cysts *(arrows) in the left panel* and increased echogenicity consistent with nephrocalcinosis *(arrowhead) in the right panel*

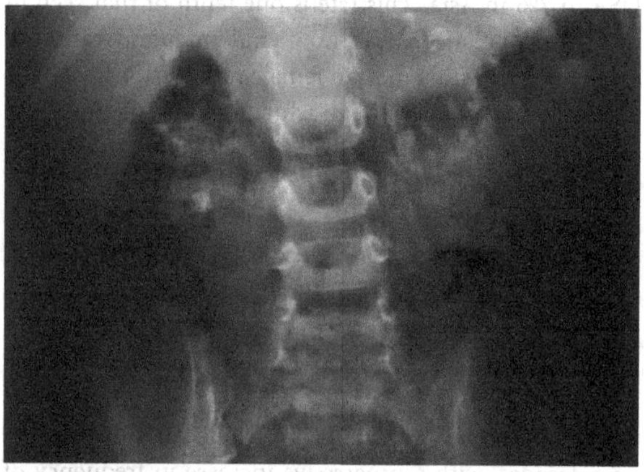

Figure 308.2
Plain abdominal radiographs demonstrating bilateral nephrocalcinosis

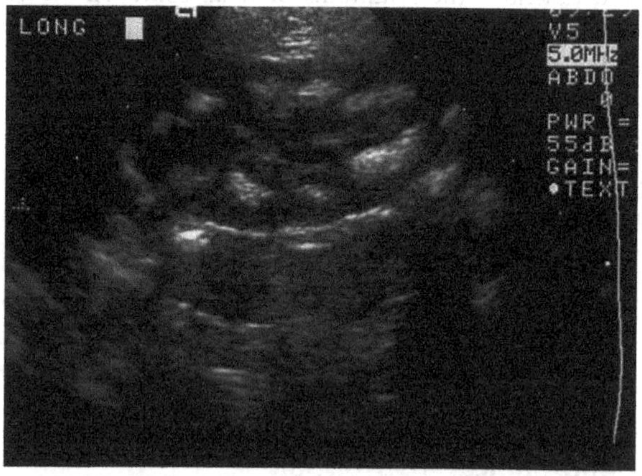

Figure 308.3
Renal ultrasound scan showing bilateral dense nephrocalcinosis with mild left pelvicalyceal dilatation (anterior-posterior diameter 7 mm)

Iran, India, China, Indochina, and Indonesia. Although the incidence is proportionally decreasing as social conditions improve. This trend defined as "stone wave" has been explained in terms of changing social conditions and the consequent changes in eating habits. In Europe, Northern America, Australia, Japan, and, more recently, Saudi Arabia, affluence has spread to all social classes and with it the tendency for individuals to increase protein intake in large quantities.

The Afro-Asian stone-sucess forming belt stretches from Sudan, the Arab Republic of Egypt, Saudi Arabia, the United Arab Emirates, the Islamic Republic of Iran, Pakistan, India, Myanmar, Thailand, and Indonesia to the Philippines (➋ *Fig. 308.5*). In this area of the world, the disease affects all age groups, from less than 1 year old to more than 70 years old, with a male-to-female ratio of 2 to 1. The prevalence of calculi ranges from 4% to 20%. The higher prevalence of urolithiasis in many of those countries is possibly determined by the high consanguinity that prevails among ethnic groups that live in those geographical areas.

Other risk factors involved in this geographical pattern are cultural practices such as the chewing of betel quid, which is common in many countries of the world, particularly in Southeast Asia. The quid consists of a preparation of areca nut, betel leaf, and calcium hydroxide "lime" paste, which produces a high incidence of hypercalciuria and hypocitraturia.

In the north Indian population, the absence of Oxalobacter formigenes, an intestinal oxalate degrading bacteria, can lead to a significant increase in the risk of absorptive hyperoxaluria.

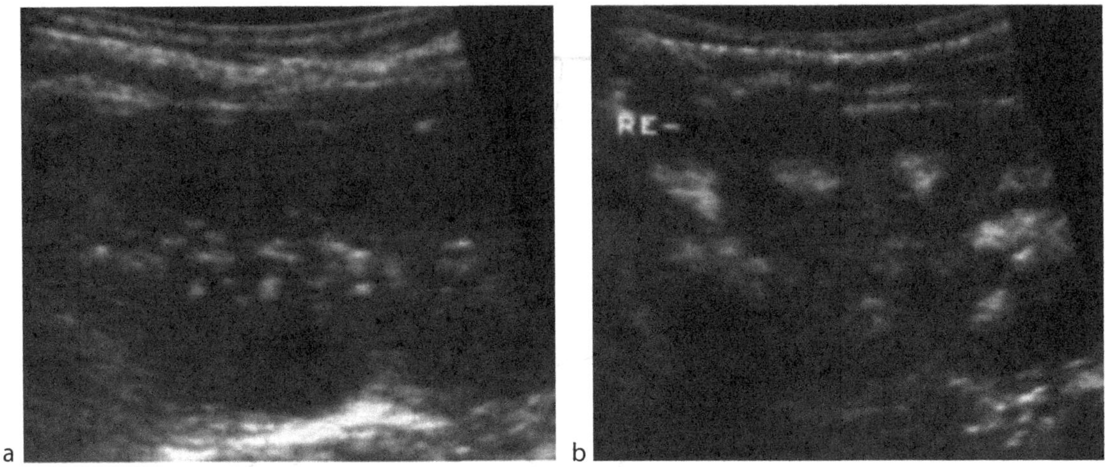

Figure 308.4
(a) Renal ultrasound of a preterm neonate with moderate nephrocalcinosis, with small white flecks in the tip of the pyramids. (b) Ultrasound of kidney of a preterm neonate with severe nephrocalcinosis. White dots almost entirely fill the pyramids

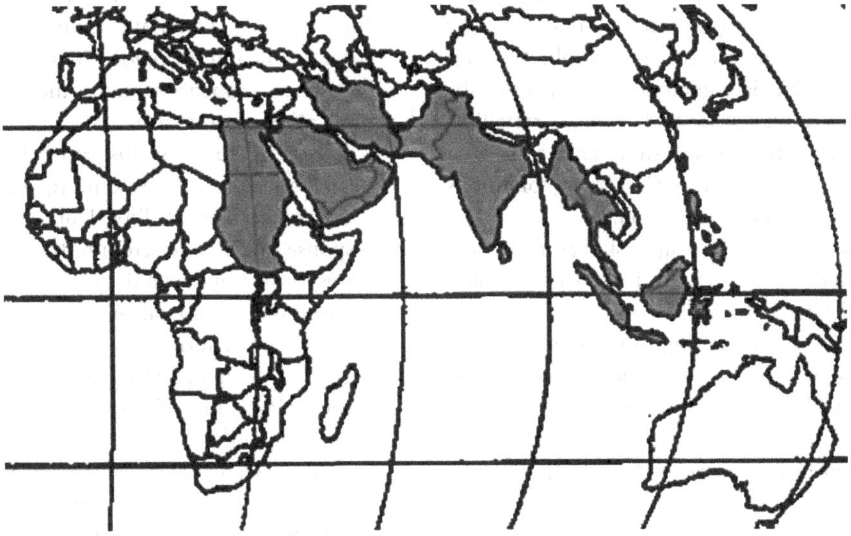

Figure 308.5
North African–Asian stone belt

Urolithiasis is most common in the southeastern region of USA, where the states of Virginia, North Carolina, Georgia, Tennessee, and Kentucky are described collectively as the North American "stone belt" (*Fig. 308.6*).

In summary, the epidemiology of renal stones with regard to stone composition is continuing to change all over the world toward a predominance of calcium oxalate stones. Major differences in the frequency of the other constituents, particularly uric acid and struvite, reflect particular eating habits and infection risk factors specific to certain population.

Pathogenesis

Stone formation is due to imbalance between *promoter* (which increases the tendency to form stone) and *inhibitor* (which increases solubility of stone constituents).

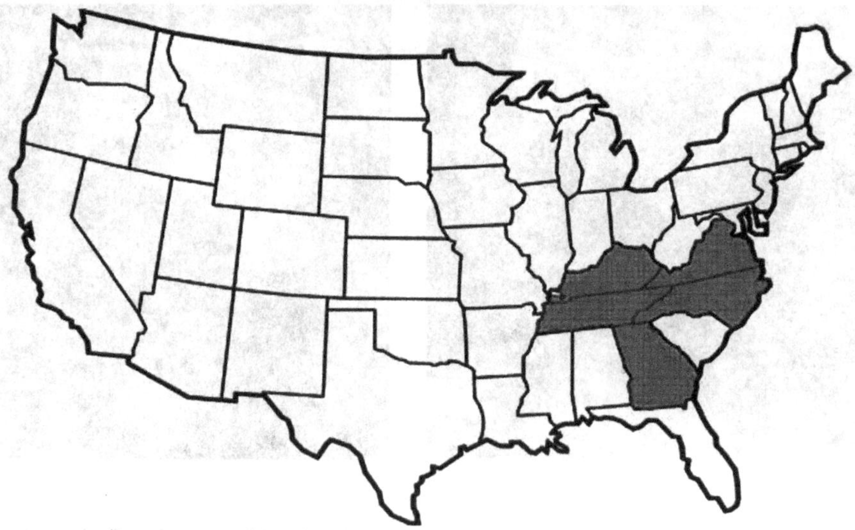

Figure 308.6
North American stone belt

The first step in the pathogenesis of nephrolithiasis is the formation of crystal nuclei. This occurs when the concentration of a salt exceeds the solubility limit "supersaturation." This is sometimes accompanied by a deficit of the protective substances known as crystallization inhibitors (e.g., citrate, magnesium, potassium etc.) The term "urinary stone risk factor" refers to conditions that promote the crystallization of a salt.

Widely recognized urinary stone risk factors are low urinary volume and increase in salt urinary excretion, and an excessively alkaline urinary pH (>7.0), or excessively acid urinary pH (<5.5), according to the type of stone. Alternatively if the urine is very concentrated due to decreased fluid intake a stone is most likely to be produced, and this is why a stone is most likely to occur in hot weather or in people who do not drink much fluid.

Etiology

There are different causes of renal stone, majority in children being metabolic causes. We can elaborate some of those causes as follows:

1. Hypercalciuria:

   Hypercalciuria is the most important pathophysiologic risk factor in calcium stone formation.

   Types of hypercalciuria:

   Absorptive hypercalciuria:

   Occurs in approximately 20–40% of stone formers, and is characterized by increased intestinal absorption of calcium. The positive calcium balance suppresses parathyroid hormone (PTH) secretion and increases the renal filtered load of calcium, leading to increased urinary calcium excretion. It was deduced that the 4q33-qter segment contains the putative gene for absorptive hypercalciuria.

   A severe form of absorptive hypercalciuria has been mapped to chromosome 1q23.3-q24.

   It is classified as Type I or II, according to the response to dietary calcium restriction. Type I is diet-unresponsive and Type II, urinary calcium normalizes in response to a low calcium diet.

   Renal Hypercalciuria:

   Secondary to Impaired renal tubular reabsorption of calcium. Renal loss of calcium reduces serum calcium and secondarily stimulates PTH secretion. Consequently, increased intestinal calcium absorption caused by enhanced 1,25-[OH]2D synthesis and mobilization of calcium from bone caused by increased PTH lead to hypercalciuria. The pathogenesis of renal calcium leak is unknown. Renal hypercalciuria is relatively uncommon, occurring in approximately 5–8% of stone formers.

   Resorptive hypercalciuria:

   Rare cause of stone disease, 3–5%, that is most commonly associated with primary hyperparathyroidism. Excessive PTH secretion from a parathyroid adenoma leads to bone resorption, increased renal synthesis of 1,25-[OH]2D (calcitriol), and enhanced intestinal absorption of calcium.

   Other causes of hypercalciuria

   A number of conditions like hypercalciuria associated with special inherited diseases, see Table 308.3,

Table 308.1

Frequency of urolithiasis according to age, stone location, gender, and stone composition in populations of different socioeconomic levels

Variable	Socioeconomic level	
	Low	High
Overall frequency in children	High	Low
Bladder stones (%)	>40	<10
Female patients (%)	<20	>25
Calcium oxalate (%)	<40	>60
Uric acid (%)	>30	<20

History, epidemiology and regional diversities of urolithiasis
Source: López M, Hoppe B (2010) Pediatr Nephrol doi: 10.1007/s00467-008-0960-5

granulomatous diseases, including sarcoidosis, tuberculosis, and histoplasmosis, have been reported to cause hypercalcemia; bedridden patients like cerebral palsy if not discovered early will have bone resorption and hypercalciuria, in which conditions weight bearing exercises and increased fluid intake can be of help.

2. Hypocitraturia
Citrate is the most abundant organic anion in human urine, and is a well-recognized inhibitor of stone formation. Hypocitraturia is a well-known risk factor for calcium nephrolithiasis, and has been identified in 20–60% of calcium stone formers.

   Citrate complexes with calcium in solution forms a soluble complex and decreases urinary saturation of stone-forming calcium salts (CaOx and calcium phosphate).

   By that it inhibits crystallization, aggregation, and agglomeration of CaOx and calcium phosphate, thereby further reducing stone formation. Acid load promotes proximal tubular reabsorption of citrate and reduced citrate synthesis, leading to hypocitraturia, whereas alkali load reduces tubular reabsorption and enhances citrate synthesis, thereby increasing urinary citrate excretion. A variety of pathology associated with acidosis leads to hypocitraturia. Distal renal tubular acidosis (RTA) is associated with systemic acidosis, and is characterized by high urine pH, and low serum bicarbonate and potassium.

   Chronic diarrhea is associated with systemic acidosis because of alkali loss in the stool. Excessive animal protein provides an acid load that promotes bone loss and causes hypocitraturia. Other causes of acidosis associated with hypocitraturia are thiazide-induced hypokalemia, which produces intracellular acidosis, and vigorous exercise, which produces lactic acidosis. Overweight status in children might be associated with an elevated risk of stone formation in both sexes owing to the alterations in urine composition, with status of hypocitraturia. Finally, idiopathic hypocitraturia may represent an isolated abnormality, unrelated to an acidotic state.

3. Hyperoxaluria
Is thought to increase the risk of stone formation by increasing urinary saturation of CaOx. The effect of oxalate on stone formation depends on the interaction between calcium and oxalate that takes place in the intestine and urine.

   In the intestine, oxalate absorption is modulated by dietary oxalate and the formation of a poorly absorbed calcium-oxalate complex. In the setting of dietary calcium restriction, calcium-oxalate complex formation is reduced, thereby increasing luminal free oxalate that is absorbed from the intestine and excreted in the urine.

   Hyperoxaluria can be associated with primary disorders in biosynthetic pathways (primary hyperoxaluria), or high substrate levels (excessive vitamin C).

   Primary hyperoxaluria is caused by a rare inherited autosomal recessive disorder in glyoxalate metabolism by which the normal conversion of glyoxalate to glycine is prevented, leading to oxidative conversion of excess glyoxalate to oxalate, an end product of metabolism. Systemic oxalosis ensues, and leads to excretion of markedly high levels of urinary oxalate. The risk of stone formation is increased when urine oxalate exceeds 0.4 mmol/L, especially if urine calcium concentration is elevated (i.e., more than 4 mmol/L), leading to the formation of monohydrated calcium oxalate (whewellite) crystals, causing stone formation and nephrocalcinosis (*Fig. 308.7*). At diagnosis, 54% of hyperoxaluric patients have had stones and 30% had nephrocalcinosis. Without treatment, end stage renal failure occurs in 50% of patients by age 15 years, with an overall mortality ~30%.

   Two forms of primary hyperoxaluria have been identified: primary hyperoxaluria type 1 (PH1) [online Mendelian Inheritance in Man (MIM) 259900] is an autosomal recessive disorder (~1:120,000 live births per year in Europe), and alanine-glyoxalate aminotransferase (AGT) activity is either absent or mistargeted to the mitochondria. Primary hyperoxaluria type 2 (PH2) (MIM 260000) has been documented in fewer than 50 patients, which differ in the enzyme defect responsible for the disease,

Table 308.2
Genetics of disorders presenting with urolithiasis and/or nephrocalcinosis

Group of defects	MIM	Locus, gene	Inheritance	Gene product	Phenotype
Hypercalciuria-induced urolithiasis/nephrocalcinosis					
Autosomal dominant hypocalcemic hypercalciuria	146200; 601199	3q13.3-q21, CASR	AD	CASR	Hypercalciuria Hypocalcemia CRF
Familial hypomagnesemia with hypercalciuria and nephrocalcinosis (FHHNC)	248250; 603959	3q27, 1p34.2, CLDN16, CLDN 19	AR	Paracellin 1, (Claudin 16, 19)	Hypercalciuria, hypercalcemia, hypomagnesemia, dRTA, CRF, hypermagnesuria, polyuria, tetany seizures
Dent's disease, (Dent 1)	300009; 310468; 300008	Xp11.22, CLCN5	XLR	CLC-5	Hypercalciuria, renal phosphate leak (variable), LMW proteinuria, hypophosphatemia (variable)
Lowe syndrome, (Dent 2)	309000	Xq.25–26, OCRL1	XLR	OCRL1 protein	Hypercalciuria, megalin deficiency, phosphate leak, Fanconi syndrome
Bartter's syndrome type 1	600839	15q15-q21.1, NKCC2	AR	SLC12A1	Salt wasting, hypokalemic metabolic alkalosis, and hypercalciuria, nephrocalcinosis
Bartter's syndrome type 2	600359	11q24, ROMK	AR	KCNJ1	Salt wasting, hypokalemic metabolic alkalosis, and hypercalciuria, nephrocalcinosis
Infantile Bartter's syndrome with sensorineural deafness	602522; 606412; 602024; 602023	1p31, 1p36, BSND CLCNKB	AR		Salt wasting, hypokalemic metabolic alkalosis, and hypercalciuria, nephrocalcinosis
Williams–Beuren syndrome	194050; 130160; 601329; 600404	contiguous gene deletion syndrome 7q11.23, ELN, LIMK1, RFC2	AD	Elastin, LIMkinase1	Hypercalcemia, hypercalciuria, mental retardation "happy party manner," aortic stenosis, "Elfin-faces", Nephrocalcinosis
Nephrolithiasis and osteoporosis associated with hypophosphatemia due to mutation in the type 2 sodium phosphate co-transporter	182309	5q.35	Unknown	NPTZa	Renal phosphate leak, hypercalciuria, osteoporosis, 1,25 dihydroxy-vitamin D
Hyperoxaluria-induced urolithiasis/nephrocalcinosis					
Primary hyperoxaluria, type I	259900; 604285	2q.37.3, AGXT	AR	AGT	Hyperoxaluria, hyperglycolic aciduria, CRF, systemic oxalosis
Primary hyperoxaluria, type II	260000; 604296	9q.11, GR/HPR	AR	GR/HPR	Hyperoxaluria, L-gylceric aciduria, CRF
Cystinuria and urolithiasis					
Cystinuria type A	104614	2p q.16.3, SLC3A1	AR	r BAT	Elevated urinary excretion of cystine (and other dibasic amino acids) Urine microscopy: hexagonal cystine crystals, recurrent

Table 308.2 (Continued)

Group of defects	MIM	Locus, gene	Inheritance	Gene product	Phenotype
Cystinuria type B	604144	19 q.13.1/ SLC7A9	Inc AR	B α + AT	Elevated urinary excretion of cystine (and other dibasic amino acids) Urine microscopy: hexagonal cystine crystals, recurrent urolithiasis, (CRF)
Cystinuria type A/B	220100	SLC3A1/SLC7A1			
Purine/pyrimidine-induced urolithiasis/nephrocalcinosis					
Lesch–Nyhan syndrome	300322	Xq26, HPRT	XLR	HPRT	Hyperuricosuria, gout, automutilation, recurrent urolithiasis
Partial HPRT deficiency	308000	Xq.26–27.2, HPRT	XLR	HPRT	Hyperuricosuria
Glycogenosis type 1a	232200	17q.21, G6PC	AR	Glucose-6-phosphatase	Hyperuricosuria
Glycogenosis type 1b	232220	11q.23, SLC37A4	AR	Transporter	Hyperuricosuria
Phosphoribosylphosphate synthetase 1 superactivity	311850	Xq21, PRPS1	XL		Hyperuricosuria
APRT deficiency	102600	16q.24.3, APRT	AR	APRT	8 dihydroxy-adeninuria, recurrent crystalluria (round + brown), urolithiasis (radiolucent), rarely renal failure from crystal nephropathy
Xanthinuria (classical)	278300	2p.22, XDH	AR	Xanthine oxydoreductase or dehydrogenase	Xanthinuria, hypouricemia
Distal renal tubular acidosis					
Renal tubular acidosis autosomal dominant	179800; 109270	17q.21–q.22, SLC4A1,AE1	AD	AE1	Hypocitric aciduria, hypercalciuria, hypokalemia, osteomalacia
Autosomal recessive dRTA with hearing loss	267300; 192132	2cen-q13, ATP6B1	AR	B1	Hypercalciuria, hypocitric aciduria, hypokalemia,rickets, hearing loss
Autosomal recessive dRTA	602722; 605239	7q.33-34, SLC4A1	AR	A4	Hypercalciuria, hypocitric aciduria, hypokalemia

Source: Hoppe B, Kempe MJ (2010) Diagnostic examination of the child with urolithiasis or nephrocalcinosis. Pediatr Nephrol 25:403–413

glyoxylate reductase/hydroxypyruvate reductase (GR/HPR), and absence of GR/HPR activity both in the liver and lymphocytes. The median age at onset is 1–2 years, and the classical presentation is urolithiasis (whewellite), including hematuria and obstruction, but stone-forming activity is lower than in PH1. GFR is usually maintained during childhood, and systemic involvement is exceptional. The biochemical hallmark is the increased urinary excretion of L-glycerate, but the definitive diagnosis requires DNA analysis and screening of the most frequent mutation (c.103delG). PH1 is the most common and the most challenging form. The median age of patients when symptoms first appear is 5–6 years, and end-stage renal disease (ESRD) is reached between 25 years and 40 years of age in half of the patients. It is responsible for less than 0.5% of ESRD in children in Europe and 10–13% in countries with a high rate of consanguineous marriages. Along with progressive decline of glomerular filtration rate (GFR < 30–50 mL/min per 1.73 m^2) due to renal parenchymal involvement, continued overproduction of oxalate by the liver and reduced oxalate excretion by the kidneys lead to systemic involvement (oxalosis), bone becomes the major compartment of the poorly soluble oxalate pool. The combination of both clinical and sonographic signs is a strong argument for PH1, i.e., the association of renal calculi, nephrocalcinosis, and renal impairment; in addition, family history may bring additional information. PH1 grossly fits five presentations: (1) infantile form with early nephrocalcinosis and kidney failure; (2) recurrent urolithiasis and progressive renal failure, leading to a diagnosis of PH1 in childhood or adolescence; (3) late-onset form with occasional stone passage in adulthood; (4) diagnosis given by post-transplantation recurrence; and (5) presymptomatic subjects with a family history of PH1. Crystalluria and infrared spectroscopy are of major interest for identification and quantitative analysis of crystals and stones showing whewellite (*Fig. 308.7*).

Currently, a polymerase chain reaction using a serum sample can identify the three most common mutations in the involved genes. The AGXT gene is located on chromosome 2q37.3; numerous mutations and polymorphisms have been identified. Prenatal diagnosis can be performed from DNA obtained from chorionic villi or amniocytes. Indeed, one study reported that 66% of patients who had hyperoxaluria were diagnosed without the need for liver biopsy. The diagnosis of primary hyperoxaluria should be suspected in any calcium stone-forming child, because nephrolithiasis is the most common presenting symptom of the disease. Transplantation of the kidney and/or liver is generally required.

Malabsorptive state is the most common cause of hyperoxaluria with intestinal disease–associated stone formers. In the setting of fat malabsorption, saponification of fatty acids with luminal calcium reduces

Table 308.3
Steps in diagnosis

Steps	Diagnostic findings
History including family history	Diet, fluid intake, medications, vitamin supplementation, chronic disease? Malabsorption syndrome? immobilization?
Clinical findings	Pain, hematuria, vomiting, UTI, passage of stones, gravel
Imaging	Ultrasonography, plain film, non-contrast-enhanced CT, (MRI) intravenous urography
Urine	Density, specific gravity, osmolality, pH, glucose, protein, sediment, culture, spot urine (molar creatinine ratio of calcium, oxalate, uric acid, citrate, magnesium, cystine screening {nitroprusside test, amino acid screen}), 24 h urine (volume, pH, lithogenic and stone-inhibitory parameters, calculation of urinary saturation).
Blood/serum	Electrolyte, calcium, phosphorus, magnesium, creatinine, urea, uric acid, alkaline phosphatase, (PTH, Vitamin D/A, plasma oxalate, serum Vitamin B6 level)
Stone analysis	Infrared spectroscopy or X-ray diffraction
Indication for metabolic stone valuation	Recurrent stone formers
	Intestinal disease (particularly chronic diarrhea)
	Pathologic skeletal fractures
	Osteoporosis
	History of urinary tract infection with calculi
	Personal history of gout
	Infirm health (unable to tolerate repeated stone episodes
	Solitary kidney
	Anatomic abnormalities
	Renal insufficiency
	Stones composed of cystine, uric acid, or struvite

Source: Hoppe B, Kemper MJ (2010) Pediatr Nephrol 25:403–413

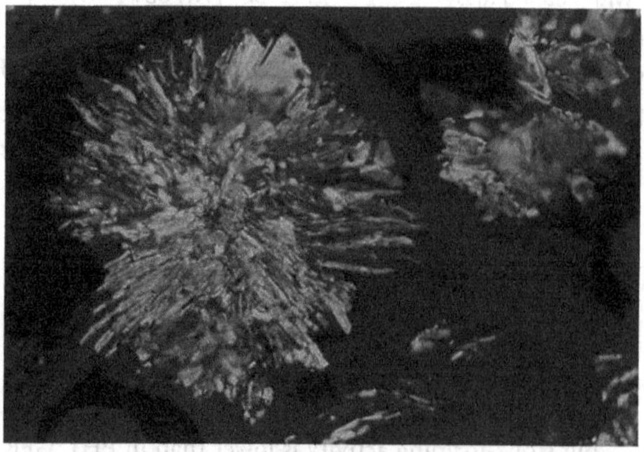

Figure 308.7
Bone biopsy in an adolescent with primary hyperoxaluria type 1. Examination under polarized light shows calcium oxalate crystals

calcium-oxalate complex formation in the gut, increasing the pool of unbound oxalate available for absorption.

Hyperoxaluria can occur from excessive dietary intake of oxalate-rich foods such as nuts, chocolate, brewed tea, spinach, and rhubarb. Severe calcium restriction may reduce intestinal oxalate binding, thereby increasing intestinal oxalate absorption. Excessive vitamin C intake has also been shown to increase oxalate excretion by in vivo conversion of ascorbate to oxalate. Oxalate-degrading bacteria such as Oxalobacter formigenes have been shown to colonize the intestine of normal individuals, and may reduce intestinal oxalate; absence of these bacteria has been linked to increased urinary oxalate levels.

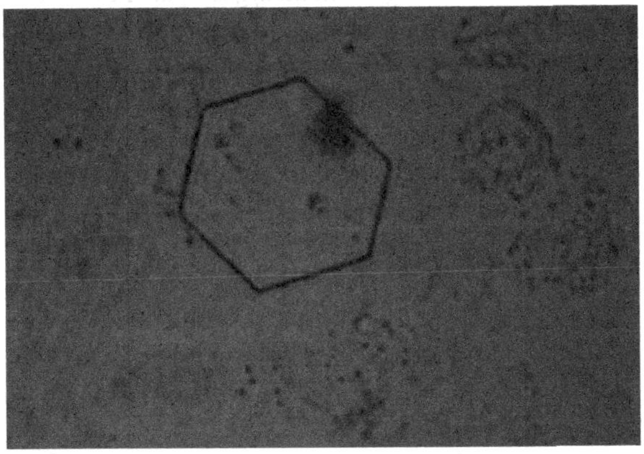

Figure 308.8
Examination of urinary sediment discloses a hexagonal crystal of cystine

4. Hyperuricosuria
   Hyperuricosuria can lead to CaOx stone formation by heterologous nucleation on the surface of monosodium urate crystals. The most common cause of hyperuricosuria is increased dietary purine intake, as uric acid is the end product of purine metabolism.

   Numerous hereditary (see *Table 308.3*) and acquired diseases can lead to hyperuricosuria, including gout, myelo- and lymphoproliferative disorders, multiple myeloma, hemolytic disorders, and hemoglobinopathies. The pathophysiology of hyperuricosuric CaOx nephrolithiasis is intimately related to urinary pH. At pH less than 5.5, poorly soluble undissociated uric acid precipitates, leading to uric acid or CaOx stone formation. At pH greater than 5.5, uric acid is found predominantly in its dissociated form. In special cases of excessive uric acid formation, increased urinary saturation of monosodium urate ensues, promoting CaOx stone formation through heterogeneous nucleation.
5. Cystinuria:
   Cystinuria (MIM 220100) is an autosomal recessive inherited aminoaciduria that leads to recurrent nephrolithiasis, accounting for approximately 6% of metabolic stones in the pediatric population with prevalence varying throughout different global locations but is approximately 1 in 7,000 in the general population of Europe and the United States. Newborn screening programs have estimated the disease frequency at 1:100,000 in Sweden. On the other hand, high frequency of the disease has been reported for Libyan Jews living in Israel with a prevalence rate of 1/2,500. In Turkey in Sivas province, the prevalence of cystinuria is 1/772; this prevalence ratio is the highest ever among those

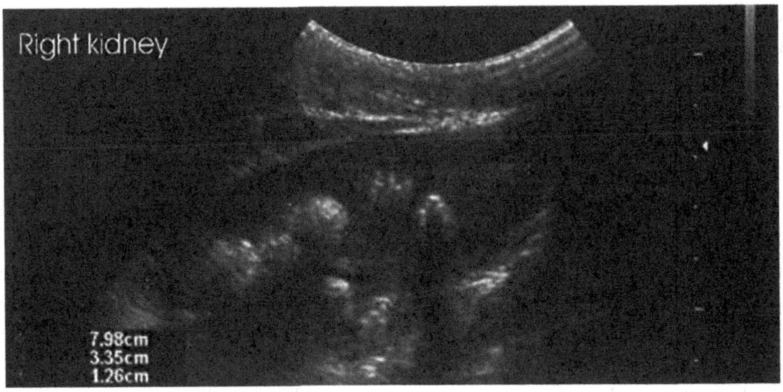

Figure 308.9
Ultrasound: staghorn urolithiasis of the right kidney

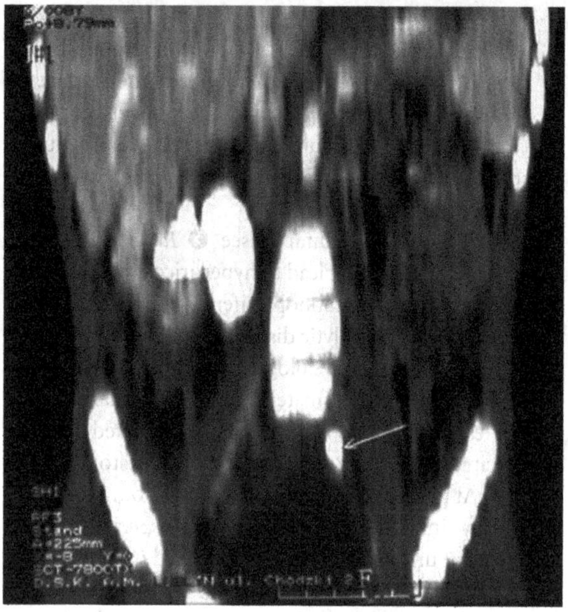

◘ Figure 308.10
CT scan: staghorn urolithiasis of the right kidney and stones in the left ureter (*arrow*). Stones within the left kidney are not visible on this scan

reported for other countries. Three different types of cystinuria (types I, II and III) have been described. This classification has been modified as type I and non-type I (divided clinically as types II and III). In1994, a cystinuria gene (*SLC3A1*) was cloned and mapped on chromosome 2p16.3. The gene encodes the protein rBAT, a b0, +AT transporter-related protein expressed in the renal and intestinal epithelium. The glycoprotein rBAT causes cystinuria type I. It is thought that b0, +AT represents the catalytic subunit of the transporter complex and that rBAT is mainly involved in the trafficking and possible stabilization of the transporter in the brush border membrane. rBAT may also modify the functional transport properties of the complete transporter complex. The transporter functions as a tertiary active exchanger taking up cystine, arginine, lysine, and ornithine from urine in exchange for neutral amino acids. To date, more than 80 mutations in *SLC3A1* have been documented as cited by Škopková et al. The International Cystinuria Consortium has described a new classification system based on the chromosomal localization of the mutation, with type A cystinuria (45% of patients with cystinuria), mutations of the SLC3A1 gene on chromosome arm 2p encoding the rBAT protein called (type I) before.

Type B cystinuria (53% of patients with cystinuria), mutations of the SLC7A9 gene on chromosome 19, was called (non-type I) previously.

Type AB with mutations on both chromosomes is found in 2% of patients with cystinuria. Homozygous, compound heterozygous, and obligate heterozygous subtypes have been described, with homozygotes excreting the greatest amount of cystine; affected individuals demonstrate excretion of cystine and the dibasic amino acids ornithine, arginine and lysine in the proximal tubule. Due to a pH drop in the collecting duct, cystine (soluble at normal urinary pH) exceeds the solubility limit in urine and forms typical crystals and eventually kidney stones; diminished reabsorption of these amino acids in the intestine is not pathologic because these are not essential amino acids and their di-peptide forms are still transported.

By 1 year of age, a homozygous patient's urinary excretion of cystine is usually more than 1,000 mmol/g creatinine with a mean excretion rate of 4,500 mmol/g creatinine. At usual urine volumes, this excretion rate exceeds its solubility. Life-long recurrent stone formation is a characteristic of patients with the homozygous forms of cystinuria.

Heterozygote carriers may also form stones because they have been shown to excrete up to 2,400 mmol/g creatinine; parents of cystinuria Type A have normal levels of cystine and lysine excretion. Therefore, this type was also referred to as the fully recessive form. In type B, elevated levels of cystine and lysine are observed in obligate heterozygotes. It is currently well established that the clinical manifestations of cystinuria are exclusively renal. Their early recognition is important for timely treatment and genetic counseling.

Cystinuria may be diagnosed by the finding of hexagonal crystals (➋ *Fig. 308.8*).

A prenatal approach to cystinuria has been suggested by the presence of hyperechoic colon during the third trimester of pregnancy, which may be due to the presence of large amounts of cystine in the colon wall.

The follow-up of these patients is based on urine volume (urine specific gravity target <1,010), urine pH (target ~7.5 – < 8), free urine cystine concentration (target < 1 mmol/L or < 100 μmol/mol creatinine), renal ultrasonography and, sometimes, urinary sodium (in order to estimate sodium intake), and crystal volume assessment (target $< 3{,}000\ \mu m^3/mm^3$).

6. Infection:
   Children with a history of multiple urinary tract infections may be at risk of nephrolithiasis (struvite stones), especially if the organisms contain the enzyme urease, which results in a high urine pH that promotes the supersaturation of urine with struvite and calcium phosphate apatites. Patients with surgically augmented bladders are at risk of developing bladder stones, most commonly struvite stones.

Clinical Manifestations

The most common findings of urolithiasis in pediatric age groups are abdominal pain and hematuria; they might have vomiting and dysuria. The observation of a 33% hematuria rate in the metabolic group and a 26% dysuria rate in the infection group is clinically significant. Many studies reported that urine oxalate, uric acid, and calcium cause hematuria by damaging the uroepithelium, and in these cases urinary N-acetyl-glucoseaminoglycan (NAG) levels, as a marker of tubular injury, were elevated . These previous findings support the association of metabolic etiology and hematuria. Recent studies from various countries reported a mean age for urolithiasis of 4.2–8.2 years. The mean ages of the groups with metabolic etiology and infectious etiology were found to be lower compared with the other groups; a family history of urolithiasis was reported in 11.8–21.9% of patients. Diagnosis is often only made when nephrocalcinosis is incidentally noted on an imaging study performed for other reasons or when symptoms of reduced concentrating capacity of the renal tubules are obvious. The underlying pathological condition is not always evident and requires a detailed history and workup. Renal colic has been reported in some infants with nephrocalcinosis, but it is more likely due to passage of tiny calculi than to nephrocalcinosis per se. It is not unusual for nephrocalcinosis to be diagnosed during systematic renal ultrasound examination of high-risk infants or as part of the diagnostic evaluation of urinary tract infection. The first clinical symptoms, if any, are gross or microscopic hematuria and/or sterile leukocyturia that may be misdiagnosed as urinary tract infection. Single family member involvement was found more than multiple involvements. Stone occurrence was more in the immediate family members than distant relatives, especially brothers of affected patients. Study of stone risk in the family members should be centered on brothers and sons of stone patients.

Diagnosis

We should start with good history including immediate close relatives (brothers and sons), medications, possible risk factors like malabsorption, and immobilizations.

Clinical findings may not be very informative, but finding of hematuria, leukocyturia, passage of stone, abdominal pain, and dysuria may be of some help.

Laboratory evaluation can help especially in metabolic caused stones:

Serum levels of uric acid, electrolytes, creatinine, calcium, phosphorus, and bicarbonate should be measured. Serum parathyroid hormone level should be obtained in children who have hypercalciuria, hypercalcemia, or hypophosphatemia, vitamin A (for patients with hypercalciuria), serum vitamin B6 levels, and plasma oxalate (for patients with primary hyperoxaluria) and, of course, molecular genetic testing will later be necessary (➋ *Table 308.3*).

Elevated serum alkaline phosphatase may indicate possible bone resorption. Twenty-four hour urine collection for sodium, calcium, urate, oxalate, cystine, citrate, and creatinine [determine tubular reabsorption of phosphate (TRP) or tubular maximum for phosphate corrected for glomerular filtration rate (TmP/GFR)] should be evaluated. Since many urinary components are influenced by dietary intake, 24 h urine collections (to exclude diurnal fluctuations related to intake of food and beverages) provide the best information and also provide an objective assessment of the child's daily intake of fluid. Advise the patient or the parent to maintain the normal fluid intake and the normal dietary habits, before 24 h urine collected (avoid urine sampling under parenteral infusions). Also keep in mind that stones in situ may diminish the excretion of urinary lithogenic material, as these substances may concurrently be absorbed by the stone. For urine collection, a preservative should ideally be placed directly into the sampling bottle; however, urine may be collected without initial preservation, so long as it is kept cool (at 4°C) and adequately preserved within 24 h. Ideally, the urine collection is to be obtained at least 6 weeks after the passage of a stone. Collecting two 24-h samples may be recommended. Determination of urinary supersaturation for calcium oxalate, calcium phosphate, and urate may be helpful (➋ *Table 308.4*). Most children with elevated supersaturation values had urine volumes $\leq$ 1 mL/kg/h. The urinary creatinine excretion rate may be used to verify an adequate urine collection, with most children excreting ~15 to 20 mg/kg/24 h. If the creatinine excretion is significantly more or less, it may indicate either an over- or undercollection.

If a 24-hour collection is difficult, especially in younger children, urinary standards based on single specimens, corrected to urine creatinine concentration, have been developed (➋ *Tables 308.4* and ➋ *308.5*).

The calcium-to-creatinine ratio changes with age. If hypercalciuria is suspected on a single random sample, confirmation with 24-hour urine collection is needed.

A urine culture should be considered to exclude the possibility of acute or chronic urinary tract infection. Urinalysis may be helpful, particularly if crystals are noted. Cystine crystals are colorless, flat, and hexagonal, and if they are found in the urine, they are diagnostic for cystinuria. Cystine is screened for by nitroprusside test or by chromatography for amino acids.

Since the pH of the urine is a major factor in the formation of many stones, its measurement, preferably by glass electrode, or, if a pH electrode is not available, by pH paper with the specific and adequately distinguishable range of pH 2 to 9, is of utmost importance. Sometimes, it is advisable to determine a daily profile of both the pH and the density (specific gravity or osmolality) of the urine. This may also be used for follow-up, e.g., to assess the effect of the administration of alkali or to check the patient's compliance regarding sufficient fluid intake. To discriminate the primary from the secondary forms of hyperoxaluria, a [13 C2] oxalate absorption test can be performed, which is safe and reliable in children, as in adults. Intestinal oxalate absorption is normal in patients with primary hyperoxaluria and would be significantly increased in those with dietary or enteric hyperoxaluria. Also, a stool analysis for the absence of oxalate-degrading

Table 308.4
Normal values for 24 h urine

Chemical component	Value
Calcium	<4 mg (0.1 mmol)/kg per 24 h
Sodium	<3 mEq (3 mmol)/kg per 24 h
Potassium	>3 mEq (3 mmol)/kg per 24 h
Magnesium	>88 mg (44 mmol)/1.73 m^2 per 24 h
Citrate	>180 mg (94 µmol/g (8.84 mmol) creatinine
Oxalate	<52 mg (593 mmol)/1.73 m^2 per 24 h
	<2 mg (23 mmol)/kg per 24 h
Cystine	<60 mg (0.5 mmol)/1.73 m^2 per 24 h
Uric Acid	<815 mg (4.9 mmol)/1.73 m^2 per 24 h
	<35 mg (0.21 mmol)/kg per 24 h
Xanthine	30–90 µg (20–60 µmol)/24 h

Source: Alon US (2009) Pediatr Nephrol. doi 10.1007/s00467-007-0740-7

Table 308.5
Normal values for spot urine samples

Parameter age	Ratio of solute to creatinine mol/mol	mg/mg	Remarks
Calcium			
<12 months	<2	0.81	Highest Ca excretion with breast milk feeding, ratio increasing after meals (up to 40%),by loop diuretics, immobilization and steroids
1–3 years	<1.5	0.53	
1–5 years	<1.1	0.39	
5–7 years	<0.8	0.28	
>7 years	<0.6	0.21	
Oxalate			
0–6 months	<325–360	288–260	Primary hyperoxaluria types I/II for constant excessive elevation, check also urinary glycolate, L-glycerate, and plasma oxalate. Secondary hyperoxaluria: determine intestinal oxalate absorption and stool. Oxalobacter formigenes colonization
7–24 months	<132–174	110–139	
2–5 years	<98–101	80	
5–14 years	<70–82	60–65	
>16 years	<40	32	
Citrate			
0–5 years	>0.25	0.42	Low with tubular dysfunction: RTA, prematurity, hypokalemia, renal transplantation
>5 years	>0.15	0.25	
Magnesium			
	>0.63	> 0.13	For <2 years, no reliable data
Uric acid			
>2 years	<0.56 mg/dL (33 µmol/L) per GFR (ratio × plasma creatinine)		Higher than in adults throughout childhood; no reliable data for age <2 years

Source: Hoppe B, Kemper MJ (2010) Pediatr Nephrol 25:403–441

bacteria, especially Oxalobacter formigenes, will give further evidence of the existence of a secondary reason for hyperoxaluria.

Qualitative analysis of the stone obtained after intervention or spontaneous stone passage is one of the most important diagnostic measures. The methods of choice are infrared spectroscopy or X-ray diffraction. Even amounts of ≤ 1 mg can be analyzed. Chemical stone analysis is inappropriate, as it is prone to errors and is obsolete. The analytic principle of X-ray diffraction is based on the crystal structure of the stone substances. With infrared spectroscopy the loss of energy in the infrared spectrum due to the circulation of the activated chemical molecules is determined.

Recurrent stones should be analyzed again, since the stone composition may change. After lithotripsy only stone fragments are available, and these can be recovered by straining the urine. All fragments should be sent for analysis to allow additional tests, if needed.

Radiologic Evaluations

Ultrasound of the kidney and bladder can show nephrocalcinosis and renal or pelvic stone; KUB does not add significant diagnostic utility above clinical evaluation with symptoms of renal colic; helical CT is the best method of testing for urinary tract stones, more sensitive and safer method than IV pyelography (IVP). The appearance on imaging studies depends upon the stone's composition. Those composed of calcium oxalate or calcium phosphate have a very dense image on conventional radiographs and on CT scans. Struvite (magnesium ammonium phosphate) and cystine stones are of intermediate density, and small stones of all compositions can be difficult to appreciate by conventional radiography. Uric acid stones are radiolucent on radiographs, requiring the administration of contrast agents for adequate visualization, and have a low density image on CT scans. Stones of all composition, with the exception of drugs (e.g., indinavir) and matrix (protein), have distinguishing characteristics of echogenicity and shadowing on ultrasonography.

Ultrasonography has the additional advantages of wide availability, avoidance of ionizing radiation, ready detection of hydronephrosis, and ability to define some aspects of the anatomy of the urinary tract; it is not as sensitive as CT is for the detection of small (smallest size between 1.5–2 mm in diameter) stones in the ureter.

Most stones can be imaged without the use of contrast agents. However, when obstruction is a concern, when radiolucent or low density stones require careful delineation, or when details of urinary tract anatomy are needed (such as confirmation of a duplicated collecting system), contrast agents (CT urography, intravenous pyelography, or retrograde ureteroscopy/pyelography, or orthograde pyelography) are usually required.

For the detecting and monitoring of nephrocalcinosis, high-resolution ultrasonography is the optimal imaging method (➋ *Fig. 308.11*).

Some pitfalls in the renal ultrasonography of neonates, and especially preterm infants, have to be noted: Tamm–Horsfall protein (THP) deposits within the renal calyces may look like nephrocalcinosis (➋ *Fig. 308.11*). THP deposition, however, disappears within 1–2 weeks, and follow-up will show completely normal kidneys. Furthermore, the echogenicity of the renal cortex in neonates is physiologically increased, hence detection of cortical nephrocalcinosis can be difficult and may become evident only some weeks later when a rim of cortical calcification becomes visible. However, diffuse cortical nephrocalcinosis may already be detectable shortly after birth in patients with suspected primary hyperoxaluria, and it is directly visible both by US and X-ray.

Treatment

Non-specific Treatment

Acute episode: During the acute phase when the stone is being passed, management is directed toward pain control, and facilitating passage or removal of the stone(s).

The acute management of nephrolithiasis depends upon the severity of the pain, and the presence of obstruction or infection. In some patients, outpatient medical management with oral analgesics and hydration is possible. However, in others, especially those with nausea, vomiting, and severe pain, hospitalization is required for parenteral fluid and pain medication. Other indications for hospitalization include urinary obstruction and infection.

Pain control: Both nonsteroidal antiinflammatory drugs (NSAIDs) and opioid therapy are used to control pain associated with nephrolithiasis. In studies of adult patients, both classes of analgesics are effective in pain relief. Combination therapy of the two has also been reported to be effective and in some cases superior to either agent alone.

Urologic removal of stones may be required in patients with unremitting severe pain that is refractory to analgesic therapy, or in those with obstruction or infection.

Prevention of recurrent disease: Aim for medical treatment is to decrease or prevent stone formation or growth,

Table 308.6
Diet variables with different sodium concentrations

Category	High sodium food	Low sodium alternative
Meats, poultry, fish, eggs	Burritos, pizzas, canned meat, ham, salted nuts	Fresh beef, fish or pork; Low sodium peanut butter; dry beans
Dairy products	Butter milk, cottage cheese, regular cheese	Milk, mozarella cheese, ice cream
Bread, grains, cereals	Salted bread, biscuits, pancakes, pasta	Non-salted breads, muffins; unsalted popcorn, pretzels
Soups	Canned and dehydrated soup	Low sodium canned soup; home-made soup without salt
Desserts and sweets	Bottled salad dressings, salted butter, instant cake	Unsalted butter, low sodium salad dressings, homemade cake

and decrease need for surgical intervention. This includes an evaluation to identify any underlying cause or risk factors for stone formation. Based upon this assessment, interventions are tailored to reduce the risk of recurrent stone formation.

Dietary and Fluids Management

Dietary management can reduce urinary excretion of stone constituents or increase urinary inhibitors. In low-risk stone formers, dietary measures alone may be sufficient to prevent stone recurrence without the need for drug therapy. A number of factors have been shown to influence stone formation, including fluids, sodium, potassium, animal protein, calcium, and oxalate.

Fluids

A high fluid intake will cause increased urine output, which will reduce urinary saturation of stone-forming calcium salts. Keeping urine flow of >1 mL/kg per hour is needed to decrease risk of supersaturation for calcium oxalate, calcium phosphate, and uric acid, thus protecting from the formation of the corresponding kidney stones. Long-term compliance with an increased fluid regimen is often poor. Coffee and tea were shown in observational studies to reduce the risk of stone formation. Potassium-rich fruit juices such as orange or lemonade juice but not potassium-poor juices, like cranberry juice, provide organic anions that are metabolized to

Table 308.7
Diet variables with different potassium concentrations

Foods high in potassium		
Group of food	**Serving size**	**Potassium (mg)**
Cereals		
Kellogg's All Bran	1/2 cup	532
Nabisco 100% Bran	1/2 cup	354
Bran Flakes	1 cup	251
Shredded Wheat	1 cup	155
Fruit		
Orange juice	1 cup	479
Dried apricots	1/4 cup	454
Cantaloupe	1/4 medium	412
Primes	1/4 cup	353
Banana	1 small	338
Grapefruit juice (canned)	1 cup	360
Tomato juice	1 cup	552
Avocado	1/2	510
Peaches, dried	4 medium halves	330
Raisins	3 tablespoons	225
Cooked beans		
Pinto beans	1/2 cup	531
Kidney beans	1/2 cup	452
Lentils	1/2 cup	374
Black beans	1/2 cup	309
Canned beans	1/2 cup	332
Vegetables		
Baked potato	1 medium	593
Baked winter squash	1 cup	590
Baked sweet potato	3/4 cup	528
Beet greens	1/2 cup	417
Chard (large leaves)	1/2 cup	563
Peas (cooked)	1/2 cup	296
Spinach (fresh)	1/2 cup	440
Lima beans (canned or frozen)	1/2 cup	473
Other		
Canned tomato sauce	1/2 cup	459
Blackstrap molasses	2 tablespoons	1,218
Sardines (canned in oil)	3 oz	459
Chocolate (unsweetened/bitter)	1 oz	249

Source: Adapted in part from the Canyon Ranch Dietary Department (1994)

Table 308.8

Diet variables with different oxalate concentrations

Food	Oxalate content
Artichokes (French)	Moderate = 5.0–9.9 mg
Baker's yeast	
Bananas	
Basil	
Broccoli, raw	
Brussell sprouts, raw	
Cabbage, green, steamed	
Carrots, boiled	
Celeriac, canned	
Chick peas	
Collard greens, boiled	
Cornstarch	
Eggplant	
Garbanzo beans	
Grape juice, red	
Lentils, boiled	
Lima beans	
Limes	
Mandarin oranges	
Mung beans	
Oats	
Papayas	
Pears, unpeeled	
Peppers, green	
Potatoes, red, peeled	
Tomato juice	
Green tea	
Broccoli, steamed	High = 10.0–14.9 mg
Brussels sprouts, steamed	
Chili peppers	
Chocolate milk	
Cinnamon	
Date sugar	
Dates	
Gooseberries	
Kidney beans	
Lemon Peel	
Lime peel	
Orange pee	
Oranges	
Oregano	
Pepper, black (spice)	
Peppercorn	
Persimmons	
Pistachio nuts	
Raspberries, red	
Tomato paste, canned; tomato purée, canned; tomato sauce, canned	
Almonds	Very high = 15.0 mg & up
Beets	
Black beans	
Blackberries	
Carrots, raw	
Carrots, steamed	
Cashews	
Celery, raw	
Chocolate	
Cocoa powder	
Durum flour	
Figs, dried; figs, fresh	
Filberts (Hazelnuts)	
Flour (Wheat)	
Hazelnuts (Filberts)	
Kiwi fruit	
Macadamia nuts	
Olives, black; olives, green	
Peanut butter	
Peanuts	
Pecans	
Pine nuts	
Pinto beans	
Potatoes, peeled; potatoes, unpeeled	
Rhubarb	
Rye	
Sesame oil	
Sesame seeds	
Soy	
Soybean milk, soybeans	
Spinach, fresh; spinach, frozen	
Sweet potatoes	
Turmeric	
Walnuts	
Wheat	

alkali, thereby increasing urinary pH and citrate. Grape fruit juice may cause concomitant increase in urinary oxalate.

Approximate fluid per day at different ages are as follows:

Infants – ≥ 750 mL
Small children below 5 years of age – ≥ 1,000 mL
Children between 5 and 10 years of age – ≥ 1,500 mL
Children greater than 10 years of age – ≥ 2,000 mL

Sodium

A high salt intake increases stone risk by reducing renal tubular calcium reabsorption and increasing urinary calcium.

High urinary sodium increases urinary saturation of monosodium urate, and reduces urinary citrate via sodium-induced bicarbonate loss. Consequently, inhibitory activity against CaOx and calcium phosphate is reduced, monosodium urate-induced CaOx crystallization is enhanced, and urinary saturation of CaOx and calcium phosphate is increased.

Furthermore, high urinary sodium reduces the efficacy of thiazide treatment for hypercalciuria by blunting the hypocalciuric effect.

A low sodium diet is allowing less than 1 teaspoon per day. The majority of sodium consumed comes from sodium chloride (NaCl), better known as salt. The average American gets 6% of their total salt added at the table, 5% added during cooking, and natural sources in food another 11%, and the remaining comes from prepared foods. Many packaged meats, canned and frozen foods, contain a surprising amount of salt, as a preservative, adds flavor to foods, and helps to keep foods from drying out. Most canned vegetables have a much higher salt content than the same fresh vegetable, in general, salt intake should be limited.

Optimal daily intake of sodium according to ages is as follows: 1.2–1.9 g for ages 4–8 years and, 1.5–2.3 g for ages 9–18 years.

Most Americans consume between 3,000 and 5,000 mg of sodium per day. The National Academy of Sciences' Institute of Medicine advises that children under the age of 11 should not be given more than 2.4 g of sodium in a day. There are few rules to be followed when following a low sodium diet for children.

Start the diet by removing salty foods (packaged foods) from the child's diet.

Lower the amount of seasoning salt used in cooking.

Use different herbs and spices like black pepper or basil to enhance the taste of certain eatables.

For few dishes, natural fruit juices can also enhance the flavor of certain meals.

Use moderate amount of soy sauce and ketchup. They contain high amounts of sodium

Measuring the urine sodium/potassium ratio, which optimally should be below 2.5, assesses compliance with the dietary recommendations related to sodium and potassium.

Potassium

High potassium intake decreases urine calcium. The optimal daily potassium intake, provided mostly in the form of fruit, vegetable, and dairy products is 3.8 g at ages 4–8 years and 4.5 g at ages 9–18 years.

Animal Protein

Animal protein provides an acid load because of the sulfur-containing amino acids. A high protein intake reduces urine pH and citrate, and enhances urinary calcium excretion via bone resorption and reduced renal calcium reabsorption; the purine load potentially increases urinary uric acid. Restriction of animal protein (red meat, fish, poultry) to two servings daily is recommended.

Calcium

Hypercalciuric patients may be optimally treated with a program of modest calcium and oxalate restriction, along with pharmacologic therapy. Severe calcium restriction should always be avoided so as to prevent a negative calcium balance; however, mild calcium restriction (less than one serving of dairy daily) should be part of a program of broad dietary modification in patients who have hypercalciuria. Normocalciuric patients do not benefit from dietary calcium restriction, and therefore, a liberal calcium intake is recommended in this group of patients.

Oxalate

The relative contribution of dietary oxalate and endogenous oxalate production to urinary oxalate is controversial. Dietary oxalate has been estimated to account

Table 308.9
Suggested therapy for urolithiasis caused by metabolic abnormalities

Metabolic abnormality	Initial treatment	Second-line treatment
Hypercalciuria	Reduction of dietary Na+	Potassium citrate
	Dietary calcium at RDA	Neutral phosphate
		Thiazides
		Alendronate (bisphosphonate) esp. in resorptive hypercalciuria
Hyperoxaluria	Adjustment of dietary oxalate	Neutral phosphate
		Potassium citrate
		Magnesium
		Pyridoxine
		Oral ingestion of Oxalobacter formigenes
Hypocitric aciduria	Potassium citrate	Bicarbonate
Hyperuricosuria	Alkalinization	Allopurinol
Cystinuria	Alkalinization	Tiopronin (Thiola)
	Reduction of dietary Na+	D-penicillamine (+pyridoxine)
		Captopril
		The goal of treatment is to keep urinary cystine concentration ≤ 250 mg (1 mmol/L.)

Source: From Milliner DS (2004). Urolithiasis. In: Pediatric nephrology. Lippincott Williams & Wilkins, Philadelphia, p 1104

for 10–50% of urinary oxalate, depending on dietary calcium and oxalate intake, and the bioavailability of oxalate in foods. In general, restriction of oxalate-rich foods, such as nuts, chocolate, tea, and dark roughage is recommended. Vitamin C has been implicated in calcium stone formation because of in vivo conversion of ascorbic acid to oxalate. Limitation of vitamin C supplements is recommended.

Other Diet Components

Other nutrients, such as sucrose, fructose, may be associated with higher risk for kidney stone disease, whereas phytate and magnesium may decrease it.

Drug Therapy

For those patients in whom conservative dietary measures fail or those who have more aggressive stone disease or identifiable metabolic abnormalities, pharmacologic therapy, along with dietary management, should be initiated.

Thiazide Diuretics

Thiazide diuretics are reserved for patients who have severe hypercalciuria not responding to conservative measures.

Doses can be divided according to ages: <6 months: 1–3 mg/kg/day in 2 divided doses;

>6 months to 2 years: 1–3 mg/kg/day in 2 divided doses; maximum: 37.5 mg/day

>2–17 years: Initial: 1 mg/kg/day; maximum: 3 mg/kg/day (50 mg/day).

Its mechanism resorts in enhancing sodium and calcium reabsorption in the distal renal tubule leading to a reduction in urinary calcium excretion. The diuresis induced may be accompanied by a fall in urinary calcium excretion of as much as 50–150 mg (1.3–3.8 mmol) per day This hypocalciuric effect is reduced if sodium intake is not limited. Stone recurrences can decrease from 50% (untreated) to 20% (treated) over 5 years. Thiazides have many other effects on the body. They increase serum calcium and uric acid levels while decreasing urinary citrate levels. Hyperuricemia or acute gout rarely develops in individuals receiving thiazides. A risk of dehydration, hypokalemia, and hyponatremia exists. They can cause magnesium loss and increase cholesterol. Adverse effects occur in about one third of patients but are usually mild. The most bothersome clinical adverse effect is lethargy, but muscle aches, depression, decreased libido, generalized weakness, and malaise also can occur. About 20% of patients stop thiazide therapy because of these adverse effects. These medications originally were intended solely for use as diuretics for hypertension. They have become the primary medical treatment for hypercalciuria because of their unique ability to remove calcium from the urine and return it to the general circulation. They can be used in virtually any type of hypercalciuria, with the possible exception of resorptive hypercalciuria, in which they can exacerbate hypercalcemia.

Potassium Citrate

Potassium citrate is effective in the treatment of patients who have calcium stones providing an alkali load, (potassium or sodium citrate, 100–150 mg/kg per day in 3–4 divided doses) increased urinary pH and citrate, thereby increasing urinary inhibitory activity especially for urate stone, cystine, and also Hypercalciuric patients. Potassium citrate can reduce stone recurrence rates by 75% among hypocitraturic stone former. It is recommended that the urine pH should not exceed 8.5, a high alkaline urine promotes formation of calcium phosphate stones.

Allopurinol

In calcium stone formers, who have moderate to severe hyperuricosuria and in whom other conservative measures fail, including high fluid intake, alkalinaization of urine and in older children diet modification, allopurinol has been shown to reduce urinary uric acid levels and prevent recurrent stone formation. Allopurinol is a xanthine oxidase inhibitor that prevents the conversion of hypoxanthine to xanthine, the precursor of uric acid, which decreases in about 2 to 3 days, in both serum and urine. Allopurinol should be discontinued at first appearance of skin rash or any sign of adverse reactions.

The skin rash may be followed by more severe hypersensitivity reactions such as exfoliative, urticarial, or purpuric lesions, as well as Stevens-Johnson syndrome (erythema multiforme) and, very rarely, a generalized vasculitis that may lead to irreversible hepatotoxicity and death. There have been occasional reports of reduction in the number of circulating-formed elements of the blood, including bone marrow suppression, granulocytopenia, and thrombocytopenia, usually in association with renal and/or hepatic disorders or in whom concomitant drugs have been administered that have a potential for causing these reactions.

Periodic liver function tests, renal function tests and complete blood cell counts should be performed in all patients on allopurinol.

Observe patients with impaired renal or hepatic functions carefully during the early stages of allopurinol administration and withdraw the drug if increased abnormalities in hepatic or renal function appear.

In cases of patients using diuretics, such as Thiazides and ethacrynic acid, when given with allopurinol, it may increase serum oxypurinol concentrations and may thereby increase the risk of serious allopurinol toxicity, including hypersensitivity reactions, particularly in patients with decreased renal function.

Allopurinol should not be given to children except those with hyperuricemia secondary to malignancy or with Lesch–Nyhan syndrome, because safety and effectiveness have not been established in other conditions.

Since allopurinol and its metabolites are excreted by the kidney, drug accumulation can occur in renal failure and the initial dose of allopurinol should consequently be reduced. In children with recurrent renal stone >10 years and adults – Oral dose: 200–300 mg daily is divided or single daily dosage.

Pyridoxine

Promotes the conversion of glyoxalate to glycine, thereby reducing the substrate for oxalate production. Pyridoxine is used for treatment of PH1, not all patients of PH1 respond to Pyridoxine, a test dose of 5–10 mg/kg per day is given. It is likely to be of limited value in patients of enteric hyperoxaluria.

Specific Treatment

Stone Removal

Indications for stone removal – severe pain, infection, severe obstruction, growth of calculus, nonprogression, interference with lifestyle, any stone can be removed by open procedure (rarely done), percutaneous nephrostomy (for kidney and upper ureter), large calculi fragmented first by ultrasound, electrohydraulic (EHL, spark in water tub) or laser lithotripters, (more effective for simple renal stones than branched or ureteral calculi), transurethral removal (calculi below pelvic rim) use basket for removal.

Extracorporeal Shock Wave Lithotripsy (ESWL)

According to the guidelines of the European Association of Urology, ESWL should be the first surgical choice for most renal pediatric stones. The underlying function of all types of ESWL machines is to generate and focus shockwave energy at a focal point that is clustered at the calculus. Ideally, the impact of the shock wave disintegrates the stone so the fragments can pass the ureter.

ESWL may not be as effective as ureteroscopic management of ureteric stones, but associated with fewer complications, comparing ESWL versus ureteroscopic management, 73% vs. 90% stone-free rate. ESWL is

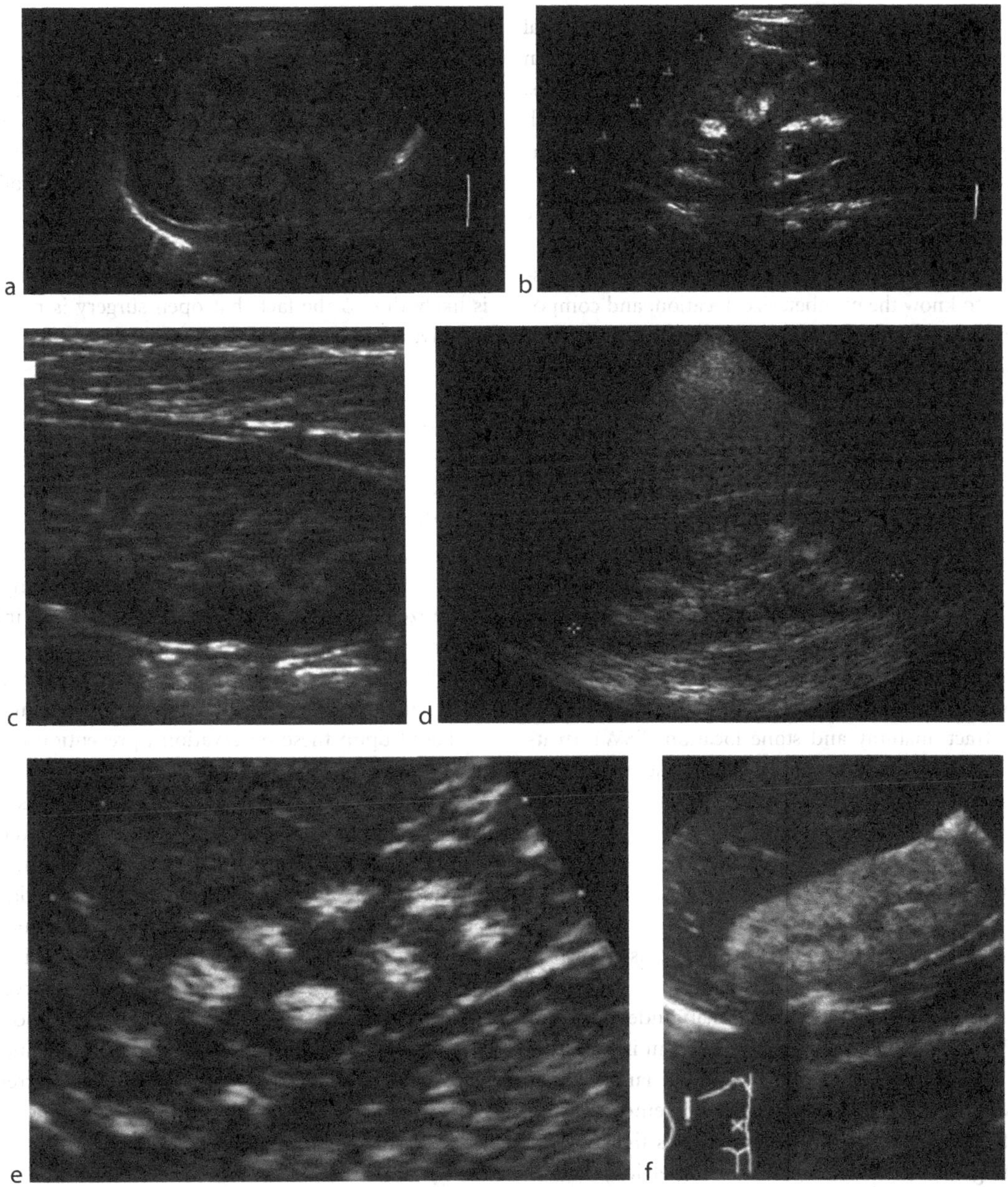

Figure 308.11

(a) Normal, still hyperechoic kidney of a preterm infant. (b) Tamm–Horsfall kidney. (c)Medullary nephrocalcinosis (NC) grade I (mild increase of echogenicity around the pyramidal border). (d) Medullary NC grade II (mild increase of echogenicity at whole pyramid). (e) Medullary NC grade III (more severe hyperechogenicity of entire pyramid). (f) Diffuse corticomedullary NC

associated with shorter length of hospital stay. Studies demonstrated that there are short-term effects such as perirenal hematomas, hematuria, and reduced GFR directly after ESWL therapy. However, there has been no evidence for long-term damage in children.

It is of utmost importance that no stone material is left behind, no matter what therapy is employed, as recurrence rates are higher than in adults. Thirty-three percent of patients with small remaining stone fragments after extracorporeal shock-wave lithotripsy (ESWL) (<3 mm), which were formerly called clinically insignificant residual fragments (CIRFs) in the early era of ESWL, had an increasing stone mass on median follow-up of 24 months.

Compared with stone-free individuals, patients with residual fragments had an increased risk for adverse clinical outcome, with an odds ratio (OR) of 3.9.

If an underlying metabolic disorder was existent, the OR for growth of residual fragments was 11.4.

Before choosing the appropriate treatment, it is indispensable to know the number, size, location, and composition of a stone, and in addition, any information about the urinary tract below the stone.

ESWL is the preferred treatment in pediatric urolithiasis patients with calculi <20 mm. Stone-free rates after ESWL in children range between 57% and 92%.

In suspected cystine stones, the maximum diameter should not exceed 15 mm because of the hardness of the stone. Hardness of cystine stones, a ureteroscopic or minipercutaneous nephrolithotomy approach is coequal, if not the new first-line therapy. Thus, large and hard stones, such as cystine and whewellite, decrease ESWL success rates.

Another important aspect in treatment planning is urinary tract anatomy and stone location. ESWL treatment of stones in lower calices has a lower success rate due to the special anatomy and gravity situation.

Minipercutaneous Nephrolithotomy

A percutaneous approach (PCNL) could be used for bigger and more complex calculi.

Although there are no international guidelines as to when PCNL should be the primary treatment in children, there are relative indications, such as large stones (>1.5 cm) or >1 cm for lower-pole concrements. Especially if there are anatomical abnormalities that prevent good fragment clearance (i.e., ureteropelvic junction obstruction, calyceal diverticulum, ureter stricture), and depending on stone composition, PCNL can be the treatment of choice. Although PCNL is an invasive treatment, it achieves excellent stone free rates and comes with a relatively low risk in experienced hands.

Ureterorenoscopy

URS is ideally suited for calculi in the mid and distal ureter; this procedure has become a first-line treatment for ureteral stones and can even be considered a good treatment option for renal calculi.

Laparoscopic Surgery/Open Surgery

In developed countries, open surgery remains the treatment of choice for 0.3–5.4% of children. In general patients with anatomical abnormalities i.e., ureteropelvic junction obstruction, obstructive megaureter, urolithiasis will receive open surgery if stone removal and anatomical correction can be combined in one operation. In developing countries, open surgery is used in 14% of cases, which is likely due to the fact that open surgery is more cost-effective in those countries.

Prevention

The best treatment both for calcium containing stones and for other stones remains prevention. A stone requires supersaturation, a nidus, and time to form. Thus, ample hydration, avoidance of infection, and good voiding habits minimize the chance of stone formation, whether initial or recurrent.

Once a stone has formed, however, there is more than a 50% chance that a second stone will form at some point.

Based upon these observations, prevention of recurrent stone disease should be a major clinical goal. Preventive measures are directed toward reducing risk factors associated with stone formation. In all children with nephrolithiasis, adequate fluid intake is a key component to reducing the risk of recurrent stones. High fluid intake increases the urine flow rate and lowers the urine solute concentration, thereby reducing the likelihood of new stone formation. The therapeutic preventive interventions are based upon the underlying metabolic condition.

Surgical success based on less complication and complete removal of the stone to reduce risk of recurrence.

Prognosis

Ninety percent of patients will pass the stone if < 4 mm in distal ureter, 50% 4–6 mm, only 20% > 6 mm pass stones. Small non-uric acid stones in upper pole appear least likely to progress; most lower pole calyceal stones < 20 mm can be adequately cleared with extracorporeal shock wave lithotripsy (ESWL); asymptomatic lower pole caliceal stones may be safe to observe.

In recent articles a recurrence rate of 67% during a mean follow-up of 59 months is quoted. Despite the excellent response to treatment noted in most children with urolithiasis, long-term nephrologic care is indicated, particularly for children who have more complex forms of renal stone disease, because renal insufficiency or end-stage renal disease may develop.

In general, increased water intake can be used for primary prevention of urinary calculi; reducing soft drink consumption reduced risk of stone recurrence among men; greater increase in urine volume associated with reduced risk of recurrence among patients who had stones, low-animal-protein, low-salt diet may prevent recurrent stones in selected patients, thiazides and allopurinol reduced 3-year recurrence rate from 55% to 15–25% in randomized trials. Restricted animal protein and salt with normal calcium intake is more effective than low-calcium diet in preventing recurrent stones in men with recurrent calcium oxalate stones and hypercalciuria.

References

Alon US (2009) Medical treatment of pediatric urolithiasis. Pediatr Nephrol 24:2129–2135

Am J Med 1982 Jan;72(1):17 in ACP J Club 1993 Jan-Feb;118(1):15

American College of Radiology (ACR) (2007) Practice guideline for performance of percutaneous nephrostomy

Bak M (2009) The metabolic etiology of urolithiasis in Turkish children. Int Urol Nephrol 41:453–460

Borghi L et al (2002) Comparison of two diets for the prevention of recurrent stones in idiopathic hypercalciuria. N Engl J Med 346(2):77

Borghi L et al (2006) Dietary therapy in idiopathic nephrolithiasis. Nutrition Rev 64:301

BMC Urol 2003 Jan 21;3:1

Churchill DN (1987) Medical treatment to prevent recurrent calcium urolithiasis. A guide to critical appraisal Miner Electrolyte Metab 13(4):294 in ACP J Club 1993 Jan–Feb;118(1):15

Cochat P et al (2010) Nephrolithiasis related to inborn metabolic diseases. Pediatr Nephrol 25:415–424

Commentary, ACP J Club 2002 Sep-Oct;137(2):62

Commentary, J Fam Pract 2002 Apr;51(4):305

Commentary, N Engl J Med 2002 May 23;346(21):1667

Durkee CT, Balcom AH (2006) Surgical management of urolithiasis. Pediatr Clin N Am 53:465–477

Editorial in N Engl J Med 2002 Jan 10;346(2):74

Elmaci MA, Unal E, Peru H (2007) The real diagnosis of cystinuria. Urol Int 78(4):363

Eur Urol 2000 Mar;37(3):339 in QuickScan Reviews in Fam Pract 2000 Nov;25(9);13

Eveline A et al (2010) Nephrocalcinosis in preterm neonates. Pediatr Nephrol 25:221–230

Fazil Marickar YM, Salim A, Vijay A (2008) Pattern of family history in stone patients. Urol Res 36:157–232

Hoppe B, Kempe MJ (2010) Diagnostic examination of the child with urolithiasis or nephrocalcinosis. Pediatr Nephrol 25:403–413

Imamura K et al (1998) 4q33-qter deletion and absorptive hypercalciuria: report of two unrelated girls. Am J Med Genet 78:52–54

Inci K, Sahin A, Islamoglu E et al (2007) Prospective long-term follow-up of patients with asymptomatic lower pole caliceal stones. J Urol 177(6):2189

J Clin Epidemiol 1992 Aug;45(8):911 in ACP J Club 1993 Jan-Feb;118(1):15

J Endourol 2004 Aug;18(6):534 in QuickScan Reviews in Fam Pract 2005 Feb 21;30(9):22

J Urol 1999 Sep;162(3 Pt 1):688 in J Watch 1999 Oc1;19(19):152

Kemper MJ, Mü ller-Wiefel DE (1996) Nephrocalcinosis in a patient with primary hyperoxaluria type 2. Pediatr Nephrol 10:442–444

Lemann J Jr et al (1985) Hydrochlorothiazide inhibits bone resorption in men despite experimentally elevated serum 1,25-dihydroxyvitamin D concentrations. Kidney Int 28(6):951–958

López M, Hoppe B (2010) Pediatr Nephrol 25:49–59. doi:10.1007/s00467-008-0960-5

Martens K, Jaeken J, Matthijs G, Creemers JWM (2008) Multi-system disorder syndromes associated with cystinuria Type-I. Curr Mol Med 8:544–550

Milliner DS (2004) Urolithiasis. In: Avner ED, Harmon WE, Niaudet P (eds) Pediatric nephrology, 5th edn. Lippincott Williams and Wilkins, Philadelphia, p 1091

Moudgil A et al (2000) Nephrocalcinosis and renal cysts associated with apparent mineralocorticoid excess syndrome. Pediatr Nephrol 15:60–62

Nicoletta JA, Lande MB (2006) Medical evaluation and treatment of urolithiasis. Pediatr Clin N Am 53(3):479–491

Pahari A et al (2003) Neonatal nephrocalcinosis in association with glucose-galactose malabsorption. Pediatr Nephrol 18:700–702

Reed BY, Heller HJ, Gitomer WL, Pak CY (1999) Mapping a gene defect in absorptive hypercalciuria to chromosome 1q23.3-q24. J Clin Endocrinol Metab 84(11):3907–3913

Reference – systematic review last updated 2006 Nov 13 (Cochrane Library 2007 Issue 1:CD006029)

Sarica K et al (2009) Role of overweight status on stone-forming risk factors in children: a prospective study. Urology 73:1003–1007

Sikora P et al (2006) Acute renal failure due to bilateral xanthine urolithiasis in a boy with Lesch-Nyhan syndrome. Pediatr Nephrol 21:1045–1047

Spivacow FR, Negri AL (2008) Metabolic risk factors in children with kidney stone disease. Pediatr Nephrol 23:1129–1133

Straub M et al (2010) Pediatric urolithiasis: the current surgical management. Pediatr Nephrol 25:1239–1244

Systematic review last updated 2004 Apr 25 (Cochrane Library 2004 Issue 3:CD004292)

Tanzer F, Ozgur A, Bardakci F (2007) Type I cystinuria and its genetic basis in a population of Turkish school children international. Int J Urol 14:914–917

Wein. Campbell-walsh urology. 9th edn

309 Interstitial Nephritis and Primary Hyperoxaluria

Pierre Cochat

Tubulointerstitial Nephritis

The definition of tubulointerstitial nephritis (TIN) is based on histopathological findings, so kidney biopsy remains the only definitive diagnostic investigation. TIN may be due to various causes and is probably underdiagnosed both in adults and children.

Acute Tubulointerstitial Nephritis (ATIN)

Presentation

Children with ATIN usually present with non-oliguric acute renal failure without edema, sometimes with loin pain, which develops over a period of days to several weeks; in case of drug-induced ATIN, symptoms typically begin 3–5 days after drug (re)exposure. Renal presentation may also include leukocyturia, and various degree of tubular impairment (polyuria, glucosuria, tubular proteinuria). Blood pressure is normal and there is neither hematuria nor heavy proteinuria. Renal ultrasonography may show normal or enlarged kidneys with increased echogenicity.

According to the primary disease, extrarenal signs such as low-grade fever, maculopapular rash, mild arthralgias, anemia, weight loss, and malaise may be associated (in 50% of cases). In the case of drug-induced ATIN, hypereosinophilia and eosinophiluria may be found. More specific organ involvement may be of major interest, and ophthalmologic examination should be recommended in most cases looking for uveitis. However it is likely that many patients with mild ATIN are often clinically silent.

Etiology

ATIN accounts for 5–10% of acute renal failure in the pediatric setting, and may have various causes, which are summarized in *Table 309.1*. However, the role of drug-related ATIN seems to be increasing during the recent years both in children and adults.

A few biological investigations are of interest: erythrocyte sedimentation rate, urinary β-2 microglobulin, antitubular cell antibodies, serum immunoglobulins, etc. In difficult cases, serum sample should be stored at −20°C for further immunological assessment.

Pathology

Renal biopsy may be useful in some patients but is not required for all. ATIN prevalence was 11.3% of biopsy-confirmed acute renal failure in a recent large series that included both children and adults.

Light microscopy shows interstitial edema with inflammatory cellular infiltrate (majority of T cells, together with macrophages and plasma cells), sometimes with granulomatous lesions or eosinophils according to etiology (mainly drug-induced ATIN). Patients with diffuse infiltrate had a worse prognosis than those with focal interstitial infiltrate. Tubes and capillaries may be sometimes involved.

Immunofluorescence staining for antibodies and complement uses to be negative, but linear or granular deposits of immunoglobulin G or M may be occasionally present along the tubular basement membranes.

Treatment

The overall outcome of ATIN is usually good without any specific treatment; the mean recovery time to the nadir creatinine level is 1–2 months. When drug-induced ATIN is suspected, the presumed causative drug should be withdrawn first, and rechallenge must be excluded.

In adults, 58% of cases require acute renal replacement therapy. According to pathological features and etiology, early short course oral corticosteroid therapy may be indicated but results are controversial. The best results have been obtained with TINU syndrome and some drug-induced (antibiotics, non-steroidal anti-inflammatory drugs) ATIN.

Abdelaziz Y. Elzouki (ed.), *Textbook of Clinical Pediatrics*, DOI 10.1007/978-3-642-02202-9_309,

Table 309.1
Etiologies of acute tubulointerstitial nephritis

Drugs and toxins +++	Hypersensitivity to drugs (acyclovir, indinavir, tenofovir; beta-lactams, cephalosporins, ciprofloxacin, rifampicin, isoniazid, sulfonamides, vancomycin, macrolides; non-steroidal anti-inflammatory drugs; frusemide, thiazides, triamterene; allopurinol; phenytoin, carbamazepine; ranitidine, cimetidine; omeprazole; bisphosphonates; alpha interferon; azathioprine)
	Mushrooms (*Cortinarius*)
	Creatine
Crystal-induced ATIN	Drugs (acyclovir, indinavir, triamterene)
	Uric acid
	Calcium salt (phosphate, oxalate)
Infections ++	Acute pyelonephritis (*Escherichia coli*)
	Systemic bacterial infection (streptococcus, staphylococcus, leptospirosis)
	Mycoplasma infection
	Viral infection (Epstein-Barr, HIV, Hantaan, BK polyoma, adenovirus)
Systemic disorders	Sarcoidosis, Sjögren syndrome, systemic lupus, inflammatory bowel disease
	Vasculitides
	"TINU" syndrome (idiopathic TubuloInterstitial Nephritis with Uveitis)
	Lymphoma, leukemia
Primary ATIN	Isolated idiopathic tubulointerstitial nephritis

Chronic Interstitial Nephritis (CTIN)

CTIN develops over months or years and is a common unspecific feature, which may also have specific causes.

Presentation

CTIN is often diagnosed late because clinical signs are usually limited. Patients present with progressive chronic kidney disease, variable degrees of arterial hypertension, tubular dysfunction (tubular proteinuria, polyuria, enzymuria, increased natriuresis, acidosis), leukocyturia, hematuria, and hyporeninemic hypoaldosteronism. Small kidneys with increased echogenicity and anemia are suggestive of a long-standing process.

Etiology

CTIN may have various causes, which are summarized in *Table 309.2*. Some specific biological investigations may be of interest: erythrocyte sedimentation rate, urinary β-2 microglobulin, antitubular basement membrane antibodies, anti-tubulointerstitial nephritis antibodies, serum immunoglobulins, etc. In difficult cases, serum should be stored at −20°C for further immunological assessment.

Pathology

CTIN associates various degrees of interstitial inflammatory infiltrate (lymphocytes, monocytes, macrophages), tubular involvement (tubular atrophy, flattened epithelial cells, tubular dilation, tubular basement membrane thickening), glomerulosclerosis, and interstitial fibrosis; vessels may also be involved.

Immunofluorescence microscopy is usually negative, except in systemic diseases. The extent of disease on renal biopsy inversely correlates with renal function and may accurately predict renal prognosis.

Treatment

In case of drug- or toxin-induced nephropathy, the causative agent should be ruled out. In most other cases, nephroprotection is recommended, such as conservative management of electrolyte disturbances, blood pressure control, angiotensin-converting enzyme inhibitor, and angiotensin-2 receptor antagonist.

Primary Hyperoxaluria

Hyperoxaluria may be either a secondary or a primary disease. Two autosomal recessive inherited enzyme defects of glyoxylate metabolism are related to type 1 and type 2 primary hyperoxalurias (PH), that is, alanine: glyoxylate aminotransferase (AGT; *AGXT* gene located on chromosome 2q37.3) and glyoxylate reductase/hydroxypyruvate reductase (GRHPR; *GRHPR* gene on chromosome 9q11), respectively. A gene for PH3 has been recently identified. Among all PH patients, type 1 accounts for ~80%, type 2 for ~10%, and non-type 1 non-type 2 for ~10%.

Patient information: www.ohf.org – www.oxaleurope.com

Table 309.2
Etiologies of chronic tubulointerstitial nephritis (CTIN)

Infections	Renal scarring post-acute pyelonephritis
	Bacterial infections
	Viral infections (Epstein Barr, BK polyoma)
Drugs and toxins	Antibiotics
	Non-steroidal anti-inflammatory drugs
	Diuretics
	Calcineurin inhibitors (cyclosporin, tacrolimus)
	Alkylating agents (iphosphamide, cis-platinum)
	Bisphosphonates
	Analgesic nephropathy
	Anorexia nervosa (hypokalemia due to diuretic and/or laxative)
	Heavy metals (cadmium, lead, lithium)
	Aristolochic acid (Chinese herbs, Balkan nephropathy) [adult]
	Radiation nephritis
Immunological disorders	CTIN due to anti-tubular basement membrane antibodies
	Systemic lupus and other immune-mediated glomerulonephritis
	T cell-induced CTIN (renal allograft rejection, TINU syndrome)
Genetic diseases	Nephronophthisis
	Cystinosis
Nephrocalcinosis	Inherited (hypercalciuria, distal tubular acidosis, hyperoxaluria)
	Acquired (drug-induced, cortical necrosis, HIV)

Primary Hyperoxaluria Type 1

Pathophysiology

The functional defect of AGT leads to oxalate overproduction by the liver. Since calcium oxalate is insoluble in urine, PH1 usually presents with symptoms referable to the urinary tract. The median age at initial symptoms is 5–6 years and end-stage renal disease (ESRD) is reached between 25 and 40 years of age in half of the patients. Along with progressive decline of glomerular filtration rate (GFR), oxalate deposition occurs in many organs, leading to systemic involvement (named "oxalosis") and bone is the main compartment of the insoluble oxalate pool.

Presentation

The combination of both clinical and renal sonographic findings is a strong argument for PH1, that is, the association of renal calculi, nephrocalcinosis, and renal impairment; in addition, family history may bring additional information.

PH1 grossly fits five presentations: (i) infantile form with early nephrocalcinosis and kidney failure, (ii) recurrent urolithiasis and progressive renal failure, leading to a diagnosis of PH1 in childhood or adolescence, (iii) late-onset form, with occasional stone passage, in adulthood, (iv) diagnosis given by post-transplantation recurrence, and (v) presymptomatic subjects with a family history of PH1.

Diagnosis

The diagnosis is based on urine crystals analysis (calcium oxalate monohydrate, i.e., whewellite), infrared spectroscopy and concomitant hyperoxaluria (urine oxalate >1 mmol/1.73 m^2/day, normal <0.5). In patients with well-defined phenotype, genotyping (DNA sequencing) can be further proposed in order to screen the most common mutations according to local background. Prenatal diagnosis can be performed from DNA obtained from crude chorionic villi or amniocytes.

The assessment of oxalate burden is a major issue when GFR falls to below 30–50 mL/min/1.73 m^2. It is mainly based on repeated plasma oxalate assessment, fundus examination, bone imaging and sometimes bone biopsy examination.

Management

Conservative measures should be started as soon as the diagnosis has been suspected. The aims are to increase urinary solubility of calcium oxalate and to decrease oxalate production (*Table 309.3*).

The treatment of stones should avoid open and percutaneous surgery because further renal lesions will alter renal function, so that the use of extracorporeal shock wave lithotripsy is an available option in selected patients. In patients with repeated renal colic, stone removal can be

Table 309.3

Supportive treatment for patients with primary hyperoxaluria type 1 with preserved renal function

Mode of action	Compound	Dose (per 24 h)
Urine dilution +++	Water	2–3 L/m^2
Crystallization inhibitor	Potassium/sodium citrate	100–150 mg/kg
Normalize urine calcium	Hydrochlorothiazide	0.5–2.0 mg/kg
Decrease oxalate production	Pyridoxine (AGT cofactor)	5–10 mg/kg

attained by ureteroscopy and a ureteral JJ stent may be helpful for pain control and protection of renal damage.

Dialysis is unsuitable for patients who have reached ESRD because it cannot overcome the continuous excess production of oxalate by the liver in spite of its small molecular mass. Peritoneal dialysis alone is unable to clear enough oxalate and is rather contraindicated in such patients. Conventional maintenance long-term hemodialysis is also associated with unacceptable quality of life and may be a life-threatening option in the long term. Therefore, daily hemodialysis is currently the preferred option despite technical challenges in infants, and it may be combined with PD in most children in order to enhance overall oxalate clearance and therefore minimize systemic involvement prior to transplantation.

There are different approaches to organ transplantation strategy, which may be influenced by the local allocation system. The largest experience has been obtained with a one-step combined liver-kidney transplantation leading to acceptable results. The option of a two-step procedure (liver transplantation followed by renal transplantation) should be kept in mind according to local experience and when the prospective waiting time is long enough to jeopardize both patient quality of life and survival. Patient survival after combined liver and kidney transplantation approximates 80% at 5 years and 70% at 10 years. Isolated kidney transplantation is not recommended due to ~100% disease recurrence, and preemptive isolated liver transplantation has limited indications due to ethical reasons.

Non-type-1 Primary Hyperoxaluria

In patients with overt hyperoxaluria, the pattern of urinary metabolites is indicative but no longer a diagnosis of PH. In patients with a clinical picture of PH1, 10–30% have normal AGT activity that may lead to a diagnosis of PH2 or of another inherited disorder causing hyperoxaluria. The overall long-term prognosis is better than for PH1.

References

Arimura Y, Tanaka H, Yoshida T et al (1999) Anorexia nervosa: an important cause of chronic tubulointerstitial nephritis. Nephrol Dial Transplant 14:957–959

Bacchetta J, Dubourg L, Juillard L, Cochat P (2009) Non-drug induced nephrotoxicity. Pediatr Nephrol 24(12):2291–2300 [Epub 2009 April 28]

Baker RJ, Pusey CD (2004) The changing profile of acute tubulointerstitial nephritis. Nephrol Dial Transplant 19:8–11

Braden GL, O'Shea MH, Mulhern JG (2005) Tubulointersitial diseases. Am J Kidney Dis 46:560–572

Clarkson MR, Giblin L, O'Connell FP et al (2004) Acute interstitial nephritis: clinical features and response to corticosteroid therapy. Nephrol Dial Transplant 19:2778–2783

Cochat P, Fargue S, Harambat J (2009) Primary hyperoxaluria. In: Avner ED, Harmon WE, Niaudet P, Yoshikawa N (eds) Pediatric nephrology, 6th edn. Springer, Heidelberg

Daudon M, Jungers P (2004) Clinical value of crystalluria and quantitative morphoconstitutional analysis of urinary calculi. Nephron Physiol 98:31–36

Diallo O, Janssen F, Hall M, Avni F (2004) Type 1 primary hyperoxaluria in pediatric patients: renal sonographic patterns. Am J Roentgenol 183:1767–1770

Fargue S, Harambat J, Gagnadoux MF et al (2009) Effect of conservative treatment on the renal outcome of children with primary hyperoxaluria type 1. Kidney Int 76:767–773

González E, Gutiérrez E, Galeano C et al (2008) Early steroid treatment improves the recovery of renal function in patients with drug-induced acute interstitial nephritis. Kidney Int 73:940–946

Leumann E, Hoppe B (2005) Primary hyperoxaluria type 1: is genotyping clinically helpful? Pediatr Nephrol 20:555–557

López-Gómez JM, Rivera F, Spanish registry of glomerulonephritis (2008) Renal biopsy findings in acute renal failure in the cohort of patients in the Spanish Registry of Glomerulonephritis. Clin J Am Soc Nephrol 3:674–681

Verghese PS, Luckritz KE, Eddy AA (2008) Interstitial nephritis. In: Geary DF, Schaefer F (eds) Comprehensive pediatric nephrology. Mosby Elsevier, Philadelphia

Vohra S, Eddy A, Levin AV et al (1999) Tubulointerstitial nephritis and uveitis in children and adolescents. Four new cases and a review of the literature. Pediatr Nephrol 13:426–432

Zhou B, Nelson TR, Kashtan C et al (2000) Indentification of two alternatively spliced forms of human tubulointestitial nephritis antigen. J Am Soc Nephrol 11:658–668

310 Urinary Tract Infection

Sean E. Kennedy · Andrew R. Rosenberg

Background

Urinary tract infection (UTI) is one of the commonest bacterial infections in children. A single UTI may lead to significant acute morbidity and often recurs. Rare but serious long-term sequelae of UTI include hypertension and chronic kidney disease. The knowledge that a significant number of young children with UTI will have an underlying anomaly of the urinary tract, most commonly vesicoureteral reflux (VUR), and that those with more severe anomalies are more likely to suffer recurrent infections and chronic injury, has led to considerable research and ongoing debate. Whilst much progress has been made in understanding the links between UTI, VUR, and chronic kidney injury, many unanswered questions remain.

Definitions

The term urinary tract infection (UTI) is used to describe both symptomatic infections as well as situations when bacterial growth is detected in children who lack any other signs or symptoms of UTI. This latter situation, known as asymptomatic bacteriuria, is a benign condition that does not require treatment unless the patient has a kidney transplant or is pregnant. In the rest of this chapter UTI refers to growth of microorganisms in the urinary tract coexistent with signs and/or symptoms of infection.

UTI can be further classified based on site of infection. Pyelonephritis is the term used for infections involving one or both kidneys. Cystitis is a lower urinary tract infection confined to the bladder.

The distinction between pyelonephritis and cystitis is usually based on clinical signs and symptoms. The classical features of pyelonephritis are fever, loin pain, and tenderness. However pain and tenderness can only rarely be elicited in young children and infants. Therefore the clinical diagnosis of pyelonephritis rests upon the presence of fever $\geq 38^\circ C$ in a child with a UTI. The presence of infection in the kidney is suggested by elevated circulating inflammatory markers such as procalcitonin and may be confirmed by dimercaptosuccinic acid (DMSA) scanning at the time of infection (see below).

A recurrent UTI is any UTI occurring after an initial infection has been fully treated.

Etiology

Gram-negative organisms cause the majority of UTI, with *Escherichia coli* accounting for at least 75% of first infections. Other common organisms include *Klebsiella* and *Proteus* species. Less common pathogens include *Enterobacter*, *Citrobacter*, and *Enterococci*.

Staphylococcus saprophyticus has been reported to cause between 7% and 15% episodes of cystitis in young women but is only rarely isolated in young children.

Staphylococcus aureus and *Pseudomonas* species are uncommon causes of UTI that are more likely to be found in children with anatomical or functional abnormalities of the urinary tract.

Chronic or recurrent infections with urease producing organisms, particularly *proteus*, may lead to precipitation of struvite (magnesium ammonium phosphate) which can form stag horn calculi. *Proteus mirabilis* can be grown from the periurethral areas of >22% of uncircumcised male infants.

Other uncommon causes of UTI in children include viruses (e.g., adenovirus) and fungi (e.g., *Candida* spp.). Adenovirus typically causes a haemorrhagic cystitis that may present as macroscopic haematuria. Fungal UTI usually occurs in association with risk factors such as long-term urinary catheterization and immunosuppression.

Tuberculous infection should be considered in a child from an area where TB is endemic who has otherwise unexplained pyuria. Tuberculous infections of the kidney and urinary tract usually occur as a result of haematogenous spread of mycobacteria. The renal infection begins in the glomeruli and, although usually asymptomatic, can cause progressive renal injury and scarring. Lower tract infection may arise secondary to shedding of mycobacteria in urine.

Abdelaziz Y. Elzouki (ed.), *Textbook of Clinical Pediatrics*, DOI 10.1007/978-3-642-02202-9_310,

Chronic infection with *schistosoma haematobia* is associated with bladder granulomata and may present as dysuria, frequency, and terminal haematuria.

Epidemiology

The incidence of UTI differs according to age and gender. Up to 10% of girls will have had a UTI by adulthood with the majority of cases occurring after the age of 2 years. On the other hand, only 2–3% of boys will be diagnosed with a UTI during childhood and more than 60% of these occur before the age of 2. UTIs are an uncommon occurrence in boys older than 4 years of age.

UTI is the cause of up to 10% of all episodes of fever without focus in children younger than 2 years of age. Uncircumcised male infants have a higher incidence of UTI than circumcised boys and UTIs cause up to 20% of febrile episodes in uncircumcised boys less than 3 months of age.

Children with UTI are more likely to have a family history of UTI in first-degree relatives than children without UTI.

Other risk factors for UTI include previous UTI, constipation, voiding dysfunction, neurogenic bladder, and structural anomalies of the urinary tract including vesicoureteral reflux (VUR). VUR is present in at least 20–30% of children having their first UTI compared to only 1–3% of the general pediatric population.

Voiding dysfunction is a broad term used to describe a urination pattern abnormal for the child's age. It may present with symptoms, including urgency, frequency, and incontinence, with onset after daytime continence has been achieved at about 4–5 years of age. Voiding dysfunction is associated with VUR but often occurs independently.

Voiding dysfunction is caused by abnormal (or immature) regulation of bladder filling and emptying, and can be classified as:

- Overactive bladder (also known as unstable bladder, or urge incontinence)
- Underactive bladder
- Dysfunctional voiding, marked by uncoordinated relaxation of the muscles of the external sphincter

Voiding dysfunction may be suggested by a history of incontinence or urgency. Overactive bladder typically is seen in young girls who have urgency and often adopt postures to prevent micturition, such as crossing of legs or squatting. It is frequently associated with constipation, and the presence of the two conditions is labelled dysfunctional elimination syndrome.

Underactive bladder is also more often seen in girls than boys and is characterized by infrequent voiding often associated with constipation. Incomplete bladder emptying may result from hypoactive detrussor function and UTI may ensue.

Neurogenic dysfunction of the bladder is most commonly due to spinal dysraphism, often as an open myelomeningocoele (*spina bifida*). Closed or occult spinal lesions may also affect bladder function. Other spinal causes of neurogenic bladder include sacral agenesis, tethered spinal cord associated with imperforate anus, cloacal malformations, and spinal cord injuries from sporting injuries. Neurogenic bladder is infrequently due to a central nervous system abnormality such as cerebral palsy.

Nonneurogenic neurogenic bladder (or Hinman's syndrome) is a term used to describe the most severe form of dysfunctional voiding. It is often associated with recurrent UTI and constipation and may lead to chronic kidney injury. The mechanisms underlying the detrusor–sphincter incoordination are not fully understood. Management may include bladder training; however, intermittent catheterization is often required.

Pathogenesis

The urinary tract above the distal urethra is usually sterile. Most infections are caused by bowel organisms that have ascended via the urethra to colonize the bladder. Uropathogenic *E. coli* characteristically have surface fimbriae (Type II or P fimbriae) that promote attachment to urinary epithelium allowing colonization. The process of attachment involves adherence of bacterial fimbriae to specific receptors expressed on the surface of urinary epithelium. The receptor for certain uropathogenic *E. coli* is a glycosphingolipid that is also expressed on red blood cells.

The urinary tract relies on several defense mechanisms to prevent infections. The primary defense is regular and complete emptying of the bladder. Other protective mechanisms include the systemic innate immune response and inherent antibacterial properties of normal bladder cells. Toll like receptor-4 (TLR4) is intricately involved in the innate immune response to UTI.

Infants may be more susceptible to UTI because of immaturity of their immune defenses, both systemic and local to the urinary tract. Other reasons for high rates of UTI during infancy include altered gut flora and colonization of periurethral areas by pathogenic organisms.

Breast fed infants have a reduced incidence of UTI relative to formula fed infants. The reasons for the protective effect of breast milk have not been elucidated but may include the transfer of secretory IgA and other immunoactive molecules.

The presence of UTI caused by organisms that usually have a low virulence for the urinary tract, such as *S. aureus*, *Enterococci* and *Pseudomonas* species, suggests that normal host defenses have been altered. The commonest reasons for this are incomplete emptying of the urinary tract due to obstruction, high-grade VUR, or dysfunctional voiding.

UTIs are rarely the result of haematogenous spread of organisms. However this should be suspected in children with UTI secondary to an atypical organism, particularly *S. aureus*, and an otherwise normal urinary tract.

Clinical Manifestations: Symptoms, Signs

Fever is the most common presenting feature of UTI in infants and young children. Children younger than 3 months of age with UTI are more prone to develop septicaemia and severe illness including meningitis. Neonates with UTI may not develop a high fever and at times may be hypothermic.

Other clinical features of UTI differ according to age and site of infection. Nonspecific signs of UTI in the first weeks of life include drowsiness, vomiting, poor feeding, lack of weight gain, and prolonged jaundice.

Infants and young children typically do not present with localizing signs of infection, consequently fever may be the only sign. Parents will occasionally notice malodorous urine and children who are out of nappies may show urinary frequency or enuresis and, rarely, dysuria.

Older children, particularly those who are verbal and fully toilet trained are more likely to present with specific symptoms such as urinary frequency and dysuria or abdominal pain.

The physical examination of a child with a suspected or proven UTI should be thorough and aim to assess for predisposing factors and complications. Hypertension may be a sign of underlying renal disease or may be a consequence of renal scarring secondary to previous UTI. Abdominal or flank masses may indicate hydronephrosis, urinary retention, or other renal pathology. *Constipation* may be identified by finding palpable feces in the left iliac fossa. Periurethral inflammation, balanitis, or phimosis may either be a source of ascending infection or alternatively may give rise to dysuria and pyuria and masquerade as a UTI. Spinal anomalies may be suggested by midline pits, dimples, birthmarks, and hairy patches, as well as reduced anal tone, an abnormal gait, and abnormal lower limb reflexes.

Diagnosis

The diagnosis of a UTI depends on collection of an uncontaminated urine sample. An older child or adolescent may be able to provide a mid stream urine (MSU) with or without the assistance of a parent; however, the majority of children with suspected UTIs will be too young to collect an uncontaminated sample for themselves. *Table 310.1* lists the methods by which urine can be collected in young children and babies.

Prompt collection of an uncontaminated urine specimen is necessary in acutely unwell babies and children to allow empiric treatment while awaiting culture results. In these situations either suprapubic aspiration (SPA) or perurethral catheterization should be used to collect a specimen. SPA is a simple and safe procedure. It can be performed in children under 2 years of age as a full bladder in this age group normally sits above the bony pelvis. The likelihood of urine being in the bladder is increased by timing the procedure to be at least 60 min from the last void and after a feed. Many centers use an ultrasound bladder scan beforehand to confirm that urine is present in the bladder.

Urine collected by an adhesive plastic bag will be contaminated by skin or bowel flora in up to 50% of cases, therefore bag collections (even if the skin has been carefully washed beforehand) should not be used to diagnose a UTI. Another simple, noninvasive method of urine collection from babies is use of a urine collection pad, but again this method is prone to contamination and should generally not be relied upon. The usefulness of these two methods is in their ability to exclude a UTI, that is, if urine collected by bag or pad does not grow a significant growth of bacteria, then a UTI is not present.

Table 310.1
Methods of urine collection for microbiological culture

Method	Diagnostic criteria
Clean catch	$>10^5$ cfu/mL of a single organism
Suprapubic aspiration	Any growth of bacteria
Transurethral catheterization	>10,000 cfu/mL of a single organism
Adhesive bag	A negative culture excludes a UTI
Absorbant pad	A negative culture excludes a UTI

UTI is defined by a significant growth of a single organism in a clean catch urine, MSU, SPA, or catheter urine. Because each of these techniques has its own risk of contamination, the diagnostic criteria for UTI depends on collection method (➔ *Table 310.1*). Urine collected by SPA should be sterile unless a UTI is present, therefore any growth of bacteria should be considered to be significant. A significant growth of bacteria from an MSU or clean catch urine is 10^5 cfu/mL of a single organism. A mixed growth or a lower colony count (10^4–10^5 cfu/mL) may also be indicative of infection if the clinical features support a diagnosis and collection of a further specimen for culture may be warranted. The laboratory should always be informed of the method used for collection.

Urine microscopy and biochemical dipstick analysis can be used to guide decisions on initial management and the need for urine culture (➔ *Table 310.2*). The presence of organisms on microscopic examination of unspun urine and/or on Gram stain of urine is strongly suggestive of a UTI. Therefore urgent microscopy of urine should be utilized if available to diagnose UTI in young children with fever without focus.

The presence of urinary nitrites detected by dipstick in a child with a fever suggests the presence of a UTI. Urinary nitrites are produced by urease splitting organisms; however, not all UTI causing organisms convert nitrate to nitrite and urease splitting bacteria may take up to 4 h to produce detectable nitrites in urine. A positive test for nitrites is therefore highly specific but lacks sensitivity to allow the diagnosis of all UTIs (➔ *Table 310.2*).

Urinary leukocytes are usually present during a UTI, but they may also be present in a large proportion of febrile children without UTI as well as in otherwise healthy children. The diagnostic utility of urinary dipsticks is maximal when the results of leukocyte esterase and nitrite tests are considered together. If both tests are negative then it is unlikely that a UTI is present. If nitrites are present then the likelihood of a UTI being present is high (>95% positive predictive value) and this likelihood is increased further if the leukocyte esterase test is also positive (➔ *Table 310.2*). The least useful result is positive leukocyte esterase with negative nitrites, as this finding is nonspecific (➔ *Table 310.2*).

Confirmation of UTI by culture is important not only for management of the current illness but also as young children with a confirmed UTI should undergo further investigation. Culture and sensitivity results will guide antibiotic management.

Blood tests are not required to make the diagnosis of UTI but may be useful to guide management, detect complications, and possibly localize the infection. Electrolyte abnormalities (e.g., *hyponatremia, hyperkalemia* and *acidosis*) may complicate infections in infants or children with urological anomalies and require judicious management. Leucocytosis is commonly seen in febrile children. C-reactive protein and plasma procalcitonin levels may both be elevated and higher levels (procalcitonin >0.5 ng/mL) are more likely in instances of pyelonephritis.

Differential Diagnosis of UTI in Children

The differential diagnosis of febrile UTI in young children is broad and includes both minor and life threatening infections. The differential diagnosis of acute cystitis in older children and adolescents includes dysfunctional voiding, urethritis, vulvovaginitis, prostatitis, epididymoorchitis, and *nephrolithiasis*.

Treatment

Any symptomatic UTI should be treated with antibiotics. Parenteral antibiotics are indicated in children less than 3 months of age or any child who appears toxic. Parenteral antibiotics should also be considered in any child who is vomiting or who is unable to tolerate oral antibiotics for any reason, and in older children with high fever and

Table 310.2
Utility of urine microscopy and dipstick analysis for guiding decisions about management and investigations of a child with a suspected UTI

Test result	Sensitivity (%)	Specificity (%)	Interpretation
Gram stain +	93	95	UTI likely
Leukocyte −, nitrite +	50	98	UTI likely
Leukocyte +, nitrite −	83	84	UTI possible
Leukocyte +, nitrite +	72	96	UTI likely
Leukocyte −, nitrite −			UTI unlikely

marked loin tenderness. Parenteral antibiotics should be continued until the defervescence occurs and the patient is able to tolerate oral medications.

In children older than 6 months there is good evidence to suggest that oral antibiotics are as efficacious as parenteral. There is less evidence to guide the duration of antibiotic therapy. Pyelonephritis is usually treated with 7–10 days of antibiotics. Antibiotic therapy should be reviewed in any child with a UTI whose fever does not settle after 48 h of appropriate therapy or if fever recurs later in the course of therapy.

Empiric antibiotics should be commenced promptly in infants that appear toxic, generally after a collection of specimens for culture, which may include cerebrospinal fluid.

Older children and those with less severe presentation should have empiric antibiotics commenced if there is a strong clinical suspicion of UTI based on presenting features, risk factor assessment, and/or urinary dipstick analysis or microscopy (➋ *Table 310.2*).

Empiric antibiotics should be active against *E. coli* and other common uropathogens (➋ *Table 310.3*). The choice of specific antibiotics should be guided by local patterns of bacterial resistance. Uropathogenic *E. coli* in most areas have a high degree of resistance to amoxicillin; therefore this antibiotic should generally be avoided for empiric use. The susceptibility of *E. coli* to first generation cephalosporins and trimethoprim/sulphamethazole varies widely.

Empiric parenteral therapy should include agents with good tissue penetration. In seriously ill young children a second agent should be added to broaden antibacterial coverage. Antibiotics that are likely to be active against *enterococci* (e.g., ampicillin) should be used empirically in children less than 3 months or those with known urological anomalies. Oral antibiotics that are excreted in the urine but do not achieve therapeutic serum levels (e.g., nitrofurantoin) should not be used to treat UTI in febrile infants and young children in whom pyelonephritis is likely.

Antibiotic therapy should be rationalized once culture results and antibiotic sensitivities are known.

The clinical condition of most patients, including normalization of temperature, improves within 24–48 h of initiation of appropriate antibiotic therapy. Repeat urine culture to confirm the success of therapy is not required if a child responds well to antibiotics and completes the full course. Non-adherence with a full course of therapy is common and may lead to inadequate treatment and relapsing infection.

Table 310.3
Empiric antibiotics for suspected UTI

Clinical features	Suitable empiric antibiotics[a]	Management guide
Age <6 months or toxic at any age	Cefuroxime 50 mg/kg 8 hourly	Parenteral antibiotics until afebrile for 48 h. Then continue appropriate oral antibiotic for a total of 7–10 days
	Cefotaxime 50 mg/kg 6 hourly	
	Ceftriaxone 100 mg/kg 24 hourly	
	Gentamicin 2.5 mg/kg 8 hourly[a] with the addition of Ampicillin 25 mg/kg 6 hourly	
Age >6 months and fever ≥38°C or other signs/symptoms of pyelonephritis	Parenteral agents as above or the following oral agents	Continue appropriate antibiotic for a total of 7 to 10 days
	Cefixime 8 mg/kg 24 hourly	
	Amoxycillin/clavulanate 12.5 mg/kg 12 hourly[b]	
	Cefuroxime 15 mg/kg 12 hourly	
	Cephalexin 12.5 mg/kg 6 hourly	
	Sulphamethoxazole/trimethoprim 4 mg/kg[c] 12 hourly	
Temp <38°C and symptoms of cystitis	Oral agents as above	Oral antibiotics for 3–5 days in total

[a]Choice of empiric antibiotics should be based on local patterns of antibiotic resistance
[b]Once daily gentamicin 7 mg kg^{-1} day^{-1} may be an alternative
[c]Dosage based on amoxicillin component
[d]Dosage based on trimethoprim component

Suppurative Complications

One uncommon complication of pyelonephritis is acute focal bacterial nephritis (also referred to as lobar nephronia or focal pyelonephritis) – a well-localized renal infection without frank abscess formation. If inadequately treated it may progress to abscess formation. At least a 3-week course of appropriate antibiotic therapy is recommended for treatment.

The presence of acute focal bacterial nephritis or abscess should be suspected if fever persists after 4 days of appropriate antibiotic treatment. The diagnosis is usually made by ultrasonography. Findings on ultrasound include appearance of an ill-defined mass with disruption of the corticomedullary junction and lack of vascularity (➋ *Fig. 310.1*).

CT scanning (with and without contrast) may be used to confirm the diagnosis and potentially to discriminate between a complex abscess and a malignancy. Findings suggestive of renal abscess include a poorly defined, wedge-shaped, hypodense area that may involve liquefaction and does not enhance after contrast administration.

Renal Scarring

Renal scarring is the primary sequelae of pyelonephritis. A scar is a discrete area of tubular atrophy, tubulointerstitial fibrosis, and chronic inflammation. Between 5% and 30% of young children will develop a renal scar after an initial febrile UTI. Risk factors for scarring include: age less than 4 years, recurrent febrile UTI, delay in treatment of UTI, dysfunctional elimination, and VUR.

New scars rarely develop in children older than 4 years of age, except in those with neurogenic bladder, severe anatomical anomalies, or transplanted kidneys. Studies of kidney transplants suggest that scarring is possible if VUR is present, regardless of age.

The most sensitive imaging technique for diagnosis of scarring is the 99m-dimercaptosuccinic acid (DMSA) scan (➋ *Fig. 310.2*). A scar is shown by diminished radioisotope uptake in a discrete area. Acute pyelonephritis is also associated with photopenia on DMSA scanning, which will resolve over time. Therefore a scar should only be diagnosed if an abnormality is detected on DMSA scan performed after a wait of at least 3 months from the time of UTI (6 months is generally preferred).

More severe degrees of renal scarring may be evident on renal ultrasonography. A clue to scarring is an unusually small kidney or a discrepancy in size between left and right kidney on ultrasound. A left kidney longer than the right by more than 10 mm or a right kidney longer than the left by 7 mm or more suggests the presence of a DMSA abnormality.

The reported long-term consequences of renal scarring are variable. Small discrete scars do not cause an appreciable impairment of renal function but may increase the risk of hypertension. Early studies suggested that up to 10% of children with renal scars will develop hypertension by early adulthood. However these studies were small and probably included more severely damaged kidneys detected by intravenous pyelograms. Larger long-term studies, including children with lesser degrees of

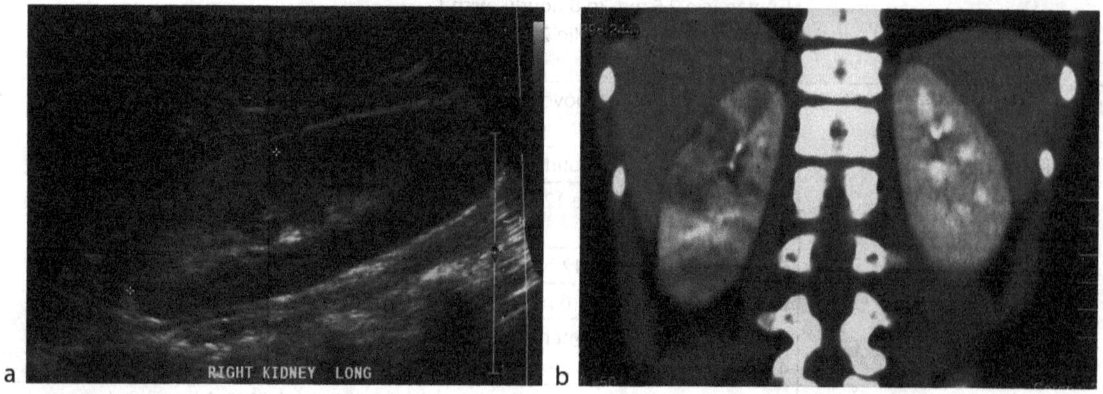

Figure 310.1

Acute focal bacterial nephritis due to E. coli in a 7 year old girl who presented with fever, right iliac fossa pain and psoas muscle spasm. (a) Ultrasound of right kidney showing a focal area of increased echogenicity and poor corticomedullary differentiation in the upper pole between markers. (b) Post-contrast CT scan of same patient showing patchy enhancement of right kidney particularly involving the lateral aspect of the upper pole, the lower pole is also affected

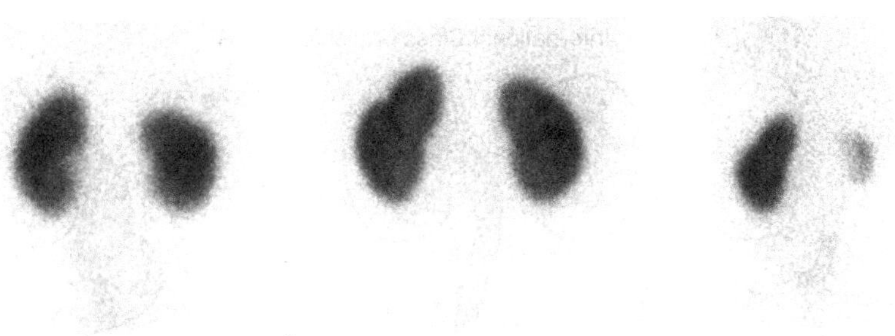

Figure 310.2
Renal DMSA Scans performed 6 months after UTI. (a) Normal scan showing symmetrical renal function and smooth renal outlines. (b) Abnormal scan of a 5-year-old girl with a history of recurrent UTIs showing a discrete cortical scar in the upper pole of the left kidney. (c) Abnormal scan from a 15-month-old boy who had a febrile UTI at age 9 months. Scan shows a small right kidney with an irregular outline and poor function. This appearance is consistent with congenital reflux nephropathy. Further investigations revealed grade IV right sided vesicoureteral reflux

scarring detected by DMSA, have failed to show similar rates of hypertension. Renal scarring increases the risk of complications during pregnancy including hypertension and pre-eclampsia.

Children with severe scarring may develop chronic kidney disease; this outcome is known as reflux nephropathy and is described below.

Vesicoureteral Reflux

VUR is the retrograde flow of urine from the bladder into one or both ureters. It is diagnosed by micturating cystourethrogram (MCUG) and is stratified into five grades of severity, depending on the radiological appearance (*Fig. 310.3*). Radionucleotide cystourethrogram is an alternative imaging modality with less radiation exposure but it provides less anatomical detail. VUR cannot be reliably diagnosed by ultrasonography.

VUR is usually an isolated finding which occurs because the submucosal tunnel through which the ureter attaches to the bladder is short and does not close on voiding.

VUR has a genetic basis and can be detected in 30% of first-degree relatives of an index case; the concordance rate in monozygotic twins is 80–100%. Inheritance patterns are usually consistent with autosomal dominant transmission with incomplete penetrance, but a causative gene/s has not been identified.

Children with neurogenic bladder, dysfunctional voiding, or bladder outlet obstruction (e.g., *posterior urethral valves*) are at risk for developing secondary VUR.

VUR is detected in 25–40% of preschool children who have had a UTI. The true prevalence of VUR in the normal population is uncertain; the most often quoted figure is 1% of all infants, but the true frequency may be higher. The prevalence of VUR is increased in children with the dysfunctional elimination syndrome.

Most children diagnosed with VUR after a UTI have low-grade reflux (grades 1 and 2) and the natural history is for resolution over time. Most low-grade cases and up to 50% of higher-grade cases will resolve by 4 years of age. VUR is less likely to resolve if it is associated with other anomalies of the urinary tract.

VUR potentially increases the risk for UTI by allowing incomplete voiding and may increase the risk of pyelonephritis by promoting passage of infected urine to the upper tract. The presence of VUR is probably the strongest single determinant of whether a child will develop a scar after pyelonephritis. However, VUR is not a prerequisite for scarring.

Surgical correction of VUR has traditionally been by ureteral re-implantation, with the aim of producing a longer intramural segment of ureter. The success rate of this surgery is 95–99%. Re-implantation surgery may reduce the risk of recurrent pyelonephritis. Whether or not this confers protection from scarring has not been established.

An alternative approach to antireflux surgery is the endoscopic injection of a bulking agent into the subureteral region of the bladder wall (subureteric transurethral injection [STING]). The rate of reflux correction overall may be less than with re-implantation surgery and the procedure appears best suited to less severe cases. A recent multicenter randomized controlled trial showed that endoscopic antireflux treatment reduced the recurrence rate of febrile UTI in young girls with high grade VUR.

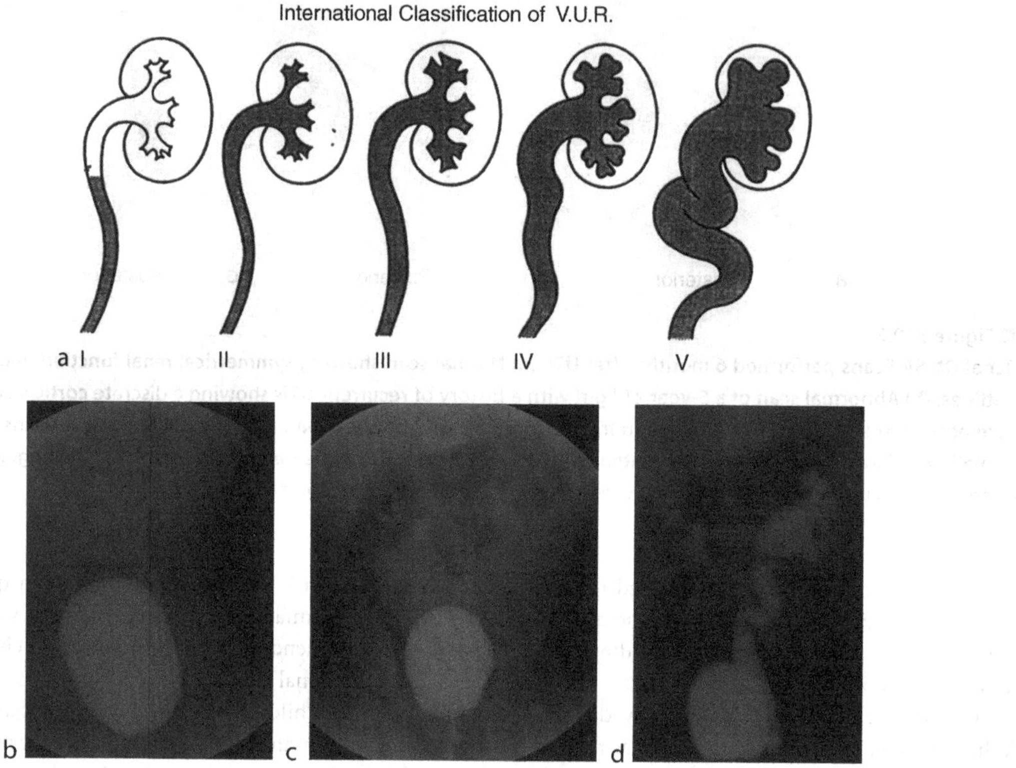

Figure 310.3
Vesicoureteral reflux. (a) Grading system proposed by the International Reflux Study Committee 1981 (Report of the International Reflux Study Committee: Medical versus surgical treatment of vesicoureteral reflux: a prospective international reflux study in children. (1981) Pediatrics 67: 392). (b) Micturating cystourethrogram (MCUG) performed after a febrile UTI in a 9 month old girl. Left sided grade II VUR. The renal ultrasound was normal. (c) MCUG performed after a febrile UTI in another 9-month-old girl. Left sided grade III VUR is demonstrated by reflux of radiocontrast into a dilated ureter. The renal ultrasound was normal. (d) MCUG performed after a febrile *Escherichia coli* UTI in a 2-week-old male infant. Bilateral high-grade VUR, grade IV on *right* and grade V on *left*. Ultrasound demonstrated bilateral ureteric dilation and mild left pelvicalyceal dilatation. DMSA showed scarring of right kidney

Reflux Nephropathy

Reflux nephropathy is the term originally proposed to describe renal scarring associated with VUR and UTI and replaced the misleading label of chronic pyelonephritis. Reflux nephropathy itself is something of a misnomer, as it is now recognized that scarring can develop after UTI without VUR being present. On the other hand, children with high-grade reflux may have abnormal kidneys without ever having a UTI.

Reflux nephropathy causes 2–5% of cases of end-stage kidney disease (ESKD). However the vast majority of children with UTI do not proceed to ESKD, reflecting the fact that reflux nephropathy includes a wide range of pathology, from small functionally insignificant scars through to badly damaged kidneys and ESKD.

The more severe end of the spectrum of reflux nephropathy includes children who have dysplastic and/or hypoplastic kidneys at birth, coexistent with VUR that is usually high grade.

Proteinuria and hypertension may be signs of reflux nephropathy. Strict blood pressure control and treatment with Angiotensin converting enzyme inhibitors may delay progression of kidney impairment.

Investigations After UTI

Most occurrences of UTI will occur in children with anatomically normal urinary tracts and will not lead to any significant complications. However, up to 30% of children will develop irreversible renal damage (scar) after a UTI and in a significant minority UTI will be the first sign of a serious urological anomaly, early detection of which may allow appropriate management and limit further renal damage. Furthermore, approximately one third of children will have recurrent UTI and detection of risk factors such as VUR can be used to direct preventative therapy. Therefore, investigation of children after an initial or recurrent UTI has two main goals:

1. Detection of underlying urological anomalies
2. Detection of complications

Several guidelines and consensus statements have been published advising on investigations after an initial UTI, these have been developed in light of considerable uncertainties about the significance of renal scarring and a lack of evidence with regard to the effectiveness of preventative strategies. Therefore the advice has ranged from the interventional approach proposed by the American Academy of Pediatrics (perform ultrasound and micturating cystogram in all young children after an initial UTI) to the relatively minimalist approach of the United Kingdom's National Institute of Clinical Excellence (www.nice.org.uk/cg54).

Routine imaging with ultrasound should be performed in any child after an initial UTI with the possible exception of adolescent girls who have cystitis on clinical grounds. Ultrasound may be avoided if a good quality antenatal ultrasound, performed after 30-week gestation, did not detect any renal anomaly. Renal ultrasound should be performed during the initial course of antibiotics to assess for obstruction or acute focal bacterial nephritis if there is a lack of response to appropriate antibiotics.

The approach to further investigation of any child should be guided by the ultrasound appearance as well as the child's age, clinical features and local resources. Urological anomalies are more likely to be present in children with UTI caused by pathogens other than *E. coli* and in children who would otherwise be considered to have a low risk of UTI (e.g., boys older than 2 years).

An MCU is often performed after resolution of the acute infection to assess for VUR. VUR is more likely to be present and significant in children who are younger, have infection with an organism other than *E. coli*, have had recurrent infections, have pyelonephritis, and/or have an abnormal ultrasound (e.g., ureteric or pelvicalyceal dilatation, or abnormal size kidneys). Evidence of pyelonephritis is provided by high plasma procalcitonin levels and by an abnormal DMSA scan at the time of infection; if either of these are present there is a greater chance of grade 3–5 VUR.

Two suggested approaches to imaging after UTI in young children are outlined in ➋ *Fig. 310.4*. Imaging of older children should be individualized based on risk factors for recurrent infections, renal scarring, and VUR.

Prevention

Recurrent UTI occurs in between 15% and 40% of children after a first infection. The majority of recurrences occur during the following 2 years after the initial UTI. Factors that are associated with recurrence include young age at first UTI, female gender, anomalies of the urinary tract including VUR, and voiding dysfunction.

Voiding dysfunction can be managed by encouraging regular and complete bladder emptying (e.g., scheduled voiding every 2–3 h) with or without the addition of anticholinergic agents. Older children may be amenable to bladder training. *Constipation* should be treated by dietary and behavioral modifications as well as laxatives as required.

Prophylactic Antibiotics

The results of two large randomized controlled trials in children recently published confirm that prophylactic antibiotics confer a small but significant degree of protection from recurrent UTI. Antibiotic prophylaxis may be of particular benefit in young girls with high grade VUR as a recent study found prophylactic antibiotics reduced the rate of recurrent febrile UTI and new scar development in this population. Once-daily therapy with antibiotics such as cotrimoxazole, trimethoprim, or nitrofurantoin has been found to be safe; however, there is some concern about prophylactic antibiotics promoting growth of resistant organisms.

Prophylactic therapy is usually discontinued when the risk of severe infection and scarring is judged to be low.

Cranberry Juice

Cranberry juice may prevent recurrent UTI in women and older girls but as yet there is no evidence to show it is effective in younger children. The mechanism of action of cranberry juice is uncertain; it appears that substances in the berries may interfere with the adherence of *E. coli* to uroepithelium. The most effective dose and formulation of cranberry juice have not been established. Cranberry juice should not be used for treating a UTI.

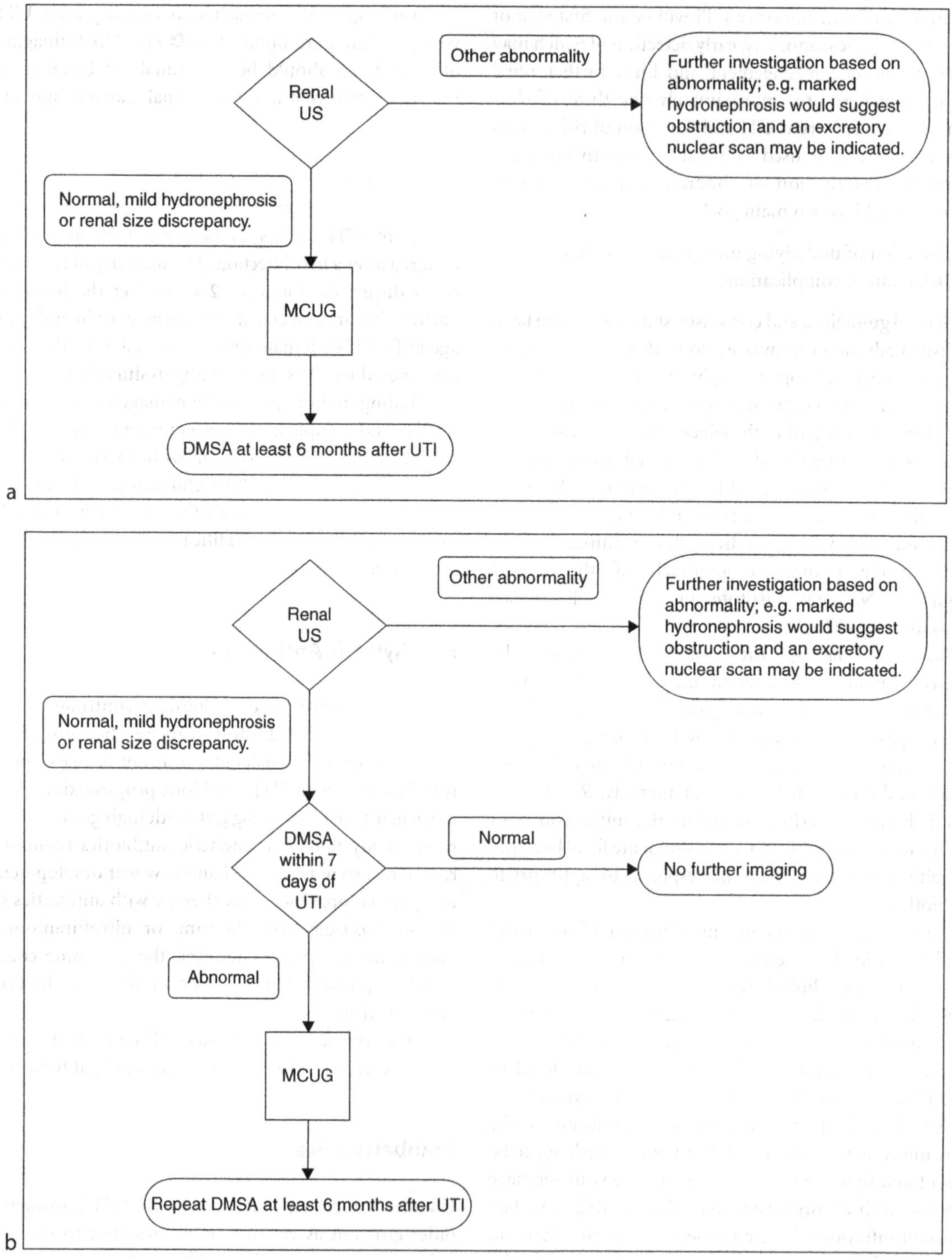

◻ Figure 310.4
Investigation after UTI of children less than 2 years of age. (a) Suggested approach to screen all young children with UTI for vesicoureteral reflux (VUR). (b) Alternative approach using an acute DMSA as a screening modality. Such an approach could lead to about a 50% reduction in MCUG rates. An abnormal acute DMSA will be present in >90% of cases of dilating VUR

Probiotics

There is no good evidence to support the use of probiotics as a preventive strategy for UTI.

Circumcision

Circumcised males have a lower rate of UTI during childhood than uncircumcised males. Given the low incidence of UTIs in boys, the vast majority of uncircumcised boys will not develop a UTI and more than 100 circumcisions would be needed to prevent one UTI. The risk: benefit ratio does not justify circumcision of all boys, but circumcision could be considered as a means to prevent UTI in boys with recurrent UTI or those at high risk of recurrence and scarring because of underlying urological abnormalities.

Antireflux Surgery

Surgical intervention to correct VUR should be considered in children with VUR, recurrent infections (despite prophylactic antibiotics), and renal damage.

Prognosis and Follow-up

Parents of children who have had a UTI should be educated about the signs of UTI to allow prompt treatment of any recurrences.

The overall prognosis for children after UTI is favorable; however, a small number, particularly those with high-grade VUR and bilateral renal damage, are at risk of *hypertension* and *chronic kidney disease*. Any child with renal scarring should have annual review for blood pressure measurement. Children who have bilateral renal scarring should be monitored for signs of progression of renal disease including proteinuria and appropriate management should be initiated for hypertension or impaired glomerular filtration rate.

References

Aggarwal VK, Verrier Jones K, Asscher AW, Evans C, Williams LA (1991) Covert bacteriuria: long term follow up. Arch Dis Child 66:1284–1286

Al-Mardeni RI, Batarseh A, Omaish L, Shraideh M, Batarseh B, Unis N (2009) Empirical treatment for pediatric urinary tract infection and resistance patterns of uropathogens, in Queen Alia hospital and prince A'Isha military center–Jordan. Saudi J Kidney Dis Transpl 20:135–139

Al-Orifi F, McGillivray D, Tange S, Kramer MS (2000) Urine culture from bag specimens in young children: are the risks too high? J Pediatr 137:221–226

American Academy of Pediatrics, Committee on Quality Improvement, Subcommittee on Urinary Tract Infection (1999) Practice parameter: the diagnosis, treatment, and evaluation of the initial urinary tract infection in febrile infants and young children. Pediatrics 103:843–852

Anatoliotaki M, Galanakis E, Schinaki A, Stefanaki S, Mavrokosta M, Tsilimigaki A (2007) Antimicrobial resistance of urinary tract pathogens in children in Crete, Greece. Scand J Infect Dis 39:671–675

Andrade SS, Sader HS, Jones RN, Pereira AS, Pignatari AC, Gales AC (2006) Increased resistance to first-line agents among bacterial pathogens isolated from urinary tract infections in Latin America: time for local guidelines? Mem Inst Oswaldo Cruz 101:741–748

Brandstrom P, Esbjorner E, Herthilius M, Swerksson S, Jodal U, Hansson S (2010) The Swedish reflux trial in children: III. Urinary tract infection pattern. J Urol 184:286–291

Brandstrom P, Neveus T, Sixt R, Stokland E, Jodal U, Hansson S (2010) The Swedish reflux trial in children: IV. Renal damage. J Urol 184:292–297

Cheng CH, Tsai MH, Huang YC, Su LH, Tsau YK, Lin CJ, Chiu CH, Lin TY (2008) Antibiotic resistance patterns of community-acquired urinary tract infections in children with vesicoureteral reflux receiving prophylactic antibiotic therapy. Pediatrics 122:1212–1217

Cheng CH, Tsau YK, Chen SY, Lin TY (2009) Clinical courses of children with acute lobar nephronia correlated with computed tomographic patterns. Pediatr Infect Dis J 28:300–303

Chertin B, Puri P (2003) Familial vesicoureteral reflux. J Urol 169:1804–1808

Chowdhury P, Sacks SH, Sheerin NS (2004) Minireview: functions of the renal tract epithelium in coordinating the innate immune response to infection. Kidney Int 66:1334–1344

Coulthard MG, Keir MJ (2006) Reflux nephropathy in kidney transplants, demonstrated by dimercaptosuccinic acid scanning. Transplantation 82:205–210

Coulthard MG, Lambert HJ, Keir MJ (1997) Occurrence of renal scars in children after their first referral for urinary tract infection. BMJ 315:918–919

Coulthard M, Verber I, Jani J, Lawson G, Stuart C, Sharma V, Lamb W, Keir M (2009) Can prompt treatment of childhood UTI prevent kidney scarring? Pediatr Nephrol 24:2059–2063

Craig JC, Simpson JM, Williams GJ, Lowe A, Reynolds GJ, McTaggart SJ, Hodson EM, Carapetis JR, Cranswick NE, Smith G, Irwig LM, Caldwell PH, Hamilton S, Roy LP (2009) Antibiotic prophylaxis and recurrent urinary tract infection in children. N Engl J Med 361:1748–1759

Estrada CR Jr, Passerotti CC, Graham DA, Peters CA, Bauer SB, Diamond DA, Cilento BG Jr, Borer JG, Cendron M, Nelson CP, Lee RS, Zhou J, Retik AB, Nguyen HT (2009) Nomograms for predicting annual resolution rate of primary vesicoureteral reflux: results from 2,462 children. J Urol 182:1535–1541

Farajnia S, Alikhani MY, Ghotaslou R, Naghili B, Nakhlband A (2009) Causative agents and antimicrobial susceptibilities of urinary tract infections in the northwest of Iran. Int J Infect Dis 13:140–144

Farrell DJ, Morrissey I, De Rubeis D, Robbins M, Felmingham D (2003) A UK multicentre study of the antimicrobial susceptibility of bacterial pathogens causing urinary tract infection. J Infect 46:94–100

Feldman AS, Bauer SB (2006) Diagnosis and management of dysfunctional voiding. Curr Opin Pediatr 18:139–147

Friedman S, Reif S, Assia A, Mishaal R, Levy I (2006) Clinical and laboratory characteristics of non-E. coli urinary tract infections. Arch Dis Child 91:845–846

Glennon J, Ryan PJ, Keane CT, Rees JP (1988) Circumcision and periurethral carriage of Proteus mirabilis in boys. Arch Dis Child 63:556–557

Gordon KA, Jones RN (2003) Susceptibility patterns of orally administered antimicrobials among urinary tract infection pathogens from hospitalized patients in North America: comparison report to Europe and Latin America. Results from the SENTRY Antimicrobial Surveillance Program (2000). Diagn Microbiol Infect Dis 45:295–301

Gorelick MH, Shaw KN (1999) Screening tests for urinary tract infection in children: a meta-analysis. Pediatrics 104:e54

Group TET (2009) Strict blood-pressure control and progression of renal failure in children. N Engl J Med 361:1639–1650

Guidoni EB, Berezin EN, Nigro S, Santiago NA, Benini V, Toporovski J (2008) Antibiotic resistance patterns of pediatric community-acquired urinary infections. Braz J Infect Dis 12:321–323

Haller M, Brandis M, Berner R (2004) Antibiotic resistance of urinary tract pathogens and rationale for empirical intravenous therapy. Pediatr Nephrol 19:982–986

Hansson S, Brandström P, Jodal U (2009) Recurrent febrile urinary tract infections in children randomized to prophylaxis, endoscopic injection or surveillance. Results from the Swedish Reflux Study. Pediatr Nephrol 24:1792

Hernandez-Porras M, Salmeron-Arteaga G, Medina-Santillan R (2004) Microbial resistance to antibiotics used to treat urinary tract infections in Mexican children. Proc West Pharmacol Soc 47:120–121

Hewitt IK, Zucchetta P, Rigon L, Maschio F, Molinari PP, Tomasi L, Toffolo A, Pavanello L, Crivellaro C, Bellato S, Montini G (2008) Early treatment of acute pyelonephritis in children fails to reduce renal scarring: data from the Italian Renal Infection Study Trials. Pediatrics 122:486–490

Hiraoka M, Hori C, Tsukahara H, Kasuga K, Ishihara Y, Kotsuji F, Mayumi M (1999) Vesicoureteral reflux in male and female neonates as detected by voiding ultrasonography. Kidney Int 55:1486–1490

Hoberman A, Charron M, Hickey RW, Baskin M, Kearney DH, Wald ER (2003) Imaging studies after a first febrile urinary tract infection in young children. N Engl J Med 348:195–202

Hodson EM, Willis NS, Craig JC (2007) Antibiotics for acute pyelonephritis in children. Cochrane Database Syst Rev:CD003772

James-Ellison M, Roberts R, Verrier-Jones K, Williams J, Topley N (1997) Mucosal immunity in the urinary tract: changes in sIgA, FSC and total IgA with age and in urinary tract infection. Clin Nephrol 48:69–78

Jodal U, Smellie JM, Lax H, Hoyer PF (2006) Ten-year results of randomized treatment of children with severe vesicoureteral reflux. Final report of the International Reflux Study in Children. Pediatr Nephrol 21:785–792

Jones ME, Karlowsky JA, Draghi DC, Thornsberry C, Sahm DF, Bradley JS (2004) Rates of antimicrobial resistance among common bacterial pathogens causing respiratory, blood, urine, and skin and soft tissue infections in pediatric patients. Eur J Clin Microbiol Infect Dis 23:445–455

Khazaei MR, Mackie F, Rosenberg AR, Kainer G (2008) Renal length discrepancy by ultrasound is a reliable predictor of an abnormal DMSA scan in children. Pediatr Nephrol 23:99–105

Kirsch AJ, Perez-Brayfield M, Smith EA, Scherz HC (2004) The modified sting procedure to correct vesicoureteral reflux: improved results with submucosal implantation within the intramural ureter. J Urol 171:2413–2416

Lau SM, Peng MY, Chang FY (2004) Resistance rates to commonly used antimicrobials among pathogens of both bacteremic and non-bacteremic community-acquired urinary tract infection. J Microbiol Immunol Infect 37:185–191

Lee JH, Son CH, Lee MS, Park YS (2006) Vesicoureteral reflux increases the risk of renal scars: a study of unilateral reflux. Pediatr Nephrol 21:1281–1284

Leroy S, Romanello C, Galetto-Lacour A, Smolkin V, Korczowski B, Rodrigo C, Tuerlinckx D, Gajdos V, Moulin F, Contardo M, Gervaix A, Halevy R, Duhl B, Prat C, Borght TV, Foix-l'Helias L, Dubos F, Gendrel D, Breart G, Chalumeau M (2007) Procalcitonin to reduce the number of unnecessary cystographies in children with a urinary tract infection: a European validation study. J Pediatr 150:89–95

Mantadakis E, Plessa E, Vouloumanou EK, Karageorgopoulos DE, Chatzimichael A, Falagas ME (2009) Serum procalcitonin for prediction of renal parenchymal involvement in children with urinary tract infections: a meta-analysis of prospective clinical studies. J Pediatr 155:875–881, e871

Marild S, Jodal U (1998) Incidence rate of first-time symptomatic urinary tract infection in children under 6 years of age. Acta Paediatr 87:549–552

Marild S, Hansson S, Jodal U, Oden A, Svedberg K (2004) Protective effect of breastfeeding against urinary tract infection. Acta Paediatr 93:164–168

Martinell J, Claesson I, Lidin-Janson G, Jodal U (1995) Urinary infection, reflux and renal scarring in females continuously followed for 13-38 years. Pediatr Nephrol 9:131–136

Mor Y, Leibovitch I, Zalts R, Lotan D, Jonas P, Ramon J (2003) Analysis of the long-term outcome of surgically corrected vesico-ureteric reflux. BJU Int 92:97–100

Mulvey MA (2002) Adhesion and entry of uropathogenic Escherichia coli. Cell Microbiol 4:257–271

Preda I, Jodal U, Sixt R, Stokland E, Hansson S (2007) Normal dimercaptosuccinic acid scintigraphy makes voiding cystourethrography unnecessary after urinary tract infection. J Pediatr 151:581–584, 584 e581

Prelog M, Schiefecker D, Fille M, Wurzner R, Brunner A, Zimmerhackl LB (2008) Febrile urinary tract infection in children: ampicillin and trimethoprim insufficient as empirical mono-therapy. Pediatr Nephrol 23:597–602

Rao S, Bhatt J, Houghton C, Macfarlane P (2004) An improved urine collection pad method: a randomised clinical trial. Arch Dis Child 89:773–775

Rosenberg AR, Rossleigh MA, Brydon MP, Bass SJ, Leighton DM, Farnsworth RH (1992) Evaluation of acute urinary tract infection in children by dimercaptosuccinic acid scintigraphy: a prospective study. J Urol 148:1746–1749

Schneider PF, Riley TV (1996) Staphylococcus saprophyticus urinary tract infections: epidemiological data from Western Australia. Eur J Epidemiol 12:51–54

Shaikh N, Morone NE, Bost JE, Farrell MH (2008) Prevalence of urinary tract infection in childhood: a meta-analysis. Pediatr Infect Dis J 27:302–308

Silva JM, Santos Diniz JS, Marino VS, Lima EM, Cardoso LS, Vasconcelos MA, Oliveira EA (2006) Clinical course of 735 children and adolescents with primary vesicoureteral reflux. Pediatr Nephrol 21:981–988

Singh-Grewal D, Macdessi J, Craig J (2005) Circumcision for the prevention of urinary tract infection in boys: a systematic review of randomised trials and observational studies. Arch Dis Child 90:853–858

Tessema B, Kassu A, Mulu A, Yismaw G (2007) Predominant isolates of urinary tract pathogens and their antimicrobial susceptibility patterns in Gondar University Teaching Hospital, northwest Ethiopia. Ethiop Med J 45:61–67

Uzunovic-Kamberovic S (2006) Antibiotic resistance of coliform organisms from community-acquired urinary tract infections in Zenica-Doboj Canton, Bosnia and Herzegovina. J Antimicrob Chemother 58:344–348

Vernon SJ, Coulthard MG, Lambert HJ, Keir MJ, Matthews JN (1997) New renal scarring in children who at age 3 and 4 years had had normal scans with dimercaptosuccinic acid: follow up study. BMJ 315:905–908

Wheeler D, Vimalachandra D, Hodson EM, Roy LP, Smith G, Craig JC (2003) Antibiotics and surgery for vesicoureteric reflux: a meta-analysis of randomised controlled trials. Arch Dis Child 88:688–694

Whiting P, Westwood M, Watt I, Cooper J, Kleijnen J (2005) Rapid tests and urine sampling techniques for the diagnosis of urinary tract infection (UTI) in children under five years: a systematic review. BMC Pediatr 5:4

Williams G, Fletcher JT, Alexander SI, Craig JC (2008) Vesicoureteral reflux. J Am Soc Nephrol 19:847–862

Wiswell TE, Miller GM, Gelston HM Jr, Jones SK, Clemmings AF (1988) Effect of circumcision status on periurethral bacterial flora during the first year of life. J P\ediatr 113:442–446

Wu CY, Chiu PC, Hsieh KS, Chiu CL, Shih CH, Chiou YH (2004) Childhood urinary tract infection: a clinical analysis of 597 cases. Acta Paediatr Taiwan 45:328–333

Yuksel S, Ozturk B, Kavaz A, Ozcakar ZB, Acar B, Guriz H, Aysev D, Ekim M, Yalcinkaya F (2006) Antibiotic resistance of urinary tract pathogens and evaluation of empirical treatment in Turkish children with urinary tract infections. Int J Antimicrob Agents 28:413–416

Zhanel GG, Hisanaga TL, Laing NM, DeCorby MR, Nichol KA, Palatnik LP, Johnson J, Noreddin A, Harding GK, Nicolle LE, Hoban DJ (2005) Antibiotic resistance in outpatient urinary isolates: final results from the North American Urinary Tract Infection Collaborative Alliance (NAUTICA). Int J Antimicrob Agents 26:380–388

Zorc JJ, Levine DA, Platt SL, Dayan PS, Macias CG, Krief W, Schor J, Bank D, Shaw KN, Kuppermann N (2005) Clinical and demographic factors associated with urinary tract infection in young febrile infants. Pediatrics 116:644–648

Wesson HE, Miller [illegible], Helston H [illegible], Jones RK, Hemmings [illegible] (1988) Effect of [illegible] status on periodontal bacterial flora using the [illegible] Health 11:44[illegible]

[illegible] (2004) [illegible] 357 cases [illegible]

[illegible] (2004) Antibiotic [illegible] use of [illegible] and [illegible] treatments [illegible] Antimicrob [illegible]

[illegible] M, [illegible] MR [illegible] A [illegible]

[illegible] B, Koston [illegible] A, [illegible] C (2007) Real-time [illegible] susceptibility [illegible] Med 1[illegible]

[illegible]

311 Obstructive Nephropathy

Stephanya Shear · Martin A. Koyle

Introduction

Congenital obstructive nephropathy represents a spectrum of disease from the partially obstructive ureteropelvic junction to severe bilateral disease associated with posterior urethral valves (PUVs). In this latter situation, the renal manifestations can lead to the extreme situation of bilateral renal dysplasia, oligohydraminos, and resultant pulmonary dysplasia resulting in Potters syndrome and fetal demise. In between these extremes lie the majority of patients who may or may not have long-term renal function deterioration. We are challenged in determining those patients who will have long-term renal damage, especially those where this deterioration can be minimized by appropriate investigation and therapy.

To date, we have no markers or studies that indicate which children will benefit from early intervention, especially in utero. In fact, many studies would argue that intervention does not change the natural history of the disease; indeed damage is more likely to have occurred during renal development and has early in gestation, determined that the kidney will carry on a path of dysplasia.

As the clinical use of prenatal ultrasound has increased to at least 80% of pregnancies in the United States, the incidence of early detection of urinary anomalies has increased. Only 1% of prenatal ultrasounds will have any anomaly, with all genitourinary anomalies composing only 20% of that 1%. The overall percentage of obstructive urinary abnormalities is thus more likely to be present in 0.04–0.3% of all antenatal evaluations by ultrasound.

As noted earlier, there is very little evidence that fetal intervention improves outcomes in renal units or infant pulmonary morbidity. However, if intervention for antenatal hydronephrosis is to be considered, the following parameters would need to be present: (1) normal chromosomes in a male fetus, with (2) no other existing urologic or non-urological abnormalities, and (3) evidence of increasing hydronephrosis with corresponding decreases in amniotic fluid level late in pregnancy. This scenario is most often associated in a male with PUV and the goal of intervention is to restore amniotic fluid with the hope of allowing improved lung maturation.

Obstructive nephropathy describes renal damage and pathology secondary to obstruction and is distinct from hydronephrosis. Hydronephrosis is a "generic" radiographic finding, meaning "water on the kidney," that can be a sign of obstructive renal damage; however hydronephrosis is not synonymous with obstructive nephropathy. Most cases of hydronephrosis are associated with a benign clinical course. The majority of fetuses will fall into the category of mild hydronephrosis; with renal pelvis diameters less than 1 mm or Society for Fetal urology (SFU) grade I-2see (➋ *Table 311.1*). Very few of these kidneys will require intervention after birth. Thirty percent of infants with AP diameters greater than 7 mm at 33 weeks gestation will have normal renal ultrasounds at 5 days of age.

Renal Damage and Hydronephrosis

The pathogenesis of renal damage after obstruction has been the subject of many well-crafted animal studies; however the natural history is poorly understood in humans, although there has been increasingly more knowledge regarding the cellular changes in renal units after obstruction.

Renal Damage, Renal Insufficiency, and Hypertension

In obstructed units, it is not the delay in emptying or hydronephrosis per se that is the primary concern. Instead, it is the resulting compromise of renal function that might lead to renal insufficiency and possibly renal failure.

The consequences of obstruction on renal function have been elucidated using animal models. When counseling patients and families, it may be useful to answer questions regarding the types of damaged obstructed

Abdelaziz Y. Elzouki (ed.), *Textbook of Clinical Pediatrics*, DOI 10.1007/978-3-642-02202-9_311,

Table 311.1
Society for Fetal Urology (SFU) grading system for Antenatal Detected Hydronephrosis (ANH) J Pediatr Urol (2010) 6, 212–231

Grade	Description
0	No hydronephrosis
1	Slight dilation of renal pelvis; normal calyces
2	Moderate renal pelvis dilation; mild caliectasis
3	Large renal pelvis with calyceal dilation but preserved renal parenchyma
4	Very large renal pelvis with severe caliectasis and thinning of renal parenchyma

kidney can incur, but care must be made when translating animal models to the human patient. Animal models differ from human natural history of the disease in time of the obstruction and species specific variations in gene expression. Chronic partial urinary obstruction has been shown to cause tubular atrophy, interstitial fibrosis, and retarded renal growth. Marked inflammation is also seen. Early relief of obstruction can restore nephrogenesis and reduce progression of renal damage with the potentially greatest ability before nephrogenesis is complete in the antenatal period. However some damage, such as fibrosis, may continue even after obstruction is alleviated. Results from these studies have both supported early intervention in the infant period as well as theories that damage in

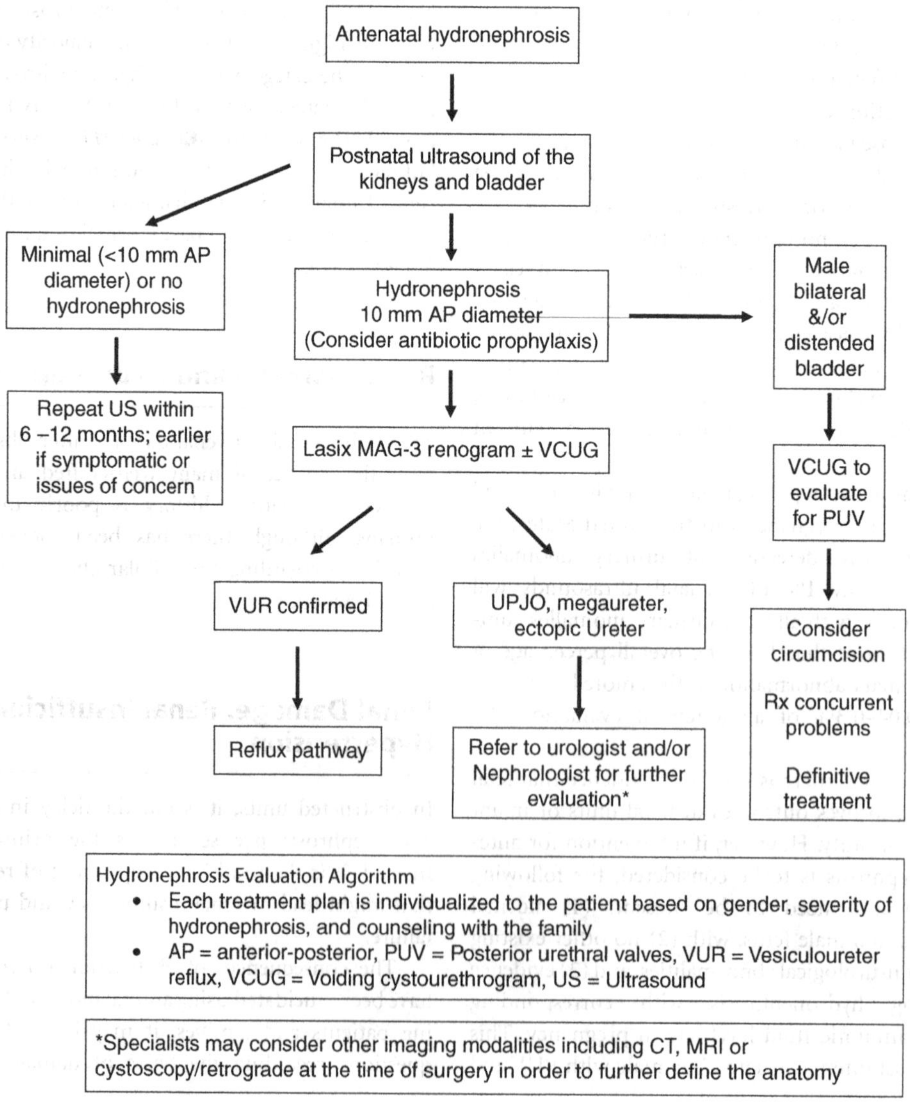

utero has already destined those poorly functioning kidneys to fail and intervention postnatally does not alter their course.

Since congenital obstruction is thought to be particularly damaging to the maturing kidney, researchers have looked for evidence of renal dysplasia in children affected with obstruction. It is still unknown to what extent obstruction in utero results in the parenchymal maldevelopment and what histological finding predicts renal function. Huang et al. performed 70 biopsies on 61 patients undergoing open pyeloplasty for ureteropelvic junction obstruction. They found epithelial proliferation, glomeruli sclerosis, and cystic dilatation; however, the degree of these changes did not correlate with hydronephrosis, age, or renogram split function levels. When comparing obstructed kidneys to autopsy controls that found in obstructed kidneys decreased proximal tubules size and a decrease concentration of distal tubules independent of glomeruli injury. Tubules were seen to have atrophy with and without overt fibrosis. The decrease in size of the proximal tubule may represent immaturity of these structures and they found a correlation between smaller proximal tubule size and longer washout times. Other studies while showing histological changes at the time of pyeloplasty, these changes correlate poorly to the differential function of the affected kidney.

Renal insufficiency is a worrisome complication in patients with congenital urinary obstruction. The true incidence of renal insufficiency is difficult to obtain since many studies of obstruction use surrogate marker such as wash out times or split function of renograms as a measurement of renal function before or after intervention. In one study, of the most severe cases of PUV, a quarter of boys have chronic renal insufficiency. In recent long-term studies, again 25% of patients may have renal insufficiency and some of those boys progress to ESRD by young adulthood. It is also true that in children with PUV with initial normal renal function from ages 5 to 11 may progress to renal insufficiency and ESRD. The degree to which this deterioration may be ameliorated by surgery is debated. One study showed no significant difference in renal outcomes based on initial surgical technique. Looking at 100 patients, chronic renal disease was seen in 51% of the boys by the age of 20 years and 40% had ESRD. Similar proportions in each surgical group had evidence of chronic disease and renal failure. Childhood cases of ESRD were rare, and insufficiency before the age of 10 was seen only in one third of patients. These results speak to theories that in utero obstruction of the kidneys sets up a path toward significant renal impairment. It also underscores the need for long-term follow-up in these children to assess renal function.

Some patients, especially those with PUV, can have hypertension. Those patients with bilateral obstruction more commonly have hypertension. Although several studies of PUV found evidence of chronic renal insufficiency (CRI), no study reports significant numbers of children with hypertension. In spite of the relatively large numbers of studies in the ureteropelvic junction obstruction (UPJO) and PUV populations, no study has directly studied the incidence of hypertension as predictive of clinical outcome.

Radiological Evaluation

Patients with suspected obstructed renal systems will be evaluated radiographically. The timing of these studies, as well as which studies are performed, may differ depending on the clinical and radiological evaluations. Although some general comments can be made, there is great variability in the frequency of studies and the merits of the various imaging modalities differ see (➋ *Fig. 311.1*) (➋ *Table 311.2*).

Unless PUV or severe obstruction is suspected, a renal and bladder ultrasound is usually performed after 72 h following birth, and in healthy infants, initial studies can be deferred until the second month of life. The delay in the neonate allows for the improved hydration and lessens the chance of missing hydronephrosis due to depleted volume status. Serial ultrasounds can be performed thereafter, depending on the diagnosis and patient's clinical picture. Ultrasounds are components of the routine management and are advantageous in that they are easy to perform, noninvasive, tolerated well by children, do not expose the child to radiation, reproducible, and relatively inexpensive.

A voiding cystourethrogram might be considered if dilatation is seen on the initial ultrasounds is suggestive of obstruction due to PUV; voiding cystourethrogram (VCUG) can also diagnose ureteroceles and ectopic ureters. Unfortunately, a VCUG exposes the patient to radiation and catheterization. Sedation is usually not required in infants but may be considered in older children.

Nuclear renal scans are used to measure obstruction, evaluate renal scars, and determine relative split renal function, and are currently the most commonly used studies used to evaluate obstruction. Current nuclear scans employ technetium-99. A comparison of the various nuclear renal scans is shown below (➋ *Table 311.3*). As

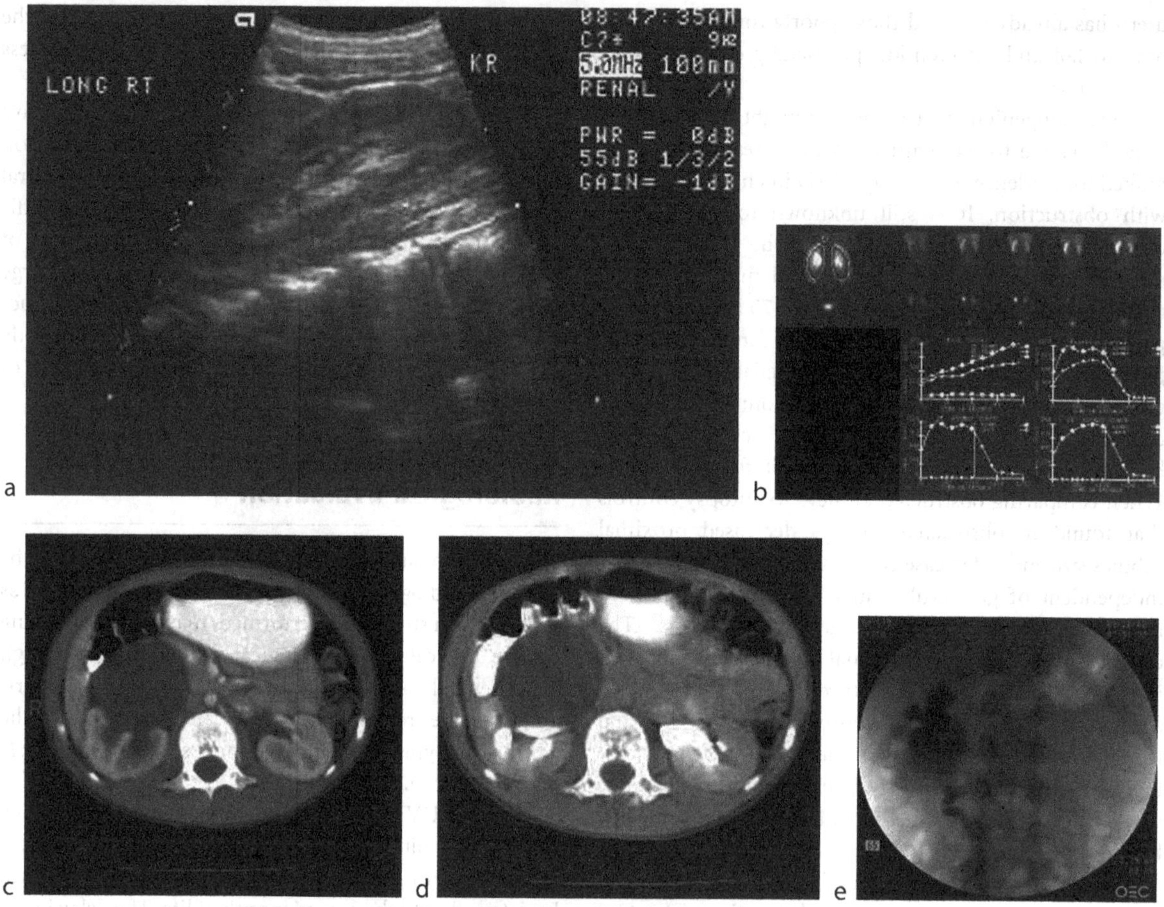

◘ Figure 311.1
This case illustrates the imperfection of imaging in detecting intermittent obstruction. This 3-year-old child had been seen for repeated bouts of abdominal pain. The ultrasound (a) and nuclear imaging study (b) demonstrate a normal right kidney, without hydronpehrosis, and with excellent function and drainage. The CT scan performed without (c) and with contrast (d) 2 weeks later when the child presented with abdominal pain, reveals marked pelviectasis and moderate caliectasis. A retrograde pyelogram (e) performed at the time of pyeloplasty further substantiates a ureteropelvic junction

with ultrasounds, there is significant variability in the use of these scans and there is significant variability in interpretation. All nuclear renal scan expose the child to significant radiation exposure and some require bladder catheterization. The child does not require sedation. Different radiopharmaceuticals are utilized depending on the information desired. When evaluating for obstruction, MAG-3 (mercaptoacetyltriglycine), which is predominately excreted by the tubules, is the preferred agent (➋ *Table 311.3*). If MAG-3 is unavailable, DTPA or GC can be used (➋ *Table 311.3*).

CT scans are ideal for imaging the parenchyma. Excretory CT scans can be used as a method to detect obstruction. However, CT scans have considerable higher radiation exposure that plain radiography and require children unable to lie still for 20 min be sedated. They also do not provide quantitative measurements regarding relative renal function.

MRI renograms are not used routinely for baseline or follow-up studies. Although they do not expose the child to radiation, they require sedation, are expensive, and like CT scans do not provide quantitative information. They do offer information about detailed anatomy but can be extremely helpful in complex circumstances, such as diagnosing ectopic ureters and duplex collecting systems. Ongoing work with this modality has been promising in

Table 311.2
Imaging techniques utilized in the evaluation of suspected obstructed hydronephrosis

Study	Utility
VCUG	Selectively utilized to diagnose posterior urethral valves, reflux and intravesical abnormalites such as diverticulcum and ureterocele.
IVP	Rarely utilized today.
Ultrasound	Almost always the initial anatomical *screening test* due to lack of radiation, rapidity of study, reproducibility, and cost. Very little functional information provided.
Renography	May be *dynamic* (MAG-3 with furosemide), to study for obstruction, or *static* (DMSA), where more precise determination of function can be elucidated. DMSA may require sedation.
CT scanning	May be useful because of anatomical detail but suffers because of significant radiation dose.
MR urography	Provides superb anatomic detail and can also provide functional information. In younger patients it may require sedation or general anesthesia and hence cost is an issue that prohibits routine use.
Invasive techniques	Cystoscopy and retrograde pyelography can be used to more clearly define an anatomical problem such as ectopic ureter, ureterocele, ureterovesical or ureteropelvic junction obstructions, and are generally performed at the time of definitive repair. Interventional radiology can be helpful in the diagnosis and treatment of come complicated obstructive pathologies. The Whithaker or pressure- flow study is rarely used in selective cases of obstructive uropathy.

Table 311.3
Basic technetium scans and their characteristics

	Technetium-99 (^{99m}TC) nuclear renal scans	
Scan	Agent	Characteristics
MAG-3	Mercaptoacetyltriglycine	Tubular clearance
		Lower radiation exposure
		High quality
		Not influenced by GFR
DPTA	Diethylenetriamine pentaacetic acid	Requires the highest concentration of ^{99m}TC
		Rapidly cleared from system
		Measures GFR
		Poor quality to measure obstruction
DMSA	Dimercaptosuccinic acid	Binds tightly to tubular cells
		Best study to assess renal cortex
		Reflect renal mass
		Partially influenced by GFR
GC	Glucoheptonate	Influenced by GFR but cannot measure
		Tubular secretion
		Visualizes cortex
		Cannot measure obstruction

not only demonstrating complex anatomy with extraordinary clarity, but also as a functional, dynamic instrument that might ultimately surpass the current nuclear medicine studies.

With modern imaging, it is rare that cystoscopy and retrograde pyelography are utilized as a routine, separate diagnostic procedure. If performed, it is often done by some pediatric urologists at the time of a definitive procedure. Likewise, the intravenous pyelogram or urogram is rarely useful.

Use of Antibiotics and Circumcision

Prescribing of antibiotic prophylaxis for all uropathies has undergone scrutiny and many question the utility of antibiotic use, even in cases of reflux. In patients with obstruction and concomitant vesicoureteral reflux, antibiotics may be of some benefit in reducing febrile urinary tract infections in some cases. Until better controlled trials yield results that define their true role, antibiotic prophylaxis should be utilized after assessing the pros and cons with the family, for those children with obstruction and reflux, ureteroceles, and/or megaureters. In essence, until studies clarify the currently conflicting data, practitioners should question their utility of prophylactic antibiotics and should manage each child individually.

Another area of practice variation is routine circumcision. Historically, in the United States, all boys with signs of neonatal uropathies, obstruction included, underwent routine neonatal circumcision as a prophylactic measure. Just as the use of antibiotics has been scrutinized, so has circumcision. The PUV population has generated the most information on the value of circumcision. It is more difficult to make statements of benefit in cases of ureteropelvic junction obstruction, megaureter, or ureterocele. Urinary tract infections can be reduced by circumcision, and the clinical benefit of the procedure is the greatest in patients with a high risk for febrile infection such as boys with PUV. The incidence of urinary tract infection may be reduced by as much as 83%. Families should be counseled in order to make an informed decision regarding circumcision, as with antibiotic prophylaxis, as part of the management options.

Major Causes of Obstruction

Ureteropelvic Junction Obstruction

Ureteropelvic junction obstruction (UPJO) is the most common cause of congenital urinary obstruction. Current theories to the cause of obstruction include deposition of collagen causing internal constriction, presence of crossing vessels that compress the pelvis, or obstructing polyps. Inherited differences in peristaltic function may contribute to the range of disease phenotypes seen in UPJO. Regardless of the cause of UPJO, the significant outcomes are hydronephrosis and presumed impact on renal function due to back pressure from the obstruction.

Prior to the widespread use of prenatal ultrasounds, children with UPJO presented in infancy with palpable abdominal masses, failure to thrive, urinary tract infections, and/or renal failure. Older children presented with flank pain usually accompanied with emesis. Although infants and children continue to present for evaluation in this manner, an increasingly greater number of children are diagnosed as a result of prenatal ultrasounds.

The use of prenatal ultrasound in the early detection and diagnosis of obstruction has increased over the last 3 decades as the use of ultrasound has become a routine part of prenatal care in the United States. Sensitivity for detection increases as ultrasounds are performed in later trimesters resulting in 1% of pregnancies indicating urinary abnormalities. Hydronephrosis is the most common finding. Most cases of prenatally detected hydronephrosis do not persist post partum. Large series indicate up to 50% of cases of prenatal hydronephrosis will resolve within 16 months of the postnatal period.

Ureteropelvic junction obstruction accounts for over 65% of the cases of prenatal hydronephrosis. Prenatal ultrasound has become the primary mode of diagnosing UPJO. Concerns arose that widespread use of prenatal ultrasound would lead to an increase in unnecessary surgery. Indeed, early detection and diagnosis has lead to earlier intervention. It is debatable to whether early detection has manifested in significant long-term outcomes. Patients with prenatal diagnosis have similar outcomes in regards to renal function when compared to patients presenting with symptoms. Both groups have similar gain of renal function, and pyeloplasty did not significantly improve renal function.

Indications for surgical intervention are a subject of debate with practitioners using consistent but different criteria for surgical correction. The use of diuretic (Lasix) renal scans has provided additional information for the clinician but interpretation and execution of tests may be confusing. Mercapto-acetyl tri glycine (MAG-3), a technetium-99 labeled compound that is secreted by the renal tubules, has significant fidelity regardless of underlying renal function, and is considered the best current agent for estimating renal obstruction and function. Since these studies are open to interpretation, these studies are best conducted as part of a comprehensive management strategy by surgeons or nephrologists.

Many children can be followed conservatively with 10–25% ultimately requiring surgical correction usually within the first 2 years of life. And some studies show that even when requiring surgical correction, delay in surgery does not impair recovery of renal function.

Important to the practicing general pediatrician is that these children need to be followed closely in order to detect clinical and radiographic changes that may indicate renal deterioration. Blood pressure measurements, urine analysis, and repeated ultrasounds or renograms maybe recommended while under the care of an urologist and/or a nephrologist. Early consultation with these specialties will insure close follow-up. It is controversial whether children without a history of UTIs or vesicoureteral reflux need to be maintained on prophylactic antibiotics and many current physicians will not routinely use them.

Posterior Urethral Valves

Posterior urethral valves (PUV) are a congenital urethral anomaly seen in boys due to an obstructing membrane. PUV accounts for 3–9% of all cases of hydronephrosis. The degree of obstruction varies and the resulting phenotype can be from mild dilation to severe obstruction affecting both the bladder and kidneys. Obstructing urine can produce a distended, poorly contractile bladder and significant bilateral vesicoureteral reflux that dilates ureters and the renal collecting system. Oligohydraminos can be associated with sever obstruction that ultimately impacts lung maturity of the developing fetus. Although less common than UPJO, it represents a significant cause of morbidity and mortality from obstruction from both a respiratory and renal perspective. Mortality was as high as 35% in the 1960s. Now, 90% of boys with PUV survive infancy. Improved outcomes are due both to aggressive antenatal care in intensive care units as well as the developments of renal dialysis and transplantation. Sever obstruction is a neonatal medical emergency requiring urinary tract drainage respiratory support, and when indicated, correction of electrolyte imbalances. Severely affected newborns may require some form of renal replacement therapy. Presence of PUV is often suspected antenatally, but is confirmed by a postnatal voiding cystourethrogram (VCUG). Bladder drainage via the urethral catheter remains in place until the child is both stable and large enough to undergo endoscopic resection of the valves or urinary diversion.

Endoscopic ablation of the valves has a high rate of success; however ablation must be confirmed by post-procedure VCUG. Boys, especially those of low birth weight, with presumed small urethras drainage can also be managed by performing a cutaneous vesicostomy that allows the bladder to drain through the abdominal wall bypassing the obstructed urethra or cutaneous ureterostomies where the ureters are brought out to the skin. Some groups suggest a stepwise approach to treat as many patients with valve ablation and then proceed to diversion if decompression of the urinary system is not achieved by ablation alone; however limited evidence exists that this alters the progression of renal damage.

Patients with significant sequela from PUV require close follow-up usually with both nephrologists and urologists. However, with aggressive management of the newborn and experience in renal dialysis and transplantation, mortality for all children with PUV is less than 5% (Parkhouse). Early aggressive measures have not changed the rate of renal insufficiently or renal failure. Ureteral dilatation and reflux are often present even after valve ablation and patients are maintained on prophylactic antibiotics. The degree of obstructive nephropathy can be significant ranging from chronic renal insufficiency, requirements for dialysis, and potential end-stage renal disease culminating in renal transplantation. As many as 35% of boys with PUV may go onto renal failure. Risk factors for renal failure include late diagnosis of PUV and bilateral reflux. Many patients have small, poorly compliant bladders that lack adequate contractile capability. Patients have varying degrees of bladder dysfunction and may need to perform clean intermittent catheterization to empty their bladders, require bladder augmentation for an adequate capacity, or need the creation of catheterizable channels. Progression of bladder dysfunction will require urodynamic evaluation as part of ongoing urological follow-up.

Bladder function remains an ongoing challenge in the management of these patients and contributes to both significant morbidity and reduced quality of life. Without aggressive management of the valve bladder, renal transplantation is associated with lower graft survival. The increasing success of renal transplantation has been one of the major factors in the recent lower mortality rates for patients with PUV.

Obstructing Megaureter

Megaureter is a descriptive term applied to all ureters that have significant dilatation (greater than 0.7–1 cm). Only a small portion of megaureters are truly obstructing. Distinguishing dilated ureters that are obstructed from those that are merely dilated is an important step. Some clinicians rely on drainage pattern from diuretic renograms. However, dilated ureter empty less efficiently and thus a delayed time to empty could potentially represent only a capacious ureter. Ultrasound findings of a progressively increasing hydronephrosis or dilatation to a level near the bladder that then sharply tapers off, is also used by some for evidence for obstruction. Those megaureters that are both obstructing and refluxing can be diagnosed by voiding cystourethrograms where the ureter is seen to taper significantly as it approaches the bladder. And as with UPJO, the insult potentially resulting in the obstruction has been linked to increased collagen deposition. In the cases of megaureter, the location of collagen deposition is near or at the ureterovesical junction. As with other causes of obstruction, many megaureters are diagnosed by prenatal ultrasounds. Prior to the widespread use of ultrasound, children presented with failure to thrive, urinary track infections, and hematuria. Although the true natural history of megaureters is unknown, many prenatally detected megaureters can be managed conservatively, at least initially. Management is similar to ureteropelvic junction obstruction in that patients are followed expectantly with serial ultrasounds and renograms. Greater controversy exists on what modality to use to determine obstruction in the cases of megaureter. Given the tortuousity and dilation of the megaureter, there is often delayed emptying of the ureter such that time to emptying becomes a less reliable marker of obstruction. Instead many physicians will use serial split renal function or sonographic evidence of thinning parenchyma as indication for intervention. Many patients are maintained on prophylactic antibiotics. Patients are more likely to undergo surgical correction when high grades of hydronephrosis are seen in combination with diminished renal function. Break through urinary tract infections while on prophylaxis is also a reason for intervention; however it is unclear if surgery decreased the incidence of further infections. Prior studies do not show significant regain of renal function after surgical correction.

Surgical repair of obstructing megaureters has consisted of separation of the ureter from the bladder, removal of the affected segment, tapering of the ureter and reimplantation into the bladder. Although the ureter may empty more efficiently after surgical correction, dilatation of the ureter may persist. Goals of the surgery are focused on alleviating obstruction so as to disrupt the continued pressure on the renal segment. As with other patients with obstructing nephropathy, these patients with megaureters are followed long term to assess their renal function and urinary tract function.

Ureteroceles

Ureteroceles are seen when the distal portion of a ureter is dilated sometimes distorting the bladder. Obstruction is thought to be caused by an anomaly at the ureteral orifice. It is not clear if this anomaly represents a partially obstructing membrane or an error in the normal development of the ureteric bud in utero. The anomaly is found four times more often in females and is associated with ureteral duplication in 80% of the time. In cases of renal duplication, the upper pole moiety is most often associated with the ureterocele. Ureteroceles are often associated with ectopic insertion of the ureteral orifice. In girls insertion can occur at the bladder neck, vagina, or urethra. In boys, ectopic insertion occurs in the urethra, seminal vesicles, prostate, or vas deferens. Up to 50% of children with ectopic ureters will have reflux into the ipsilateral lower pole kidney. Even those ureteroceles that are not ectopic can be quite large and may obstruct the bladder neck. A patient with an ureterocele most commonly presents with urinary tract infections and/or sepsis. Patents can present with urinary obstruction due to the extension of ureterocele beyond the bladder neck, or incontinence in the case of ectopic insertion. In recent years, more ureterocele are diagnosed with prenatal ultrasounds, but still a significant number are detected symptomatically. Although early detection has not altered renal function, it has been shown to decrease the morbidity associated with ureteroceles by instituting early use of antibiotic prophylaxis and resulting lower rates of UTI.

Treatment of the ureterocele is tailored to the individual patient in regards to symptoms, age, presence or absence of duplication, relative function of the upper pole moiety if present, presence or absence of reflux, location of insertion of the ureter, renal function, and history of infection. Asymptomatic patients, most often those diagnosed prenatally, can be managed conservatively with serial renal ultrasounds; however limited information is available to whether this represents a course for most patients. Various surgical options are available with the goal of treatment being assuring adequate drainage, minimizing the risk for infection, preservation of renal function, and management of reflux if present. Surgical techniques include endoscopic incision of the ureterocele, upper pole heminephrectomy with or without lower tract reconstruction, ureteroureterostomy, and complete nephroureterectomy. Increasingly, treatment plans have maintained renal tissue by performing ureteroureterostomies with only limited indications for heminephrectomy.

References

Bajpai M, Dave S, Gupta D (2001) Factors affecting outcome in the management of posterior urethral valves. Pediatr Surg Int 17:11–15

Baskin L, Zderic S, Snyder H, Duckett J (1994) Primary dilated megaureter: long term follow up. J Urol 152:618–621

Bieri M, Smith C, Smith A, Borden T (1998) Ipsilateral ureteroureterostomy for single ureteral reflux or obstruction in a duplicate system. J Urol 159:1016–1018

Capilicchio G, Leonard M, Wong C, Jednek R, Brezezinski A, Pippi-Salle JL (1999) Prenatal diagnosis of hydronephrosis: impact on renal function and its recovery after pyeloplasty. J Urol 162:1029–1032

Chako J, Koyle M, Mingin G, Furness P (2007) Ipsilateral ureteroureterostomy in the surgical management of the severely dilated ureter in ureteral duplication. J Urol 178:1689–1692

Chen F (2009) Plumbing the depths of urinary tract obstruction by using murine models. Organogenesis 5:297–305

Chertin B, Fridmans A, Knizhnik M, Hadas-Halpern I, Hain D, Farkas A (1999) Does early detection of ureteropelvic junction obstruction improve surgical outcome in terms of renal function? J Urol 162:1037–1040

Chertin B, Rabinowitz R, Pollack A, Koulikov D, Fridmans A, Hadas-Halpern I, Hain D, Farkas A (2006) Does prenatal diagnosis influence the morbidity associated with left in situ nonfunctioning or poorly functioning renal moiety after endoscopic puncture of ureterocele. J Urol 173:1349–1352

Chertin B, Pollack A, Koulikov D, Rabinowitz R, Shen O, Hain D, Hadas-Halpern I, Farkas A (2008) Long term follow up of antenatally diagnosed megaureters. J Pediatr Urol 4:188–191

Chevalier R (2006) Pathogenesis of renal injury in obstructive uropathy. Curr Opin Pediatr 18:153–160

Chevalier R, Thornhill B, Change A, Cachat F, Lackey A (2002) Recovery release of ureteral obstruction in the rat: relationship to nephrogenesis. Kidney Int 61:2033–2043

Close C, Carr M, Burns M, Mitchell M (1997) Lower urinary tract changes after early vale ablation in neonates and infants: is early diversion warranted? J Urol 157:984–988

Conlin M, Skoog S, Tank E (1995) Current management of ureteroceles. Urology 45:357–362

Cooper C, Passerini-Glazel G, Hutcheson J, Iafrate M, Camuffo C, Milani C, Snyder H (2000) Long-term Follow up of Endoscopic Incision of Ureteroceles: Intravesical versus Extravesical. J Urol 164:1097–1100

Coplen D, Barthold J (2000) Controversies in the management of ectopic ureteroceles. Urology 56:665–668

Coplen D, Duckett J (1995) The modern approach to ureteroceles. J Urol 153:166–171

Cromie W, Lee K, Houde K, Holmes K (2001) Implications of the prenatal ultrasound screening in the incidence of major genitourinary malformations. J Urol 165:1677–1680

Dhillon HK (1998) Prenatally diagnosed hydronephrosis: the great ormand street experience. Br J Urol 81:34–44

Direnna T, Leonard M (2006) Watchful waiting for prenatally detected ureteroceles. J Urol 175:1493–1495

Elder J (1997) Antenatal hydronephrosis: fetal and neonatal management. Pediatr Clin N Am 44:1299

Elder J (2002) Early postnatal intervention for congenital hydronephrosis in congenital urinary tract obstruction. In: Chevalier R, Peters C (eds) Proceedings of the State-of-the-Art Strategic Planning Workshop-National Institutes of Health, Bethesda, Maryland 11–12 March 2002. Reprinted in 2003 Pediatr Nephrol 18:576–606

Ellsworth P, Sitnikova L (2005) Impact of prenatal ultrasonography in the detection, evaluation, management and outcome of genitourinary anomalies. AUA Update Ser 24:246–251

Farnham S, Adams M, Brock J, Pope J (2005) Pediatric urological causes of hypertension. J Urol 173:697–704

Fefer S, Ellsworth P (2006) Prenatal hydronephrosis. Pediatr Clin N Am 53:429–447

Ghanen M, Wolffenbuttel K, Vyler A, Njman R (2004) Long term bladder dysfunction and renal function in boys with posterior urethral valves based on urodynamic findings. J Urol 171:2409–2412

Gonzales R, Schimke CM (2001) Ureteropelvic junction obstruction in infants and children. Pediatr Clin N Am 46:1505–1518

Gran C, Kopp B, Cheng E, Kropp K (2005) Primary lower urinary tract reconstruction for nonfunctioning renal moieties associated with obstructing ureteroceles. J Urol 173:198–201

Grattan-Smith J, Jones R (2008) MR urography: technique and results for the evaluation of urinary obstruction in the pediatric population. Magn Reson Imaging Clin N Am 16:643–660

Grisoni E, Gaudere M, Wolfson R, Izant R (1986) Antenatal ultrasonography: the experience in a high risk perinatal center. J Pediatr Surg 21:358–361

Herd D (2008) Anxiety in children undergoing VCUG: sedation or no sedation? Adv Urol 498614 (online):1–9

Holmdahl G, Sillen U (2005) Boys with posterior urethral valves: outcome concerning renal function, bladder function and paternity at ages 31 to 44. J Urol 174:1031–1034

Huang W, Peters C, Zurakowski D, Borer J, Diamond D, Bauer S, McLellan M, Rosen S (2006) Renal biopsy in congenital ureteropelvic junction obstruction: evidence for parenchymal maldevelopment. Kidney Int 69:137–143

Husmann D, Ewalt D, Glenski W, Bernier P (1995) Ureterocele associated with ureteral duplication and a non functioning upper pole segment: management by partial nephoureterectomy alone. J Urol 154:723–726

Husmann D, Strand B, Ewalt D, Clement M, Kramer S, Allen T (1999) Management of ectopic ureterocele associated with renal duplication: a comparison of partial nephrectomy and endoscopic decompression. J Urol 162:1406–1409

Ismaili K, Avni F, Hall M, and for the Brussels Free University Perinatal Nephrology (BFUPN) Study Group (2002) Results of systematic voiding cystourethrography in infants with antenatally diagnosed renal pelvis dilation. J Pediatr 141:21–24

Ito K, Chen J, El Chaar M, Stern J, Seshan S, Khodadadian J, Richardson I, Hyman M, Vaughan E, Poppas D, Felsen D (2004) Renal damage progresses despite improvement of renal function after relief of unilateral ureteral obstruction in adult rats. Am J Physiol Ren Physiol 287:F1283–F1293

Jee L, Rickwood A, Williams M, Anderson P (1993) Experience with duplex system anomalies detected by prenatal ultrasonography. J Urol 149:808–810

Koff S, Campbell K (1992) Nonoperative management of unilateral neonatal hydronephrosis. J Urol 148:525–531

Lee BR, Silver RI, Partin AW, Epstein J, Gearhart J (1998) A quantitative histologic analysis of collagen subtypes: the primary obstructed and refluxing megaureter of childhood. Urology 51:820–823

Lim DJ, Park JY, Kim JH, Paick SH, Oh SJ, Choi H (2003) Clinical characteristics and outcomes of hydronephrosis detected by prenatal ultrasound. J Korean Med Soc 18:859–862

Liu H, Dhillon H, Yeung C, Diamond D, Duffy P, Ransley P (1994) Clinical outcomes and management of prenatally diagnosed primary megaureters. J Urol 152:614–617

McKenna P (2002) Epidemiology: incidence and prevalence in congenital urinary tract obstruction. In: Chevalier R, Peters C (eds) Proceedings of the State-of-the-Art Strategic Planning Workshop-National Institutes of Health, Bethesda, Maryland, 11–12 March 2002. Reprinted in Pediatr Nephrol 18:576–606

Mukherjee S, Joshi A, Carroll D, Chandran H, Parashar K, McCarthy L (2009) What is the effect of circumcision on risk of urinary tract infection in boys with posterior urethral valves? J Pediatr Surg 44:417–421

Nguyen H, Peters C (1999) The long-term complications of posterior urethral valves. Br J Urol Int 83(Supplement 3):23–28

Palmer L, Maizels M, Cartwright P, Fernbach S, Conway J (1998) Surgery versus observation for managing obstructive grade 3 to 4 unilateral hydronephrosis: report from the society of fetal urology. J Urol 159(1):222–228

Parkhouse H, Woodhouse C (1990) Long-term status of patients with posterior urethral valves. Urol Clin N Am 17:373–378

Peters C (1995) Urinary tract obstruction in children. J Urol 154:1874–1884

Peters C (1997) Obstruction of the fetal urinary tract. J Am Soc Nephrol 8:653–663

Podesta M, Ruarte A, Gargiulo C, Medel R, Castera R, Herrera M (2002) Bladder function associated with posterior urethral valves after primary valve ablation or proximal urinary diversion in children and adolescents. J Urol 168:1830–1835

Ransley P, Dhillon H, Duffy G, Dillon M, Barratt T (1990) The postnatal management of hydronephrosis diagnosed by prenatal ultrasound. J Urol 144:584–587

Rosen S, Peters C, Chevalier R, Huang W (2008) The kidney in congenital ureteropelvic junction obstruction: a spectrum from normal to nephrectomy. J Urol 179:1257–1263

Shekarriz B, Updhyay J, Fleming P, Gonzalez R, Barthold J (1999) Long term outcome based on the initial surgical approach to ureterocele. J Urol 162:1072–1076

Shi Y, Pedersen M, Li C, Wen J, Thomsen K, Stødkilde-Jørgensen H, Jørgensen T, Knepper M, Nielsen S, Djurhuus J, Frøkiaer J (2004) Early release of neonatal ureteral obstruction preserves renal function. Am J Physiol Ren Physiol 286:F1087–F1099

Shokeir A (2008) Role of urinary biomarkers in the diagnosis of congenital upper urinary tract obstruction. Indian J Urol 24:313–319

Shokeir A, Nijman R (2002) Ureterocele: an ongoing challenge in infancy and childhood. Br J Urol Int 90:777–783

Shukla A, Cooper J, Patel R, Carr M, Canning D, Zderic S, Snyder H (2005) Prenatally detected primary megaureter: a role for extended followup. J Urol 173:1353–1356

Singh-Grewal D, Macdessi J, Craig J (2005) Circumcision for the prevention of urinary tract infection in boys: a systematic review of randomized trials and observational studies. Arch Dis Child 90:853–858

Smith G, Canning D, Schulman S, Snyder H, Duckett J (1996) The long term outcome of posterior urethral valves treated with primary ablation and observation. J Urol 155:1730–1734

Tan BJ, Smith AD (2004) Ureteropelvic junction obstruction repair: when, how, what? Curr Opin Urol 14:55–59

Thornhill B, Burt L, Chen C, Forbes S, Chevalier R (2005) Variable chronic partial ureteral obstruction in the neonatal rat: a new model of ureteropelvic junction obstruction. Kidney Int 67:42–52

Ulman I, Jayanthi VR, Koff SA (2000) The long-term follow-up of newborns with severe unilateral hydronephrosis initially treated nonoperatively. J Urol 164:1101–1115

Wang G, Topeu S, Ring T, Wen J, Djurhuus JC, Kwon TH, Nielsen S, Frokiaer J (2009) Age dependent renal expression of acid-base transporters in neonatal ureter obstruction. Pediatr Nephrol 24: 1487–1500

Wiener JS, Emmert GK, Mesrobian HG, Whitehurst H, Smith R, King L (1995) Are modern imaging techniques over diagnosing ureteropelvic junction obstruction? J Urol 154:659–661

312 Acute Kidney Injury

Hui-Kim Yap

Definition

Acute renal failure occurs when there is a rapid decline in glomerular filtration rate, resulting in impairment of excretion of nitrogenous waste product, and loss of water and electrolyte regulation as well as acid-base regulation. This is reflected clinically by an abrupt increase in serum creatinine, and/or an abrupt decrease in urine output. Although oliguria, defined as urine volume less than 400 mL/m^2 per day, is common in acute renal failure, non-oliguric renal failure in which urine volume is normal is a well-recognized entity occurring in conditions such as aminoglycoside toxicity.

More recently, the Acute Kidney Injury Network (AKIN) proposed to use the term "acute kidney injury" (AKI) to redefine the entire spectrum of acute renal dysfunction, encompassing early and mild forms all the way to severe forms requiring renal replacement therapy. In adults, a classification system known as the RIFLE criteria, to define the severity of AKI, has been proposed by the Acute Dialysis Quality Intitiative. This defines risk, injury, and failure based on changes in serum creatinine and/or urine output, combined with the clinical outcome classes based on persistence of renal failure, namely, loss and end-stage kidney disease. Studies in the adult intensive care setting suggest that use of the RIFLE criteria conveys significant prognostic information, and may therefore aid in clinical decision making, especially the timing to institute renal replacement therapy. Similarly, modified criteria for pediatric patients have been proposed based on estimated creatinine clearances and urine output (➋ *Fig. 312.1*), although there are concerns regarding the validity of estimated glomerular filtration rates when plasma creatinine is not in equilibrium as is the case in AKI.

Etiology

Causes of acute kidney insufficiency in children can be broadly classified into pre-renal, renal, and post-renal causes (➋ *Table 312.1*).

Pre-renal vasomotor causes are potentially reversible if hypoperfusion can be corrected before tubular damage is established. Hypoperfusion may result from intravascular volume depletion as seen in blood loss, severe dehydration, or "third-spacing" in intestinal obstruction, as well as hypotension following sepsis or shock, and ineffective circulatory volume as in cardiac failure or states of severe hypoproteinemia. Failure to adequately reverse these predisposing conditions will result in hypoxic-ischemic AKI. Recognizing that various "toxins" can cause AKI is important, as there is evidence that preventive measures may be effective. These nephrotoxic compounds include intravascular radiocontrast agents, aminoglycoside antibiotics, amphotericin B, chemotherapeutic agents such as ifosfamide and cisplatin, acyclovir, acetaminophen, and calcineurin inhibitors.

Renal causes include the rapidly progressive forms of glomerulonephritis, including post-infectious glomerulonephritis, lupus nephritis, Henoch-Schönlein nephritis, membranoproliferative glomerulonephritis, anti-neutrophil cytoplasmic antibody-associated glomerulonephritis, and anti-glomerular basement membrane disease. Thrombosis of the renal vessels, especially in the critically ill neonate, may lead to AKI. Hemolytic-uremic syndrome which may follow diarrheal illnesses or pneumococcal infection is not uncommon in young children. Other renal causes include acute pyelonephritis; acute tubulointerstitial nephritis, which may be secondary to infections or drugs such as ampicillin; and tumor infiltration such as that seen in lymphoid malignancies.

In tropical countries, infections such as falciparum malaria which cause pigment injury secondary to intravascular hemolysis, and leptospirosis associated with hepatorenal failure, are important causes of AKI. Additionally, in populations where glucose-6-phosphate dehydrogenase deficiency is prevalent, drug-induced acute intravascular hemolysis may result in renal failure. Heat stroke and exercise-induced rhabdomyolysis must be considered in adolescents presenting with AKI.

Post-renal causes especially obstructive uropathies should be excluded as these are potentially reversible causes of AKI. Bladder outlet obstruction, such as that seen in posterior urethral valves in boys and neurogenic bladder, is an important cause. Ureteral obstruction of a single functioning kidney must be considered, unless

Abdelaziz Y. Elzouki (ed.), *Textbook of Clinical Pediatrics*, DOI 10.1007/978-3-642-02202-9_312,

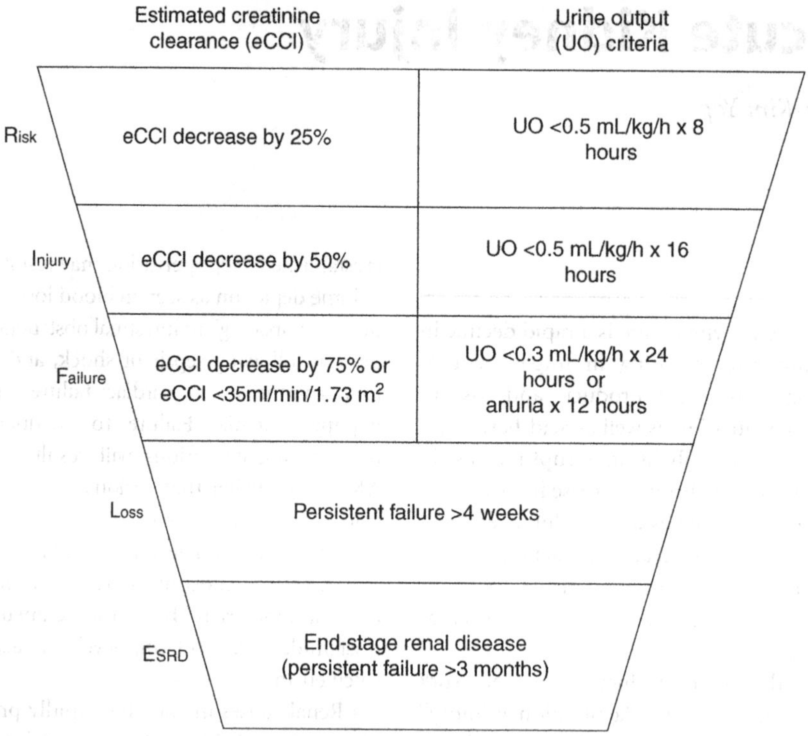

Figure 312.1
The pediatric-modified RIFLE (pRIFLE) criteria for the diagnosis of AKI. RIFLE: Risk, Injury, and Failure with the outcome classes Loss and End-stage kidney disease (Modified from Ackan-Arikan A et al., Kidney Int 10:963–964)

Table 312.1
Causes of acute kidney injury in children

Pre-renal (vasomotor nephropathy)	Renal	Post-renal
Ischemic • Hypovolemia including hemorrhage, gastrointestinal losses, burns, renal salt-wasting conditions • Hypotension • Hypoxia • Cardiac failure • Sepsis • Intestinal obstruction • Hepatorenal syndrome Toxic • Aminoglycosides • Wasp sting • Plant toxins • Snake-bite • Pigments eg hemoglobin or myoglobin • Radiocontrast agents	Glomerulonephritis (GN) • Post-infectious GN • Systemic lupus erythematosus • Henoch-Schönlein nephritis • Membranoproliferative GN • Anti-neutrophil cytoplasmic antibody-associated GN • Anti-glomerular basement membrane disease • Idiopathic rapidly progressive GN Vascular • Hemolytic-uremic syndrome • Renal artery thrombosis • Renal vein thrombosis Acute tubulointerstitial nephritis • Infections, e.g., Ebstein Barr virus and leptospirosis • Drugs including herbal preparations Acute pyelonephritis Tumor infiltration	Structural • Posterior urethral valve • Ureteric obstruction • Neurogenic bladder Crystalluria • Tumor lysis syndrome • Melamine Calculi Blood clot

obstruction occurs bilaterally. Another cause of significant obstruction in children is crystal precipitation in the renal tubules. Children with acute lymphoblastic leukemia and B-cell lymphoma are at the highest risk of AKI due to tumor lysis syndrome following chemotherapy. This results in tubular precipitation of uric acid crystals and its precursors, xanthine and hypoxanthine, as well as calcium phosphate crystals.

Epidemiology

Epidemiological data on the incidence and prevalence of AKI in children is difficult to ascertain. A retrospective review from England estimated a yearly incidence for AKI in children as 0.8 per 100,000 population. Geographic differences in the causes of AKI do exist (➲ *Fig. 312.2*). In developing countries, primary renal diseases such as post-infectious glomerulonephritis and hemolytic-uremic syndrome are important causes of AKI. Although survival is generally better in children with primary renal disease, lack of access to medical care coupled with the poor socio-economic conditions in these countries contribute to the poor outcomes in these patients. Unfortunately the real tragedy in these areas is that AKI secondary to pre-renal causes such as gastroenteritis would have been preventable if they were able to have timely volume replacement.

Recent pediatric AKI epidemiological data for critically ill children demonstrate a shift from primary renal disease to injury secondary to other systemic illnesses and/or their treatment. With the development of pediatric intensive care in tertiary hospitals catering for specialties such as cardiac surgery, oncology, and solid organ and bone marrow transplant, a larger proportion of pediatric AKI is due to ischemic or toxic injury (➲ *Fig. 312.2*). The mortality in this group of infants and children is higher, ranging from 33% to 78%, due to the concomitant presence of multiorgan failure. The most important predictors

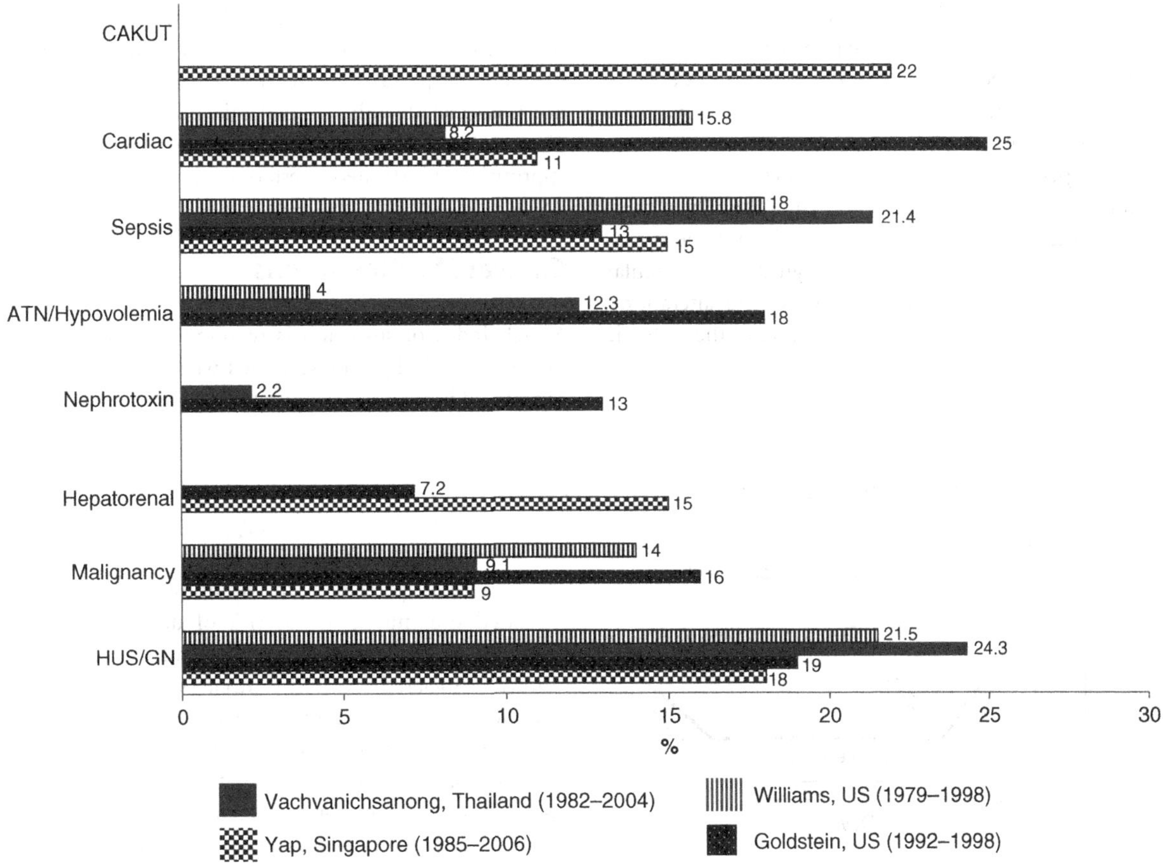

Figure 312.2
Causes of AKI worldwide. CAKUT: congenital abnormalities of the kidney and urinary tract. ATN: acute tubular necrosis

of mortality among these critically ill children include the severity of the underlying systemic illness, hemodynamic stability, and the degree of fluid overload at initiation of renal replacement therapy.

Similarly AKI affects approximately 8–24% of severely ill newborns treated in the neonatal ICU, with a mortality rate of between 10% and 61%. Data from the literature suggest that the incidence of AKI in asphyxiated newborns is high, and portends a poor outcome. Other factors associated with development of AKI in neonates include very low birth weight (less than 1,500 g), a low Apgar score, persistent arterial duct, and maternal use of antibiotics and nonsteroidal anti-inflammatory drugs.

Pathogenesis

Molitoris proposed a mechanistic classification that delineates four distinct phases in AKI: initiation, extension, maintenance, and recovery (➋ *Fig. 312.3*). In the "initiation phase," numerous ischemic insults, alone or in synergistic combination with nephrotoxins, initiate epithelial and vascular cell injury, resulting in patchy tubular necrosis and a rapid decline in glomerular filtration rate. Hypoxic or ischemic AKI is characterized by early vasoconstriction followed by patchy tubular necrosis. Following reperfusion, loss of endothelial cell function with distorted peritubular pericapillary morphology occurs. Possible mechanisms of cellular injury include perturbation in endothelin or nitric oxide regulation of vascular tone, ATP depletion with resultant cytoskeletal alterations, changes in heat shock proteins, induction of the systemic inflammatory response, and the generation of reactive oxygen and nitrogen molecules.

The "extension phase" immediately follows the "initiation phase," where multiple interrelated events lead to a worsening of epithelial and endothelial cell injury and cell death, primarily in the cortico-medullary region. A phase of stabilization of injury known as the "maintenance phase" precedes the "recovery phase" where cellular repair, division, and redifferentiation occurs, resulting in improved epithelial and endothelial cell function and recovery of the glomerular filtration rate. Previously, it was thought that recovery from hypoxic-ischemic and nephrotoxic AKI was complete with normalization of renal function; however, recent studies have shown that recovery may be partial and patients may be at higher risk for chronic kidney disease.

This pathogenetic concept provides an important framework upon which therapy can be based. (➋ *Fig. 312.3*). Utilizing this approach, it is easy to understand why studies that initiate therapy during the maintenance phase have proven uniformly unsuccessful. On the other hand, significant progress has been made in the prevention of ischemic AKI, especially with regards to the high-risk population, defined as children with conditions associated with hypovolemia or underlying renal disease. Finally, renal replacement therapy should be appropriately instituted in established AKI.

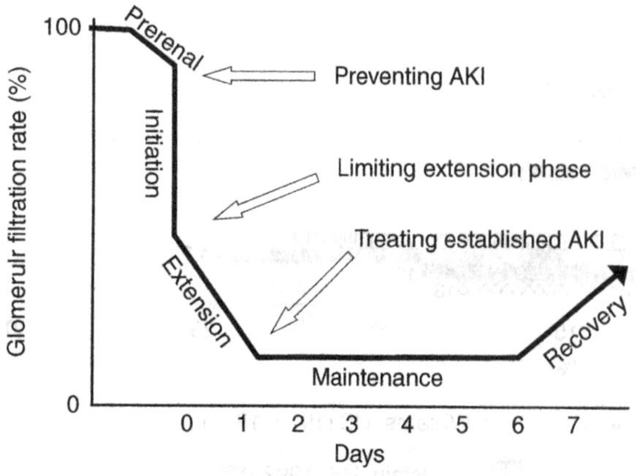

Figure 312.3
Mechanistic basis for the treatment of AKI (Modified from Molitoris J (2003) J Am Soc Nephrol 14:265–267)

Clinical Manifestations

A high index of suspicion is required to diagnose AKI. There are typically four scenarios where AKI should be considered in infants or children with oliguria.

Children Presenting with Conditions Associated with Severe Hypovolemia

Children who present with vomiting, diarrhea, and decreased oral intake are at risk of developing severe hypovolemia and AKI. On the other hand, in some conditions associated with polyuria, such as diabetic ketoacidosis, renal tubular acidosis and chronic tubulopathies, these children can develop severe hypovolemia and pre-renal AKI if their fluid intake is insufficient for any reason to keep up with the urine loss. Physical signs of hypovolemia are prominent, such as tachycardia, poor capillary refill, decreased skin turgor, dry mucous membranes, sunken eyes, and orthostatic blood pressure changes.

Children Presenting Acutely with Symptoms Suggestive of Renal Disease

Acute onset of oliguria, edema, and gross hematuria, with a preceding history of pharyngitis or impetigo, is consistent with post-infectious glomerulonephritis, where AKI requiring dialysis occurs in less than 1%. Bloody diarrhea with oliguria or anuria suggests diarrhea-associated hemolytic-uremic syndrome, whereas in children with pneumonia, development of oliguria accompanied by anemia and thrombocytopenia is indicative of pneumonia-associated hemolytic-uremic syndrome. In children with nephrotic syndrome, AKI though uncommon, should be suspected if there is severe hypovolemia with hypotension and tachycardia, accompanied by marked decrease in urine output. Systemic signs and symptoms of vasculitis, such as purpuric or malar rash, joint pain or swelling, and hemoptysis, suggest the possibility of rapidly progressive glomerulonephritis associated with systemic vasculitis.

Critically Ill Children with Predisposing Factors for Multiorgan Failure

Critically ill children with sepsis and hypotension frequently have multiorgan failure resulting in AKI with oligoanuria, especially with the use of inotropes such as noradrenaline or adrenaline. Often these children are immunosuppressed or neutropenic such as in oncology patients undergoing chemotherapy or bone marrow transplantation. A history of nephrotoxic medications is often present, including antibiotics such as aminoglycosides or amphotericin-B, chemotherapeutic agents such as cisplastin, and calcineurin inhibitors.

Newborn Infants with Oliguria or Anuria

Oliguria in the newborn beyond 72 h is worrying and should be investigated. In the absence of ischemic injury, anuria or oliguria suggests a major congenital malformation such as posterior urethral valves, or genetic disease such as autosomal recessive polycystic kidney disease. In the sick neonate with hematuria, bilateral renal vein thrombosis should be suspected.

Diagnostic Approach

The modified RIFLE criteria for pediatric patients (➋ *Fig. 312.1*) will help in standardizing the definition of AKI so that the appropriate therapeutic decisions can be made. These criteria are based importantly on either the degree of oliguria over a timed period or a change in the estimated creatinine clearance.

Having defined the presence of AKI, the next step is to differentiate the various causes using several noninvasive methods. Early diagnosis of pre-renal and obstructive causes is important as prompt corrective measures may prevent the onset of established renal injury.

Urinary Sediment

The urinary sediment should be examined for the presence of cells, crystals, cellular debris, and casts. The presence of hematuria associated with dysmorphic red cells and red cell casts suggests a diagnosis of glomerulonephritis, while renal tubular epithelial cells, tubular cell casts, or coarsely granular pigmented casts suggest acute tubular necrosis. Pyuria may suggest pyelonephritis, although tubulointerstitial disorders may present with sterile pyuria. Moreover, the presence of eosinophils is highly suggestive of acute allergic interstitial nephritis. Crystals in the urine such as uric acid or calcium oxalate crystals may be useful indicators of the underlying etiology in the appropriate clinical setting with AKI, namely, tumor lysis syndrome and ethylene glycol poisoning, respectively. If there are scant findings on microscopy examination of the urine, this may be consistent with pre-renal or obstructive causes of AKI.

Blood and Urinary Indices to Differentiate Between Pre-renal and Established Renal Failure

Blood and urinary indices used to differentiate between pre-renal and established acute renal failure are based on the premise that the proximal renal tubular transport mechanisms are still able to respond to the hypovolemic stimulus in pre-renal failure, as compared to the failure of these transport mechanisms in acute tubular necrosis. The serum urea/creatinine ratio has been used to distinguish between pre-renal and established renal failure, in older children and adolescents with hypovolemia. This ratio is usually high in pre-renal disease due to increased urea reabsorption following enhanced proximal transport of sodium and water. A ratio greater than 20:1 for urea and creatinine measured in mg/dL or 0.10 for urea measured in mmol/L and creatinine in μmol/L is seen in pre-renal disease. Unfortunately, in conditions of increased catabolism, gastrointestinal hemorrhage and corticosteroid administration, the ratio can be elevated. Conversely, a normal ratio can be seen in liver disease or protein malnutrition.

Urinary indices derived from measurements on simultaneous random urine and plasma specimens, in the absence of diuretic use, can help differentiate pre-renal versus established renal failure (➋ *Table 312.2*). In hypovolemia, there is marked urinary sodium reabsorption and concentration of the urine, whereas in irreversible tubular injury, the tubules are unable to appropriately conserve sodium. As urinary sodium concentration can also be low as a result of dilution, the fractional excretion of sodium (FeNa) is a better index to take into account renal water handling. In conditions where there is relative renal hypoperfusion such as hypovolemic dehydration, nephrotic syndrome, congestive cardiac failure, or cirrhosis, the FeNa is less than 1%. In contrast, tubular damage results in FeNa ranging from 2% to 3%. As the renal tubules in newborns are relatively immature compared to older infants and children, the corresponding FeNa in newborns with hypovolemia is less than 2.5%. However, in patients given diuretics, and in salt-losing conditions, such as Bartter's syndrome, interstitial nephritis, and chronic renal disease, urinary sodium may be high, thus obviating the value of indices based on urinary sodium excretion. In these situations, the fractional excretion of urea (FeUN) has been proposed as a better index to distinguish between pre-renal failure and established tubular necrosis. The FeUN should be less than 35% in conditions of hypovolemia, whereas in acute tubular necrosis, the value is greater than 50%.

Table 312.2
Use of urinary indices to differentiate pre-renal and intrinsic renal causes of AKI

	Pre-renal cause*	Intrinsic renal cause*
Urine sodium (mmol/L)	<20 (<20)	>40 (>50)
Urine osmolality (mOsm/kg)	>500 (>400)	<350 (<400)
Urine/plasma urea	>8	<3
Urine/plasma osmolality	>1.15 (>1.2)	<1.1 (<1.2)
Urine/plasma creatinine	>40	<20
Fractional sodium excretion (FeNa)	<1 (<2.5)	>1 (>2.5)
Fractional urea excretion (FeUN)	<35%	>50%

FeNa = (urine sodium/plasma sodium) × (plasma creatinine/urine creatinine) × 100%
FeUN = (urine urea/plasma urea) × (plasma creatinine/urine creatinine) × 100%
These indices must be used with caution in premature neonates less than 32 weeks gestation, since a high urinary sodium excretion is commonly observed
*Values in parenthesis are the criteria for neonates

Other Laboratory Tests

Other laboratory tests may provide some clues as to the underlying etiology of the AKI. The complete blood count is important to look for anemia and thrombocytopenia, suggestive of hemolytic-uremic syndrome or a vasculitis-associated glomerulonephritis. The peripheral blood smear should also be done to look for schistocytes in hemolytic-uremic syndrome, or spherocytes in lupus nephritis. The urine should be tested for hemoglobin or myoglobin to exclude pigment nephropathy, if the history is suggestive of intravascular hemolysis or rhabdomyolysis. Decreased serum complement levels (C3 with or without C4), elevated anti-nuclear antibodies, anti-neutrophil cytoplasmic antibodies, and anti-glomerular basement membrane antibodies are useful to distinguish the various glomerular diseases resulting in AKI. The serum complement C3 is low at presentation in post-infectious glomerulonephritis, lupus nephritis, and membranoproliferative glomerulonephritis. Specific patterns of biochemical abnormalities may be seen in certain causes of AKI. Hypocalcemia, hyperphosphatemia, and hyperuricemia occur in tumor lysis syndrome, while in rhabdomyolysis, there is additional elevation of the serum creatine kinase levels. An increase in anion and osmolar gaps in the presence of AKI is suggestive of ethylene glycol poisoning.

Novel Biomarkers of AKI

Serum creatinine is a poor marker of early renal dysfunction, especially in AKI where the patients are not in steady state. Substantial elevation in serum creatinine is often not witnessed until 48–72 h after the initial insult to the kidney. The tools of modern science have provided promising novel plasma and urinary biomarkers for AKI, with potentially high sensitivity and specificity. These include a plasma panel comprising neutrophil gelatinase-associated lipocalin (NGAL) and cystatin C, and a urine panel comprising NGAL, interleukin-18 (IL-18), and kidney injury molecule-1 (KIM-1).

Cystatin C is a cysteine protease inhibitor that is produced at a constant rate, freely filtered by the kidneys, and is almost completely reabsorbed by the proximal renal tubular cells. Prospective studies have shown that an increase in cystatin C levels occurred 1½ days before AKI developed.

Circulating NGAL is normally reabsorbed in the proximal tubule. Following kidney injury, NGAL is secreted in the thick ascending limb of the loop of Henle, and is found in the urine, and the NGAL protein is detected in the blood and urine very early in the course of AKI. In a prospective study of children undergoing cardiopulmonary bypass, plasma and urinary NGAL levels were elevated within 2–6 h of surgery, and was able to predict the development of AKI, compared to serum creatinine levels which rose by at least 50% only 1–3 days after surgery. However, NGAL is also increased in infections, inflammatory conditions, and malignancies, and thus may have limited value in predicting AKI in these clinical situations.

Urinary IL-18 is a pro-inflammatory cytokine that is induced and cleaved in the proximal tubule. It is detected in the urine following ischemic AKI, but not in chronic kidney disease, urinary tract infections, nephrotic syndrome, or pre-renal failure. In the intensive care setting, urine IL-18 measurements were able to predict AKI about 2 days prior to the rise in serum creatinine, and was an independent predictor of mortality in these critically ill children with AKI.

KIM-1 is a type 1 transmembrane protein that is not detectable in normal kidney tissue or urine, but is expressed at very high levels in dedifferentiated proximal tubule epithelial cells in human kidneys after ischemic or toxic injury. Earlier studies have shown that KIM-1 measurement was able to distinguish between ischemic AKI from pre-renal azotemia and chronic kidney disease. More recently, urinary KIM-1 levels were shown to be predictive of AKI in children undergoing cardiopulmonary bypass. In fact, urinary KIM-1 performed best as an early marker of AKI compared to other urinary biomarkers such as N-acetyl-beta-D-glucosaminidase (NAG), NGAL, IL-18, cystatin C, and alpha-1 microglobulin. However, urinary KIM-1 measurements may be also induced in a variety of chronic proteinuric, inflammatory, and fibrotic disease states, as well as upregulated by nephrotoxins, including cyclosporine, cisplatin, and gentamicin, thus limiting its value in predicting AKI in the presence of these confounding factors.

Imaging

Imaging of the urinary tract is important in the diagnostic workup of children with AKI, as it is crucial for the exclusion of obstructive uropathies. In addition, assessment of kidney size is a useful indicator of the chronicity of the renal failure. Enlarged kidneys standardized to patient's age and size is suggestive of AKI, whereas small contracted kidneys suggest chronic renal failure. These imaging modalities include ultrasonography, CT urogram, radionuclide imaging, magnetic resonance imaging, and, occasionally, plain film of the abdomen.

Ultrasonography should be the initial imaging modality in the diagnostic workup of children with AKI to detect bilateral upper tract obstruction, bladder outlet obstruction, or obstruction of a solitary functioning kidney. Dilatation of the pelvicalyceal system can be detected within 24–36 h of the onset of acute urinary obstruction. It is important to realize that dilatation of the upper tract may not be seen in the acute stage of ureteral obstruction if this is accompanied by a decrease in urine output. In lower tract obstruction, ureteral dilatation, bladder size, and wall hypertrophy, as well as the presence of associated lesions such as ureterocele can be identified by ultrasonography. An increase in echogenicity is seen in both acute and chronic kidney disease. In neonates with renal vein thrombosis, Doppler flow scanning will be able to demonstrate decreased blood flow.

Radionuclide imaging using ^{99m}Tc mercaptoacetyltriglycine (MAG3) or ^{131}I-iodohippurate is used to assess blood flow and the severity of functional obstruction. Noncontrast CT scans are able to demonstrate the renal pelvis and proximal ureter, and may be helpful in identifying sites of ureteral obstruction, stones, tumors, or congenital abnormalities. Contrast-enhanced scans will add functional information of the individual kidney; however, this should be avoided in AKI due to the risk of contrast nephropathy. Magnetic resonance urogram, both static and gadolinium enhanced, is a useful study to identify collecting system morphology in obstructive uropathies, regardless of excretory fuction. Unfortunately, infants and young children require sedation for this study. Moreover, the risk of nephrogenic systemic fibrosis following gadolinium-based contrast agents in patients with renal failure limits the use of the dynamic scan in AKI.

Renal Biopsy

Renal biopsy should be considered if there is clinical suspicion of a rapidly progressive form of glomerulonephritis or acute allergic interstitial nephritis. A definitive histological diagnosis in these instances will be important as immunosuppressive therapy can alter the outcome of the disease.

Clinical Management

Medical Management

The main aim in managing AKI is to maintain homeostasis, while awaiting improvement in renal function, either spontaneously or while the underlying cause is being treated. Because of the availability and efficacy of dialysis, patients with AKI often succumb not due to AKI, but to other comorbidities. The main goals in medical management are therefore to maintain adequate renal perfusion, prevent fluid overload and hypertension, maintain normal electrolytes and acid-base status, and ensure adequate nutrition.

Maintaining Adequate Renal Perfusion

In severely ill patients who are at risk of ischemic AKI, correction of pre-renal factors such as dehydration, poor cardiac output, hypovolemia, and acid-base and electrolyte abnormalities is important to prevent development of AKI (➋ *Fig. 312.4*). Unless contraindicated due to fluid overload or cardiac failure, a child with clinical evidence of hypovolemia and oliguria should be administered an intravenous fluid challenge over 20–30 min, with either crystalloid solutions such as normal saline (10–20 mL/kg) or colloid solutions such as 5% albumin if hypotensive. This can be repeated if the child is still hypovolemic. Restoration of adequate urine flow and improvement in renal function with fluid resuscitation is consistent with pre-renal disease. However, if urine output does not increase and renal function fails to improve with

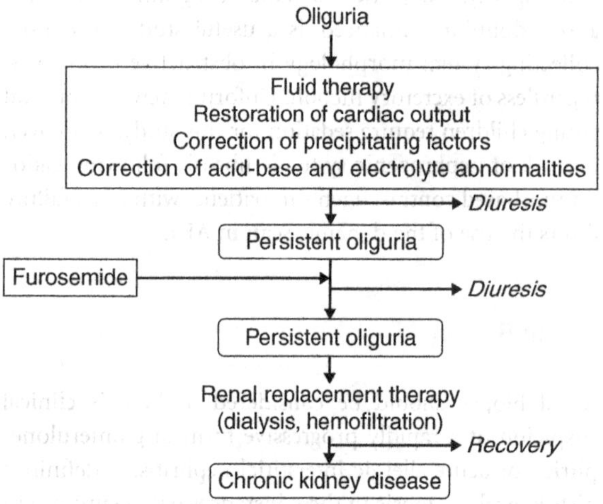

Figure 312.4
Algorithm for intervention in vasomotor nephropathy

restoration of intravascular volume, invasive monitoring may be required to adequately assess the child's fluid status and help guide further therapy.

If oliguria persists despite adequate correction of pre-renal factors, a trial of loop diuretics such as furosemide (2–5 mg/kg) may be attempted to promote diuresis, converting the child from oliguric to non-oliguric renal failure, thus facilitating fluid balance without the need for dialysis. Low dose dopamine infusion (1–5 mcg/kg per hour) is thought to promote renal vasodilatation, however, the evidence that this has a beneficial effect in limiting or preventing established AKI is lacking. Fenoldopam, a potent, short-acting, selective, dopamine-1 receptor agonist that decreases vascular resistance while increasing renal blood flow, has been shown in a meta-analysis to decrease the incidence of AKI and the need for renal replacement therapy in critically ill adults. Although there are some good results with its use in children, additional studies need to be performed to determine its value. On the other hand, use of vasoactive agents in hypotensive patients to maintain adequate blood pressure may improve renal perfusion.

Preventing Fluid Overload and Hypertension

In general, infants and children with AKI are not severely uremic, but their major problem is fluid overload following oliguria or anuria. Fluid overload is potentially fatal in AKI due to pulmonary edema, and the first line of treatment in these oliguric or anuric patients is fluid restriction and intravenous diuretics. Fluid volume should be restricted to insensible water loss calculated at 400 mL/m^2 per day, in addition to replacing urine, gastrointestinal, and other losses. Therapy should be aimed at decreasing the body weight by 0.5–1% daily.

Fluid overload may aggravate hypertension in patients with glomerulonephritis, resulting in hypertensive urgencies or emergencies. These children are symptomatic with complaints of nausea, headache, and blurred vision. Uncontrolled hypertension often leads to acute end-organ injury such as posterior reversible encephalopathy syndrome with altered mental state and seizures, cerebral infarction, cerebral hemorrhage, left heart failure, and grade III–IV retinopathy with exudates, hemorrhage, and papilledema. It is important to treat these hypertensive emergencies with intravenous antihypertensive agents that can produce a controlled reduction of blood pressure in order to avoid worsening of the cerebral edema due to disruption of cerebral autoregulation.

Maintaining Normal Electrolytes and Acid-Base Status

The common electrolyte disorders in AKI are hyperkalemia, hyponatraemia, hypocalcemia, and hyperphosphatemia. Hyperkalemic emergencies, where serum potassium levels are greater than 7 mmol/L accompanied by electrocardiographic changes such as peaked T waves, flattened P waves, increased PR interval, and widening of the QRS complex, can be managed with intravenous calcium (0.5 mL/kg up to a maximum of 20 mg given slowly over 15 min) to stabilize the cardiac membrane, followed by nebulized (2.5 mg for body weight less than 25 kg or 5 mg for body weight 25 kg or more) or intravenous salbutamol (4 mg/kg) or intravenous insulin (1 IU/5 g dextrose) and dextrose (0.5 g/kg) to temporarily lower the serum potassium levels, prior to dialysis. Less urgent elevations of serum potassium (6–7 mmol/L) can be managed with oral or rectal kayexylate (1 g/kg to a maximum of 30 g) or other ion exchangers, and correction of concomitant acidosis. Hyponatraemia due to fluid overload can be corrected with fluid restriction and loop diuretics. If there is renal salt wasting, then sodium supplementation may be necessary. Hypocalcemia and hyperphosphatemia can be managed with calcium-based phosphate binders. Severe metabolic acidosis where serum bicarbonate is less than 15 mmol/L or pH less than 7.2 may be corrected with oral sodium citrate or intravenous sodium bicarbonate. The latter has the adverse effect of hypernatremia, and exacerbating fluid overload, necessitating dialysis.

Ensuring Adequate Nutrition

Ensuring adequate nutrition is often a real challenge in the critically ill patient. Energy balance studies on patients with AKI have demonstrated that cumulative energy deficits are associated with increased mortality. In infants and children with AKI, given their limited reserves, these nutritional issues will be further amplified. Because of the necessity for fluid restriction, increasing the concentration of the enteral feeds or parenteral hyperalimentation will improve caloric delivery. However, this is often limited by the consequent increase in osmolarity of the feeds. Early institution of dialysis will allow better optimization of nutrition in these patients.

Acute Renal Replacement Therapy

The traditional indications for renal replacement therapy in AKI include severe hyperkalemia unresponsive to conservative therapy, uncontrolled acidosis that cannot be safely corrected because of risk of sodium or volume overload, severe volume overload with uncontrolled hypertension, pulmonary edema or cardiac failure, progressive uremia with deterioration in the general condition, and hypercatabolic states with increase in blood urea by greater than 10 mmol/L per day.

The critically ill child is often on a downward spiral, with sepsis, shock, acute respiratory distress syndrome, often leading to multiorgan failure which forms the final common pathway of lethal infective and non-infective complications. In this setting, where there is hypotension, effective hypovolemia, hypoxemia, hypercapnia, and hypothermia, coupled with the use of a multitude of vasoactive and nephrotoxic drugs, AKI is inevitable. This is often associated with a poor outcome. In general, these children may not be severely uremic, but their major problem is fluid overload and electrolyte perturbations especially acidosis, hyponatremia, and hyperkalemia. Conservative management with severe fluid restriction is not the answer, as this has its attendant problems of inadequate nutrition, propensity to hypoglycemia, insufficient volume space for blood products, and difficulty in drug delivery, such as inotropic support and antibiotic infusions. Therefore, early institution of dialysis is important in these critically ill children with AKI to maintain homeostasis and create enough volume space so that the nutritional and therapeutic needs may be met.

There are various strategies for the dialytic treatment of children with AKI, including peritoneal dialysis (PD), intermittent hemodialysis (HD), and continuous renal replacement therapy (CRRT). Choice of dialysis modality is largely influenced by the age and size of the child or infant, clinical presentation, presence or absence of multiorgan system failure, indication for renal replacement therapy, experience of the center, and the available resources (➋ *Table 312.3*).

Acute Peritoneal Dialysis

Acute PD is still the modality of choice in many countries, especially in the developing world. It is a relatively cheap form of dialysis, and does not require sophisticated equipment or complicated technical expertise. Acute PD is associated with less hemodynamic instability, and has the advantage of avoiding the need for vascular access and blood priming. It can be done in very young infants, and does not require anticoagulation in the child with disseminated intravascular coagulopathy.

Table 312.3
Comparison of different dialytic modalities in AKI

Variable	PD	HD	CRRT
Continuous therapy	Yes	No	Yes
Hemodynamic stability	Yes	No	Yes
Fluid balance achieved	Variable	Yes (intermittent)	Yes
Optimal nutrition	No	No	Yes
Metabolic control	Yes	Yes (intermittent)	Yes
Easy to perform	Yes	No	No
Anticoagulation	Not required	Heparin anticoagulation or heparin free	Heparin or citrate anticoagulation
Vascular access required	No	Yes	Yes

Although PD has certain advantages over filter dependent procedures, there are several problems that make PD difficult especially in the small infant. Catheter problems are common such as leakage into the subcutaneous tissue and hernia sites, especially inguinal. Drainage is frequently a problem because of catheter malposition, kinking, omental wrapping, and fibrin clot. In young infants, it is often not possible to increase the dwell to the desired volume due to splinting of the diaphragm in the critically ill infants with acute respiratory distress syndrome. The slow and relatively inefficient removal of all types of molecules, as well as unreliable ultrafiltration, represents a considerable drawback compared to other modalities of acute dialysis, especially in patients with hypotension and poor peritoneal perfusion. Hence, acute PD may not provide adequate clearances in the hypercatabolic patient with severe hyperkalemia and hyperphosphatemia. Moreover, acute PD is contraindicated in patients with recent abdominal surgery, necrotizing enterocolitis, and presence of ventriculo-peritoneal shunts. Therefore acute PD is currently best for "uncomplicated" or medical causes of AKI.

Intermittent Hemodialysis

Intermittent HD is still the mainstay of dialysis for AKI in older children and is performed in adult centers in many countries. Its main advantage is the rapid removal of uremic toxins and fluid volume. Therefore it is indicated in the emergency treatment of hyperkalemia, lactic acidosis and myoglobinuria. However, HD in young children is notoriously difficult in view of the smaller blood volumes. This is especially accentuated in the critically ill child, where inotropes are usually required to support the systemic blood pressure. Moreover, these children often have acute respiratory distress syndrome, and are hypoxemic, resulting in hemodynamic instability during intermittent HD. Rapid HD may also result in dialysis dysequilibrium. In view of the difficulties of HD in the critically ill pediatric patient, this dialytic modality is generally limited to children with "uncomplicated" AKI.

Continuous Renal Replacement Therapy (CRRT)

This decade has seen much enthusiasm for the use of CRRT for the critically ill child. CRRT encompasses a wide range of strategies, which include slow continuous ultrafiltration, continuous venovenous hemofiltration, continuous venovenous hemodialysis, to a combination of continuous venovenous hemodiafiltration. There are many advantages of continuous modalities of dialysis in the critically ill patient. Despite removal of large volumes of fluid by ultrafiltration, the critically ill patient on CRRT remains hemodynamically stable. In a large randomized controlled trial comparing CRRT with intermittent HD in critically ill patients, CRRT resulted in more efficacious solute clearances. Studies have also shown that inflammatory mediators, cytokines, and toxins may be removed by continuous hemofiltration in patients with sepsis, not only by adsorption to certain hemofilter membranes, but also through the ultrafiltrate, providing a rationale for the use of high volume ultrafiltration.

Some of the disadvantages of CRRT include bleeding complications following the use of heparin. Citrate anticoagulation is now widely used to circumvent this problem. Other problems include temperature instability, requiring warming of either the dialysate or blood returning to the patient. Small molecular sized nutrients such as oligosaccharides, peptides, and amino acids, and electrolytes such as phosphate and magnesium can be lost through the hemofilter, and therefore need to be replaced. The bradykinin release syndrome is an important complication seen specifically with the commonly used polyacrylonitrile (AN69) membranes. Blood contact with the AN69 membrane results in generation of bradykinin, especially in the presence of acidosis. Hence priming of the dialysis lines with banked blood should be avoided.

Prognosis

The prognosis of AKI is highly dependent on the underlying etiology. Mortality is high in critically ill children with multiorgan failure. Recovery from intrinsic renal disease is also highly dependent on the underlying etiology. Children with nephrotoxic AKI and hypoxic/ischemic AKI usually recover normal renal function; however, those who have suffered substantial nephron loss, such as in hemolytic-uremic syndrome or rapidly progressive glomerulonephritis, may progress to chronic kidney disease. Therefore these children need to be followed up in the long-term for blood pressure monitoring and development of proteinuria.

References

Ackan-Arikan A, Zappitelli M, Loftis LL, Washburn KK, Jefferson LS, Goldstein SL (2007) Modified RIFLE criteria in critically ill children with acute kidney injury. Kidney Int 10:1028–1035

Agarwal R, Brunelli SM, Williams K, Mitchell MD, Feldman HI, Umscheid CA (2009) Gadolinium-based contrast agents and nephrogenic systemic fibrosis: a systematic review and meta-analysis. Nephrol Dial Transplant 24:856–863

Andreoli SP (1991) Reactive oxygen molecules, oxidant injury and renal disease. Pediatr Nephrol 5:733–742

Andreoli SP (2004) Acute renal failure in the newborn. Semin Perinatol 8:112–123

Andreoli SP (2009) Acute kidney injury in children. Pediatr Nephrol 24:253–263

Andreoli SP, McAteer JA (1990) Reactive oxygen molecule mediated injury in endothelial cells and renal tubular epithelial cells in vitro. Kidney Int 38:785–794

Askenazi DJ, Feig DI, Graham NM, Hui-Stickle S, Goldstein S (2006) 1–5 year longitudinal follow-up of pediatric patients after acute renal failure. Kidney Int 69:184–189

Basile DP (2007) The endothelial cell in ischemic acute kidney injury: implications for acute and chronic function. Kidney Int 72: 151–156

Bellomo R, Ronco C, Kellum JA, Mehta RL, Palevsky P (2004) Acute Dialysis Quality Initiative workgroup. Acute renal failure – definition, outcome measures, animal models, fluid therapy and information technology needs: the second international consensus conference of the Acute Dialysis Quality Initiative (ADQI) Group. Crit Care 28:R204–R212

Bellomo R, Kellum JA, Ronco C (2007) Defining and classifying acute renal failure: from advocacy to consensus and validation of the RIFLE criteria. Intensive Care Med 33:409–413

Brivet FG, Kleinknecht DJ, Loirat P, Landais PJ (1996) Acute renal failure in intensive care units – causes, outcome, and prognostic factors of hospital mortality: a prospective, multicenter study. Crit Care Med 24:192–198

Brophy PD, Mottes TA, Kudelka TL, McBryde KD, Gardner JJ, Maxvold NJ, Bunchman TE (2001) AN-69 membrane reactions are pH-dependent and preventable. Am J Kidney Dis 38:173–178

Bunchmann TE, McBryde KD, Mottes TE, Gardner JJ, Maxvold NJ, Brophy PD (2001) Pediatric acute renal failure: outcome by modality and disease. Pediatr Nephrol 16:1067–1071

Carvounis CP, Nisar S, Guro-Razuman S (2002) Significance of the fractional excretion of urea in the differential diagnosis of acute renal failure. Kidney Int 62:2223–2229

Cataldi L, Leone R, Moretti U, De Mitri B, Fanos V, Ruggeri L, Sabatino G, Torcasio F, Zanardo V, Attardo G, Riccobene F, Martano C, Benini D, Cuzzolin L (2005) Potential risk factors for the development of acute renal failure in preterm newborn infants: a case controlled study. Arch Dis Child Fetal Neonatal Ed 90:514–519

Coca1 SG, Yalavarthy R, Concato J, Parikh CR (2008) Biomarkers for the diagnosis and risk stratification of acute kidney injury: a systematic review. Kidney Int 73:1008–1016

Cole L, Bellomo R, Silvester W, Reeves JH (2000) A prospective, multicenter study of the epidemiology, management, and outcome of severe acute renal failure in a "closed" ICU system. Am J Respir Crit Care Med 162:191–196

Coleman BG (1985) Ultrasonography of the upper genitourinary tract. Urol Clin North Am 12:633–644

Devarajan P (2007) Neutrophil gelatinase-associated lipocalin: new paths for an old shuttle. Cancer Ther 5:463–470

Ellis EN, Arnold WC (1982) Use of urinary indexes in renal failure in the newborn. Am J Dis Child 136:615–617

Fiaccadori E, Lombardi M, Leonardi S, Rotelli CF, Tortorella G, Borghetti A (1999) Prevalence and clinical outcome associated with preexisting malnutrition in acute renal failure: a prospective cohort study. J Am Soc Nephrol 10:581–593

Goligorsky MS, Brodsky SV, Noiri E (2002) Nitric oxide in acute renal failure: NOS versus NOS. Kidney Int 61:855–861

Gong WK, Tan TH, Murugasu B, Yap HK (2001) 18 years experience in pediatric acute dialysis: analysis of predictors of outcome. Pediatr Nephrol 16:212–215

Grootendorst AF, van Bommel EF (1993) The role of hemofiltration in the critically-ill intensive care unit patient: present and future. Blood Purif 11:209–223

Han WK, Bailly V, Abichandani R, Thadhani R, Bonventre JV (2002) Kidney injury molecule-1 (KIM-1): a novel biomarker for human renal proximal tubule injury. Kidney Int 62:237–244

Han WK, Waikar SS, Johnson A, Betensky RA, Dent CL, Devarajan P, Bonventre JV (2008) Urinary biomarkers in the early diagnosis of acute kidney injury. Kidney Int 73:863–869

Heinzelmann M, Mercer-Jones MA, Passmore JC (1999) Neutrophils and renal failure. Am J Kidney Dis 34:384–399

Herget-Rosenthal S, Marggraf G, Husing J, Goring F, Pietruck F, Janssen O, Philipp T, Kribben A (2004) Early detection of acute renal failure by serum cystatin C. Kidney Int 66:1115–1122

Himmelfarb J, Ikizler TA (2007) Acute kidney injury: changing lexicography, definitions, and epidemiology. Kidney Int 10:971–976

Himmelfarb J, McMonagle E, Freedman S, Klenzak J, McMenamin E, Le P, Pupim LB, Ikizler TA, The PICARD Group (2004) Oxidative stress is increased in critically ill patients with acute renal failure. J Am Soc Nephrol 15:2449–2456

Hui-Stickle S, Brewer ED, Goldstein SL (2005) Pediatric ARF epidemiology at a tertiary care center from 1999 to 2001. Am J Kidney Dis 45:96–101

Kaye M, Gagnon RF (2008) Acute allergic interstitial nephritis and eosinophiluria. Kidney Int 73:980

Kellum JA, Johnson JP, Kramer D, Palevsky P, Brady JJ, Pinsky MR (1998) Diffusive vs. convective therapy: effects on mediators of inflammation in patient with severe systemic inflammatory response syndrome. Crit Care Med 26:1995–2000

Kellum J, Leblanc M, Venkataraman R (2006) Acute renal failure. Clin Evid 15:1–24

Kelly KJ, Williams WW, Colvin RB, Bonventre JV (1994) Antibody to intercellular adhesion molecule-1 protects the kidney against ischemic injury. Proc Natl Acad Sci USA 91:812–817

Knoderer CA, Leiser JD, Nailescu C, Turrentine MW, Andreoli SP (2008) Fenoldopam for acute kidney injury in children. Pediatr Nephrol 23:495–498

Kraut JA, Kurtz I (2008) Toxic alcohol ingestions: clinical features, diagnosis, and management. Clin J Am Soc Nephrol 3:208–225

Kwon O, Corrigan G, Meyers BD, Sibley R, Scandling JD, Dafoe D, Alfrey E, Nelson WJ (1999) Sodium reabsorption and distribution of Na+K+ATPase during post-ischemic injury to the renal allograft. Kidney Int 55:963–975

Landoni G, Biondi-Zoccai GGL, Tumlin JA (2007) Beneficial impact of fenoldopam in critically ill patients with or at risk for acute renal failure: a meta-analysis of randomized clinical trials. Am J Kidney Dis 49:56–68

Lauschke A, Teichgraber UKM, Frei U, Eckardt KU (2006) "Low-dose" dopamine worsens renal perfusion in patients with acute renal failure. Kidney Int 69:1669–1674

Liangos O, Tighiouart H, Perianayagam MC, Kolyada A, Han WK, Wald R, Bonventre JV, Jaber BL (2009) Comparative analysis of urinary biomarkers for early detection of acute kidney injury following cardiopulmonary bypass. Biomarkers 14:423–431

Liano F, Pascual J, the Madrid Acute Renal Failure Study Cluster (1996) Epidemiology of acute renal failure: a prospective, multicenter, community-based study. Kidney Int 50:811–818

Martin-Ancel A, Garcia-Alix A, Gaya F, Cabañas F, Burgueros M, Quero J (1995) Multiple organ involvement in perinatal asphyxia. J Pediatr 127:786–793

Mathew OP, Jones AS, James E, Bland H, Groshong T (1980) Neonatal renal failure: usefulness of diagnostic indices. Pediatrics 65:57–60

Mehta RL, Chertow GM (2003) Acute renal failure definitions and classification: time for change? J Am Soc Nephrol 14:2176–2177

Mehta RL, McDonald B, Gabbai FB, Pahl M, Pascual MT, Farkas A, Kaplan RM, Collaborative Group for Treatment of ARF in the ICU (2001) A randomized clinical trial of continuous versus intermittent dialysis for acute renal failure. Kidney Int 60:1154–1163

Mercado-Deane MG, Beeson JE, John SD (2002) US of renal insufficiency in neonates. Radiographics 22:1429–1438

Mishra J, Qing M, Prada A, Zahedi K, Yang Y, Barasch J, Devarajan P (2003) Identification of NGAL as a novel early urinary marker for ischemic renal injury. J Am Soc Nephrol 14:2534–2543

Mishra J, Dent C, Tarabishi R, Mitsnefes MM, Ma Q, Kelly C, Ruff SM, Zahedi K, Shao M, Bean J, Mori K, Barasch J, Devarajan P (2005) Neutrophil gelatinase-associated lipocalin (NGAL) as a biomarker for acute renal injury after cardiac surgery. Lancet 365:1231–1238

Moghal NE, Brocklebank JT, Meadow SR (1998) A review of acute renal failure in children: incidence, etiology and outcome. Clin Nephrol 49:91

Molitoris BA (1997) Putting the actin cytoskeleton into perspective: pathophysiology of ischemic alterations. Am J Physiol 272:F430–F433

Molitoris B (2003) Transitioning to therapy in ischemic acute renal failure. J Am Soc Nephrol 14:265–267

Morgan DB, Carver ME, Payne RB (1977) Plasma creatinine and urea-creatinine ratio in patients with raised plasma urea. Br Med J 2:929–932

Newman DJ, Cystatin C (2002) Ann Clin Biochem 39:89–104

Nolte-Ernsting CCA, Adam GB, Gunther RW (2001) MR urography: examination techniques and clinical applications. Eur Radiol 11:355–372

Oda S, Hirasawa H, Shiga H, Nakanishi K, Matsuda K, Nakamura M (2002) Continuous hemofiltration/hemodiafiltration in critical care. Ther Apher 6:193–198

Parikh CR, Jani A, Melnikov VY, Faubel S, Edelstein CL (2004) Urinary interleukin-18 is a marker of human acute tubular necrosis. Am J Kidney Dis 43:405–414

Patel HP (2006) The abnormal urinalysis. Pediatr Clin North Am 35:958–962

Pickering JW, Endre ZH (2009) GFR shot by RIFLE: errors in staging acute kidney injury. Lancet 373:1318–1319

Prandota J (2001) Clinical pharmacology of furosemide in children: a supplement. Am J Ther 8:275–289

Ruschitzka F, Shaw S, Gygi D, Noll G, Barton M, Luscher TF (1999) Endothelial dysfunction in acute renal failure: role of circulating and tissue endothelin-1. J Am Soc Nephrol 10:953–962

Schaefer JH, Jochimsen F, Keller F, Wegscheider K, Distler A (1991) Outcome prediction of acute renal failure in medical intensive care. Intensive Care Med 17:19–24

Sotsiou F, Dimitriadis G, Liapis H (2002) Diagnostic dilemmas in atypical postinfectious glomerulonephritis. Semin Diagn Pathol 19:46–59

Sutton TA, Fisher CJ, Molitoris BA (2002) Microvascular endothelial injury and dysfunction during ischemic acute renal failure. Kidney Int 62:1539–1549

Vachvanichsanong P, Dissaneewate P, Lim A, McNeil E (2006) Childhood acute renal failure: 22-year experience in a university hospital in southern Thailand. Pediatrics 118:e786–e791

Van Biljon G (2008) Causes, prognostic factors and treatment results of acute renal failure in children treated in a tertiary hospital in South Africa. J Trop Pediatr 54:233–237

van Timmeren MM, van den Heuvel MC, Bailly V, Bakker SJ, van Goor H, Stegeman CA (2007) Tubular kidney injury molecule-1 (KIM-1) in human renal disease. J Pathol 212:209–217

Van Why SK, Mann AS, Ardito T, Thulin G, Ferris S, Macleod MA, Kashgarin M, Siegel NJ (2002) Hsp27 associates with actin and limits injury in energy depleted renal epithelial. J Am Soc Nephrol 13:2667–2680

Warady BA, Bunchman T (2000) Dialysis therapy for children with acute renal failure: survey results. Pediatr Nephrol 15:11–13

Washburn KK, Zappitelli M, Arikan AA, Loftis L, Yalavarthy R, Parikh CR, Edelstein CL, Goldstein SL (2007) Urinary interleukin-18 is an acute kidney injury biomarker in critically ill children. Nephrol Dial Transplant 23:566–572

Williams DM, Sreedhar SS, Mickell JJ, Chan JCM (2002) Acute kidney failure: a pediatric experience over 20 years. Arch Pediatr Adolesc Med 156:893–900

Zarich S, Fang LS, Diamond JR (1985) Fractional sodium excretion of sodium. Exceptions to its diagnostic value. Arch Intern Med 145:108–112

Zhou Y, Vaidya VS, Brown RP, Zhang J, Rosenzweig BA, Thompson KL, Miller TJ, Bonventre JV, Goering PL (2008) Comparison of kidney injury molecule-1 and other nephrotoxicity biomarkers in urine and kidney following acute exposure to gentamicin, mercury, and chromium. Toxicol Sci 101:159–170

Zuk A, Bonventre JV, Brown D, Matlin KS (1998) Polarity, integrin and extracellular matrix dynamics in the post ischemic rat kidney. Am J Physiol 275:C711–C731

313 Chronic Kidney Disease (CKD)

Lesley Rees

Definition

Chronic kidney disease (CKD) means any abnormality of the renal parenchyma that will not recover. A progressive decline in kidney function may occur, but only if both kidneys are abnormal.

Classification

Staging of CKD

CKD is divided into stages according to its severity (➋ *Table 313.1*). As renal function declines, uremia, electrolyte disturbances and anemia become more common, and lead to uremic complications such as lethargy and poor appetite, sodium retention and hypertension, acidosis, bone disease and vascular calcification. By CKD stage 5, renal replacement therapy (RRT) may become necessary, but some children who maintain good urine output may manage without for many years with a glomerular filtration rate (GFR) as low as this. Renal function may remain stable or even show some improvement in infancy and early childhood. Decline in renal function occurs thereafter, particularly, in the peripubertal years.

Etiology

The commonest cause of CKD in childhood is renal dysplasia, representing up to 70% of cases. Renal dysplasia is due to abnormal renal development, either because of intra uterine obstruction or in association with vesicoureteric reflux, syndromes, genetic defects such as branchio-oto-renal syndrome or renal coloboma syndrome, or causes as yet undefined. In boys, most cases are due to a posterior urethral valve. Abnormal urinary tract drainage will predispose to urinary tract infection (UTI), which can cause further renal damage.

Renal cystic diseases are the second commonest cause. Autosomal recessive polycystic kidney disease (ARPKD) is often diagnosed antenatally or is recognized in infancy when palpable kidneys, hepatosplenomegaly and hypertension are found. Autosomal dominant PKD (ADPKD) rarely causes problems in childhood, unless there is disruption of TSC2 and the adjacent PKD1 gene (contiguous gene syndrome), as in 2% of patients with tuberose sclerosis. Patients with Bardet–Biedel Syndrome may have cystic kidney disease and there may be (but not always) cysts with nephronophthisis. Nephronophthisis may occur in isolation or in association with retinitis pigmentosa (Senior-Loken Syndrome). Glomerulocystic disease is becoming a more frequent diagnosis with the identification of the renal cysts and diabetes syndrome due to HNF1β gene mutations.

The next commonest causes are the nephrotic syndromes (NS), including congenital NS, which presents in infancy, and focal segmental glomerulosclerosis (FSGS). FSGS is a unifying term used to describe steroid resistant NS with a particular histological appearance that is due to different genetic abnormalities. Another NS, membranoproliferative glomerulonephritis, is a less common cause of CKD.

Other causes include renal vascular events (particularly neonatal arterial and venous thromboses), atypical Hemolytic Uremic Syndrome (HUS), renal stone diseases, subsequent to acute kidney injury (AKI) due to any cause (including rapidly progressive glomerulonephritis, HUS, dehydration with cortical necrosis), hereditary nephropathies, systemic diseases such as SLE and the vasculitides, renal diseases that occur in association with syndromes, and in some patients the cause is not known. As time goes by, more and more genes that cause CKD are being identified.

Epidemiology

Although the identification of CKD in children has improved due to antenatal screening programs, the true incidence is unknown and may be higher than suspected. Studies suggest an annual acceptance rate for new pediatric patients with a GFR < 75 ml/min.1.73 m^2 of around 12 cases per million child population. It is easier to be more precise about the incidence of children needing to enter RRT programs because such data are collected by national registries, being 9 per million child population per year in the UK, 10 in Australia and New Zealand, and 15 in the USA.

Abdelaziz Y. Elzouki (ed.), *Textbook of Clinical Pediatrics*, DOI 10.1007/978-3-642-02202-9_313,

Table 313.1
Staging of CKD

Stage	GFR ml/min/1.73 m^2	Features
1	>90	Renal parenchymal disease present
2	60–90	Usually no symptoms but may develop biochemical abnormalities at the lower end of the GFR range
3	30–60	Biochemical abnormalities and anemia and in addition may develop poor growth and appetite
4	15–30	Symptoms more severe
5	<15	Renal replacement therapy may be required

Pathogenesis

Although the etiologies of CKD are multiple, progressive destruction of renal tissue occurs through a common pathway regardless of the cause. Intrarenal pathology leads to abnormal hemodynamics, chronic hypoxia, inflammation, cellular dysfunction and the activation of fibrogenic biochemical pathways. The end result is the replacement of normal structures with extracellular matrix, culminating in fibrosis.

Clinical Manifestations

Presentation of CKD: Symptoms and Signs

The commonest way for CKD to present is during antenatal scanning. Around 50% of children are diagnosed antenatally; some can be missed if there has not been a third trimester ultrasound scan. The next commonest way is with a complicating episode of AKI, which can be precipitated by infection or dehydration. Children may also present with nonspecific symptoms, such as anorexia and lethargy, which may be severe enough to cause failure to grow normally. Diseases that predominantly affect the renal tubular concentrating mechanisms, such as juvenile nephronophthisis or renal dysplasia, may present with polydipsia and polyuria. Less commonly, children may present with hypertension or with an incidental finding of proteinuria, or to orthopedic surgeons with bony abnormalities such as knock knees or bow legs. They may be detected by screening because of another affected family member.

Case No 1

A male infant was diagnosed antenatally with one bright kidney and one hydronephrotic kidney with oligohydramnios. He was delivered prematurely due to the spontaneous onset of labor and developed respiratory distress and a pneumothorax. Subsequent imaging showed a posterior urethral valve, which was ablated urethrally. He had bilateral renal dysplasia. His renal function progressively declined throughout childhood and declined rapidly during puberty, so that he needed a renal transplant at the age of 16.

Diagnosis

Investigations

Assessment of Renal Function

The easiest way to assess renal function on a day-to-day basis is to use the plasma creatinine. Creatinine is produced at a constant rate from the breakdown of creatine phosphate from muscle and is excreted by filtration without reabsorption; therefore, it is a good representation of renal function. There are pitfalls in the interpretation of the plasma creatinine: first, plasma levels do not rise until renal function has halved; second, as creatinine levels increase progressively with muscle bulk and, therefore growth, the level has to be interpreted according to age; third, levels will be lower than expected in a child who is malnourished. This means that formulae used to calculate the GFR may give results that are higher than the true result. One such formula is shown below:

$$\mathrm{GFR} = \frac{40 \times \text{height (cm)}}{\text{creatinine } (\mu\text{mol/l})}$$

GFR can be more accurately assessed by measuring the rate of disappearance from the plasma of a substance that is freely filtered by the glomerulus but not reabsorbed by the tubules, but in practice this is rarely needed. It can also be calculated by measuring the clearance of creatinine, but as a timed urine collection is needed for this, it is not often undertaken in childhood.

Investigation of the Cause of CKD; Differential Diagnosis

The History and Examination

It is always important to find out the results of antenatal scans, amniotic fluid status (as this represents fetal urine production), and the neonatal and family history. The physical examination should include a general examination, but should focus on growth, the BP, and look for evidence of bone disease.

Investigations

There are two investigations that are crucial for the diagnosis of the cause of CKD: ultrasound (US) and urine stick testing for protein. The appearances of the kidneys (i.e., renal sizes, the presence of cysts, and evidence of obstruction or calculi) on US (➋ *Table 313.2*) will then guide further more selective investigations. Additional imaging may be necessary if a structural or cystic lesion or calculi are the cause and will depend on the US appearances.

Urine stick testing can also be very helpful: heavy proteinuria suggests a nephrotic syndrome; proteinuria and hematuria suggest a glomerulonephritis or familial nephropathy; and no proteinuria may be present with cystic diseases and dysplasias. However, proteinuria may result from any cause due to hyperfiltration, when reduced nephron number leads to increased glomerular pressure within the remaining glomeruli. Proteinuria may be tubular in cases of tubulopathy, when urinary retinol binding protein and N-acetyl glucosaminidase levels will be raised.

Complement levels, anti-DNA antibodies, anti-neutrophil cytoplasmic antibodies and IgA levels should be measured if glomerulonephritis is suspected; plasma and urine calcium, oxalate and purines if calculi; and urine pH and white cell cystine if a tubulopathy is suspected. Genetic analysis may be available for some conditions. Renal biopsy may be necessary if the cause of CKD remains unclear.

Case No 2

A 12 year old boy presented with a 3 month history of bone pain, loss of appetite, lethargy, and vomiting. He had a long history of polydipsia and polyuria. His younger brother was taller than him. On examination he was on the second centile for height, he was pale, his BP was normal, and there were no other abnormalities. Investigations showed his hemoglobin to be 8 gm/dl, creatinine 1,200 mcmol/l, potassium normal, calcium low, and phosphate high. He had no proteinuria. His kidneys were normal sized and bright with poor cortico-medullary differentiation and some small cysts at the corticomedullary junction. Nephronophthisis was suspected and this was confirmed by DNA analysis for the presence of the commonest gene for this condition, which has been designated NPHP1, rendering renal biopsy unnecessary.

Measurements to be Made at Each Clinic Visit

Height and weight, and head circumference in young children and pubertal stage in older ones, should be plotted on a growth chart and BP checked at each clinic visit. Early morning urine should be tested for albumin to creatinine ratio. Routine blood tests include a full blood count, urea, electrolytes, bicarbonate, creatinine, calcium,

Table 313.2

Appearance of kidneys on renal ultrasound

Cystic	Small	Normal sized	Obstruction	Calculi
Dysplasia	Dysplasia ± vesico-ureteric reflux	Glomerulo-nephritides	Dysplasia with posterior urethral valves	Recurrent UTIs ± obstruction/reflux
Autosomal recessive polycystic kidney disease	Vascular insults (venous or arterial)	Familial nephropathies	Dysplasia with VUJ obstruction	Calcium disorders
Autosomal dominant polycystic kidney disease	All causes may result in small kidneys by Stage 5 CKD	Nephrotic syndromes	Dysplasia with PUJ obstruction	Hyperoxaluria
Tuberose Sclerosis		Nephronophthisis (may be cystic)	Neuropathic bladder	Purine disorders
Glomerulocystic diseases		Tubulopathies		Cystine

phosphate, alkaline phosphatase, intact PTH, and albumin. Fasting HDL and LDL cholesterol and triglycerides and iron status may be checked less often.

One very important aspect of the management of the child with CKD is care of the blood vessels. The use of antecubital veins should be avoided when possible as they will be needed in the future for fistula formation. Similarly damage resulting in stenosis of the subclavian veins would preclude creation of a fistula in that arm.

Treatment

Prevention of Progression of CKD

The first aim of management of CKD is to reduce its progression as far as is possible. Progression can be attenuated by the maintenance of the BP within the normal range for age and height, and by the use of an ACE inhibitor (e.g., ramipril) ± an AT1 receptor blocker (e.g., losartan) to dilate the glomerular afferent arteriole, reduce intraglomerular pressure and, therefore, reduce proteinuria, which is thought to contribute to the development of fibrosis. Dyslipidemia may play a role in the progression of CKD. Increased LDL cholesterol is a particular problem for children with nephrotic syndrome. Hypertriglyceridemia and abnormal apolipoprotein metabolism is a feature of CKD. Dietary intervention may be necessary, and some children (particularly those with nephrotic syndrome) may need lipid lowering agents.

Growth, Nutrition, and Electrolytes

Growth retardation occurs in up to 50% of children with CKD stages 3–5. Children with congenital nephropathies are particularly severely affected. This is because growth in the first 2 years of life is as high as 25 cm/year at birth, falling to 18 cm/year at 1 year and 10 cm/year at the age of 2, by which time half of the final adult height has been achieved. It is, therefore, possible to lose considerable height potential at that age, which can be as much as 2SD in the first 6 months of life in infants with severe CKD. The calorie and protein requirement is extremely high during this period of rapid growth, and an adequate nutritional intake can be very difficult to maintain. After this age, when the role of growth hormone (GH) becomes more important, the rate of growth can be normal. Growth may also be adversely affected at the time of puberty, which may be delayed, with an attenuated pubertal growth spurt. Growth retardation increases with the severity of CKD. However, it has to be remembered that there are children with CKD who have associated syndromes that in themselves affect growth. Successful renal transplantation can normalize growth in some children, but may be counteracted by corticosteroid therapy used as immunosuppression and poor transplant function.

There are many different causes for poor nutritional intake: CKD is characterized by a predisposition to anorexia and vomiting. Poor appetite may be due to abnormal taste sensation, the requirement for multiple medications, the preference for water in the polyuric child, and elevated circulating cytokines such as leptin, TNF-α and IL-1 and -6, which act through the hypothalamus to affect appetite and satiety. Vomiting may result from gastroesophageal reflux and delayed gastric emptying in association with increased polypeptide hormones, and may be so profound that as much as one third of feed can be lost. Other factors that contribute to insufficient nutrition include episodes of fasting surrounding surgical procedures and episodes of sepsis, which may have a significant effect on growth, principally in the infant. Importantly, many children with severe CKD have associated co-morbidities that influence feeding and growth in their own right.

The child on dialysis has even more issues that affect their nutritional intake. They are likely to be on a fluid restriction, appetite may be affected by the presence of a full abdomen and constipation in patients on peritoneal dialysis (PD), and there may be considerable losses of protein in the dialysate in PD and amino-acids in hemodialysis (HD).

Ensuring adequate nutrition is one of the most important aspects of care of the child with CKD. As well as its obvious importance in promoting adequate growth, nutritional manipulation can control symptoms and prevent complications, particularly uremia and bone disease, such that it is possible to delay the need for dialysis.

Case No 3

A boy was referred at age 2 with prune belly and CKD stage 5 (creatinine 400 mcmol/l). He was lethargic and refusing food and was on the second centile for height. A gastrostomy was placed and provision of adequate calories and protein allowed catch-up growth to the 25th centile. He continued to grow along that centile and symptomatically improved. Dialysis was not needed until nearly 6 years of age despite a creatinine in the high 500s mcmol/l.

The type of diet recommended depends on the cause and severity of CKD and mode of RRT. If dietary intake is inadequate, the first thing is to try an oral dietary supplement in addition to a normal diet. There are various types of supplements, with different ratios of calories and protein. In the young child with vomiting it is possible to increase the feed concentration and, therefore, decrease the feed volume. However, the rate-limiting step for this is that vomiting may worsen and diarrhea can occur with increasing feed density. Medications such as prokinetic agents (domperidone), H2-receptor antagonists (ranitidine), proton pump inhibitors (lansoprazole), and 5HT3 receptor antagonists (ondansetron) may be of benefit. The stress on the family of trying to feed an anorexic child cannot be overestimated, and this, along with a declining rate of growth, can only be resolved by the use of enteral feeding.

A nasogastric tube is acceptable for a short time, and is the method of choice in the infant weighing <4 kg, but most families prefer the placement of a gastrostomy as it is hidden under clothing. Enteral feeding via any route, but particularly gastrostomy, is associated with decreased vomiting and improved appetite, nutrition, and growth. The tube has the additional benefit of its potential use in the administration of medications, and the large fluid volumes that may be prescribed post transplant.

Overall, calorie and protein allowances should be the same as for the normal child. However, as CKD progresses it may become necessary to ensure that the protein intake is not above requirements, aiming to keep the serum albumin in the normal range with a plasma urea below 20 mmol/l. Above this level of urea, nausea, lethargy, itching, and worsening anemia may occur. The child on PD absorbs up to 12 kcal/kg/day from the dialysate, but may lose protein in the dialysate effluent. The child on HD may lose amino acids in the same way. Supplements of protein of up to 50% of the dietary requirements may, therefore, be needed in very young children on PD, who have the highest protein losses.

Structural renal diseases have a predominant effect on the renal tubule, so that reabsorption of sodium bicarbonate and water from the glomerular filtrate is inadequate. Therefore, these children are often polyuric and polydipsic, and need salt and bicarbonate supplementation and free access to water. However, children with CKD due to predominantly glomerular disease may retain salt and develop hypertension. Such children should be managed with a salt restricted diet and medications as necessary. A low potassium diet is usually only necessary at CKD stage 5.

Recombinant human growth hormone is effective in some children with CKD, and can be considered when growth has failed to respond to correction of inadequate diet and biochemical abnormalities and optimization of dialysis, and, for children on steroid therapy, when the dose of steroids has been reduced to the lowest possible.

Anemia

The anemia of CKD is normochromic and normocytic, with a low reticulocyte count. It is important to exclude iron, vitamin B12, or folate deficiency, which may play a role due to the anorexia of CKD. However, when the GFR falls below 35 ml/min/1.73 m^2, decreased production of erythropoietin is common and responds well to subcutaneous injection of this hormone, which can usually be administered weekly or even less often with some newer erythropoietin preparations. Uremia itself may cause decreased red cell survival and bone marrow inhibition. Bone marrow fibrosis occurs with severe hyperparathyroidism (osteitis fibrosa). Blood loss occurs during HD and the anticoagulation required during the HD process can result in chronic blood loss from the gastro-intestinal tract.

Chronic Kidney Disease – Mineral and Bone Disorder (CKD-MBD)

Effects of CKD on Mineral Metabolism

CKD leads to abnormal calcium, phosphate, parathyroid hormone (PTH), and vitamin D metabolism resulting not only in disordered bone turnover, mineralization and growth, but also cardiovascular and soft tissue calcification. For this reason, the term CKD-MBD is now used to encompass all these abnormalities, and the term renal osteodystrophy should be reserved for the bony abnormalities that are seen on histology.

Calcium absorption and, therefore, plasma calcium levels are usually low in untreated CKD. Calcium absorption is under the control of vitamin D, levels of which are also usually low in CKD. This is for two reasons. First, there is deficiency of the substrate 25(OH)D due to poor appetite and protein and dairy food restriction, reduced production in the skin due to reduced outdoor activity and, therefore, sunlight exposure, and loss of vitamin D binding protein in the urine. Second, there is decreased 1α hydroxylation in the kidney of 25(OH)D to the active form of vitamin D, 1,25-dihydroxyvitamin D (1,25$(OH)_2$D). Another contributory factor is that dietary calcium is reduced for similar reasons to vitamin D.

Conversely, it would be expected that phosphate levels would be high, due to decreased renal phosphate excretion. Although this is the case as CKD progresses, in early

CKD normophosphatemia is maintained. This is because the high phosphate load stimulates the production of fibroblast growth factor 23 (FGF23), a phosphaturic hormone produced by the osteocyte. FGF23 induces a negative phosphate balance in two ways: it decreases renal tubular phosphate reabsorption, and decreases the production of 1,25 $(OH)_2D$; 1,25$(OH)_2D$ increases gut phosphate absorption as well as calcium.

As CKD progresses, FGF23 is no longer able to prevent hyperphosphatemia, so phosphate levels rise. This, along with low plasma calcium and 1,25$(OH)_2D$ levels, stimulate PTH secretion through the calcium sensing receptors and vitamin D receptors in the parathyroid gland. All the actions of PTH are to restore the plasma calcium to normal. It effects this by mobilizing calcium from bone, increasing tubular reabsorption of calcium, increasing hydroxylation of 25(OH)D, thereby promoting gut absorption of calcium and decreasing tubular reabsorption of phosphate.

The Role of PTH in CKD-MBD

PTH is thought to be the main player in the evolution of CKD-MBD: persistent stimulation of the parathyroid glands leads to hypertrophy, progressing to nodular hyperplasia, and culminating in the need for parathyroidectomy. The logic, therefore, has to be that prevention of the process starting must be beneficial.

PTH and Renal Osteodystrophy

The effect of PTH on the skeleton is to increase the activity of osteoclasts and osteoblasts such that high PTH levels cause high turnover (osteitis fibrosa), and low levels low turnover (adynamic) bone disease. Both types lead to bone pain, fractures, and growth problems. They can also lead to cardiovascular and soft tissue calcification because of hypercalcemia and hyperphosphatemia: in high turnover bone disease, calcium and phosphate are removed from bone into the circulation, and in low turnover, bone is unable to buffer changes in plasma calcium and phosphate.

Aims of Management of CKD-MBD

The aim of management of CKD-MBD is to maintain normal bone turnover and, therefore, prevent symptoms of bone pain and fractures, allow normal growth and prevent vascular disease and soft tissue calcification. It is important to intervene early in the course of CKD to prevent escape of the parathyroid glands from normal control mechanisms.

Phosphate Control

Plasma phosphate levels fall progressively from birth to the age of 3 and then remain stable. Maintenance of a normal age-related plasma phosphate is crucial to the prevention of hyperparathyroidism. Dietary phosphate is principally in protein containing foods, and dairy products in particular, and these foods should be restricted if the phosphate is above normal.

Reduction in phosphate load results in a reduction in FGF23 and an increase in 1,25$(OH)_2D$, which increases calcium absorption and plasma calcium and, therefore, suppresses PTH. However, 1,25$(OH)_2D$ increases phosphate absorption to as much as 80–90% of dietary intake, so it is usually the case that phosphate binders, which latch on to phosphate in the gut and prevent its absorption, are needed. The principal phosphate binders contain calcium Calcium carbonate is the cheapest and most used, followed by calcium acetate. If required in large quantities such binders present a large calcium load; calcium free phosphate binders are available if there are problems with hypercalcemia. Phosphate, being predominantly intracellular, is poorly removed by dialysis. It is one of the most toxic molecules that circulates in excess in CKD, and plays an important role in vascular calcification. Maintenance of the plasma phosphate well below the upper limit of the age-related normal range is, therefore, crucial.

Calcium

The requirement for calcium varies with age, from 0.4 to 1 g daily, and is relatively higher when growth is fastest, that is, in the first 2 years of life. Plasma calcium is, like phosphate, age dependent, falling over the first 3–4 years of life. Interpretation of the plasma calcium requires adjustment for the albumin and pH, or ionized calcium can be used.

Vitamin D

The benefits of vitamin D extend beyond its effect on bone disease, as it has anti-inflammatory properties and beneficial effects on the cardiovascular system. Conversely, this has to be balanced against the risks of hypercalcemia and its depressive effect on the chondrocyte. If it is possible to measure 25(OH)D, and this proves to be low, ergo, or cholecalciferol should be prescribed. If the PTH remains high, the smallest possible dose of 1,25$(OH)_2D$ to suppress the PTH can then be added. If hypercalcemia develops, the 1,25$(OH)_2D$ should be stopped.

PTH

Guidelines for the management of CKD-MBD hinge on the need to keep the PTH level within a fixed range, which is one that maintains normal bone turnover. European guidelines recommend maintaining the PTH in the normal range until dialysis, when up to 3 × the upper limit of normal (ULN) is acceptable. KDOQI recommends the normal range until CKD 4, when 1–2 × ULN is recommended and then 3–5 × ULN for patients on dialysis, in order to allow for skeletal resistance to PTH as CKD evolves. These guidelines were written as the understanding of the interplay with cardiovascular disease was emerging. They are predominantly opinion-based as they are extrapolated from adult studies and a small number of pediatric studies, and are largely out-of-date. When hyperparathyroidism becomes tertiary, with persistent hypercalcemia and radiological changes, new therapies that block the calcium sensing receptor are beneficial in adults and have been successfully used in children. Severe, uncontrolled hyperparathyroidism may necessitate parathyroidectomies.

Radiological Changes

Radiological changes of CKD-MBD include rickets, hyperparathyroidism, and osteosclerosis. Features include periosteal erosions and elevation and widening of the zone of provisional calcification with a coarse trabecular pattern. Vertebral collapse, alternating with areas of osteosclerosis, gives the appearance called rugger jersey spine. Radiological changes occur late and may be normal even with moderate hyperparathyroidism.

Vascular Calcification

Vascular calcification has been demonstrated in children on dialysis. Disorders of phosphate, calcium, PTH, and vitamin D have all been shown to contribute. Large epidemiological studies in adults have shown that mortality rises exponentially as the plasma phosphate rises; the risk of death increases by 6% for every 0.3 mmol/l rise in plasma phosphate. Mortality also increases exponentially as the calcium × phosphate product rises above 5 $mmol^2/l^2$. PTH itself is a risk actor for vascular disease in several studies of children on dialysis. The most risk is when the level is >2 × ULN. Vitamin D has a bimodal effect, such that vitamin D levels above and below the normal range are associated with vascular calcification.

Prognosis

The diagnosis of CKD implies progressive decline in renal function, but whether mild impairment progresses, is unknown. Studies have shown that the probability of kidney survival at 20 years of age with a diagnosis of a GFR in early childhood of 51–75 ml/min.1.73 m^2 is 63%, 30% in those with a GFR of 25–50, and 3% in those with a GFR <25 mL/min/1.73 m^2. The diagnosis of CKD has implications for survival: the overall mortality rate has been estimated to be 1.4% for children before RRT is needed, but much higher for children on dialysis, when lifespan is reduced by 40–60 years.

Prevention

Prevention of CKD is the Holy Grail for the nephrologist. At present, however, there are only a few situations where prevention is possible, such as relief of urinary tract obstruction or prevention of infection. It is important to identify children with CKD as early as possible because the mainstay of treatment is to attenuate the rate of progression of CKD by normalization of BP and reduction of proteinuria. Careful attention to nutrition, electrolytes, and anemia is essential to maintain well-being and growth.

References

Ardissino G, Daccò V, Testa S, Bonaudo R, Claris-Appiani A, Taioli E, Marra G, Edefonti A, Sereni F, ItalKid project (2003) Epidemiology of chronic renal failure in children: data from the ItalKid project. Pediatrics 111(4 Pt 1):e382–387

Hadtstein C, Schaefer F (2008) Hypertension in children with chronic kidney disease: pathophysiology and management. Pediatr Nephrol 23(3):363–371

http://www.kidney.org/professionals/KDOQI/'KDOQI (2009) Clinical practice guideline for nutrition in children with chronic kidney disease: 2008 update. Am J Kidney Dis 53(3 Suppl 2):S1–124

http://www.kidney.org/professionals/kdoqi/guidelines_pedbone/index.htm

Kari JA, Gonzalez C, Ledermann SE, Shaw V, Rees L (2000) Outcome and growth of infants with chronic renal failure. Kidney Int 57(4):1681–1687

Keithi-Reddy SR, Singh AK (2009) Hemoglobin target in chronic kidney disease: a pediatric perspective. Pediatr Nephrol 24(3):431–434

Klaus G, Watson A, Edefonti A, Fischbach M, Rönnholm K, Schaefer F, Simkova E, Stefanidis CJ, Strazdins V, Vande Walle J, Schröder C, Zurowska A, Ekim M, European Pediatric Dialysis Working Group (EPDWG) (2006) Prevention and treatment of renal osteodystrophy in children on chronic renal failure: European guidelines. Pediatr Nephrol 21:151–159

Moe S, Drüeke T, Cunningham J, Goodman W, Martin K, Olgaard K, Ott S, Sprague S, Lameire N, Eknoyan G (2006) Kidney disease: improving global outcomes (KDIGO). Definition, evaluation, and classification of renal osteodystrophy: a position statement from kidney disease: improving global outcomes (KDIGO). Kidney Int 69:1945–1953

National Kidney Foundation (2002) Clinical practice guidelines for chronic kidney disease: evaluation, classification and stratification. K/DOQI clinical practice guidelines. Am J Kidney Dis 39:S1–S266

Rees L (2007) Chronic renal failure investigations. In: Rees L, Webb N, Brogan P (eds) Paediatric Nephrology. Oxford University Press, Oxford, p 397

Rees L (2008) What parathyroid hormone levels should we aim for in children with stage 5 chronic kidney disease; what is the evidence? Editorial. Pediatr Nephrol 23(2):179–184

Rees L, Shaw V (2007) Nutrition in children with CRF and on dialysis. Pediatr Nephrol 22(10):1689–1702

Schwartz GJ, Muñoz A, Schneider MF, Mak RH, Kaskel F, Warady BA, Furth SL (2009) New equations to estimate GFR in children with CKD. J Am Soc Nephrol 20(3):629–637

Shroff RC, Donald AE, Hiorns MP, Watson A, Feather S, Milford D, Ellins EA, Storry C, Ridout D, Deanfield J, Rees L (2007) Mineral metabolism and vascular damage in children on dialysis. J Am Soc Nephrol 18(11):2996–3003

Shroff R, Egerton M, Bridel M, Shah V, Donald AE, Cole TJ, Hiorns MP, Deanfield JE, Rees L (2008) A bimodal association of vitamin D levels and vascular disease in children on dialysis. J Am Soc Nephrol 19(6):1239–1246

Vimalachandra D, Hodson EM, Willis NS, Craig JC, Cowell C, Knight JF (2006) Growth hormone for children with chronic kidney disease. Cochrane Database Syst Rev (3):CD003264

Waller S, Reynolds A, Ridout D, Cantor T, Gao P, Rees L (2003) Parathyroid hormone and its fragments in children with chronic renal failure. Pediatr Nephrol 18:1242–1248

Warady BA, Chadha V (2007) Chronic kidney disease in children: the global perspective. Pediatr Nephrol 22(12):1999–2009

314 Dialysis in Children

Bradley A. Warady

Incidence, Prevalence and Causes of End-Stage Renal Disease in Children

End-stage renal disease (ESRD) is an uncommon disorder in children, with an incidence rate in the USA of approximately 14 patients per million children of similar age. The incidence varies within the pediatric population with a rate of 29 per million for children 15–19 years, in contrast to a rate of 9 per million for children 0–4 years. The incidence in children is also significantly different from that which is experienced by adults in whom rates of 127 per million and 625 per million characterize the 20–44 and 45–64 year age groups, respectively. Similarly, pediatric patients only account for a small percentage of the total dialysis population. In 2007, of a total of 354,753 patients on dialysis in the USA, only 2,177 (0.6%) were younger than 20 years (➋ *Table 314.1*). Approximately one-half of children who initiate chronic dialysis have a congenital or hereditary disorder, such as aplastic/hypoplastic/dysplastic kidneys or obstructive uropathy (e.g., posterior urethral valves), whereas the remainder have an acquired cause of ESRD such as focal segmental glomerulosclerosis (FSGS). In all cases, the development of ESRD, as defined by an estimated glomerular filtration rate (eGFR) of 8 mL/min/ 1.73 m^2 or the development of treatment-resistant signs and symptoms of uremia (e.g., lethargy, recurrent emesis, poor growth, anemia, elevated blood pressure, acidosis, fluid overload, poor school performance), mandate the provision of renal replacement therapy in the form of dialysis or transplantation. Although kidney transplantation is the nearly universal goal for children who develop ESRD, approximately 75% of patients initially receive chronic peritoneal dialysis (CPD), hemodialysis (HD), or both, prior to receipt of a kidney transplant.

Choice of Dialysis Modality in Children

The percentage of children that receive one form of chronic dialysis versus the other varies globally. For instance, nearly 80% of prevalent pediatric (0–19 years) dialysis patients in Russia receive HD, in contrast to Spain where almost 60% receive CPD. The choice is most often made based on patient age and size, dialysis center experience and philosophy, family preference, assessment of whether the individual patient and family can be adherent with a home dialysis regimen, and the availability of the specific modality. Careful evaluation of the family's social, psychological, and economic background, ideally by a multiprofessional team including the family physician and nephrologist, dialysis nurse, psychologist, and social worker, is mandatory if a fully informed decision regarding modality selection is to be made. The quality of life (QOL) of the patient and family and the potential impact of the dialysis modality on this parameter also assumes great importance in the decision process. In all cases, HD is the modality of choice when the family is unwilling or unable to conduct dialysis at home. Although few in number, absolute contraindications to CPD include the presence of the following:

- Omphalocele
- Gastroschisis
- Bladder extrophy
- Diaphragmatic hernia
- Obliterated peritoneal cavity and peritoneal membrane failure

At present, there is no clear evidence that one form of dialysis is preferable over another for most children with ESRD. In all cases, patients and families should understand that, at some point during the clinical management with dialysis, a change in modality may be necessary as a result of compromised efficacy and/or the development of complications associated with their current therapy.

Chronic Peritoneal Dialysis

Peritoneal dialysis is frequently the preferred initial dialysis modality in pediatric programs, primarily for psychosocial reasons. CPD, which is characteristically performed at home following the training of patients/parents/caregivers by dialysis staff, permits flexibility of the treatment schedule and normal attendance at school, does not

Abdelaziz Y. Elzouki (ed.), *Textbook of Clinical Pediatrics*, DOI 10.1007/978-3-642-02202-9_314,

Table 314.1
Prevalent dialysis patients (Data from US patients in 2007)

Age	HD	PD
0–19	1,253	860
20–44	46,105	5,842
45–64	133,637	11,510
65–74	74,674	4,748
75+	72,084	3,122

require venipuncture during the dialysis procedure, and allows for a reasonable fluid intake because dialysis is conducted on a daily basis.

Peritoneal dialysis makes use of the peritoneal membrane as a natural dialyzing membrane. The dialysis solution is instilled and dwells within the peritoneal cavity, during which time bloodstream derived solutes (e.g., urea, creatinine) move down a concentration (electrochemical) gradient based on the principle of diffusion. At the same time, the osmotic component of the dialysis solution, typically glucose, causes fluids to move from blood to dialysate (e.g., ultrafiltration) as a result of the osmotic gradient. Peritoneal dialysis solutions are commercially available in standard dextrose concentrations of 1.5%, 2.5%, and 4.25%. The inflow, dwell, and drainage of dialysate characterize a single dialysis cycle or exchange.

A reliable peritoneal catheter is the cornerstone of successful CPD. Most long-term catheters are constructed of either silastic or polyurethane. The Tenckhoff catheter is the one most commonly used and, like all CPD catheters, is comprised of an intraperitoneal and an extraperitoneal portion. The former contains holes through which the dialysis solution flows into the peritoneal cavity and then subsequently drains. A portion of the extraperitoneal segment of the catheter is tunneled subcutaneously within the abdominal wall and has one or two Dacron cuffs that primarily fix the catheter's position at its exit site.

The CPD prescription takes into account the amount and dextrose concentration of the dialysis solution to be used for each cycle and the length of the cycle. In part, the prescribed cycle length is determined by the time it takes for solute and osmotic equilibration to take place between plasma and dialysate such that the infusion of fresh dialysis solution would be advantageous. The speed with which solutes and water move across the peritoneal membrane (e.g., transport capacity) can be determined clinically by performance of the peritoneal equilibration test (PET). Continuous ambulatory peritoneal dialysis (CAPD) is a manual form of CPD in which the patient or caregiver attaches and instills a bag of sterile dialysis solution into the peritoneal cavity four times per 24 h, with each of the three daytime exchanges lasting approximately 5 h and the nighttime exchange, 9 h. In contrast, the most frequently used CPD modality for children in many countries, automated peritoneal dialysis (APD), uses an automated device which can measure, heat, deliver, drain, remeasure, and discard dialysate in patterns determined by the prescribing team. The greatest percentage of children receiving APD utilize a regimen consisting of 6–12 exchanges over 8 to 10 h per night with a daytime dwell consisting of approximately 50% of the nocturnal exchange volume. Guidelines for the performance of CPD in children recommend an individual exchange volume of 1,000–1,200 mL/m^2 for patients >2 years of age; younger patients should be prescribed a lower initial volume (600–800 mL/m^2) to promote tolerance. The efficacy or "adequacy" of CPD has historically been characterized by the measurement of small solute clearance, most commonly in terms of the Kt/V_{urea}. However, recently published guidelines by the National Kidney Foundation emphasize the clinical status of the patient as an important qualitative target and state that "adequate dialysis is likely provided if the patient's clinical status is characterized by adequate growth, blood pressure control, and nutritional status; avoidance of hypovolemia (or hypervolemia) and sodium depletion; and adequate psychomotor development." Factors that might contribute to inadequate CPD include:

- Loss of residual native kidney function
- Reduced peritoneal surface area caused by intra-abdominal adhesions
- Loss of membrane solute transport capacity/ultrafiltration capacity because of peritonitis
- Noncompliance with CPD prescription
- Poorly functioning PD catheter

Complications of CPD

The single most common complication that occurs in children maintained on CPD is peritonitis. Peritonitis contributes to significant morbidity and can lead to irreversible technique failure. The frequency of peritonitis in children regularly exceeds that in adults. The most recent annual report of the North American Pediatric Renal Trials and Collaborative Studies (NAPRTCS) includes information on 3,999 episodes of peritonitis in 6,008 years of follow-up for an annualized rate of 0.67 (one episode every 18.0 months). Young patient age and catheter

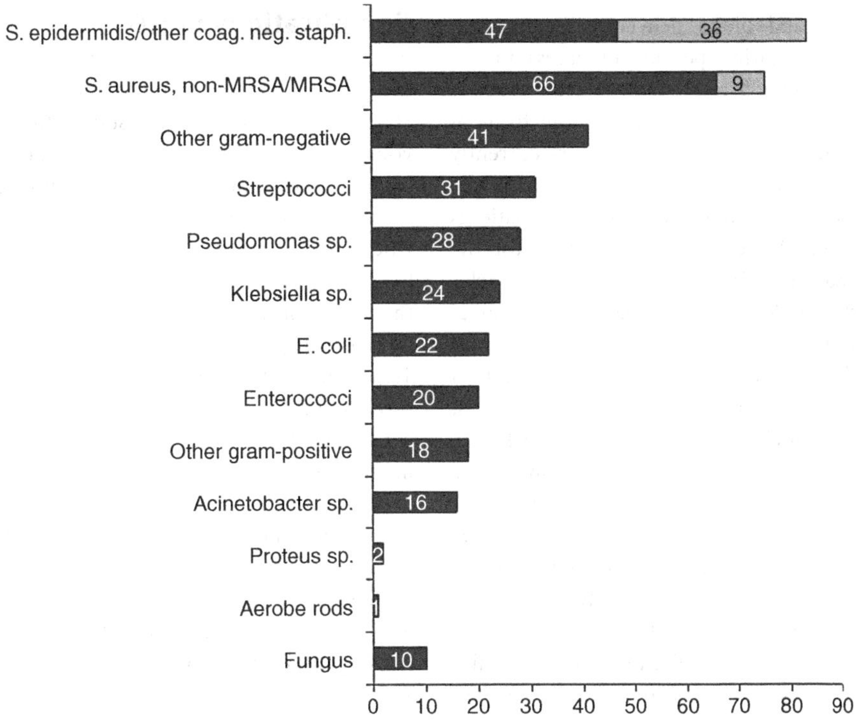

Figure 314.1
Distribution of peritonitis (n = 350) causative organisms in children receiving peritoneal dialysis

exit-site and tunnel infections, often secondary to *Staphylococcus* or *Pseudomonas*, are important risk factors for peritonitis. Approximately 50% of peritonitis episodes are caused by Gram-positive bacteria, particularly *Staphylococcus epidermidis* and *Staphylococcus aureus*, 20–30% by Gram-negative organisms, with the cultures remaining negative in a substantial percentage (<20%) of episodes (*Fig. 314.1*). Peritoneal dialysis patients presenting with abdominal pain and/or cloudy drained dialysis fluid (effluent) should be presumed to have peritonitis and should be evaluated for this infection. The diagnosis is confirmed when the effluent white blood cell (WBC) count is $>100/mm^3$ and at least 50% of the WBCs are polymorphonuclear leukocytes. When peritonitis is suspected and following collection of dialysate effluent for culture and cell count, empiric antibiotic therapy should be administered through the intraperitoneal route and consist of a combination of a first generation cephalosporin or a glycopeptide, with a third-generation cephalosporin or an aminoglycoside. To minimize the risk for antibiotic-related toxicity associated with the use of either vancomycin or an aminoglycoside, maintenance antibiotic therapy with alternative choices should be instituted as soon as the antibiotic susceptibilities are known.

Chronic Hemodialysis

Hemodialysis is currently the dialysis modality used by nearly 60% of prevalent pediatric patients in the USA and in almost all cases, is performed in a dialysis center. A HD system consists of a blood circuit, a dialysate circuit, and a dialyzer. Blood is pumped from the patient's vascular access to the dialyzer (the "arterial segment") and uremic toxins and water are removed. A separate pump delivers anticoagulants to prevent clotting within the extracorporeal circuit. The clearance of solutes is a function of the blood and dialysate flow rates and the permeability of the dialyzer's membrane to the solutes as clearance occurs by diffusion down a concentration gradient between plasma and dialysate. Ultrafiltration occurs because a transmembrane hydrostatic gradient is created from the blood to the dialysate compartment. The dialyzed blood is subsequently recirculated to the patient through the "venous segment" of the circuit. Throughout this process, ultrafiltration control systems and monitors that evaluate pressures within the blood lines and airleaks are engaged and alert the dialysis staff if adjustments are needed.

The vascular access is a crucial aspect of the blood circuit as the efficiency of HD is in large part dependent on access function and blood delivery. HD access is divided into two categories: permanent access in the form of an arteriovenous fistula (AVF) or arteriovenous graft (AVG) and semipermanent access in the form of catheters with a subcutaneous cuff. Catheters currently serve as the most common form of access for children receiving HD, being present in more than 60% of patients at dialysis initiation. While these devices allow for the blood flow necessary for HD in patients who have relatively small vessels that do not permit the surgical connection between the native artery and vein necessary for an AVF or AVG, catheters have a much greater complication rate than either of the permanent accesses. For this reason, it is recommended that children more than 20 kg who are expected to receive HD for more than 1 year should be evaluated for permanent vascular access placement.

The HD prescription incorporates the size of the dialyzer to be used, the blood and dialysate flow rates and the length of the treatment. To prevent hemodynamic instability, the extracorporeal circuit should not exceed 10% of the patient's blood volume, a requirement that often dictates dialyzer size. Blood flow rates are generally less than 400 mL/min/1.73 m^2 to minimize the risk for cardiovascular compromise and the dialysate rate is >1.5 times the blood flow rate to prevent dialysate saturation and the associated limitation of clearance. In most cases, HD is provided three times weekly, with each session lasting 3.5–4 h. Recent positive experiences with frequent HD (e.g., >5 days weekly) suggest that this approach may become more common. The urea reduction ratio is an approximation of the fraction of blood urea nitrogen (BUN) removed in a single dialysis session and is a method of quantitating HD adequacy. It is determined in the following manner:

$$\mathrm{URR} = (\mathrm{preBUN} - \mathrm{postBUN})/\mathrm{preBUN} \times 100\%$$

Although simplistic, the URR has a number of shortcomings: most importantly, the inability to provide any information about a patient's nutritional status. As a result, Kt/V has become the preferred method for measuring delivered dialysis as it more accurately reflects urea removal than does URR, and it provides information on patient nutrition by allowing for the calculation of the protein catabolic rate. Like in adults, the Kt/V in children should be >1.2 per dialysis session. Factors that might contribute to inadequate HD include:

- Underprescription
- Inadequate vascular access
- Shortened treatment time
- Dialyzer clotting

Complications of HD

Hypotension is the most common acute complication of HD and often arises as a result of the removal of large volumes of fluid by ultrafiltration and depletion of the intravascular volume during the dialysis session. At times, this may be accompanied by muscle cramps, nausea, dizziness, or headache. Noninvasive monitoring of the hematocrit within the dialysis circuit may help "predict" this complication since changes in hematocrit are inversely proportional to changes in intravascular volume. Treatment consists of stopping (or slowing) ultrafiltration, providing saline as deemed necessary to maintain blood pressure and minimize symptoms, and placing the patient in the Trendelenburg position. Adjusting the timing of antihypertensive medications on dialysis days and decreasing fluid gain between dialysis sessions are often effective preventative measures.

The most common complication associated with dialysis catheter usage is infection and sepsis. Infection rates of catheters are 60% higher than the rates for AVF and AVGs and often require removal/replacement of the access along with systemic antibiotic therapy. Catheter usage can also be complicated by the development of vascular stenosis and the inability to create a permanent vascular access.

Additional Clinical Issues for the Pediatric Dialysis Patient

Optimal management of the dialysis patient requires attention to a variety of clinical manifestations for which treatment guidelines do exist. Issues to be addressed include anemia management with iron and erythropoiesis stimulating agents (ESA), nutrition, growth and the possible use of recombinant growth hormone therapy (rhGH), bone-mineral management with phosphate binders and vitamin D therapy, blood pressure management, education, and health-related quality of life (HRQOL). In all cases, centers providing chronic dialysis to children should have access to the expertise needed to address these important concerns.

References

Chadha V, Warady BA (2005) Epidemiology of pediatric kidney disease. Adv Chronic Kidney Dis 12(4):343–352

Chadha V, Schaefer FS, Warady BA (2009) Dialysis-associated peritonitis in children. Pediatr Nephrol 24(3):463–474

National Kidney Foundation (2006) KDOQI Clinical Practice Guidelines and Clinical Practice Recommendations for 2006 updates: hemodialysis adequacy. peritoneal dialysis adequacy and vascular access. Am J Kidney Dis 48(suppl 1):S1–S322

North American Pediatric Renal Trials and Collaborative Studies (NAPRTCS) 2008 Annual Report. www.naprtcs.org

U.S. Renal Data System, USRDS 2007 Annual Data Report: Atlas of Chronic Kidney Disease and End-Stage Renal Disease in the United States, National Institutes of Health, National Institute of Diabetes and Digestive and Kidney Diseases, Bethesda, MD, 2007

U.S. Renal Data System, USRDS 2008 Annual Data Report: Atlas of Chronic Kidney Disease and End-Stage Renal Disease in the United States, National Institutes of Health, National Institute of Diabetes and Digestive and Kidney Diseases, Bethesda, MD, 2008

Warady BA, Schaefer F, Holloway M, Alexander S, Kandert M, Piraino B, Salusky I, Tranaeus A, Divino J, Honda M, Mujais S, Verrina E, The International Society for Peritoneal Dialysis (ISPD) Advisory Committee on Peritonitis Management in Pediatric Patients (2000) Consensus guidelines for the treatment of peritonitis in pediatric patients receiving peritoneal dialysis. Perit Dial Int 20:610–624

Warady BA, Feneberg R, Verrina E, Flynn JT, Müller-Wiefer DE, Besbas N, Zurowska A, Aksu N, Fischbach M, Sojo E, Donmez O, Sever L, Sirin A, Alexander SR, Schaefer F, The International Pediatric Peritonitis Registry (IPPR) (2007) Peritonitis in children who receive long-term peritoneal dialysis: a prospective evaluation of therapeutic guidelines. J Am Soc Nephrol 18:2172–2179

Warady BA, Alexander SR, Schaefer F (2009a) Peritoneal dialysis in children. In: Khanna R, Krediet RT (eds) Nolph and Gokal's textbook of peritoneal dialysis, 3rd edn. Springer, New York, pp 803–859

Warady BA, Jabs K, Goldstein SL (2009b) Chronic dialysis in children. In: Henrich WL (ed) Principles and practice of dialysis, 4th edn. Lippincott Williams & Wilkins, Philadelphia, pp 613–640

315 Pediatric Kidney Transplantation

Peter F. Hoyer

Introduction

Dr. Murray performed the first successful kidney transplantation more than 50 years ago among identical twins. At that time immunological and immunosuppressive concepts did not exist. About 15 years later, transplantation became an accepted treatment modality for adults with renal failure but was regarded as unethical for children. Today kidney transplantation is the preferred treatment for renal replacement therapy in children.

Major side effects of chronic renal failure like growth retardation, developmental delay, anemia, renal osteodystrophic bone disease as well as poor school attendance improve dramatically after successful kidney transplantation. Contraindications against kidney transplantations are few, i.e., malignancies or chronic infections. A major problem is still shortage of suitable and compatible organs. Unsolved challenges remain the preservation of renal function, prevention of infections, long-term cardiovascular problems, side effects of chronic drug administration, and long-term rehabilitation.

Underlying Diseases Leading to Kidney Transplantation

Underlying diseases leading to kidney transplantation are in one-third urinary tract malformations, one-third nephronophthisis and cystic kidney disease, and one-third acquired diseases like non genetic hemolytic uremic syndrome (HUS) and other glomerulopathies (➋ *Table 315.1*). Multiorgan diseases, which may deteriorate after transplantation, are important for the prognosis after transplantation. Syndromatic diseases with mental retardation require very intensive and long-term care.

Pretransplant Assessment and Preparing for the Waiting List

Outcome after transplantation clearly depends on careful pretransplant evaluation and preparation. Infections after transplantation are a major problem due to chronic immunosuppression. Therefore, care must be given to get all information about previous vaccinations and to complete missings recommended vaccinations. Especially life-attenuated vaccines should be completed before immunosuppression starts.

Complete assessment of the recipient includes a general physical status, evaluation of organ functions, mental and cognitive status. The immunological status includes blood groups and human leukocyte antigens, i.e., HLA antigens, and in case of autoimmune disease activity parameters including complement, anti-DNA antibodies or ANCAs. Chronic infections like tuberculosis must be excluded. In case of urinary tract malformation, a careful planning together with the pediatric urologist is mandatory; this may include nephrectomy of chronic infected kidneys as well as evaluation of the bladder by urodynamic studies. A miction cysturethrogram is recommended for almost all patients in order to diagnose a relevant vesicoureteral reflux.

Attention must be given to medications, which inhibit or enhance the drug metabolizing system cytochrome p450 of the liver, because this might have a tremendous effect on doses and drug levels of calcineurin inhibitors (➋ *Table 315.2*).

Living Transplantation Versus Deceased Donor Organ Transplantation

Nowadays most families wish to contribute to the treatment of renal failure by offering living transplantation to their children. It is important to inform the families as early as possible about such options, but very balanced information about the pros and cons is necessary. The pros for living-related transplantation are a short waiting time or even a preemptive transplantation, optimal timing of the transplantation, early and excellent graft function, almost no delayed graft function and fewer rejection episodes (➋ *Fig. 315.1*). In general, in the long-term run the prognosis of a living-related kidney is superior to a deceased donor organ (➋ *Fig. 315.2*). On the other hand, ethical issues have to be addressed. It is absolutely mandatory, that the transplantation is self-motivated and

Abdelaziz Y. Elzouki (ed.), *Textbook of Clinical Pediatrics*, DOI 10.1007/978-3-642-02202-9_315,

Table 315.1
Underlying diseases in pediatric kidney transplant recipients (NAPRTCS 2008)

Recipient and transplant characteristics	*N*	%
Total	9,854	100.0
Sex		
Male	5,853	59.4
Female	4,001	40.6
Primary diagnosis		
Aplasia/hypoplasia/dysplasia kidney	1,564	15.9
Obstructive uropathy	1,538	15.6
Focal segmental glomerulosclerosis	1,154	11.7
Reflux nephropathy	515	5.2
Chronic glomerulonephritis	328	3.3
Polycystic disease	287	2.9
Medullary cystic disease	271	2.8
Hemolytic uremic syndrome	260	2.6
Prune belly syndrome	254	2.6
Congenital nephrotic syndrome	254	2.6
Familial nephritis	225	2.3
Cystinosis	201	2.0
Pyelonephritis/interstitial nephritis	173	1.8
Membranoproliferative glomerulonephritis – Type I	171	1.7
Idiopathic crescentic glomerulonephritis	171	1.7
SLE nephritis	150	1.5
Renal infarct	136	1.4
Berger's (IgA) nephritis	127	1.3
Henoch-Schonlein nephritis	110	1.1
Membranoproliferative glomerulonephritis – Type II	81	0.8
Wegener's granulomatosis	55	0.6
Wilms' tumor	52	0.5
Drash syndrome	52	0.5
Oxalosis	52	0.5
Membranous nephropathy	44	0.4
Other systemic immunologic disease	32	0.3
Sickle cell nephropathy	16	0.2
Diabetic glomerulonephritis	11	0.1
Other	962	9.8
Unknown	608	6.2

Table 315.2
Drugs inducing or inhibiting the metabolizing system *Cytochrome P450 3A4* in the liver with the consequence of lowering or increasing blood levels of calcineurin inhibitors

Induction (CNI level down)	Inhibition (CNI level up)
Phenobarbital	Erythromycin
Phenytoin	Clarithromycin
Carbamacepin	Ketoconazole
Rifampicin	Fluconazole
Gluco-corticosteroids	Itraconazole
St. John´s wort etc.	Verpamil
	Diltiazem
	Grapefruit etc.

a free decision without any coercion. A careful clinical, laboratory and radiological evaluation of the donor is a prerequisite for transplantation. The safety of the donor has a high priority and donors with diseases that are occasionally unknown before evaluation must be excluded from living donation. In general, 30–50% of parents are acceptable as donors. Unrelated living donor transplantation has become an option if a clear relationship among donor and recipient is granted but any commercial organ transplantation has to be rejected.

Access to Transplantation and the Waiting List

In almost all countries, possible transplant recipients have to be registered on a waiting list in a local organ sharing network like in the *Eurotransplant foundation, UK Transplant, Scandinavian Transplant* network, or in the *UNOS* network in the United States. Waiting time for a transplant is by no means uniform and several factors are taken into consideration for an algorithm for organ allocation. ABO blood types continue to have a major effect and also HLA typing and histocompatibility are still considered as a major predictor for transplant success. Specific cytotoxic antibodies have to be measured on a regular basis. In case of competing for a same organ because of equal histocompatibility, time on a waiting list and medical urgency play a major role. Patients with special medical risk factors get some priority. In some countries, children get a preference on the waiting list, while in other countries this is not the case. Recently, data from UNOS suggest that children should preferentially receive organs from donors younger than 35 years and that HLA matching has less impact on outcome for a first transplant.

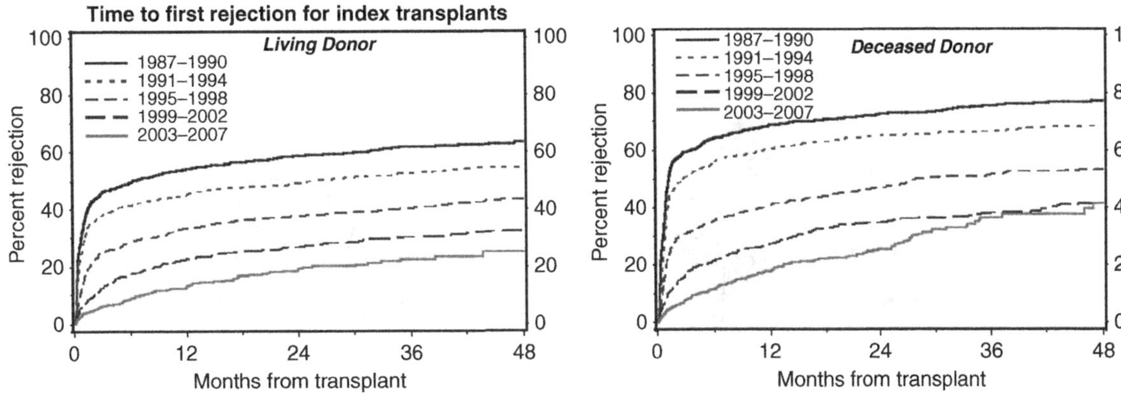

Figure 315.1
Time to first rejection episode in living donor transplantation and in deceased donor transplantation. There is a remarkable improvement over time (NAPRTCS 2008)

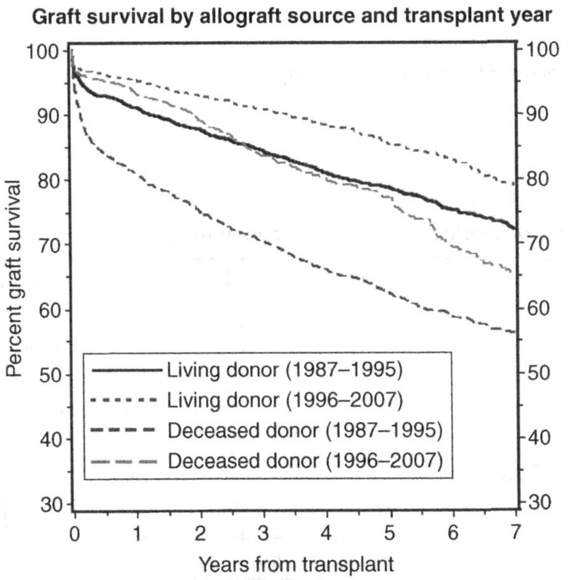

Figure 315.2
Improvement of graft survival over time in living and deceased donor transplantation. Five year graft survival after living donor transplantation is now in the order of 90% (NAPRTCS 2008)

Technical Aspects of Kidney Transplantation

In most children, the transplant kidney is placed like in adults in the right or left fossa iliaca with an anastomosis to the iliac artery and iliac vein. However, in the very young, large kidneys have not enough space and blood supply from the iliac artery may be insufficient. Therefore, the vascular anastomosis should be placed between the aorta and caval vein in the middle of abdomen (*Fig. 315.3*). Careful consideration has to be given to the kidney size and the recipient's size because a large transplanted kidney may require a high blood supply, which will not be achievable in very small recipients. Therefore, most centers recommend to transplant a kidney to a recipient with a minimum weight of 8–10 kg and to take into consideration the diameter of the aorta.

Perioperative Management

The perioperative management of kidney transplantation is standardized. Successes are clearly related to a center experience, which includes pretransplant preparation, experienced anesthesiology, specially trained transplant surgeons, as well as postoperative care. Adequate hydration should be measured by a central venous line, and fluid and electrolytes have to be balanced according to circulatory parameters and urine output. Most centers have a standard operation procedure with the administration of diuretics such as furosemide and infusion of mannitol before the anastomoses are opened. Dopamine infusion is widely accepted to enhance kidney perfusion and to maintain blood pressure adequately high; however, this recommendation has never been tested in a prospective trial in children.

Postoperative application of Doppler sonography in the operation room is important in order to exclude organ compression or early thrombosis. Urine output via transurethral catheter or suprapubic catheter should be checked hourly and any obstruction must be detected early in order to prevent a leakage of the vesicoureteral anastomosis.

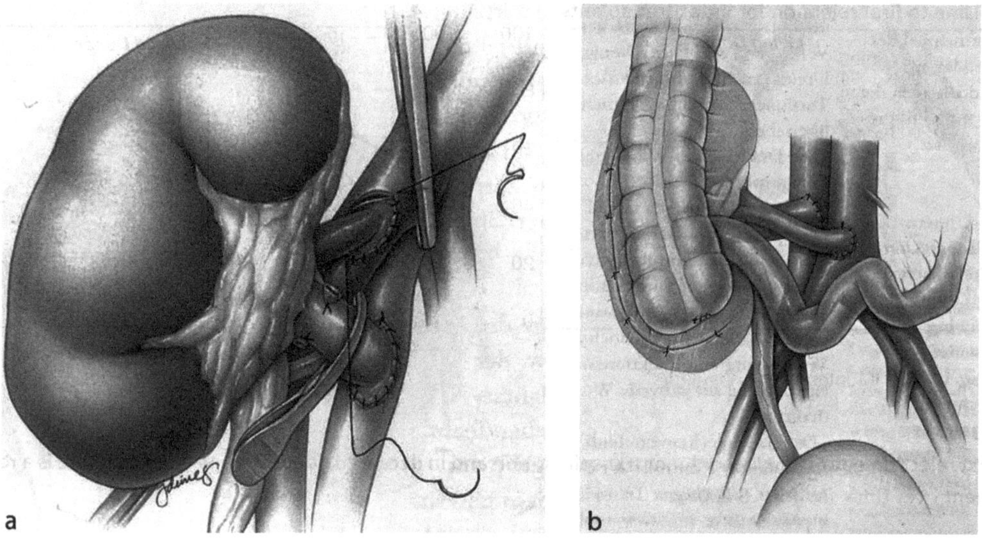

Figure 315.3
Surgical technique in the standard situation panel a and in small children panel b. In panel b, the renal artery is anastomosed to the aorta and the renal vein to the caval vein (Courtesy of Professor Paul, Clinic for Transplantation Surgery University Clinic Essen)

Immunosuppression

Immunosuppressive drugs can be classified in different categories:

- Steroids
- Lymphocyte-directed antibodies such as ATG, OKT3, thymoglobulin or IL2 receptor antibodies
- Calcineurin inhibitors like cyclosporine or tacrolimus
- mTOR-inhibitors (mammalian target of rapamycin): sirolimus and everolimus
- Antiproliferative agents like azathioprine or mycophenolic acid

Newer agents like co-stimulatory pathway blocking agents are used in adults but have not been tested in children so far. Major side effects of immunosuppressive drugs are listed in *Table 315.3*.

Steroids have been used as a basic drug in transplantation long time before newer drugs were developed. Most protocols still include steroids. Because of the major side effects, especially on growth in pediatric transplantation a search for steroid avoidance protocols or steroid withdrawal is going on. First trials without steroid treatment seem promising; however, a translation into daily routine outside from studies needs further confirmation.

The monoclonal antibodies OKT3 and ATG have been recommended as induction therapy by the NAPRTCS registry some years ago, but the superiority to treatment without the induction antibodies have not been demonstrated. The monoclonal antibody basiliximab, which is directed against the alpha chain of the interleukin 2 receptor on activated lymphocytes, should be in theory synergistic to treatment with calcineurin inhibitors. In large trials and meta-analysis, a reduction in early acute rejection episodes has been demonstrated but no benefit with

Table 315.3
Major specific side effects of immunosuppressive drugs

Steroids	Obesity, arterial hypertension, growth retardation
Cyclosporine A	Nephrotoxicity, hypertrichosis, gingival hyperplasia, elevated lipids
Tacrolimus	Nephrotoxicity, beta cell toxicity, EBV infectious problems
mTOR inhibitors	Elevated lipids, wound healing problems, enhancing cyclosporine toxicity, hypergonadotropic hypogonadism
MMF; MPA	Gastrointestinal tract, diarrhea, leucopenia, anemia, viral infections
IL2 R-AB	Antibody development, impact on CD4+CD25+ T_{regs}?

MMF mycophenolate mofetil, *MPA* mycophenolate acid, *IL2R-AB* interleukin 2 receptor antibody, T_{regs} regulatory T-cells regard to long-term outcome. In a prospective randomized double blind trial basiliximab was tested versus placebo with a standard immunosuppression consisting of cyclosporine steroids and mycophenolate mofetil. In this trial, no benefit with regard to rejection episodes was visible for basiliximab, however, the overall data were extremely good compared to results which are analyzed by registries (➋ *Fig. 315.1*) and which are much inferior. Therefore, a benefit of a monoclonal antibody against the IL2-receptor cannot be excluded under standard situation.

Cyclosporine A has become a corner stone in kidney transplantation in the late 1980s. Major side effects are nephrotoxicity, hypertrichosis, gingival hyperplasia, and elevated lipids. The calcineurin inhibitor tacrolimus is more powerful in terms of dosis and blood levels, but has the same nephrotoxic side effects. In addition to that, some beta cell toxicity has been reported in trials with adult patients and higher doses are associated with PTLD, especially in patients who are EBV naïve before transplantation. With regard to cosmetic side effects and compliance in young adolescents, tacrolimus is gaining preference by many centers.

mTOR inhibitors were introduced with the promise to lead to less nephrotoxicity and improved kidney function. However, high lipids early after transplantation, wound healing problems, and enhanced cyclosporine toxicity has reduced the enthusiasm. A recent trial by NAPRTCS combining sirolimus with tacrolimus has lead to unacceptable high PTLD rates. Nevertheless, mTor inhibitors with their specific profile have a place in a subgroup of patients with special problems. Mycophenolate mofetil (MMF) and the compound mycophenolic acid are the most widely used immunosuppressive drugs in about 80% of patients. Generally, they are used in combination with calcineurin inhibitors allowing a substantial reduction of these nephrotoxic compounds. MMF has become a substitute for azathioprine over the last 15 years. However, in terms of cost-effectiveness and long-term benefit azathioprine needs new consideration.

Due to the importance of the immunosuppressive therapy most drugs require a pharmacokinetic monitoring. The therapeutic window is rather small; undertreatment may lead to rejection and graft loss while overtreatment to toxicity or severe infections. In addition to that, many drugs may interfere with metabolism of calcineurin inhibitors (➋ *Table 315.2*) and also mycophenolate acid. The average dose of drugs used in various combinations after transplantation has been evaluated by NAPRTCS (➋ *Fig. 315.4*). It is of note that a combination of tacrolimus and MMF requires about half the dose of MMF, which is required with the combination of cyclosporine and MMF. Drug levels are measured as predose trough level or at certain time points to calculate drug exposure as area under the curve (AUC). This is essential to adjust drug dosing.

Reasons for Graft Failure

Under the current immunosuppressive therapies, graft loss due to rejection has become less important. The NAPRTCS registry reported in 2006 that the leading cause of graft failure are thrombosis with 21%, chronic rejection 20%, acute rejection 10%, death 8%, recurrence of original disease 9%, and all other different reasons 32%. Therefore, prevention of graft thrombosis has the major impact on outcome. Although there are no prospective trials, several factors may reduce the risk for thrombosis: meticulous surgical techniques with anastomosis guarantee in high kidney perfusion are of major importance. Identification of a hypercoagulable state with APC resistance, or a previous history of multiple thrombotic events may point to an increased risk after transplantation. While some centers report almost no graft thrombosis by prophylactic use of heparin, others have not seen a benefit. However, these results are difficult to interpret, because immediate postoperative monitoring of anticoagulation is not always reported and some publications are biased by large historical data.

Acute Rejection Episodes

Most acute rejection episodes are observed during the first 3 months after transplantation. The percentage of patients who are treated for acute rejections during the first year after transplantation has continued to decline from 30% to 20–15%. An acute rejection is defined as an acute deterioration of the graft function associated with specific pathologic changes. These pathologic changes have been classified by the Banff consortium (➋ *Table 315.4*).

The gold standard for diagnosing a rejection episode is a kidney biopsy. An ultrasound-guided kidney biopsy is a safe procedure and has the advantage to provide a clear diagnosis and to prevent unnecessary treatment. Other causes for functional deterioration of the graft can also be described by a kidney biopsy, i.e., drug toxicity (➋ *Fig. 315.5a*), unspecific tubular injury, recurrence of original diseases, and chronic allograft nephropathy (➋ *Fig. 315.5b*).

In case of acute rejection, steroid therapy usually can reverse rejection episodes. Steroid-resistant rejection is a rare event, which may require intensified immunosuppression

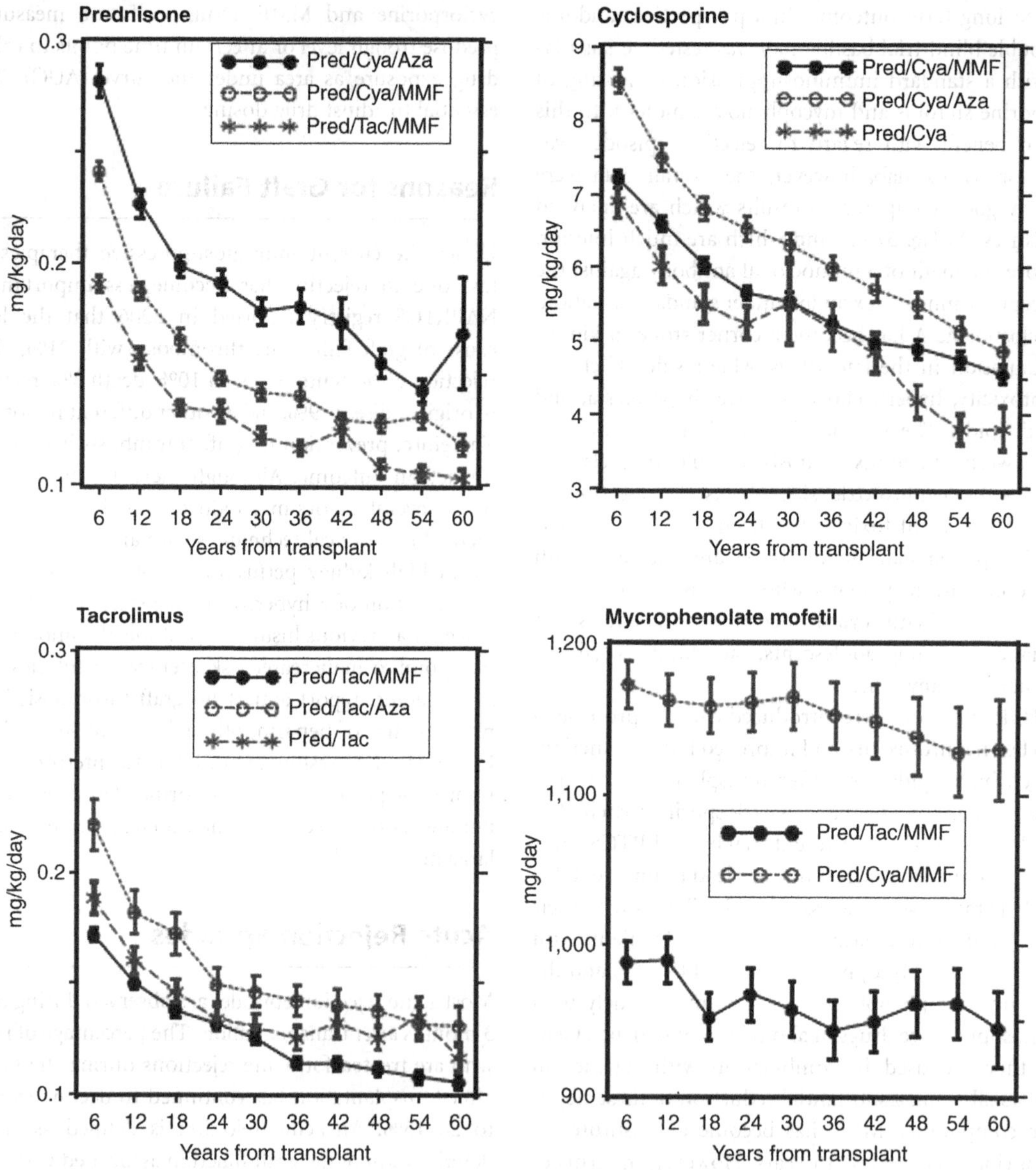

Figure 315.4
Mean drug concentrations used after transplantation in relation to combined drug therapies (NAPRTCS 2008)

with antibody therapy. In case of acute rejection, inadequate immunosuppression induced by poor drug absorption or noncompliance must be excluded. Switching to other drug combinations may be advisable.

Chronic Allograft Dysfunction

Chronic allograft dysfunction is an unsolved problem in kidney transplantation. While rejection episodes are rare events in younger children, poor compliance in adolescence may lead to chronic inadequate immunosuppression. Other reasons for chronic allograft nephropathy are not well-defined chronic immunologically mediated injury, arterial hypertension, chronic calcineurin inhibitor toxicity, the senescence of renal cells, and de novo diseases in the kidney such as transplant glomerulopathy or tubular interstitial nephritis by recurrent urinary tract infection.

Table 315.4
Banff 2005 diagnostic categories for renal allograft biopsies (2005 revision)[a]

1. Normal
2. AMR
Acute AMR (C4d$^+$) type
(a) ATN-like
(b) Capillary margination and/or thrombosis
(c) Arterial
Chronic active AMR[b]
glomerular double contours, peritubular capillary basement membrane multilayering. interstitial fibrosis, tubular atrophy, fibrous intimal thickening
3. Borderline changes
4. T cell–mediated rejection
Acute
• (a) Significant interstitial infiltration (<25% of parenchyma) and moderate tubulitis
(b) Significant interstitial infiltration (>25% of parenchyma) and severe tubulitis
• (a) Mild to moderate intimal arteritis
(b) Cases with severe intimal arteritis comprising >25% of the luminal area
• Transmural arteritis
Chronic active T cell–mediated rejection[b]
5. Interstitial fibrosis and tubular atrophy, no evidence of any specific cause
Grade
(a) Mild (<25% of cortex)
(b) Moderate (26–50% of cortex)
(c) Severe (>50% of cortex)
6. Other: Categories not considered to be due to rejection; may coincide with categories 2 through 5

[a]Adapted from reference
[b]Changes in the updated Banff 2005 schema
AMR = antibody mediated rejection

Infections After Transplantation

Infections after transplantation may be related to the disease of organs, to the recipient's immune status or to the immunosuppression itself. In a recent prospective trial with cyclosporine, MMF and basiliximab almost any infection was encountered in 95.4%, a cytomegalovirus infection in 12.8%, EBV virus infection in 9.2%, gastroenteritis in 23.9%, herpes simplex 10.1%, pyelonephritis 9.2%, rhinitis 21.1%, upper respiratory tract infection in 34.9%, and urinary tract infection 34.9%. Since CMV infection has an impact on graft function, the CMV recipient donor constellation is of great importance. In general, studies suggest a prophylactic gancyclovir therapy for at least 3 months in case of CMV mismatch, i.e., a positive donor in a negative recipient. In addition to that, monitoring of cytomegalovirus replication by measuring PP65 is established in many pediatric transplant programs.

EBV infection has also an impact on outcome. EBV infection rates increases with the amount of immunosuppression. EBV naïve children are at risk to develop an infection with a high viral DNA load and a prolonged course. Some studies reported coincidence with a cyclomegalovirus infection. A primary EBV infection in an EBV naïve recipient is a risk factor for the development of posttransplant lymphoproliferative disease (PTLD). The EBV viral load is measured in many centers, since it may point to a risk for PTLD, but there seems to be no definite correlation.

Urinary tract infections are common problems in patients with obstructive uropathy or bladder dysfunction. There is a high risk that this problem continues after transplantation. Operative removal of the recipient's diseased kidney and ureters, evaluation of the bladder

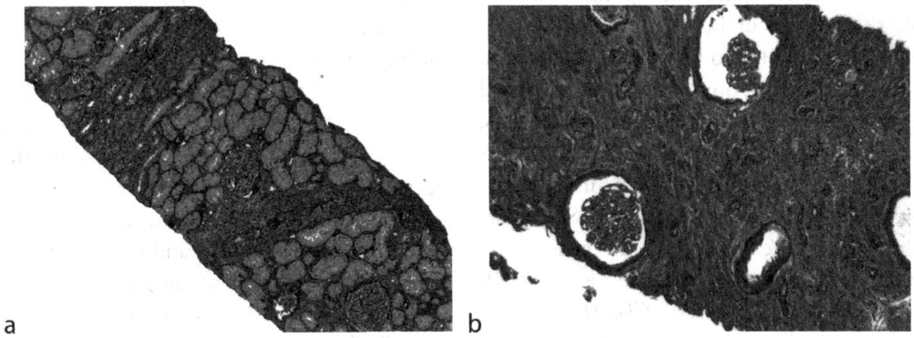

Figure 315.5
(a) Kidney biopsy with a striped form of interstitial fibrosis as can be seen as sign of calcineurin inhibitor toxicity or perfusion injury. (b) Chronic allograft dysfunction. Biopsy with severe interstitial fibrosis

function as well as treatment of bladder dysfunction should ameliorate the situation. Some cases can only be managed by continuous prophylactic antibiotic therapy.

Besides these classical infections, chronic immunosuppression may pose the patients to the risk of fungal infections or pneumocystis carini pneumonia (PCP). Due to a high fatality rate of PCP, intensive immunosuppressive protocols should get PCP prophylaxis with trimethoprim sulfamethoxazole.

Long-Term Problems After Organ Transplantation

After successful organ transplantation many problems may interfere with a good rehabilitation. These problems may be categorized as follows:

- Recurrence of original disease
- Progress of extra renal complications of the disease
- Consequences of chronic immunosuppression, i.e., direct toxicity of immunosuppressive drugs or consequences of over immunosuppression
- Cardiovascular diseases
- Progressive deterioration of the graft function

Recurrence of Original Diseases

With a transplantation of a new organ as a substitute to a failing organ, there is a hope, that the problem is cured. A look to the underlying diseases leading to renal transplantation makes clear, that different original diseases may not be cured in the same way by renal transplantation. A recurrence of original diseases after kidney transplantation is a relevant problem (➋ *Table 315.5*).

FSGS has been described for a long time to have a considerable risk to reoccur in a transplanted organ. Up to 30% have been reported to lose their organ due to recurrent FSGS. Treatment options that have been tried are intensified immunosuppression and plasmapheresis. The increasing knowledge about the etiology of FSGS allows a new perspective on this problem. In pediatric patients, about one-third of cases with FSGS may have an underlying gene mutation in genes that have been described to lead to FSGS, i.e., *NPHS1, NPHS2* (podocine), *NPHS3, Wt1, CD2AP, TRPC6, Laminin beta 2,* etc. By discriminating genetic and non-genetic FSGS it has been demonstrated, that genetic FSGS has a very low risk to reoccur in a transplanted organ while the rate of recurrence in non-genetic FSGS is high. These findings are very important for counseling parents who wish to donate a kidney.

Table 315.5
Recurrences of original diseases after kidney transplantation in children

	Recurrence (%)	Grade	Loss of kidney transplant (%)
HUS, atypic	>40	++	>50
FSGS	25–30	++	>50
MPGN I	70	+	12–30
MPGN II	100	(+)	10–20
Lupus erythematodes	5–40	(+)	5
IgA nephritis	55–85	+	5–20

HUS hemolytic uremic syndrome, *FSGS* focal segmental glomerulosclerosis, *MSGN* membrano proliferative glomerulonephritis

In Alport syndrome, mutations in the collagen gene (*X-linked Col4A5 and autosomal Col4A3/Col4A4*) have been described. After successful transplantation, deafness may progress. Some rare cases may develop a picture like a Goodpasture syndrome. An explanation for this is that a patient with a mutated collagen will receive a new antigen by a transplanted kidney which then causes anti-GBM antibodies.

Hemolytic uremic syndrome is one of the most common causes for acute renal failure. While the shigatoxine-associated HUS has a good chance for full recovery, the so-called atypical HUS, which is not caused by shigatoxine, may have a high risk for recurrence after transplantation. Various mutations in the complement/factor H system have been described to cause atypical HUS. In these cases, the kidney is a target for uncontrolled complement activation. While the transplantation procedure itself may activate the complement system, an insufficient inhibitory potential may then lead to the recurrence of the HUS in the transplanted kidney. Therefore, patients with atypical HUS should have an intensive workup to look for mutations in factor H, factor I, and factor B or to detect antibodies against factor H. The prognosis of recurrent HUS after transplantation is poor. Intensive plasmapheresis and plasma infusion may be an option in some patient. Besides recurrence of atypical HUS, a de novo HUS in a transplanted kidney has been described and explanations point toward a possible rule of calcineurin inhibitors.

In lupus nephritis, recurrence of the original disease is a rare event. Other immunological diseases like Wegner's granulomatosis or pauci-immune glomerulonephritis may have some risk for relapses after transplantation.

Data on the recurrence of Henoch Schönlein Purpura after transplantation are not conclusive.

In IgA nephropathy, IgA deposits in the mesangium can be demonstrated in almost all transplanted kidneys. However, this cannot be correlated with a further deterioration of the graft function.

In primary hyperoxaluria, the transplanted kidney may still be a target for continuous calcium oxalate deposition and early graft failure. In patients with primary hyperoxaluria, combined kidney liver transplantation should be considered, before a high oxalate load may worsen the general prognosis.

Progress of extra renal manifestation of systemic diseases is important in patients with autosomal recessive polycystic kidney disease (ARPKD). A liver involvement with liver fibrosis is obligatory. In addition to that, some patients have cholangiodysplastic features. The consequence of liver fibrosis is the development of portal hypertension, splenomegaly, and hypersplenism. Cholangiodysplasia may lead to cholangitis. Some patients with ARPKD may need a liver transplantation later in their course after kidney transplantation, in other patients; the liver involvement requires early combined liver kidney transplantation.

Patients with autosomal dominant polycystic kidney disease (ADPKD) rarely need a renal replacement therapy during childhood or adolescence phase. Some patients may develop liver cysts or mitral ballooning. Cerebral aneurisms have not been reported in pediatric patients.

Juvenile nephronophthisis is a common cause for chronic renal failure and transplantation in children. The disease may be very complex and many subtypes have been described. Major problems due to the progress of underlying disease are liver involvement with cholangiodysplasia and liver fibrosis, or tapetoretinal degeneration like in Senior–Loken syndrome.

Rare diseases with multiorgan involvement, which continue to be a problem after transplantation, are Joubert syndrome, Jeune syndrome, spondyloepiphyseal dysplasia, Bardet–Biedl syndrome, or juvenile cystinosis. Long-term problems are cerebellar ataxia, mental retardation, failure to growth, cerebral ischemia, or vision loss in case with tapetoretinal degeneration. Patients with cystinosis suffer from crystal deposition in the cornea, diabetes, and hypergonadotropic hypogonadism.

Malignancies After Organ Transplantation

The rate of malignancy is correlated to the intensity of immunosuppression. Lymphoproliferative diseases have been described in 2–5% of patients. First infection with EBV early after transplantation may be a risk for further development of PTLD (➲ *Fig. 315.6a*). PTLD may appear as polymorphic or monomorphic lymphoma (➲ *Fig. 315.6b*). While in milder cases, stopping of calcineurin inhibitor therapy may lead to tumor regression, others with monoclonal elements and CD20 expression (➲ *Fig. 315.6c*) improve after therapy with rituximab. Patients with undifferentiated lymphoproliferative diseases have a much less favorable prognosis despite intensive chemotherapy. Lymphomas, which appear beyond the early transplant phase after 1 or 2 years, are more likely to be Non-Hodgkin lymphomas. Then a standard chemotherapy is required. All children with chronic

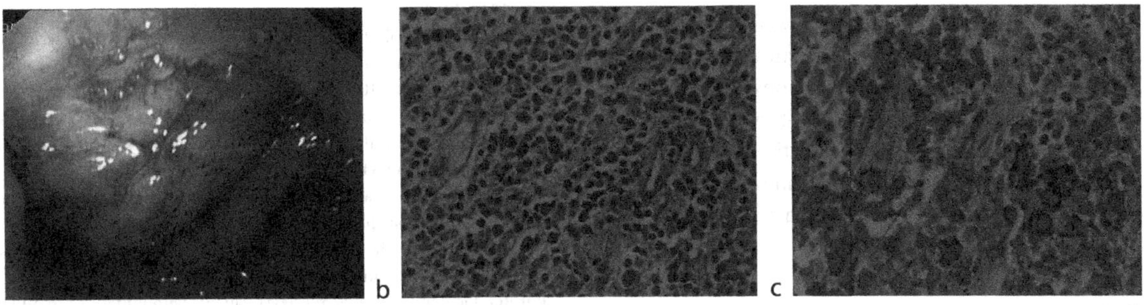

a b c

Figure 315.6
(a) Six years old boy 8 months after transplantation. Endoscopy of the distal esophagus: polypous swelling in the cardia region. (b) HE staining of the biopsy reveals a monomorphic lymphoma. (c) Biopsy of the lymphoproliferation with positive staining for the marker CD20

immunosuppressive therapy have an increased risk to develop skin cancer. Therefore, special attention must be given to suspicious skin lesions.

Cardiovascular Problems

An unsolved problem after solid organ transplantation is a high cardiovascular mortality. Major risk factors for that are long time on dialysis, chronic hyperphosphatemia, hyperlipidemia, arterial hypertension, and long-term administration of steroids and calcineurin inhibitors. Recent studies have shown calcifications in the coronary arteries in young adults and an increased arterial stiffness in patients with renal insufficiency on dialysis and also after transplantation. Future research for long-term rehabilitation for patients with chronic renal failure and transplantation should address the high impact of cardiovascular disease on patient's survival.

Noncompliance

Worldwide there are reports of high rejection rates and up to 20% of organ losses in young adolescents. Patients who are transferred to adult units are at highest risk. This age group has been described not to follow the multidrug regimes. Adolescents have an increased readiness for risks and decreased capability to estimate the future consequences of their acts and omissions. They are teenagers and they want to behave like teenagers. Pediatrics transplant centers pay increasing attention to this problem and many programs are under development to improve the noncompliance in young adolescents.

Summary

Pediatric kidney transplantation is a well-established therapy for chronic renal failure. Sophisticated surgical techniques and modern drug combinations lead to excellent short-term results; however, long-term problems like deterioration of graft function, infections, and cardiovascular morbidity beyond the child and adolescent phase remain challenges for future research activities.

References

Benfield MR, Tejani A et al (2005) A randomized multicenter trial of OKT3 mAbs induction compared with intravenous cyclosporine in pediatric renal transplantation. Pediatr Transplant 9(3):282–292

Caprioli J, Noris M et al (2006) Genetics of HUS: the impact of MCP, CFH, and IF mutations on clinical presentation, response to treatment, and outcome. Blood 108(4):1267–1279

Ciancio G, Burke GW et al (2008) Randomized trial of mycophenolate mofetil versus enteric-coated mycophenolate sodium in primary renal transplant recipients given tacrolimus and daclizumab/thymoglobulin: one year follow-up. Transplantation 86(1):67–74

Gritsch HA, Veale JL et al (2008) Should pediatric patients wait for HLA-DR-matched renal transplants? Am J Transplant 8(10):2056–2061

Harmon W, Meyers K et al (2006) Safety and efficacy of a calcineurin inhibitor avoidance regimen in pediatric renal transplantation. J Am Soc Nephrol 17(6):1735–1745

Hildebrandt F, Zhou W (2007) Nephronophthisis-associated ciliopathies. J Am Soc Nephrol 18(6):1855–1871

Hoyer PF, Vester U (2004) The impact of cyclosporine on the development of immunosuppressive therapy–pediatric transplantation using cyclosporine. Transplant Proc 36(2 Suppl):197S–202S

Kliem V, Fricke L et al (2008) Improvement in long-term renal graft survival due to CMV prophylaxis with oral ganciclovir: results of a randomized clinical trial. Am J Transplant 8(5):975–983

Kranz B, Vester U et al (2006) Outcome after kidney transplantation in children with thrombotic risk factors. Pediatr Transplant 10(7):788–793

Loirat C, Fremeaux-Bacchi V (2008) Hemolytic uremic syndrome recurrence after renal transplantation. Pediatr Transplant 12(6):619–629

Maecker B, Jack T, Zimmermann M, Abdul-Khaliq H, Burdelski M, Fuchs A, Hoyer P, Koepf S, Kraemer U, Laube GF, Müller-Wiefel DE, Netz H, Pohl M, Toenshoff B, Wagner HJ, Wallot M, Welte K, Melter M, Offner G, Klein C (2007) CNS or bone marrow involvement as risk factors for poor survival in post transplantation lymphoproliferative disorders in children after solid organ transplantation. J Clin Oncol 25(31):4902–4908

Mitsnefes MM (2004) Hypertension and end-organ damage in pediatric renal transplantation. Pediatr Transplant 8(4):394–399

Mitsnefes MM (2005) Cardiovascular morbidity and mortality in children with chronic kidney disease in North America: lessons from the USRDS and NAPRTCS databases. Perit Dial Int 25(Suppl 3):S120–S122

NAPRTCS (2008) Annual report 2008. http://spitfire.emmes.com/study/ped/annlrept/Annual Report – 2008.pdf

Offner G, Toenshoff B et al (2008) Efficacy and safety of basiliximab in pediatric renal transplant patients receiving cyclosporine, mycophenolate mofetil, and steroids. Transplantation 86(9):1241–1248

Oh J, Wunsch R et al (2002) Advanced coronary and carotid arteriopathy in young adults with childhood-onset chronic renal failure. Circulation 106(1):100–105

Opelz G, Dohler B (2007) Effect of human leukocyte antigen compatibility on kidney graft survival: comparative analysis of two decades. Transplantation 84(2):137–143

Pape L, Ehrich JH et al (2004) Cyclosporine in pediatric kidney transplantation. Transplant Proc 36(2 Suppl):203S–207S

Pondrom S (2009) The AJT report: news and issues that affect organ and tissue transplantation. Am J Transplant 9(9):1969–1970

Ruf RG, Lichtenberger A et al (2004) Patients with mutations in NPHS2 (podocin) do not respond to standard steroid treatment of nephrotic syndrome. J Am Soc Nephrol 15(3):722–732

Santoro D, Bellinghieri G et al (2005) Evolution of the classification of acute and chronic transplant rejection. G Ital Nefrol 22(Suppl 33):S65–S70

Sarwal M, Pascual J (2007) Immunosuppression minimization in pediatric transplantation. Am J Transplant 7(10):2227–2235

Smith JM, Ho PL et al (2002) Renal transplant outcomes in adolescents: a report of the North American Pediatric Renal Transplant Cooperative Study. Pediatr Transplant 6(6):493–499

Smith JM, Stablein D et al (2006) Decreased risk of renal allograft thrombosis associated with interleukin-2 receptor antagonists: a report of the NAPRTCS. Am J Transplant 6(3):585–588

Smith JM, Stablein DM et al (2007) Contributions of the transplant registry: the 2006 annual report of the North American Pediatric Renal Trials and Collaborative Studies (NAPRTCS). Pediatr Transplant 11(4):366–373

Terasaki PI, Cecka JM et al (1995) High survival rates of kidney transplants from spousal and living unrelated donors. N Engl J Med 333(6):333–336

Weber LT, Hocker B et al (2003) Mycophenolate mofetil in pediatric renal transplantation. Minerva Urol Nefrol 55(1):91–99

Webster AC, Playford EG et al (2004) Interleukin 2 receptor antagonists for renal transplant recipients: a meta-analysis of randomized trials. Transplantation 77(2):166–176

Blood Diseases

Michael Recht

316 Practical Approach to Anemia in Children

Ahmad A. Mallouh

Introduction

Like any other health problem, the etiologic diagnosis of anemia depends on interpreting information obtained from history, physical examination, and appropriately ordered laboratory tests. Before embarking on an extensive and expensive "laundry list" of laboratory testing, the physician needs to determine if the patient is truly anemic, taking into consideration the normal values for age, sex, and ethnicity (➋ *Table 316.1*).

Classification of Anemia in Children

Anemia is classified into two ways: erythrokinetic (physiologic) and morphologic classification.

Erythrokinetic (Physiologic) Classification

This classification utilizes the pathophysiology of anemia, whether it resulted from (a) underproduction (bone marrow suppression or infiltration), (b) shortened red blood cell (RBC) survival (hemolysis), (c) blood loss, or (d) the combination of more than one factor. A normal or low reticulocyte count indicates bone marrow suppression (aplasia or hypoplasia), infiltration (malignancy or storage disease), replacement (myelofibrosis or osteopetroses), deficient or poor utilization of iron (iron deficiency, anemia of chronic disease) or acute blood loss or early acute hemolysis (before the bone marrow has the time to respond), while a high reticulocyte count and/or the presence of nucleated RBCs in the peripheral circulation indicate an active bone marrow, such as hemolysis, recovery from transient aplasia, response to anemia caused by acute blood loss, or response to iron therapy in iron deficient patients (➋ *Table 316.2*).

Morphologic Classification

Based on the RBC morphology, anemia is classified according to the RBC size (mean corpuscular volume or MCV), mean hemoglobin concentration (MCHC), or mean hemoglobin content (MCH). Morphologically, anemia can be classified as normocytic (normal MCV), microcytic (low MCV), or macrocytic (high MCV). Depending on the hemoglobin concentration and content, anemias can be classified as normochromic (normal MCHC and MCH) or hypochromic (low MCHC and MCH). Development changes of these parameters should be taken in to consideration (➋ *Tables 316.1* and ➋ *316.3*).

Clinical Findings

History, physical examination, results from a complete blood count (CBC), and inspection of a well-prepared blood smear are the essential first steps in the workup for anemia. A systematic analysis of the information obtained in such a way enables the physician to establish a correct diagnosis in some cases and narrow the differential diagnosis for others, thus limiting the number of the needed specific tests.

History

Age, gender, ethnicity, dietary history, history of acute or repeated blood loss, dark colored stools, history suggestive of associated or causative diseases (fever, arthritis, skin rash, weight loss), history suggestive of inflammatory bowel disease, prolonged menstruation in teenaged girls, history of pica, history of drug or toxin exposure, past history of blood transfusion, present or past history of jaundice and red colored urine, family history of anemia, blood transfusion, splenectomy, or cholecystectomy represent only a short list of important information which direct the workup of children with anemia. These factors, alone or in various combinations, can direct the investigation toward or away from a possible diagnosis. Inherited anemias usually present early in childhood. RBC membrane disorders (hereditary spherocytosis, hereditary elliptocytosis, hereditary pyropoikilocytosis, etc.),

Abdelaziz Y. Elzouki (ed.), *Textbook of Clinical Pediatrics*, DOI 10.1007/978-3-642-02202-9_316,

Table 316.1
Normal hematologic values at various ages

Age	Hemoglobin (g/dl)	RBC (×10^{12}/l)	Hematocrit (%)	MCV (ft)	MCH (pg)	MCHC (%)	Reticulocytes
Cord blood	16.6	5.25	63	120	34	31.7	3.2
1 day	19.0	5.14	61	119	36.9	31.6	3.2
3 days	18.7	5.11	62	116	36.5	31.1	3.8
7 days	17.9	4.86	56	115	36.2	32.0	0.5
2 weeks	17.3	4.80	54	112	36.8	32.1	0.5
3 weeks	15.6	4.20	46	111	37.1	33.9	0.8
4 weeks	14.2	4.00	43	1–5	35.5	33.5	0.6
2 months	10.7	3.40	31	93	31.5	34.1	1.8
3 months	11.3	3.70	33	88	30.5	34.8	0.7
6 months	12.3	4.60	36	78	27	34	1.4
8 months	12.1	4.60	36	77	26	34	1.1
10 months	11.9	4.60	36	77	26	34	1.0
1 year	11.6	4.60	36	78	25	33	0.9
2 years	11.7	4.70	38	79	25	33	1.0
4 years	12.6	4.70	38	80	27	34	1.0
6 years	12.7	4.70	39	81	27	33	1.0
8 years	12.9	4.70	40	83	27	33	1.0
10–12 years	13.0	4.80	40	83	27	33	1.0
Men	16.0	5.40	47	87	29	34	1.0
Women	14.0	4.80	42	87	29	34	1.0

RBC red blood cells, *MCV* mean corpuscular volume, *MCH* mean corpuscular hemoglobin, *MCHC* mean corpuscular hemoglobin concentration

disorders of alpha globin chain (α-thalassemia), and RBC enzymopathies (G6PD, pyruvate kinase deficiency) may present in the neonatal period, while beta globin chain disorders (sickle cell disease, β-thalassemia) do not manifest clinically until at least 2–3 months of age. X-linked anemias, such as G6PD deficiency, affect mainly boys. However, it should be kept in mind that homozygous females are not uncommon in communities with high rates of consanguineous marriage. Race and ethnicity help in directing the investigations toward certain disease entities. Sickle cell disease is common in people of African origin, parts of the Arabian Peninsula, and parts of India. β-thalassemia is common in people of Mediterranean origin. α-thalassemia is common in people of African origin, Arabs in the Gulf area and in Southeast Asia. Hemoglobin E is common in Southeast Asian origin and parts of the Indian subcontinent. G6PD deficiency is common in people of Mediterranean origin (Greek, Arabs, Sardinians), in people of African origin, and in Southeast Asia. Nutritional anemia (iron deficiency, folate deficiency) and chronic lead poisoning are more common in children of low socioeconomic class. Iron deficiency is common in exclusively breast-fed infants and those taking non-iron-fortified formulas. Folate deficiency may occur in infants exclusively fed on goat's milk. Vitamin B12 deficiency may occur in vegetarians. Acute blood loss is usually evident and can be a cause of significant anemia depending on the amount of the lost blood. Chronic and repeated blood loss, on the other hand, can be missed without a specific and detailed history. Heavy menstrual periods, upper or lower gastrointestinal tract bleeding, manifesting as hemopytisis, melena, or fresh blood in the stools (esophageal varices, peptic ulcer, Meckle's diverticulum, intestinal hemangioma) might be the cause of iron deficiency anemia. A history of jaundice and/or dark colored urine suggests an acute hemolytic anemia. Hemolytic anemia after ingestion of fava beans, sulfa drugs, or antimalarial medications suggests the diagnosis G6PD deficiency. Aplastic anemia may result from ingestion of benzene, chemotherapeutic drugs, or myelosuppresive medication, i.e., chloramphenicol. Exposure to certain "folk medications" may lead to chronic lead poisoning.

Table 316.2
Erythrokinetic classification of anemia

Decreased or absent production of red blood cells
Aplastic/hypoplastic anemia
Congenital aplastic/hypoplastic anemia
Fanconi anemia
Diamond–Blackfan anemia
Dyskeratosis congenital
Schwachman–Diamond syndrome (pancreatic insufficiency and bone marrow failure syndrome)
Paroxysmal nocturnal hemoglobinuria, acquired aplastic/hypoplastic anemia
Acquired constitutional aplastic anemia (idiopathic or secondary to known causes, i.e., post hepatitis)
Transient erythroblastopenia of childhood (TEC).
Aplastic anemia secondary to Parvovirus B 19 in patients with chronic hemolytic anemia
Bone marrow failure due to drugs, toxins, irradiation, or infection
Bone marrow replacement malignancies (leukemia, lymphoma, disseminated solid tumor)
Myelofibrosis
Osteopetrosis
Myelodysplasia
Deficiency syndromes due to deficiency of substance needed for red blood cell production
Iron deficiency
Vitamin B12 deficiency
Folate deficiency
Copper deficiency
Zinc deficiency
Pyridoxine deficiency
Thiamine deficiency
Protein deficiency
Anemia secondary to erythropoietin deficiency
Chronic renal failure
Anemia of prematurity
Chronic malnutrition
Hypothyroidism, hypopituitarism
Ineffective erythropoiesis
Dyserythropoietic anemias
Vitamin B12 and folate deficiencies
Sideroblastic anemia
Chronic lead poisoning
Thalassemia syndrome
Thiamine-responsive megaloblastic anemias

Table 316.2 (Continued)

Orotic aciduria with megaloblastic anemia
Ineffective utilization of iron by bone marrow
Chronic inflammatory diseases
Acute or chronic infection
Viral diseases
Excessive red blood cell destruction (shortened red blood cell survival)
Hemolytic anemias
Congenital hemolytic anemias
Hemoglobinopathies (sickle cell disease, hemoglobin C, hemoglobin E, etc.)
Thalassemia syndrome (α and β thalassemia)
Unstable hemoglobin mutation
Red blood cell membrane disorders (hereditary spherocytosis, hereditary elliptocytosis, hereditary pyropoikilocytosis, hereditary pyknocytosis, hereditary stomatocytosis, and paroxysmal nocturnal hemoglobinuria)
Red blood cells, enzyme deficiency (glucose-6-phosphate dehydrogenase deficiency, pyruvate kinase deficiency)
Acquired hemolytic anemias
Immune hemolytic anemia
Autoimmune hemolytic anemia
Allo-immune hemolytic anemia
Drug-induced immune hemolytic anemia
Immune hemolytic anemia associated with collagen-vascular diseases, lymphoma, or infections
Nonimmune acquired hemolytic anemia
Disseminated intravascular coagulopathy (DIC)
Hemolytic–uremic syndrome (HUS)
Thrombotic thrombocytopenic purpura (TTP)
Kasabach–Merritt syndrome (KMS)
Hemolytic anemia associated with bacterial or parasitic infection
Microangiopathic hemolytic anemia associated with congenital heart disease or prosthetic heart valves
Hypersplenism
Acute splenic sequestration (in sickle cell disease)
Anemia due to blood loss

Associated symptoms can direct investigation to certain diagnostic entities. History of recurrent painful attacks suggests sickle cell disease. History of petecheal rash, echymosis, epistaxis, or easy bruisability may indicate thrombocytopenia. History of severe or recurrent infection may indicate the presence of severe neutropenia

Table 316.3
Morphologic classification of anemia

Microcytic anemias
Iron deficiency anemia
Thalassemia syndromes
Chronic lead poisoning
Sideroblastic anemia
Pyridoxine deficiency/dependency
Anemia of chronic inflammatory disease
Some anemias associated with unstable hemoglobins
Macrocytic anemia
A. With megaloblastic features
Vitamin B1 deficiency
Folate deficiency
Orotic aciduria
Thiamine-responsive megaloblastic anemia
Drug-induced megaloblastic anemia (methotrexate, 6MP, anticonvulsants, Bactrim)
B. Without megaloblastic features
Reticulocytosis
Aplastic/hypoplastic anemia (may be normocytic or macrocytic)
Dyserythropoietic anemia
Liver disease
Hypothyroidism
Normocytic anemia
Aplastic anemia
Hemoglobinopathies
Red blood cell membrane disorders
Red blood cell enzymopathies
Immune hemolytic anemia
Microangiopathic hemolytic anemia
Acute blood loss
Hypersplenism
Anemia associated with acute infection
Anemia of chronic renal failure

either as a separate entity or in association with pancytopenia, i.e., aplastic anemia or hypersplenism. A history of systemic disease may give a clue to the etiologic diagnosis of the anemia. A history of chronic disease may cause anemia either by improper utilization of iron by the bone marrow, malabsorption, poor diet intake, or occult blood loss. A past history of blood transfusion suggests a chronic or recurrent process. A history of neonatal jaundice and/or anemia may suggest an inherited disease. A past history of cholelithiasis suggests a chronic hemolytic process. A family history of a specific type of anemia suggests a similar diagnosis in the child. Family history of splenectomy or cholelithiasis at a young age suggests an inherited chronic hemolytic anemia. Family history of a hypochromic microcytic anemia not responding to iron therapy in a parent or sibling suggests the diagnosis of thalassemia.

Physical Examination

The clinical manifestations of anemia are nonspecific. They are related to the severity and acuteness of the anemia. Pallor, tachycardia, and lethargy may be present in severe anemia; however, these are not sensitive, especially in chronic anemia. Anemia is often diagnosed on routine CBC done prior to a surgical procedure, routine clinic visit, or on hospitalization for other medical problems. Associated findings may suggest the etiologic diagnosis:

- Hepatosplenomegaly and chronic hypochromic microcytic hemolytic anemia together with family history or certain ethnic background suggests the diagnosis of β-thalassemia major
- Splenomegaly with chronic hemolytic anemia and family history of splenectomy or cholecystectomy suggest hereditary spherocytosis
- Lymphadenopathy with or without hepatosplenomegaly associated with a petecheal rash may suggest hematologic malignancy
- Jaundice and/or dark colored urine suggest a hemolytic process
- A petecheal rash and/or ecchymoses suggest pancytopenia
- Various dysmorphic features may suggest a specific type of anemia, i.e., Fanconi anemia, Blackfan–Diamond syndrome, or thalassemia major

Complete Blood Count and Inspection of the Blood Smear

The physician needs to look at and try to interpret every item in the CBC. RBC indices form the bases of the morphologic classification of anemia (*Table 316.3*). The degree of bone marrow activity forms the basis of the erythrokinetic classification of anemia (*Table 316.2*). Some types of anemia can be diagnosed simply by inspecting a peripheral blood smear (RBC membrane disorders and microangiopathic anemias). Target cells are suggestive of hemoglobinopathies. The presence of hypersegmented neutrophils is suggestive of folic acid or vitamin B12 deficiency. Abnormal malignant cells (blasts) are suggestive of leukemia. Basophilic stippling of the RBCs suggests chronic lead poisoning (although, it must be remembered that basophilic stippling may be present in other disease entities such as congenital nonspherocytic hemolytic anemias and unstable hemoglobins). Thrombocytopenia and/or neutropenia indicate involvement of other cellular blood elements rather than isolated anemia.

Diagnosis of Anemia

Once it is decided that a patient has anemia, several questions must be answered prior to a plan for specific laboratory testing is pursued:

- Does the patient have isolated anemia or pancytopenia?
- Is the anemia due to underproduction (bone marrow failure), hyperdestruction (hemolysis) or underproduction on top of hyperdestruction (aplastic crisis in patients with chronic hemolytic anemia)?
- Is the anemia acute or chronic?
- Is there a family history of a similar condition?
- Are there any dysmorphic features present on physical exam?
- Are the RBCs microcytic, normocytic, or microcytic?

Further investigations should be planned using the answers to these questions and using the morphologic and erythrokinetic classification.

Hypochromic Microcytic Anemia

For practical purposes, the differential diagnosis of hypochromic microcytic anemia in children includes: iron deficiency anemia, β-thalassemia trait, hemoglobin E disease, α-thalassemia trait, chronic lead poisoning, anemia of chronic disease, and the sideroblastic anemias (➲ *Tables 316.4* and ➲ *316.5*). Hemoglobin electrophoresis is the preferred diagnostic test for β-thalassemia trait. A high hemoglobin A2 level is diagnostic. Hemoglobin A2, however, can be normal if β-thalassemia trait is associated with severe iron deficiency, δ/β-thalassemia, or α-thalassemia. Hemoglobin F is also often elevated in β-thalassemia trait. Hemoglobin electrophoresis also is diagnostic for other hemoglobinopathies with microcytic anemia, i.e., Hb E, Hb C, Hb D, and Hb H. Low serum iron, high total iron binding capacity (TIBC), and low serum ferritin are characteristic of iron deficiency. The serum ferritin level is the most sensitive and specific none invasive test, as it is a reflection of iron stores. Serum

Table 316.4
Differential diagnosis and expected laboratory values for microcytic hypochromic anemia

Laboratory value[a]	Iron deficiency	β-thalassemia trait	α-thalassemia trait	Hemoglobin H disease	Chronic lead poison	Sideroblastic anemia	Chronic disease
MCV	↓	↓	↓	↓	↓	↓ or N	↓ or N
RDW	↑	N	N	↑	N	↑	N
Parents' MCV	N	↓ One parent	↓ One parent	↓ One parent	N	N	N
Serum iron	↓	N	N	↑	N	↓ or N	↓
TIBC	↑	N	N	↑	N	↓ or N	↓ or N
Serum ferritin	↓	N	N	↑	N	↑ or N	↓
FEP	↑	N	N	N	N	↑ or N	↑
Hemoglobin electrophoresis	N	↑A_2 ↑F	N	Hb H present	N	N	N
Brilliant crystal blue stain	Neg	Neg	Neg	Neg	Neg	Neg	Neg

[a]*MCV* mean corpuscular volume, *RDW* red blood cell distribution width index, *TIBC* total iron-binding capacity, *FEP* free erythrocyte protoporphyrin

Table 316.5
Laboratory values in iron deficiency anemia versus anemia of chronic disease

	Normal range	Iron deficiency (mean)	Chronic disease (mean)
Iron (μg/dl)	70–190	≤30	>30
TIBC (μg/dl)	250–400	≥450	>200
Transferrin saturation	30	≤7	≤14
Ferritin	20–220	≤10	≤150
Macrophage iron in marrow	2+	0	3+

TIBC total iron-binding capacity

ferritin, however, is an acute phase reactant and can be normal if iron deficiency is associated with inflammatory disease, infection, hepatitis, or pregnancy. A therapeutic trial of iron therapy can be used as a diagnostic and therapeutic test. A significant rise in the reticulocyte count after 5–7 days or a significant rise of hemoglobin (1–1.5 gms/dl) after one month of oral iron therapy are diagnostic of iron deficiency. Failure to respond almost always exclude iron deficiency. It should be remembered; however that noncompliance is one of the most causes of failure to respond. Isolated iron malabsorbtion is extremly rare. The RDW and Mentzer index (MCV/RBC) are useful in differentiating iron deficiency from thalassemia trait. A higher RDW (>20) and high Mentzer index (>13) are suggestive of iron deficiency. α-thalassemia is diagnosed by exclusion, except for hemoglobin H disease which can be diagnosed by supravital stain (brilliant cresyle blue) and hemoglobin electrophoresis. The presence of high levels of hemoglobin Barts in newborn blood is diagnostic of α-thalassemia trait.

Chronic lead poisoning is characterized by hypochromic microcytic anemia and basophilic stippling of the RBCs. High whole blood lead level is diagnostic. The sideroblastic anemias are rare in children. Bone marrow examination is required for diagnosis. The presence of ringed sideroblasts in the bone marrow is diagnostic. Anemia of chronic disease can be differentiated from iron deficiency by (in addition to the clinical picture) normal to high serum iron and serum ferritin and normal TIBC.

Macrocytic Anemias

Macrocytosis denotes large red blood cells (high MCV). While megaloblastic anemia is the most common cause of macrocytosis and while megaloblasts are by definition macrocytes, not every macrocyte is a megaloblast. Megaloblastic anemia results from impaired DNA synthesis resulting in large RBCs. Bone marrow RBC precursors are dysblastic with the maturation of the nucleus, and cytoplasm is asynchronous. Macrocytic anemias can be divided into two subtypes: the megaloblastic anemias and the nonmegaloblastic macrocytic anemias.

Megaloblastic Anemia

Megaloblastic anemias are characterized by macrocytic RBCs, macro-ovalocytes, hypersegmented neutrophils, and megaloblastic erythroid precursors in the bone marrow. The most common causes of megaloblastic anemia are folate deficiency (diagnosis is confirmed by low RBC folate level) and vitamin B12 deficiency (diagnosis is made by low serum vitamin B12 level).

Further studies are needed to confirm the diagnosis of megaloblastic anemia and to identify an etiology (e.g., the Schilling test, anti-parietal cell antibodies, anti-intrinsic factor antibody). Several drugs interfere with DNA synthesis and cause megaloblastic changes in the RBC precursors with or without anemia. These drugs include anticonvulsants (phenytoin, phenobarbital), chemotherapeutic agents (methotrexate, 6-mercaptopurine, hydroxyurea), and trimethoprim-sulfamethoxazole. Diagnosis in these cases is clearly based on the history of drug intake. Several inborn errors of metabolism can cause megaloblastic anemia (orotic aciduria, homocystinuria, methylemalonic aciduria). Patients affected by these conditions have complex clinical manifestations. The diagnosis depends on the clinical picture and specific tests for the suspected disease. Thiamine-responsive anemia is usually associated with sideroblastc anemia. The diagnosis is suggested by the exclusion of other causes of megaloblastosis and response to thiamine therapy.

Non-megaloblastic Macrocytic Anemia

Macrocytic anemia without megaloblastic bone marrow changes can be due to reticulocytosis, aplastic anemia, Blackfan–Diamond anemia, myelodysplastic syndromes, and dyserythropoietic anemias. Reticulocytes are large cells. A high reticulocyte count can be the cause of an elevated MCV. The diagnosis of aplastic anemia is suggested by reticulocytopenia and is confirmed by the examination of bone marrow biopsy. Myelodysplastic syndromes and dyserythropoietic anemias require bone marrow examination for diagnosis.

Normocytic Anemias

Normocytic anemias are due to either RBC underproduction or hyperdestruction (hemolysis):

1. Anemias due to underproduction (bone marrow failure): This group includes the aplastic anemias (congenital or acquired), bone marrow infiltration (leukemia, lymphoma, disseminated malignant solid tumors etc.), myelofibrosis, and osteopetrosis. In addition to the clinical picture, which may suggest the diagnosis in some cases, these anemias are characterized by a low reticulocyte count. The diagnosis is confirmed by bone marrow examination.
2. Anemias due to hyperdestruction (hemolytic anemias): These anemias are characterized by laboratory evidence of hyperactive bone marrow (high reticulocytes count and/or the presence of nucleated RBCS in the peripheral circulation). They include:
   (a) Red blood cells membrane disorders such as hereditary spherocytosis, hereditary elliptocytosis, and hereditary pyropoikilocytosis. A family history of one of these diseases, a family history of splenectomy and/or cholelithiasis at a young age may suggest the diagnosis. These diagnoses are confirmed by inspection of a well-prepared blood smear. Specific tests such as the osmotic fragility may be required to confirm the diagnosis.
   (b) Hemoglobinopathies (sickle cell disease, Hb C, Hb D) are diagnosed by hemoglobin electrophoresis.
   (c) Red blood cells enzymopathies (G6PD deficiency, pyruvate kinase deficiency) are diagnosed by specific enzyme assays.
   (d) Autoimmune hemolytic anemia is diagnosed by a positive direct anti-globulin test.
   (e) The microangiopathic hemolytic anemias (DIC, hemolytic uremic syndrome) are diagnosed by inspection of the peripheral blood smear. Thrombocytopenia and schistocytes (fragmented RBCs) are often present.

References

Bessman JD, Gilmer PR, Gardner FH (1983) Improved classification of anemia by MCV and RDW. Am J Clin Pathol 80:322–326

Brown RG (1991) Determining the cause of anemia: general approach with emphasis on microcytic hypochromic anemias. Postgrad Med 89:161–164

D'Onofrio G, Chirillo R, Zini G et al (1995) Simultaneous measurement of reticulocytes and red blood indices in healthy subjects and patients with microcytic anemia. Blood 85:818–823

Irwin JJ, Kirchner JT (2001) Anemia in children. Am Fam Phys 64:1379–1387

Kohli-Kumar M (2001) Screening for anemia in children: AAP recommendation – a critique. Pediatrics 108:e56

Novak RW (1987) Red blood cell distribution width in pediatric microcytic anemias. Pediatrics 80:251–254

Richardson M (2007) Microcytic anemia. Pediatr Rev 28:5–14

Robins EB, Blum S (2007) Hematologic reference values for African American children and adolescents. Am J Hematol 82: 611–614

Walters MC, Abelson HT (1996) Interpretation of the complete blood count. Pediatr Clin N Am 43:599–622

Yip R, Dallman PR (1984) Age-related changes in laboratory values used in the diagnosis of anemia and iron deficiency. Am J Clin Nutr 39:427–436

317 Immune Hemolytic Disease of the Newborn

Jason Glover · Bill H. Chang

Definition/Classification

Hemolytic disease of the newborn (HDN) is a form of IgG-mediated red blood cell (RBC) destruction whereby maternal antibodies cross the placenta and cause hemolytic anemia in the newborn. It is classified as a congenital anemia due to peripheral destruction of the red blood cells.

Etiology

The first description of HDN is thought to have been in 1609 by a French midwife named Louyse Bourgeois about a twin birth. The first infant died of hydrops fetalis and the second died of jaundice and opisthotonis a few days later. It was not until 1932 when Diamond et al. coined the term "erythroblastosis fetalis" as a syndrome linking congenital anemia, jaundice, and hydrops fetalis with evidence of extramedullary hematopoiesis and erythroblastemia. During the 1930s and 1940s, Landsteiner and Weiner described the Rhesus (Rh) blood groups, while Levine and associates described the link between the Rh groups and HDN. This description involved a case of a woman who had a recent delivery of a hydropic stillborn then had a severe transfusion reaction to her husband's blood. Levine postulated that she had become sensitized to her husband's blood from the fetus. They later showed that the mother was Rh-negative and her husband was Rh-positive. Later, Chown's description of how Rh-negative mothers could be sensitized by a transplacental hemorrhage led to clinical trials in both the UK and the US suppressing allo-immunization. Women given anti-D IgG intramuscularly at the time of delivery had a dramatic decrease in the risk of HDN. Therefore, the history and management of HDN have led to many breakthroughs including immunoprophylaxis using human antibodies and development of screening programs for maternal blood group antibodies.

Epidemiology

Prior to immunoprophylaxis, HDN due to the Rh was a major source of long-term morbidity and early mortality in the developing fetus and newborn. Since the majority of HDN is due to Rh allo-immunization, the incidence is closely linked with the proportion of a population who are Rh-negative. For example, about 10% of live births in the UK were of Rh-positive children to Rh-negative mothers. It is thought that about 1 pregnancy in 200 is susceptible to hemolytic disease of the newborn with a historical mortality rate of 1 in 400. Prior to the use of immunoprophylaxis, approximately 16% of Rh-negative women became sensitized in their first ABO compatible Rh-positive pregnancy and one half would have detectable anti-D immunoglobulin 6 months after delivery. This usually occurs as a result of exposure to fetal antigens during pregnancy. Although fetal cells can be detected in maternal blood during all trimesters of most pregnancies, the largest exposure to fetal blood occurs in the third trimester and delivery. Interestingly, about 25% of D-negative women will either not become sensitized or will become tolerant. Partial protection can also come from ABO incompatibility by unknown mechanisms. By their fifth pregnancy the probability of sensitization is about 50%. With the advent of Rh immunoprophylaxis, the incidence of HDN due to Rh has decreased to approximately 1.8% of susceptible pregnancies.

Pathogenesis

The Rh blood group system is a complex system comprised of a tetramer of several proteins. Rh-positive blood type is mainly comprised of one D subunit, one CE subunit, and two RhAg subunits, whereas Rh-negative blood type consists only of two CE subunits and two RhAg subunits. Therefore, sensitization occurs due to exposure of the RhD subunit. At first exposure a primary

Abdelaziz Y. Elzouki (ed.), *Textbook of Clinical Pediatrics*, DOI 10.1007/978-3-642-02202-9_317,

weak IgM response will not affect the fetus because IgM does not cross the placenta. The subsequent IgG response will then affect the fetus causing hemolysis. After a primary response, a subsequent exposure produces a rapid IgG response that then crosses the placenta. Therefore, repeated exposures increase the severity of HDN in subsequent pregnancies. The fundamental cause of erythroblastosis is an immune-mediated red cell destruction causing increased erythropoiesis. Due to peripheral red cell destruction, extramedullary erythropoiesis can be found in the liver, spleen, kidneys, skin, intestines, and adrenal glands with subsequent immature nucleated RBCs found in the peripheral blood.

Other rare causes of varying degrees of HDN are due to at least 26 other blood group systems. These molecules include transporter and channels such as Diego or Kidd, pathogen receptors such as Duffy, adhesion molecules, enzymes such as ABO and Kell, structural proteins, and complement receptors. With the advent of immunoprophylaxis and decreasing family sizes, the incidence of HDN due to Rh has been decreasing whereas other causes appear to be slightly increasing. Of the multitude of antibodies that have been reported to cause HDN, most have been single case reports or cause a mild form of the disease. In contrast, disease caused by antibodies to Kell has been described as severe. It is second to RhD in its immunizing potential. Since this antigen is expressed in early erythroid progenitors, it may suppress erythrogenesis causing early hydrops. HDN due to ABO incompatibility accounts for approximately 5% of infants with jaundice. It usually causes a milder form of HDN except in southeast Asia, Africa, and Latin America for unknown reasons.

Pathology

Once sensitization occurs, the factors affecting the severity of HDN include the placental transfer of antibody, the characteristics of the antibody and antigen, the maturation of the spleen, and fetal erythropoiesis. All four IgG subclasses can be transported across the placenta with fetal levels reaching the mother's levels by 17–20 weeks' gestation. Typically, in Rh HDN, antibodies do not fix complement. Instead, Fc-mediated pathways lead to opsonization of the RBCs. Anti-D coated RBCs adhere to macrophages in rosettes, especially in the spleen. The RBCs are then consumed by the macrophages, or their membranes become damaged and fragile leading to lysis. Antibody-dependent cellular toxicity also accounts for some RBC destruction through myeloid and NK cell activity.

On occasion antibodies that bind to the RBCs can fix complement (as in ABO incompatible transfusion reactions). If a high enough concentration fixes complement, red cell extravascular destruction occurs which can lead to hemoglobinemia, shock, and disseminated intravascular coagulopathy. End products of red cell destruction are then predominantly cleared by the liver. Antigens such as Rh and Kell are restricted to the erythroid cells expressed in the fetus and neonate. Therefore, infants with this disease can present in hydrops due to early severe anemia.

Clinical Manifestation

Since the 1950s, degrees of severity of HDN have been used to assist in classification, research, and treatment of the disease. Mild HDN is described as having antibody-coated red cells that are identifiable by Coomb's test, without an associated anemia. This group accounts for close to 50% of the affected fetuses and requires almost no treatment. Infants with moderate HDN have elevated bilirubin and are at risk for neural toxicity and kernicterus without treatment. They will have signs of anemia without acidosis or signs of hydrops. Peripheral blood will show polychromasia, anisocytosis, and reticulocytosis. This group accounts for approximately 30% of affected fetuses and requires intensive phototherapy and exchange transfusion to manage the jaundice. Severe HDN present with severe anemia, hydrops, or impending hydrops and can die before, during, or after birth without intensive management (including intrauterine transfusion). If untreated, one half will develop hydrops between 18 and 34 weeks' gestation with polyhydramnios. Ascites, pleural, and pericardial effusions may develop with subsequent compression hypoplasia of the lungs making respiration difficult at birth.

Diagnosis

Initial prenatal diagnosis for infants at risk of Rh-mediated HDN can be performed by blood type and antibody screen on the mother. A thorough prenatal history should include whether the mother had previous pregnancies and/or blood transfusions. Maternal antibody screening and typing for both ABO and D-antigen is the standard of care at the first prenatal visit. This should include elective abortions, due to the sensitization of the mother and risk of HDN to complicate future pregnancies. In a mother who is Rh-negative and an initial antibody screen is weak or negative, testing should be repeated at 24–28 weeks into the pregnancy, prior to the administration of anti-D immunoglobulin. Mothers with maternal serum red cell antibody titers ≥1:16 should then undergo Doppler ultrasound for peak systolic blood flow of the middle cerebral artery to predict moderate to severe anemia. Fetuses diagnosed with early anemia should undergo prenatal treatment.

In 1997, Lo et al. were able to identify the presence of free fetal DNA from a maternal blood sample. This discovery had obvious implications in reducing the need for invasive procedures such as chorionic villus sampling and amniocentesis to determine a fetus' blood type. The fetal DNA obtained from the mother's serum can be used to determine the fetal blood group phenotype for the D-antigen as well as the minor antigens c, E, C, K. Prenatal determination of fetal D-antigen status may reduce the rate of unnecessary anti-D immunoglobulin injections (40% of D-negative mothers will have a D-negative fetus). Typing of all D-negative mothers has been determined to be feasible and will likely become standard of care.

HDN in the newborn is typically diagnosed through clinical symptoms and laboratory tests that are common to any hemolytic process. Clinical symptoms include jaundice, pallor, hepatosplenomegaly, and may progress to tachycardia. The jaundice associated with HDN often presents within the first 24 h of life. A thorough laboratory evaluation would include complete blood counts with differential, manual examination of the smear for schistocytes, and increased reticulocytes. An elevated unconjugated serum bilirubin can aid in establishing the diagnosis of HDN from other types of jaundice, assessing the degree of hemolysis, and estimating the risk of developing kernicterus. Microspherocytes may be seen in HDN due to ABO incompatibility but is usually not seen in HDN due to Rh incompatibility.

Either the direct antiglobulin test (Coomb's) or the indirect antigen test may be used to detect an antibody-mediated HDN. The direct antiglobulin test is utilized to show the presence of maternal antibody on the child's red blood cells. The maternal antibody will cause agglutination of the child's red blood cells in a standard serum that is known to contain antibodies to IgG. An indirect antiglobulin test is used to screen for very low concentrations of IgG antibodies present in the mother's serum that can cross the placenta. The Kleihauer-Betke test can be used to estimate the degree of fetal hemoglobin transferred from either placental hemorrhage, or the normal transfer of the fetal components of the placenta.

Differential Diagnosis

The differential diagnosis of HDN is dependent on the severity of the disease. Causes of hydrops fetalis in the fetus or newborn include other blood disorders such as severe iron deficiency anemia; alpha thalassemia; cardiac dysrhythmias such as supraventricular tachycardia; metabolic disorders such as lysosomal storage diseases; genetic disorders such as Turner's (XO) Syndrome; maternal infections such as syphilis and parvovirus B19; and tumors such as teratomas.

Neonatal jaundice can be subdivided into indirect (unconjugated) and direct (conjugated) hyperbilirubinemia. Causes of unconjugated hyperbilirubinemia, if left untreated may develop into kernicterus, including HDN, bacterial and viral sepsis, normal physiologic jaundice, dehydration, cephalohematomas, hypothyroidism, or metabolic disorders such as Crigler–Najjar syndrome and Gilbert's Syndrome. The etiology of hemolysis in a newborn (➋ *Table 317.1*) should also include the broad categories of sepsis/infection, red blood cell membrane defects, red blood cell enzyme deficiencies, hemoglobinopathies, and medication associated red cell destruction.

Treatment

Maternal Treatment

Attempts to suppress the maternal immune response in cases with a prior history of HDN have been attempted. Although Rh-immune globulin is effective in preventing the mother's immune response, it is known to be ineffective in stopping a response once it has begun. Plasma exchange of the mother has also been attempted to lower the maternal antibody levels. However, this decrease is only transient, and higher rebound can occur. The procedure is costly, can be painful, and vascular access is necessary. Administration of pooled IVIG to the mother has also been attempted in cases of expected severe disease, although the exact mechanism of action is not well defined. Clinical research trials are continuing to investigate IVIG's safety and efficacy.

Fetal Treatment

Prior to immunoprophylaxis, 8% of fetuses would develop hydrops before 32 weeks making early intervention important for the outcome of the fetus. Early attempts at intraperitoneal fetal transfusion proved to be efficacious.

Table 317.1
Causes of hemolytic anemias in the newborn

General etiologies	Specific etiologies	Special features
Immune-mediated	– Rh incompatibility – ABO incompatibility – Minor antigen mismatch: Kell, Duffy	– The most common cause of severe early jaundice
Sepsis	– Bacterial – Viral sepsis (such as herpes simplex viremia)	Jaundice may be conjugated and unconjugated, due to hemolysis- and endotoxin-mediated reduction of bile secretion
RBC membrane defect	– Hereditary spherocytosis – Hereditary elliptocytosis – Hereditary stomatocytosis – Hereditary ovalocytosis	– Family history may be positive for anemia and gallstones at an age <40 years
RBC enzyme deficiency	– Glucose-6-phosphate – Pyruvate kinase – Hexokinase – Glucose-6-phosphate isomerase – Phosphofructokinase – Aldolase – Triose phophate – Glyceraldehyde-3-phophate isomerase – Phosphoglycerate	– Rare other than G6PD – Associated with metabolic and severe neurologic disorders
Hemoglobinopathies	– Thalassemias – Sickle cell diseases	β-thalassemia may present with significant severe hemolysis
Drug-induced	– Oxytocin – Drugs that cause oxidative stress in G6PD	– May be worsened by drug passage in the breast milk – May increase the hemolysis in G6PD

Later, fetal intravascular transfusion became the preferable procedure as it dramatically reversed hydrops and increased survival. This procedure is usually performed under ultrasound guidance into the umbilical vein at its insertion into the placenta. Intraperitoneal fetal transfusion remains a technique used for the severely affected fetus with small cord vessels, or more commonly, the older fetus where fetal size and placement of the placenta preclude access to the umbilical vessels.

Neonatal Treatment

General Care

Fortunately, in the post-Rh-immunoprophylaxis era, cases of severe hydrops fetalis are rare. This has made the study of interventions in the management of severe HDN in clinical trials difficult. Many of the procedures such as drainage of pleural and peritoneal effusions, and what level to perform exchange transfusion remain studied in small numbers. Standard treatment of issues from prematurity such as surfactant administration need to be more aggressive in the child with HDN as they may compound systemic problems. Top-up transfusions should be considered in anemic neonates who are acidotic, hypoxic, and hypotensive. However, if multiple top-up transfusions are needed then iron studies should be followed for signs of overload, especially in cases of liver dysfunction.

Infants with mild to moderate disease should undergo early and aggressive phototherapy with both spotlights and a fiber-optic blanket. A bilirubin level at which to institute phototherapy is largely arbitrary; however, it is accepted that premature infants should start phototherapy at a much lower level. The rate of rise of the bilirubin may be more concerning than a stably high level. Although dehydration is a potential risk of phototherapy, it is less compared to the risks associated with exchange transfusion.

Feeding should be encouraged early as long as exchange transfusion is not anticipated, given exchange transfusion's increased risk of necrotizing enterocolitis.

Although breast milk and colostrum contain Rh antibodies, very little antibody is absorbed across the intestine of the infant. Folate supplementation may be necessary in children who have had exchange transfusion from adult sources which have a lower folate level. Folic acid supplementation (100–200 μg/day) is recommended for several weeks after exchange transfusion. Iron supplementation is not needed in cases of HDN as the iron will be reabsorbed, and additional transfusion may cause overload. Vitamin B12 is usually adequate in the mother's breast milk.

Exchange Transfusion

Originally performed in the 1920s through the anterior fontanelle, exchange transfusion is now performed using umbilical catheterizations. This technique not only replaces the antigen-coated RBCs of the newborn with fresh RBCs, but also corrects the anemia, prevents hyperbilirubinemia, and modestly removes unbound anti-D antibody. Exchange transfusion can produce a significant drop in neutrophil levels and a reduction in platelets that are both generally well tolerated. Other complications include apnea and bradycardia, hypocalcemia, bleeding, and catheter-associated thrombosis. These complications are mostly mild and asymptomatic but rarely can be catastrophic leading to the death of the patient. Because of these risks, there are no specific thresholds for the indication of exchange transfusion. Instead, most providers will perform the procedure on their experience for significant anemia or when conservative measures do not control the bilirubin. Since the risk of serious complications are higher in the ill patient versus the mildly symptomatic patient, early exchange may be warranted.

IVIG

Several small studies have examined the use of IVIG on the infant to potentially treat HDN. However, there is a lack of evidence to indicate the safety and efficacy of IVIG. Therefore, IVIG should only be recommended in a well-defined clinical trial.

Prognosis

Both the morbidity and mortality of the disease is dependent on the successful treatment of the hemolysis and anemia. With successful prevention and treatment there should be minimal long-term effects from this disease. Patients with mild HDN (about 50% of cases) will most likely suffer no long-term effects. Newborns with moderate disease (about 30% of cases), however, are at risk for kernicterus if they do not receive treatment. Again, with successful treatment of the anemia and hyperbilirubinemia, minimal sequelae should occur. The maternal anti-D-titers of these infants are usually >1:64. They will have some degree of a symptomatic anemia but are not usually hydropic. In the past they would have received exchange transfusion, however, with current aggressive management with intense phototherapy this may be avoided. Cases of severe HDN have hydrops or are progressing toward hydrops in utero. They will die in utero or shortly after birth if aggressive interventions such as fetal intravascular transfusion are not undertaken. Polyhydramnios may be the first sign in utero of a hydropic infant. Anasarca, ascites, pleural, and peritoneal effusions may develop and cause hypoplasia of crucial organ formation such as the lungs.

Prevention

Prevention of Rh sensitization hinges on immunoprophylaxis by injecting anti-RhD immunoglobulin to the recipient. Originally tested to prevent sensitization in males, successful trials were undertaken in which Rh-negative, unsensitized females were given anti-D intramuscularly after delivery of an Rh-positive infant. Post-natal Anti-D prophylaxis of 200–300 μg given within 72 h of pregnancy lowered the incidence of RhD alloimmunization 6 months after delivery and in subsequent deliveries. Further, prenatal administration of 100 μg (500 international units) of anti-D at 28 weeks and 34 weeks' gestation to women in their first pregnancy can reduce the risk to about 0.2%. Therefore, most guidelines recommend routine administration of Rh immunoglobulin to all D-negative pregnant women in the early and mid-third trimester. Both pre- and post-natal prophylaxis will prevent 96% of RhD isoimmunization. Earlier antenatal prophylaxis for women who are likely to abort or undergo amniocentesis or chorionic villus sampling is safe and may reduce further sensitization. Although small amounts of anti-D may cross the placenta, there appears to be no adverse effects to the fetus. In rare occasions, a large fetal-to-maternal transplacental hemorrhage may occur at the time of delivery needing prompt assessment and a titrated dose of anti-D.

References

(1966) Prevention of Rh-haemolytic disease: results of the clinical trial. A combined study from centres in England and Baltimore. Br Med J 2(5519):907–914

Bowman JM (1988) The prevention of Rh immunization. Transfus Med Rev 2(3):129–150

Bowman JM, Chown B et al (1978) Rh isoimmunization during pregnancy: antenatal prophylaxis. Can Med Assoc J 118(6):623–627

Chown B (1954) Anemia from bleeding of the fetus into the mother's circulation. Lancet 1:1213

Chown B (1969) Prevention of Rh immunization. Can Med Assoc J 100(18):869

Daniels G, Finning K et al (2009) Noninvasive prenatal diagnosis of fetal blood group phenotypes: current practice and future prospects. Prenat Diagn 29(2):101–107

Darrow R (1938) Icterus gravis (erythroblastosis neonatorum). An example of etiologic considerations. Arch Pathol 25:378

Diamond LK, Blackfan KD et al (1932) Erythroblastosis fetalis and its association with universal edema of the fetus, icterus gravis neonatorum and anemia of the newborn. J Pediatr 1:269–309

Grannum PA, Copel JA et al (1988) The reversal of hydrops fetalis by intravascular intrauterine transfusion in severe isoimmune fetal anemia. Am J Obstet Gynecol 158(4):914–919

Hartwell EA (1998) Use of Rh immune globulin: ASCP practice parameter. American Society of Clinical Pathologists. Am J Clin Pathol 110(3):281–292

Jackson JC (1997) Adverse events associated with exchange transfusion in healthy and ill newborns. Pediatrics 99(5):E7

Landsteiner K, Wiener A (1940) An agglutinable factor in human blood recognized by immune sera of rhesus blood. Proc Soc Exp Biol Med 43:223

Levine P, Stetson R (1939) An unusual case of intra-group agglutination. JAMA 113:126

Levine P, Katzin E et al (1941) Isoimmunizatoin in pregnancy: its possible bearing on the etiology of erythroblastosis foetalis. JAMA 116:825

Liley HG (2003) Immune hemolytic disease. In: Nathan DG, Orkin SH, Ginsburg D, Look AT (eds) Nathan and Oski's hematology of infancy and childhood, 6th edn. vol 1. Elseiver, pp 56–85

Lo YM, Corbetta N et al (1997) Presence of fetal DNA in maternal plasma and serum. Lancet 350(9076):485–487

Maayan-Metzger A, Schwartz T et al (2001) Maternal anti-D prophylaxis during pregnancy does not cause neonatal haemolysis. Arch Dis Child Fetal Neonatal Ed 84(1):F60–F62

Mari G, Deter RL et al (2000) Noninvasive diagnosis by Doppler ultrasonography of fetal anemia due to maternal red-cell alloimmunization. Collaborative Group for Doppler Assessment of the Blood Velocity in Anemic Fetuses. N Engl J Med 342(1):9–14

Medearis AL, Hensleigh PA et al (1984) Detection of fetal erythrocytes in maternal blood post partum with the fluorescence-activated cell sorter. Am J Obstet Gynecol 148(3):290–295

Pollack W, Gorman JG et al (1968) Results of clinical trials of RhoGAM in women. Transfusion 8(3):151–153

Vaughan JI, Manning M et al (1998) Inhibition of erythroid progenitor cells by anti-Kell antibodies in fetal alloimmune anemia. N Engl J Med 338(12):798–803

318 Iron Metabolism and Iron Deficiency Anemia

Heather Bradeen · Samir Shehab · Michael Recht

Background

Anemia is defined as a reduction in red blood cell mass or blood hemoglobin concentration. In practice, these are most often signaled by reductions of either the hemoglobin, a measure of the concentration of hemoglobin in the whole blood expressed as grams per 100 mL (dL), or hematocrit, the fractional volume of a whole blood sample occupied by red blood cells. The age variation for the hemoglobin and hematocrit varies widely in the pediatric population. It is particularly important to use age- and sex-adjusted norms when evaluating a pediatric patient for anemia. Iron deficiency is the most common nutritional deficiency in children. The World Health Organization estimates that anemia, largely caused by iron deficiency, affects between 500 million and two billion people worldwide. In some developing countries, up to 50% of preschool children and pregnant mothers have iron deficiency anemia (IDA). In the United States, the prevalence of IDA among children has been declining as a result of improved dietary iron supplementation.

Iron Metabolism

Iron is an abundant element in the natural world. Iron plays a critical role in mammalian cells. It is essential for oxygen delivery as well as numerous enzymatic systems. However, excess iron is toxic to cells and a deficiency of iron impairs cellular functions. Iron homeostasis is tightly regulated. Its excretion from the body is limited either through blood loss or sloughing of mucosal cells of the gastrointestinal lining. There are no known pathways for regulated iron excretion. Complex systems control iron absorption from dietary sources. Efficient recycling of iron is necessary to maintain its balance in the body. Disturbances to iron homeostasis have a significant impact on children's health. Insufficient iron intake leads to iron deficiency anemia, the most common pediatric hematology disorder worldwide. An excess of iron also causes problems particularly in children receiving chronic blood transfusions. Iron overload causes serious chronic organ dysfunction particularly in the liver, the heart, and the endocrine glands.

Normal Iron Endowment

Full term infants are born with approximately 350 mg of total body iron. By adulthood, an individual's iron endowment increases to 3–5 g. Normal adult men usually absorb 0.5–1 mg of iron each day from the diet. Menstruating women absorb more, approximately 1–2 mg of iron each day, to account for iron losses through blood loss. In pregnancy, iron absorption increases to approximately 2–4 mg daily to support the iron needs of the developing fetus. Approximately 75% of the total iron is within the erythrocyte and erythrocyte precursor population, and 10–20% is in storage form in the body. The remaining iron is utilized iron-dependent enzymatic pathways and biochemical reactions.

Iron Absorption

Total iron absorption depends on the bioavailability of dietary iron as well as regulation of iron absorption from the intestinal cells (➔ *Fig. 318.1*).

Dietary Iron

Animal sources provide iron in the form of heme iron. Heme iron is a component of hemoglobin and myoglobin. It is the most bioavailable form of iron and is efficiently absorbed from the diet. Heme iron passes into the cytoplasm unchanged, where the iron molecule is then released. Nonheme iron, in the form of an insoluble ferric salt, is less bioavailable than heme iron. Nonheme iron is absorbed using a different cellular pathway. The ferric iron must first be converted to ferrous form, and then it is transported through the intestinal cell membranes with

Abdelaziz Y. Elzouki (ed.), *Textbook of Clinical Pediatrics*, DOI 10.1007/978-3-642-02202-9_318,

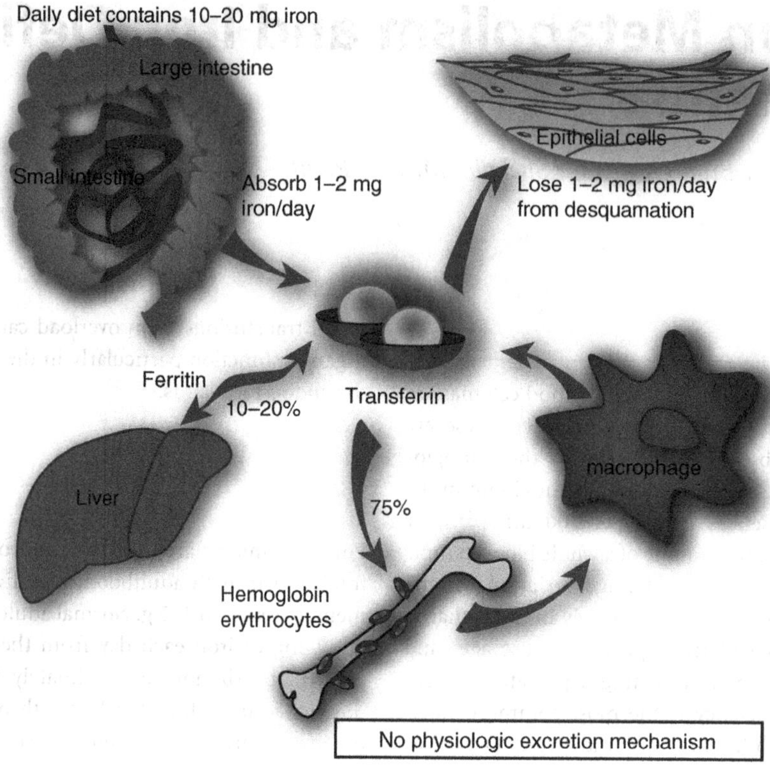

Fig. 318.1
Iron absorption

iron transport proteins. A variety of factors influence the absorption of nonheme iron. Acidic foods such as food rich in vitamin C enhance conversion of iron in the ferric form to the soluble ferrous form. The presence of dietary meat proteins in the intestinal lumen also enhances the absorption of nonheme iron. On the other hand, certain foods can impede absorption, such as tannates (tea and coffee), phosphates, antacids, and egg yolks. The decreased bioavailability of nonheme iron puts the vegan at risk for developing iron deficiency. Human breast milk, although low in total iron content, contains iron in a highly bioavailable form.

Intestinal Iron Absorption

Iron is absorbed in the proximal duodenum. Intestinal iron absorption is controlled at the level of mucosal transport and absorption. When total body iron stores are low, iron absorption is increased. Hypoxia and increased erythropoietic demand increase intestinal iron absorption. Both inflammation and increases in body iron have an opposing effect and decrease iron absorption.

Iron Storage and Recycling

Most of the body's iron is within a closed loop involving circulating transferrin, the erythroid bone marrow, senescent erythrocytes, and the reticuloendothelial macrophages. There is additional gain and loss through the intestinal mucosa. Excess iron is stored as ferritin in the liver. Smaller amounts of iron are utilized in muscle by myoglobin (not shown). The potential reactivity of iron molecules necessitates mechanisms for its safe transport and storage. Several important proteins are required for the safe handling of iron.

- Transferrin is the plasma transport protein for iron. Transferrin binds iron with extremely high affinity and prevents iron from reacting with other molecules so that iron may be delivered to tissues in a nontoxic form.
- Ferritin is a protein that stores iron and prevents it from reacting with other molecules. Iron stored as ferritin is relatively available for iron metabolism when iron needs arise. The liver is the primary location for ferritin. Plasma ferritin measurement is related to cellular iron stores.

- Hemosiderin is another form of stored iron, but its iron is much less available and is difficult to mobilize in the regulation of iron hemostasis. Its primary role is probably to keep iron from causing damage to surrounding molecules.

Iron Deficiency Anemia

Prevalence

In the United States, about 9% of toddlers have iron deficiency, with 3% affected by iron deficiency anemia. Rates decrease with advancing age until adolescence, when up to 16% of girls develop iron deficiency and 3% have iron deficiency anemia. The overall rate of iron deficiency in young children has declined only slightly during the past 4 decades. In the United States, iron deficiency is higher among children living at or below the poverty level, and in Black and Hispanic children. Other risk factors for IDA include childhood obesity and a history of prematurity or low birth weight. These findings demonstrate the need for ongoing surveillance and early intervention to prevent iron deficiency during infancy and early childhood, particularly among high-risk groups.

Clinical Features

Although iron deficiency anemia is often asymptomatic, the ability to recognize its clinical signs and symptoms is essential to preventing long-term neurodevelopmental delay. Additionally, appropriate therapy for those who are otherwise symptomatic has been shown to effectively treat symptoms as well as correct the underlying deficiency. Although its correlation with the severity of anemia is poor, pallor is the most easily recognizable sign of iron deficiency anemia. It is most prominent in the conjunctivae, gingiva, palmar creases, and nailbeds. Physical exam often also reveals tachycardia and systolic flow murmurs, and, less commonly, glossitis, stomatitis, koilonychias, and blue sclerae.

Children with mild to moderate iron deficiency anemia, defined as having hemoglobin concentrations of 6–10 g/dL, may be asymptomatic as a result of effective compensatory mechanisms. However, when iron deficiency becomes severe, with hemoglobin concentrations <5 g/dL, irritability, fatigue, and anorexia are common. Pica (which may also be a sign of lead toxicity) and pagophagia (craving and eating ice) are relatively common behavioral indicators of iron deficiency anemia. Older children and adolescents may present with exercise intolerance and shortness of breath. Of note, iron replacement therapy has been shown to improve symptoms even before laboratory values reflect changes.

In early infancy, iron deficiency anemia has been correlated with lower scores on mental and motor developmental assessments, although the exact mechanism by which this occurs has yet to be fully elucidated. Evaluations of toddlers have demonstrated similar results. Adolescent females are at a particularly high risk for iron deficiency. Poor dietary intake in this population as well as increased iron demand due to menstruation, rapid growth, and vigorous exercise contribute to this phenomenon. Anemia in teenage girls has been linked to impairments in verbal memory and learning, which can improve with iron replacement therapy, and girls with iron deficiency with and without anemia have been shown to score below average in math assessments. Of note, the cognitive sequelae of iron deficiency may precede the anemia itself as CNS iron is decreased before red blood cell production is impaired.

Populations at Risk for Iron Deficiency Anemia

Neonatal and Infant Iron Deficiency Anemia

Neonates of mothers with iron deficiency are at increased risk for IDA in early infancy. During the first 5–6 months of life, the normal term infant is iron replete. However, several conditions in the newborn period can lead to the development of IDA:

- Prematurity
- The administration of erythropoietin for anemia of prematurity
- Fetal-maternal hemorrhage
- Twin–twin transfusion syndrome
- Other perinatal hemorrhagic events
- Insufficient dietary intake

Premature infants are at increased risk for IDA in early infancy because of a smaller total blood volume at birth, increased loss through phlebotomy, and poor gastrointestinal absorption. Dietary issues contribute significantly to the evolution of IDA in infancy and early childhood. Common factors leading to IDA include the following:

- Insufficient iron intake
- Decreased absorption because of poor dietary sources of iron

- Early introduction of whole cow's milk
- Occult blood loss secondary to cow's milk intolerance
- Medications
- Malabsorption states

Recommendations for the prevention of iron deficiency in infants include the following:

- Encourage breast-feeding for the first 4–6 months; after this time, consider adding iron-fortified cereals. Two or more servings a day meet an infant's requirement for iron.
- For breast-fed preterm or low-birth weight infants, begin iron supplementation (1–2 mg/kg/day) at 1 month and continue until 12 months.
- For infants younger than 12 months of age who are not breast-fed or are partially breast-fed, use only iron-fortified formulas.
- At 6 months of age, encourage one feeding per day of foods rich in vitamin C.
- After 6 months of age, or when developmentally ready, consider introducing pureed meats, which increase the absorption of nonheme iron.
- Avoid low iron formulas or cow's milk until 12 months of age.
- Children aged 1–5 years should consume no more than 600 mL (20 oz) of milk daily. They should consume an adequate amount of iron-containing foods to meet daily requirements.

Toddler Iron Deficiency Anemia

Although the rapid growth rates of infancy are complete, iron deficiency anemia is most prevalent at this stage of development, particularly between 1 and 2 years of age. Many children have low iron stores early in the toddler years, particularly those who have received whole cows' milk throughout many months of infancy. Further, the dietary forms of iron consumed during these ages are often the nonheme forms of iron salts, iron that is much less bioavailable. Although insufficient stores and poor dietary intake are common in this age group, microcytic anemia presenting after the age of 3 years must be further investigated. Further investigation should aim to exclude malabsorption, bleeding, or chronic illnesses with true or apparent iron deficiency. Inflammatory bowel disease may occasionally present in toddlers. Ulcerative colitis presents as bloody diarrhea with incidental anemia. Crohn's disease is often more insidious, sometimes only vague ill heath and anemia are found.

Adolescent Iron Deficiency Anemia

The Third National Health and Nutrition Examination Survey (NHANES III) found a 9% incidence of iron deficiency and a 2% incidence of iron deficiency anemia among American females between the ages 12 and 15 years; the respective values were 11% and 3% in girls between the ages of 16 and 19 years. Less than 1% of adolescent males had iron deficiency. Studies in other countries have found higher rates of iron deficiency in male and female adolescents. Adolescents with chronic illness, heavy menstrual blood loss (>80 mL/month), or who are underweight or malnourished are at increased risk for iron deficiency and should be screened during health supervision or specialty clinic visits. Overweight and obese adolescents also appear to be at increased risk for iron deficiency and should undergo screening. Obesity was a risk factor for iron deficiency anemia in both boys and girls, but rates were approximately three times higher in girls. In addition, adolescent athletes, particularly those participating in endurance training, following alternative diets (vegetarian), or females at menarche, appear to be at risk for iron deficiency and should be screened as part of the pre-sport physical examination.

Differential Diagnosis

The differential diagnosis of microcytic anemia must be considered when iron deficiency anemia is suspected. Most commonly, microcytosis results from either iron deficiency, alpha or beta thalassemia trait, or heterozygous hemoglobin E disease. Hemoglobin electrophoresis is useful in differentiating and diagnosing thalassemias and hemoglobinopathies. Less common causes include inflammation, lead toxicity, thalassemia major, and sideroblastic anemia. Infection and anemia of chronic disease, while usually associated with normocytic anemia, may cause a mild microcytic anemia as well.

Blood loss must also be ruled out in children presenting with features of anemia. Most frequently, a dietary history of foods not fortified with iron and/or excessive cow's milk intake (>24 oz/day) may be elicited in these patients, especially those between the ages of 6 months and 2 years. Cow's milk iron is poorly absorbed in comparison to human breast milk, and excessive consumption results in early satiety and delayed gastric emptying. This, in turn, leads to decreased intake of iron-rich foods. Additionally, cow's milk often causes microscopic blood loss and may cause gross blood loss if a significant milk-protein inflammatory colitis develops. It is therefore recommended that children ideally consume <16 oz of cow's milk daily and eat iron-fortified foods. Other sources of blood loss, such as gastrointestinal abnormalities or infections, should also be considered. Peptic ulcers, polyps, Meckel diverticula, hemangiomas, and inflammatory bowel disease may present with anemia. Hookworm infestation and *Helicobacter pylori* infection are important infectious causes of iron deficiency anemia and should be considered in geographic areas in which these infections are prevalent. Consideration of the patient's ethnicity may be useful in differentiating the causes of anemia. Alpha thalassemia is found in children of African, Chinese, and Southeast Asian descent. Beta thalassemia occurs in those of Mediterranean, African, and Asian origins. Glucose-6-phosphate dehydrogenase (G6PD) deficiency is more commonly found in children of Mediterranean descent. Hemoglobinopathies, such as sickle cell disease and sickle cell thalassemia, are found more frequently in those of African descent.

Laboratory Features

Red Blood Cell Indices

Even before anemia occurs, the red cell indices fall and they fall progressively as the anemia becomes more severe. The blood film shows hypochromic, microcytic cells with occasional target cells. The reticulocyte count is low in relation to the degree of anemia. The platelet count is often moderately raised in iron deficiency, particularly when hemorrhage is ongoing.

Serum Iron and Total Iron-Binding Capacity

The serum iron falls and the total iron-binding capacity (TIBC) rises so that the TIBC is less than 10% saturated. This contrasts both with the anemia of chronic disorders when the serum iron and TIBC are both reduced and with other hypochromic anemias, where the serum iron is normal or even raised.

Serum Transferrin Receptor

Transferrin receptor is shed from cells into plasma. The level of serum transferrin receptor is increased in iron deficiency anemia but not in the anemia of chronic conditions or thalassemia trait. The level is also raised if the overall level of erythropoiesis is increased.

Serum Ferritin

A small fraction of body ferritin circulates in the serum, the concentration being related to tissue, particularly reticuloendothelial, iron stores. The normal range in men is higher in men than in women. In iron deficiency anemia, the serum ferritin is low. A raised serum ferritin indicates iron overload. Other causes of increased ferritin include excess release of ferritin from damaged tissues or an acute phase response (e.g., inflammation). The serum ferritin is normal or increased in the anemia of chronic disorders.

Therapy

For infants and children presenting with a mild microcytic anemia and a presumptive diagnosis of IDA, the most cost-effective strategy is a therapeutic trial of oral iron supplementation. Ferrous sulfate (3–6 mg/kg of elemental iron, once or twice daily between meals) should produce a rise of more than 1 g/dL in patients with IDA. For infants with confirmed IDA, ferrous sulfate (3–6 mg/kg/day of elemental iron) remains the standard therapy. Iron-fortified formulas and iron supplementation at these doses are infrequent causes of gastrointestinal symptoms. In children with severe IDA, a reticulocyte response may be seen within 72 h. If a child does not respond to adequate oral iron supplementation, potential causes for refractory IDA include the following:

- Failure to adhere to recommendations
- Intolerance to medication
- Ongoing gastrointestinal blood loss
- Chronic inflammatory disease
- Pulmonary hemosiderosis
- Incorrect diagnosis

Parenteral iron therapy should be reserved for patients with severe, persistent anemia who have proven intolerance to oral supplements, malabsorption, or poor compliance to oral therapy. Parenteral iron should be used with caution because there is a 2–3% risk for anaphylaxis, some cases of which result in death. Iron dextran is the parenteral form most commonly used preparation for pediatric patients. Sodium ferric gluconate and iron sucrose are also available, but these were developed for use in dialysis patients and are not approved by the US Food and Drug Administration for use in children.

Transfusion therapy is rarely necessary for severe IDA, even with hemoglobin concentrations of 4–5 g/dL. Transfusions should be reserved for patients in distress (heart rate greater than 160/min, respiratory rate greater than 30/min, lethargy, not feeding well). Transfusions should be administered with caution to such patients, giving transfusion volumes of 5 mL/kg over 3–4 h to avoid inducing heart failure.

Follow-up

Follow-up is essential because of the effects of iron deficiency on neurodevelopment. Unfortunately, failure to follow up is a common occurrence, even among children who present with severe anemia. It is essential that the health care provider develop a proactive plan to ensure adequate compliance and follow-up of these patients during a critical time of neurodevelopment.

References

Andrews N (2008) Pathology of iron metabolism. In: Hoffman R (ed) Hematology: basic principles and practice, 5th edn. Churchill Livingstone, Philadelphia

Andrews N, Schmidt P (2007) Iron homeostasis. Annu Rev Physiol 69:69

Booth IW, Aukett MA (1997) Iron deficiency anemia in infancy and early childhood. Arch Dis Child 76:549

Finberg FE (2009) Iron-refractory iron deficiency anemia. Semin Hematol 46:378

Glader B (2007) Iron-deficiency anemia. In: Kleigman RM, Behrman RE, Jenson HB, Stanton BF (eds) Nelson textbook of pediatrics, 18th edn. WB Saunders, Philadelphia

Halterman JS, Kaczorowski JM, Aligne CA et al (2001) Iron deficiency and cognitive achievement among school-aged children and adolescents in the United States. Pediatrics 107:1381

Oski FA (1993) Iron deficiency in infancy and childhood. N Engl J Med 329:190

Richardson M (2007) Microcytic anemia. Pediatr Rev 28:5

Segel GB (1988) Anemia. Pediatr Rev 10:77–88

Will A (2006) Disorders of iron metabolism: iron deficiency, iron overload and the sideroblastic anemias. In: Arceci R, Hann I, Smith O (eds) Pediatric hematology, 3rd edn. Blackwell, Oxford

319 Autoimmune Hemolytic Anemia

Veronica H. Flood · Michael Recht

Definition/Classification

Autoimmune hemolytic anemia (AIHA) is a condition in which red blood cell (RBC) destruction occurs due to antibody formation directed against self RBC antigens. In children, AIHA typically occurs following viral infection. AIHA can be due to either warm or cold antibodies, with the temperature referring to the optimal binding temperature of the antibody. AIHA is less likely to be chronic in children than in adults, but the anemia may be severe on initial presentation. In adults, the incidence of AIHA is approximately 1–3/100,000. Warm AIHA is more common than cold AIHA, accounting for about 90% of adult cases. The prevalence of cold AIHA in adults is 16/million. In children, the incidence is unknown, but mild AIHA may be more frequent, with some cases never coming to medical attention.

Pathology

Warm AIHA is due to IgG antibodies directed against RBC membrane proteins (➋ *Table 319.1*). These antibodies bind maximally at body temperature (37°C), causing extravascular hemolysis. Most RBC destruction occurs via splenic macrophages, although liver sequestration may occur. Pediatric AIHA is thought to result from antecedent viral infection inducing anti-RBC antibodies, possibly through molecular mimicry as has been described for infection-associated ITP. Additional mechanisms include self-ignorance, loss of tolerance, polyclonal T or B cell activation, and immunoregulatory disorders.

Antibodies may be directed against any RBC antigen, but anti-Rh antibodies are the most common, usually anti-e or anti-c. Epitope mapping studies performed for the Rh D autoantigen have identified specific peptides important in IL10-mediated T cell response, although the clinical significance is not yet defined. Glycophorin is another common antigenic site. In addition, antibodies have been reported against Wr^b, En^a, LW, U, Ge, Sc1, Kell, and band 3. Warm AIHA antibodies are usually polyclonal.

Evans syndrome refers to those patients with both AIHA and ITP. The disorders may occur sequentially or simultaneously, and relapse is frequent. Underlying immune dysregulation may be present, with new evidence suggesting Evans syndrome is part of a spectrum with autoimmune lymphoproliferative disease (ALPS). Seif and colleagues studied 45 children with Evans syndrome and diagnosed 47% with ALPS. Treatment of refractory Evans syndrome and ALPS differs from that of isolated pediatric AIHA in that these patients may require additional immune modulatory agents. Many, however, do respond to corticosteroids.

Cold AIHA is due to IgM antibodies, also referred to as cold agglutinins. These antibodies bind at lower temperatures, with maximal reactivity typically at 4°C. Mycoplasma infection is the most frequent triggering agent for cold AIHA in children. Antibody specificity is usually anti-I or anti-i. Cold AIHA antibodies are usually monoclonal and hemolysis is primarily intravascular.

Paroxysmal cold hemoglobinuria (PCH) is caused by IgG antibodies that bind at cold temperatures but cause RBC lysis at warmer temperatures. These are often referred to as Donath-Landsteiner antibodies. The Donath-Landsteiner antibody is directed against the P antigen. The classic presentation of PCH in adults is associated with syphilis, but in children viral infections are the most common cause. Many different viral and bacterial pathogens have been reported in childhood PCH, including *Staphylococcus aureus*, *Haemophilis influenzae*, and adenovirus.

Clinical Manifestations

Hemolytic anemia is the hallmark of AIHA. Patients may present with fatigue or pallor due to the anemia. Dizziness, headache, and shortness of breath are signs of more severe anemia. Jaundice or scleral icterus may be noted due to elevated bilirubin from extravascular hemolysis. Dark, cola colored urine occurs in the presence of intravascular hemolysis. Fever may also be seen, particularly with viral illnesses as the precipitating factor. On exam, patients may demonstrate splenomegaly, but spleen size may also be

Abdelaziz Y. Elzouki (ed.), *Textbook of Clinical Pediatrics*, DOI 10.1007/978-3-642-02202-9_319,

Table 319.1
Classification of AIHA

Type	Antibody	Temperature	Specificity
Warm AIHA	IgG	37°C	Anti-Rh most common
Cold AIHA	IgM	0–4°C	Anti-I or anti-i
PCH	IgG	0–4°C	Anti-P

AIHA autoimmune hemolytic anemia, *PCH* paroxysmal cold hemoglobinuria

Table 319.2
Laboratory workup for AIHA

Initial testing	Confirmatory testing
Complete blood count	Direct antigen test (Coombs)
Review of peripheral blood smear	Donath-Landsteiner testing
Reticulocyte count	
Lactate dehydrogenase	
Bilirubin (total and indirect)	
Haptoglobin	
Urinalysis	

normal. Tachycardia may be present, particularly if the anemia is of recent onset. Lymphadenopathy is common in patients with viral infections. Cold AIHA may present with acrocyanosis similar to that seen in Raynaud's syndrome.

Diagnosis

Diagnosis of AIHA involves a variety of laboratory tests, with the typical workup summarized in *Table 319.2*. A complete blood count will show anemia, typically with a normal MCV. The RDW is usually high due to concurrent elevation in the reticulocyte count. Except in the setting of marrow suppression due to parvovirus, there is usually a brisk reticulocytosis. Review of the peripheral blood smear should show spherocytes, formed when part of the antibody-coated RBC membrane is removed by the spleen, resulting in spherocytes rather than the classic biconcave disk shape. Increased hemolysis will result in increased spherocytosis. Cold AIHA may result in RBC agglutination on the peripheral smear. Erythrophagocytosis may also be observed (*Fig. 319.1*).

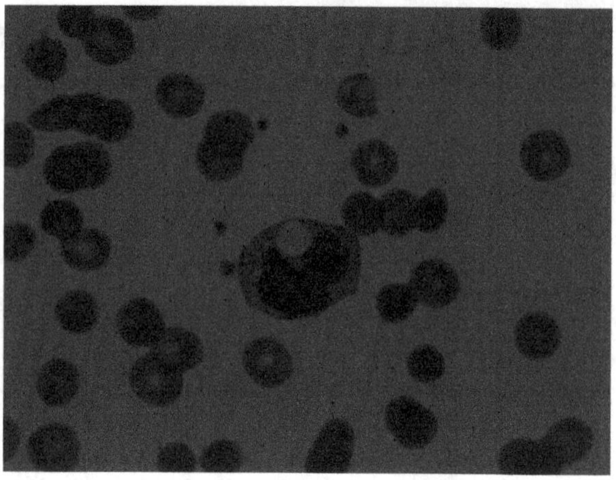

Figure 319.1
Peripheral smear demonstrating spherocytes and erythrophagocytosis (courtesy of Dr. Gabriela Gheorghe, Medical College of Wisconsin)

Blood chemistries will show elevated unconjugated bilirubin levels. Conjugated bilirubin should be normal in AIHA. Lactate dehydrogenase is also elevated due to increased RBC turnover. Haptoglobin will be decreased due to scavenging of free hemoglobin. Hemoglobinuria is uncommon in warm AIHA but frequently seen in cold AIHA and paroxysmal cold hemoglobinuria.

The pathognomonic test for AIHA is the direct Coombs test, or direct antiglobulin test (DAT). The DAT detects IgG antibodies or complement (C3) bound to the patient's RBCs. In warm AIHA, the IgG DAT will be positive, while in cold AIHA, the complement DAT will be positive, demonstrating the presence of complement on the RBC surface. The DAT is performed by incubating patient RBCs with reagents containing either anti-IgG or anti-complement to detect bound antibodies. Occasionally, symptoms of AIHA will be present with a negative DAT. Rare patients will have a positive DAT without symptoms. Thermal amplitude testing may be helpful, particularly for cold AIHA. Testing is performed at 4°, 22°, 30°, and 37°C to determine at what temperature maximal agglutination occurs.

Donath-Landsteiner testing should be performed when paroxysmal cold hemoglobinuria is suspected. If patient serum is incubated with normal RBCs at 0°C or 37°C, no lysis is observed, but when the incubation first occurs at 0°C and is then moved to 37°C, lysis will occur. Thermal amplitude may vary, with some antibodies binding at intermediate temperatures.

Table 319.3
Treatment options for AIHA

First line treatment	Second line treatment	Third line treatment
Corticosteroids	Rituximab	Plasmapheresis
Transfusion	Splenectomy	Cytotoxic agents Cyclophosphamide 6-Mercaptopurine Azathioprine 6-Thioguanine Danazol
IVIG		Immune suppressive agents Cyclosporine Mycophenolate mofetil

Differential Diagnosis

AIHA is due to antibody-mediated RBC destruction. Other causes of hemolysis should be considered and excluded on the basis of patient and family history as well as laboratory testing. Hereditary spherocytosis (HS) can present with anemia and spherocytosis, although the DAT should be negative in HS. Enzymopathies and other RBC membrane defects may also present with anemia and hemolysis. Family history may be useful in evaluation for the presence of inherited RBC defects, as many patients will have affected parents or other family members. Dark urine due to intravascular hemolysis is common in cold AIHA, but may also be a presenting feature of paroxysmal nocturnal hemoglobinuria (PNH). Anemia and hemolysis are also seen in microangiopathic disorders such as hemolytic uremic syndrome (HUS) and thrombotic thrombocytopenic purpura (TTP) although thrombocytopenia and schistocytes on the peripheral blood smear should help to differentiate these from the anemia of AIHA.

In addition, AIHA may be secondary to other underlying disorders. Systemic lupus erythematosis has been associated with AIHA as has lymphoma. Infections such as HIV may also be responsible for AIHA. Hemolytic anemias may occur following solid organ or bone marrow transplant when there is an ABO mismatch between donor and recipient, with antibodies produced either by the grafted marrow or organ against recipient RBCs, or by the recipient against the donor RBCs. Adults are more likely to have AIHA secondary to an underlying condition than young children.

Drug-induced hemolytic anemia has been reported following administration of numerous medications, including penicillins, cephalosporins, and methyldopa. While original reports of drug-induced immune hemolysis were common with penicillin and methyldopa, cephalosphorins are now responsible for the majority of cases. Reactions have been reported with other frequently used medications, including NSAIDs and trimethoprim.

Treatment

Transfusion may be required in severe AIHA. Symptomatic patients should receive the least incompatible unit available, but extensive testing should not delay transfusion when clinically indicated. Most children with AIHA are previously healthy, and are unlikely to have previous exposures such as pregnancy or transfusions that could have led to the development of an underlying alloantibody. Since most AIHA antibodies are directed against common RBC antigens such as the Rh epitope, finding a perfectly compatible unit may be impossible. In such instances, slow RBC transfusion is acceptable, with close monitoring for a possible transfusion reaction. Survival of the transfused cells will likely be affected by the autoantibody as well, but may suffice to reduce symptoms while other therapeutic measures are employed. Some clinicians recommend using the "least incompatible" unit but transfusion guidelines at present support transfusion regardless of the crossmatch results once a significant alloantibody has been ruled out. Hemoglobin levels less than four merit transfusion, as do children with significant symptoms, particularly with concurrent reticulocytopenia. For cold AIHA, a blood warmer should be used to maintain a temperature of 37°C. Additional treatment options are summarized in *Table 319.3*.

Steroids are the mainstay of AIHA treatment. In warm AIHA, steroids decrease RBC sequestration and antibody formation. Glucocorticoids are thought to inhibit clearance of RBCs via the Fc receptors. Their effect, however, is not instantaneous, as improvement in symptoms usually takes several days. Dosing varies widely in pediatrics, with typical dosing of prednisone at 1–4 mg/kg/day given for at least 5 days or until the hemolysis slows. Most clinicians will then wean steroids over several weeks but no standard protocol exists. IV methylprednisolone may be used in severe cases. Response rates to oral steroids are excellent, with typical response rates of 80% in both adults and children. Relapses are infrequent in children, but may occur, so close monitoring following recovery is warranted. Parents should be counseled regarding signs and symptoms of anemia.

Cold avoidance is important in paroxysmal cold hemoglobinuria. Since these antibodies bind only at cold temperatures, preventing binding will reduce hemolysis. Room temperature should be raised as high as comfortable. In addition, patients should avoid cold foods, such as ice cream and popsicles, as these may precipitate a bout of hemolysis. Warm clothes, including hats and gloves, should be worn when outside, and extreme cold temperatures avoided if possible. IV fluids and medications, including RBC transfusions, should be administered via a blood warmer.

IVIG may be useful, either alone or in combination with steroids. Trials of IVIG in adult patients demonstrated a response rate of 40%. Early pediatric trials showed a response in 3 of 4 children. A larger study demonstrated a response rate of 40%, but children tended to fare better than adults. IVIG may work by several mechanisms, including Fc receptor blockade or decrease in antibody production. Cold AIHA is thought to be generally less responsive to IVIG than warm AIHA.

Splenectomy is generally reserved for those children refractory to medical therapy for two reasons. First, the risk of infection following splenectomy in children is not insubstantial, and therefore should be avoided in younger children if at all possible. Second, the response rate to splenectomy is only about 60%, with at present no clear indication of which patients will respond best to splenectomy. In theory, removing the spleen will remove the site of RBC destruction, but some patients have continued hemolysis, suggesting that alternate sites of RBC removal are present.

Recently, the monoclonal anti-CD20 antibody rituximab has been used for a variety of autoimmune conditions, including AIHA. Rituximab is a chimeric antibody composed of human IgG heavy and light chains fused to a murine variable region. It binds to CD20, removing B cells from circulation and thus decreasing antibody production. Reactivation of hepatitis B has been reported following rituximab treatment. The risk of serious infection, however, appears to be low despite B cell depletion. Some clinicians administer IVIG following rituximab, but there are no strong data to support its use. Adult trials suggest approximately 50% will respond to rituximab, and those who relapse following rituximab may respond to retreatment. One pediatric trial showed response in 13 of 15 patients, although 3 of the responders later relapsed. Response rates in children appear to be greater than those in adults, with over 90% remission in a collection of case reports. Publication bias, however, must be taken into account, as it is likely there are many non-responders that have not shown up in case reports. At present, rituximab and splenectomy are both considered second line treatment following steroids and/or IVIG.

Plasmapheresis may be of some utility in cold AIHA to remove the inciting IgM antibody. A blood warmer should be utilized to keep blood products at 37°C. Plasmapheresis has also been utilized in warm AIHA. No clinical studies exist, but case reports in adults with severe AIHA suggest a response rate of around 65%. The necessity of catheter placement limits this procedure to pediatric intensive care units in most hospitals, and plasma exchange may not be rapidly available for small children, limiting the use of this therapeutic modality. However, it may be beneficial in refractory cases.

Numerous other cytotoxic agents have been utilized in refractory AIHA, including cyclophosphamide, 6-mercaptopurine, azathioprine, 6-thioguanine, and danazol. Immune suppressants such as cyclosporine or mycophenolate mofetil have been tried with some success. In pediatric AIHA patients, a recent study by Sobota and colleagues in 29 refractory AIHA patients demonstrated an 83% response rate to 6-mercaptopurine. Consideration of immune suppressive agents for refractory patients should take into account cost and convenience of administration as there is at present no clear order of precedence given the limited data available on these medications in pediatric AIHA.

Summary

AIHA is not uncommon in children. Although warm AIHA is observed most frequently, cold AIHA and PCH may also occur in this age group. Viral infections are thought to be the initiating agent in pediatric AIHA. Children typically present with anemia, reticulocytosis, and signs of hemolysis. The diagnosis of AIHA relies on the ability to demonstrate the presence of anti-RBC antibodies, typically through a positive DAT. Treatment may be required, with steroids the mainstay of AIHA therapy. Alternate treatment options are available for refractory patients.

References

Akpek G, McAneny D, Weintraub L (1999) Comparative response to splenectomy in Coombs-positive autoimmune hemolytic anemia with or without associated disease. Am J Hematol 61(2):98–102

Allgood JW, Chaplin H Jr (1967) Idiopathic acquired autoimmune hemolytic anemia. A review of forty-seven cases treated from 1955 through 1965. Am J Med 43(2):254–273

Arndt PA, Garratty G (2005) The changing spectrum of drug-induced immune hemolytic anemia. Semin Hematol 42(3):137–144

Barker RN, Casswell KM, Reid ME, Sokol RJ, Elson CJ (1992) Identification of autoantigens in autoimmune haemolytic anaemia by a non-radioisotope immunoprecipitation method. Br J Haematol 82(1):126–132

Berentsen S, Ulvestad E, Langholm R et al (2006) Primary chronic cold agglutinin disease: a population based clinical study of 86 patients. Haematologica 91(4):460–466

Coombs RR, Mourant AE (1947) On certain properties of antisera prepared against human serum and its various protein fractions; their use in the detection of sensitisation of human red cells with incomplete Rh antibody, and on the nature of this antibody. J Pathol Bacteriol 59(1–2):105–111

Dacie JV (1968) Autoimmune haemolytic anaemia. Introduction and perspectives. Proc R Soc Med 61(12):1307–1309

Dacie JV (1970) Autoimmune haemolytic anaemias. Br Med J 2(5706):381–386

Dacie SJ (2001) The immune haemolytic anaemias: a century of exciting progress in understanding. Br J Haematol 114(4):770–785

Dervite I, Hober D, Morel P (2001) Acute hepatitis B in a patient with antibodies to hepatitis B surface antigen who was receiving rituximab. N Engl J Med 344(1):68–69

Eder AF (2005) Review: acute Donath-Landsteiner hemolytic anemia. Immunohematology 21(2):56–62

Emilia G, Messora C, Longo G, Bertesi M (1996) Long-term salvage treatment by cyclosporin in refractory autoimmune haematological disorders. Br J Haematol 93(2):341–344

Flores G, Cunningham-Rundles C, Newland AC, Bussel JB (1993) Efficacy of intravenous immunoglobulin in the treatment of autoimmune hemolytic anemia: results in 73 patients. Am J Hematol 44(4): 237–242

Fries LF, Brickman CM, Frank MM (1983) Monocyte receptors for the Fc portion of IgG increase in number in autoimmune hemolytic anemia and other hemolytic states and are decreased by glucocorticoid therapy. J Immunol 131(3):1240–1245

Garratty G (2005) Immune hemolytic anemia associated with negative routine serology. Semin Hematol 42(3):156–164

Garvey B (2008) Rituximab in the treatment of autoimmune haematological disorders. Br J Haematol 141(2):149–169

Gehrs BC, Friedberg RC (2002) Autoimmune hemolytic anemia. Am J Hematol 69(4):258–271

Giulino LB, Bussel JB, Neufeld EJ (2007) Pediatric and platelet immunology committees of the TMH clinical trial network. Treatment with rituximab in benign and malignant hematologic disorders in children. J Pediatr 150(4):338–344, 344.e1

Gottsche B, Salama A, Mueller-Eckhardt C (1990) Donath-Landsteiner autoimmune hemolytic anemia in children. A study of 22 cases. Vox Sang 58(4):281–286

Gupta S, Piefer CL, Fueger JT, Johnson ST, Punzalan RC (2010) Trimethoprim-induced immune hemolytic anemia in a pediatric oncology patient presenting as an acute hemolytic transfusion reaction. Pediatr Blood Cancer 55(6):1201–1203

Hall AM, Ward FJ, Vickers MA, Stott LM, Urbaniak SJ, Barker RN (2002) Interleukin-10-mediated regulatory T-cell responses to epitopes on a human red blood cell autoantigen. Blood 100(13):4529–4536

Heddle NM (1989) Acute paroxysmal cold hemoglobinuria. Transfus Med Rev 3(3):219–229

Hilgartner MW, Bussel J (1987) Use of intravenous gamma globulin for the treatment of autoimmune neutropenia of childhood and autoimmune hemolytic anemia. Am J Med 83(4A):25–29

Howard J, Hoffbrand AV, Prentice HG, Mehta A (2002) Mycophenolate mofetil for the treatment of refractory auto-immune haemolytic anaemia and auto-immune thrombocytopenia purpura. Br J Haematol 117(3):712–715

Jandl JH, Kaplan ME (1960) The destruction of red cells by antibodies in man. III. Quantitative factors influencing the patterns of hemolysis in vivo. J Clin Invest 39:1145–1156

Johnson ST, Fueger JT, Gottschall JL (2007) One center's experience: the serology and drugs associated with drug-induced immune hemolytic anemia–a new paradigm. Transfusion 47(4):697–702

King KE (2007) Review: pharmacologic treatment of warm autoimmune hemolytic anemia. Immunohematology 23(3):120–129

King KE, Ness PM (2005) Treatment of autoimmune hemolytic anemia. Semin Hematol 42(3):131–136

Leddy JP, Falany JL, Kissel GE, Passador ST, Rosenfeld SI (1993) Erythrocyte membrane proteins reactive with human (warm-reacting) anti-red cell autoantibodies. J Clin Invest 91(4):1672–1680

Moyo VM, Smith D, Brodsky I, Crilley P, Jones RJ, Brodsky RA (2002) High-dose cyclophosphamide for refractory autoimmune hemolytic anemia. Blood 100(2):704–706

Naithani R, Agrawal N, Mahapatra M, Kumar R, Pati HP, Choudhry VP (2007) Autoimmune hemolytic anemia in children. Pediatr Hematol Oncol 24(4):309–315

Ness PM (2006) How do I encourage clinicians to transfuse mismatched blood to patients with autoimmune hemolytic anemia in urgent situations? Transfusion 46(11):1859–1862

Norton A, Roberts I (2006) Management of Evans syndrome. Br J Haematol 132(2):125–137

Packman CH (2008) Hemolytic anemia due to warm autoantibodies. Blood Rev 22(1):17–31

Petz LD (2004) A physician's guide to transfusion in autoimmune haemolytic anaemia. Br J Haematol 124(6):712–716

Petz LD (2008) Cold antibody autoimmune hemolytic anemias. Blood Rev 22(1):1–15

Pignon JM, Poirson E, Rochant H (1993) Danazol in autoimmune haemolytic anaemia. Br J Haematol 83(2):343–345

Ramsey G, Nusbacher J, Starzl TE, Lindsay GD (1984) Isohemagglutinins of graft origin after ABO-unmatched liver transplantation. N Engl J Med 311(18):1167–1170

Reardon JE, Marques MB (2006) Laboratory evaluation and transfusion support of patients with autoimmune hemolytic anemia. Am J Clin Pathol 125(Suppl):S71–S77

Reff ME, Carner K, Chambers KS et al (1994) Depletion of B cells in vivo by a chimeric mouse human monoclonal antibody to CD20. Blood 83(2):435–445

Schreiber AD, Parsons J, McDermott P, Cooper RA (1975) Effect of corticosteroids on the human monocyte IgG and complement receptors. J Clin Invest 56(5):1189–1197

Schwartz R, Dameshek W (1962) The treatment of autoimmune hemolytic anemia with 6-mercaptopurine and thioguanine. Blood 19:483–500

Seif AE, Manno CS, Sheen C, Grupp SA, Teachey DT (2010) Identifying autoimmune lymphoproliferative syndrome in children with Evans syndrome: a multi-institutional study. Blood 115(11):2142–2145

Semple JW, Freedman J (2005) Autoimmune pathogenesis and autoimmune hemolytic anemia. Semin Hematol 42(3):122–130

Sewell WA, Jolles S (2002) Immunomodulatory action of intravenous immunoglobulin. Immunology 107(4):387–393

Sniecinski IJ, Oien L, Petz LD, Blume KG (1988) Immunohematologic consequences of major ABO-mismatched bone marrow transplantation. Transplantation 45(3):530–534

Sokol RJ, Booker DJ, Stamps R (1999) Erythropoiesis: paroxysmal cold haemoglobinuria: a clinico-pathological study of patients with a positive Donath-Landsteiner test. Hematology 4(2):137–164

Sokol RJ, Stamps R, Booker DJ et al (2002) Posttransplant immune-mediated hemolysis. Transfusion 42(2):198–204

Toriani-Terenzi C, Fagiolo E (2005) IL-10 and the cytokine network in the pathogenesis of human autoimmune hemolytic anemia. Ann NY Acad Sci 1051:29–44

Valent P, Lechner K (2008) Diagnosis and treatment of autoimmune haemolytic anaemias in adults: a clinical review. Wien Klin Wochenschr 120(5–6):136–151

von Baeyer H (2003) Plasmapheresis in immune hematology: review of clinical outcome data with respect to evidence-based medicine and clinical experience. Ther Apher Dial 7(1):127–140

Wheeler CA, Calhoun L, Blackall DP (2004) Warm reactive autoantibodies: clinical and serologic correlations. Am J Clin Pathol 122(5):680–685

Wikman A, Axdorph U, Gryfelt G, Gustafsson L, Bjorkholm M, Lundahl J (2005) Characterization of red cell autoantibodies in consecutive DAT-positive patients with relation to in vivo haemolysis. Ann Hematol 84(3):150–158

Wright JF, Blanchette VS, Wang H et al (1996) Characterization of platelet-reactive antibodies in children with varicella-associated acute immune thrombocytopenic purpura (ITP). Br J Haematol 95(1):145–152

Zecca M, Nobili B, Ramenghi U et al (2003) Rituximab for the treatment of refractory autoimmune hemolytic anemia in children. Blood 101(10):3857–3861

320 Glucose-6-Phosphate Dehydrogenase Deficiency

Hassan M. Yaish

> ▶ The indiscriminate selection of a battery of hematologically oriented tests, such as obtaining a Coomb's test and levels of serum iron, Vitamin B12, and folic acid in every anemic patient is wasteful, unwise, and unnecessary.
>
> Maxwell Wintrobe, 1930

Among the various red cell enzymes disorders, glucose-6-phosphate dehydrogenase (G6PD) deficiency is by far the most common and most significant clinical entity. The several disorders resulting from this enzymopathy affect more than 400 million people worldwide and probably twice as many heterozygous girls. The highest incidence is encountered in the tropics or the subtropics where malaria was endemic in the past. A highest incidence of G6PD deficiency is found around the Mediterranean region, affecting Southern Europeans, Middle Easterners, and North Africans. Both the rate of incidence and the type of G6PD may vary from one region to another in the same country. More than 50% of the populations of certain oases in the Eastern Province of Saudi Arabia, for instance, were found to have G6PD deficiency, in contrast to less than 2% in the central region. G6PD deficiency is also encountered in certain parts of India and Southeast Asia.

G6PD Function

This enzyme catalyzes the first reaction in the oxidative pentose phosphate pathway, through which less than 5% of the red cells' glucose is metabolized. It is clear, therefore, that the main function of this pathway is not glucose metabolism but to provide a continuous supply of the reduced nicotinamide dinucleotide phosphate (NADPH) necessary for conversion of the oxidized form of glutathione (GSSG) to the reduced form (GSH), in a second reaction mediated by glutathione reductase (➋ *Fig. 320.1*). Reduced glutathione, in turn, plays a critical role in the detoxification and reduction of the various oxidants accumulating in the red cells, such as hydrogen peroxide and other oxygen radicals. For this reason, G6PD was classified as a "housekeeping" enzyme. The last reaction in this pathway is usually mediated by glutathione peroxidase and is crucial for the protection of the integrity of the red cell, which is already handicapped by the lack of a nucleus and mitochondria that render it unable to produce G6PD. In addition, the red cell's oxygen load represents an occupational hazard for the cell itself. It acts as a continuous source for oxidants with damaging potential for the cell integrity. These red cell characteristics explain why, among all cells that lack G6PD activity, red blood cells are the most vulnerable. Many children with G6PD deficiency develop episodic hemolysis upon exposure to oxidants.

G6PD Polymorphism

The G6PD gene (Gd) is located on the long arm of chromosome X in close proximity to the color blindness and the classic hemophilia A genes. Inherited as an X-linked disorder, it affects primarily hemizygous boys (Gd−), homozygous girls (Gd−/Gd−), and occasionally heterozygous girls (Gd−/Gd+). More than 400 different variants of G6PD have been identified so far. Almost all such variants are the results of point mutations rather than actual deletions. Amino acid substitutions at different points of the G6PD gene's polypeptide chain characterize the various mutants, similar to the substitutions encountered in the different hemoglobinopathies. The G6PD enzyme mutants include:

G6PD B+: Refers to the normal enzyme found in most populations.

G6PD A+: Designation for another normal enzyme mutant present in people of African origin.

G6PD A−: The designation for the African mutant once activity drops to 5–15% of normal.

G6PD B− (Mediterranean): Designation for the variant exhibited by people of Mediterranean, North African, and Far East descent with activity less than 5% of normal.

Abdelaziz Y. Elzouki (ed.), *Textbook of Clinical Pediatrics*, DOI 10.1007/978-3-642-02202-9_320,

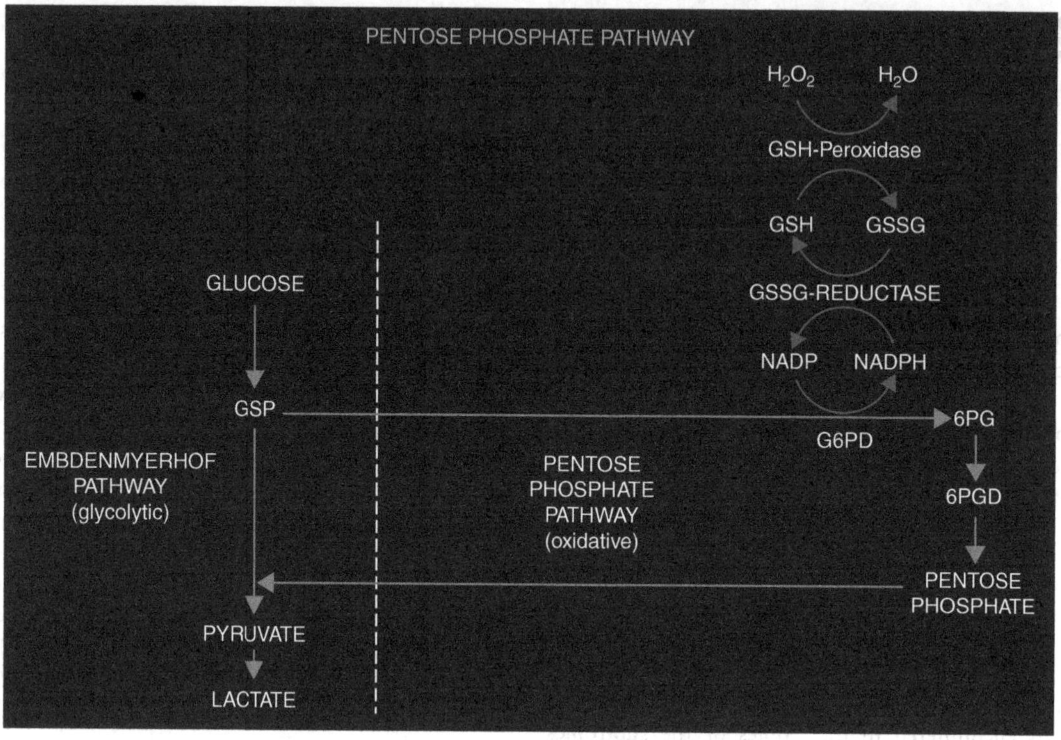

Figure 320.1

Chronic Nonspherocytic Hemolytic Anemia

Small minorities of individuals with G6PD deficiency tend to manifest a variable degree of hemolysis that can be easily detected at all times. Such patients are constantly symptomatic with anemia that ranges from slight to transfusion dependent. Reticulocytosis, jaundice, and splenomegaly are frequent findings. The hemolysis is extravascular, and the picture is that of a chronic hemolytic anemia. Various G6PD mutants are now known to cause congenital nonspherocytic hemolytic anemia (CNSHA), many of which have had their molecular defect and amino acid substitutions elucidated. The reason for the peculiar clinical behavior of this entity remains largely unexplained.

Patients are invariably males and the condition is encountered anywhere in the world especially in Europe and Japan. Symptoms may present at birth with neonatal jaundice (NNJ), which does not clear later on. The condition is caused by special G6PD mutations, commonly clustered in exon 10. Such mutations do not require a triggering exogenous factor to induce hemolytic crisis, hence anemia and hemolysis are always present. Acute exacerbation of hemolysis, however, may occur after exposure to the same oxidative agents that cause acute hemolytic anemia (AHA) in patients with the more common forms of G6PD deficiency. Several mutants of G6PD deficiency are known to manifest CNSHA, which may explain the variation in the severity of the condition.

Red cell morphology is usually normal; anemia, hyperbilirubinemia, low haptoglobin, and elevated LDH are frequently encountered. Lack of hemoglobinuria suggests that the hemolysis is extravascular and splenomegaly is frequently present.

G6PD Deficiency and Malaria

The "malaria hypothesis" was formulated nearly half a century ago based on the observation of the striking correlation between the world distribution of G6PD deficiency and *Plasmodium falciparum* malaria. Several epidemiologic and clinical studies since then have confirmed that G6PD deficiency confers some degree of protection from the potentially lethal malaria parasite. Even though all the clinical studies have agreed that such protection exists, nevertheless there was no agreement on who is protected. Some studies have shown that the protection involves only the G6PD deficient male, while others concluded that the heterozygous female shows resistance to the parasite. Several factors have been suggested as a potential explanation for such differences. The mechanism of this phenomenon is not fully understood. One of the theories indicates that macrophages are able to recognize the parasite-infected G6PD deficient red blood cells more efficiently, accelerating the removal of the cells (suicidal infection).

Clinical Manifestations of G6PD Deficiency

Symptoms in G6PD-deficient individuals vary significantly in their severity depending on the particular G6PD variant involved. Red cell life span is always somewhat shortened in all types of G6PD deficiency, even though, in most cases, this finding is subclinical and not easily detected. For this reason, it is probably appropriate to describe the clinical manifestations separately for each clinical entity in G6PD-deficient children. Three clinical entities are encountered in patients with G6PD deficiency: acute hemolytic anemia, neonatal jaundice, and chronic nonspherocytic hemolytic anemia. The first two are the most common with AHA usually presenting as an episodic crisis upon exposure to oxidants, or in the neonatal period as jaundice mostly without anemia. The third form however is characterized by chronic life-long hemolytic process.

Acute Hemolytic Anemia

This condition is usually triggered by exposure to certain drugs such as the antimalarials, some sulphonamides, analgesics, and antimicrobials. Of interest, there have been reports of hemolytic reactions due to the use of the cosmetic dye henna applied to different parts of the body in certain populations around the world. Infections such as hepatitis, pneumonia, typhoid fever, and brucellosis were all incriminated in inducing hemolysis in G6PD deficient individuals. Ingestion of fava beans or inhalation of its pollen have caused significant hemolytic crisis in some deficient individuals resulting in the condition known as favism.

Except for the CNSHA mutant, described earlier, children with G6PD deficiency in the steady state are usually asymptomatic and hematologically normal. A hemolytic crisis can begin within a few hours to 3 days after the exposure to the responsible agent. The length of the interval as well as the severity of the reaction is both functions of the offending factor as well as the type of the deficient enzyme. G6PD B– (Mediterranean), for instance, is characterized by a disease that is more severe than G6PD A– (African), with intervals of hours rather than days and the potential of being fatal in rare occasions, rather than self-limited because of the extreme short half-life of the enzyme, even in the newly produced reticulocytes.

Diagnosis

The diagnosis is straight forward if the patient with a history of fava bean ingestion or exposure to its pollen develops hemoglobinuria. Rarely, a hemolytic crisis can occur in breast-feeding infants whose mothers have ingested fava beans. In the absence of such history, however, and in patients with hemoglobinuria, one should consider other forms of hemolytic anemia. A coomb's test is positive in autoimmune hemolytic anemia. Malaria and babesiosis need also to be considered in epidemic regions.

Favism

Ingestion of fava beans by the child with G6PD B– may result in the condition known as favism. This is a term used to describe the harmful effects of fava beans (*Vicia faba*) in certain individuals with G6PD deficiency. The condition has been known for centuries, probably dating from the early Greek and Roman times, as reflected by the observations attributed to Hippocrates and Pythagoras who warned his disciples against dangers of eating fava beans. The etiology of favism remained a mystery, however, until the mid-1950s, when the cause of acute hemolysis in African-American soldiers who were given antimalarial drugs was identified and attributed to the deficient G6PD enzyme. This condition occurs most often in people of Mediterranean, Middle Eastern, or Far Eastern origin. It is described as an episodic intravascular hemolysis associated with hemoglobinuria, described by the parents or the patients as dark urine resembling the color of dark tea or cola. Jaundice, abdominal pain, and vomiting are sometimes described. Laboratory findings reveal anemia with hemoglobins measured as low as 2–3 g/dL, hemoglobinemia, and hemoglobinuria early in the process. The presence of Heinz bodies (➋ *Fig. 320.2*) on supravital stain or reticulocyte stain preparations supports

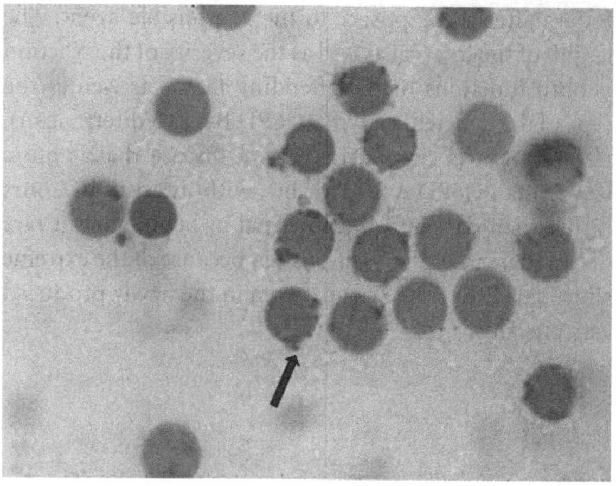

Figure 320.2

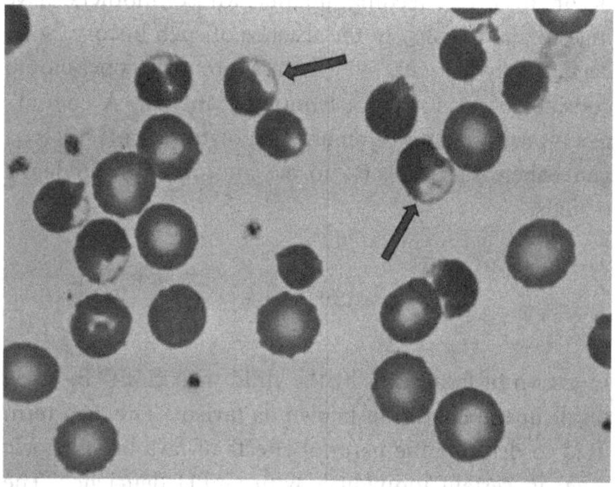

Figure 320.3

the diagnosis. Heinz bodies represent precipitated hemoglobin that is quickly pinched off by the spleen, leaving the characteristic blister or basket-shaped cell (*Fig. 320.3*). The morphology of the red blood cell is striking in that marked anisocytosis, contracted, and spherocytic-like cells are usually seen. Reticulocytes peak may be as high as 30% or more. Even though many patients require red blood cell transfusion, in many others the hemolytic crisis is self-limited and resolves spontaneously.

Not all deficient individuals develop favism upon ingestion of fava beans or inhaling the bean pollen. Furthermore, many individuals have eaten fava beans frequently before and after their first hemolytic crises without any similar episodes. This indicates that other etiologic factors are involved even though they have never been documented.

Neonatal Jaundice

The issue of hyperbilirubinemia in G6PD-deficient neonates of different ethnic groups has been a subject of debate for many years. At the present time, there is enough evidence to suggest that more neonates with G6PD deficiency of any type develop hyperbilirubinemia than do non-deficient ones. Earlier studies have confirmed such findings in newborns with G6PD B− (Mediterranean) and only the premature baby with G6PD A−. A recent report, however, demonstrated that despite the low incidence of hyperbilirubinemia in African-American newborns, 25% of children who develop kernicterus occur in this population of newborns. Sixty percent of the cases were due to G6PD deficiency while 40% were caused by preterm births and ABO hemolytic disease. In almost all such instances, no offending agent was identified and the etiology of the hyperbilirubinemia, which had presented as an exaggerated physiologic jaundice. Once a responsible agent becomes active, however, the potential response is expected to occur in any infant regardless of term or ethnicity. In such circumstances, the clinical picture may present more like hemolytic anemia and hyperbilirubinemia rather than exaggerated jaundice without anemia.

Evidence of cholestasis with significant elevation of conjugated bilirubin without any evidence of hepatobiliary disease was reported in a neonate with novel mutation resulting in CNSHA. A new, previously unrecognized agent has been incriminated as a cause of hemolysis and jaundice in newborns in certain regions of the world, mainly the Middle East, India, and North Africa. Neonatal hyperbilirubinemia of G6PD deficiency is rarely manifested at birth, and it usually peaks between days 3 and 4 of age, which coincides with time of discharge or after being discharged home.

Testing for G6PD Deficiency

All tests for G6PD activity are based on the detection of the presence of NADPH in the red cell by spectrophotometric methods. Leukocytes, which have much higher level of G6PD than erythrocytes, should be removed from the hemolysate for accurate measurements. Two kinds of tests are usually utilized: a screening test designed to identify deficient individuals and a quantitative method that measures the rate of formation of NADPH by spectrophotometric means. Dye decolorization, methemoglobin reduction, and the fluorescence spot test as well are all used for screening purposes. Once a positive test is identified, confirmation by a quantitative method is required.

Samples with less than 30% activity are considered deficient since any level that exceeds 30% is usually asymptomatic. G6PD activity in normal mature red cells is in the range of 7–10 IU/g of hemoglobin. In order to appropriately evaluate the results of G6PD testing, one should be aware of two major causes of false-negative results in deficient individuals at the time of testing. First, because leukocytes and platelets have higher G6PD activity than mature erythrocytes, when these cells contaminate the specimen, artificially elevated G6PD activity will be seen. Secondly, when G6PD is measured in a reticulocyte-rich specimen, levels can be artificially elevated.

Preventive Medicine in G6PD Deficiency

Universal screening for the deficiency is neither feasible nor recommended except in a very few circumstances where the condition is common and the symptomatology is relatively severe. Cord blood screening is currently utilized in several countries of the world where the condition is very common. Once an infant is identified as deficient, oxidant drugs, chemicals, and cosmetics (henna) are to be avoided. In addition, close monitoring for at least the first 4–5 days of life will ensure appropriate and timely management of any otherwise unexplained hyperbilirubinemia. The parents are instructed to avoid certain medications and chemicals in the older child, and to ask the child to give up eating fava beans or any foods that have fava bean as an ingredient (e.g., falafel). The physician should also know that most of the newly introduced drugs, regardless of the indications for its use, are not tested and may carry a potential risk for the deficient child.

It is known that hemolytic anemia and neonatal jaundice are the most common and well-recognized clinical manifestations in G6PD deficient individuals. Many other indirect effects of the deficiency are now being described. High blood sugar in patients with type 2 diabetes have been incriminated in inhibiting G6PD expression causing increased oxidative stress leading to gradual loss of beta cells in patients with diabetes.

The more pronounced effect of the enzyme deficiency on the RBCs is attributed to the fact that the cell is anucleated and unable to produce the enzyme. The eye lens is another example of an organ composed of non-nucleated cells, which might be the site of developing juvenile cataracts in young people with G6PD deficiency. Nucleated cells in the deficient individuals however retain the ability to produce some limited amounts of the enzyme as found in the granulocytes which may maintain a level of 30% of normal compared to only 5% in the RBCs. Despite this fact, some types of G6PD deficiency have been associated with increased incidence of infections, and poor healing after trauma as a result of leukocytes dysfunction.

Treatment

In acute hemolysis that develops after exposure to drugs or chemicals, particularly in patients with the G6PD A− mutant, the course is frequently mild and self-limited. On the other hand, in the G6PD B− (Mediterranean) type of G6PD deficiency, the hemolysis is frequently more severe and intervention is usually required. In many of the Middle Eastern countries, as is true elsewhere, blood transfusion has been used indiscriminately. To avoid such practice and minimize the various risks of blood transfusion, the physician is urged to evaluate the patient's clinical status carefully before blood transfusion is administered. On many occasions, the child presents to the physician toward the end of the course of illness with reticulocytes already rising, urine clearing, and none of the classic morphologic findings (blister cells, Heinz bodies) present. Such patients, even with their hemoglobin at 6–7 g/dL, can be closely observed for 24–48 h. On the other hand, a child with severe anemia and a hemoglobin causing symptoms, or in the face of ongoing hemolysis, should be considered for transfusion. All other acute episodes in between these two extremes should be evaluated carefully and treated accordingly.

Even though renal failure rarely occurs in children, one should always be aware of such a complication. In neonatal jaundice, on should always exclude other causes of hyperbilirubinemia and manage the baby according to the severity of the condition. Phototherapy has decreased the need for exchange transfusion in many neonates with hyperbilirubinemia. In such infants, one is rarely faced with severe anemia similar to the condition observed in hemolytic disease of the newborn. In most cases such infants are usually hyperbilirubinemic rather than anemic, and, unless they were exposed to an oxidant, they do not show any of the classic morphologic findings.

In CNSHA, the treatment depends on the severity of the anemia, which may be very mild, requiring only monitoring of the hemoglobin level and avoiding any oxidant that may exaggerate the existing anemia. Severe transfusion-dependent anemias are also encountered in such patients, and, based on the frequency of the transfusions, iron chelation might be required. Splenectomy was shown to be effective in some children in either decreasing the frequency of transfusions or to treat a hypersplenic state. Genetic counseling and prenatal diagnosis should be considered in severe cases.

References

GM, Fico A, Martini G et al (2010) Discussion on pharmacogenetic interaction in G6PD deficiency and methods of identifying potential hemolytic drugs. Cardiovasc Hematol Disord Drug Targets 1(E Pub)

Harley JD, Agar NS, Yoshida A et al (1978) Glucose-6-phosphate dehydrogenase variants: Gd(+) Alexandra associated with neonatal jaundice and Gd(−) Camperdown in a young man with lamellar cataracts. J Lab Clin Med 91:295–300

Kordes U, Richter A, Santer R et al (2010) Neonatal cholestasis and glucose-6-phosphate dehydrogenase deficiency. Pediatr Blood Cancer 54(5):758–760

McDade J, Abramamova T, Mortier N et al (2008) A novel G6PD mutation leading to chronic hemolytic anemia. Pediatr Blood Cancer 51(16):816–819

Meloni L, Manca MR, Loddo I et al (2008) Glucose-6-phosphate dehydrogenase deficiency protects against coronary heart diseases. J Inherit Metab Dis 31(3):412–417, E Pub

Naizi GA, Adeyokunno A, Westwood B et al (1996) Neonatal jaundice in Saudi newborns with G6PD Aures. Ann Trop Paediatr 16(1):33–37

Pamuk GE, Dogan Celik A, Uyanik MS et al (2009) Brucellosis triggering hemolytic anemia in glucose-6-phosphate dehydrogenase deficiency. Med Princ Pract 18(4):329–331, E Pub

Spolaris Z, Siddiqi M, Siegel JH et al (2001) Increased incidence of sepsis and altered monocyte function in severely injured type A- glucose-6-phosphate dehydrogenase deficient African American trauma patients. Crit Care Med 29:728–736

Tinely KE, Loughlin AM, Jepson A et al (2010) Evaluation of a rapid qualitative enzyme chromatographic test for glucose-6-phosphate dehyadrogenase deficiency. Am J Trop Med Hyg 82(2):210–214

Watchko JF(2009) Hyperbilirubinemia in African American neonates : clinical issues and current challenges. Semin Fetal Neonatal Med

Yaish HM, Naizi GA, Al-Shaalan M et al (1991) Increased incidence of hyperbilirubinemia in unchallenged G6PD deficiency in term Saudi newborns. Ann Trop Paediatr 11:259–266

Zhang Z, Liew CW, Handy DE et al (2009) High glucose inhibits glucose-6-phosphate dehydrogenase leading to increased oxidative stress and beta-cells apoptosis. FASEP J

321 Other Red Cell Enzymopathies

Ahmad A. Mallouh

Introduction

Congenital nonspherocytic hemolytic anemia was described for the first time by Dacie in 1952. In addition to a variable degree of hemolytic anemia, these disorders are characterized by the absence of spherocytes in the peripheral blood and normal osmotic fragility of the Red Blood Cells (RBCs). The term "Congenital NonSpherocytic Hemolytic Anemia" (CNSHA) is used to describe a heterogeneous group of congenital hemolytic anemias that results from the inherited deficiency of RBC glycolytic enzymes of the Embden-Meyerhof or pentose phosphate metabolic pathway. As these are anaerobic pathways, in which glucose is catabolized to pyruvate and lactate and thus produce Adenosine TriPhosphate (ATP), deficiency of any enzyme in this pathway results in decreased level or complete absence of ATP in the RBCs. ATP plays a major role in maintaining the red blood cells' membrane integrity. Glucose-6-Phosphate Dehydrogenase (G6PD) deficiency, the most common red blood cells enzyme deficiency, affects around 100 million people around the world. Pyruvate Kinase (PK) deficiency, the second most common red cell enzyme deficiency, affects a few thousand individuals globally. All the other red cell enzyme deficiencies affect a few hundred persons.

Pyruvate Kinase Deficiency

The production of the pyruvate kinase enzyme in human is controlled by two genes. The M gene (located on chromosome 15q22) is responsible for PK production in muscle, brain, white blood cells and platelets, while the L gene (located on chromosome 1q21) is responsible for the enzyme production in the red blood cell and liver. Hemolytic anemia with PK deficiency is limited to the L gene mutation that results in quantitative or qualitative deficiency in the red blood cell and liver with normal enzyme level in other tissues. Several (around 180) mutations of the L gene in association with PK-deficient hemolytic anemia have been identified. Clinically significant hemolytic anemia occurs in patients who are homozygous for the same gene mutation or doubly heterozygous for two different mutations. Heterozygous persons have intermediate level of the enzyme in the red blood cells and they are clinically and hematologically normal without evidence of hemolysis.

Pathophysiology

Pyruvate kinase is involved in the anaerobic glycolytic pathway which results in the production of ATP and lactate. Blockage of this pathway in the pyruvate kinase deficient patients leads to markedly decreased level or absent ATP in the red blood cells. ATP is thought to be essential to maintaining the red blood cell milieu. Reduced or absent levels or activity of PK lead to potassium and water leak from the RBCs resulting in dehydrated, shrunken and spiculated cells (echynocytes) and shortened red cell survival (hemolysis). In vitro, addition of ATP to incubated PK deficient red blood cells corrects this defect, while addition of glucose fails to do so. ATP deficiency, however, is not sufficient to explain the mechanism of hemolysis. It is difficult to demonstrate ATP deficiency in some patients with severe hemolysis, while hemolysis is not found in some disorders with more severe ATP deficiency. PK deficiency results in an increased level of 2,3 diphosphoglycerate (2,3-DPG), which leads to a rightward shift of the oxygen dissociation curve. This shift results in better oxygen delivery to the tissues, which explain the adequate exercise tolerance despite significant anemia in those affected by PK deficiency.

The pyruvate kinase deficiency phenotype is thought to be more common among people of the northern European extraction, with prevalence ranging between 0.14 to more than 1%. Other reports, however, have demonstrated a higher prevalence in other ethnic groups (Indians, Chinese, Saudi Arabs, Turks and Iranians). The prevalence of clinically significant anemia (homozygous or doubly heterozygous) is expected to be higher with high rate of consanguinity.

Clinical Picture

Pyruvate kinase (PK) deficiency is the most common cause of congenital nonspherocytic anemia (CNSHA).

Abdelaziz Y. Elzouki (ed.), *Textbook of Clinical Pediatrics*, DOI 10.1007/978-3-642-02202-9_321,

It affects males and females equally because it is inherited as a recessive trait. The severity of anemia is highly variable, ranging from a severe transfusion dependent hemolytic anemia beginning at birth to a well-compensated asymptomatic hemolytic process recognized in later life because of the worsening of anemia (aplastic or hemolytic crisis) or because of the development of complications (cholelithiasis). In some extreme conditions, the anemia is severe enough to cause non-immune hydrops fetalis. The degree of severity is typically similar within a family with PK deficiency. The severity is probably related to influence of the L gene and the compensatory effect of the M2 gene, which is widely distributed in various tissues including the red blood cells. Absence of this compensatory mechanism results in severe life threatening anemia. In severe cases, patients present, at birth, with evidence of hemolysis (pallor, jaundice and splenomegaly). Reticulocytes are usually extremely high (40–70%), especially after splenectomy. This interesting phenomenon of increased reticulocytes after splenectomy is thought to be due to the interaction between the PK deficient reticulocytes and some unknown factor in the splenic environment (possibly hypoxia due to hemostasis). The anemia and hyperbilirubinemia might be severe enough to require phototherapy with or without simple or exchange blood transfusion. Patients may present with one or more complications of disease, which include hepatosplenomegaly, gallbladder stones, transient aplastic crisis caused by parvovirus B19, megaloblastic anemia due to folic acid deficiency or a hyper-hemolytic event.

Diagnosis

Diagnosis of PK deficiency is based on clinical and laboratory findings described above and confirmed by the assay of the red blood cells' PK enzyme level. Specific gene mutation can be identified in specialized laboratories.

Treatment

Treatment of PK deficiency consists of supportive care, splenectomy, treatment or prevention of complications, stem cell transplantation and gene therapy. Intra-uterine transfusion is indicated for severe anemia with hydrops. Newborn infants with severe anemia and/or hyperbilirubinemia should be treated with phototherapy, simple transfusion, or exchange transfusion as appropriate. Infants and children who have severe anemia may require repeated transfusions. Transfusion may be sporadically required in patients with mild disease during transient aplastic or hemolytic events. As with all chronic hemolytic anemias, folic acid supplementation is recommended. Splenectomy is recommended for children with severe, transfusion-dependent anemia. Splenectomy results in the amelioration of the hemolytic process leading to either the abolishment or greatly decreasing the need for transfusion. Splenectomy should be delayed until 5–6 years of age to avoid post-splenectomy sepsis, unless otherwise absolutely necessary. Complications which require treatment and/or prevention include cholelithiasis, which often requires surgery. Post splenectomy sepsis by the encapsulated organisms (streptococcus pneumoniae, haemophilus influenzae and neisseria meningitidis) can be prevented by pre splenectomy immunization and post splenectomy antibiotic prophylaxis. Iron overload caused by blood transfusion may require chelation therapy. Hematopoietic stem cell transplantation has been successfully performed in some severe cases. Gene therapy is still experimental.

Deficiencies of Other Glycolytic Enzymes

Congenital nonspherocytic hemolytic anemia had been reported with several other glycolytic erythrocyte enzyme deficiencies, including hexokinase, glucose-6 phosphate isomerase, glyceraldehyde-3-phosphate isomerase, phosphofructokinase, triosephosphate isomerase, aldolase and phosphoglycerate kinase deficiencies. These rare inherited enzymopathies have in common, an autosomal recessive mode of inheritance and a nonspherocytic hemolytic anemia with variable severity, which usually starts in infancy. The anemia in the newborn might be severe enough and may be associated with hyperbilirubinemia that require phototherapy and simple or exchange transfusion. The anemia during infancy and childhood may be compensated and asymptomatic, or severe transfusion dependant. The anemia may be exacerbated with transient bone marrow aplasia or acute hemolytic event in association with infection. Red blood cell morphology is normal and osmotic fragility is normal. However, spiculated red cells and target red blood cells might be seen in some patients. The reticulocyte count is elevated, especially after splenectomy. Clinical manifestations are those of hemolytic anemia and its complications. Pallor, jaundice and splenomegaly are present in patients with severe disease. Gallbladder stones may develop early in childhood. Of interest is the reported association of these disorders with other hematologic, neurologic, metabolic, or glycogen storage diseases. Hexokinase deficiency was reported with Fanconi aplastic anemia, triosephosphate isomerase deficiency with progressive neurologic disorder, phosphofructokinase deficiency with myopathy, phosphoglycerate kinase deficiency with mental retardation and aldolase deficiency with disorders of glycogen metabolism. Diagnosis of these disorders is confirmed by the enzymatic assay. Treatment is mainly supportive with blood transfusion as needed, phototherapy and/or exchange transfusion for severe neonatal anemia and hyperbilirubinemia, folic acid supplementation and cholecystectomy for symptomatic gallbladder stones. Splenectomy resulted in amelioration, but not complete resolution of hemolysis. After splenectomy, transfusion requirements is decreased or completely abolished.

References

Abu-Melha AM, Ahmed MAM, Knox-Macaulay H et al (1991) Erythrocyte pyruvate kinase deficiency in newborns of Eastern Saudi Arabia. Acta Haematol 85:192

Akin H, Baykal-Erkilic A, Aksu A et al (1997) Prevalence of erythrocyte kinase deficiency and normal values of enzyme in a Turkish population. Hum Hered 47:42

Ayi K, Min Oo, Serghides L, Crokckett M et al (2008) Pyruvate kinase deficiency and malaria. N Engl J Med 358:1805

Beutler E, Gelbart T (2000) Estimating the prevalence o pyruvate kinase deficiency from the gene frequency in the general white population. Blood 95:3585

Bowman H, McKusick V, Dronamraju K (1965) Pyruvate kinase deficient hemolytic anemia in an Amish Isolate. Am J Hum Genet 17:1

Dacie JV, Mollison PL, Richardson N et al (1953) Atypical congenital hemolytic anemia. Q J Med 22:79

Demina A, Varughese K, Barbot J et al (1998) Six previously undescribed pyruvate kinase deficiency mutation causing enzyme deficiency. Blood 15:647

Diez A, Gilsanz F, Martinez J et al (2005) Life-threatening nonspherocytic hemolytic anemia in a patient with null mutation in the PKLR gene and no compensatory PKM gene expression. Blood 106:1851

Ferreira P, Morais L, Costa R et al (2000) Hydrops fetalis associated with erythrocyte pyruvate kinase deficiency. Eur J Pediatr 159:481

Fung RH, Keung YK, Chung GS (1969) Screening of pyruvate kinase deficiency and G6PD deficiency in Chinese newborn in Hong Kong. Arch Dis Child 44:373

Kedar PS, Warang P, Colah RB, Mohanty D (2006) Red cell pyruvate kinase deficiency in neonatal jaundice cases in India. Indian J Pediatr 73:985

Miwa S, Fujii H (1996) Molecular bases of erythroenzymopathies associated with hereditary hemolytic anemia: tabulation of mutant enzymes. Am J Hematol 51:122

Mohrenweiser HW (1987) Functional hemizygosity in the human genome: direct estimate from twelve erythrocyte enzyme loci. Hum Genet 77:241

Pissard S, de Montalembert M, Bachir D et al (2007) Pyruvate kinase (PK) deficiency in newborns: the pitfalls of diagnosis. J Pediatr 150:443

Sandoval C, Stringel G, Weiberger J et al (1997) Failure of partial splenectomy to ameliorate the anemia of pyruvate kinase deficiency. J Pediatr Surg 32:641

Tanaka KR, Zerez CR (1990) Red cell enzymopathies of the glycolytic pathway. Semin Hematol 27:165

Tanphaichitr VS, Suavatte V, Issaragrisil S et al (2000) Successful bone marrow transplantation in a child with red blood cell pyruvate kinase deficiency. Bone Marrow Transplant 26:689

Yavarian M, Karimi M, Shahriary M et al (2008) Prevalence of pyruvate kinase deficiency among the South Iranian population: quantitative assay and molecular analysis. Blood Cells Mol Dis 40:308

Zanella A, Fermo E, Bianchi P, Valentini G (2005) Red cell pyruvate kinase deficiency: molecular and clinical aspects. Br J Haematol 130:11

322 Red Blood Cell Membrane Disorders

Ahmad A. Mallouh

Introduction

The red blood cell (RBC) membrane is a complex structure consisting of approximately 50% proteins, 40% lipids, and 10% carbohydrates, containing 10–12 major proteins and possibly hundreds of minor ones. RBC membrane proteins are divided into those that are integral to the membrane (glycophorins A, B, C, and D that contain membrane receptors and antigens and protein 3 which is responsible for anion exchange) and those that play a role in the cytoskeleton. Spectrin is the major skeletal protein of the RBC membrane; it constitutes 50–70% of the skeletal part of the membrane. The RBC membrane has two major functions: maintenance of the structural integrity of the cell and control of cations, anions, and water permeability. As the membrane is semipermeable, water and some cations and anions can migrate passively through the RBC membrane. However, some cations (Na, K, and Ca) are transported through the membrane both passively and by an active mechanism (Na/K pump and calcium efflux pump) using energy produced by ATP. Changes in the membrane surface area in relation to the red cell volume result in changes in the shape and deformability of the cells. These changes render the abnormal RBCs susceptible to destruction by the reticuloendothelial system. Loss of surface area without loss in volume from either inherited or acquired causes results in formation of spherocytes. Following is discussion of inherited RBCs membrane disorders.

Hereditary Spherocytosis

Around 75% of hereditary spherocytosis (HS) is inherited in an autosomal dominant pattern. The remaining 25% are mostly inherited as an autosomal recessive trait. Some cases (up to 10% in some studies) are thought to be new mutation or mild cases of the dominant type. Homozygous of the dominantly inhireted HS has not been reported and is thought to be incompatible with life. The incidence of HS is about 200–300 per million in the Caucasians, but this figure is likely to an underestimation as mild cases are often not diagnosed. Some studies suggest that the true incidence is probably four to five times greater. The incidence in other ethnic groups is not known but thought to be much lower than that of the Caucasians.

Pathophysiology

The primary problem in HS is loss of the RBC membrane surface area leading to a change of the cell shape from a biconcave disk-like to a spherocyte. This change in the shape makes the cells less deformable and more susceptible to hemolysis in hypotonic solution (increased osmotic fragility). The reticulocytes and the younger red cells are not spherical. As these cell age they become more spherical and their membrane more rigid. The most common defect is spectrin deficiency. However three other abnormalities had been identified as the main causes of HS: combined spectrin and ankyrin, protein 3 deficiency, and protein 4.2 abnormality. The spherical RBCs with a rigid membrane are trapped and hemolyzed in the spleen (extravascular). The severity of anemia depends on this chronic process of intrasplenic hemolysis.

Clinical Picture

The disease is variable in severity ranging from the asymptomatic patient who is diagnosed only because of family history or because they develop cholelithiasis; to the severe patient who may be packed red cell (PRBC) transfusion dependent. Some patients present in the neonatal period with anemia, which may require PRBC transfusion, and/or jaundice, which requires phototherapy, or even exchange transfusion. In such patients, a family history of HS may be the first clue of the diagnosis. Other aspects of the family history that would raise the possibility of HS include "chronic anemia," jaundice in the neonatal period or later, splenomegaly, cholelithiasis, and/or history of HS. A child may present with severe abdominal pain and jaundice with or without fever and chills as a result of the cholelithiasis and/or cholecystitis. The degree of anemia is variable and so its manifestations. Around 5% of patients with HS have severe anemia, reticulocytosis, and significant splenomegaly. Anemia in these patients can be

Abdelaziz Y. Elzouki (ed.), *Textbook of Clinical Pediatrics*, DOI 10.1007/978-3-642-02202-9_322,

severe enough to cause hydrops fetalis and intrauterine death. Postnatally these patients often require repeated PRBCs transfusion. Up to 75% of patients with HS have moderate anemia with mild to moderate splenomegaly and moderate reticulocytosis, ranging from 5% to 10%. These patients usually, but not always, have the dominantly inherited condition. Patients with mild HS (20–30% of all patients) usually have a dominant type inheritance. As mentioned above these patients are asymptomatic and are diagnosed only on family study or when they develop complications as cholelithiasis or aplastic crisis. The spleen is palpable in 75–95% of people with HS. Splenomegaly in mild cases might be absent. In some patients (usually in the most severe ones who have a recessive type of inheritance), splenomegaly can be massive and may be the main presenting complaint. About 30–50% of adults with HS have history of jaundice. The jaundice in the newborn can be severe and may require exchange transfusion. In older children and adults it is usually mild and intermittent. In addition to the above-mentioned manifestations, patients may present with more acute complication. These include hemolytic events, aplastic events, megaloblastic events, cholelithiasis, cholecystitis, and severe neonatal hyperbilirubinemia. Hemolytic events are usually triggered by a viral infection that stimulates the reticuloendothelial system mainly in the spleen. The patient presents with anemia, jaundice, and reticulocytosis and often increased splenic size. Aplastic events are oftentimes caused by human parvovirus 19 (B19). These patients present with anemia, reticulocytopenia, and no jaundice. Megaloblastic events are due to folic acid deficiency. Therefore, folic acid supplementation is recommended for all patients with HS. Unlike the other types of events, a megaloblastic event usually develops slowly. Cholelithiasis can occur at any early age, having been reported in children as young as 3 years old. The incidence, however, increases with age; upto 75% of all patients with HS after the fifth decade of life. Most patients are diagnosed with gallstones in the second and third decade of life. Many patients with cholelithiasis are asymptomatic. However, several studies suggest that around 50% of patients with pigmented gall bladder stones have or are expected to develop symptoms of cholecystitis and/or biliary colic with jaundice.

Diagnosis

Diagnosis of HS depends on history, physical examination, and appropriately ordered laboratory tests. A family history of chronic anemia, confirmed HS, cholelithiasis at young age, or history of splenectomy is of paramount importance in suggesting the diagnosis. A history of anemia and or jaundice in the neonatal period which is not explained by other causes (blood group incompatibility) may suggest an inherited cause of hemolysis including HS. A history of previous blood transfusions in the patient or other family members might be present. Depending on the severity of anemia, patients may have exercise intolerance. Physical findings may include pallor (depending on level of anemia), jaundice, and splenomegaly. Biliary colic with jaundice may be the first presenting sign. Manifestations of cholecystitis (abdominal pain, fever, chills, and jaundice) may also be the first presenting problem. Growth retardation and delayed sexual maturation may be present in severe cases. Severe cases also may have bone marrow expansion mostly in the facial and other skull bones causing frontal bossing and dental malocclusion.

The degree of anemia is variable, ranging from compensated state with normal hemoglobin to severe, transfusion-dependent anemia. Most cases however have compensated mild to moderate anemia (hemoglobin >10 g/dl). Patients who present early during infancy usually have more severe anemia (hemoglobin 8–9 g/dl). Reticulocytosis is usually present. Its value depends on the severity of the anemia and the appropriateness of the bone marrow response. During aplastic events, reticulocytopenia is present. Unconjugated bilirubin may be high especially in jaundiced patients. Serum haptoglobin is usually low but it is not required for diagnosis. The hallmark of the disease is the presence of microspherocytes on a peripheral blood smear. The blood smear (➔ *Fig. 322.1*) should be inspected by a qualified or experienced observer.

The most commonly used test to confirm the diagnosis of HS is the osmotic fragility. This test detects hemolysis of RBCs from patients affected with HS at higher concentration of saline than those of normal RBC. The unincubated osmotic fragility test, performed on fresh RBCs, may miss up to a third of the cases. Incubation of the blood for 24 h makes the test more sensitive. A newly described flow cytometry assessment can provide a rapid and reliable diagnosis, but is not generally available. Analysis of the cell membrane for determination of the specific protein defect is available only in specialized laboratories and is of no clinical value.

Treatment

As with other chronic hemolytic anemia, daily folic acid supplementation should be given to avoid megaloblastic events. PRBC transfusion might be needed in severe cases of hemolytic events or aplastic events. Phototherapy and/or

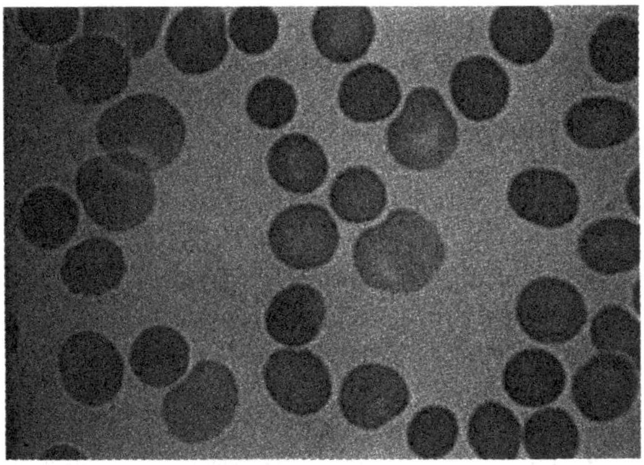

Figure 322.1
Blood smear in hereditary spherocytosis. Note the spherical RBCs without central pallor

exchange transfusion is indicated for newborn infants with severe anemia or hyperbilirubinemia.

Splenectomy usually results in complete or partial correction of the anemia associated with HS. RBCs maintain their spherical shape but their life span increases even though it is usually shorter than normal RBCs. Before proceeding with splenectomy, the following should be considered:

- Indications
- Potential benefits
- Potential risks and their prevention and/or treatment
- Type of the procedure
- Timing
- Potential failure and its causes

In patients with clinically mild HS, the only benefit of splenectomy is prevention of gall stone formation. The risk and cost of the procedure in this setting is higher than the expected benefit. If splenectomy is to be done, some studies suggest doing prophylactic cholecystectomy in the same setting. In patients with clinically severe HS, those who require repeated blood transfusion and those with moderate but symptomatic anemia, splenectomy is recommended. This procedure is expected to correct the anemia to normal values except in some patients with autosomal recessive HS, in which the anemia may be only partially corrected. In those patients with moderate but asymptomatic anemia (hemoglobin concentration from 8 to 10 g/dl), splenectomy may be indicated, even though there is a paucity of studies demonstrating benefit. The expected benefits of splenectomy include correction of anemia, prevention of development of cholelithiasis, prevention of bone marrow expansion and growth failure, decreased serum bilirubin level, and decreased reticulocyte count.

In addition to the risks of anesthesia and the surgical procedure, the most serious risk is post-splenectomy infection caused by encapsulated organisms (*Streptococcus pneumoniae, Haemophilus influenzae,* and *Neisseria meningitidis*). These infections are life threatening. Even though these infections can occur at any age they are more common when splenectomy is performed before 6 years of age. This serious problem can be minimized by:

- Delaying splenectomy until 6 years of age (unless absolutely necessary)
- Giving immunizations against the above-mentioned organism a few weeks before the procedure
- Giving antibiotic prophylaxis (usually penicillin)

The duration of the prophylaxis is not well established. Some authorities recommend a minimum of at least 3 years post splenectomy and probably for life.

Other post-splenectomy complications include an increased incidence of venous and arterial thrombosis and thromboembolism. An increased risk of arteriosclerosis later in life has been reported. Laparoscopic splenectomies are preferred by many centers because they may shorten hospital stay, decrease postoperative pain, and decrease scarring. Partial splenectomy (removing 80–90% of the spleen) results in significant improvement, but not complete resolution of the anemia. It however retains splenic function and decreases or prevents post-splenectomy sepsis. Total splenectomy is often needed later because the spleen regrows in most patients to its original size and hemolysis accordingly increases in severity. In one study near total (98%), splenectomy was found to correct anemia without significant regrowth of the spleen. In some patients, the hemolytic anemia in HS is only partially corrected or recurs after splenectomy, because of:

- The presence of a severe recessive phenotype
- Partial splenectomy
- The presence of accessory spleen which is not removed during surgery
- The presence of splenosis that results from spillage and peritoneal implantation of splenic tissue

Accessory spleens and splenosis should be suspected if Howell–Jolly bodies are not identified postoperatively. Confirmation of this diagnosis can be obtained by radiological means mainly nuclear scan.

Management of asymptomatic cholelithiasis is controversial. Some authorities recommend cholecystectomy with or without splenectomy, while the others suggest expectant observation. Performing the procedure when the patient's condition is stable and the timing is appropriate for the patient and family is warranted. Management of symptomatic cholelithiasis is urgent.

Hereditary Elliptocytosis

Hereditary elliptocytosis (HE) is a genetically phenotypically and biochemically inherited type of hemolytic anemia characterized by the presence of elliptical, oval, or elongated (rod-like) and sometimes spherical RBCS in the peripheral blood smear (➋ *Fig. 322.2*). The incidence is estimated to be from 250 to 500 per million. The mode of inheritance is autosomal dominant in most cases. However, a recessive inheritance is typical of the subtype called hereditary pyropoikilocytosis (HPP). HE results from a defect in the skeleton of the RBC membrane. Defects in several RBC membrane proteins have been identified, including spectrin, protein 3, protein 4.1, and protein 4.2 alone or in combination.

Clinical Picture

The clinical picture of HE is variable and ranges between a hematologically normal to a severe and occasionally fatal anemia. Most cases, however, are mild. The following subtypes have been described:

- Common HE: This most common type of HE is divided clinically into the following subtypes.
  - Silent carrier: These patients are clinically and hematologically normal. They have normal hemoglobin, normal RBC morphology, a normal reticulocyte count, normal LDH, and normal haptoglobin. Patients who are silent carriers of HE are usually diagnosed on family studies of an affected member.

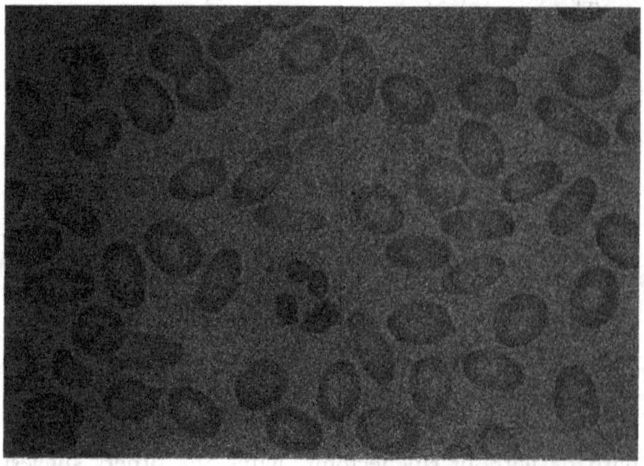

Figure 322.2
Blood smear in hereditary elliptocytosis

- Mild HE: These patients usually have a mild compensated hemolytic anemia with a mild reticulocytosis. They are clinically asymptomatic. They are diagnosed when elliptocytes are seen on a routine CBC. They may develop mild hemolytic events on exposure to certain infections.
- HE with chronic hemolysis: Several families had been reported with moderate hemolytic anemia with reticulocytosis without known trigger. Mild splenomegaly and mild RBC fragmentation can be present in these patients.
- HE with infantile poikilocytosis: In this interesting type of HE, infants have severe hemolytic anemia requiring repeated PRBC transfusions in the first 12–24 months. Their RBC morphologic and laboratory findings are similar to HPP (see below). One of the parents usually has common-type HE. The hemolytic process decreases over time. By 12–24 months of age, the clinical course is similar to those with mild HE. This type seems to be common in certain ethnic groups. The author has seen more than 100 cases in Saudi Arabian infants.
- Severe HE: In this type of HE, patients are often transfusion dependent. The disease can be fatal. Severe HE is thought to be a homozygous or doubly heterozygous form of mild HE.
- Hereditary pyropoikilocytosis (HPP): This type of recessively inherited hemolytic anemia was thought to be a specific entity, however further studies suggest that it a relatively severe subtype of HE. Both parents are often clinically and hematologically normal (silent carriers) but in other families at least one parent may have mild HE. HPP affects mostly people of African descent; however, it has been reported in other ethnic groups including a Saudi Arabian family reported by this author. HPP is characterized by moderately severe hemolytic anemia that usually starts in infancy and is lifelong. Many patients need repeated PRBC transfusions. Patients often have splenomegaly. The hallmark of this condition is the bizarre RBC morphology including spherocytes, microspherocytes, fragmented cells, cell membrane budding, schistocytes, and poikilocytosis. These morphologic changes are exaggerated with in vitro exposure to a relatively low temperature, resulting in increased fragmentation and more budding. Osmotic fragility is increased in patients with HPP. In most patients, the MCV is low, sometimes in the 50 or 60 femtoliter range.

- Spherocytic elliptocytosis: This type of HE is inherited in an autosomal dominant pattern. Spherocytic elliptocytosis has been reported only in Caucasians. The anemia is mild to moderate. Most patients have splenomegaly. Examination of the peripheral blood smear can be confusing as the number of elliptocytes can be lower than the number of spherocytes. Spherocytic elliptocytosis is considered a hybrid of ES an HS.
- Southeast Asian ovalocytosis: As the name implies, this type of HE is preset in the area of the world where malaria is or was endemic. Southeast Asian ovalocytosis is inherited in an autosomal dominant pattern. Heterozygous Southeast Asian ovalocytosis is asymptomatic, does not cause anemia, and is thought to be protective against malaria. The homozygous form is not compatible with life. Review of the peripheral blood smear is characteristic with the presence of "stomatocytic elliptocytes."

Diagnosis

Diagnosis of HE is straightforward, requiring a complete blood count, reticulocyte count, and a peripheral blood smear. Other tests (osmotic fragility, heat stability, and structural study of the RBCS membrane) are often of academic interest and rarely add any significant clinical diagnostic value. When considering the diagnosis of HE, several points should be kept in mind:

- Unaffected people may have up to 5% elliptocytes in their peripheral blood.
- Elliptocytes are increased in some acquired conditions, for example, megaloblastic anemias and iron efficiency anemia.
- Silent carrier HE can be diagnosed only with a RBC member structural study. This is rarely clinically indicated.
- HE with infantile poikilocytosis cannot be differentiated from true HPP except by time.
- Spherocytic HE can be confused with HS.

Treatment

Most patients with HE do not need any treatment except folic acid supplementation (especially when there is evidence of hemolysis) and observation for development of cholelithiasis. Blood transfusion is usually needed for severe episodes of anemia especially in homozygous common HE, HPP, infantile poikilocytosis in the first 12–24 months of life, and occasionally in the common type after a hemolytic event. Splenectomy might be needed in HPP and homozygous common HE if and when anemia is severe and repeated transfusion is required.

Hereditary Stomatocytosis

This rare RBC membrane defect is characterized by the presence of elongated RBCs with a slit-like pallor resembling a mouth (stoma). It is inherited in an autosomal dominant manner. The change in the shape of the RBCs results from a decrease in the ratio between surface area and cell volume, usually due to increased volume. The exact pathogenesis is not well understood. Alteration of the membrane permeability leads to sodium and water movement into the RBC causing increased cell volume. With increased water and sodium, the RBCs become swollen. The clinical and hematologic findings are variable. Approximately one third of the patients are asymptomatic with normal hematological values and no evidence of hemolysis. The remainder of the patients have mild to moderate and occasionally severe transfusion-dependent chronic hemolytic anemia, jaundice, and splenomegaly. Some patients with hereditary stomatocytosis have recurrent vaso-occlusive events (similar to those of sickle cell disease) and an increased incidence of thromboembolic complications especially after splenectomy. These two complications are thought to be due to increased adherence of the elongated RBC to the endothelium. Stomatocytes may be present on the blood smear of several congenital and acquired conditions. Stomatocytosis with thrombocytopenia and large platelets had been reported in people of Mediterranean origin. Stomatocytosis is associated with two hereditary diseases: cryohydrocytosis and familial pseudohyperkalemia. A syndrome of stomatocytosis with mental retardation and cataracts has been reported. Acquired stomatocytosis can occur with acute alcohol intoxication, chronic liver disease, and with administration of vinca alkaloids (vincristine or vinblastine). Stomatocytosis is often an artifact. Diagnosis of hereditary stomatocytosis is supported by the presence of a macrocytic, hypochromic hemolytic anemia with a high number of stomatocytes on the peripheral blood smear (up to 60%). Treatment is usually supportive (folic acid supplementation and blood transfusion in severe cases). Splenectomy for severe cases may be necessary and may improve the anemia. However, splenectomy may increase the risk of serious thrombotic complications.

Acanthocytosis and Echynocytosis

Acanthocytes have a small number (5–10) of irregularly spaced, long spicules that arise from the RBC membrane. Echinocytes, or crenated cells, on the other hand, have 10–30 regularly spaced, short projections that arise from the surface of red cells. Spur cells are remodeled acanthocytes in which spicules become blunt and short. Acanthocytes and echynocytes, separately or in combination, can be associated with several congenital or acquired conditions. They both are often found in end stage renal disease, advanced hepatocellular disease, and vitamin E deficiency. Echynocytes may be seen in association with pyruvate kinase deficiency. Echynocytes are commonly seen as artifact of the preparation of the peripheral blood smear. Acanthocytosis is a typical feature of abetalipoproteinemia, in which progressive ataxia, retinitis pigmentosa, and fat malabsorption are present. Acanthocytosis may be associated with hypothyroidism, myelodysplasia, having no expression of the Lutheran or McLeod blood groups, and infantile pyknocytosis. Acanthocytes are also associated with several neurological diseases including McLeod syndrome, various mitochondrial diseases, choreo-acanthocytosis, familial acanthocytosis with paroxysmal exertion-induced dyskinesias, and epilepsy and Huntington's disease. The significance and pathogenesis of this association is not understood. In most cases, the presence of acanthocytes and/or echynocytes is of no clinical significance except as a diagnostic tool for certain diseases.

Hereditary Xerocytosis

Xerocytosis is a chronic hemolytic anemia inherited as autosomal dominant trait. It is characterized by the presence of densely stained contracted and sometimes spiculated red cells. The hemoglobin may "puddle" in one part of the cell. The pathophysiology is due a defect in RBC membrane permeability, with an increased potassium efflux resulting in low potassium content. These changes lead to decreased deformability, increased rigidity, and increased susceptibility to shear cell damage. The diagnosis is based on the presence of chronic hemolytic anemia and the presence of xerocytes on peripheral smear. The MCV and MCHC are both elevated. Target cells are usually present. The osmotic fragility is decreased. The severity of anemia is variable, particularly during the newborn period, in which anemia may be severe enough to require exchange transfusion. The anemia may be exacerbated by viral infections. Transient aplastic events have been reported. A subtype of xerocytosis (called stomatocytic xerocytosis) is often difficult to differentiate from classic stomatocytosis. Both stomatocytes and dehydrated target cells are present on the peripheral blood smear. Unlike stomatocytosis, the osmotic fragility is reduced in stomatocytic xerocytosis. Like the classic form of hereditary xerocytosis, the MCV and MCHC are elevated. Treatment for xerocytosis is symptomatic. Folic acid supplementation is recommended. Splenectomy has been performed with amelioration of the anemia. However, there have been reports of an increased risk of deep venous thrombosis after this procedure in patients with this diagnosis.

Infantile Pyknocytosis

Infantile pyknocytosis is a transient hemolytic anemia that occurs in the newborn infants, particularly those born preterm. It is characterized by a hemolytic anemia and jaundice without splenomegaly. The severity of anemia is variable and may pass unnoticed. In some infants, however, the anemia is severe enough to require PRBC transfusion. The anemia peaks at 3–4 weeks of age and resolves spontaneously by 4–6 months of age. Pyknocytes are densely stained, spiculated, and irregularly contracted cells. Up to 5% of pyknocytes can be found on the peripheral blood smear in unaffected premature infants. Pyknocytes may be associated with many inherited or acquired disease including severe G6PD deficiency, neonatal hepatitis, hereditary elliptocytosis, vitamin E deficiency, and microangiopathic hemolytic anemia.

Vitamin E Deficiency

Vitamin E deficiency may occur in premature infants and in children with malabsorption disorders such as liver cirrhosis, cholestatic liver disease, cystic fibrosis, celiac disease, Crohn's disease, and pancreatic insufficiency. Hemolytic anemia, thrombocytosis, and the presence of a variable number of spiculated and contracted RBCs are the hallmark of the hematological manifestation of vitamin E deficiency. Generalized or pedal edema may be seen in severely affected infants. When suspected, measuring serum vitamin E levels makes the diagnosis. Oral vitamin E supplementation may be needed especially in premature infants. In patients with chronic malabsorption, the treatment of the original disease together with vitamin E supplementation is required.

Paroxysmal Nocturnal Hemoglobinuria

Paroxysmal nocturnal hemoglobinuria (PNH) is an acquired disorder characterized by episodes of hemolysis during sleep as well as early morning hemoglobinuria. Approximately 15% of the reported cases occur in children 6–20 years old. The basic defect is in the glycosylphosphatidylinositol (GPI) anchor. This defect leads to partial or complete absence of all GPI-linked membrane proteins, including CD59 and CD55. Occasionally CD8 expression may be decreased. These changes in the RBC-binding membrane proteins results in increased sensitivity of affected red cells to hemolysis by the activated complement system.

Clinical Presentation

Patients with PNH usually present with episodes of intravascular hemolysis that occur during sleep and lead to early morning hemoglobinuria. The anemia is variable in severity. Some patients have chronic hemolysis. Hemolysis can be induced or exacerbated by infection, whole blood transfusion, vaccine administration, iron therapy, or exercise. The severity of hemolysis is related to the size of the PNH clone, the degree of the abnormality (partial or complete absence of CD59 and CD55), and the degree of complement activation. Patients often present with other hematological or with nonhematological complications. Hematologic complications include venous or arterial thromboembolism, aplastic anemia, leukemia, myelodysplastic syndrome, and iron deficiency anemia. Venous thrombosis is much more common than arterial. Thrombosis may involve any vein, large or small. However, they most often involve the large intra-abdominal veins, particularly the hepatic, portal, and splenic veins, as well as the inferior vena cava. Thrombosis of the cerebral veins, specially the major venous sinuses, occurs less frequently than the intra-abdominal veins. Hepatic venous thrombosis may cause splenomegaly, hepatomegaly, and ascites (Budd–Chiari syndrome). Thrombosis of the small splanchnic veins may cause severe abdominal pain. The prevalence of thrombosis in Japanese patients is lower (6%) than among the American patients (38%). Aplastic anemia may develop after the diagnosis of PNH or it may be the presenting problem. The incidence is not known and it may appear years after the diagnosis of PNH. Leukemia, usually acute myeloid leukemia, develops years after the diagnosis of PNH. The reported incidence ranges from <1% up to 5%. Myelodysplastic and myeloproliferative disorders have been associated with PNH. Iron deficiency anemia is common in patients with PNH because of the urinary loss of iron caused by hemosiderinuria and/or hemoglobinuria. Nonhematological presentations include acute renal failure (from hemoglobinuria), proximal tubular dysfunction, and chronic renal failure. Esophageal spasm and erectile dysfunction has been reported in patients with PNH, though only in adults.

Diagnosis

Traditionally PNH was diagnosed by inducing in vitro hemolysis using the sucrose lysis test and the Ham acid hemolysis test. Both of these tests depend on activation of the complement system. Recently, flow cytometry using monoclonal antibodies against CD59 and CD55 has largely replaced the sucrose lysis and Ham tests for accurate diagnosis of PNH.

Treatment

The treatment of the anemia associated with PNH is supportive. Iron supplementation for iron deficiency anemia and folic acid supplementation to prevent megaloblastic anemia are indicated. PRBC transfusion should be given if clinically indicated. Caution should be given when iron or blood is given as they may induce acute hemolytic episodes. Whole blood should be avoided and only washed and preferably leukoreduced RBCs are recommended to decrease the possibility of transfusion-induced hemolysis. A humanized monoclonal antibody (eculizumab) that inhibits terminal complement activation by binding to the C5 was found to reduce hemolysis, transfusion requirements, and thromboembolic event rates. Prednisone and androgenic hormones (danazol) have been effective in diminishing anemia in some reports. Their role in PNH, however, is controversial. The thromboembolic complications should be treated in the same therapeutic modality as other patients. Hematopoietic cell transplantation (HCT) from an HLA identical sibling is indicated in the patient with severe aplastic anemia. Immunotherapy with cyclosporine and antithymocyte globulin (ATG) has been successful in some patients with aplastic anemia. Their role remains to be determent by further studies.

References

Agre P, Orringer EP (1982) Deficient red cell spectrin in severe, recessively inherited spherocytosis. N Engl J Med 306:1155

Austin RF, Desforges JF (1969) Hereditary elliptocytosis: an unusual presentation of hemolysis in the newborn associated with transient morphologic abnormalities. Pediatrics 44:196

Bader-Meunier B, Gauthier F, Archambaud F et al (2001) Long-term evaluation of beneficial effect of subtotal splenectomy for management of hereditary spherocyosis. Blood 97:399

Ballas SK, Clark MR, Mohandas N et al (1984) Red cell membrane and cation deficiency in Rh null syndrome. Blood 63:1046

Becker PS, Lux SE (1985) Hereditary spherocytosis and related disorders. Clin Haematol 14:15

Bolton-Maggs PH, Stevens RF, Dodd NJ et al (2004) Guidelines for the diagnosis and management of hereditary spherocytosis. Br J Haematol 126:455

Bossi D, Russo M (1996) Hemolytic anemia due to disorders of red cell membrane skeleton. Mol Aspects Med 17:171

Brodsky RA (2008) Narrative review: paroxysmal nocturnal hemoglobinuria: the physiology of complement-related hemolytic anemia. Ann Intern Med 148:587

Brodsky RA (2009) How I treat paroxysmal nocturnal haemoglobinuria. Blood 113:6522

Brodsky RA, Young NS, Antonioli E et al (2008) Multicenter phase 3 study of the complement inhibitor eculizumab for the treatment of patients with paroxysmal nocturnal hemoglobinuria. Blood 111:1840

Coetzer T, Palek J, Lawler J et al (1990) Structural and functional heterogeneity of alpha spectrin mutations involving the spectrin heterodimer self-association site: relationships to hematologic expression of homozygous hereditary elliptocytosis and hereditary pyropoikilocytosis. Blood 75:2235

Cynober T, Mohandas N, Tchernia G (1996) Red cell abnormalities in hereditary spherocytosis: relevance to diagnosis and understanding of the variable expression of clinical severity. J Lab Clin Med 128:259

Davidson RJ, How J, Lessels S (1977) Acquired stomatocytosis: its prevalence and significance in routine haematology. Scand J Haematol 19:47

de Latour RP, Mary JY, Salanoubat C et al (2008) Paroxysmal nocturnal hemoglobinuria: natural history of disease subcategories. Blood 112:3099

de Planque MM, Bacigalupo A, Wursch A et al (1989) Long-term follow-up of severe aplastic anaemia patients treated with antithymocyte globulin. Severe Aplastic Anaemia Working Party of the European Cooperative Group for Bone Marrow Transplantation (EBMT). Br J Haematol 73:121

del Miraglia Gindice E, Perotta S, Sannjno F et al (1994) Molecular heterogeneity of hereditary elliptocytosis in Italy. Hematologica 79:400

Delhommeau F, Cynober T, Schischmanoff P0 et al (2000) Natural history of hereditary spherocytosis during the first year of life. Blood 95:393

Eber SW, Armbrus R, Schroter W (1990) Variable clinical severity of hereditary spherocytosis: relation to erythrocytic spectrin concentration, osmotic fragility and autohemolysis. J Pediatr 117:409

Eyssette-Guerreau S, Bader-Meunier B, Garcon L et al (2006) Infantile pyknocytosis: a cause of haemolytic anaemia of the newborn. Br J Haematol 133:439

Flatt JF, Bruce LJ (2009) The hereditary stomatocytosis. Haematologica 94:1039

Gallagher PG, Lux SE (2003) Disorders of the erythrocyte membrane. In: Nathan DG, Orkin SH, Ginsburg D, Look TA (eds) Hematology of infancy and childhood. W.B. Saunders, Philadelphia, p 560

Glader BE, Fortier N, Albala MM, Nathan DG (1974) Congenital hemolytic anemia associated with dehydrated erythrocytes and increased potassium loss. N Engl J Med 291:491

Haines PG, Jarvis HG, King S et al (2001) Two further British families with the 'cryohydrocytosis' form of hereditary stomatosis. Br J Haematol 113:932

Hall SE, Rosse WF (1996) The use of monoclonal antibodies and flow cytometry in the diagnosis of paroxysmal nocturnal hemoglobinuria. Blood 87:5332

Hartmann RC, Luther AB, Jenkins DE Jr et al (1980) Fulminant hepatic venous thrombosis (Budd-Chiari syndrome) in paroxysmal nocturnal hemoglobinuria: definition of a medical emergency. Johns Hopkins Med J 146:247

Hassoun H, Palek J (1996) Hereditary spherocytosis: a review of the clinical and molecular aspects of the disease. Blood Rev 10:1

Hill A, Richards SJ, Hillmen P (2007) Recent developments in the understanding and management of paroxysmal nocturnal haemoglobinuria. Br J Haematol 137:181

Hillmen P, Lewis SM, Bessler M et al (1995) Natural history of paroxysmal nocturnal hemoglobinuria. N Engl J Med 333:1253

Hillmen P, Muus P, Duhrsen U et al (2007) Effect of the complement inhibitor eculizumab on thromboembolism in patients with paroxysmal nocturnal haemoglobinuria. Blood 110:4132

Kanzaki A, Yawata Y (1992) Hereditary stomatocytosis: phenotypical expression of sodium transport and band 7 peptides in 44 cases. Br J Haematol 82:133

Kawahara K, Witherspoon RP, Storb R (1992) Marrow transplantation for paroxysmal nocturnal haemoglobinuria. Am J Hematol 39:283

Konradsen HB, Henrichsen J (1991) Pneumococcal infections in splenectomized children are preventable. Acta Paediatr Scand 80:423

Lolascon A, Miraglia del Gindice E, Perotta S et al (1998) Hereditary spherocytosis: from the clinical to molecular defects. Hematologica 83:240

Mallouh AA, Saa'di AR, Ahmad MS et al (1984) Hereditary pyropoikilocytosis: report of two cases from Saudi Arabia. Am J Med Genet 18:413

Manno CS, Cohen AR (1989) Splenectomy in mild hereditary spherocytosis: is it worth the risk? Am J Pediatr Hematol Oncol 11:300

Marchetti M, Quaglini S, Barosi G (1998) Prophylactic splenectomy and cholecystectomy in mild hereditary spherocytosis: analyzing the decision in different clinical scenarios. J Intern Med 244:217

McMullin MF, Hillmen P, Jackson J et al (1994) Tissue plasminogen activator for hepatic vein thrombosis in paroxysmal nocturnal hemoglobinuria. J Intern Med 235:85

Medejel N, Garcon L, Guitton C et al (2008) Effect of subtotal splenectomy for management of hereditary pyropoikilocytosis. Br J Haematol 142:315

Miraglia del Giudice E, Francese M, Nobili B et al (1998) High frequency of de novo mutation in ankyrin gene (ANK1) in children with hereditary spherocytosis. J Pediatr 132:117

Mohandas N, Winardi R, Knowles D et al (1992) Molecular basis for membrane rigidity of hereditary ovalocytosis. J Clin Invest 89:686

Mooraki A, Boroumand B, Mohammad Zadeh F et al (1998) Acute reversible renal failure in a patient with paroxysmal nocturnal hemoglobinuria. Clin Nephrol 50:255

Moyo VM, Mukhina GL, Garrett ES, Brodsky RA (2004) Natural history of paroxysmal nocturnal haemoglobinuria using modern diagnostic assays. Br J Haematol 126:133

Nishimura J, Kanakura Y, Ware RE et al (2004) Clinical course and flow cytometric analysis of paroxysmal nocturnal hemoglobinuria in the United States and Japan. Medicine (Baltimore) 83:193

Palek J (1985) Hereditary elliptocytosis and related disorders. Clin Haematol 14:45

Palek J, Jarolim P (1993) Clinical expression and laboratory detection of RBC membrane protein mutations. Semin Hematol 30:249

Palek J, Lux S (1983) Red cell membrane skeletal defects in hereditary and acquired hemolytic anemias. Semin Haematol 20:189

Paquette RL, Yoshimura R, Veiseh C et al (1997) Clinical characteristics predict response to antithymocyte globulin in paroxysmal nocturnal haemoglobinuria. Br J Haematol 96:92

Parker C (2009) Eculizumab for paroxysmal nocturnal haemoglobinuria. Lancet 373:759

Parker C, Omine M, Richards S et al (2005) Diagnosis and management of paroxysmal nocturnal hemoglobinuria. Blood 106:3699

Patton ML, Moss BE, Haith LR et al (1997) Concomitant laparoscopic cholecystectomy and splenectomy for surgical management of hereditary spherocytosis. Am Surg 63:536

Ray JG, Burows RF, Ginsberg JS, Burrows EA (2000) Paroxysmal nocturnal hemoglobinuria and the risk of venous thrombosis: review and recommendations for management of the pregnant and nonpregnant patient. Haemostasis 30:103

Rees DC, Iolascon A, Carella M et al (2005) Stomatocytic haemolysis and macrothrombocytopenia (Mediterranean stomatocytosis/ macrothrombocytopenia) is the haematological presentation of phytosterolaemia. Br J Haematol 130:297

Rescorla FJ, Breitfeld PP, West KW et al (1998) A case controlled comparison of open and laparoscopic splenectomy in children. Surgery 124:670

Saso R, Marsh J, Cevreska L et al (1999) Bone marrow transplants for paroxysmal nocturnal hemoglobinuria. Br J Haematol 104:392

Schilling RF (2009) Risks and benefits of splenectomy versus no splenectomy for hereditary spherocytosis – a personal view. Br J Haematol 145:728

Silveira P, Cynobe T, Dhermy D et al (1997) RBC abnormalities in hereditary elliptocytosis and their relevance to variable clinical expression. Am J Pathol 108:391

Socie G, Mary JY, de Gramont A et al (1996) Paroxysmal nocturnal haemoglobinuria: long term follow-up and prognostic factors. French Society of hematology. Lancet 384:573

Stewart GW, Amess JAL, Eber S et al (1996) Thrombo-embolic disease after splenectomy for hereditary stomatocytosis. Br J Haematol 93:303

Stoehr GA, Stauffer UG, Eber SW (2005) Near-total splenectomy: a new technique for the management of hereditary spherocytosis. Ann Surg 241:40

Stoehr GA, Sobh JN, Luecken J et al (2006) Near-total splenectomy for hereditary spherocytosis: clinical prospects in relation to disease severity. Br J Haematol 132:791

Stoppa AM, Vey N, Sainty D et al (1996) Correction of aplastic complicating paroxysmal nocturnal hemoglobinuria: absence of eradication of the PNH clone and dependence of response on cyclosporine A admpnstration. Br J Haematol 93:42

Stoya G, Gruhn B, Vogelsang H et al (2006) Flow cytometry as a diagnostic tool for hereditary spherocytosis. Acta Haematol 116:186

Tchernia G, Bader-Meunier B, Berterottiere P et al (1997) Effectiveness of partial splenectomy in hereditary spherocytosis. Curr Opin Hematol 4:136

Tse WT, Lux SE (1999) RBC membrane disorders. Br J Haematol 104:2

van den Heuvel-Eibrink MM, Bredius RG, te Winkkel Ml et al (2005) Childhood paroxysmal nocturnal hemoglobinuria (PNH), a report of 11 cases in the Netherlands. Br J Haematol 128:571

Vicente-Gutierrez MP, Castello-Almazan I, Salvia-Roiges MD et al (2005) Nonimmune hydrops fetalis due to congenital xerocytosis. J Perinatol 25:63

Vives Corrons JI, Beson I, Aymerich M, Ayala S et al (1995) Hereditary xerocytosis report of six Spanish families with leaky red cell syndrome and increased heat stability of the erythrocyte membrane. Br J Haematol 90:817

Wiley JS (1984) Inherited red cell dehydration: a hemolytic syndrome in search of a name. Pathology 16:115

Zarkowsky HS, Mohandas N, Speaker CB et al (1975) A congenital haemolytic anemia with thermal sensitivity of the erythrocyte membrane. Br J Haematol 29:573

Stewart GW, Amess [illegible] (1990) [illegible] affer [illegible] [illegible]

Stock [illegible] [illegible] 31:40

[illegible] GA, Sohn JN [illegible] hereditary spherocytosis [illegible] specific [illegible]

Sharpe AM [illegible] [illegible] spherocytosis [illegible]

[illegible] hereditary [illegible] Haemat [illegible]

[illegible] due to [illegible]

[illegible] (1996) Hereditary [illegible] red cell [illegible]

[illegible] (1983) Red cell membrane skeletal defects in hereditary and acquired hemolytic anemias. [illegible] Hematol [illegible]

Paquette [illegible] (1979) Clinical characteristics [illegible] paroxysmal nocturnal [illegible]

Parker [illegible] [illegible]

[illegible] management [illegible]

[illegible] spherocytosis [illegible]

[illegible] nocturnal [illegible]

323 Microangiopathic Hemolytic Anemias

Ahmad A. Mallouh

Introduction

The hallmark of the microangiopathic hemolytic anemia is the presence of fragmented, distorted red blood cells (schistocytes) on the peripheral blood smear of a patient with hemolytic anemia (➋ *Fig. 323.1*). It does not represent a specific diagnostic entity, but rather a morphologic manifestation of mechanical destruction and fragmentation of the red blood cells by shear stress as they pass through fibrin strands deposited on the vascular endothelium or within small blood vessels. Its clinical value lies in narrowing the differential diagnosis in a patient with hemolytic anemia. It should be remembered that a small number of schistocytes may be present in normal individuals. Mild increase in the number of schistocytes may be seen in some diseases with no evidence of hemolysis, i.e., renal disease, prosthetic heart valve, and preeclampsia. The presence of more than 1% of schistocytes or two schistocytes per high power field on a well prepared blood smear is suggestive of microangiopathic hemolytic anemia. Several disease processes may be associated with microangiopathic hemolytic anemia (➋ *Table 323.1*). The clinical manifestations are those of the hemolytic anemia and the manifestations of the underlying precipitating condition. Following is a discussion of disease entities associated with microangiopathic hemolytic anemia.

Disseminated Intravascular Coagulation (DIC)

Introduction

Human blood remains in a fluid state without bleeding or intravascular thrombosis by a delicate balance between the vascular system and the coagulation, anticoagulation, fibrinolytic and antifibrinolytic pathways. When a blood vessel is injured, it constricts immediately to limit blood loss. This is followed by the formation of a reversible platelet plug. Local activation of the coagulation cascade results in formation of thrombin, which stabilizes the platelet plug and generates fibrin from fibrinogen forming a stable haemostatic plug. The fibrinolytic system is locally activated to remove the unneeded thrombus to keep the injured blood vessel open. As these processes are transient, localized and compensated by production of the consumed factors (platelets and coagulation factors) by the liver and bone marrow, no excessive or prolonged bleeding or harmful thrombosis occur.

Pathogenesis

Uncontrolled and excessive activation of the extrinsic pathway of the coagulation cascade produces large amounts of thrombin. Activation of the coagulation cascade results from exposure of the blood to large amounts of the tissue factor and activated factor VII (FVIIa), which results from tissue injury (by trauma), injury of the vascular endothelium (usually by endotoxin) or increased release or expression in the monocytes. Prothrombin leads to widespread intravascular coagulation and deposition of fibrin in the deferent organs causing tissue ischemia and organ damage. The fibrinolytic system is activated to dissolve the fibrin deposits producing fibrinogen degradation products (FDP) and D-Dimers. Platelets and coagulation factors (fibrinogen, prothrombin, and factors V and VIII) are depleted leading to spontaneous bleeding. Excess FDP enhances bleeding by interfering with platelets aggregation and fibrin polymerization. In addition, excessive amounts of plasmin (which is produced from plasminogen) causes degradation of the clotting factors causing further drop in their level and leading to more bleeding. Destruction of the red blood cells (RBCs) by passing through the fibrin mesh results in the classic finding of Schistocytic hemolytic anemia. Activation of the intrinsic pathway of coagulation is thought to cause hypotension but not DIC.

Etiology

Disseminated intravascular coagulation (DIC) may be triggered by a number of serious disease processes. The

Abdelaziz Y. Elzouki (ed.), *Textbook of Clinical Pediatrics*, DOI 10.1007/978-3-642-02202-9_323,

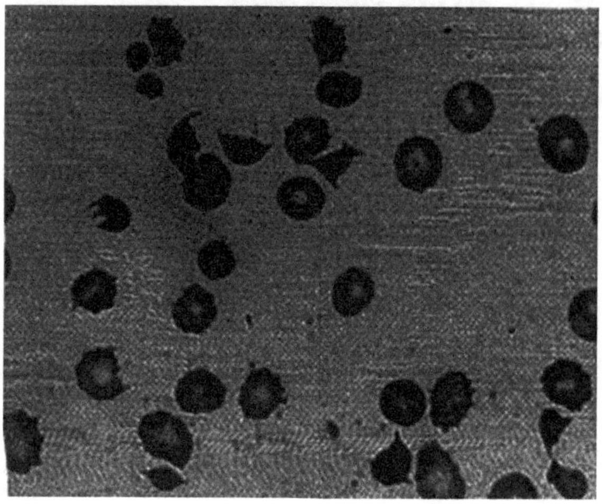

Figure 323.1
Blood smear from a patient with hemolytic-uremic syndrome showing schistocytes and other forms of deformed and fragmented red blood cells

Table 323.1
Conditions associated with microangiopathic hemolytic anemia

Disseminated intravascular coagulation (DIC)
Hemolytic-uremic syndrome (HUS)
Thrombotic thrombocytopenic purpura (TTP)
Giant hemangioma (Kasabach–Merritt syndrome)
Extracorporeal circulation (after open heart surgery)
Intracardiac prosthesis
Malignant hypertension
Strenuous exercise

most common causes are infection, trauma (accidental or surgical), and malignancy. However, it may be associated with other disease processes, including, giant hemangioma, acute hemolytic transfusion reaction, paroxysmal nocturnal hemoglobinuria (PNH), snake bites, fulminant hepatic failure, burns, severe hypoxia, shock, heat stroke, and severe metabolic disturbances. In newborn infants, septicemia, severe respiratory distress syndrome, hypoxia, shock, necrotizing enterocolitis and homozygous proteins C or S deficiency are known to cause DIC.

Severe infections, including bacterial, systemic viral (i.e., varicella), parasitic (malaria), fungus (systemic canididemia, aspergillosis) and rickettsial infections are the most common cause of DIC in children. Gram negative sepsis may be present in up to 50% of all children with DIC. Severe trauma (accidental, burn, or major surgery) is the second most common cause of DIC. The possibility of the development of DIC depends on the severity of the trauma and the extent of tissue damage. Head injury is more likely to be associated with DIC, when compared with injuries of similar extent in other organs. The severity of coagulopathy and the development of systemic inflammatory response syndrome (SIRS) are strong determinants of the outcome of trauma associated DIC. DIC develops in most patients with acute promyelocytic leukemia (APL) due to the release of the tissue factor from the blasts. Even though it may be present at presentation, it often develops after starting chemotherapy. DIC also often develops with other types of Hematologic malignancy or disseminated solid tumors.

Clinical Picture

DIC is a secondary syndrome associated with or caused by any of several serious and often clinically obvious causes. Even though the exact incidence is not known, it is estimated that around 1% of the hospitalized patients develop coagulopathy. Clinical picture is that of the triggering disease process together with bleeding tendency, disseminated thrombosis causing organ damage and microangiopathic hemolytic anemia. External (skin, mucous membranes, venipuncture site, or wounds) and/or internal (central nervous system, lungs, gastrointestinal tract, urogenital tract, or adrenal glands) bleeding are usually present. Pallor, jaundice, tachycardia, hypotension, and/or hemoglobinuria are manifestations of hemolysis and may be present depending on the severity of the anemia. Purpura fulminats with skin necrosis and/or gangrene of the fingers and toes may be present. Acute renal, hepatic, pulmonary or CNS injury may occur due to hemorrhage, and microthrombosis of feeding vessels and/or hypoperfusion due to hypotension. It should be remembered that even though activation of the intrinsic coagulation pathway dose not play a role in the pathogenesis of DIC, it may cause or exasperate hypotension and shock, which in turn exasperate tissue hypoxia and organ damage.

Chronic DIC is often associated with solid tumors. It results from release of small amounts of tissue factor and a compensatory response from the liver, which replete the consumed coagulation factors, and the bone marrow, which compensate for the consumed platelets. Patients with chronic DIC have no or minor bleeding tendency. However, they are liable to develop venous or arterial thrombosis.

Diagnosis

DIC should be suspected in any patient with increased bleeding tendency, thrombotic episodes or microangiopathic hemolytic anemia in association with severe disease, especially, the causative entities described above. Diagnosis is confirmed by a combination of laboratory findings which include thrombocytopenia or steadily falling platelets count, prolonged prothrombin (PT) and partial activated thromboplastin times (PTT), low levels of fibrinogen, and elevated levels of fibrinogen degradation product (FDP) and D-dimers. Hemolytic anemia with the characteristic schistocytes is always present. Coagulation factors (especially factors V and VIII) are usually low. Thrombin time and reptilase time are usually prolonged; however they are not usually required for diagnosis or management of DIC. Diagnosis of chronic DIC can be problematic because PT, aPTT, and platelet count may be normal, as the consumed coagulation factors and platelets are compensated for by the liver and bone marrow, respectively. In addition to the clinical picture (usually thrombosis) and the presence of the initiating disease (usually disseminated solid tumor), diagnosis depends on the presence of microangiopathic hemolytic anemia and elevated FDP and D-dimers.

Differential Diagnosis

Even though all causes of bleeding diathesis, hypercoagulable states and hemolytic anemia should be considered in the differential diagnosis, in most case scenarios, the diagnosis is clear based on the clinical findings and simple laboratory tests. Liver disease, hemolytic-uremic syndrome (HUS), thrombotic thrombocytopenic purpura (TTP) and heparin induced thrombocytopenia (HIT) are sometimes difficult to differentiate from DIC. The clinical picture, however, is often suggestive of the diagnosis. Liver disease in particular can be a difficult diagnostic problem. It should be remembered that severe liver disease may cause DIC and liver damage can be caused by the same triggering disease which causes DIC (i.e. sepsis, trauma, shock). Thrombocytopenia, microangiopathic hemolytic anemia and elevated FDP are usually absent in primary liver disease. Thrombocytopenia, however, may result from congestive splenomegaly and hypersplenism. Hemolytic-uremic syndrome and thrombotic thrombocytopenic purpura (see below) both cause thrombocytopenia and microangiopathic hemolytic anemia. They, however, usually have normal PT, aPTT, fibrinogen, and FDP. Heparin induced thrombocytopenia (HIT) can be differentiated based on the history of heparin administration in the prior few days, the absence of DIC causing diseases (sepsis, trauma, or malignancy), and normal fibrinogen and FDP. PT and aPTT might be prolonged, if the patient is still receiving heparin.

Prognosis

DIC is a serious medical problem with high morbidity and mortality. Multiple organ damage may result from the initiating disease (sepsis, trauma, malignancy, etc.) or from bleeding, thrombosis or hypoxia due to the anemia or shock. Mortality, which can be as high as 80%, depends on the original causative disease (sepsis, trauma, malignance, etc.) and its severity, the severity of the coagulopathy, organs involved and the degree of their damage, the development of systemic inflammatory response syndrome (SIRS) and the appropriateness and promptness of therapy.

Treatment

Other than treating the original initiating disease, which is essential to hope for a good outcome, treatment of DIC is mainly symptomatic. Aggressive treatment of shock is essential part of therapy. Hypo-perfusion and tissue hypoxia furthers tissue damage and mortality. Anemia is treated with packed red blood cells transfusion as required. Platelets and fresh frozen (FFP) transfusion is recommended to stop or prevent anticipated bleeding. They should not be given to correct abnormal laboratory results. Cryoprecipitate should be given if bleeding could not be stopped with platelets and FFP. The transfused elements (red cells, coagulation factors, and platelets) are consumed rapidly; however, their administration helps to stop or decrease bleeding and correct the anemia until the triggering factor is corrected. Anticoagulant therapy, mainly with unfractionated or low-molecular heparin, is often recommended in chronic DIC with major thrombosis. The use of anticoagulant in acute DIC is of questionable value and should be avoided specially in patients with CNS bleeding. Some studies showed that protein C concentrates decreases mortality in adult patients with sepsis and DIC. However further studies are needed before recommending its routine use.

Hemolytic-Uremic Syndrome

Introduction

Hemolytic-uremic syndrome (HUS) is an acquired disease characterized by an acute onset of the triad of microangiopathic hemolytic anemia, thrombocytopenia, and nephropathy. The disease is classified into two types, the typical type (shiga-like toxin associated, postdiarrheal, D+) and the atypical type (non-shiga associated, non-postdiarrheal, D-). The two types have deferent etiology, epidemiology, clinical picture, clinical course, and prognosis. The typical type constitutes around 90%, while the atypical type constitutes around 10% of the reported cases.

Pathophysiology

Endothelial damage in the capillaries and/or arterioles leading to thrombotic microangiopathy and red blood cells fragmentation is the main lesion in both types of HUS (see section "Nephrology").

Etiology

The typical type (also called classic, epidemic, postdiarrheal, D+ and shiga-like toxin associated) is caused by shiga-like toxin producing organisms. In North America, around 70% of the typical type is caused by enterohemorrhagic *E. coli*, around 80% of which is *E. coli* O157:H7. In contrast, in other countries (Australia, Germany and Austria), the majority of postdiarrheal HUS is caused by non-O157:H7 *E. coli*, while in Asia and Africa, the most common cause is *Shigella dysenteriae* type 1. The atypical type is divided into two types, the genetic and the non-genetic types. The genetic type results from deficiency of complements components (mainly C3, factors H, B, I and the so called membrane factor), Von Willebrand factor cleaving protease (ADAMTS13) or defects of vitamin B12 metabolism. Some cases are inherited, but without known complement deficiency or abnormal metabolic etiology. The atypical non-genetic type is caused by non-enteric infections. *Streptococcus pneumoniae* causes up to 40% of the non-diarrheal type and up to 14% of all HUS in children. HUS has been reported with viral infection (especially HIV), systemic lupus erythematosus, antiphospholipid syndrome, and malignancy.

Epidemiology and Incidence

HUS occurs worldwide. Its incidence, causative agents, and age distribution differ from one area to another. In North America and Western Europe, around 90% of the cases are of the typical and around 10% are of the atypical type. The annual incidence is around 2–3 per 100,000 in children less than 5 years old. The peak incidence is in the summer and fall. However, the atypical type caused by *Streptococcus pneumoniae* occurs more commonly in winter months. The inherited types have no seasonal predilection. Most cases occur sporadically; however, epidemics often occur in day care center either because of exposure to a common source of infection or due to cross infection. Cases may occur in several family members either because they are exposed to the same source of infection or due to inherited type of the disease.

Clinical Picture

Most cases of the typical (shiga-like toxin associated) type occur in children less than 5 years old. Patients usually present with prodromal symptoms of diarrhea (often bloody), abdominal pain, fever, and vomiting. The full blown picture of microangiopathic hemolytic anemia, thrombocytopenia, and acute renal failure follows in 5–10 days. Diarrhea precedes the development of HUS in over 90% of the cases. However, it is bloody only in 50–60% of the cases. Extra-gastrointestinal infection (urinary tract) with enterohemorrhagic *E. coli* may cause HUS without preceding bloody diarrhea. CNS involvement including irritability, seizures, coma, stroke, or hemiparesis occurs in one fifth to one fourth of the cases of HUS. Renal involvement, which occurs in over 95% of the cases, ranges between simple proteinuria, hematuria and severe acute renal failure. Anuria occurs in around half of the cases. The severity of renal involvement does not correlate with the severity of the prodromal symptoms, anemia, or thrombocytopenia. Hypertension occurs in around 50% of the cases. In addition to the bloody diarrhea, gastrointestinal complications may include intestinal gangrene, perforation, intussusception, or rectal prolapse. Other organs that may be involved include liver and pancreas. The atypical type is heterogeneous in its clinical presentation, severity, complications, and prognosis. It is not preceded by diarrhea. It usually presents in more insidious onset. Patients are at higher risk of severe acute renal failure, chronic renal failure, hypertension, recurrence, and death. It usually occurs at older age. However, recent studies showed that, depending on the etiology, some patients with the atypical type may present at early age and have milder course than the typical type.

Diagnosis and Deferential Diagnosis

With high index of suspicion, diagnosis is usually easily made based on the clinical picture and the presence of microangiopathic hemolytic anemia, thrombocytopenia, and evidence of renal injury. Isolating *E. coli* or *Shigella* from the stools is helpful but not essential for diagnosis. Serologic detection of the shiga toxin in the stools can be done, but it is neither essential nor available in most settings.

Deferential diagnosis in the prodromal phase includes all causes of infectious (*Shigella, Salmonella, Campylobacter, Yersinia*, ameba) and noninfectious (ulcerative colitis, Henoch–Schonlien purpura) bloody diarrhea. All causes of microangiopathic hemolytic anemia, thrombocytopenia, and acute renal failure should be included in the deferential diagnosis of HUS. Most of these cases, however, can be easily differentiated based on the clinical and laboratory finding. Patients with disseminated intravascular coagulopathy (DIC) have the triad of HUS, but they also have prolonged PT and PTT, low fibrinogen, and high FDP and low coagulation factors (mainly factors V and VIII). The typical type of childhood HUS can be differentiated from thrombotic thrombocytopenic purpura (TTP) by the presence of bloody diarrhea and the isolation of the pathogenic *E. coli.*

Treatment

The need for and modality of treatments depend on the organ/system involved and the severity of involvement. Acute renal failure and its related problems (hypertension, electrolytes disturbance, and fluid imbalance) is managed like other types of acute renal failure (see section "Nephrology"). Indications for dialysis are the same as for other forms of acute failure. It is required in around 50% of the typical type. Early dialysis, as previously suggested, does not improve the final outcome. Anemia might be severe enough to require packed red blood cells transfusion. Blood transfusion is usually recommended, if the hemoglobin drops to <6 g/dl. This indication, however, is not based on solid scientific grounds. The indication for transfusion should be individualized and be based on the clinical picture, the bone marrow activity as evidenced by the reticulocytes count, and the direction in which hemoglobin level is going (upward, downward, or stable). Platelets transfusion should be reserved for patients with uncontrolled active bleeding or those who are at risk of developing bleeding (planned surgical procedures). Careful fluid and electrolytes management is essential, especially in patients with oliguria or Anuria. Treatment of other involved organs (CNS, heart, pancreas, liver, or lungs) is similar to their treatment in other diseases. The role of plasma simple or exchange transfusion is controversial and its efficacy is doubtful in shiga-like toxin associated type. It is, however, recommended by some authorities in cases with severe CNS involvement. Plasma exchange is recommended in the atypical type. The response to this therapy, however, depends on the affected complement. Antibiotic to treat *E. coli* should be avoided, as it was shown to increase the risk of HUS without shortening the course of the gastrointestinal symptoms. Antibiotics may be used in *Shigella* associated HUS, as they do not appear to increase the risk of HUS. Renal transplantation is recommended for the typical type with end stage renal disease. Success rate is similar to other causes of end stage renal disease (ESRD). Recurrence rate is between 0% and 10%. The indication for renal transplant in the atypical type is controversial because of the high rate of recurrence.

Prognosis

Hematologic problems resolve in almost all cases of the typical type. Complete renal function recovery occurs in around 80% of the cases. However, recent long-term follow-up showed that renal dysfunction (clinical or subclinical) persists in much higher percentage (up to 30% of the cases). Around 5% of the patients die from the disease or its complications. Several bad prognostic factors were identified including prolonged oliguria or anuria, leukocytosis, the need for dialysis in the acute stage and the presence of arteriolar microangiopathy, cortical necrosis or microangiopathy involving over 50% of the glomeruli. Prognosis for the atypical type depends on the etiology or the mutated gene. *Streptococcus pneumonia* associated disease has bad early prognosis, caused mainly by death due to the infection itself (sepsis or meningitis), but it has better long-term renal function (inpatients who survive the acute phase) than the typical type. Most patients with HIV associated HUS end with ESRD. The prognosis for the inherited types depends on the mutated gene. Dominantly inherited cases have a better prognosis than the recessive cases. Mutation of factors H, I, C3, and ADAMTS 13 is usually associated with severe and progressive renal disease, while HUS associated with the mutation of membrane cofactor protein (MCP) deficiency rarely leads to ESRD.

Thrombotic Thrombocytopenic Purpura

Thrombotic thrombocytopenic purpura (TTP) is characterized by the sudden onset of microangiopathic hemolytic anemia and consumptive thrombocytopenia, often associated with neurologic dysfunction, impairment of renal function, and fever. It is primarily a disease of the adults. However, both acquired and congenital types are known to occur in children. In adults, the clinical picture and pathology TTP overlap with hemolytic-uremic syndrome (HUS). The two syndromes are usually considered as one disease (TTP/HUS) and they are managed in the same way. In children, however, the typical type (shiga toxin associated, diarrhea associated) HUS is distinct from TTP in its etiology, clinical picture, therapy, and prognosis. The atypical type (non-shiga toxin associated) can be confused with TTP.

Pathogenesis and Pathology

The hallmark of TTP is the formation of platelets-rich microthrombi in the microcirculation of deferent organs. Obstruction of the blood supply results in ischemic damage of the involved organs. The development of these microthrombi is triggered by the presence of unusually large VWF (ULVWF) multimers in the circulation. In normal individuals, these multimers are cleaved to smaller inactive form by a protease identified as ADAMTS13. Acquired or congenital ADAMTS13 deficiency results in intravascular accumulation of the ULVWF multimers. These multimers promote platelets adhesion and aggregation, causing platelets-rich microthrombi. ADAMTS13 deficiency results from an autoimmune mechanism in the acquired (idiopathic) TTP and from an autosomally inherited gene in the congenital type.

Clinical Picture

The clinical picture and prognosis of TTP depend largely on the organs involved, degree of organ damage, and the type and timing of therapy. The classic required diagnostic criteria are the pentad of microangiopathic hemolytic anemia, thrombocytopenia, neurologic abnormalities, renal dysfunction, and fever. However, because of the efficacy of early plasma exchange in inducing remission and cure in a disease with high mortality, less stringent criteria are presently accepted as a presumptive diagnosis in adult patients and those who (based on family history) are suspected to have congenital ADAMTS13 deficiency. The sudden onset of Coomb's negative microangiopathic hemolytic anemia and thrombocytopenia without an apparent cause is an indication to start therapy. CNS involvement, which is present in most cases, ranges between headache, confusion, transient ischemic attacks and seizures, hemiparesis, coma, or death. Unlike HUS, TTP involves CNS more often than the kidneys. However, both diseases can cause deferent degrees of CNS and/or renal damage.

Diagnosis

For practical purposes, diagnosis depends on the clinical picture. Treatment should be started as soon as the diagnosis is made or highly suspected. Low plasma level of DAMTS13 is important to confirm the diagnosis, but it is not essential to start therapy. ADAMTS13 may be found in normal people and diseases other than TTP, i.e., sepsis and in some cases of HUS. The diagnostic sensitivity and specificity is 89% and 91%, respectively.

Treatment

Plasma exchange is the primary treatment for TTP. It should be started as soon as the diagnosis is highly suspected. Plasma exchange is given once daily (in severe cases twice daily) until complete clinical remission and platelets recovery. In the acquired TTP, plasma exchange removes ULVWF and the auto antibodies against ADAMTS 13 and it increases the level of the deficient ADAMTS 13. In the congenital type, simple rather than exchange plasma transfusion (10–15 ml/k daily) is usually adequate.

Rituximab (an anti-CD20 antibody) is effective in achieving remission and possibly preventing relapse in some refractory or relapsing cases. Steroids, cyclosporine, and cyclophosphamide were used in refractory and relapsing cases with variable results. Splenectomy was effective in some refractory cases. However, nowadays, it is rarely needed and it should be avoided specially in children.

Prognosis

The prognosis used to be dismal with a mortality rate approaching 100. Early plasma exchange decreased mortality rate to around 20%. (It should be remembered that these therapeutic and prognostic data are extrapolated mainly from adult studies because the disease is rare in children.).

Giant Hemangioma and Thrombocytopenia (Kasabach–Merritt Syndrome)

The association of microangiopathic hemolytic anemia, thrombocytopenia with or without evidence of coagulopathy (prolonged PT and PTT, low fibrinogen level and high level of fibrinogen degradation products and D-dimers) with cutaneous or visceral kaposiform hemangioendothelioma or tufted angioma is referred to as Kasabach–Merritt Syndrome (KMS).

Pathology and Pathogenesis

Recent literature suggests that all cases of KMS are associated with kaposiform hemangioendothelioma or tufted angioma rather than the classic infantile hemangioma. This confusion is thought to be caused by imprecise definition and imprecise histological diagnosis of "hemangioma." However, some other recent literature suggests that it can be associated with other types of vascular tumors (hepatic hemangioma, splenic hemangioma, lymphangioma, and diffuse neonatal hemangioma). Thrombocytopenia results from trapping in vascular spaces of the hemangioma and activation of these platelets by the proliferating endothelium of the tumor. Platelets activation results in thrombin production, which causes local and/or disseminated fragmentation of the red blood cells leading to microangiopathic hemolytic anemia that results from the shear stress (while passing through the small blood vessels) and/or due to the consumptive coagulopathy. Thrombocytopenia and consumption of the plasma coagulation factors may cause localized or generalized bleeding.

Clinical Picture

KMS is a disease of infancy and childhood. Most cases are diagnosed in the first 5 years of age. Cutaneous "hemangioma" may be present at birth or develop or enlarge over few months or occasionally few years. Diagnosis of KMS is usually clear. An infant or a child with cutaneous hemangioma develops thrombocytopenia and microangiopathic hemolytic anemia. In patients with visceral hemangioma, unexplained thrombocytopenia and microangiopathic hemolytic anemia might be the first and the only manifestation of KMS. The clinical picture of KMS depends on the size, location and local complications of the tumor, and the severity of the thrombocytopenia and consumptive coagulopathy. "Hemangiomas" can be of any size, be located in anywhere, and can be single or multiple. The most common site is the skin. Visceral lesion may be located in the liver, spleen, retroperitoneal, mediastinum, or CNS. Clinical manifestations caused by the hemangioma may include (depending on the location, size, and infiltration of adjacent structures) obvious cutaneous lesion, abdominal distention, abnormal live function tests, respiratory compromise, seizures, bony deformity, or obstructive uropathy. High output heart failure may occur. Bleeding due to thrombocytopenia (with or without consumptive coagulopathy) may occur anywhere including skin (petechiae, bruising), mucus membranes (including epistaxis, gastrointestinal, or urogenital), CNS, or within the hemangioma itself. Bleeding in the hemangioma results in sudden increase in size of the visible mass, increased abdominal distention, increased respiratory compromise or CNS complications, i.e., seizure, coma, stroke, etc. Patients may present with complications of the hemangioma, which may include ulceration, infection or infiltration or compression of vital structures, e.g., the eye.

Diagnosis

Diagnosis is usually obvious. Most patients present with a visible subcutaneous mass, with or without evidence of bleeding. Investigations show microangiopathic hemolytic anemia and severe thrombocytopenia. PT and PTT are often high; fibrinogen may be low and FDP may be high depending on the presence and severity of DIC. MRI and/or CT scans of the visible lesion should be done to delineate the extent of the tumor and to decide if surgical removal is feasible. MRA and/or CT scans and Doppler ultrasound may identify large feeding vessels. MRI and/or CT scans of the head, chest, abdomen, and pelvis are indicated in cases of cutaneous lesions to look for multifocal lesions. The same radiological investigations are required when primary visceral hemangioma is suspected. Unexplained thrombocytopenia and microangiopathic hemolytic anemia may be the only manifestation of KMS in which a search for visceral hemangioma is indicated. Biopsy is not routinely indicated.

Deferential Diagnosis

When hemangioma is located in the skin, it is easily identified clinically. MRI or Doppler ultrasonography can differentiate visceral and ambiguous superficial hemangioma from solid tumors. Differentiating hemangioma from vascular malformation is important but often difficult. All causes of consumptive coagulopathy and thrombocytopenia are usually easily differentiated from KMS, except in the case of unrecognized visceral hemangioma in which other causes of DIC should be considered.

Treatment

Supportive treatment is required in symptomatic patients and those who are planned for surgical procedures.

It includes packed red blood cells transfusion as indicated by the severity of the anemia and the clinical picture. Platelets transfusion should be reserved for patients with active and uncontrolled bleeding or those who are planned to have a surgical procedure. Fresh frozen plasma (FFP) is indicated for patients with evidence of consumptive coagulopathy and active bleeding or prior to surgical procedures. Cryoprecipitate is indicated in an actively bleeding patient with severe hypofibrinogenemia. Treatment of the hemangioma depends on its size, site, number, and complications (KMS, bleeding, ulceration, heart failure, or infection). Most hemangiomas run their natural course of proliferative phase followed by involution. Involution usually starts after 1 year of age. Around 75% of them are completely involuted by 5–7 years of age. However, many are left with residual lesions. Asymptomatic patients or those with minimal problems need no active therapy. Surgical removal of a small single lesion or few lesions is recommended if surgically feasible without mutilation. Embolization or ligation of large feeding arteries, if present, can be done in a single or a few lesions. Most lesions are large, infiltrating or visceral and not accessible for surgical removal or embolization. Medical therapy is indicated in such cases. Systemic steroid therapy is the first line of medical therapy. Different dosing regimens were found to be effective (2–3 mg/kg/day for 4 weeks, 5 mg/kg/day for 2 weeks, and megadose of 30 mg/kg/day for 3 days). Response usually starts after few days. Around 90% of cutaneous hemangioma has a good response; however, only 30–50% of KMS patients have a good response because most, if not all, lesions are not true hemangiomas. Alternative therapies which were found to be effective in some cases include alpha interferon, vincristine, cyclophosphamide, and actinomycin-D. Antifibrinolytic, antiplatelet, and anticoagulants should be avoided as their efficacy is controversial and they might increase the chances of bleeding. Even though radiotherapy was effective in many studies, it should be used only in resistant cases with life-threatening situation.

Prognosis

Prognosis depends on the location, extent, infiltration of vital organs, severity of consumptive coagulopathy, and therapeutic intervention. Mortality is more common in visceral lesions and large infiltrating lesions and in those with severe thrombocytopenia with or without DIC. Mortality rate ranges between 10% and 37%. Morbidly includes residual tumor, scar, and residual damage in the involved organs, i.e., CNS, liver.

References

Abbas AAH, Raddadi AA, Chidid FD (2003) Haemangiomas: a review of the clinical presentation and treatment. Middle East Paediatr 8:52

Abbas K, Saad H, Kherala M et al (2008) Successful treatment of Kasabach-Merritt syndrome with vincristine and surgery: a case report and review of literature. Cases J 1:9

Barbui T, Falanga A (2001) Disseminated intravascular coagulation in acute leukemia. Semin Thromb Hemost 27:593

Barbui T, Finazzi G, Falanga A (1998) The impact of all-trans-retinoic acid on the coagulopathy of acute promyelocytic leukemia. Blood 91:3093

Bick RL (2003) Disseminated intravenous coagulation: current concept of etiology, pathophysiology, diagnosis and treatment. Hematol Oncol Clin North Am 17:149

Blei F, Karp N, Rosen R et al (1998) Successful multimodal therapy for kaposiform hemangioendothelioma complicated by Kasabach-Merritt phenomenon: a case report and review of the literature. Pediatr Hematol Oncol 15:295

Bouw MC, Dors N, van Ommen H et al (2009) Thrombotic thrombocytopenic purpura in childhood. Pediatr Blood Cancer 53:537

Buchanan GR (1986) Coagulation disorders in the neonate. Pediatr Clin N Am 33:203

Cataland SR, Jin M, Lin S et al (2007) Cyclosporine and plasma exchange in thrombotic thrombocytopenic purpura: long term follow up with serial analysis of ADAMTS 13 activity. Br J Haematol 139:486

Constantinescu AR, Bitzan M, Weiss LS et al (2004) Non-enteropathic hemolytic uremic syndrome: causes and short term course. Am J Kidney Dis 43:976

Copelovitch L, Kaplan BS (2010) Streptococcus pneumoniae-associated hemolytic uremic syndrome: classification and the emergence of serotype 19A. Pediatrics 125:e174

Elliott MA, Heit JA, Pruthi RK et al (2009) Rituximab for refractory and or relapsing thrombotic thrombocytopenic purpura related to immune-mediated severe ADMATS 13-deficiency: a report of four cases and a systemic review of the literature. Eur J Haemtol 83:365

Enjolras O, Riche MC, Merland JJ (1990) Management of alarming hemangioma in infancy: a review of 25 cases. Pediatrics 85:491

Enjolras O, Wassef M, Mazoyer E et al (1997) Infants with Kasabach-Merritt syndrome do not have "true" hemangioma. J Pediatr 130:631

Franchini M, Manzato F (2004) Update on the treatment of disseminated intravascular coagulation. Hematology 9:8

Furlan M, Robles R, Galbusera M et al (1998) Von Willebrand factor cleaving protease in thrombotic thrombocytopenic purpura and hemolytic uremic syndrome. N Engl J Med 339:1578

Gando S, Saitoh D, Ogura H et al (2008) Natural history of disseminated intravascular coagulation diagnosed based on the newly established diagnostic criteria for critically ill patients: results of a multicenter, prospective survey. Crit Care Med 36:145

Garg AX, Suri RS, Barrowman N et al (2003) Long-term renal prognosis of diarrhea-associated hemolytic uremic syndrome: a systemic review, meta-analysis and meta- regression. JAMA 290:1360

George JN (2006) Clinical practice. Thrombotic thrombocytopenic purpura. N Engl J Med 354:1927

Gerber A, Karch H, Allerberger F et al (2002) Clinical course and the role of Shiga toxin-producing Escherichia coli infection in the hemolytic-uremic syndrome in pediatric patients, 1997–2000, in Germany and Austria: a prospective study. J Infect Dis 186:493

Haisley-Royster C, Enjolras O, Frieden IJ et al (2002) Kasabach-Merritt syndrome phenomenon: a retrospective study of treatment with vincristine. J Pediatr Hematol Oncol 24:459

Hall GW (2001) Kasabach-Merritt syndrome: pathogenesis and management. Br J Haematol 112:851

Hesselmann S, Micke O, Marquardt T et al (2002) Case report: Kasabach-Merritt syndrome: a review of the therapeutic options and a case report of successful treatment with radiotherapy and interferon alpha. Br J Radiol 75:180

Horton TM, Stone JD, Yee D et al (2003) Case series of thrombocytopenic purpura in children and adolescents. J Pediatr Hematol Oncol 25:336

Lämmle B, Kremer Hovinga JA, George JN (2008) Acquired thrombotic thrombocytopenic purpura: ADAMTS 13 activity, anti-ADMAMTS 13 auto antibodies and risk of recurrent disease. Haematologica 93:172

Levi M (2004) Current understanding of disseminated intravascular coagulation. Br J Haematol 124:567

Levi M, ten Cate H (1999) Disseminated intravascular coagulation. N Engl J Med 341:586

Levi M, Toh CH, Thachil J et al (2009) Guidelines for the diagnosis and management of disseminated intravascular coagulation. Br J Haematol 145:24

Ling HT, Field JJ, Blinder A (2009) Sustained response with Rituximab in patients with thrombotic thrombocytopenic purpura: a report of 13 cases and review of the literature. Am J Hematol 84:814

Maguiness S, Guenther L (2002) Kasabach-Merritt syndrome. J Cutan Med Surg 6:335

Neuhaus TJ, Calonder S, Leumann EP (1997) Heterogeneity of atypical haemolytic uraemic syndrome. Arch Dis Child 76:518

Noris M, Remuzzi G (2005) Hemolytic uremic syndrome. J Am Soc Nephrol 16:1035

Noris M, Remuzzi G (2009) Atypical syndrome. N Engl Med 36:1676

Oakes RS, Siegler RL, McReynolds MA et al (2006) Predictors of fatality in postdiarrheal hemolytic uremic syndrome. Pediatrics 117:1656

Oakes RS, Kirkhamm JK, Nelson RD et al (2008) Duration of oliguria and anuria as predictive of chronic renal related sequelae in post-diarrheal hemolytic uremic syndrome. Pediatr Nephrol 23:1303

Outshoorn UM, Ferber A (2006) Outcome in the treatment of thrombotic thrombocytopenic purpura with splenectomy: a retrospective cohort study. Am J Hematol 81:895

Peyvandi F, Lavoretano S, Palla R et al (2008) ADAMTS 13 and anti-ADAMTS 13 antibodies as markers for recurrence of acquired thrombotic thrombocytopenic purpura during remission. Haematologica 93:232

Sarkar M, Mulliken JB, Kozakewich HP et al (1997) Thrombocytopenic coagulopathy (Kasabach-Merritt syndrome) is associated with Kaposiform hemangioendothelioma and not with common infantile hemangioma. Plast Reconstr Surg 100:1377

Scherer RU, Spangenberg P (1998) Procoagulant activity in patients with isolated head trauma. Crit Care Med 26:149

Siegler R, Oakes R (2005) Hemolytic uremic syndrome. Curr Opin Pediatr 17:200

Spero JA, Lewis JH, Hasiba U (1980) Disseminated intravascular coagulation, findings in 346 patients. Thromb Haemost 43:28

Tarr PI, Gordon CA, Chandler WL (2005) Shiga-toxin-producing Escherichia coli and hemolytic uraemic syndrome. Lancet 365:1073

Tsai HM (2003) Advances in the pathogenesis, diagnosis, and treatment of thrombotic thrombocytopenic purpura. J Am Soc Nephrol 14:1072

van Gorp EC, Suharti C, ten Cate H et al (1999) Review: infectious diseases and coagulation disorders. J Infect Dis 180:176

Vesely SK, George JN, Lämmle B et al (2003) ADAMTS 13 activity in thrombotic thrombocytopenic purpura-hemolytic syndrome: relation to presenting features and clinical outcomes in a prospective cohort of 142 patients. Blood 102:60

Wananukul S, Nuchprayoon I, Seksarn P (2003) Treatment of Kasabach-Merritt syndrome: a stepwise regimen of prednisolone, dypyridamole and interferon. Int J Dermatol 42:741

[illegible] RS, Kirkham [illegible], Nelson RD et al (2008) Duration of [illegible] as predictors of chronic renal related sequelae [illegible] post-[illegible] analysis in one environment. Pediatr Nephrol [illegible]

[illegible] Otten [illegible] [illegible] [illegible] spectrum [illegible] cohort [illegible]

[illegible] antibodies [illegible] serum [illegible]

Parker M, Mordier [illegible], Kitamura [illegible] (1997) [illegible] with [illegible] not with common [illegible]

[illegible] activity [illegible]

[illegible]

[illegible]-Koyner C, [illegible] O, Friedman T et al (2007) Kawasaki [illegible] syndrome [illegible] a retrospective study [illegible] with [illegible]

[illegible]

Hovelmann S, Wicke [illegible] Merrill [illegible] report of [illegible] alpha [illegible]

[illegible] antibodies and risk [illegible] Rheumatologica [illegible]

[illegible] (2006) [illegible]

[illegible] Minder A [illegible] combined [illegible]

[illegible]

324 Sickle Cell Disease

Ahmad A. Mallouh

Introduction

Human hemoglobin is composed of two parts: (a) the iron-containing part (heme), which is a porphyrin ring responsible for the reversible combination with and transport of oxygen, and (b) a protein part (globin), which is a tetramer made up of two α and two non-α (β, γ, or δ) polypeptide chains, each formed from a large numbers of amino acids (α = 141, β, γ, and δ = 145 amino acids) attached to each other in a linear sequence. There are three types of normal human hemoglobins:

- Hemoglobin A (α2β2) is the main hemoglobin beyond the neonatal period.
- Hemoglobin F (α2γ2) is the main hemoglobin in the fetus and the newborn. Hemoglobin F is gradually replaced by hemoglobin A after birth reaching an adult level by 9–12 months of age.
- Hemoglobin A2 (α2δ2) constitutes 2.5–3.5% of the total hemoglobin in children and adults.

Hemoglobinopathies result from the substitution of one or more amino acids in the globin chain or by the shortening or elongation of the globin chain by deleting or adding amino acids. To date, more than 800 structurally abnormal hemoglobins have been described. Most structurally abnormal hemoglobins are only of academic interest as they are physiologically normal. Others have abnormal solubility, molecular stability, and/or oxygen affinity, resulting in significant clinical problems. Hemoglobins S, C, E, D, O Arab, unstable hemoglobins, and hemoglobins M are among the clinically important types.

Sickle Cell Disease (SS)

Sickle cell disease usually refers to either homozygous (SS) disease or doubly heterozygous hemoglobin S and other abnormal hemoglobins or β-thalassemia (SC, SD, SE, S O Arab or S β-thal).

Pathophysiology

Sickle hemoglobin (Hb S) results from the substitution of the amino acid valine for glutamic acid (Glutamic acid →Valine) in position number six of the β globin chain of hemoglobin. When deoxygenated, hemoglobin S molecules polymerize, forming an elongated rope-like fiber that aligns with other fibers inside the red blood cells, eventually forming parallel bundles oriented along the axis of sickle-shaped red blood cells (RBCs). This process results in increased RBC membrane rigidity, abnormal membrane function, and deceased RBC deformability. Even though hemoglobin S polymerization is an essential event of the pathogenesis of vaso-occlusion, polymerization does not by itself explain the whole clinical picture. Previously, it was thought that the sickle-shaped cells became entangled in the small capillaries, thus occluding them. In fact, vessel occlusion often occurs in medium sized blood vessels. It is accepted now that vaso-occlusion is a complex process which includes, in addition to Hb S polymerization, increased adhesion of the RBCs to the vascular endothelium, structural and functional RBC membrane abnormalities, increased leukocyte adhesion, platelets and coagulation activation, endothelial damage, and an increased tendency to vasoconstriction. Sickle-promoting factors include hemoglobin S concentration, hypoxia, acidosis, hemoconcentration (increased blood viscosity), hemostasis, hypothermia, and hypotension. Sickling is influenced by the coexistence of hemoglobin S with other hemoglobins. Coexistence of hemoglobins F, A, C, or O Arab increases hemoglobin S solubility which explains the asymptomatic course of sickle cell trait and sickle cell-hereditary persistence of fetal hemoglobin (S-HPF) and the relatively mild course of homozygous Indian–Arabian SS disease (known to have high hemoglobin F levels) and S-C disease, S-D, and A-O Arab. In vivo, hemoglobin S-containing red blood cells undergo sickling and unsickling continuously. They sickle when they pass through the slow capillary circulation and the venous system due to local hypoxia, relative stasis, and acidosis.

Abdelaziz Y. Elzouki (ed.), *Textbook of Clinical Pediatrics*, DOI 10.1007/978-3-642-02202-9_324,

They unsickle as they return to the larger blood vessels with higher blood velocity and better oxygenation. When the process of sickling and unsickling is repeated several times, the RBC membrane becomes stiff, and the RBCs stay in an irreversible sickle form (➔ *Fig. 324.1*). The number of irreversibly sickled cells in a freshly prepared blood smear may be an indication of the severity of the disease.

Figure 324.1
Peripheral blood smear in sickle cell disease showing the sickled-shaped irreversibly sickled red blood cell (open arrow). Target cells (solid arrows) are not uncommon in sickle cell disease

Epidemiology

The sickle cell gene is prevalent in parts of the world were falciparum malaria was or is still endemic. The distribution of gene coincides with that of malaria (➔ *Fig. 324.2*). The highest incidence is in sub-Saharan Africa, where the incidence reaches around 30%. It is also common in the Middle East (southern and eastern parts of the Arabian Peninsula) and in other countries around the Persian Gulf (Eastern province of Saudi Arabia, Bahrain, Qatar, southern Iraq, and southern Iran), East and West Africa, Mediterranean countries (southern Italy, Sicily, and certain parts of Greece), and parts of the Indian subcontinent. The incidence in African American is around 8–10%. Sickle cell trait provides protection against severe falciparum infection (up to 90% protection against cerebral malaria and severe malaria-induced hemolytic anemia). Hospitalization and mortality from severe falciparum malaria infection is decreased by around 60% in patients with sickle cell trait as compared with those normal hemoglobin (HbAA). Its protection against mild malaria is controversial.

Diagnosis

The diagnosis of sickle cell disease starts with the clinical suspicion (see below). The diagnosis is then confirmed by:

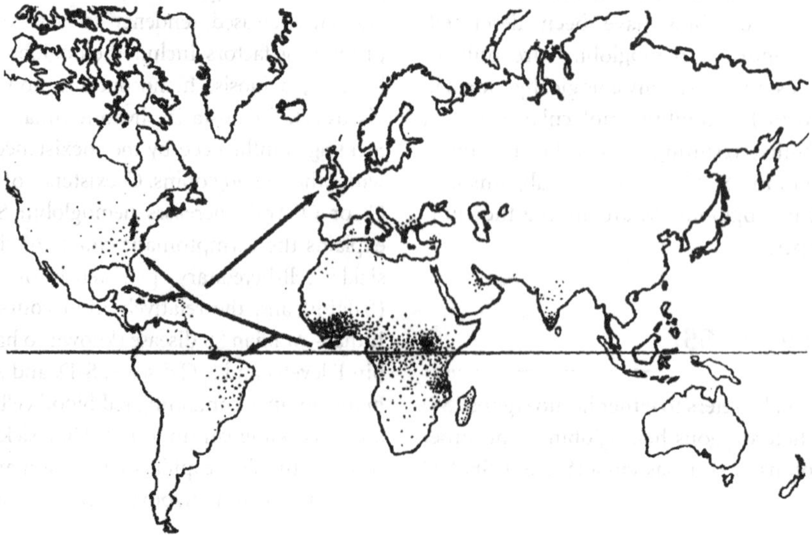

Figure 324.2
Global distribution of sickle hemoglobin gene

- The presence of sickle-shaped cells in a freshly prepared blood smear (irreversibly sickled red blood cells).
- Precipitation tests in which the red blood cells or hemoglobin is exposed to hypoxic environment. The red blood cells take sickle shape in the first, and the hemoglobin precipitates in the second. The above mentioned two methods are not sensitive and do not differentiate homozygous sickle cell disease form sickle cell trait or doubly heterozygous diseases (S-HPFH, S-C, S-D, S-O Arab, or S-E).
- Hemoglobin electrophoresis in cellulose acetate at pH 8.4. It should be kept in mind that hemoglobins S, D, and G have the same mobility in alkaline media. Electrophoresis at acid pH (citrate agar at pH 6.2) separates these hemoglobins.
- High-performance liquid chromatography (HPLC) and isoelectric focusing are sensitive and can be used to diagnose sickle cell disease. Sickle cell disease can be diagnosed in the neonatal periods with some limitation. The presence of hemoglobins S and F with no hemoglobin A is consistent with homozygous sickle cell disease (SS), sickle cell-β° thalassemia, or sickle cell-hereditary persistence of fetal hemoglobin (S-HPFH). Differentiating these diseases is made by family studies. Both parents are expected to have sickle cell trait in SS disease, while one parent has sickle cell trait in the other two entities and the other has β° thalassemia trait or HPFH, respectively. Prenatal diagnosis is technically possible using fetal blood or fetal fibroblasts, or using DNA techniques.

Clinical Manifestations

Infants born with homozygous sickle cell disease are asymptomatic at birth and in the first few months of life because of the protective effect of hemoglobin F. As the production of hemoglobin S increases and replaces hemoglobin F, clinical manifestations start appearing. Vaso-occlusive events may manifest as early as 3 months of age, while chronic hemolytic anemia is usually present by the fourth month of life. Approximately 6% of infants with homozygous sickle cell disease are symptomatic at 6 months, 32% at 1 year, 61% at 2 years, 92% at 6 years, and 96% at 8 years of age. The severity of sickle cell disease is variable. The reason/reasons for this variable clinical expression are not fully understood. However, early onset of dactylitis (hand-foot syndrome), high steady state leukocytes, and low steady state hemoglobin were found to be predictors of a more severe clinical picture. The co-inheritance of α thalassemia with sickle cell disease has been suggested to result in milder anemia; however, its effect on the whole clinical picture is variable. The clinical severity varies among sickle cell genotypes with a milder course in the Arabian-Indian and to a lesser extent in the Singhalese genotypes. This difference is due to persistently high levels of hemoglobin F in these two genotypes.

Sickle cell disease complications can involve any organ. Its clinical manifestations or complications can mimic any disease process involving almost any part of the body. Clinical manifestations can be acute, chronic, acute on top of chronic, or recurrent. They may be divided according to their etiology:

- Manifestations due anemia, whether acute, chronic, or acute on top of chronic.
- Manifestations due the vaso-occlusion phenomenon.
- Manifestations due to infection.

Manifestations due to Anemia

Patients with sickle cell disease usually have moderately severe chronic anemia with appropriate bone marrow response. Hemoglobin concentration levels range between 6 and 10 g/dl (mean 7.9 g/dl). Reticulocyte counts range between 10% and 15%. The major contributing cause of anemia is hemolysis. The mean life span of a hemoglobin S-containing (SS) RBC is approximately 17 days. Folate deficiency due to increased utilization by the hyperactive bone marrow, iron deficiency caused by urinary blood loss due to renal infarction, and erythropoietin deficiency due to renal damage may contribute to the chronic anemia. Iron deficiency was found in up to 20% of patients in some studies. Patients are usually clinically stable. The possible signs and symptoms depend on the severity and acuteness of the anemia.

Acute anemia may develop due to aplastic events, splenic sequestration, hyperhemolytic events, or delayed hemolytic transfusion reaction.

Aplastic Events (Aplastic Crises)

Aplastic events are characterized by a transient drop in the hemoglobin level with bone marrow suppression, as evidenced by reticulocytopenia and decreased erythroid cell precursors in the bone marrow. Most aplastic events are secondary to the human parvovirus B19 which has special affinity to attack the erythroid precursors. Other viruses (EpsteinBarr) or bacterial infections (*Streptococcus pneumoniae*, *Salmonella*) may cause transient aplasia in patients with sickle cell disease. Human parvovirus B19 is common among all people, especially in children less than 15 years. Because of the short duration of the bone marrow suppression and long red blood cells life span, anemia is not noticed in the population unaffected by hemolytic anemias. Patients with any chronic hemolytic anemia, whose RBC life span is shortened, may develop significant anemia. Erythroid aplasia is usually short lived, lasting a few days. Recovery is often spontaneous without a need for blood transfusion. If the anemia is severe and the patient is symptomatic, packed red blood cells transfusion is indicated. Patients often present at the end of the aplastic episode with high reticulocyte counts and jaundice from the chronic hemolysis. A hemolytic rather than aplastic event might be suggested. Combined aplastic event and splenic sequestration had been reported in association with parvovirus infection. Infection with human parvovirus B19 usually confers a long-lasting immunity. Recurrent aplastic events; however, may be caused by other infectious agents.

Splenic sequestration: Splenic sequestration is defined as a precipitous drop in the steady-state hemoglobin concentration by at least 2 g/dl, sudden enlargement of the spleen (secondary to pooling of the blood in the spleen), and a compensatory bone marrow response as evidenced by reticulocytosis and/or the presence of nucleated red blood cells in the peripheral blood. Splenic sequestration occurs mostly in infants and young children before autosplenectomy due to repeated splenic infarctions occurs. Even though it has been reported in infants as young as a few weeks of age, most cases occur in children between 8 months and 5 years old. Splenic sequestration is not unusual in older children with mild forms of sickle cell syndromes (S-C, S-β thalassemia and in genetically mild homozygous sickle cell diseases, i.e., the Arabian–Indian genotype). The exact etiology of splenic sequestration is not known. It is often associated with viral infection (human parvovirus B19) and/or bacterial infections. Splenic sequestration events often present with sudden onset of severe anemia (pallor, decreased activity, generalized weakness, tachycardia, and tachypnea), hypotension, and abdominal distention due to massive splenomegaly. Splenic sequestration is the initial presenting clinical event in approximately 20% of all infants with homozygous sickle cell disease and 30% in those below 2 years of age. It carries high mortality rates (almost 12% in a Jamaican study). Patients can die prior to presenting for medical care before the diagnosis is made. Association with acute chest syndrome occurs in up to 20% of the splenic sequestration episodes. The recurrence rate can be as high as 50% and carries the same risk of mortality as the first episode. Recurrence is not uncommon even while the patient is on chronic blood transfusion. Subacute splenic sequestration events are characterized by increased splenic size, a modest (up to 25%) drop in the hemoglobin level, and no hypotension.

Splenic sequestration is a medical emergency. Restoration of intravascular volume and improvement of oxygen delivery to various organs are the main goals of treatment. Slow and fractionated PRBC transfusion should be started as soon as possible. Rapid transfusion may lead to congestive heart failure because the sequestered blood returns from the spleen to the vascular system as normal red blood cells are given. Splenectomy is recommended by most authorities after the first episode because of the high recurrence rate and high mortality. Chronic blood transfusion to avoid recurrence and to delay splenectomy has been recommended by some. However recurrence may occur while the patient is on or after chronic transfusion is discontinued and often splenectomy is needed. Some studies showed that the incidence of bacterial infection did not increase after splenectomy in infants with homozygous sickle cell disease because these infants often have functional asplenia. This argument might not apply to the mild forms (SC, SE, SD, and the Arabian–Indian homozygous disease) of sickle cell disease in which the splenic function is maintained for long time. In these cases, splenectomy can be delayed or avoided especially if the sequestration even is of the subacute type.

Hyperhemolytic Events

Hyperhemolytic events are characterized by a sudden drop in the hemoglobin level, unconjugated hyperbilirubinemia, and reticulocytosis. Several authorities doubt its existence and believe that this presentation is due to either aplastic events presenting in the recovery state or a mild splenic sequestration. Sickle cell disease is often associated with G6PD deficiency, which might be the cause of the acute hemolytic episode. Most episodes are self-limiting and require no treatment. If anemia is severe and the patient is symptomatic, blood transfusion may be indicated.

Delayed Hemolytic Transfusion Reactions (DHTR)

Delayed hemolytic transfusion reaction is a posttransfusion hemolytic reaction characterized by hemolytic anemia, reticulocytopenia and posttransfusion hemoglobin levels lower than the pre-transfusion level. Hemolysis usually occurs 4–10 days (mean 5 days) after transfusion. Even though it has been reported in patients who have received a single transfusions, most cases occur in repeatedly transfused patient with sickle cell disease with a reported incidence of 4–11%. Severe cases can be life threatening and are often associated with other severe complications, including painful events, fever, hemoglobinuria, acute chest syndrome, DIC, pancreatitis, congestive heart failure, acute renal failure, and splenic sequestration. Mild cases can pass unnoticed. The mechanism of the anemia is thought to be due to an immune process. Most patients have a positive direct antiglobulin test (DAT) at presentation. However, 20–30% of the patients never develop detectable antibodies. It is believed that these patients have antibodies below detectable level. Hemolysis of the donor as well as recipient RBCs possibly explains the drop of hemoglobin to a level below that of the pre-transfusion level. Recipient RBC hemolysis is also suggested by the decrease in hemoglobin S percentage. Reticulocytopenia is thought to be secondary transfusion-induced bone marrow suppression. Treatment is mainly by avoiding transfusion as much as possible. Intravenous IgG (IVIg) and steroids were successful in preventing of hemolysis in some cases.

Vaso-Occlusive Events

Vaso-occlusive events are the most common manifestation of sickle cell disease (for pathophysiology see above). It can involve any organ. Repeated attacks of the same organ result in chronic organ damage.

Acute Painful Events

Commonly known as acute vaso-occlusive or thrombotic events, acute painful events are the most common manifestation of sickle cell disease, resulting in the majority of emergency room visits and hospitalizations. The frequency, severity, and anatomic location of the pain differ from one patient to another and from one episode to another in the same patient. Up to 40% of patients with homozygous sickle cell disease (SS) have no painful episodes. In one large study, one third of the patients had three to six episodes per year and one third had more than six episodes per year. Painful events may involve any part of the body. Low back, extremities, or abdomen are common sites. Multiple site involvement is not unusual. The pain may migrate from one site to another during the same episode. The events are usually self-limiting and last for only a few hours in most episodes. However, the pain can last for days and, occasionally, for weeks. Fever, localized tenderness, swelling, warmth, and limitation of joint movement may be present. When local signs are severe, differentiating painful vaso-occlusive event; involving bones; from osteomyelitis may be difficult. Abdominal vaso-occlusive events are of particular concern. Differentiating an abdominal vaso-occlusive event from a surgical abdomen is often difficult, but essential. Appendicitis, cholelithiasis, cholecystitis, and intestinal obstruction can all occur in patients with sickle cell disease and may mimic an acute painful event. Every effort should be made to differentiate vaso-occlusive events from these entities in order to plan proper management and avoid unnecessary high-risk surgical intervention.

Treatment: A first and an important step in the management of painful events is a search for a cause other than vaso-occlusion. Once the diagnosis of vaso-occlusive event is made, every effort should be made to relieve the pain using pharmacologic and/or nonpharmacologic methods. It should always be remembered that the patient is the one who is suffering, not the physician or nurse. Inadequate pain relief results in mistrust between the patient and his or her health care provider. Pain management depends on the severity of the pain and the patient's perception of it. Previous painful events may be used as a general guide to what the patient needs.

The use of pharmacologic agents for adequate pain relief is the mainstay of management of painful events. Acetaminophen, paracetamol, and other nonsteroidal anti-inflammatory drugs together with oral hydration may be tried as a home therapy in mild episodes. Opioids should be used to treat moderate to severe painful episodes. The initial suggested dose of morphine is 0.1–0.15 mg/kg IV, followed by maintenance therapy either by continuous IV infusion or patient-controlled analgesia (PCA). Repeated smaller doses (0.05–0.1 mg/kg) can be given every 15–30 min with close monitoring for respiratory depression until complete pain relieve is obtained. The morphine dosage should be individualized. History of previous painful episodes and their management can be used as a guide. Hydromorphone and fentanyl can be used as an alternative to morphine. Meperidine should be avoided because of its potential CNS toxicity. Adjuvant drugs, which may help in pain relief, include antihistamines, muscle relaxants, and antidepressants. Non-pharmacological therapies which may be helpful include local warm compresses, hypnosis, acupuncture, and behavioral techniques. A short course of steroids was found to shorten the course of the painful episodes. However, severe rebound pain occurred after discontinuation of steroids. Patients should be continued on oral medication after discharge to avoid pain recurrence. Spinal anesthesia may be required in severe cases. Patients with severe debilitating pain may be treated with chronic RBC transfusions or stem cell transplantation.

Health-care providers often avoid using opioids because of the fear of addiction. It should be stressed that this belief is unfounded. Withholding needed analgesia results in patient suffering, mistrust of health-care providers, and patient's drug-seeking behavior.

Central Nervous System Events

Cerebrovascular accidents (CVAs) are the leading cause of morbidity and mortality in both children and adult patients with sickle cell disease. Cerebrovascular accidents include ischemic stroke, hemorrhagic stroke, transient ischemic accidents (TIAs), and silent infarcts. CVAs occur in 8–15% of children with homozygous sickle cell disease. In the cooperative study of sickle cell disease of 3,647 patients, CVAs occurred in 11% of children (below 20 years of age) with homozygous sickle cell disease. Ischemic stroke (which results from occlusion or stenosis of large intracranial arteries) is most common in children between 2 and 9 years of age, while hemorrhagic stroke occurs most commonly between 20 and 29 years. Hemorrhagic stroke occurs in 3% of children below 20 years of age. Clinical manifestations are similar to those of strokes in people not affected by sickle cell anemia and depend on the location of the lesion, degree of the damage, and etiology (ischemic vs hemorrhagic stroke). Manifestations include seizures, hemiparesis, dysphasia, visual disturbances, abnormal gait, headaches, vomiting, and/or coma. The mortality rate in hemorrhagic stroke is between 25% and 50% and may reach 20% in untreated ischemic stroke. With early and aggressive therapy, mortality is low in the ischemic stroke; however, up to 70% of the survivors are expected to have significant residual neurologic defects or cognitive problems. Computerized tomography (CT) or magnetic resonance imaging (MRI or MRA) are the recommended diagnostic modalities. CT easily detects hemorrhagic lesions, although changes of an ischemic stroke may be delayed for a few hours. MRI is more sensitive in the first few hours (up to 6 h) after an ischemic infarct. MRA has replaced conventional angiography in identifying vascular lesions, e.g., moyamoya, aneurysm, and venous malformations. Conventional angiography may be required in hemorrhagic stroke if MRA is not conclusive. Care should be taken if hypertonic contrast solution is used as this may cause vascular occlusion. Lowering hemoglobin S level before the procedure is recommended.

Treatment: Patients should be managed in the intensive care unit. Treatment of seizures, fever, hypotension, hypoxia, or respiratory compromised (if present) should be managed urgently. A search for and treatment of other causes of the stroke, i.e., trauma, infection, etc. is essential. As the recurrence rate is high (44–67%), chronic blood transfusion to keep hemoglobin S levels below 30% is recommended. This practice results in reduction of recurrence rate to less than 10%. The duration for chronic transfusion is unknown. Stroke recurrence is high after discontinuing transfusion regardless of the duration of the chronic transfusion. Lifelong transfusion with iron-chelation therapy is currently the most reliable method to prevent recurrence. Some authorities recommend stopping chronic transfusion after 5 years or at the age of 18 years. Recurrence can occur while on transfusion in several of these cases hemoglobin S level was found to be higher than the recommended 30%. A recent report showed that progressive cerebral infarcts occurred in 45% (27.5% overt and 17.5% silent) in children with previous overt stroke while receiving transfusion therapy. Hematopoietic stem cell (HSC) transplantation is recommended by several authorities if a donor and resources are available (see bone marrow transplant below). Small studies have demonstrated that hydroxyurea may be effective in preventing stroke recurrence in those patients who are unable to receive blood transfusion (those who have developed alloantibodies, those who are nonadherent with chelation, etc.). However, further studies are needed before recommending its routine use. Treatment of the hemorrhagic stroke depends on the location of the bleeding and if an associated vascular abnormality is present. The benefit of exchange transfusion in the therapy of hemorrhagic stroke is not clear. However, many authorities recommend transfusion, especially if large-vessel disease or abnormal velocity is present.

Transient ischemic attacks are defined as ischemic events in which symptoms resolve in less than 24 h. They are a strong predictor of development of overt stroke. These patients should be evaluated by Transcranial Doppler (TCD) and MRI. Patients who have abnormal velocity on TCD or significant large-vessel disease on MRI/MRA should begin a chronic transfusion regimen.

Silent infarcts were found in up to 30% of children with homozygous sickle cell anemia on screening of asymptomatic patients using MRI. These patients should be evaluated and followed closely if the TCD is normal. Primary prevention using TCD ultrasonography screening is recommended to identify patients at risk of developing stroke. Screening should start at 2 years of age. Chronic transfusion is recommended for those who had abnormal results (>200 cm/s). The optimal frequency of TCD scanning is not established; however, repeating the study every 3–12 months has been recommended by most authorities.

Acute Chest Syndrome

Acute chest syndrome (ACS) is characterized by the radiographic appearance of new pulmonary infiltrates, fever, respiratory compromise (manifested by cough, tachypnea, wheezing, labored breathing and/or hypoxia), chest pain, and leukocytosis. Radiographic findings may lag behind the clinical picture. Repeat X-ray should be done 24–48 h later if the clinical picture is suggestive of ACS. Many patients (up to 60% in one study) who have fever and chest pain without clinical evidence of pulmonary problems were found to have radiographic evidence of ACS on repeat chest X-ray (➋ *Fig. 324.3*). Over 50% of ACS develops after hospitalization. Triggering factors, which cause local hypoxia and induce local sickling, include splinting in patients with acute pain involving the ribs, abdomen and/or back, respiratory depression as a result of the use of pain medications, postoperative splinting in abdominal or thoracic surgery, or due to under ventilation due to atelectasis and bronchospasm in asthmatic children. ACS is the most common cause of death in children with sickle cell disease (around 2%) and the second cause of hospitalization after acute pain events. Even though ACS occurs at any age and any time of the year, it peaks between 2 and 4 years of age and in the winter.

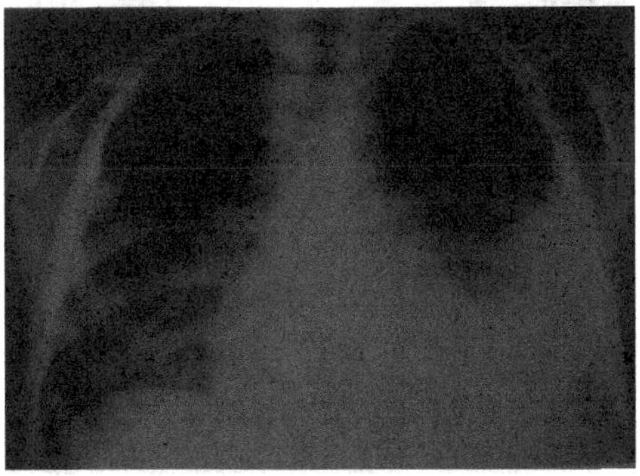

Figure 324.3
Chest X-ray of a child with sickle cell disease and acute chest syndrome (ACS)

The pathogenesis of ACS is complex and includes vasculopathy of SCD and hypoxia induced by pulmonary infection and/or the presence of one or more the sickling-promoting factors mentioned above. Early studies suggested that infection is the main causes of this syndrome in children as opposed to the adults in whom pulmonary infarction is the major mechanism of ACS. Recently, however, it has been shown that pulmonary infarction, caused by fat emboli or local hypoxia due to vaso-occlusion, is a common cause of ACS in children. Whatever the initiating process, the end result is a combination of infection and infarction. Devitalized infarcted lung tissue promotes infection, while infection causes local edema and occlusion of the small blood vessels causing local hypoxia and sickling. An infectious cause is found in 30–40% of ACS in children. Infectious agents include mycoplasma, chlamydia, viral, and bacteria. In over 50% of the cases, no specific etiology was found. Recurrence rate is high, occurring in up to 80% of the cases, especially in those who have been affected before 3 years of age. Hypoxia induced by ACS may lead to worsening of pulmonary involvement, CNS infarction, generalized vaso-occlusion or multisystem failure, and death. Repeated episodes of ACS may lead to lung fibrosis.

Treatment: Acute treatment consists of respiratory support, fluid management, antibiotics, pain management, PRBC transfusion, as well as the possible use of steroids. Long-term, preventative management can include the use of hydroxyurea and hematopoietic stem cell transplantation. Respiratory support includes oxygen supplementation to maintain arterial oxygen saturation ≥92%, incentive spirometry, and nitrous oxide. Mechanical ventilation may be required in severe cases. Dehydration and acidosis should be corrected. Overhydration should be avoided as it may cause pulmonary edema. Third generation cephalosporins and macrolides are a reasonable initial empiric antibiotic combination for coverage of expected pathogens (*Streptococcus pneumoniae*, H influenzae, mycoplasma, and chlamydia). Vancomycin should be added in severe cases or when resistant organisms are suspected or proven by culture. Simple or exchange transfusion should be started early except in the clinically and radiologically mild cases. Simple transfusion is adequate in most cases, particularly in patients with low hemoglobin. Exchange transfusion is indicated in severe cases, progressive cases, hypoxic cases, cases with multiple-lobe involvement, and in those who do not respond to simple transfusion. Hemoglobin levels should not exceed 11–12 g/dl to avoid hyperviscosity, which promotes sickling and thrombosis. With exchange transfusion, the aim is to decrease hemoglobin S level to <30%.

Pain management is important not only because it decreases the suffering and apprehension of the patient but also it controls splinting which may be a factor in increasing hypoxia and worsening the condition. Systemic steroids have been found to be beneficial in mild and moderate cases of ACS. However relapse and readmission was found to be high in patients who received steroid therapy. Further studies are needed before their routine use is recommended. Hydroxyurea is effective in reducing the frequency of recurrence. It is recommended in recurrent cases, especially severe ones (see below). Allogenic hematopoietic cell transplant is curative in 80–90% of cases of SCD. It is recommended for recurrent severe cases of ACS if a matched sibling is available.

Bones and Joints

Cortical bone infarction: Painful vaso-occlusive events are the most common manifestation of sickle cell disease. These events are thought to result from marrow infarction. A less common form of painful event is thought to result from cortical bone infarction. It manifests with local swelling, tenderness redness, hotness, imitation of movement, and fever. Bone destruction and periosteal new bone formation are common. Differentiating this type of event from osteomyelitis is often difficult. A toxic appearance and high-grade fever are suggestive but not diagnostic of osteomyelitis. Even histology can be confusing unless an organism is isolated as both may demonstrate an inflammatory process. Treatment of cortical bone infarction is similar to that of acute painful events.

Osteomyelitis and septic arthritis: Osteomyelitis may involve any bone; however, it most commonly involves the diaphysis of long bones and often involves multiple sites. Technetium bone scan, CT, and MRI are of limited value in differentiating osteomyelitis from cortical bone infarction. Isolating an organism from the local lesion or from blood culture is the only definitive diagnosis of osteomyelitis/septic arthritis. The most common cause of osteomyelitis in children with sickle cell anemia is *Staphylococcus aureus*. However, it is well known that in children with sickle cell disease who develop osteomyelitis, infection is often attributable to *Salmonella*, especially in areas where gastrointestinal infection by salmonella is common. It has been postulated that salmonella egress through microinfarcts of the intestinal wall and settle in the previously infarcted bone. Gram-negative bacilli (*E. coli*, *Klebsiella*) are relatively common causes of osteomyelitis in the sickle cell population, especially in older children and adults.

Treatment: Surgical drainage and parental antibiotic therapy are the primary therapeutic modality. The initial choice of antibiotic should include coverage for Salmonella species and coagulase-positive staphylococci. The duration of antibiotic coverage is not well established; however, 6–8 weeks are usually recommended. It has been suggested that early surgical drainage is important to assure good and early recovery and avoid chronicity and extensive bone destruction (➲ *Fig. 324.4*).

Arthritis (non-septic): Arthritis may due synovial infarction or reactive arthritis secondary to adjacent osteonecrosis. Treatment is symptomatic.

Dactylitis (hand–foot syndrome): The vast majority of dactylitis occurs in the first 2 years of life. It is uncommon after 4 years of age. It occurs in over 40% of children with homozygous sickle cell disease. It presents with bilateral swelling of the hands and/or feet. It may involve all four extremities at the same time. It may cause excessive destruction of the affected bones (➲ *Fig. 324.5*). Dactylitis in the first 2 years of life predicts a more severe clinical course of sickle cell disease. Treatment is similar to that of acute painful events. Most patients recover completely. Some may end with shortening of the involved bones.

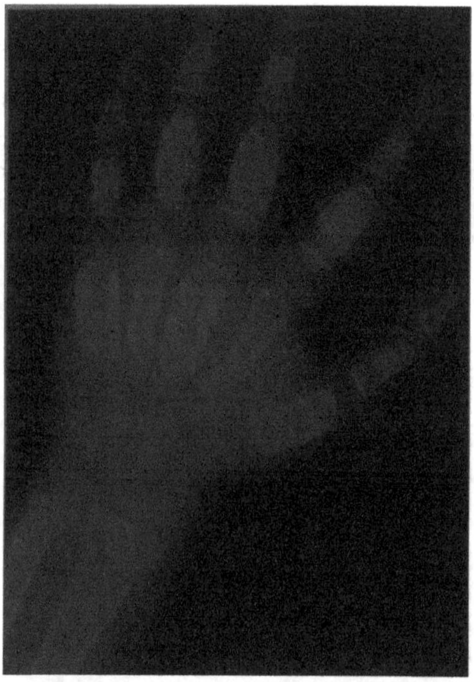

Figure 324.4
X-ray of the hand of a child with sickle cell disease with hand-foot syndrome

Figure 324.5
X-ray of the femur of a child with sickle cell disease and salmonella osteomyelitis

Avascular necrosis (AVN): Avascular necrosis of the femoral and humeral head is a common and serious complication of sickle cell disease. The true incidence is not known. In a large study, 10% of the patients were found to have AVN of the femoral head, and 5.6% of patients had AVN of the humeral head. The incidence of AVN is higher in patients with concomitant α-thalassemia. AVN may occur as early as 5 years of age. The prevalence increases with age. AVN of the femoral head is bilateral in over 50% of patients. Clinical manifestations include pain, limp, and limitation of movement. Conservative treatment of AVN in children below 12 years of age usually results in healing and remodeling of the femoral or humeral heads with good function. The natural history in older children and adults is progressive. Permanent damage is the expected result in most patients. Diagnosis can be made by plain x-ray in advanced cases. Expected early or mild lesions should be diagnosed by MRI. Treatment is conservative and includes avoidance of weight bearing (crutches and bed rest), analgesics, and nonsteroidal anti-inflammatory drugs. Surgical intervention in the form of core decompression, osteotomy, or arthroplasty has a low success rate and high rate of complication and failure. These procedures should be reserved for the most severe cases.

Bone marrow hyperplasia: Bone marrow hyperplasia is a consequence of bone marrow hyperactivity in response to the hemolytic anemia, resulting in widening of the marrow space and bone deformities such as frontal bossing, hair on end appearance of the skull x-ray, and protrusion of the incisors with associated overbite. Pathologic bone fracture may result from osteopenia and thinning of the cortex of the long bones. Vertebral collapse due to marrow necrosis and marrow hyperplasia leads to biconcave deformity. Compression fractures may cause a biconcave deformity with or without kyphosis.

Orbital compression syndrome: A rare but serious skeletal complication is the orbital compression syndrome that is caused by bone infarction around the globe. It is associated with pain, periorbital swelling with or without proptosis, ophthalmoplegia, visual impairment, and subperiosteal hematoma. The few reported cases were treated conservatively as other cases of vaso-occlusion.

Hepatobiliary System

Hepatobiliary complications of sickle cell disease include hepatomegaly, hepatic vaso-occlusive events, intrahepatic cholestasis, benign hyperbilirubinemia, hepatic sequestration events, and cholelithiasis with or without cholecystitis. Therapy of other sickle cell complications may also induce hepatobiliary complications. The frequency of hepatomegaly is not known because of different types of reporting (clinical vs radiologic vs autopsy). Hepatomegaly was found in 90% in an autopsy report. Hepatic vaso-occlusive events present with pain and tenderness in the right upper quadrant and jaundice with or without low-grade fever. Liver enzymes and bilirubin are usually modestly elevated (ALT and AST <500 IU/l, bilirubin <15 mg/dl). Treatment with analgesics and hydration is usually adequate and recovery is the rule. Intrahepatic cholestasis, as evidenced by markedly elevated liver enzymes, may end in hepatic failure. This syndrome is often associated with renal failure. The fatality rate is extremely high. Exchange transfusion and fresh frozen plasma can reverse this process. Liver transplantation is the only option for severe nonresponsive cases.

Benign hyperbilirubinemia is characterized by marked conjugated hyperbilirubinemia, modest elevation of liver enzymes with mild or no symptoms. The patient may look extremely yellow, but feels well. This process usually resolves without any treatment.

Hepatic sequestration events are less common and less severe than splenic sequestration. They present with right upper quadrant pain, a rapid drop in hemoglobin level, and significant increase in liver size. The frequency of hepatic sequestration events is possibly underestimated as mild episodes might be missed because most patients have steady state hepatomegaly. The treatment depends on the severity of the anemia and the clinical picture. Mild cases resolve spontaneously. In most cases, the liver size decreases and the hemoglobin rises as the sequestered blood returns to the circulation. Treatment of severe, symptomatic cases is similar to that of splenic sequestration and includes restoration of the intravascular volume and simple or exchange transfusion.

Cholelithiasis has been reported in children as young as 2 years old. The incidence increases with age, eventually reaching 70% in adults. Diagnosis is made by ultrasonography that shows stones, sludge, or both. Most patients are asymptomatic. However, cholelithiasis may be complicated with cholecystitis and/or common bile duct obstruction. Cholecystectomy is indicated for the symptomatic patient and for those in whom differentiating hepatic vaso-occlusion from cholelithiasis-related symptoms is not possible. Elective cholecystectomy in patients with asymptomatic cholelithiasis is suggested by some authorities to avoid potential complications at inappropriate times and to alleviate patient and family anxiety. Sludge should be followed by repeated ultrasonography as it may resolve spontaneously. Cholecystectomy is to be done in symptomatic cases. Treatment of cholecystitis is similar to the same problem in other settings and includes antibiotics and cholecystectomy after stabilizing the patient. Common bile duct stones may be removed prior to surgery by ERCP.

Renal System

Renal complications of sickle cell disease include hyposthenuria, hematuria, proteinuria, tubular acidosis, nephrotic syndrome, renal infarction, acute renal failure, urinary tract infection, and end-stage renal disease. Hyposthenuria is almost universal in patients with sickle cell disease. Sickling in the hypertonic environment and slow circulation in the renal medulla leads to poor urinary concentration. Polyuria and enuresis are common manifestation of SCD. No treatment is available or needed. However, patients should be encouraged to drink fluids sufficient to avoid dehydration. Microscopic or gross hematuria is common in both sickle cell trait and sickle cell disease. It is due to papillary necrosis caused by vaso-occlusion in the hypertonic, hypoxic, and acidic environment of the renal tubular system. Bleeding is usually painless and unilateral (most commonly from the left kidney). Hematuria is usually mild and self-limiting. Supportive care in the form of bed rest, hydration, urine alkalization, and diuretics is usually adequate. Occasionally, hematuria may be severe enough to necessitate blood transfusion. Nephrotic syndrome, acute or chronic renal failure, and renal infarction are rare but serious complications in children with sickle cell disease. Treatment is the same as the treatment of similar conditions in patients not affected by sickle cell anemia. Dialysis and renal transplantation is indicated in end-stage renal disease.

Spleen: The presence of a palpable spleen is common in infants with homozygous sickle cell disease (SS) and in young children with compound SC, S β thalassemia, and homozygous sickle cell disease with high hemoglobin F. Splenic infarction (which is more common at high altitude) presents with acute abdominal and pleuritic chest pain. Functional, reversible hyposplenia, or asplenia is found in over 90% of children with homozygous SCD (SS) between 6 months and 3 years of age. Functional hyposplenia/asplenia is due to the slow circulation and local hypoxia in the splenic sinusoids. Functional impairment of the splenic reticuloendothelial system can be demonstrated by an increased number of pocked or pitted red blood cells or by technetium liver/spleen scan. This functional asplenia can be reversed by simple or partial exchange transfusion. Anatomic irreversible asplenia is caused by repeated splenic infarctions which lead to splenic atrophy and shrinkage. The spleen becomes fibrosed or calcified. This anatomic, irreversible asplenia is evident by 5–8 years of age. Hypersplenism, as evidenced by splenomegaly and pancytopenia with evidence of bone marrow hyperplasia, may be present in some infants with homozygous sickle cell disease (SS). Hypersplenism is more common in patients with milder forms of sickle cell disease, i.e., SC, SD, Sβ thalassemia, and homozygous sickle cell disease with high hemoglobin F level. Splenectomy is recommended in patients with significant hypersplenism and massive splenomegaly.

Priapism is defined as sustained painful erection lasting for more than 2 h. Priapism is common in patients with sickle cell disease after puberty. The reported prevalence varies widely from 5% to more than 40%. Priapism in patients with sickle cell disease is a low flow type of priapism. It is due to vaso-occlusion of the venous drainage of the corpus cavernosum. Sickling in the corpus cavernosum is due to stasis, hypoxia, and acidosis. Priapism can be classified as stuttering, an episode which lasts more than few minutes but less than 3 h, and prolonged, which lasts more than 3 h. The peak incidence is 12–15 years of age (some studies showed two peaks; 13–15 and 20–29 years). Up to 90% of the first events occur before 20 years of age. Diagnosis is usually based on physical exam. The patient presents with unwanted painful erection with a rigid penis and soft glands. Doppler ultrasonography can differentiate low-flow, the usual type in SCD, from high-flow priapism. Prolonged (over 12 h) or repeated attacks may result in necrosis and fibrosis of the corpus cavernosum and erectile dysfunction and impotence in 25–35% of the patients. Conservative management, including hydration, analgesia, and frequent urination, is recommended for cases lasting more than 2 h but less than 6 h. The role of simple or exchange transfusion is controversial because of the lack of evidence of its benefit and the reported high complication rate (headache, seizures, and obtundation). Aspiration of the corpus cavernosa followed by saline irrigation has been demonstrated to be effective for those nonresponsive to conservative management and for episodes lasting more than 2 h. Instillation of α and β adrenergic agonists in the corpus cavernosa together with aspiration was effective in inducing detumescence in 95% of the cases. Surgical shunting is indicated in prolonged nonresponsive cases (over 6–12 h). Creating a shunt from the corpus cavernosa to the corpus spongiosum is the most commonly used procedure.

Skin: Leg ulcers occur mainly over the medial or the lateral malleolus and occasionally on the dorsum of the foot. The ulcers are often painful, indolent, and disfiguring. They occur in 10–20% of patients with homozygous sickle cell disease. The ulcers usually occur between 20 and 50 years of age. Ulcers are caused by skin ischemia due to hypoxic vascular occlusion and may be exaggerated by infection, trauma, or high temperature. The natural course is rapid healing in some cases, recurrent ulcerations in others, and chronic and protracted ulceration in most cases. Secondary local infection is common but systemic infection is unusual. A reasonable approach to the treatment of sickle cell–associated leg ulcers is adequate analgesia, bed rest, elastic compression, leg elevation, good local hygiene, debridement and local antiseptic, and the use of systemic antibiotics if cellulitis, lymphadenitis, or systemic infection is present. Other modalities, which had been used in resistant cases, include local and systemic zinc oxide, hyperbaric oxygen, and skin grafting.

Ophthalmologic manifestations/complications: Vaso-occlusion may involve any blood vessel in the eye or the globe. The clinical significance depends on the involved tissue and the degree of damage. Tortuosity of the conjunctival blood vessels is of diagnostic but not clinically significance. Retinopathy is classified into proliferative and nonproliferative types. Proliferative retinopathy is a serious complication which may lead to vitreous hemorrhage or retinal detachment ending in visual loss. The proliferative process starts with vaso-occlusion of the peripheral retinal arteries which stimulates neovascularization. Proliferative retinopathy is classified in five stages, including:

- Stage 1, peripheral retinal arteries occlusion
- Stage 2, arteriovenous anastomoses
- Stage 3, neovascularization
- Stage 4, vitreous hemorrhage
- Stage 5, retinal detachment

Nonproliferative retinopathy results from retinal infarction and adjacent hemorrhage. It may result in several retinal findings but rarely cause visual problems. Acute loss of vision due to central retinal artery occlusion has been reported. Hyphema may result from trauma. If untreated, it may lead to glaucoma and blindness.

Unlike hyphema in the patient not affected by sickle cell anemia, in which hypemas usually resolve spontaneously, hyphema in sickle cell disease requires immediate evacuation to avoid loss of vision. Treatment is indicated in bilateral disease, rapidly progressive disease, and in case of spontaneous hemorrhage. Laser photocoagulation is the preferred procedure with the least rate of complications. Surgical intervention is required for retinal detachment or unresolving vitreous hemorrhage.

Cardiovascular system: Cardiovascular manifestations are common in patients with sickle cell disease. Systolic heart murmurs are found in most patients and are caused by the anemia. Exercise tolerance is markedly impaired because of the anemia. Cardiomegaly is present in both children and adults and secondary to the anemia and microvascular disease. Detailed studies showed that most patients have dilatation of the ventricles and interventricular septum. However, ventricular contractility is normal in most patients. Heart failure, when it occurs, is usually due to sudden drop in hemoglobin (splenic sequestration) or fluid overload (rapid blood transfusion, especially for splenic sequestration).

Multiorgan failure: Multisystem failure syndrome, defined as failure of two or more systems (hepatic, renal, pulmonary, and cardiac), is a rare and potentially fatal complication in patients with sickle cell disease. It is often associated with severe painful vaso-occlusive event or sepsis. Aggressive exchange transfusion may be life saving.

Hearing: Sensorineural hearing loss occurs in around 10% of patients with sickle cell anemia disease. The frequency increases with age. It is caused by sickling in the cochlear vasculature, which results in destruction of hair cells.

Infection: Bacterial and viral infection is a major cause of morbidity and mortality in patients with sickle cell disease. Hyposplenia/asplenia caused by repeated splenic infarction is the main reason of increased susceptibility to the encapsulated organisms (*Streptococcus pneumoniae and Haemophilus influenzae*). Impaired opsonization and abnormal alternative complement pathway activation increases the susceptibility to *Salmonella, E. coli, Staphylococcus aureus*, and *Mycoplasma pneumoniae*. Abnormalities in neutrophil function have been demonstrated in several studies. Devascularized tissue due to vaso-occlusive episodes in the bone, lungs, or skin provides a suitable environment for bacterial invasion and growth. Microinfarcts of the wall of the gastrointestinal tract provide egress of the *Salmonella* to the circulation, causing sepsis and/or osteomyelitis. The incidence of *Streptococcus pneumoniae* and *H. influenzae* infection (sepsis, pneumonia, or meningitis) was 400–600 and 4 times more frequent, respectively, compared with children not affected by sickle cell anemia. The mortality rate is 30% and 10% for sepsis and meningitis, respectively. The incidence of and the mortality/morbidity caused by infection by these two organisms decreased significantly since the universal use of immunization and penicillin prophylaxis. A further drop in the rate of complications from these organisms is expected with the recent approval of the 13-valent pneumococcal vaccine. Infection with the two organisms, however, remains a major cause of morbidity and mortality, especially in children less than 5 years old. Infection by other organisms is less frequent and probably less fulminant than *Streptococcus pneumoniae* and *H. influenzae*. Aggressive antibiotic treatment should be started as soon as bacterial infection is suspected. The choice of the antibiotic depends on the suspected organism. Empiric antibiotics should be started immediately in a febrile child after obtaining the appropriate cultures (blood, urine, local aspirate etc.). Ceftriaxone is recommended as an empiric antibiotic by most authorities. Vancomycin should be reserved for severely sick patients (e.g., those in shock), patients suspected to have meningitis, or in areas where penicillin resistant streptococcus pneumoniae is prevalent. Macrolide antibiotics should be given for febrile patients with pneumonia/acute chest syndrome to cover for mycoplasma and Chlamydia. There is no evidence that children with the sickle cell disease are more susceptible to virus infection than their normal counterparts. The incidence of parvovirus B19 infection is similar to that of general population; however, it may cause transient but severe aplastic anemia.

Prevention: Penicillin prophylaxis was shown to decrease pneumococcal infection by 85%. However, it should be remembered that these results were obtained when almost all isolates of *Streptococcus pneumoniae* were susceptible to penicillin. Oral penicillin or amoxicillin prophylaxis is still recommended for children with SCD as soon as the diagnosis is made. The goal of newborn screening programs is to get penicillin prophylaxis started by 2 weeks of age. The duration of the prophylaxis is not known. At least one study suggested that it should be stopped at 5 years of age. A first generation cephalosporin is a good alternative. Macrolides or trimethroprim-sulfamethoxazole is recommended for patients who are allergic to penicillin. Conjugate *H. influenzae* and conjugate (PCV7) or the most recently approved 13-valent streptococcus pneumoniae are part of routine childhood immunization. Twenty-three-valent pneumococcal vaccine (PCV23) is recommended after 2 years of age and repeated once after 3–5 years. Meningococcal conjugate vaccine is recommended after 2 years of age. Hepatitis B and A vaccination are also recommended.

Psychosocial: The patient with sickle cell anemia as well as their families are under severe psychological, social, and financial stress. Recurrent painful events, frequent hospitalizations, inability to keep up with peer's exercise activities, delayed sexual and physical maturation, school absenteeism, job-related problems, financial and insurance problems, and fear of premature death puts severe pressure on the families. Comprehensive and sympathetic programs for early diagnosis, education, physical and psychological treatment, and financial support are needed. Participation of hematologists, psychologists/psychiatrists, nurses, social workers, self-help groups, and government and nongovernment organizations are essential to assure proper care for patients and their families. Special sickle cell clinics are also important.

Growth and development: The weight and height of infants with sickle cell disease is normal. This is not surprising as the levels of hemoglobin S levels are low intrauterinely as well as in the first few months of life. With increasing age and rising hemoglobin S levels, however, patients become more anemic and fall behind in weight and height. Weight is more affected than height. Growth deficits may be evident as early as 2 years of age and become more pronounced with increasing age. Sexual maturation is delayed in both sexes. Females have delayed onset of menarche. Both males and females have delays in attaining normal Tanner development stages. Development delay is multifactorial. The severe chronic anemia is probably the most important factor. Other implicated factors include, malnutrition, vitamin and mineral deficiency, infection, and the stress of chronic disease. Most patients with sickle cell disease do not require therapy for physical or sexual delays unless they have slow growth velocity.

Cognitive function: For a long time, patients with sickle cell disease were thought to have learning, neuropsychological, and cognitive problems. Recent evidence suggests that silent CNS infarction may be the major cause of these problems. MRI scans have identified several brain lesions in children without a history of clinical CNS problems.

Neonatal screening: Neonatal screening is recommended in areas where sickle cell gene is prevalent. The interpretation of screening results is shown in ➋ *Table 324.1*. Screening programs, together with close follow-up and parental education programs, have resulted in decreased mortality and morbidity and a better lifestyle in children with sickle cell disease. This improved outcome is the result of:

- Antibiotic prophylaxis
- Appropriate and timely immunization programs
- Aggressive treatment of febrile episodes
- Aggressive management of splenic sequestration events
- Comprehensive multidisciplinary sickle cell programs
- Parental education about the potential complications (splenic sequestration fever, seizures respiratory distress, etc.) and the necessity of urgent medical consultation
- Prenatal diagnosis and counseling of pregnant women
- Premarital counseling of patients with sickle cell trait
- Parental and children guidance on methods of coping with the stress of the condition and its complications

Surgery and General Anesthesia

Children with sickle cell disease are at high risk of developing severe complications with surgery and general or regional anesthesia. Postoperative complications include acute chest syndrome, painful events, infection, fever, CNS events, and death. Sickling-promoting factors that may be induced or exaggerated by surgery and anesthesia include hypoxia, dehydration, acidosis, stasis, hypotension, hypothermia or hyperthermia, hypoperfusion, and pressure on major blood vessels by tourniquets or improper positioning. These factors may be induced by medications, improper preparation, improper positioning (immobility, pressure on major blood vessels), the operating room environment (hypo or hyperthermia), the disease itself (pulmonary or cardiac disease). Generalized sickling leading to serious complications (respiratory failure) and/or death or localized sickling leading to organ damage (loss of a limb) may be the end result. Complications may occur intraoperativly or postoperatively. It is important to remember that complications occur more commonly in the recovery room when patient monitoring may be less intense.

Table 324.1
Interpretation of hemoglobin electrophones in the newborn

FA	Normal
FAS	Sickle cell trait
FS	1. Homozygous sickle cell disease (SS)
	2. Sickle-β° thalassemia
	3. Sickle hereditary persistent hemoglobin F (HPHF) disease
FS+C,D,E,O Arab, etc.	Double heterozygous of sickle with Hbs C, D, E, or O Arab, etc.
FA+C,D,E, O-Arab	Trait for hemoglobins C, D, E, or O-Arab the present Hb

Any of the above could be associated with alpha gene hemoglobinopathy, mainly α thalassemia.

These complications can be avoided by careful monitoring, adequate oxygenation, hydration, avoidance of hypotension, hypovolemia, hypothermia, local or generalized stasis, and acidosis are essential. The use of tourniquets should be avoided, and care should be taken to avoid pressure on major blood vessels due to improper positioning. These measures need to be started prior to general anesthesia and continued during surgery and through postoperative period, until the patient is fully awake. Close monitoring of temperature, blood pressure, oxygen saturation, and blood loss is essential. These measures are more important in patients with compromised pulmonary or cardiac function and in those who require surgery that compromises these organs (i.e., cardiac, CNS, or chest surgery).

The need for preoperative blood transfusion is controversial. Recent evidence suggests that transfusion may not be necessary in all patients. Preoperative blood transfusion to raise the hemoglobin level to 10 g/dl was found to be as effective as exchange transfusion to lower the level of hemoglobin S to less than 30%. Until further studies are completed, preoperative simple blood transfusion is indicated for all patients. Exchange transfusion should be reserved for patients with significant anemia (to avoid CHF), patients with compromised cardiac or pulmonary function, and those undergoing thoracic, cardiac, or CNS surgery.

Pregnancy in Sickle Cell Disease

Fetal and neonatal related issues: Complications associated with maternal sickle cell anemia include spontaneous abortion, intrauterine growth retardation, low birth weight, prematurity, and increased perinatal mortality.

These complications are mainly due to placental compromise caused by decreased uterine blood flow. Other factors which may contribute to fetal problems include maternal anemia, maternal malnutrition, and increased incidence of placenta previa and abruption placenta in mothers with sickle cell disease. Perinatal mortality was as high as 20–50%. However, improvement in obstetric care leads to a significant decrease in the perinatal mortality. Routine prophylactic blood transfusion is not recommended.

Hematopoietic stem cell transplantation (HPSC): Hematopoietic transplantation is the only curative therapy for patients with sickle cell disease. Overall survival and event-free survival range between 91–100% and 73–93%, respectively, with the higher figures in the more recent studies. Transplant early in the course of sickle cell related complications is associated with a better outcome with overall and disease free survival of 100% and 93%, respectively, as compared with 88% and 80% for transplants later in the course of the condition. The majority of the reported cases were from matched siblings. Few cases were from cord blood of matched siblings with overall and disease-free survival of 100% and 90%, respectively. The main limiting factors for HPSC transplant are the variable clinical severity and the lack of known predictors of severity of SCD. Indications for HPSC vary between transplant centers. Accepted indications include a history of stroke, repeated severe acute chest syndrome, and frequent severe and debilitating vaso-occlusive events. It should be remembered that HLA-matched siblings with sickle cell trait can be used as donors.

Augmentation of Hemoglobin F Production

Several pharmacologic agents (5-Azacytidine, 5-Azadeoxycytidine, butyric acid, arginine butyrate, and erythropoietin) have been used in animal model and/or humans to increase hemoglobin F levels. Hydroxyurea is the agent commonly used in clinical practice in patients with sickle cell anemia. Several studies in both adults and children proved its efficacy in decreasing the frequency and severity of painful events, acute chest syndrome, blood transfusion, hospitalization, and mortality. Limited observational studies with small numbers of patients provided evidence that hydroxyurea prevents primary and secondary stroke, reverses splenic function, prevents or reverses chronic organ damage, improves oxygenation, and reduces proteinuria. Currently, hydroxyurea is indicated for patients with recurrent severe painful episodes, recurrent acute chest syndrome, and recurrent hospitalizations. Further studies are needed before recommendation can be made for its use for other indications. It is generally believed that the benefits of hydroxyurea are due to the increase in hemoglobin F level. However, the improvement in many patients was noticed with minimal or no change in hemoglobin F levels. Other possible mechanisms of action include neutropenia (neutrophil count correlates with event rate), reduction of reticulocytes, and young red blood cell which have high tendency to adhere to the vascular wall and induce vaso-occlusion and generation of nitric oxide. The major limiting factor in the routine use of hydroxyurea is neutropenia. However this complication is reversible with reduction of the dose or temporally discontinuing the drug. An unproved but serious concern is the possible carcinogenic effect of hydroxyurea. This concern originated from the observation that hydroxyurea increased the incidence of malignancy in patients with polycythemia vera and myelodysplastic syndromes. These diseases, however, are monoclonal and premalignant. There is no evidence that the hydroxyurea is carcinogenic in patients with sickle cell disease. The recommended starting dose is 15 mg/kg given once daily. The dose is increased every 8 weeks to the maximum tolerated dose.

Blood transfusion in sickle cell disease: Blood transfusion is an integral tool in the treatment of patients with sickle cell disease. When used appropriately, transfusions may treat or prevent complications, prevent organ damage, alleviate suffering, and prevent death. As any patients with SCD are expected to receive repeated blood transfusion, care should be taken to avoid unnecessary transfusion and to avoid or minimize potential complications. In addition to the precaution necessary for transfusion in other patients (donor screening for infectious agents, proper cross matching, etc.), the following steps are essential:

- Donors should be screened for sickle cell disease and trait.
- Antigenic phenotypes of the patient should be known and records well kept for future reference.
- Limited matching for ABO, Rh, E, C, and Kell is essential to minimize the incidence of alloimmunization.
- The use of leukodepleted blood units reduces febrile reactions, platelet refractoriness, infections, and cytokine-induced complications.

The indications for blood transfusion is not precisely defined and most recommendations are based on experience or uncontrolled studies. Most patients with sickle cell disease tolerate their anemia. Indications for packed red blood cell transfusion include:

- Severe symptomatic anemia (splenic sequestration event, aplastic event, hypersplenism, and hyperhemolytic event). The indication of transfusion in these cases depends on the clinical picture (real or pending heart failure, hypotension, tachypnea, tachycardia or pallor hypoactivity, and generalized weakness), degree of the drop in hemoglobin level (2 g/dl) and bone marrow activity as evidenced by reticulocyte count and/or the presence of NRBCS in the peripheral blood. These patients should receive simple transfusion.
- *Acute chest syndrome*: Most patients with ACS present with low hemoglobin. Simple transfusion is usually adequate in mild and moderate case of ACS. Partial or total exchange transfusion is recommended in severe, progressive cases and those patients with high hemoglobin level.
- Preparation for general anesthesia (see "➋ Surgery and General Anesthesia").
- *Stroke*: Immediate exchange transfusion is indicated for ischemic stroke. Chronic transfusions with iron-chelating therapy are recommended for primary and secondary stroke prevention and for patients with recurrent debilitating painful event.
- *Multisystem failure*: Exchange transfusion might be life saving.

Controversial indications include priapism, skin ulcers, preparation for infusion of contrast media, and silent CNS infarction. Some authorities recommend chronic transfusion in infants with ASSC to delay splenectomy. Recent literature, however, suggests that splenectomy does not increase the chances of serious bacterial infection in children with sickle cell disease because these children have functional asplenia. The hematocrit should not exceed 36% in any kind of transfusion. Higher levels result in exponential increase in blood viscosity, leading to painful events. Potential complications of transfusion should be kept in mind when considering such therapy. In addition to the known complications, patients with sickle cell disease have a higher incidence of alloimmunization and delayed hemolytic transfusion reactions. Alloimmunization occurs in 8–35% (mean, 25%) of transfused sickle cell disease patients.

Mild Sickle Cell Disease

An interesting and relatively mild form of homozygous sickle cell disease is known to occur in the Shiite Muslims population of the Arabian Gulf area. These patients have a less severe course, a higher percentage of splenomegaly and normal splenic function in most patients; at least in young children and adolescents, a lower incidence of pneumococcal infection, and a longer life expectancy. The reasons for the relatively mild course are not fully understood. High levels of hemoglobin F, which is common in this population and the common association with the α-thalassemia gene, may be the major contributing factors. This kind of sickle cell disease is not completely benign (as previously reported) as many patients develop serious complications, such as sepsis, meningitis, osteomyelitis, aseptic necrosis of femoral and humeral heads, ACS, and cerebrovascular accidents.

Sickle Cell Trait (AS)

Patients with sickle cell trait are clinically, hematologically, and developmentally normal. Around 40% of their hemoglobin is sickle hemoglobin (hemoglobin S). Hematuria and hyposthenuria are common. Extreme conditions including severe hypoxia may lead to sickling and even death. Flying in an unpressurized plane, strenuous exercise at high altitude, and severe pulmonary or cardiac disease are examples of situations in which complications and death have been reported. During general anesthesia, tourniquets and pressure on major blood vessels should be avoided to prevent severe hypoxia distal to the tourniquet, which may result in sickling and loss of an extremity.

Compound heterozygous sickle cell disease: The term "sickle cell disease" is usually used to describe patients with homozygous sickle cell disease (SS) and compound (doubly) heterozygous disease which results from co-inheritance of hemoglobin S and another abnormal hemoglobin or thalassemia. SC, SD, S/O-Arab, and SE diseases are discussed in the chapter on "hemoglobinopathies other than sickle cell disease."

Sickle cell β thalassemia: Compound heterozygous sickle cell-beta thalassemia results from inheritance of a sickle cell gene from one parent and β thalassemia gene from the other. The clinical manifestations are extremely variable ranging from asymptomatic to a clinical picture similar to that of homozygous sickle cell disease. The clinical severity depends on the amount of hemoglobin A produced. Sickle-β+ thalassemia is usually milder than homozygous sickle cell disease and sickle-β° thalassemia. However, both sickle-β° thalassemia and Sickle-β+ thalassemia have a higher incidence of splenomegaly than homozygous sickle cell disease. Retinopathy is more common in sickle-β+ thalassemia than homozygous sickle cell disease and sickle-β° thalassemia. Patients with sickle-β+ thalassemia tends to have a higher hemoglobin concentration (10–12 g/dl) and lower reticulocyte count than that of sickle-β° thalassemia (8–10 g/dl) who, in turn, have a higher hemoglobin concentration and lower reticulocyte count than those affected by homozygous sickle cell disease. The anemia in sickle-β° thalassemia and sickle-β+ thalassemia is hypochromic and microcytic. Hemoglobin electrophoresis of sickle-β° thalassemia is similar to that of homozygous sickle cell disease with higher hemoglobin A2 level (4–5%) and with no hemoglobin A. Hemoglobin electrophoresis in sickle-β+ thalassemia reveals hemoglobin S, with variable amounts of hemoglobins A, F, and A2. One parent has sickle cell trait while the other has β thalassemia and hypochromic, microcytic red blood cells.

Homozygous Sickle Cell Disease with α Thalassemia

The association of α-thalassemia with homozygous sickle cell disease (SS) results in a hypochromic microcytic anemia. The red blood cells of the newborn infant are usually microcytic (mean corpuscular volume <94 fl). Results of hemoglobin electrophoresis later in life are similar to those of homozygous sickle cell disease (SS). The anemia is usually less severe, and the reticulocyte count is lower than those of sickle cell disease (SS). The clinical effects are variable. Some studies showed that the increased frequency of painful vaso-occlusion is related to the higher hemoglobin level which is usually found in patients with sickle cell/α thalassemia. The incidence of acute chest syndrome was higher in some studies and lower in others. Some studies suggested an increased incidence of avascular necrosis of the femoral head and decreased incidence of leg ulcers.

Sickle cell with hereditary persistence of fetal hemoglobin (HPFH): Two types of HPFH have been described. One type (deletion type) results in higher levels and a pancellular distribution of hemoglobin F. Patients who coinherit this type of HPFH with sickle cell gene (sickle cell trait) are usually asymptomatic and have normal hematologic parameters. The second type (non-deletion) results in a heterogeneous distribution of hemoglobin F. The clinical picture in these patients is variable and depends on hemoglobin F level and the pattern of its distribution. Parents' studies should show that one parent has sickle cell trait, while the other has high hemoglobin F level.

Sickle cell/Hb Lepore disease: Co-inheritance of sickle cell gene with hemoglobin Lepore is rare. The clinical severity is similar to sickle-β+ thalassemia.

References

Abboud MR, Cure J, Granger S et al (2004) Magnetic resonance angiography in children with sickle cell disease and abnormal transcranial Doppler ultrasonography findings enrolled in the STOP study. Blood 103:2822

Adams RJ (2000) Lessons from the stroke prevention trial in sickle cell anemia (STOP) study. J Child Neural 15:344

Adams RJ, Brambilla D (2005) Discontinuing prophylactic transfusion used to prevent stroke in sickle cell disease. N Engl J Med 353:2769

Adams RJ, McKie VC, Hsu L et al (1998) Prevention of a first stroke by transfusion in children with sickle cell anemia and abnormal results on transcranial Doppler ultrasonography. N Engl J Med 339:5

Adekile AD, Gupta R, Yacoub F et al (2001) Avascular necrosis of the hip in children with sickle cell disease and high Hb F: magnetic resonance imaging findings and influence of alpha-thalassemia trait. Acta Haematol 105:27

Almeida A, Roberts I (2005) Bone involvement in sickle cell disease. Br J Haematol 129:482

Armstrong FD, Thompson RJ Jr, Wang W et al (1997) Cognitive functioning and brain magnetic resonance imaging in children with sickle cell disease. Neuropsychology Committee of the Cooperative Study of Sickle Cell Disease. Pediatrics 97:864

Aygun B, Padmanabhan S, Paley C et al (2002) Clinical significance of RBC alloantibodies and autoantibodies in sickle cell patients who received transfusion. Transfusion 42:37

Bainbridge R, Higgs DR, Maude GH et al (1985) Clinical presentation of homozygous sickle cell disease. J Pediatr 106:881

Balkaran B, Char G, Morris IS et al (1992) Stroke in a cohort of patients with homozygous sickle cell diseased. J Pediatr 120:360

Berger E, Saunders N, Wang L et al (2009) Sickle cell disease in children: differentiating osteomyelitis from vaso-occlusive event. Arch Pediatr Adolesc Med 163:251

Bernini JC, Rogers ZR, Sandler ES et al (1998) Beneficial effect of intravenous Dexsamethasone in children with mild to moderately severe acute chest syndrome complicating sickle cell disease. Blood 139:3082

Bunn HF (1997) Pathogenesis and treatment of sickle cell disease. N Engl J Med 337:762

Burnett MW, Bass JW, Cook BA (1998) Etiology of osteomyelitis complicating sickle cell disease. Pediatrics 101:296

Castro O, Brambilla DJ, Thorington B et al (1994) The acute chest syndrome in sickle cell disease: incidence and risk factors. Blood 84:643

Chadebech P, Habibi A, Nzouakou R et al (2009) Delayed hemolytic transfusion reaction in sickle cell disease patients: evidence of an emerging syndrome with suicidal red blood cell death. Transfusion 49:1785

Chambers JB, Forsythe DA, Bertrand SL et al (2000) Retrospective review of osteoarticular infection in a pediatric sickle cell age group. J Pediatr Orthop 20:682

Chang JC, Kan YW (1982) A sensitive new prenatal test for sickle cell anemia. N Engl J Med 307:30

Cheung AT, Chen PC, Larkin EC et al (2002) Microvascular abnormalities in sickle cell disease: a computer-assisted intravital microscopy study. Blood 99:3999

Dalton OP, Drummond DS, Davidson RS et al (1996) Bone infarction versus infection in sickle cell disease in children. J Pediatr Orthop 16:540

De Montalember M, Brousse V, Elie C et al (2006) French Study Group on Sickle cell Disease. Long term hydroxyurea treatment in children with sickle cell disease: tolerance and clinical outcome. Haematologica 91:125

Dean D, Neumayr L, Kelly DM et al (2003) Chlamydia pneumoniae and acute chest syndrome in patients with sickle cell disease. J Pediatr Hematol Oncol 25:46

Downes SM, Hambleton IR, Chuang EL et al (2005) Incidence and natural history of proliferative sickle cell retinopathy: observations from a cohort study. Ophthalmology 112:1869

Embury SH, Dozy AM, Miller J et al (1982) Concurrent sickle cell anemia and alpha thalassemia: effect on severity of anemia. N Engl J Med 306:270

Emond AM, Collis R, Darvill D et al (1985) Acute splenic sequestration in homozygous sickle cell disease: natural history and management. J Pediatr 107:201

Haberkern CM, Neumayr LD, Orringer EP et al (1997) Cholecystectomy in sickle cell anemia patients: perioperative outcome of 364 cases from the National Preoperative Transfusion Study. Preoperative Transfusion in Sickle Cell Disease Study Group. Blood 89:58

Halasa NB, Shankar SM, Talbot TR et al (2007) Incidence of invasive pneumococcal disease among individuals with sickle cell disease before and after the introduction of the pneumococcal conjugate vaccine. Clin Infect Dis 44:1428

Hankins JS, Ware RE, Rogers ZR et al (2005a) Long-term hydroxyurea therapy for infants with sickle cell anemia: the HUSOFT extension study. Blood 106:2269

Hankins J, Jeng M, Harris S et al (2005b) Chronic transfusion therapy for children with sickle cell disease and recurrent acute chest syndrome. J Pediatr Hematol Oncol 27:158

Heeney MM, Ware RE (2008) Hydroxyurea for children with sickle cell disease. Pediatr Clin N Am 55:483

Hernigou P, Galacteros F, Bachir D et al (1991) Deformities of the hip in adults who have sickle cell disease and had avascular necrosis in childhood. A natural history of fifty two patients. J Bone Joint Surg Am 73:8

Hsieh MM, Kang EM, Fitzhugh CD et al (2009) Allogeneic hematopoietic stem-cell transplantation for sickle cell disease. N Engl J Med 361:2309

Hulbert ML, McKinstry RC, Lacey JL et al (2011) Silent cerebral infarcts occur despite regular blood transfusion therapy after first strokes in children with sickle cell disease. Blood 117:772

Keeley K, Buchanan GR (1982) Acute infarction of long bones in children with sickle cell anemia. J Pediatr 101:170

Kizito ME, Mworozi E, Ndugwa C et al (2007) Bacteraemia in homozygous sickle cell disease in Africa: is pneumococcal prophylaxis justified? Arch Dis Child 92:21

Kogan SC, Doherty M, Gitschier J (1987) An improved method of amplified DNA sequences. N Engl J Med 317:985

Koren A, Segal-Kupershmit D, Zalman L et al (1999) Effect of hydroxyurea in sickle cell anemia: a clinical trial in children and teenagers with severe sickle cell anemia and sickle cell beta-thalassemia. Pediatr Hematol Oncol 16:221

Kwiatkowski JL, Zimmerman RA, Pollock AN et al (2009) Silent infarcts in young children with sickle cell disease. Br J Haematol 146:300

Mallouh AA, Asha MI (1988) Beneficial effect of blood transfusion in children with sickle cell chest syndrome. Am J Dis Child 142:178

Mallouh AA, Qudah A (1993) Acute splenic sequestration together with aplastic event caused by human parvovirus B19 in patients with sickle cell disease. J Pediatr 122:593

Mallouh AA, Qudah A (1995) An epidemic of aplastic event caused by human B19. Pediatr Infect Dis J 14:31

Mallouh AA, Salamah MM (1985) Pattern of bacterial infection in homozygous sickle cell disease: a report from Saudi Arabia. Am J Dis Child 139:820

Mantadakis E, Cavender JD, Rogers ZR et al (1999) Prevalence of priapism in children and adolescents with sickle cell anemia. J Pediatr Hematol Oncol 21:518

McCarville MB, Goodin GS, Fortner G et al (2008) Evaluation of a comprehensive transcranial Doppler screening program for children with sickle cell anemia. Pediatr Blood Cancer 50:818

Mekeel KL, Langham MR Jr, Gonzalez-Peralta R et al (2007) Liver transplantation in children with sickle cell disease. Liver Transpl 13:505

Miller ST, Sleeper LA, Pegelow CH et al (2000) Prediction of adverse outcome in children with sickle cell disease. N Engl J Med 342:83

Miller ST, Wright E, Abboud M et al (2001) Impact of chronic transfusion on incidence of pain and acute chest syndrome during the Stroke Prevention Trial (STOP) in sickle cell anemia. J Pediatr 139:785

Nietert PJ, Abboud MR, Silverstein MD et al (2000) Bone marrow transplantation versus periodic prophylactic blood transfusion in sickle cell patients at high risk of ischemic stroke: a decision analysis. Blood 95:3057

Ohene-Frempong K (2001) Indications for red blood cell transfusion in acute chest syndrome of sickle cell disease. Semin Hematol 38:5

Ohene-Frempong K, Weiner SJ, Sleeper LA et al (1998) Cerebrovascular accidents in sickle cell disease: rates and risk factors. Blood 91:288

Okuonghae HO, Nwankwo MU, Offor EC (1993) Pattern of bacteraemia in febrile children with sickle cell anaemia. Ann Trop Paediatr 13:55

Orkin SH, Little PF, Kazazian HH et al (1982) Improved detection of sickle mutation by DNA analysis: application to prenatal diagnosis. N Engl J Med 307:32

Platt OS (2000) The acute chest syndrome of sickle cell disease. N Engl J Med 342:1904

Poillon WN, Kim BC, Castro C (1998) Intracellular hemoglobin S polymerization and the clinical severity of sickle cell anemia. Blood 91:1777

Quinn CT, Rogers ZR, Buchanan GR (2004) Survival of children with sickle cell disease. Blood 103:4023

Quinn CT, Shull LA, Ahmad N et al (2007) Prognostic significance of early vaso-occlusive complications in children with sickle cell anemia. Blood 111:544

Rao SP, Miller ST, Cohen BJ (1992) Transient aplastic event in patients with sickle cell disease. B19 parvovirus studies during a 7-year period. Am J Dis Child 146:1328

Raphael JL, Shetty PB, Liu H et al (2008) A critical assessment of transcranial Doppler screening rates in a large pediatric sickle cell center: opportunities to improve health care quality. Pediatr Blood Cancer 51:647

Rogers ZR (2005) Priapism in sickle cell disease. Hematol Oncol Clin North Am 19:917

Rosse WF, Gallagher D, Kinney TR et al (1990) Transfusion and alloimmunization in sickle cell disease. The Cooperative Study of Sickle Cell disease. Blood 76:14

Sadat-Ali M (1998) The status of acute osteomyelitis in sickle cell disease. A 15-year review. Int Surg 83:84

Scott JP (2010) Hydroxyurea and sickle cell disease: its been a long, long coming. Pediatr Blood Cancer 54:185

Serjeant BE, Hambleton IR, Kerr S et al (2001) Haematological response to parvovirus B19 infection in homozygous sickle cell disease. Lancet 358:1779

Skagges DL, Kim SK, Greene NW et al (2001) Differentiation between bone infarction and acute osteomyelitis in children with sickle cell disease with use of sequential bone marrow and bone scan. J Bone Joint Surg Am 83-A:1810

Talano JA, Hillery CA, Gottschall JL et al (2003) Delayed hemolytic transfusion reaction/hyperhemolysis syndrome in children with sickle cell disease. Pediatrics 111:e661

Telen MJ (2001) Principles and problems of transfusion in sickle cell disease. Semin Hematol 38:315

Telen MJ (2007) Role of adhesion molecules and vascular endothelium in the pathogenesis of sickle cell disease. Hematology Am Soc Hematol (ASH) Education program 2007(1):84–90

The Management of sickle cell disease. National Institute of Health; National Heart, Lung and Blood Institute, Division of Blood diseases and resources. NIH publication 2004; pp 7–204.

Vichinsky EP, Haberkern CM, Neumayr L et al (1995) A comparison of conservative and aggressive transfusion regimens in the perioperative management of sickle cell disease. The Preoperative Transfusion in Sickle Cell Disease Study Group. N Engl J Med 333:206

Vichinsky EP, Styles LA, Colangelo LH et al (1997) Acute chest syndrome in sickle cell disease: clinical presentation and course. Cooperative Study of Sickle Cell Disease. Blood 89:1787

Vichinsky EP, Neumayr LD, Earls AN et al (2000) Causes and outcomes of the acute chest syndrome in sickle cell disease. National Acute Chest Syndrome Study Group. N Engl J Med 342:1855

Walker TM, Hambllton IR, Serjeant GR (2000) Gallstones in sickle cell disease: observations from the Jamaican Cohort study. J Pediatr 136:80

Ware RE, Aygun B (2009) Advances in the use of hydroxyurea. In: Hematology (American Society of Hematology Education Book)., p 62

Win N, New H, Lee E et al (2008) Hyperhemolysis syndrome in sickle cell disease: a case report (recurrent episode) and literature review. Transfusion 48:1231

Zimmerman SA, Schultz WH, Davis JS et al (2004) Sustained long-term hematologic efficacy of hydroxyurea at the maximum tolerated dose in children with sickle cell disease. Blood 103:2039

325 Hemoglobinopathies-Non-Sickle Cell

Ahmad A. Mallouh

Introduction

The globin part of the normal human hemoglobins (Hb A, F, and A2) consists of two alpha and two non-alpha chains (β in hemoglobin A, γ in hemoglobin F and δ in hemoglobin A2). Hemoglobinopathies result from genetic mutations causing structural changes in one of the globin chains by adding, deleting, or exchange of one or more amino acid. Over 800 mutations have been identified. The majority of these mutant hemoglobins are innocuous. A few of them, however, cause lifelong serious and sometimes fatal health problems. The following hemoglobinopathies will be discussed in this chapter, either because of high prevalence in certain ethnic groups or geographical area and/or their clinical severity either alone or in co-inheritance with sickle cell disease or thalassemia:

- Hemoglobin C
- Hemoglobin E
- Hemoglobin D
- Hemoglobin O Arab
- Unstable hemoglobins
- High oxygen affinity hemoglobins

Hemoglobin C

Pathogenesis and Incidence

Hemoglobin C results from a genetic mutation, resulting in the replacement of glutamic acid with lysine in the β chain subunit at position 6. It is less soluble than hemoglobin A. It precipitates into hexagonal crystals inside the RBCs. The red blood cells (RBCs) become less deformable and are easily removed by the spleen. The prevalence of Hemoglobin C is approximately 40–50% in West Africa, 3.5% in Carribbeans of African descent, 3% in African Americans, and 1–10% in North Africa. It has been also reported in other countries, for example, Italy and Turkey. This geographic distribution is probably due its protective effect against falciparum malaria.

Clinical Picture

Patients with hemoglobin C trait (Hgb AC) are asymptomatic with normal hematological values, except for a mild microcytosis and target red blood cells. Homozygous patients (Hb CC) usually have a mild, compensated hemolytic anemia and splenomegaly. Like other chronic hemolytic anemias, patients affected by homozygous hemoglobin C may develop cholelithiasis. Parvovirus infection may induce a transient aplastic crisis.

Co-inheritance with Thalassemia or Other Hemoglobinopathy

Patients with double heterozygous hemoglobin S/hemoglobin C (Hb SC) disease have a clinical picture similar but usually milder than homozygous hemoglobin S (Hb SS). Approximately 2% of these patients have severe disease. Aseptic necrosis of the femoral head and proliferative retinopathy are, in particular, common in patients with SC disease. Patients with C/β-0 thalassemia usually have a thalassemia intermedia-like picture. Those with C/β+ thalassemia usually have a mild, compensated hemolytic anemia. Patients with C/E, C/Lepore, and C/δ β thalassemia have a moderate hemolytic anemia. Patients with C/O Arab usually have a mild, compensated hemolytic anemia.

Diagnosis

Heterozygous hemoglobin C is usually diagnosed on hemoglobin electrophoresis either as a part of neonatal screening or as part of the investigation of a patient with mild chronic hemolytic anemia. The blood indices typically demonstrate a mild microcytosis. Target cells are seen on the peripheral blood smear of patients with hemoglobin C trait. The peripheral blood smear has a high number of target red blood cells with the presence of xerocytes and hexagonal crystals, inside the red blood cells. Hemoglobin C has the

Abdelaziz Y. Elzouki (ed.), *Textbook of Clinical Pediatrics*, DOI 10.1007/978-3-642-02202-9_325,

same mobility as hemoglobins E, O Arab, and A2 in alkaline media. Hemoglobin electrophoresis in acid citrate agar or high performance liquid chromatography (HPLC) is required for definitive diagnosis. The electrophoresis pattern of C/β-0 thalassemia is similar to that of Hb CC disease. Both demonstrate a high Hb C levels (over 95%) and no hemoglobin A. Hb C/β-0 thalassemia, however, has a marked microcytosis. At least one parent would have β thalassemia trait.

Treatment

No specific therapy is needed for patients with AC or CC. Parvovirus induced aplastic crisis anemia is usually mild and compensated. Folic acid supplementation is recommended in homozygous or doubly heterozygous patients (SC, C/β thalassemia, etc.). Treatment of SC disease is similar to that for SS disease. Treatment for C/β thalassemia depends on the severity of the anemia and may require blood transfusion. Splenectomy is rarely required in CC disease, but might be necessary in SC or Hb C/β thalassemia disease.

Hemoglobin E

Pathophysiology and Incidence

Hemoglobin E results from substitution of glutamic acid by lysine in position 26 of the β globin chain. The β chain of Hb E is synthesized at a slower rate compared with that of Hb A. This leads to imbalance of globin chain synthesis which results in a thalassemia-like morphology of the RBCs. Hemoglobin E is the second most common hemoglobinopathy worldwide. The highest prevalence of Hb E is found in South East Asia (Thailand, Cambodia, and Laos), where the prevalence reaches 20–30%. It is also common in the Indian subcontinent (India, Pakistan, Bangladesh, and Sri Lanka), Vietnam, Nepal, China, Turkey, Malaysia, and the Phillipines. This distribution is probably due to its protective function against falciparum malaria. It has been brought to North America and Europe through immigration.

Clinical Picture

Heterozygous patients (Hb AE) have normal hematologic values except for a mild microcytosis and target cells identified on the peripheral blood smear. Homozygous patients (Hb EE) have a mild compensated hypochromic microcytic anemia. Mild splenomegaly may be present. Co-inheritance of Hb E with β-thalassemia is the major concern for patients with Hb E. Patients with E/β-thalassemia disease have a highly variable clinical and hematologic manifestations ranging from mild thalassemia trait-like hypochromic, microcytic anemia to severe transfusion-dependant hemolytic anemia. Around 50% of the patients are phenotypically similar to β-thalassemia major. The severity seems to be influenced by several factors including the type of the inherited β gene (E/β0 vs E/β+ disease), associated inheritance of α-thalassemia, and possibly environmental factors. Co-inheritance with Hb S (ES) results in a phenotypically mild sickle cell disease. Patients have fewer problems with vaso-occlusive crisis, splenic sequestration crisis, and increased susceptibility to infection than patients with Hb SS.

Diagnosis

Hemoglobin E should be considered in a patient with hypochromic, microcytic anemia, especially if the family history or ethnicity is suggestive of the gene inheritance. It has the same mobility as Hb C and Hb A2 in alkaline medium. It can be differentiated from Hb C by electrophoresis at acid pH, in which its mobility is the same as Hb A and Hb A2. High performance liquid chromatography separates Hb E from hemoglobins A and C.

Treatment

No treatment is needed for Hb E. Treatment for E/β-thalassemia depends on the severity of the anemia and its complications. Mild cases require no therapy except folic acid supplementation. Treatment of severe case is the same as β-thalassemia major. ES disease is managed as patients with SS disease.

Counseling

Patients with heterozygous and homozygous Hb E should be counseled when having children with individuals who have β-thalassemia, Hb SS, β-thalassemia trait, or sickle cell trait.

Hemoglobin D

There are a number of hemoglobins termed "hemoglobin D". Hemoglobin D-Punjab (also called Hb Los

Angeles) and hemoglobin Ibadan are the most common ones. Hemoglobin D-Punjab is a mutant hemoglobin that results from the genetic substitution of glutamic acid by glutamine at position 121 in the β globin chain. It occurs most commonly in the Punjab part of the Indian subcontinent and Iran, where the reported prevalence is around 2%. It is also reported in the Turkish, Algerian, West African, Saudi Arabian, African American, Native American, English, and Irish population. The occurrence of the gene in the United Kingdom and Ireland is mostly a result of immigration from and intermarriage with people from the Indian subcontinent.

Clinical Picture

People with hemoglobin D trait (Hb AD) are asymptomatic and they have normal hemoglobin level and normal red blood cells indices. Homozygous disease (Hb DD) is extremely rare. Patients usually have normal hemoglobin level and normal red blood cells indices. Co-inheritance with hemoglobin S (Hb SD) results in a mild form of sickle cell disease. Patients usually have fewer problems with vaso-occlusive crisis, infection, organ damage or splenic sequestration crisis than Hb SS patients. Some patients, however, develop serious complications including stroke. Co-inheritance with β-thalassemia (Hb D/β-thal) results in mild to moderate hypochromic, microcytic anemia.

Diagnosis

Hemoglobin D has the same mobility as hemoglobin S in alkaline media. It can be differentiated from hemoglobin S by their distinct mobility in acid media, in which hemoglobin D migrates with hemoglobin A and by the fact that hemoglobin D does not sickle. An increased number of target cells is seen on review of the peripheral blood smear. Red blood cells' osmotic fragility is decreased. Differentiating Hb DD from D/β-0thal can be a problem, as both have over 95% hemoglobin D with no hemoglobin A. Red blood cells in patients affected by Hb D/β0-thal are hypochromic and microcytic. At least one parent is expected to have β-thalassemia or β-thalassemia trait.

Treatment

No treatment is needed for Hb AD or Hb DD except for folic acid supplementation, as the patients are clinically and hematologically normal. Patients with Hb SD and Hb D/β-thal are treated as those with Hb SS and β-thalassemia intermedia or thalassemia major, respectively. Therapy depends on the severity and/or complications of the disease.

Counseling

Patients with either heterozygous or homozygous hemoglobin D should be counseled when having children with individuals who have β-thalassemia, Hb SS, β-thalassemia trait, or sickle cell trait.

Hemoglobin O Arab

Hemoglobin O Arab results from genetic substitution of lysine for glutamic acid at position121 in the β globin chain. It is mainly found in the Middle East, the Balkans, Greece, North Africa, West Africa, and in African Americans.

Clinical Picture

Persons with hemoglobin O-Arab trait (Hb A/O Arab) are asymptomatic and have normal hemoglobin levels and normal or mildly microcytic red blood cells. Homozygous disease is extremely rare. Patients are asymptomatic with normal hemoglobin or mild compensated hemolytic anemia. Red blood cells are microcytic with high MCHC. Co-inheritance with hemoglobin S (S/O Arab) results in a moderate sickle cell disease–like clinical picture with variable severity. Patients may have vaso-occlusive events, splenomegaly, jaundice, and reticulocytosis. Hemoglobin level ranges betweem7 and 8 g/dl. Co-inheritance with β-thalassemia results in a thalassemia intermedia picture.

Diagnosis

The red blood cells in patients with heterozygous or homozygous hemoglobin O-Arab are either morphologically normal or mildly microcytic. Hemoglobin O Arab migrates with Hb C in alkaline media and it migrates between hemoglobins A and S in acid media. It can be identified by high performance liquid chromatography.

Treatment

No treatment (except folic acid supplementation) is needed for Hg A/O Arab or Hb O Arab/O Arab, as the patients are clinically and hematologically normal. Patients with Hb S/O Arab and Hb O Arab/β-thal are treated as those with Hb SS and β-thalassemia intermedia or thalassemia major, respectively. Therapy depends on the severity and/or complications of the disease.

Unstable Hemoglobins

Unstable hemoglobins are inherited structurally abnormal hemoglobins characterized by decreased solubility, resulting in intracellular hemoglobin precipitation forming intracorpuscular Heinz bodies and shortened red blood cells survival.

Pathophysiology

Unstable hemoglobins result from substitution or deletion of amino acids in one of the globin chains. (α, β, or γ). Decreased solubility of the unstable hemoglobins results from the weak binding between globin and heme parts of the hemoglobin and from interference with the tertiary and quaternary structure of the subunits. As a result, hemoglobin is denatured and precipitated inside the red blood cell as Heinz bodies. Heinz bodies attach to the cell membrane and make red blood cells susceptible to destruction by the spleen.

Clinical Picture

Unstable hemoglobins are rare. They are mostly inherited as dominant disorders. Approximately, 250 mutations have been identified so far. Chronic hemolytic anemia of variable severity is the main clinical manifestation. The severity of anemia and the age of its onset depend on the type of the mutation and are modified by extrinsic factors. Mutations involving the γ chain (Hb Poole) are associated with transient hemolytic anemia and jaundice in the newborn, which lasts for the first few months of life. It resolves as hemoglobin A replaces hemoglobin F. Mutations involving the α chain (Hb Hasharon) presents with anemia and jaundice in the neonatal period and persists lifelong. People who inherit an unstable hemoglobin involving the β chain (Hb Koln and Hb Zurich) are hematologically normal at birth. Anemia and dark colored urine (pigmenturia) develop at 2–4 months of age, as hemoglobin F is replaced with hemoglobin A. Patients may develop acute hemolytic episodes triggered by infection or exposure to oxidant drugs and may develop transient aplastic crisis with parvovirus B19 infection. As in other chronic hemolytic anemia, patients may develop cholelithiasis. Patients with the rare types of unstable hemoglobin named "hyperunstable hemoglobin" have a thalassemia intermedia-like clinical and hematologic picture. They have moderately severe hypochromic, microcytic anemia with or without splenomegaly.

Diagnosis

Diagnosis should be suspected in a patient with hemolytic anemia and RBC Heinz bodies found using supravital stains. Diagnosis is confirmed by the heat stability test or isopropanol stability test. Hemoglobin electrophoresis is usually not useful for diagnosis of the unstable or hyperunstable hemoglobins. In these cases, globin chain sequencing using DNA based methods is required to confirm the diagnosis.

Treatment

Treatment is mainly supportive with folic acid and avoidance of oxidant drugs. Blood transfusion is rarely needed as most patients are asymptomatic or have compensated anemia. Splenectomy may be required in the very few severe cases. Splenectomy does not always ameliorate anemia.

High Oxygen Affinity Hemoglobins

Over 200 variants of high oxygen affinity hemoglobins have been described. The oxygen dissociation curve in these patients is shifted to the left. Oxygen delivery to the tissues is poor resulting in tissue hypoxia, increased erythropoietin level and secondary erythrocytosis. Individuals with these hemoglobin variants are usually asymptomatic and require no therapy. However, they should be considered in the differential diagnosis of erythrocytosis.

References

Adekile AD, Kazanetz EG, Leonova JY et al (1996) Co-inheritance of Hb D-Punjab (codon 121; GAA –> CAA) and β0 thalassemia (IVS-II-1; G–> A). J Pediatr Hematol Oncol 18:151–153

Agarwal S, Gupta UR, Kohli N et al (1989) Prevalence of haemoglobin D in Uttar Pradesh. J Med Res 90:39–43

Agarwal A, Guindo A, Cissoko Y et al (2000) Hemoglobin C associated with protection from severe malaria in the Dogon of Mali, a West African population with low prevalence of hemoglobin S. Blood 96:2358–2363

Agarwal N, Mojica-Henshaw MP, Simmons ED et al (2007) Familial polycythemia caused by a novel mutation in the beta globin gene: essential role of P50 in evaluation of familial polycythemia. Int J Med 4:232–236

Ashtiani MT, Monajemzadeh M, Sina AH et al (2009) Prevalence of haemoglobinopathies in 34,000 healthy adults in Tehran, Iran. J Clin Pathol 62:924–925

Atalay EO, Koyuncu H, Turgut B et al (2005) High incidence of Hb D-Los Angeles (β121(GH4) GLU – >Gln) in Denizli province, Aegean region of Turkey. Hemoglobin 29:307–310

Athanasiou-Metaxa M, Economou M, Tsatra I et al (2002) Co-inheritance of hemoglobin D-Punjab and hemoglobin S: a case report (letter). J Pediatr Hematol Oncol 24:421

Bachir DD, Galacteros F (2004) Hemoglobin C, Orphanet Encyclopedia www.orpha.net/data/patol/GB/uk. November

Bain BJ (2009) C/beta0 thalassemia. Am J Hematol 84:749

Brugnara C, Kopin AS, Bunn HF et al (1985) Regulation of cation content and cell volume in hemoglobin erythrocytes from patients with homozygous hemoglobin C disease. J Clin Invest 75:1608–1617

Cario H (2005) Childhood polycythemia/erythrocytosis: classification, diagnosis, clinical presentation and treatment. Ann Hematol 84:137–145

Chernoff AI (1958) The hemoglobin D syndrome. Blood 13:116–127

Efremov GD, Simjanovska L, Plaseska-Karanfilska D et al (2007) Hb Jambol: a new hyperunstable hemoglobin causing severe hemolytic anemia. Acta Haematol 117:1–7

Fairhurst RM, Fujioka H, Hayton K et al (2003) Aberrant development of Plasmodium falciparum in hemoglobin CC red cells: implications for the malaria protective effect of the homozygous state. Blood 101:3309–3315

Fort JA, Graham-Pole JR, Chopik J (1988) Vaso occlusion with homozygous hemoglobin C disease. Am J Pediatr Hematol Oncol 10:323–325

Fucharoen S, Winichagoon P (2000) Clinical and hematologic aspects of hemoglobin E beta-thalassemia. Curr Opin Hematol 7:106–112

Fucharoen S, Ketvichit P, Pootrakul P et al (2000) Clinical manifestation of beta thalassemia/hemoglobin E disease. J Pediatr Hematol Oncol 22:552–557

Hafsia R, Gouider S, Ben Moussa S et al (2007) Hemoglobin O Arab: about 20 cases. Tunis Méd 85:637–640

Kishore B, Khare P, Gupta RJ et al (2007) Hemoglobin E disease in North Indian population: a report of 11 cases. Hematology 12:343–347

Mantovani A, Figinin I (2008) Sickle cell-hemoglobin C retinopathy: transient obstruction of retinal and choroidal circulations and transient drying out of retinal neovessels. Int Ophthalmol 28:135–137

Masiello D, Heeney MM, Adewoye AH et al (2007) Hemoglobin SE disease a concise review. Am J Hematol 82:643–649

Masmas TN, Garly ML, Lisse IM et al (2006) Inherited hemoglobin disorders in Guinea- Bissau, West Africa: a population study. Hemoglobin 30:355–364

Olivieri NF, Muraca GM, O'Donnell A et al (2008) Studies in haemoglobin E – beta thalassemia. Br J Haematol 141:388–397

Owaidah TM, Al-Saleh MM, Al-Hellani AM (2005) Hemoglobin D/beta-thalassemia and beta-thalassemia major in a Saudi family. Saudi Med J 26:674–677

Papadopoulos V, Vassiliadou D, Xanthopoulidis G et al (2003) The implications of haemoglobin O-Arab mutation. Haema 6:479–485

Papadopoulos V, Dermitzakis E, Konstantinidou D et al (2005) Hb O-Arab mutation originated in the Pomak population of Greek Thrace (letter). Haematologica 90:255–257

Pegelow CH, Mack AK (1989) Incidence of hemoglobins S and C in infants born in Miami to recent Haitian immigrants. Trop Geogr Med 41:316–319

Percy MJ, Butt NN, Crotty GM et al (2009) Identification of high oxygen affinity hemoglobin variant in the investigation of patients with erythrocytosis. Haematologica 94:1321–1322

Perea FJ, Casas-Castaneda M, Villalobos-Arambula AR et al (1999) Hb D-Los Angeles associated with Hb S or beta-thalassemia in four Mexican Mestizo families. Hemoglobin 23:231–237

Petkov GH, Simjanovska L, Tchakarova P et al (2005) Hb Stara Zagora: a new hyper-unstable hemoglobin causing severe hemolytic anemia. Hemoglobin 29:249–256

Prehu C, Pissard S, Al-Sheikh M et al (2005) Two French Caucasian families with dominant thalassemia-like phenotypes due to hyperunstable hemoglobin variant: Hb Sainte Seve [codon 118(-T)] and codon 127 (CA→TAG [Gln→Stop]). Hemoglobin 29:229–233

Premawardhena A, Fisher CA, Olivieri NF et al (2005) Hemoglobin E beta thalassemia in Sri Lanka. Lancet 366:1467–1470

Rachmilewitz EA, Tamari H, Liff F et al (1985) The interaction of hemoglobin O Arab with HbS and beta+ thalassemia among Israeli Arabs. Hum Genet 70:119–125

Richet P, Flori L, Tall F (2004) Hemoglobin C is associated with reduced Plasmodium falciparum parasitemia and low risk of malaria attack. Hum Mol Genet 13:1–6

Rivera-Ruiz M, Varon J, Sternbach GL (2008a) Acute splenic sequestration in an adult with hemoglobin S-C disease. Am J Emerg Med 26(1064):e5–e8

Rivera-Ruiz M, Varon J, Sternbach GL (2008b) Acute splenic sequestration in an adult with hemoglobin S-C disease. Am J Emerg Med 26(1064):e5–e8

Sangare A, Sango M, Meite M et al (1992) Hemoglobin O Arab in Ivory Coast and Western Africa. Med Trop 52:163–167

Thomburg CD, Zimmerman SA, Schultz WH et al (2001) An infant with homozygous hemoglobin D-Iran. J Pediatr Hematol Oncol 23:67–68

Vichinsky E (2007) Hemoglobin E syndrome. Hematol Am Soc Hematol Educ Program 2007:79–83

Vichinsky EP, MacKlin EA, Waye JS et al (2005) Changes in the epidemiology of thalassemia in North America: a new minority disease. Pediatrics 116:e818–e825

Wajcman H, Galacteros F (2005) Hemoglobins with high oxygen affinity leading to erythrocytosis. New variants and new concept. Hemoglobin 29:91–106

Wajcman H, Traeger-Synodinos J, Papassotiriou I et al (2008) Unstable and thalassemic alpha chain hemoglobin variants: a cause of Hb H disease and thalassemia intermedia. Hemoglobin 32:327–349

Ware OJF, RE SWH et al (1994) Hemoglobin C in infancy and childhood. J Pediatr 125:745–747

Weatherall DJ (2000) Introduction to the problem of hemoglobin EB thalassemia. J Pediatr Hematol Oncol 22:551

Williamson D (1993) The unstable haemoglobins. Blood Rev 7:146–163

Zimmerman SA, O'Branski EE, Rosse WF et al (1999) Hemoglobin S/O Arab: thirteen new cases and review of the literature. Am J Hematol 60:279–284

326 Thalassemia

Nameeta P. Richard · Kristina M. Haley · Michael Recht

General Considerations

A red blood cell (RBC) contains approximately 640 million hemoglobin molecules, which allow the red cell to perform its essential function of oxygen delivery in exchange for carbon dioxide. Alteration of the hemoglobin molecule can result in various forms of anemia and their subsequent long-term complications. Hemoglobin abnormalities can be a result of synthesis of abnormal hemoglobin as in Sickle Cell Disease, or abnormalities can result from reduced synthesis of normal hemoglobin, as in thalassemia.

Hemoglobin synthesis, a process that predominantly occurs in the mitochondria of the cells, changes as a fetus develops, is born, and becomes an adult. At any point of hemoglobin development, though, a hemoglobin molecule is made up of four polypeptide chains. In order to accommodate for differences in oxygen delivery requirements as a fetus develops and enters extrauterine life, different polypeptide chains come together to create hemoglobin molecules with oxygen affinity specific for their current environment. The genes for the polypeptide chains are located on chromosomes 11 and 16, and the genes result in the synthesis of six different globin chains: alpha, beta, gamma, delta, epsilon, and zelta. Pairs of these globin chains come together to form tetramers, resulting in functional hemoglobin molecules. In embryonic development, the predominant hemoglobin molecules are $\zeta_2\varepsilon_2$ (Hemoglobin Gower 1), $\zeta_2\gamma_2$ (Hemoglobin Portland), and $\alpha_2\varepsilon_2$ (Hemoglobin Gower 2). Hemoglobin F ($\alpha_2\gamma_2$) is the most prevalent hemoglobin in later fetal development, while the primary hemoglobin in an older infant and an adult is Hemoglobin A1 ($\alpha_2\beta_2$), with small portions of Hemoglobin F as well as Hemoglobin A2 ($\alpha_2\delta_2$) (➋ *Fig. 326.1*). In the first 3–6 months of life, the amount of β chain production increases, and the γ-chain is mostly replaced by β-chain (➋ *Fig. 326.2*). Eventually, the cell synthesizes α-chains in proportion to β-chains in order to match the two together and create adult hemoglobin.

Problems arise when the cells are unable to synthesize the normal amount of α- or β-chain as the two will become mismatched, resulting in decreased synthesis of normal, adult hemoglobin. The general-term thalassemia refers to a group of genetic anemias that are a result of inadequate or absent synthesis of normal globin chains. Thus, in contrast to Sickle Cell Anemia where an abnormal hemoglobin is created, thalassemia is a *quantitative defect* in hemoglobin synthesis. The clinical picture of a patient with thalassemia depends on which chain is affected and how many genes are deleted or mutated.

Epidemiology

The genes producing the different types of thalassemia can be found throughout the world, but they are concentrated in the Mediterranean area, Southeast Asia, India, and Middle East (➋ *Fig. 326.3*). It appears that the heterozygote state provides increased resistance to *falciparum* malaria, much like the genes for Sickle Cell Anemia and Glucose-6-Phosphate Dehydrogenase Deficiency.

Categories of Thalassemia

The thalassemias are a heterogeneous group of anemias resulting from a reduced or absent rate of production of one or more of the globin chains. This quantitative decrease in globin chain synthesis results in the microcytic, hypochromic anemias, called α-thalassemia and β-thalassemia. The classification of thalassemias can be based on which globin chain is decreased or absent.

α-Thalassemia

General Information

The majority of α-thalassemia is a result of deletion of one or more of the α-globin genes. Normal cells have four α-globin genes, and the clinical variability seen in α-thalassemia is in direct relation to the number of genes deleted (➋ *Fig. 326.4*). Deletion of one gene results in a silent carrier state of α-thalassemia. If two genes are deleted (on either chromosome), then the patient has α-thalassemia trait. Hemoglobin H disease refers to the state of three genes being deleted, and results in

Abdelaziz Y. Elzouki (ed.), *Textbook of Clinical Pediatrics*, DOI 10.1007/978-3-642-02202-9_326,

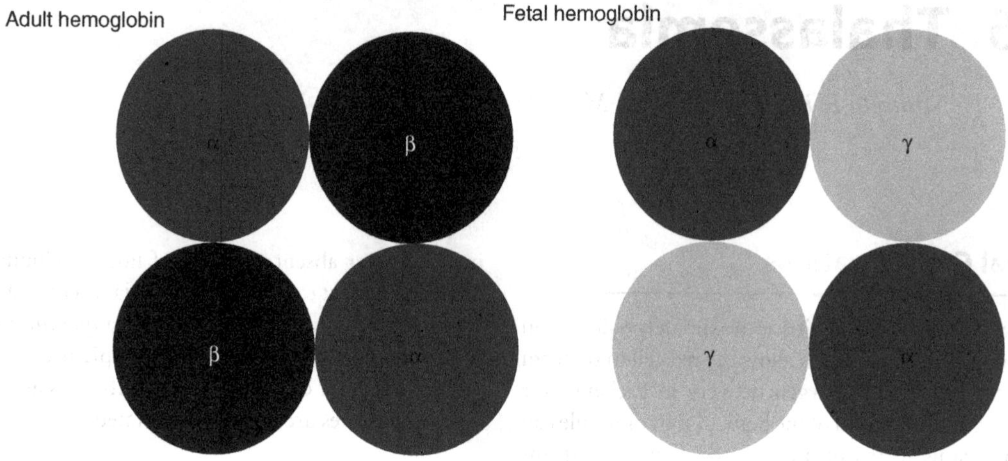

Figure 326.1

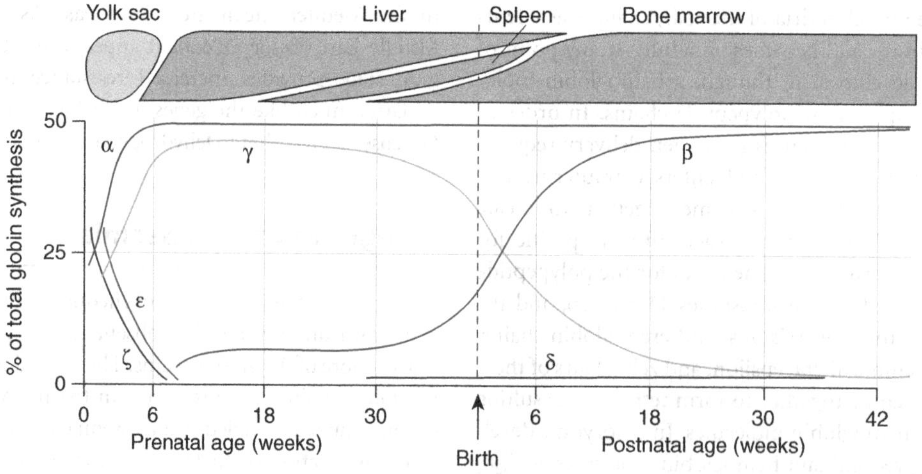

Figure 326.2

a moderately severe anemia. Deletion of all four genes results in hydrops fetalis and is incompatible with extra-uterine life.

Clinical Characteristics

As stated previously, the clinical features seen in α-thalassemia are directly related to the number of genes deleted. See *Table 326.1* for a summary of α-thalassemia syndromes, clinical features, and hemoglobin electrophoresis findings.

Individuals who have three α-globin genes present are asymptomatic and have normal hemoglobin levels and mean corpuscular volume (MCV). These silent carriers may come to the pediatrician's attention as a result of a newborn screen report of Hemoglobin Bart's (*Fig. 326.5*). Hemoglobin Bart's is a type of hemoglobin made of four γ-globin chains. Silent carriers show 0–3% hemoglobin Bart's during the newborn period. Eventually, as the γ-chain is replaced by β-chain, the Hemoglobin Bart's disappears. A follow-up hemoglobin electrophoresis at 6 months of age would be normal but is largely unnecessary.

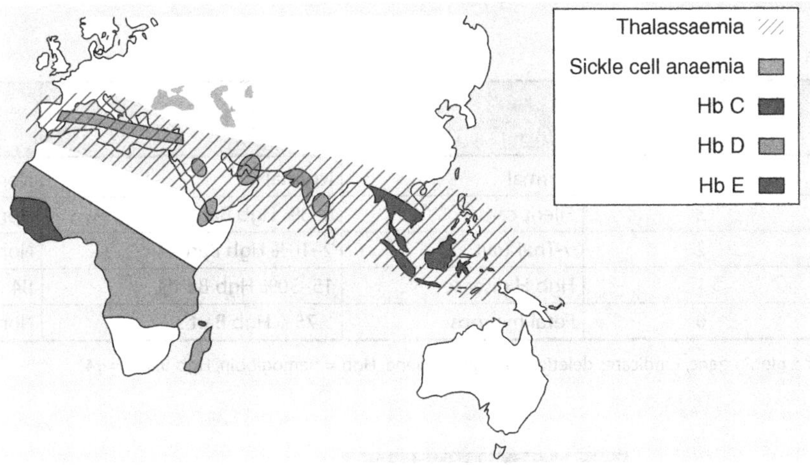

Figure 326.3
Caption missing

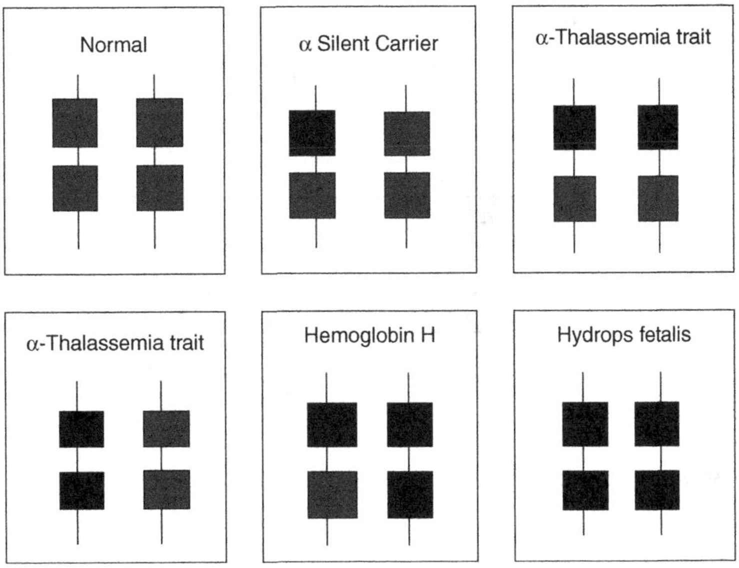

Figure 326.4
The genetics of α-thalassemia. ■ = normal genes ■ = gene deletions

Individuals with only two α-globin genes present are usually asymptomatic as well, and this is termed α-thalassemia trait. As an infant, the MCV will likely be <100, the hemoglobin may be slightly low, and the peripheral smear will appear slightly hypochromic with few target cells. On hemoglobin electrophoresis, α-thalassemia trait patients have 2–10% hemoglobin Bart's at birth, but the electrophoresis is normal after >6 months of age.

When three out of the four α-globin genes are deleted, an individual will have mild to moderately severe microcytic, hypochromic anemia (Hgb 7–11g/dL). This is known as hemoglobin H disease. Hemoglobin H is created when excess β-globins come together to form a tetramer (β_4). Hemoglobin H can aggregate within a red blood cell, forming an inclusion body and resulting in hemolysis. The peripheral blood smear shows

Table 326.1
The α thalassemias

Genotype	# of α genes present	Clinical characteristics	Hgb electrophoresis at birth	Hgb electrophoresis >6 months
αα / αα	4	Normal	Normal	Normal
-α / αα	3	Silent carrier	0–3% Hgb Bart's	Normal
- - / αα or -α/-α	2	α-Thal trait	2–10% Hgb Bart's	Normal
- - / - α	1	Hgb H disease	15–30% Hgb Bart's	β4
- - / - -	0	Fetal hydrops	>75% Hgb Bart's	None

α refers to presence of α globin gene, - indicates deletion of α globin gene, Hgb = hemoglobin, Hgb Bart's = γ4

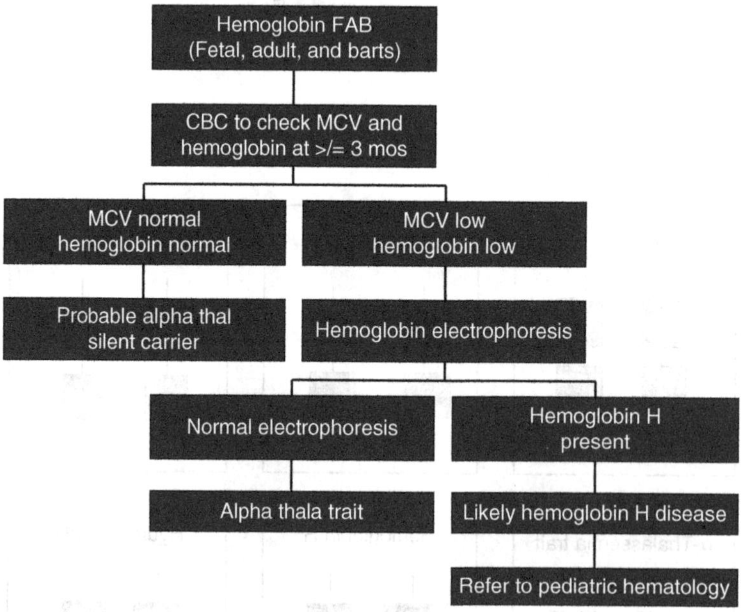

Figure 326.5
α-thalassemia newborn screen results

microcytosis, hypochromia, and poikilocytosis (abnormal cell shape). On hemoglobin electrophoresis, patients with hemoglobin H disease have 15–30% hemoglobin Bart's at birth. As older infants and children, hemoglobin H will continue to be present on electrophoresis. Patients with Hemoglobin H disease generally do well in the first decade of life and do not require many transfusions. However, they will likely show evidence of chronic hemolysis with hepatosplenomegaly, elevated indirect bilirubin, and increased susceptibility to aplastic crisis. In addition, because of ineffective eythropoiesis, patients may have skeletal abnormalities and hepatosplenomegaly, which is less severe than in β-thalassemia (see "Clinical Characteristics" in β-Thalassemia). As the patient ages, they may require more frequent and eventually chronic transfusions and begin to experience the consequences of iron overload (see "Complications" in β-Thalassemia). Finally, Hemoglobin H is readily oxidized and makes the patient especially susceptible to oxidative stress as in Glucose-6-Phosphate Dehydrogenase Deficiency, and oxidative stressors should be avoided.

Individuals with deletion of all four α-globin chains have intrauterine anemia and hydrops fetalis, which is incompatible with extrauterine life. This is the most severe form of α-thalassemia. On hemoglobin electrophoresis, these patients have mostly Hemoglobin Bart's and absent fetal or adult hemoglobin.

Differential Diagnosis

Patient's with α-thalassemia trait will have evidence of microcytosis, and other causes of microcytic anemia should be considered such as iron deficiency, lead exposure, β-thalassemia minor, and other hemoglobinopathies. When compared to children with iron deficiency anemia, patients with α-thalassemia trait have normal or increased ferritin and serum iron. When compared to children with β-thalassemia minor, patients with α-thalassemia trait have normal hemoglobin electrophoresis as older infants and children. Newborns with Hemoglobin Bart's on newborn screen may be a silent carrier of α-thalassemia, may have α-thalassemia trait, or may have α-thalassemia. In an infant with hydrops fetalis, one must also consider other causes of intrauterine anemia such as alloimmunization.

Complications

A common scenario seen in patients with α-thalassemia is unnecessary prescription of oral iron because a child has microcytic anemia thought to be due to iron deficiency. Patients with hemoglobin H disease may require blood transfusions when exposed to oxidant stressors or as they age. Chronic transfusions may result in iron overload and subsequent cardiac, hepatic, endocrine, pulmonary, and renal effects. Mothers of infants with fetal hydrops have complications such as hemorrhage after delivery, and if possible, should be counseled on therapeutic termination of pregnancy.

Treatment and Prognosis

Children with α-thalassemia trait generally do not require treatment and lead a normal life. Similar to patients with G6PD deficiency, individuals with hemoglobin H disease should take folic acid and avoid medications which cause oxidant stress. In addition, hemoglobin H patients may require splenectomy due to the development of hypersplenism. However, the prognosis for most patients with Hemoglobin H disease is excellent, but there are some exceptions that require more extensive treatment and experience more severe complications. Finally, mothers of children with fetal hydrops should have genetic counseling in order to plan for future pregnancies.

β Thalassemia

General Information

In β-thalassemia, the genetic abnormality is most commonly a result of a point mutation. Normal cells, in contrast to the α-globin genes, have only two β-globin genes. Similar to α-thalassemia, though, the phenotypic heterogeneity is a result of the number of normal genes present. If the gene is altered in such a way that no β-globin is produced, then it is termed β^0. If instead the gene is altered in a way that results in a deficit of β-globin, then it is termed β^+. An individual may be heterozygote or homozygote for the altered β gene. Patients that are heterozygotes and produce enough β-globin chain to not develop clinically significant disease typically have β-thalassemia minor. Homozygotes may have β-thalassemia major (also known as Cooley Anemia) or thalassemia intermedia, depending on if they are β^0 or if they are β^+ with a more significant deficiency (➲ *Fig. 326.6*). In addition to the anemia that results from decreased normal adult hemoglobin synthesis, there can be marked hemolysis as the result of precipitation of unpaired α-globin chains.

Clinical Characteristics

Individuals with β-thalassemia minor are asymptomatic, but their complete blood count will be significant for microcytosis with or without a mild anemia. The peripheral blood smear shows hypochromia, target cells, and basophilic stippling (as a result of α-globin chain precipitation). The hemoglobin electrophoresis at birth will be normal, but after 6 months of age, it will show elevated hemoglobin A_2 and hemoglobin F.

Patients with β-thalassemia intermedia fall somewhere between β-thalassemia minor and β-thalassemia major and have varying degrees of anemia. The anemia is typically significant but does not require transfusions as frequently as β-thalassemia major. However, a patient with anemia and a marked microcytosis with splenomegaly and skeletal changes consistent with bone marrow expansion should raise suspicion for β-thalassemia intermedia.

Individuals with β-thalassemia major are normal at birth because β-globin gene production is not necessary for embryonic or fetal hemoglobin. However, it is unlikely for these patients to be missed because the newborn screen will be abnormal as no hemoglobin A will be present. At 3–6 months of life, the infant will become symptomatic as γ-globin production switches to β-globin production.

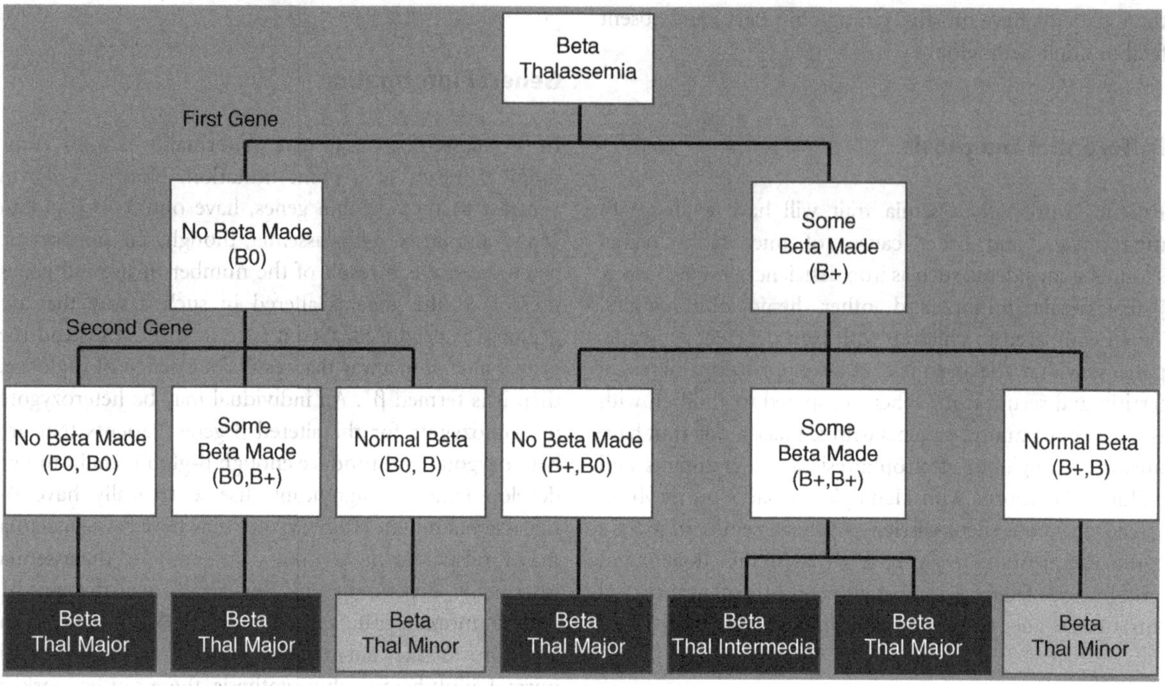

Figure 326.6
Genetics of Beta Thalassemia. The genetic abnormality seen in Beta Thalassemia is a result of a point mutation, which means that the gene is present but altered. The alteration determines, when the gene is expressed, how much Beta globin is made. There can be a variety of Beta globin production when some Beta is expressed as in Beta +. The phenotype of Beta thalassemia can vary for a given genotype

Because little to no β-globin chains will be produced, excess α-globin accumulates. These excess α-globin chains precipitate in red cells at all stages of their development and result in ineffective erythropoiesis and hemolysis. Thus, severe anemia is present because of deceased hemoglobin production as well as destruction of red cells. Similarly, symptoms are present both because of inadequate hemoglobin synthesis as well as hemolysis. The peripheral blood smear of these patients shows severe hypochromic, microcytic anemia with anisocytosis (variety of cell size) and poikilocytosis (abnormal cell shape). A plethora of target cells is a hallmark of the β-thalassemia peripheral blood smear.

The clinical features of β-thalassemia major are many and affect nearly every organ system. As a result of red blood cell destruction, there is extensive extramedullary hematopoiesis within the liver, spleen, kidneys, and entire skeletal system. Hepatomegaly develops and changes in the liver are similar to those seen in viral hepatitis and can result in variable liver dysfunction. Splenomegaly further accentuates the anemia by resulting in increased red cell destruction as well as red cell pooling. Some patients require splenectomy, which places them at increased risk for serious bacterial infection with encapsulated organisms. The expansion of bones for additional hematopoiesis leads to the characteristic thalassemia facies with bossed skull, prominent frontal and parietal bones, and enlarged maxilla. A skull x-ray in β-thalassemia major shows a "hair-on-end" appearance because of extramedullary hematopoiesis. Other bones may be at increased risk of fracture due to thinning of the cortex.

Chronic hemolysis results in elevated indirect bilirubin with subsequent gallstone formation, elevated LDH, increased susceptibility to aplastic crisis (as in Parvovirus B19 infection), and hypersplenism. In addition, patients with β-thalassemia major can experience high-output cardiac failure if frequent transfusions are not administered.

Patients with β-thalassemia major are typically managed with chronic transfusions. The iron overload that results from chronic transfusions is compounded by the fact that patients with β-thalassemia major have increased dietary iron absorption. Iron overload in these patients affects many different organ systems and is further discussed in the ➔ "Complications".

Differential Diagnosis

The differential for microcytic, hypochromic anemias includes iron deficiency anemia, α-thalassemia, β-thalassemias, lead poisoning, and other hemoglobinopathies. One way to begin to differentiate iron deficiency and thalassemia is to calculate the Mentzer Index (mean corpuscular volume divided by red blood cell number). Individuals with β-thalassemia minor have a Mentzer Index <13, while iron deficient patients typically have a Mentzer Index >13. An elevated hemoglobin A_2 is diagnostic for β-thalassemia minor, but a normal hemoglobin A_2 level can be misleading since it can be decreased in iron deficiency. In order to differentiate the most common cause of transfusion dependent anemia worldwide, β-thalassemia major, from hemoglobin E/β-thalassemia, one should obtain a hemoglobin electrophoresis.

Treatment

Children with β-thalassemia minor should not receive long-term iron therapy and do not require folic acid supplementation. The two main treatments for β-thalassemia major are chronic transfusions with iron chelation therapy and bone marrow transplantation. Due to the severity of their anemia, children with β-thalassemia intermedia and major need referral to a pediatric hematologist in early childhood to manage issues such as chronic transfusions, prevention of iron overload with chelation therapy, and management of hypersplenism. Children with β-thalassemia major and hemoglobin <6 g/dL should receive chronic transfusions with usual target hemoglobin of 10 g/dL to maintain growth and decrease frequency of infections. Chelation therapy options to avoid iron overload include IV deferoxamine or oral deferasirox (Exjade), which prevents or, at least, limits cardiac, liver, and endocrine complications such as congestive heart failure, hepatic failure, diabetes mellitus, osteoporosis, and delayed puberty. The addition of Vitamin C increases the excretion of iron produced by deferoxamine.

Complications

Like α-thalassemia minor, the most common complication of β-thalassemia minor is the unnecessary prescription of oral iron because a child has microcytic anemia thought to be due to iron deficiency. The most significant complication in β-thalassemia major is iron overload as a result of chronic transfusion and increased iron absorption. Iron overload affects nearly every body system. In the liver, iron accumulates in the Kupffer cells and eventually will result in hepatic fibrosis and potentially end-stage liver disease. Endocrine dysfunctions from chronic iron overload include hypogonadism, growth failure, diabetes, and hypothyroidism. Iron often infiltrates the cardiac muscle in overload states and can result in a restrictive cardiomyopathy and arrhythmias. Iron deposition can also occur in the skin and result in a gray skin color. However, without blood transfusions, these children will suffer from inadequate growth, increased susceptibility to infections, and high-output cardiac failure. Many patients will develop splenomegaly and hypersplenism, which may necessitate splenectomy. In patients undergoing splenectomy, pneumococcal and *Haemophilus* influenza type B vaccine should be administered prior to surgery. After splenectomy, these children should remain on prophylactic penicillin and seek immediate medical attention for febrile illnesses.

Prognosis

Life expectancy for β-thalassemia depends on the severity of the anemia and requirement for chronic blood transfusions. Specifically, without bone marrow transplantation, children with β-thalassemia major will likely die in their third decade of life as a result of complications from chronic blood transfusions and iron overload symptoms.

Other Thalassemias

In addition to α- and β-thalassemia, there are many other abnormalities of globin chains, which can result in the thalassemia phenotype either alone or in combination with α- or β-thalassemia. Furthermore, a patient can be affected simultaneously by both a qualitative abnormality of hemoglobin synthesis as well as a quantitative defect. Although gene deletions are the most common cause of α-thalassemia, some cases of α-thalassemia are a result of point mutations. Hemoglobin Constant Spring is a result of a mutation that alters termination of translation causing an elongated, unstable α-globin chain. If a patient with two alpha gene deletions also has Hemoglobin Constant Spring, they will have a clinical syndrome similar to Hemoglobin H disease but may require more frequent transfusions. Hemoglobin E is a result of an amino acid substitution on the β-chain, and this mutation results in activation of an mRNA splice site and subsequent reduced β-chain synthesis. Hemoglobin E/β-thalassemia is common in Southeast Asia and typically results in a β-thalassemia major phenotype, and the patient requires chronic transfusions. In addition, β-thalassemia can combine with Sickle Cell Anemia in a variety of clinical scenarios that largely depend on the extent of β-gene production.

Future Directions

Current treatment for thalassemia involves chronic transfusions and therapy to prevent or treat the complications of iron overload. However, transfusions treat the symptoms of the disease, not the disease itself. If there were more fetal hemoglobin present, then the need for adult hemoglobin would be reduced. In Sickle Cell Disease, Hydroxyurea has become a commonly used agent to increase the proportion of fetal hemoglobin made. Hydroxyurea has been shown in clinical trials to increase hemoglobin and MCV and reduce the need for transfusions in patients with thalassemia intermedia and thalassemia major. However, further work needs to be done prior to Hydroxyurea becoming a mainstay of thalassemia treatment. Bone Marrow Transplant is currently the only known cure for thalassemia, however; bone marrow transplant requires that the patient be healthy enough to undergo the myeloablative pre-transplant conditioning and that there is an available donor source. Extensive work-up must be done prior to transplant in order to assess pre-transplant morbidity, and the family must be well counseled on the possible complications of transplant, including but not limited to graft rejection, graft failure, graft versus host disease, and death. Despite these complications, there have been many successful matched related donor transplants for thalassemia patients. Finally, gene therapy has been proposed as a cure for thalassemia major. The idea of replacing the abnormal β-globin gene with a normal β-globin gene transported via an autologous Hematopoietic stem cell transplant seems plausible, but this therapeutic strategy has met a variety of challenges and has not yet become a part of thalassemia treatment.

In summary, the microcytic, hypochromic anemia that results from the quantitative defects of hemoglobin production seen in thalassemia have a wide range of clinical significance. Disease severity is a function of the number of absent or abnormal genes as well as the aggregation of excess globin chains. Many patients will be brought to the pediatrician's attention as a result of an abnormal newborn screen, but the diagnosis should be included in the differential for any patient who presents with a microcytic anemia. In taking care of patients with more significant disease states, it is important to recognize the signs and symptoms of hemolysis and chronic iron overload.

References

Ambruso DR, Hays T, Goldenberg NA (2009) Hematologic disorders. In: Hay WW Jr, Levin MJ, Sondheimer JM, Deterding RR (eds) Current diagnosis & treatment, pediatrics, 19th edn. McGraw Hill, USA

Hillman RS, Ault KA, Leporrier M, Rinder HM (2011) Thalassemia. In: Hematology in clinical practice, 5th edn. McGraw Hill, China

Hoffbrand AV, Moss PAH, Pettit JE (2006) Genetic disorders of haemoglobin. In: Essential haemotology, 5th edn. Wiley-Blackwell, MA

327 Polycythemia

Hassan M. Yaish

Polycythemia is a condition characterized by an increase in both the total red blood cells mass and blood volume, resulting in hemoglobin and hematocrit levels significantly higher than normal for the patient's age. It is divided into three types: (1) Primary polycythemia, or polycythemia vera (PV), a condition classified as myeloproliferative disease (MPD) and is rarely encountered in children. (2) Secondary polycythemia, resulting from: physiologically appropriate increase in production of erythropoietin in response to hypoxia of various causes or inappropriate secretion of erythropoietin by a tumor, hemoglobinopathy associated with hemoglobin of low oxygen affinity, and decreased level 2–3 DPG in the red blood cells. (3) Relative polycythemia. In the first two types, the red blood cell mass is increased, while in the third type, the plasma volume is decreased, causing relative rather than real increase in red blood cell counts while red blood cell mass is normal.

Primary Polycythemia

Definition: Primary polycythemia, or polycythemia vera (PV), is a myeloproliferative disease resulting from the clonal expansion of an abnormal multipotent stem cell that produces erythroid progenitors which can proliferate without the presence of erythropoietin (EPO), a feature which is frequently utilized as a diagnostic mean for PV. This multipotent stem cell is unlike the normal fetal progenitor stem cells and those cells with a mutation in the EPO receptor in that they still require erythropoietin for clonal expansion.

Incidence and epidemiology: The prevalence of PV has not been well documented in the USA. In 2003, a study from Connecticut demonstrated an incidence of PV of 22 per 100,000 people. Generalized to the population of the USA, this would reflect approximately 65,243 patients with PV in the USA. The median age at presentation of PV is 60 years. Less than 1% of the patients are less than 25 years of age.

Pathology and laboratory findings: The condition is characterized by polycythemia, leukocytosis, thrombocytosis, and a hypercellular bone marrow.

Signs and Symptoms: Patients with erythrocytosis may develop cardiac and CNS related symptoms such as dyspnea, hypertension, paresthesias, and dizziness. Thrombocytosis may result in thrombosis and bleeding. Pruritus and GI symptoms are frequently seen in adults with PV. They are thought to be the result of increased histamine turnover due to granulocytes proliferation. Patients frequently have splenomegaly.

Prognosis: It is common to see long survivors of PV, even though spontaneous remissions are very rare. Disease-related morbidities are mainly the result of vascular occlusion, bleeding, marrow fibrosis, and leukemia transformation.

Diagnosis: In the past, the diagnosis of PV used to be a diagnosis of exclusion. Both secondary as well as relative polycythemias have to be excluded. At the present time, however, a newly described somatically acquired clonal V617F mutation in the Janus 2 kinase (Jak2) as found to be positive in 90% of adults with PV. The incidence of Jak-2 mutation is significantly less in children. A proportion of children with PV were misdiagnosed as a result of relying on the presence of the Jak-2 mutation. This emphasizes the need for separate diagnostic criteria in children (➲ *Table 327.1*). CD 117, polycythemia rubra vera-1 RNA (PRV-1 RNA) over-expression is another myeloproliferative marker found more frequently in children with PV and sporadic ET. In contrast to the acquired nature of the mutation leading to PV, inborn mutations have been described resulting in what is known as primary familial and congenital polycythemia (PFCP). This condition was shown to be a result of erythropoietin receptor mutation as was described in a report on two new such mutations. The condition, also known as familial erythrocytosis, is characterized by elevated red blood cell mass, low serum erythropoietin, normal oxygen affinity, and autosomal dominant inheritance. Other mutations involving exon 12 of the Jak2 were described in patients with PV and negative Jak2 V617F mutation. A variant of the primary familial and congenital polycythemia (PFCP) is known as Chuvash polycythemia. It was first described in an endemic Russian population and was found to be caused by a mutation in the Von Hippel- Landau (VHL) gene. This gene is associated with mutation in oxygen-sensing

Abdelaziz Y. Elzouki (ed.), *Textbook of Clinical Pediatrics*, DOI 10.1007/978-3-642-02202-9_327,

Table 327.1
Suggested criteria for childhood polycythemia vera (the presence of both major and one minor are required for the diagnosis)

Major criteria: elevated red cell mass
No cause of secondary erythrocytosis, including:
(a) Absence of familial erythrocytosis (e.g., hereditary mutations of erythropoietin (EPO) receptor)
(b) No elevation of EPO caused by
• Hypoxia (arterial po2 < 92%)
• High oxygen affinity hemoglobin
• Truncated EPO receptor
• Inappropriate EPO production by tumor
Minor criteria
(a) Presence of JAK2 V617F mutation
(b) Endogenous erythroid colony formation
(c) Hypercellular bone marrow with trilineage proliferation
(d) Low serum EPO levels

pathway that regulates EPO synthesis. Children with similar conditions outside Russia is referred to as, primary proliferative polycythemia.

Treatment: The goal of PV treatment is to reduce the numbers of the proliferating cells so as to prevent the symptoms associated with high RBCs, platelets, and WBCs. Phlebotomy or isovolemic erythropheresis, are the most commonly used procedures to achieve this goal. Iron replacement is essential to prevent hyperviscosity associated with iron deficiency. Low dose aspirin can also be beneficial. Among agents known to control cell counts, hydroxyurea is thought to be safer and have less side effects than other agents, especially in children. Anagrelide, an agent that targets megakaryocytes differentiation and proliferation, has proven effective in eliminating the thrombocythemia-related symptoms in 80% of patients with PV. Erlotinib, a specific inhibitor of *Jak2* mutation, is currently undergoing clinical trials in PV and other myeloproliferative disorders. Stem cell transplantation has been successfully utilized in some patients.

Secondary Polycythemia

Definition: Secondary polycythemia is defined as a reactive polycythemia as a result of any clinical condition associated with chronic decreased tissue oxygenation, which in turn triggers the physiologic reaction of excess erythropoietin production. Cyanotic congenital heart disease with right-to-left shunts and various chronic pulmonary diseases compromising proper oxygenation are the most common causes of secondary polycythemia. Living at high altitudes, congenital methemoglobinemia, and abnormal hemoglobin with increased oxygen affinity are some of the other common causes of secondary polycythemia. Certain vascular or renal tumors are associated with polycythemia due to erythropoietin secretion by the tumor itself.

Signs and Symptoms: Cyanosis, hyperemia of the sclera and mucous membranes, and clubbing of the fingers are the most frequently encountered clinical manifestations. The oxygen saturation of arterial blood is decreased, and, as the hematocrit rises above 65%, symptoms of hyperviscosity may develop, requiring frequent phlebotomy. To maintain such a high hemoglobin level, and as a result of frequent phlebotomies, iron deficiency develops. In the presence of high viscosity and the rigid iron-deficient red blood cells, the risk of intracranial thrombosis has been reported to be increased. As indicated earlier, iron therapy is recommended despite the high hemoglobin level.

Prognosis: the prognosis of secondary polycythemia is that of the original disease process which have resulted in this condition.

Relative Polycythemia

In contrast to the first two types, relative polycythemia is not associated with true increase in red cell mass, but instead a decrease in plasma volume. Dehydration and burns are classic causes of this type of polycythemia. It is a preventable condition and could be corrected by hydration or treatment of the precipitating cause.

References

Kralovics R, Indrak K, Stopka T et al (1977) Two new EPO receptor mutations: trunculated EPO receptors are most frequently associated with primary familial and congenital polycythemias. Blood 90(5):2057–2061

Li Z, XU M, Xing S et al (2007) Erlotinib effectively inhibits Jak 2V617F activity and polycythemia vera cell growth. J Biol Chem 282:3428–3432

Ma X, Vanasse G, Cartmel B et al (2008) Prevalence of polycythemia vera and essential thrombocythemia. Am J Hematol 83(5):359–362

Orkin S, Fisher D, Look T et al (2009) Oncology of infancy and childhood. W.B. Saunders, Philadelphia

Petrides PE, Beykirch MK, trapp OM et al (1998) Anagrelides, a novel platelets lowering option in essential thrombocythemia treatment experience in 48 patients in Germany. Eur J Haematol 61:71–76

Tefferi A, Thiele J, Orazi A et al (2007) Proposal and rationale for revision of the world health organization diagnostic criteria for polycythemia vera, essential thrombocythemia, and primary myelofibrosis: recommendations from an ad hoc international expert panel. Blood 110:1092–1097

Teofili L, Giona F, Martini M et al (2007a) The revised WHO diagnostic criteria for ph-negative myeloproliferative diseases are not appropriate for diagnostic screening of childhood polycythemia vera and essential thrombocythemia. Blood 110(9):3384–3386

Teofili L, giona F, Martini M et al (2007b) Markers of myeloproliferative diseases in childhood polycythemia vera and essential thrombocythemia. J Clin Oncol 25(9):1048–1053

Vardiman JW, Harris NL, Brunning RD (2002) The world Health Organization (WHO) classification of the myeloid neoplasms. Blood 100:2292–2302

328 Transfusion of Blood and Blood Products

Trisha E. Wong · Meghan Delaney

Our knowledge of blood compatibility and safety has come a long way since the first documented blood transfusion from a sheep to a human in 1667. In developed countries, transfusions are primarily used to support patients undergoing invasive procedures and complex medical treatments for diseases such as cancer and complex surgical procedures. In developing countries, blood is given mostly to children with anemia and women with pregnancy-related complications. Transfusion of blood products can significantly reduce morbidity and mortality, but still carries risks. Children undergoing complicated therapies often depend on transfusions for survival. As the demand for blood component transfusions increase, so must the inventory of safe blood components and the knowledge of transfusion medicine.

Blood Groups

Blood groups are determined by inherited antigenic molecules on the surface of blood cells. These antigens can be proteins, carbohydrates, glycoproteins, or glycolipids depending on the blood group system. A total of 308 blood group antigens are currently recognized, 270 of which are clustered into 30 blood group systems, ➋ *Table 328.1.* Once exposed to foreign red blood cells, the immune system can form alloantibodies against blood group antigens that are not present on the recipient's own red blood cells (RBCs). In general, red cell alloantibodies can only be formed following exposure to another person's red blood cells through blood transfusion or pregnancy. Subsequent transfusion of incompatible blood can cause these pre-formed antibodies to trigger hemolysis of transfused cells. Unlike alloantibodies, ABO antibodies are "naturally occurring" and are formed as a result of exposure to A and B-like substances from bacteria, plants, and other exogenous material in the gastrointestinal tract. The most clinically relevant groups will be discussed here.

ABO is the most important blood group for transfusion because nearly all people have naturally occurring ABO antibodies capable of causing hemolysis of incompatible red cells. Each person's RBCs demonstrate A antigens (type A), B antigens (type B), both (type AB), or neither (type O), ➋ *Table 328.2.* A person will only make antibodies to ABO antigens that they are lacking; for example, a group A person makes anti-B antibody, ➋ *Table 328.2.* ABO antibodies are both IgG and IgM class and can fix complement, which leads to brisk hemolysis. Transfusion of ABO-incompatible RBCs is likely to cause severe morbidity or death. Thus, it is imperative that safety procedures are followed to ensure patient safety. ABO incompatibility is the most common cause of maternal-fetal incompatibility, but it is rarely a cause of severe hemolytic disease of the fetus and newborn (HDFN). ABO antigens are not fully developed in infants <4 months of age and infants do not form natural ABO antibodies until approximately 6 months of age.

The Rh system contains at least 50 antigens of which the major antigens are D, C, E, c, and e coded on two distinct genes. The D antigen (RhD) has greater immunogenicity than any other non-ABO RBC antigen. Antibodies to Rh antigens are mostly IgG and do not bind complement. Therefore, they tend to lead to extravascular hemolysis and can cause mild to severe delayed transfusion reactions. Anti-D antibodies made by multiparous, RhD-negative mothers are able to cross the placenta and are capable of causing HDFN in RhD-positive fetuses.

Hundreds of other blood cell antigen groups have been described. Antibodies to the clinically significant blood groups such as ABO, Rh, Kell, Duffy, Kidd, and Ss are capable of causing HDFN. Antibodies to other blood groups can also cause HDFN if the antibody is IgG and can cross the placenta. In neonates, certain classes of antigens are not fully expressed, including the Lewis system, I, P, Lutheran, and Xg systems. Expression of all blood groups can usually be detected around 1 year of age.

Blood Donation

Blood transfusions would be impossible without a consistent, reliable pool of blood products. Until blood

Abdelaziz Y. Elzouki (ed.), *Textbook of Clinical Pediatrics*, DOI 10.1007/978-3-642-02202-9_328,

Table 328.1
International Society of Blood Transfusion defined blood group systems (system symbol)

ABO (ABO)	Yt (YT)	Cromer (CROM)
MNS (MNS)	Xg (XG)	Knops (KN)
P (P1)	Scianna (SC)	Indian (IN)
Rh (RH)	Dombrock (DO)	Ok (OK)
Lutheran (LU)	Colton (CO)	RAPH (RAPH)
Kell (KEL)	Landsteiner- Weiner (LW)	John Milton Hagen (JMH)
Lewis (LE)	Chido-Rogers (CH/RG)	I (I)
Duffy (FY)	Hh (H)	Globoside (GLOB)
Kidd (JK)	Kx (XK)	Gil (GIL)
Diego (DI)	Gerbich	RhAg (RHAG)

Table 328.2
ABO antigens, antibodies, and compatible blood products

Patient blood type	ABO antigen(s) on RBCs	Antibodies in plasma	Compatible RBCs	Compatible plasma products
A	A	Anti-B	A, O	A, AB
B	B	Anti-A	B, O	B, AB
AB	A, B	None	AB, A, B, O	AB
O	None	Anti-A, Anti-B	O	O, A, B, AB

can be manufactured using synthetic materials, living human donors are the only source. From the time the donor presents for blood collection until the blood is transfused into the recipient, dozens of carefully regulated steps are completed to ensure the safety and efficacy of the blood product.

Donor Screening

Screening donors to identify those at high risk for transfusion-transmitted disease is the first and most cost-effective step in maintaining a safe blood supply. There is a higher frequency of transfusion-transmitted infections when donors are compensated for their donation with monetary or material incentives. As a result, the World Health Organization advocates making all blood donation voluntary. Unfortunately, there are not enough voluntary donors to meet the needs of the blood supply in many developing countries, which still rely on family members and replacement or paid donors. An ideal donor is a healthy adult free of viral disease who does not participate in high-risk behaviors (intravenous drug use, multiple sex partners, etc.) and is willing to donate blood for free. In the United States, donated blood undergoes testing for transfusion-transmitted infectious diseases, including cytomegalovirus (CMV), human immunodeficiency virus (HIV), hepatitis B, hepatitis C, human T-cell lymphotropic virus 1 and 2 (HTLV-1,2), West Nile Virus, *Trypanosoma cruzi*, syphilis, and bacteria (*Table 328.5*).

Autologous Donation

Prior to an elective procedure, a patient may donate blood for their own use during or after surgery. Autologous donations increase the risk of pre-operative anemia and can carry risk if the unit is contaminated ex vivo or if it is transfused to the wrong patient. In addition, autologous donation for a pediatric patient is difficult for ethical and logistical reasons. The child may be unable to consent or assent to phlebotomy and/or the child's size may limit the amount of blood that can be collected. Intraoperative blood salvage, in which blood is removed from the surgical field, washed, and returned to the patient, is another method of transfusing a patient with their own blood.

Directed Donation

Directed blood donation is uncommon in developed countries, but is a common source of blood in developing countries. The strength of directed donation is the ease of identifying a donor. In many places, directed donation is logistically complex. Generally, directed donation is discouraged in places that have access to a safe, volunteer blood supply, as research has shown that directed donation increases blood wastage and carries a higher rate of donor deferral for increased infectious disease risks. Moreover, all red cell and platelet donations from blood relatives must be irradiated to prevent transfusion-associated graft versus host disease (TA-GVHD), a rare but fatal complication of transfusion (see further discussion about TA-GHVD below). If maternal blood is given to her newborn, it should also be washed to prevent antibodies in her serum from reacting to the infant's RBCs. If paternal blood is given to an infant, it may express cognate antigens to clinically significant antibodies which the infant received passively from the mother prior to birth, which could lead to a severe hemolytic reaction.

Collection

In most developed countries, the collection of blood is highly regulated by the government. In other countries, collection processes follow the recommendations of health organizations such as the AABB (formerly known as American Association of Blood Banks), World Health Organization, or American Red Cross or a local government or hospital.

There is a worldwide initiative to use only volunteer blood donors. In the absence of sufficient volunteers, alternate donors are often used. In places where it is expensive to collect a unit of blood and the prevalence of viral disease is high, pre-donation viral testing is done. Once a donor is cleared for donation, whole blood is collected into a sterile storage container containing anticoagulant, buffer, and preservative. To minimize the risk of contamination, the system of needles, tubes, and containers must remain closed, ensuring no contact with the environment. Generally, the maximum amount of blood that can be collected from each donor is 10.5 ml/kg, or around 500 ml. The most common adverse reaction to donating blood is a bruise or hematoma at the site of the venipuncture. A vasovagal event, ranging from lightheadedness to complete loss of consciousness, is seen in 2–3% of donations. Donors experiencing this complication should be kept either supine or in trendelenburg position and provided with electrolyte-containing fluids until they have recovered.

Storage

Preparation and storage of blood components will vary based on the regulations that apply in different countries. In general, whole blood is separated into components to make efficient use of the donor pool and to allow clinicians the flexibility to transfuse only the component(s) needed by the patient. Each unit must be tested for ABO and RhD type and infectious agents prior to release. Once testing is completed and the unit is deemed eligible, it is stored at the proper temperature until it is needed for transfusion or until it expires, ➲ *Table 328.3*. The expiration date of packed red blood cells (PRBCs) varies with the storage solution of the component. The use of additive

Table 328.3
Storage temperature and expiration date for blood components

Product	Storage temperature	Expiration (additive solution)
Whole blood	1-6°C	21 days (CPD)
		35 days (CPD-A)
Packed RBCs	1-6°C	21 days (CPD)
		35 days (CPD-A)
		42 days (AS-1,3,5)
FFP and cryoprecipitate	≤−18°C	24 h after thawing
Platelets	20–24°C	4–7 days
Granulocytes	20–24°C	24 h
RBCs frozen in 40% glycerol	≤−65°C	24 h after deglycerolizing
RBCs frozen in 20% glycerol	≤ −120°C	

solutions lengthens the time for red cell unit storage and has allowed blood banks to maintain larger inventories and minimize the risk of blood shortages. Detailed records of the entire process are maintained for every blood component in order to ensure that each was processed under appropriately controlled conditions. These records are also required so that look-back studies can be done if a unit needs to be recalled or tracked for any reason.

Compatibility

In the United States, tests done routinely to determine donor and recipient compatibility are forward and reverse typing to determine the patient's ABO and RhD type, antibody screen, and crossmatching. To determine the forward ABO-typing (also known as "front type"), reagent antisera is used to test for the presence of A or B antigens on the RBC surface. Reverse ABO-typing ("back type") is done using reagent red cells to test for the presence of ABO antibodies in the serum. The front and back type should always agree. If not, the underlying reason for the discrepancy must be determined prior to transfusion. Red cell antigens other than ABO and RhD are not determined on a routine basis. Exceptions may include chronically transfused patients, such as those with sickle cell disease or women of childbearing age. In the United States, the standard of care for sickle cell disease patients is to provide ABO, RhD, RhCE and Kell blood group antigen matched red cells to prevent alloimmunization.

The antibody screen tests for the presence of red cell alloantibodies in the plasma. The test methodology is an indirect antiglobulin test (IAT), ➋ *Fig. 328.1*. The recipient's plasma is incubated separately with at least two reagent RBCs that express a known phenotype of common red cell antigens. Antihuman globulin (AHG or "Coombs reagent") is added to help magnify the agglutination reaction to detect any RBC alloantibody that is present in the recipient's serum. If a clinically significant red cell alloantibody is detected, it is identified by further IAT testing of the serum using more extensive reagent red cell panels. Once identified, antigen negative, crossmatch-compatible RBCs must be transfused.

The direct antiglobulin test (DAT), also called the direct Coombs test, is typically done if autoimmune hemolysis is suspected. The DAT determines if a recipient's RBCs are coated with antibody, ➋ *Fig. 328.1*. This evaluation is done by mixing the recipient's red blood cells with Coombs reagent and scoring the reaction for agglutination. If the DAT is positive, follow-up testing requires identification of the antibody using IAT as

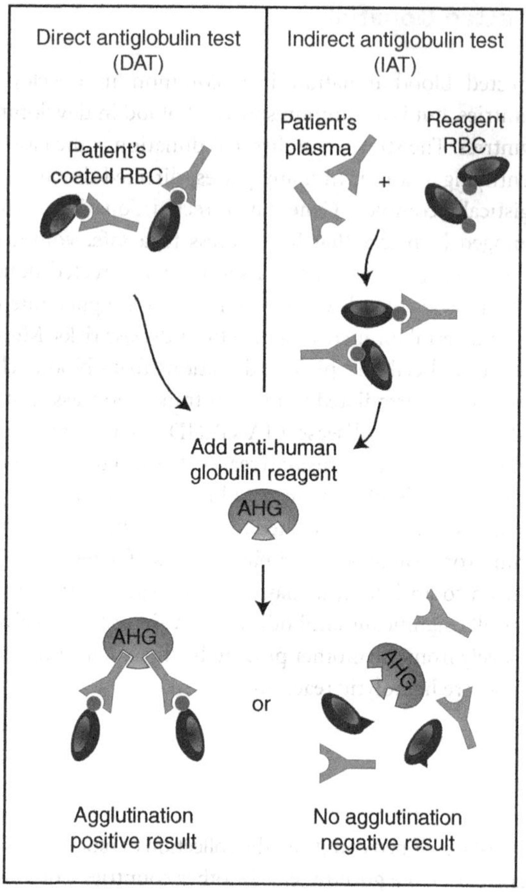

Figure 328.1
Comparison of the direct and indirect antiglobulin tests. The indirect antiglobulin test is also known as an antibody screen. If the antigen and corresponding antibody are present in the reaction, AHG reagent will agglutinate the red cells resulting in visible clumping. If the corresponding antibody or antigen is not present, the antibody cannot bind and agglutination will not occur

described above. In neonates, the DAT is routinely performed using only anti-IgG reagent since any antibody found in the neonate is an IgG antibody that was passively transferred from the mother.

Once a unit of blood is identified for possible transfusion, the patient's plasma is mixed with the donor red cells to ensure that they are compatible; this is called a crossmatch. In emergency situations, the physician may choose to use uncrossmatched group O, RhD-negative blood. Since no compatibility testing is conducted, this should only be done when there is insufficient time to conduct crossmatching. In order of descending preference, the RBC products that should be used during an emergency are crossmatch compatible RBCs, ABO/RhD-type specific RBCs, and uncrossmatched group O RBCs. Physicians must weigh the risk of a hemolytic transfusion reaction against the need for blood transfusion in a hemorrhaging patient. In these situations, crossmatching can be conducted post-transfusion. Neonates <4 months old typically do not require a crossmatch as long as group O RBCs are given and the antibody screen is negative. If anything other than group O cells are intended, a crossmatch is done to determine if the neonate passively received anti-A or anti-B from the mother.

Causes of incompatibility between donor and patient include red cell alloantibodies, passive maternal immunoglobulin in neonates, recipients of plasma or IVIG, hematopoietic stem cell transplant, laboratory or phlebotomist error, or cold or warm autoantibodies. In most countries, patients require a repeat crossmatch sample every 3 days to detect the development of new red cell alloantibodies. Neonates are unlikely to form alloantibodies, thus only require compatibility testing once per hospitalization when under the age of 4 months. This approach lessens the amount of blood phlebotomized from neonatal patients.

Blood Products

Whole Blood

Whole blood (WB) is rarely used in developed countries because individual component therapy is better tailored to the needs of the patient and more efficiently uses the blood supply. Fresh WB contains RBCs, plasma, clotting factors, platelets, and leukocytes. However, following 24 h of storage at 4°C, the platelets are non-functional. Granulocyte function is also not reliable in WB transfusions. Activity of coagulation proteins will decrease over the duration of the 21 days storage. When large-volume transfusion is necessary, such as in trauma or in exchange transfusion, WB may be used to minimize dilutional coagulopathy. Because WB contains a relatively large amount of plasma containing ABO antibodies, it must be ABO-identical to the recipient to prevent hemolytic reactions.

Packed Red Blood Cells

Packed red blood cell (PRBC) transfusion is indicated to increase the oxygen carrying capacity to vital organs. A unit of PRBCs is made by centrifuging a unit of WB and removing most of the plasma and platelets. PRBCs have a hematocrit of 50–80%, and therefore must be infused slowly due to the high viscosity. In pediatric patients, 10–15 ml/kg is transfused over 2–4 h for routine transfusion. If the patient is not losing blood concurrently, 10 ml/kg should raise the hemoglobin by 1–2 g/dl or the hematocrit by 3–6%. As with every transfusion, the benefit of increased red cell mass must be vigilantly weighed against the risks of exposure.

Platelets

Platelet transfusion is indicated in some patients with thrombocytopenia or platelet function defects, ➲ *Table 328.4.* Platelet units can be collected from a single donor during an apheresis procedure or extracted from multiple units of whole blood. The shelf life of platelets is usually limited to 5–7 days because platelets must be kept at room temperature in order to remain viable and efficacious. The risk of bacterial growth is approximately 1 in 5,400 units in the United States and is significantly increased with storage beyond 5 days. This risk has been decreased in some countries by the use of pathogen inactivation protocols.

Typically 10–15 ml/kg of platelets is transfused over 30–60 min. This should increase the platelet count by

Table 328.4
Indications for platelet transfusion in children

Platelet count < 10,000 and decreased platelet production, without other risk factors for bleeding
Platelet count < 20,000 and planned minor procedure, such as lumbar puncture
Platelet count < 50,000 with DIC, active bleeding, or planned major procedure in patient with decreased platelet production
Platelet count < 100,000 with multiple traumas, CNS bleeding, or undergoing surgery in critical sites, such as CNS or eyes

Table 328.5
Estimated prevalence of transfusion-transmitted viruses by country

	Sub-Saharan Africa	United States	Japan
HIV	1:1,000	1 : 2,135,000	1 : 11,000,000
HBV	1:4,300	1 : 205,000	1 : 340,000 – 1 : 450,000
HCV	1:2,500	1 : 1,935,000	1 : 22,000,000

approximately 50,000/μl. However, patients with sepsis, splenomegaly, bleeding, drug-induced thrombocytopenia, disseminated intravascular coagulopathy (DIC), or other illnesses may have lower than expected post-transfusion platelet recovery. Platelets express ABO, but not RhD antigens. Transfusion of ABO-compatible platelets are preferred as they result in improved posttransfusion platelet recovery and reduced rates of alloimmunization. In addition, platelets should be compatible with the patient's RhD type since platelet units contain small amounts of red blood cells. If Rh-positive platelets must be given to a Rh-negative patient, a dose of Rh Immune Globulin (RhIG) may be given to prevent RhD alloimmunization as per the institution's policy. Rather than provide RhIG to all RhD-negative patients who received RhD-positive platelets, some centers choose to give it only to females of child-bearing potential. One 300 ug dose of RhIG neutralizes 15 ml of RBCs, which contains sufficient anti-D to cover several adult-sized transfusions of contemporary platelets derived from whole blood, plateletphersis, or buffy coats.

Platelets express many membrane antigens, including HLA class I antigens. As a result, patients who have been pregnant or exposed to multiple blood donors are at risk of HLA-alloimmunization. Once a patient is HLA alloimmunized, the antibodies may cause the transfused platelets to be destroyed rapidly and the post-transfusion platelet count will not rise as expected. This is called platelet transfusion refractoriness. Three options exist for platelet refractory patients: (a) select HLA-compatible donors from an HLA-typed registry of apheresis donors; (b) identify HLA-antibody specificities and select antigen-compatible apheresis donors; and (c) perform platelet cross-match testing to select compatible platelets.

Plasma Products

Fresh Frozen Plasma

Plasma is the liquid, acellular portion of WB which contains proteins, colloids, nutrients, crystalloids, hormones and vitamins. Plasma can be prepared and stored in several ways resulting in numerous types of plasma products, but fresh frozen plasma (FFP) is most commonly used. FFP is frozen within 8 h of collection to maintain the optimal activity of the coagulation factors. Once thawed, FFP should be given within 24 h. However, plasma used within 5 days of thawing is still considered efficacious for treatment of coagulation factor deficiencies, though there is slightly decreased activity of clotting factors (F) V and VIII. As plasma is rich in clotting factors, the main indication of plasma transfusion is to increase clotting factor levels in a coagulopathic patient. The typical dose of 10–20 ml/kg is expected to increase the coagulation factor concentrations by 30% in a non-bleeding patient. Plasma must be ABO-compatible but does not require Rh-compatibility, crossmatching, or product modifications such as irradiation or leukoreduction because it is acellular.

Cryoprecipitate

When plasma is frozen and subsequently thawed in a refrigerator, an insoluble precipitate forms that is very rich in FVIII, von Willebrand factor (VWF), FXIII, and fibrinogen. Historically, cryoprecipitate was used to treat patients deficient in VWF (von Willebrand disease) or FVIII (hemophilia A). Today, it is primarily used to replete fibrinogen, especially in patients with DIC or dilutional coagulopathy. One pool of cryoprecipitate (six to ten donors) will typically increase the fibrinogen level by 60–100 mg/dl in an adult. The equivalent pediatric dose is one unit of cryoprecipitate for every 10 kg of patient weight.

Albumin

Albumin is the most abundant protein in plasma. Commercially-available human albumin is purified using cold ethanol fractionation, pooled, and sold in either a 5% or 25% solution. The main indication is to increase oncotic pressure in patients with low albumin levels, such as those with liver disease or nephrotic syndrome.

Intravenous Immunoglobulin

Intravenous immunoglobulin (IVIG) is a commercial product prepared by purifying and pooling immunoglobulins from human plasma. Indications for IVIG include idiopathic thrombocytopenia purpura, severe combined immunodeficiency, acquired immunodeficiencies, and Kawasaki syndrome. Its mechanism of action in these disease processes is poorly understood. Mild flushing, headache, rash, and allergic reactions are common following infusion of IVIG. More serious side effects, including renal failure, aseptic meningitis, and pulmonary edema, can occur. Because IVIG contains small amounts of all immunoglobulin classes, anaphylaxis has been described in patients with absence of IgA.

Clotting Factors

For patients with a congenital deficiency of a clotting factor, plasma was once the only source of clotting factors. Cryoprecipitate offered a more efficient clotting factor source for those deficient in FVIII and VWF. As technology advanced, various purification techniques allowed for individual clotting factor concentrates to be isolated with minimal contamination by other clotting factors. Recombinant or plasma-derived clotting factor concentrates are the preferred treatment for hemophilia and VWD patients worldwide. With new viral deactivation techniques, plasma-derived products are considered extremely safe but still possess a theoretical risk of transmitting an emerging infectious agent.

Granulocytes

The main indication for infusing granulocytes is a refractory bacterial, yeast, or fungal infection in a severely neutropenic patient. In most cases of granulocyte transfusions, volunteer donors are mobilized with corticosteroids and/or granulocyte colony stimulating factor (G-CSF) to increase their peripheral white blood cell count prior to undergoing donor apheresis. The goal is to maintain the recipient's granulocyte count above 500 granulocytes/ul. Adverse effects are common and include fever, shaking chills, dyspnea, wheezing, and pulmonary infiltrates. Prophylactic granulocyte transfusions are not recommended in patients who are neutropenic without overt signs of serious infection. Granulocytes must be stored at room temperature and given within 24 h of collection in order to preserve granulocyte function. Because granulocytes contain significant amounts of red blood cells, they must be crossmatch-compatible and irradiated in order to decrease the risk of transfusion-associated graft versus host disease (TA-GVHD).

Product Preparation

Upon completion of compatibility testing for cellular components, the most appropriate blood product must be identified for each patient. Factors to consider when selecting a unit for transfusion include using autologous or directed donor cells if available, ABO/RhD typing, antibody screen results, diagnosis, age, transfusion history, volume of blood component needed, and time and date the blood is required. As discussed here, the treating physician may also request specific attributes of cellular blood products depending on the patient's age, diagnosis, and transfusion history.

Leukocyte Reduction

Reducing the number of leukocytes in cellular blood components, such as platelets or red cells, is accomplished by filtration. Indications for leukocyte reduction include prevention of recurrent febrile non-hemolytic transfusion reactions, prevention of primary HLA-alloimunization, and to decrease transfusion-transmitted cytomegalovirus (CMV) infections in immunocompromised patients. As per the standards of the AABB, leukoreduced products must contain fewer than 5×10^6 white blood cells for apheresis platelets and PRBC and fewer than 8.3×10^5 for pooled platelets. Some blood banks universally leukoreduce cellular components while others do so at the discretion of the ordering physician.

CMV-Negative Components

Transfusion-associated cytomegalovirus (CMV) infection is usually of no clinical significance in immunocompetent recipients. However, CMV can result in serious morbidity and even mortality in immunocompromised patients, young children, and fetuses. At-risk people may include fetuses, neonates with immature immune systems, patients with a congenital or acquired immunodeficiency, patients on immunosuppressive medications as part of treatment for cancer or a solid organ or hematopoietic stem cell transplant. Leukocytes are the only hematopoietic reservoir for CMV, thus transfusion of leukoreduced blood products is considered an acceptable substitute to blood products from a CMV-seronegative donor. However, transfusing blood from patients who are CMV-negative may be safer for patients most at risk.

Irradiated

Blood products are irradiated to prevent transfusion-associated graft versus host disease (TA-GVHD), an often fatal transfusion reaction. TA-GVHD occurs when lymphocytes in the blood unit escape detection by the recipient's immune system. The donor lymphocytes then proliferate, detect the recipient's antigens as foreign, and mount an inflammatory reaction that can cause severe morbidity and mortality. In pediatrics, irradiation is indicated for fetuses receiving intrauterine transfusions, patients with lymphoma or a congenital immunodeficiency, or recipients of granulocyte transfusions or a hematopoietic stem cell transplant. Less evidence supports irradiation of blood products given to premature or term infants, or those receiving immunosuppressants for a hematologic malignancy, solid tumor, or solid organ transplant. In addition, irradiation is indicated for blood products from blood-related donors or in populations with restricted HLA diversity, as their histocompatibility may be similar enough as to go undetected by the competent immune system.

Volume Reduced

Plasma in which red cells or platelets are suspended may be removed from the blood product for several reasons. Volume reduction is accomplished by centrifugation and discarding the plasma from the unit. Plasma may be reduced from RBCs to obtain a concentrated product (hematocrit >90%), which can be used for patients who require tight regulation of volume, such as neonates or patients with congenital cardiac defects. Incompatible plasma can be removed when ABO-incompatible platelets must be transfused. Other indications include reducing the risk of recurrent, moderate allergic transfusion reactions or circulatory overload.

Washed

Washing PRBCs or platelets is done by volume reduction and subsequent suspension of the cells in saline or albumin. There are very few indications for washing cellular blood products. Blood components transfused to patients with congenital absence of IgA should be washed prior to transfusion to avoid anaphylactic reactions triggered by donor IgA. Other indications include removal of residual plasma following recurrent, severe allergic or anaphylactic reactions, reducing potassium accumulated in blood units prior to large-volume transfusions (>25 ml/kg), removing plasma in the case of neonatal alloimmune thrombocytopenia, or removing additive solution prior to transfusion. Routine washing is not recommended because it can lead to loss of cells or functional impairment. When washing cannot be accomplished for potassium or additive solution removal, volume reduction may be an alternative choice. Use of PRBC products without additives (PRBC in CPD solution, ➋ *Table 328.2*) can also be used to avoid transfusion of large quantities of additives to small pediatric patients.

Satellite Packs

Sick neonates and small children may require repeated, small-volume units of red cell transfusions. To limit the exposure to different donors, transfer systems that remain closed to the environment can be used to divide a single blood donation into four to eight small aliquots. The aliquots from one donor can be designated for one neonate. By minimizing donor exposure, the risks of transfusion-transmitted infections and alloimmunization are minimized. Satellite packs waste less blood and are proven to be cost-effective. Because these units are given in small doses, the risk of hyperkalemia or other adverse effects of storage are minimal.

Complications

Infectious Complications

The three most clinically significant transfusion-transmitted infectious agents are human immunodeficiency virus (HIV), hepatitis B (HBV), and hepatitis C (HCV). Though the risk of HIV, HBV, or HCV viral transmission via transfusion is low in the United States, such is not the case worldwide, ➋ *Table 328.5*. Additionally, many other known or potential pathogens are transmissible by blood, ➋ *Table 328.6*. Certain opportunistic infections, such as human parvovirus B19, cytomegalovirus (CMV), and other herpesviruses, may cause serious disease in immunocompromised transfusion recipients. Fortunately, advances in virology, donor screening techniques, and viral detection assays have resulted in a worldwide decrease in the incidences of these and other transfusion-transmitted infections in the last decades. However, vigilance must continue in order to ensure that the blood supply remains free of known and emerging infectious agents.

Non-infectious Complications

Non-infectious complications of transfusion are equally as important as infectious complications and far more common. ➋ *Table 328.7* briefly describes the majority of clinically-significant transfusion reactions.

Table 328.6
Categories of transfusion-transmitted infectious agents by AABB

Agents for which donors are routinely screened
Hepatitis B virus
Human immunodeficiency virus
Hepatitis C virus
Human T-cell lymphotropic virus
West Nile virus
Bacteria
Trypanosoma cruzi (Chagas disease)
Cytomegalovirus
Agents with scientific evidence of risk and potential for severe clinical outcome, but not currently screened
Human variant Creutzfeldt-Jakob disease
Dengue viruses
Babesia species
Agents with sufficient scientific evidence of risk that might support elevation to a higher priority in future
Chikungunya virus
St. Louis encephalitis virus
Leishmania species
Plasmodium species
Agents with absent or low scientific evidence of risk but public and/or regulatory concern present
Chronic wasting disease prion
Human herpesvirus 8
HIV variants
Human parvovirus B19
Influenza A virus, subtype H5N1
Simian foamy virus
Borrelia burgdorferi (Lyme disease)
Hepatitis A virus
Agents to monitor but do not currently represent risk or concern
Hepatitis E virus
Anaplasma phagocytophilum (Human granuloyctyic anaplasmosis)
Others – AABB monitoring 51 other low risk prion, viral, rickettsial, and protozoan agents
Agents currently with unclear scientific evidence of risk
Xenotropic Murine Leukemia Virus-Related Virus (XMRV)

Human error in drawing, labeling, and administration of blood is the leading cause of ABO-incompatible hemolytic transfusion reactions, underscoring the importance of maintaining strict and clear procedures during all phases of transfusion. When a transfusion reaction is suspected, the transfusion should be stopped and supportive care instated immediately. The unit label and patient identification should be re-checked to detect possible errors in patient identification. The unit of blood should be sent to the blood bank along with a post-transfusion blood sample from the patient. The blood bank will conduct testing to identify potential causative factors, such as clerical errors, hemolysis, or bacterial contamination.

Transfusion-related acute lung injury (TRALI) is a rapid onset of non-cardiogenic pulmonary edema within 6 h of transfusion and is the leading cause of death from transfusion in the United States. There are three proposed mechanisms for TRALI: (a) donor-derived anti-granulocyte or (b) anti-HLA antibodies, and (c) biologic response modifiers such as cellular membrane fragments of donor cells that stimulate an inflammatory response in the recipient's pulmonary vasculature. These etiologies lead to hypoxic respiratory failure that is not responsive to diuretics. Supportive care is only required for the recipient. TRALI investigations are intended to help the blood center manage their donor pool since a donor with granulocyte or HLA antibodies, most of which are multiparous women, should be deferred from further donations of high plasma-volume components. To this end, the United Kingdom implemented a policy in 2003 to minimize the donations of FFP and platelets from females. This strategy has yielded a significant decrease in the rate of reported cases of probable TRALI.

Some adverse effects are more commonly associated with the pediatric population. Rapid infusion may cause fluid shifts in the intravascular compartment and can cause significant metabolic derangements. As RBCs age during storage, potassium levels increase in the supernatant. Large-volume transfusions of older red cell units to small children can result in hyperkalemic cardiac arrest and death. Hyperkalemia can be avoided by using fresher units, washing the cells, reducing the plasma volume before transfusion, or transfusing red cells slowly. Because blood products contain citrate, a calcium-binding anticoagulant, hypocalcemia may result from rapid infusion of blood products. In order to avoid hypothermia during large volume transfusions, blood can be passed through a blood warmer. Red cell additive solutions contain adenine, which carry a low risk of renal or liver insult when infused at high doses; plasma reduction or washing may decrease the risk. Hyperosmolality, hyperglycemia, hypernatremia, and hyperphosphatemia are theoretical concerns in children based on calculations of these constituents in storage media.

Table 328.7
Non-infectious transfusion reactions

Adverse effect	Etiology	Symptoms	Treatment or prophylaxis
Acute (<24 h) transfusion reactions, immunologic			
Acute hemolytic transfusion reaction	Immune destruction of transfused RBCs by a naturally occurring ABO-antibody or an alloantibody produced following immunization from a previous transfusion or pregnancy	Chills, fever, hemoglobinuria, renal failure, DIC, back pain, pain along infusion catheter, anxiety, shock. Gross hemoglobinemia in vitro	Supportive treatment
Febrile, non-hemolytic transfusion reaction	Accumulated cytokines or antibody to donor white cells	Fever, chills/rigors, headache, vomiting, exacerbation of cardiovascular or respiratory distress	Leukocyte reduction, premedication with acetaminophen
Urticarial transfusion reaction	Antibody to donor plasma proteins	Urticaria, pruritis, flushing	Antihistamine. May restart transfusion if symptoms resolve
Anaphylactic transfusion reaction	Antibody to donor plasma proteins, cytokines	Hypotension, urticaria, bronchospasm, angioedema, anxiety	Fluids, epinephrine, antihistamine, corticosteroids, beta-2-agonists, IgA deficient components
Transfusion Related Acute Lung Injury (TRALI)	Donor-derived antibodies to granulocytes or HLA antigens; or other WBC-activating agent	Hypoxemia, respiratory failure, hypotension, fever, bilateral pulmonary edema	Supportive care until recovery, defer implicated donor(s) if implicated antibody detected
Acute (<24 h) transfusion reactions, non-immunologic			
Sepsis	Bacterial contamination	Fever, chills, hypotension, shock	Supportive care, empiric broad spectrum antibiotics until sensitivity testing completed
Circulatory Overload	Volume overload due to transfused blood products	Dyspnea, orthopnea, cough, tachycardia, hypertension, headache	Upright posture, oxygen, IV diuretics, rarely phlebotomy
Non-immune hemolysis	Physical or chemical destruction of blood (heating, freezing, hemolytic drug or solution)	Hemoglobinuria, hemoglobinemia, jaundice	Identify and eliminate underlying cause
Air embolus	Infusion of air bubble	Sudden dyspnea, acute cyanosis, pain, cough, hypotension, arrhythmia	Place patient on left side with legs elevated above chest and head
Hypocalcemia	Rapid citrate infusion (massive transfusion)	Parasthesia, arrhythmia, tetany	Oral calcium for mild symptoms, slow IV calcium with close monitoring for more severe reactions
Hypothermia	Rapid infusion of cold or room temperature blood	Arrhythmia	Warm patient and use a blood warmer
Hyperkalemia	Leak of potassium into supernatant plasma from RBCs as they age. Pediatric and renal failure patients most at risk	Arrhythmia	Transfuse slowly. Transfuse fresh, washed, or volume reduced units to at-risk patients. Treat same as hyperkalemia from other causes (ie: IV calcium, insulin/glucose)

Table 328.7 (Continued)

Adverse effect	Etiology	Symptoms	Treatment or prophylaxis
Delayed (>24 h) transfusion reactions, immunologic			
Alloimmunization, HLA antigens	Exposure to foreign HLA antigens on WBC or platelet through prior transfusions or pregnancies	Platelet transfusion refractoriness	Avoid unnecessary blood, leukoreduction, transfuse HLA-matched or crossmatched platelet products
Delayed hemolytic transfusion reaction	Anamnestic immune response to RBC antigen; alloantibody titer increases after re-stimulation	Positive antibody screen in vitro following exposure to red cell transfusion, fever, hemolysis, jaundice in vivo 7–14 days after transfusion	Identify antibody, transfuse antigen negative, crossmatch compatible RBCs as needed
Transfusion-assocaiated graft-vs-host disease	Donor lymphocytes engraft in recipient and mount attack on tissues (see section on irradiation of blood components)	Fever, erythroderma, maculopapular rash, anorexia, nausea, vomiting, diarrhea, hepatitis, pancytopenia	Prevent with irradiation of blood components for at-risk patients. Stem cell transplant, corticosteroids, cytotoxic agents
Posttransfusion purpura (PTP)	Recipient-derived antibodies to human platelet antigens (HPA system) destroy donor *and* autologous platelets after re-exposure to platelet fragments (usually through a red cell transfusion)	Thrombocytopia and severe bleeding typically 8–10 days following RBC transfusion	IVIG, plasmapheresis, corticosteroids, antigen-negative platelets preferred
Delayed (>24 h) transfusion reactions, non-immunologic			
Iron overload	Storage of iron in organs and tissues in chronically transfused patients	Diabetes, cirrhosis, cardiomyopathy	Avoid unnecessary transfusions, phlebotomy if possible, iron chelation

Special Considerations

Massive Transfusion

The use of blood products has decreased mortality in hemorrhaging patients. A massive transfusion is defined as replacement of a patient's entire blood volume in 24 h, transfusion of more than ten PRBC units in adults, or replacement of more than 50% of the circulating blood volume within 3 h. In children <1 year, one adult-sized red cell unit can constitute massive transfusion. PRBCs are transfused rapidly to maintain adequate blood pressure and oxygen carrying capacity. For females of childbearing potential, group O, RhD-negative products should be used to protect against sensitization to RhD in cases of emergency, which could later cause HDFN. In the case of life threatening bleeding, however, group O PRBCs of any RhD type are acceptable, and may actually be preferentially used for male patients if medical center policy allows. A blood sample must be drawn early during resuscitation so that the sample reflects the patient's blood type prior to replacement with donated blood products. This is essential if the bleeding patient is to be switched to ABO-type specific products to preserve the inventory of universal donor products (group O RBC and group AB plasma products) in the blood bank.

Many institutions have a massive transfusion protocol that mandates a set ratio of the number of plasma and platelet components transfused per number of PRBC units transfused. This ratio is used to treat active hemorrhage and prevent dilutional coagulopathy. Alternatively, ABO/RhD-specific whole blood can be used if available. Due to a lack of controlled trials, no specific recommendation has been set for the ratio of PRBCs to platelets and plasma, so medical centers must create their own. All patients undergoing massive transfusion should have hematocrit, platelet count, prothrombin time, and fibrinogen checked regularly to assess coagulation status and to guide component therapy. Children undergoing massive transfusion should have electrolytes monitored as they are at higher risk of metabolic derangements including hyperkalemia, hypoglycemia, hypothermia, hypocalcemia, and fluid overload. Because hypothermia and acidosis can inactivate clotting factors, it is imperative that these be tightly regulated to control bleeding effectively.

Exchange Transfusion

The more common indications for red cell or whole blood exchange transfusion include HDFN with kernicterus, sickle cell crisis, malaria, and hyperleukoctyosis seen in acute leukemia. Exchange transfusions can be accomplished by manual or automated techniques. Warmed, fresh, whole blood or PRBCs reconstituted with compatible plasma should be used to avoid the risks that accompany massive transfusion in whole blood exchange. The reported rate of mortality is 0–3.6% and adverse effects occur in 4–15.3% of patients. Complications includes sepsis, bradycardia, thrombocytopenia, apnea, cyanosis, hypocalcemia, hypoglycemia, and central catheter-related thrombi. Two times the blood volume is usually exchanged, ➋ *Table 328.8*. For the treatment of HDFN, this will replace about 75–90% of the recipient's RBCs, and remove 50% of the bilirubin and 75–90% of the causative antibody.

Chronic Transfusions

Some patients require RBC transfusions on a regular basis. The goal of chronic transfusions for patients with hemoglobinopathies (thalassemia or sickle cell disease) is to increase oxygen-carrying capacity, replace the defective red cells with normal RBCs, and to suppress erythropoiesis. Patients with a pure quantitative defect, such as Diamond Blackfan anemia, require transfusions to correct a qualitative defect while patients with myelodyplastic syndrome may have both quantitative and qualitative RBC defects. These patients may require lifelong transfusions if unable to obtain more definitive treatment. The most significant consequence of chronic transfusion is the deposition of iron into organs such as the liver and heart, which can lead to end-organ dysfunction. The effects of iron overload can be ameliorated by conducting exchange transfusion instead of simple transfusions or by starting iron chelation therapy. Neither of these options is without adverse effects, thus the risks and benefits must be heavily considered. Those receiving chronic transfusions also have a higher risk of alloimmunization and of contracting transfusion-transmitted infections based on the number of donors they are exposed to throughout life.

Table 328.8
Estimated blood volume

Age group	Approximate blood volume
Preterm neonate	100 ml/kg
Term neonate	85 ml/kg
>1 month	75 ml/kg

Extracoporeal Circuits Requiring Blood Products

Extracoporeal membrane oxygenation (ECMO), cardiopulmonary bypass (CPB), and automated apheresis are medical therapeutics that require significant blood bank participation. All of these treatment modalities use a circuit with an inline pump which draws blood out, processes it, and infuses it back into the patient. The modalities differ in clinical utility and methodology, as discussed below.

ECMO and CPB both provide artificial oxygenation and cardiac output. CPB is used by pediatric anesthesia during cardiac surgery in order to circulate blood while providing a bloodless, asystolic heart. ECMO is reserved for patients with potentially reversible respiratory and/or cardiac failure who have failed more conventional, less invasive techniques. Automated apheresis is a technique used to separate a cellular component or antibody from the blood and remove it. Apheresis can be used to remove blood cells (cytapheresis) in the case of polycythemia, thrombocythemia, sickle cell disease, or leukocytosis. Plasma can be removed via plasmapheresis and replaced with donor plasma and/or albumin. This is typically used to deplete a pathological IgG immunoglobulin in immune-mediated or malignant disease.

Although these techniques can potentially save lives and improve health, they are invasive, complex procedures that require hospital resources and carry risks. A variety of commercial instruments are available for each technique but each require specialized personnel to operate. Donor blood is usually necessary to prime the circuit in each scenario for small children. An anticoagulant, typically heparin or citrate, is added to the circuit to minimize the risk of a clot forming in the circuit tubing during operation. This can increase the risk of bleeding and/or hypocalcemia in patients. Any of these extracorporeal techniques can cause significant shifts of fluid. In addition, these techniques subsume all the infectious, immunological, and thrombotic risks due to the necessity of an indwelling central line and exposure to multiple blood donors.

Summary

Transfusions of blood and blood products have significantly reduced morbidity and mortality in children worldwide. A readily-available, safe supply of blood is now available to more physicians around the world, although significant disparities in testing and capabilities still exist between regions. Despite the advances, the potential complications of blood transfusion can be significant. The benefits and risks of the transfusion to individual patients must also be weighed against the conservation of the precious community resource. Efficacy and safety will continue to improve as the knowledge of pediatric transfusions increases.

References

AABB (2010) Recommendation on chronic fatigue syndrome and blood donation. http://www.aabb.org/pressroom/Pages/cfsrecommendation.aspx. Accessed 20 March 2011

Abu-Ekteish F, Daoud A, Rimawi H, Kakish K, Abu-Heija A (2000) Neonatal exchange transfusion: a Jordanian experience. Ann Trop Paediatr 20:57–60

Aster RH (1965) Effect of anticoagulant and ABO incompatibility on recovery of transfused human platelets. Blood 26:732–743

Auf der Maur C, Hodel M, Nydegger UE, Rieben R (1993) Age dependency of ABO histo-blood group antibodies: reexamination of an old dogma. Transfusion 33:915–918

Behjati S, Sagheb S, Aryasepehr S, Yaghmai B (2009) Adverse events associated with neonatal exchange transfusion for hyperbilirubinemia. Indian J Pediatr 76:83–85

Bowden RA, Slichter SJ, Sayers M, Weisdorf D, Cays M, Schoch G, Banaji M, Haake R, Welk K, Fisher L, McCullough J, Miller W (1995) A comparison of filtered leukocyte-reduced and cytomegalovirus (CMV) seronegative blood products for the prevention of transfusion-associated CMV infection after marrow transplant. Blood 86:3598–3603

British Committee for Standards in Haematology, Blood Transfusion Task Force (2003) Guidelines for the use of platelet transfusions. Br J Haematol 122:10–23

Burks AW, Sampson HA, Buckley RH (1986) Anaphylactic reactions after gammaglobulin administration in patients with hypogammaglobulinemia. Detection of IgE antibodies to IgA. N Engl J Med 314:560–564

Carr R, Hutton JL, Jenkins JA, Lucas GF, Amphlett NW (1990) Transfusion of ABO-mismatched platelets leads to early platelet refractoriness. Br J Haematol 75:408–413

Castro O, Sandler SG, Houston-Yu P, Rana S (2002) Predicting the effect of transfusing only phenotype-matched RBCs to patients with sickle cell disease: theoretical and practical implications. Transfusion 42:684–690

Chapman CE, Stainsby D, Jones H, Love E, Massey E, Win N, Navarrete C, Lucas G, Soni N, Morgan C, Choo L, Cohen H, Williamson LM, Serious Hazards of Transfusion Steering Group (2009) Ten years of hemovigilance reports of transfusion-related acute lung injury in the United Kingdom and the impact of preferential use of male donor plasma. Transfusion 49:440–452

Chen CH, Hong CL, Kau YC, Lee HL, Chen CK, Shyr MH (1999) Fatal hyperkalemia during rapid and massive blood transfusion in a child undergoing hip surgery – a case report. Acta Anaesthesiol Sin 37:163–166

Daniels GL, Fletcher A, Garratty G, Henry S, Jorgensen J, Judd WJ, Levene C, Lomas-Francis C, Moulds JJ, Moulds JM, Moulds M, Overbeeke M, Reid ME, Rouger P, Scott M, Sistonen P, Smart E, Tani Y, Wendel S, Zelinski T, International Society of Blood Transfusion (2004) Blood group terminology 2004: from the International Society of Blood Transfusion committee on terminology for red cell surface antigens. Vox Sang 87:304–316

Daniels G, Castilho L, Flegel WA, Fletcher A, Garratty G, Levene C, Lomas-Francis C, Moulds JM, Moulds JJ, Olsson ML, Overbeeke M, Poole J, Reid ME, Rouger P, van der Schoot E, Scott M, Sistonen P, Smart E, Storry JR, Tani Y, Yu LC, Wendel S, Westhoff C, Yahalom V, Zelinski T (2009) International Society of Blood Transfusion Committee on terminology for red blood cell surface antigens: Macao report. Vox Sang 96:153–156

Delaflor-Weiss E, Mintz PD (2000) The evaluation and management of platelet refractoriness and alloimmunization. Transfus Med Rev 14:180–196

Eastlund T (1998) Monetary blood donation incentives and the risk of transfusion-transmitted infection. Transfusion 38:874–882

Eder AF, Kennedy JM, Dy BA, Notari EP, Weiss JW, Fang CT, Wagner S, Dodd RY, Benjamin RJ, American Red Cross Regional Blood Centers (2007) Bacterial screening of apheresis platelets and the residual risk of septic transfusion reactions: the American Red Cross experience (2004–2006). Transfusion 47:1134–1142

FDA (2010) Guidance for industry: implementation of acceptable full-length donor history questionnaire and accompanying materials for use in screening donors of blood and blood components. http://www.fda.gov/downloads/BiologicsBloodVaccines/BloodBloodProducts/ApprovedProducts/LicensedProductsBLAs/BloodDonorScreening/UCM213552.pdf. Accessed 20 March 2011

FDA (2010) Fatalities reported to FDA following blood collection and transfusion: annual summary for fiscal year 2009. http://www.fda.gov/BiologicsBloodVaccines/SafetyAvailability/ReportaProblem/TransfusionDonationFatalities/ucm204763.htm. Accessed 20 March 2011

Hillyer CD, Strauss RG, Luban NL (eds) (2004) Handbook of pediatric transfusion medicine. Elsevier Academic Press, San Diego

Hilsenrath P, Nemechek J, Widness JA, Cordle DG, Strauss RG (1999) Cost-effectiveness of a limited-donor blood program for neonatal red cell transfusions. Transfusion 39:938–943

Hoffmeister KM, Felbinger TW, Falet H, Denis CV, Bergmeier W, Mayadas TN, von Andrian UH, Wagner DD, Stossel TP, Hartwig JH (2003) The clearance mechanism of chilled blood platelets. Cell 112:87–97

Hosking MP, Beynen FM, Raimundo HS, Oliver WC Jr, Williamson KR (1990) A comparison of washed red blood cells versus packed red blood cells (AS-1) for cardiopulmonary bypass prime and their effects on blood glucose concentration in children. Anesthesiology 72:987–990

Ibojie J, Greiss M, Lloyd DJ, Urbaniak SJ (2003) Donor exposure rate to transfusion ratio: a better discriminator of improvement in neonatal transfusion practice. Transfus Med 13:287–291

Jackson JC (1997) Adverse events associated with exchange transfusion in healthy and ill newborns. Pediatrics 99:E7

Jayaraman S, Chalabi Z, Perel P, Guerriero C, Roberts I (2010) The risk of transfusion-transmitted infections in sub-Saharan Africa. Transfusion 50:433–442

Keenan WJ, Novak KK, Sutherland JM, Bryla DA, Fetterly KL (1985) Morbidity and mortality associated with exchange transfusion. Pediatrics 75:417–421

Luban NL, Strauss RG, Hume HA (1991) Commentary on the safety of red cells preserved in extended-storage media for neonatal transfusions. Transfusion 31:229–235

Menitove JE (2002) Immunoprophylaxis for D-patients receiving platelet transfusions from D+ [correction of D-] donors? Transfusion 42:136–138

Newman BH (1997) Donor reactions and injuries from whole blood donation. Transfus Med Rev 11:64–75

Nichols WG, Price TH, Gooley T, Corey L, Boeckh M (2003) Transfusion-transmitted cytomegalovirus infection after receipt of leukoreduced blood products. Blood 101:4195–4200

Nunez TC, Dutton WD, May AK, Holcomb JB, Young PP, Cotton BA (2010) Emergency department blood transfusion predicts early massive transfusion and early blood component requirement. Transfusion 50(9):1914–1920

Osby M, Shulman IA (2005) Phenotype matching of donor red blood cell units for nonalloimmunized sickle cell disease patients: a survey of 1182 North American laboratories. Arch Pathol Lab Med 129:190–193

Otsubo H, Yamaguchi K (2008) Current risks in blood transfusion in Japan. Jpn J Infect Dis 61:427–433

Patra K, Storfer-Isser A, Siner B, Moore J, Hack M (2004) Adverse events associated with neonatal exchange transfusion in the 1990s. J Pediatr 144:626–631

Phan HH, Wisner DH (2010) Should we increase the ratio of plasma/platelets to red blood cells in massive transfusion: what is the evidence? Vox Sang 98:395–402

Price TH (ed) (2008) Standards for blood banks and transfusion services. AABB, Bethesda

Pruss A, Kalus U, Radtke H, Koscielny J, Baumann-Baretti B, Balzer D, Dorner T, Salama A, Kiesewetter H (2004) Universal leukodepletion of blood components results in a significant reduction of febrile non-hemolytic but not allergic transfusion reactions. Transfus Apher Sci 30:41–46

Reid ME, Lomas-Francis C (2004) The blood group antigen: factsbook. Academic, San Diego

Roback JD, Combs M, Grossman BJ, Hillyer CD (eds) (2008) Technical manual. AABB, Bethesda

Ruhl H, Bein G, Sachs UJ (2009) Transfusion-associated graft-versus-host disease. Transfus Med Rev 23:62–71

Sanpavat S (2005) Exchange transfusion and its morbidity in ten-year period at King Chulalongkorn Hospital. J Med Assoc Thai 88:588–592

Schiffer CA, Anderson KC, Bennett CL, Bernstein S, Elting LS, Goldsmith M, Goldstein M, Hume H, McCullough JJ, McIntyre RE, Powell BL, Rainey JM, Rowley SD, Rebulla P, Troner MB, Wagnon AH, American Society of Clinical Oncology (2001) Platelet transfusion for patients with cancer: clinical practice guidelines of the American Society of Clinical Oncology. J Clin Oncol 19:1519–1538

Schuster KM, Davis KA, Lui FY, Maerz LL, Kaplan LJ (2010) The status of massive transfusion protocols in United States trauma centers: massive transfusion or massive confusion? Transfusion 50:1545–1551

Sidhu RS, Le T, Brimhall B, Thompson H (2006) Study of coagulation factor activities in apheresed thawed fresh frozen plasma at 1-6 degrees C for five days. J Clin Apher 21:224–226

Simon TL, Snyder EL, Solheim BG, Stowell CP, Strauss RG, Petrides M (eds) (2009) Rossi's principles of transfusion medicine. Blackwell, Chichester

Smith HM, Farrow SJ, Ackerman JD, Stubbs JR, Sprung J (2008) Cardiac arrests associated with hyperkalemia during red blood cell transfusion: a case series. Anesth Analg 106:1062–1069, able of contents

Stramer SL, Hollinger FB, Katz LM, Kleinman S, Metzel PS, Gregory KR, Dodd RY (2009) Emerging infectious disease agents and their potential threat to transfusion safety. Transfusion 49(Suppl 2):1S–29S

Strauss RG, Connett JE, Gale RP, Bloomfield CD, Herzig GP, McCullough J, Maguire LC, Winston DJ, Ho W, Stump DC, Miller WV, Koepke JA (1981) A controlled trial of prophylactic granulocyte transfusions during initial induction chemotherapy for acute myelogenous leukemia. N Engl J Med 305:597–603

Strauss RG, Villhauer PJ, Cordle DG (1995) A method to collect, store and issue multiple aliquots of packed red blood cells for neonatal transfusions. Vox Sang 68:77–81

Strauss RG, Burmeister LF, Johnson K, James T, Miller J, Cordle DG, Bell EF, Ludwig GA (1996) AS-1 red cells for neonatal transfusions: a randomized trial assessing donor exposure and safety. Transfusion 36:873–878

The Trial to Reduce Alloimmunization to Platelets Study Group (1997) Leukocyte reduction and ultraviolet B irradiation of platelets to prevent alloimmunization and refractoriness to platelet transfusions. N Engl J Med 337:1861–1869

Tilley L, Green C, Poole J, Gaskell A, Ridgwell K, Burton NM, Uchikawa M, Tsuneyama H, Ogasawara K, Akkok CA, Daniels G (2010) A new blood group system, RHAG: three antigens resulting from amino acid substitutions in the Rh-associated glycoprotein. Vox Sang 98:151–159

Vamvakas EC (1998) Meta-analysis of randomized controlled trials of the efficacy of white cell reduction in preventing HLA-alloimmunization and refractoriness to random-donor platelet transfusions. Transfus Med Rev 12:258–270

Vamvakas EC, Blajchman MA (2010) Blood still kills: six strategies to further reduce allogeneic blood transfusion-related mortality. Transfus Med Rev 24:77–124

Vamvakas EC, Pineda AA (1997) Determinants of the efficacy of prophylactic granulocyte transfusions: a meta-analysis. J Clin Apher 12: 74–81

van Rhenen D, Gulliksson H, Cazenave JP, Pamphilon D, Ljungman P, Kluter H, Vermeij H, Kappers-Klunne M, de Greef G, Laforet M, Lioure B, Davis K, Marblie S, Mayaudon V, Flament J, Conlan M, Lin L, Metzel P, Buchholz D, Corash L, euroSPRITE trial (2003) Transfusion of pooled buffy coat platelet components prepared with photochemical pathogen inactivation treatment: the euroSPRITE trial. Blood 101:2426–2433

Wales PW, Lau W, Kim PC (2001) Directed blood donation in pediatric general surgery: is it worth it? J Pediatr Surg 36:722–725

Westhoff CM (2007) The structure and function of the Rh antigen complex. Semin Hematol 44:42–50

World Health Organization (2009) Fact File on Blood Transfusion. http://www.who.int/bloodsafety/FactFile2009.pdf%202010

World Health Organization Voluntary blood donation. 2010

Wu Y, Zou S, Cable R, Dorsey K, Tang Y, Hapip CA, Melmed R, Trouern-Trend J, Wang JH, Champion M, Fang C, Dodd R (2010) Direct assessment of cytomegalovirus transfusion-transmitted risks after universal leukoreduction. Transfusion 50:776–786

Yu MY, Alter HJ, Virata-Theimer ML, Geng Y, Ma L, Schechterly CA, Colvin CA, Luban NL (2010) Parvovirus B19 infection transmitted by transfusion of red blood cells confirmed by molecular analysis of linked donor and recipient samples. Transfusion 50(8):1712–1721

329 Care of the Child Refusing Blood Products

Lynn Boshkov

Background: Jehovah's Witnesses and Prohibitions on Transfusion of Blood

The Watch Tower Bible and Tract Society web site (http://www.watchtower.org/e/statistics/worldwide_report.htm accessed January 29, 2011) indicates that in 2009, there were over 7.3 million Jehovah's Witnesses in 236 countries worldwide. The greatest number of these (over 1.1 million) live in the USA, with numbers in excess of 100,000 being found in other countries in North America (Canada, Mexico), South America (Argentina, Brazil, Columbia, Peru), Eurasia (France, Germany, Great Britain, Poland, Russia, Spain), the Far East (Japan, Philippines), and Africa (Congo, Nigeria, Zambia). Thus, it is likely that the medical practitioner treating children almost anywhere in the world will come into contact with a Jehovah's Witness family.

Jehovah's Witnesses believe that the Bible prohibits ingesting blood and do not accept transfusion of whole blood or any of its four primary components – red cells, platelets, plasma, or white cells. This prohibition applies even in clinical contexts where such refusal may result in serious harm or death. The transfusion prohibition also extends to predonation and storage of a patient's own blood for later transfusion back to the patient. However, it is worth noting that Jehovah's Witnesses are not one of the religious groups who shun medical care generally, and that acceptability of sophisticated medical interventions where their own blood is kept in contact with the body (cardiopulmonary bypass, dialysis), as well as receipt of organ transplants, are considered "matters of conscience" to be decided by each individual Witness. Other "matters of conscience" to Witnesses are intraoperative blood salvage where the blood is kept in contact with the body ("Cell Saver" type devices, perioperative hemodilution) and a range of "minor fractions" of blood (discussed in greater detail below). While most countries legally permit refusal of medical interventions by adults, the desire of Jehovah's Witness parents and guardians to extend refusal of blood therapy to their minor children often results in legal and ethical tensions between the family and health-care providers treating the child, as those providers are most often both legally obligated to provide medical intervention that will save life or prevent serious harm, and also obligated to do so by personal ethical imperatives. This tension may be particularly acute in the case of patients who are "mature minors," and who are themselves also refusing blood.

Faced with such a conflict, what is the best way to proceed? Several general guiding precepts may be helpful:

1. Work in partnership with the patient and family and Jehovah's Witness community; act as the patient's and the family's advocate.
2. Know and explore the acceptability of the full range of "matters of conscience" minor fractions and non-blood therapeutic options with the patient and family and use them prior to resorting to unacceptable interventions.
3. Act preemptively if possible to prevent anemia and coagulopathy and use combined interventions to treat these.
4. Realize physiological tolerance of anemia is generally greater than one might think.
5. Make the family aware of the legal obligation to transfuse a minor to prevent serious harm or death.

If the treating physician truly adheres to these guiding precepts, even though the child ends up receiving a blood product, tensions are minimized to the extent this is possible and the therapeutic relationship is served. Elaborating on these guiding precepts:

Work in partnership with the patient and family and Jehovah's Witness community; act as the patient's and the family's advocate.

In difficult cases, it is especially useful to have access to other physicians who have managed Jehovah's Witness cases (hospitals with Bloodless Medicine and Surgery programs are good places to start), and, if possible, to work in partnership with a local Jehovah's Witness Hospital Liaison Committee Elder. The Hospital Information Services (HIS) branch of the Watch Tower Society, headquartered in Brooklyn, New York, has as its mandate provision of education and facilitation of bloodless medicine and

Abdelaziz Y. Elzouki (ed.), *Textbook of Clinical Pediatrics*, DOI 10.1007/978-3-642-02202-9_329,

surgery. HIS has a web site (http://www.watchtower.org/e/vcnr/article_01.htm, accessed January, 2011) with videos showing transfusion alternatives; it also has a contact phone number for physicians listed on that web site: 1-718-560-4300. When HIS was contacted by this writer regarding a contact number for physicians using this chapter they also suggested their e-mail address: his@jw.org.

HIS services also include Hospital Liaison Committees (HLCs) with specially trained Jehovah's Witness HLC Elders whose function is to support the patient and family and to work in cooperation with treating health-care professionals. There are 131 HLCs in the USA and 1,650 worldwide in over 200 countries. HLC Elders can be contacted through inquiries directed by the Witness family to leaders at their local centers of worship; HLC Elders can also be reached through contact with HIS. HLCs have access to a large database of medical literature on bloodless medicine and surgery and preprinted general information on management of the surgical patient, the critically ill patient, the ob/gyn patient, etc. HLC Elders will often bring such literature to the attention of the treating physician for his or her perusal regarding relevance to the case at hand. More importantly to the treating practitioner, HLC Elders also have access through HIS to a worldwide network of physicians who have extensive experience in treating Jehovah's Witness patients and who are often willing to provide timely telephone and electronic (pertinent papers, etc.) consultation to less-experienced health-care providers. Simply seeing interaction between their treating health-care providers and HLC Elders is often tremendously reassuring to families, and these Elders can also help with support of the family and the child if transfusion is ultimately necessary. Health-care providers are frequently fearful that the transfused child will be ostracized by the Jehovah's Witness community. In this writer's extensive Canadian and US experience, this has not been the case.

Know and explore the acceptability of the full range of "matters of conscience" minor fractions and non-blood therapeutic options with the patient and family and use them prior to resorting to unacceptable blood options, time permitting.

In the Developing World, the only blood product available may be whole blood, and this is unacceptable to Witnesses. Also unacceptable are the four primary components of whole blood (red cells, platelets, plasma, white cells) which are usually prepared by simple centrifugation of whole blood or some modification of this. However, once primary components of whole blood are further sub-separated into their constituent parts, receipt of the resulting "fraction" is considered a "matter of conscience." For example, from a 500 ml whole blood donation, a 250–300 ml unit of plasma may be separated. Neither the whole blood nor the plasma is acceptable to Witnesses. However, if that unit of plasma is chilled, and the flocculent white precipitate is centrifuged out to prepare a unit of cryoprecipitate (usually about 10–15 ml), that cryoprecipitate "fraction" is considered to be a matter of conscience – as is the fibrin glue that can be further prepared from a pool of cryoprecipitate activated with bovine thrombin.

The use of cryoprecipitate, if acceptable, can be helpful in avoiding transfusion of unacceptable blood components. As a unit of cryoprecipitate contains, in very concentrated form, about half the Von Willebrand Factor (important in platelet adhesion), half the Factor VIII, and half the fibrinogen in the original unit of plasma, cryoprecipitate given at ~1 unit/5–10 kg can often help improve platelet function and provide at least some crucial coagulation factors necessary for hemostasis.

Large plasma pools (~2,000–20,000 donors) may also be fractionated into a variety of plasma derivatives such as albumin, plasma-derived clotting proteins (FVIII, FIX, fibrinogen, antithrombin, and others), intravenous immune globulins, Rh immune globulin, and many others. Such plasma derivatives may also be used to make local fibrin glue or topical thrombin hemostatic agents. Such plasma "fractions" are all considered to be "matters of conscience" to individual Witnesses and all may be useful in avoiding transfusion of unacceptable primary components in selected situations.

It is worth noting that many adult Witnesses in the USA and elsewhere carry "Advance Directives." These are concise statements of the individual's wishes regarding medical interventions and end-of-life care and include a section dealing with blood and blood fractions. Usually, if one blood fraction is acceptable, all are. However, it is often helpful for the practitioner to be able to explain where the fractions come from in relation to whole blood, as many Advance Directives state the patient might be willing to accept fractions but needs to know more about them.

In explaining fractions to Jehovah's Witness, several things may be helpful. First, the practitioner should make it explicit that the "fraction" discussion is being motivated not by a desire to coerce, but rather to use the full armamentarium of products and interventions available and acceptable to the patient to improve medical outcome and to prevent administration of unacceptable products and interventions. Second, it may be helpful to emphasize plasma's general role as a sort of "carrier river," not only for cellular blood elements made in the bone marrow (red cells, white cells, and platelets), but also for blood sugar, hormones, waste products, liver and kidney function enzymes, and for clotting proteins made in the liver and linings of the blood vessels (such as Von Willebrand Factor, fibrinogen, and other clotting factors), and for albumin (a protein made in the liver which helps blood stay in vessels and stabilizes many hormones). Third, that use of fractions can truly spare use of unacceptable products at times and even be lifesaving – for example, although neither platelets nor plasma is acceptable to Witnesses, cryoprecipitate can help platelets work better, fibrin glue and topical thrombin hemostatic agents can help make local clots when used during surgery or invasive procedures, and albumin can help blood stay in the vessels. Fourth, it may be helpful to note that while cellular blood elements do not normally traffic across the placenta, the other fractions do. (This was a personal observation made to this writer by a HLC Elder when queried regarding his own "matters of conscience" beliefs, and used with his permission subsequently in explaining fractions to other Jehovah's Witness patients). Lastly, it is also worth noting that HLC Elders can often assist in explaining fractions and transfusion-sparing interventions where the blood is kept in contact with the body (Cell Saver, perioperative hemodilution) to patients and families. They can also help provide the patient and family with information – written, videos – explaining these.

As the whole issue of acceptability of different fractions and interventions can vary greatly according to the individual conscience of a particular Witness family, it can be useful for hospitals and transfusing institutions to have a special "Blood Refusal" Form which concisely summarizes these. As a model, the Oregon Health & Science University "Transfusion Blood Refusal" form is shown in ➋ *Fig. 329.1.*

Interestingly, hemoglobin-based oxygen carriers (HBOCs), derived from human or animal red cells, are also considered "fractions" and "matters of conscience" by Witnesses. Only one HBOC (Hemopure by Biopure) was ever licensed worldwide and then only in South Africa, although several have been available on a "Compassionate Release" basis in the past, with the Compassionate Release Programs being made available by the companies and overseen by national regulatory agencies such as the US FDA. Compassionate Release Programs exclude minors, however, and, as of this writing (January 2011), to this writer's knowledge, no Compassionate Release Programs currently exist anywhere worldwide. Also, to this writer's knowledge, manufacture of essentially all HBOCs has currently been terminated or suspended due to unfavorable phase 3 trial outcomes and such products were no longer available anywhere worldwide as of January 2011, apart from residual stores in South Africa.

As mentioned, other "matters of conscience" to Witnesses are intraoperative blood salvage where the blood is kept in contact with the body ("Cell Saver"–type devices, perioperative hemodilution). These interventions are generally not suitable for small children. The "Cell Saver" is most useful in large volume "clean" losses (no infection or malignancy present) such as vascular surgery. Perioperative hemodilution is generally most useful in patients with high starting hematocrits and large volume losses, and may be used in malignancy cases.

Act preemptively if possible to prevent anemia and coagulopathy and use combined interventions to treat these.

Routine supplementation of Witness patients with hematinics, especially in the context of hospitalization and perisurgically is often advisable. This should include consideration of full marrow repletion doses of iron preferably given IV, as oral iron may be poorly tolerated and often cannot be given quickly enough in large enough doses. The iron sucrose preparations and other iron preparations associated with very low reaction rates are recommended. It should be noted that in sick patients, iron studies and ferritin are unreliable and that normal ferritins do not rule out absent bone marrow iron stores. Daily folate either PO or IV should also be given. Vitamin K supplementation PO or IV twice weekly is also often helpful.

The issue of use of erythroid-stimulating agents (ESAs) such as erythropoietin (epo) and darbepoietin (darbe) should be considered. There is more experience with the use of epo in pediatric patients and it alone may be approved for pediatric use. Although neither epo nor darbe is derived from blood, epo is stabilized with traces of albumin and may therefore be unacceptable to certain Witnesses, whereas darbe is albumin free. Iron repletion is essential for ESAs to act most effectively and should be assured prior to ESA administration. ESAs are most effective given preoperatively as there is antagonism to the effect of ESAs mediated by inflammatory cytokines postoperatively and in the context of intercurrent illness. To obtain a reticulocyte rise with ESAs usually takes 3–4 days (rises of five- to tenfold above baseline are usual), and to obtain a meaningful increase in the hemoglobin (>1 g/dl) usually takes 10–14 days. To significantly augment the hemoglobin (Hb) preoperatively with an ESA can therefore take 3–4 weeks. Weekly doses of epo at 300–500 U/kg (or equivalent doses of darbe) are recommended for this purpose, preferably given SQ rather than IV. In the postoperative setting, and in the setting of illness, there is usually inflammatory cytokine-mediated (IL-1, TNF, and

Oregon Health & Science University
Hospitals and Clinics

MR1418

TRANSFUSION BLOOD REFUSAL

Page 1 of 1

ACCOUNT NO.
MED. REC. NO.
NAME
BIRTHDATE

Patient Identification

Please check one: ( ) I myself or
( ) My minor child (aged_____) or
( ) The person I am signing this Refusal for because: ____________

____

am one of **Jehovah's Witnesses** and refuse transfusion of whole blood or any of its primary components (red cells, white cells, platelets or plasma). Jehovah's Witnesses consider a number of fractions of primary components to be matters of conscience. Other matters of conscience are erythropoietin and intra-operative blood salvage. I am indicating below whether any of these blood fractions or blood alternatives are acceptable to me (or person I am signing for).

Blood Fraction or Transfusion Alternative	Acceptable	Unacceptable
Erythropoietin (EPO) (stabilized with traces of albumin)	( )	( )
Intra-operative blood salvage where the blood is kept in contact with my body ("Cell-Saver," perioperative hemodilution)	( )	( )
Cryoprecipitate	( )	( )
Fibrin Glue	( )	( )
Plasma derived clotting factor concentrates	( )	( )
Albumin	( )	( )
Rh immune globulin, intravenous gamma globulin and other gamma globulin preparations	( )	( )
Topical Thrombin Hemostatic Agents	( )	( )

( ) I am not a Jehovah's Witness but refuse the following blood products:

____

The risk attendant to my refusal has been explained to me, and I understand that my refusal may in some cases seriously reduce my chances of regaining normal health or even threaten my life. I further understand that every effort will be made to deliver highest quality medical care using all available means despite my refusal; also that I am free to modify this refusal at any time. I release the Hospital, its personnel and other persons participating in my care from any responsibility for respecting and following my express wishes and directions.

Refusal of Blood transfusion for a minor. As the parent/guardian of a minor child I understand that the doctor(s) treating my child will make every effort to respect my beliefs regarding the transfusion of blood products as indicated above. However I also recognize that my child's physicians have a legal obligation not to withhold therapy the think is necessary to keep my child alive or to keep him/her from serious harm or permanent injury or disability. I understand therefore that, if the treating physician believes transfusion, after evaluating alternative non-blood medical management, is necessary to save my child's life, or to prevent serious irreversible harm, my child may be transfused, although every effort will be made to avoid this.

____________ ____________

Patient's Parent's Guardian's Consenter's (circle one) Signature **Date and time**

If Consenter specify relationship to patient: ____________

____________ ____________

Signature of Witness to this Refusal **Date and time**

The staff physician should notify the Multnomah County Juvenile Court at (503) 988-3460 (M-F, 8am – 5pm) and ask to speak to someone in the Intake Department regarding an emergency medical court order, after 5pm and on weekends call (503) 988-3489 or (503) 988-3475 and ask to speak to someone in the Custody Intake Department regarding an emergency medical court order.

ONLINE 9/08 (Supersedes 6/07) **MR-1418**

Figure 329.1

others) resistance to the action of epo. This can often be at least partially overcome by pharmacological doses of epo (300–500 U/kg SQ daily).

ESA use in adults with critical illness and with malignancy is associated with increased thrombogenicity (blood clots, heart failure, myocardial infarction, stroke). It is unclear if this is also the case in pediatrics. In older children requiring sustained high dose epo therapy, consideration should be given to prophylactic doses of antithrombotics. In the case of cancer in adult populations, use of ESAs is also associated with increases in mortality independent of thrombogenicity and possibly mediated by tumor receptors for ESAs and promotion of angiogenesis. The US Food and Drug Administration (FDA) issued a block box warning for ESAs in 2007 prompting a series of revised clinical guidelines and, as of 2010, the FDA is requiring that all ESAs given to patients with malignancy be prescribed under a Risk Evaluation and Mitigation Strategy (REMS) which includes a medication guide to explain risks to patients and caregivers, and the ESA APPRISE (Assisting Providers and cancer Patients with Risk Information for the Safe use of ESAs) Oncology Program (http://www.fda.gov/Drugs/DrugSafety/PostmarketDrugSafetyInformationforPatientsandProviders/ucm200297.htm, accessed January 29, 2011). Thus, in pediatric patients with cancer, careful weighing of the risk benefit of ESA administration needs to be done.

Regarding management of thrombocytopenia or thrombocytopathy in Witnesses refusing platelet transfusion, cryoprecipitate, if acceptable, at 1 U/5–10 kg is often effective in the treatment of petechaie and minor platelet-type bleeding in patients, and this dose may be administered prophylactically daily if the platelet count is under 10×10^{-9}/l. Adult anecdotal and published experience, and anecdotal pediatric experience, suggests administration of either aminocaproic acid or tranexamic acid may also be helpful in preventing and treating bleeding if the platelet count is $<10^{-30} \times 10^{-9}$/l. Tranexamic acid if available is a more potent antifibrinolytic agent than aminocaproic acid. Consideration may also be given to the use of thrombopoietin (tpo) mimetics if available (romiplostim, eltrombopag).

It should be noted that Witnesses have no issues with the use of a variety of non-blood-derived and non-albumin-stabilized pharmacological hemostatic agents such as ddAVP, antifibrinolytics, and recombinant factor VIIa. As well, as discussed in the section on fractions above, fibrin glues and topical thrombin-based hemostatic agents may be acceptable and transfusion-sparing in the setting of surgery or invasive procedures.

Realize physiological tolerance of anemia is generally greater than one might think.

Tolerance of anemia is determined by multiple factors including chronicity of development, underlying cardiovascular status, age, and oxygen demands. Animal studies suggest the lower limit of tolerance to sustained anemia in animals with a normal cardiovascular system is a Hb of around 3–5 g/dl and in those animals with coronary stenosis is a Hb around 7–10 g/dl. The largest published series of morbidity and mortality in the perioperative setting in adult patients refusing blood transfusion suggests that survival with a Hb < 2 g/dl is very infrequent and that both morbidity and mortality rise substantially when the Hb falls to less than 5–6 g/dl. That said, the Transfusion in Critical Care (TRICC) trial indicates that in adult ICU patients, there is at least an equivalent outcome in patients randomized to a restrictive (target Hb 7–9 g/dl) rather than liberal (target Hb 10–12 g/dl) transfusion strategy. This has recently also been confirmed in the pediatric critical care setting. Thus, as a general rule, concerns regarding adverse effects of anemia should probably begin to rise only when the Hb falls below 7 g/dl, and the decision to intervene subsequently needs to be tempered by the anticipated chronicity of further fall in the Hb, the underlying cardiovascular status of the patient, and the anticipated oxygen demands the patient will face (sepsis, surgery, etc.). In children, it is probably unwise to wait to transfuse until frank florid physiological decompensation as children appear to manifest signs and symptoms of impending decompensation later than adults.

Make the family aware of the legal obligation to transfuse a minor to prevent serious harm or death.

Witnesses generally abide by the law despite strong objection at times to its dictates (transfusion of minor children). In the USA, in the case of impending serious irreversible harm or death, traditionally "court orders" have been obtained mandating transfusion of minor children whose Jehovah's Witness parents or guardians have refused to sign permission for blood transfusion. Court orders are often traumatic to Witness families not only because of the transfusion itself, but because court orders are usually subsets of child abuse laws, and when a court order is obtained the child is made a ward of the court, and a court-appointed representative thereafter legally signs permission for surgeries, dialysis, etc. If a court order is obtained therefore it is advisable to ask that it be limited only to blood. At the author's institution, Oregon Health & Science University (OHSU), the Transfusion Blood Refusal Form (➋ *Fig. 329.1.*) tries to avoid court orders by incorporating specific language indicating that the parent or guardian, while not giving permission for the transfusion, nonetheless recognizes the legal obligation of the treating physician to transfuse to save life or prevent irreversible harm. If the parent or guardian signs this form, it is the opinion of both OHSU Legal and Risk Management that a court order is not necessary, and very few have been obtained subsequent to this form's adoption.

References

Avvisati G, Bfiller HR, Ten Cate JW et al (1989) Tranexamic acid for control of haemorrhage in acute promyelocytic leukemia. Lancet 334(8655):122–124

Brown NM, Keck G, Ford PA (2008) Acute myeloid leukemia in Jehovah's Witnesses. Leuk Lymphoma 49(4):817–820

Carson JL, Noveck H, Berlin JA et al (2002) Mortality and morbidity in patients with very low postoperative Hb levels who decline blood transfusion. Transfusion 42:812–818

Fergusson DA, McIntyre L (2008) The future of clinical trials evaluating blood substitutes. J Am Med Assoc 299(19):2324–2326. doi:10.1001/jama.299.19.jed80027

Hebert PC, Wells G, Blajchman MA et al (1999) A multicenter, randomized controlled trial of transfusion requirements in critical care. N Engl J Med 340:409–417

LaCroix J, Hebert PC, Hutchison JS et al (2007) Transfusion strategies for patients in pediatric intensive care units. N Engl J Med 356:1609–1619

Mitka M (2007) FDA sounds alert on anemia drugs. J Am Med Assoc 297(17):1868–1869

Monk TG (2005) Acute normovolemic hemodilution. Anesthesiol Clin North Am 23:271–281

Natanson C, Kern S, Lurie P et al (2008) Cell-free hemoglobin based blood substitutes and risk of myocardial infarction and death: a meta-analysis. J Am Med Assoc 299(19):E1–E9. doi:10.1001/jama.299.19.jrv80007

Rizzo JD, Brouwers M, Hurley P et al (2010) American Society of Hematology/American Society of Clinical Oncology clinical practice guideline update on the use of epoetin and darbepoetin in adult patients with cancer. Prepublished online as Blood First Edition paper, 25 Oct 2010, DOI: 10.1182/blood-201008-300541

330 Disorders of Heme Biosynthesis

Thomas G. DeLoughery

Porphyria

The porphyrias are a group of rare diseases of heme metabolism (➋ *Table 330.1*). They have a protean array of symptoms and can represent a diagnostic challenge. Although rare, diagnosis is important as a mainstay of therapy for most porphyria is avoidance of precipitating factors.

Symptoms

One fundamental principle is that the pathogenesis of symptoms of porphyria is due to accumulations of the metabolites of heme synthesis (➋ *Fig. 330.1*). These metabolites can be neurotoxic (ALA, PGB), acutely toxic to the skin (protoporphyrins), or chronically toxic to the skin (uropophyrinogen and coproporphyrinogen) (➋ *Table 330.2*). Thus, there are three basic ways porphyria can present:

1. Neurovisceral – The neurovisceral symptoms consist of autonomic neuropathies (constipation, colicky abdominal pain, vomiting, hypertension), peripheral neuropathy (most often motor), seizures, delirium, coma, and depression. The abdominal pain is severe and lasts for several days. Severe abdomen pain of short (less than one day) duration or chronic abdominal pain is unusual. The sequence of events in attacks is usually: first abdominal pain, then psychiatric symptoms such as hysteria, and then the peripheral neuropathies. Most patients are completely free of symptoms between attacks. Hyponatremia due to SIADH can be seen in severe cases. These symptoms can be seen with AIP, HCP, and VP.
2. Acute cutaneous – Symptoms occur quickly (minutes) of being exposed to the sun – redness, edema, and itching and is seen with EP, CEP, and HP.
3. Chronic cutaneous – The cutaneous manifestations are characterized by bullae formation in sun exposed areas, fragile skin, and hypertrichosis and is seen with PCT, HCP, VP, CEP, and HP.

Most porphyrias present at puberty or older. The exceptions are the rare ALA dehydratase porphyria, congenital erythropoietic porphyria, or hepateoerythropoietic porphyria which present soon after birth. Also, symptoms of EP can start in childhood.

Diagnosis

The diagnosis of any porphyria is based on both the clinical presentation and the demonstration of excessive porphyrin excretion in relation to these symptoms. The essential procedure in ascribing any neurovisceral symptoms to porphyria is to establish that there is an increase in porphyrin precursors at the time of these problems. These precursors are PorphoBilinoGen (PBG) and AminoLevulinic Acid (ALA). A common mistake in diagnosing porphyria is to observe just an elevated level of porphyrins (not precursors) in the urine or stool and label the patient as having porphyria. Neurovisceral attacks are only associated with over-excretion of PGB and ALA. This is most common in AIP, but can be seen in VP and HCP. Another difficulty in diagnosing porphyria is many patients have minor (less than 3–5 times) elevation of urine and/or stool porphyrins. This can be a normal variant or seen in fasting, iron deficiency, ingestion of meat, or any illness. The chronic cutaneous porphyrias – PCT, HCP, and VP – have classic dermatological manifestations. The key testing is urine and stool for the formed porphyrins such as uropophyrinogen. There is an entity known as "Pseudoporphyria" where patients have the skin manifestations of porphyria but urine and stools demonstrate normal porphyrin excretion. This can be seen as a complication of certain medications such as naproxen or in dialysis patients. The acute cutaneous porphyrias are diagnosed by finding increased erythrocyte porphyrins.

A very simple bedside assay for acute porphyrias is examination of a fresh urine sample. It is clear at first, but will darken with exposure to the sun. If available, the presence of PBG can be confirmed by adding Ehrlich's aldehyde reagent in a 1:1 ratio to the urine; the presence of a pink color confirms the presence of PBG. Definitive

Abdelaziz Y. Elzouki (ed.), *Textbook of Clinical Pediatrics*, DOI 10.1007/978-3-642-02202-9_330,

Table 330.1
The porphyria

	Presentation	Urine	Stool	RBC	Inheritance
Neurovisceral porphyria		PBG, ALA, porphyrins			
Acute intermittent porphyria (AIP)	Acute attacks				AD
Neurovisceral +/– cutaneous					
Coproporphyria (HCP)	Acute attacks, skin blisters	PBG, ALA, porphyrins	Copro		AD
Variegate porphyria (VP)	Acute attacks, skin blisters	PBG, ALA, porphyrins	Proto IX > Copro		AD
Cutaneous					
Porphyria cutanea tarda (PCT)	Skin blisters	Uro, Hepta	Isocopro, hepta		AD
Photosensitivity					
Erythropoietic protoporphyria (EP)	Acute photosensitivity	Normal	Proto IX	Free proto	AD
X-linked protoporphyria	Acute photosensitivity	Normal	Proto IX	Free and Zn proto	X-Linked
Recessive					
ALA dehydratase porphyria	Neuropathy	ALA, copro	Normal	Proto IX	AR
Congenital erythropoietic porphyria (CEP)	Severe photosensitivity	Uro, Copro	Copro	Uro, copro	AR
Hepateoerythropoietic porphyria (HP)	Severe photosensitivity	Uro, Hepta	Isocopro, hepta	Proto IX	AR

PBG porphobilinogen, *ALA* aminolevulic acid, *copro* coporphyrin, *uro* uroporphyrin, *isocopro* isocoproporphyrin, *proto* protoporphyrin, *AD* autosomal dominant, *AR* autosome recessive

diagnosis of the different porphyrias requires analysis of urine, stool, and blood samples for the specific porphyrins and their precursors. In theory, since most porphyrias are due to mutations in the genes encoding the enzymes for heme synthesis, DNA analysis or assays of enzymes active would be useful. But given the low penetrance of the porphyria, this testing is useful only in selected cases.

Acute (Neurovisceral) Porphyrias

Acute intermittent porphyria has onset in puberty with only neurovisceral symptoms. Many more patients have the genetic defect than express clinical disease. Most patients will only have one attack. Attacks are provoked by anything that leads to increase in the heme synthesis pathway. The classics are starvation (glucose suppresses heme synthesis) and a multitude of drugs. The classic drugs are estrogen, barbiturates, and ethanol. There are lists of "safe" and "unsafe," easily found on the Internet. http://www.drugs-porphyria.org and http://www.porphyriafoundation.com are the two most researched and complete websites.

Diagnosis is by a demonstrated increase – greater than tenfold – in urine porphobilinogen. Levels can remain raised for years after the attack. One can verify by checking the activity level of PBG deaminase, but this will be normal in 10% of patients as only the hepatic form is affected and not the form measured in the circulating red cells.

The therapy of the neurovisceral symptoms of AIP is based on shutting down the heme synthesis pathway to prevent accumulation of the toxic precursors. High doses of glucose (300 g/day) can mildly inhibit the pathway and is used for mild attacks. Hematin, which is intravenous preparation of heme, is used for severe attacks to stop the heme synthesis pathway. Either heme-arginine (250 mg × 5 days) or hematin (4 mg/kg × 4 days) can be used to suppress the heme synthetic pathway and is effective for severe acute attacks or attacks associated with neurological defects. These agents are well tolerated but can lead to

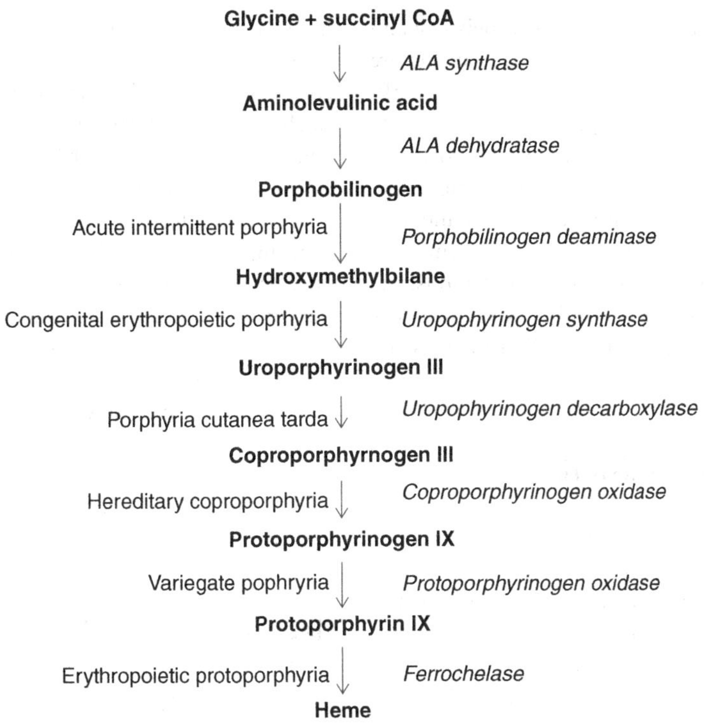

Figure 330.1
Heme synthesis

Table 330.2
The porphyrias: symptoms and therapy

	Therapy
Neurovisceral	Acute: increase glucose, hematin Chronic: avoid fasting and precipitating drugs
Acute intermittent porphyria (AIP)	
Coproporphyria (HCP)	
Variegate porphyria (VP)	
Cutaneous	Phlebotomized to reduce ferritin, avoid sun exposure, avoid precipitating medications
Porphyria cutanea tarda (PCT)	
Photosensitivity	Avoid sun exposure, beta-carotene
Erythropoietic protoporphyria (EP)	
X-linked protoporphyria	
Recessive	
ALA dehydratase porphyria	Hematin
Congenital erythropoietic porphyria (CEP)	Stem cell transplant
Hepateoerythropoietic porphyria (HP)	Avoid sun exposure

thrombophlebitis and often need to be given via central venous access. Rarely, there can be a severe sympathetic crisis manifesting with severe hypertension and seizures. Patients with repeated attacks can be treated with weekly heme infusions. In patients with severe intractable symptoms, liver transplantation can be considered. Prevention of future attacks is by avoiding precipitating factors such as fasting, medications, and alcohol.

Hereditary coproporphyria has both neurovisceral and skin manifestations (described under PCT). Patients are rarely symptomatic. Diagnosis is by demonstrating markedly increased urine and stool coproporphyrinogens. As noted above, mild elevations of coproporphyrinogens is common and not pathogenic. Treatment is the same as AIP.

Variegate porphyria has both neurovisceral and skin manifestations (described under PCT). Patients are sporadically symptomatic. Diagnosis is by demonstrating markedly increased urine and stool coproporphyrinogen and protoporphyrinogen. Treatment is the same as AIP.

Chronic Cutaneous (Blistering) Porphyrias

Porphyria cutanea tarda presents with skin disease in sun exposed areas. The first signs are fragile skin with, then, the formation of blisters and bulla that can take weeks to heal. This over time leads to chronic skin damage with increased pigmentation and hair growth. Given the relationship with sun exposure, the skin involved is on the upper hands, face, and neck. Most patients have an acquired inhibitor of uropophyrinogen decarboxylase, with only a minority (~25%) having a mutation in the gene encoding for this enzyme; but even, patients with the mutation will only manifest symptoms with acquitted risk factors. The risk factors for PCT are liver damage – from alcohol – iron overload and hepatitis, estrogens, and HIV. Iron overload appears to be crucial given the relationship of the hemochromatosis genotype and iron overload with PCT.

Diagnosis is the combination of the classic skin findings and demonstration of excess urine uropophyrinogen and stool isocoproporphyrinogen. Therapy is by reduction of iron stores. Phlebotomy with a goal ferritin of under 50 mg/L is very effective. Patients must be cautious that their skin disease resolution can lag by months, as the porphyrin laden skin must be shed for symptoms to abate. Chloroquine (100–200 mg two times weekly) can also be effective especially in the rare patient who cannot be phlebotomized. Also helpful is avoidance of risk factors such as excess sun exposure, estrogen, or alcohol.

Acute Cutaneous (Photosensitive) Porphyrias

Erythropoietic protoporphyria has early onset of acute photosensitive. Patients noticed with sun exposure will have a burning, stinging sensation in their skin. This can be accompanied by swelling and redness. Cold water or compression can bring symptom-relief. Over time, there can be chronic skin damage with skin thickening, crusting, and waxy-changes. In ~10% of patients, there can be liver disease due to accumulation of protoporphyrins that, over time, can lead to liver failure. Diagnosis is established by showing increased levels of stool and red cell protoporphyrins. The vast majority of patients have mutations in the ferrochelase gene, but about 2% have an X-linked mutation in the ALA synthase gene.

Therapy is by protecting the skin from sunlight. Clothing, large hats, and sun screen can be used. Beta-carotene (75–200 mg/day) can help symptoms in some patients. Patients need to be screened yearly for liver disease, for which liver transplantation may sometimes be required.

Neonatal Porphyrias

ALA dehydratase porphyria is extremely rare but can cause neurovisceral attacks in children. Diagnosis is made by demonstrating marked over-excretion of ALA in the urine. Therapy is with hematin, but some patients have had a progressive course despite therapy.

Congenital erythropoietic porphyria is marked by severe photosensitivity starting at an early age that can lead to mutilating changes and disfigurement with loss of appendages. Teeth can be pink to red due to accumulation of porphyrins. Patient can have bone disease leading to fractures. Many patients have a hemolytic anemia that can be severe with associated large spleen.

Diagnosis can be suggested by the clinical findings and red urine in the diapers. Diagnosis is established by finding excess isomer I of uropophyrinogen and coproporphyrin in urine, stool, and red cells.

Curative therapy is with stem cell transplantation. If this cannot be done, then supportive care can be tried with avoidance of sun exposure and splenectomy if hypersplenism is present.

Hepateoerythropoietic porphyria can lead to a severe PCT syndrome in childhood. The main differential diagnosis is CEP, but the skin disease tends to be more scarring than mutilating. The defect is a homozygous mutation in the uropophyrinogen decarboxylase gene and diagnosis is made by demonstrating excess urine uropophyrinogen and stool isocoproporphyrinogen. Therapy is supportive with avoiding sun exposure. Unlike PCT, reduction of iron stores and chloroquine are not effective.

References

Anderson KE, Bloomer JR, Bonkovsky HL, Kushner JP, Pierach CA, Pimstone NR, Desnick RJ (2005) Recommendations for the diagnosis and treatment of the acute porphyrias. Ann Intern Med 142(6):439–450

Bonkovsky HL (2005) Neurovisceral porphyrias: what a hematologist needs to know. Hematology Am Soc Hematol Educ Program 24–30

Puy H, Gouya L, Deybach JC (2010) Porphyrias. Lancet 375(9718):924–937

Sarkany RP (2008) Making sense of the porphyrias. Photodermatol Photoimmunol Photomed 24(2):102–108

331 Platelet Structure, Function, and Disorders

Daniel Greenberg

Introduction

Platelets are anucleate cells that circulate in the bloodstream. They are essential for normal hemostasis, and patients with a very low concentration of circulating platelets or disorders that result in severe platelet dysfunction have serious bleeding disorders. They are also essential for normal clot retraction and wound healing. Conversely, platelet adhesions to vascular atherosclerotic lesions are a major cause of myocardial infarction and ischemic stroke. Over the past several years, numerous elegant experimental observations suggest platelets also play a key role in angiogenesis and in pathological processes such as infection and cancer metastasis.

Platelets are derived from bone marrow progenitor stem cells in a process known as thrombopoiesis. During this process, the pluripotent marrow stem cell first undergoes a transformation into a giant cell with a large cytoplasm and a polyploid nucleus, called a megakaryocyte. Platelets are created when the cytoplasm of the megakaryocyte divides into thousands of individual platelets that are released into the circulation through the bone marrow sinusoids (see ➲ *Fig. 331.1*). Accordingly, platelets can be thought of little packages of the megakaryocyte cytoplasm wrapped up in a specialized membrane. Thrombopoiesis is regulated, in large part, by the hepatic production of the cytokine thrombopoietin (TPO). TPO is homologous with erythropoietin (EPO); however, the TPO receptor (Mpl) is primarily expressed by stem cells and megakaryocytes in the bone marrow, whereas the EPO receptor is primarily expressed by erythroblasts and developing erythroid cells. Although TPO is not known to have a direct biological effect on mature platelets, TPO is cleared from the plasma by platelets through the process of receptor-induced endocytosis. The concentration of TPO in the plasma and its biological effect of inducing thrombopoiesis are largely regulated by the platelet count through this negative feedback pathway: Because of the clearance of TPO by platelets, a high platelet count has the effect of decreasing the concentration of biologically active TPO. Conversely, a low concentration of platelets results in an increased concentration of free TPO in the plasma. For almost all normal individuals, this feedback mechanism results in circulating a platelet concentration between 150,000 and 350,000/μl of whole blood.

During normal hemostasis, platelets are recruited to a site of vascular injury where they become activated to form a plug over the disrupted vessel(s). This process of platelet activation is mediated by complex array of membrane receptors and other integral membrane and cytoskeleton proteins which are essential for normal platelet activation and hemostasis. The receptors present on the platelet plasma membrane range from specialized adhesive receptors that recognize complex polymeric proteins such as fibrinogen, collagen, and Von Willebrand Factor to specific single molecule receptors (e.g., ADP, thrombin, and collagen) that mediate platelet activation through intracellular signal transduction pathways. ➲ *Figure 331.2* shows a schematic representation of platelets adhering to the sub-endothelium by VWF and aggregating in the presence of fibrinogen. The aggregated platelet plug provides a surface for the coagulation proteins to form fibrin (secondary phase of hemostasis).

Most clinical laboratory testing of platelet activation relies on the ability of platelets to aggregate in the presence of fibrinogen after the platelets are stimulated with a platelet agonist such as thrombin, collagen, or ADP. These agonists act on specific platelet receptors (see below) all of which end up causing the activation of the platelet fibrinogen receptor to recognize and bind fibrinogen. Fibrinogen is a large hetero-heximeric protein that forms bridges between activated platelets piled one on top of another to form a stable aggregate. In the commonly practiced platelet aggregation test, a solution containing the patient's platelets (either platelet rich plasma or whole blood) is treated with the appropriate agonists in the presence of fibrinogen. The solution is then analyzed to determine the extent to which the platelets have aggregated into clumps relative to a standard, positive control. Full activation of platelet function requires, but is not limited to, platelet aggregation. As discussed below, platelet activation involves much more than the ability to

Abdelaziz Y. Elzouki (ed.), *Textbook of Clinical Pediatrics*, DOI 10.1007/978-3-642-02202-9_331,

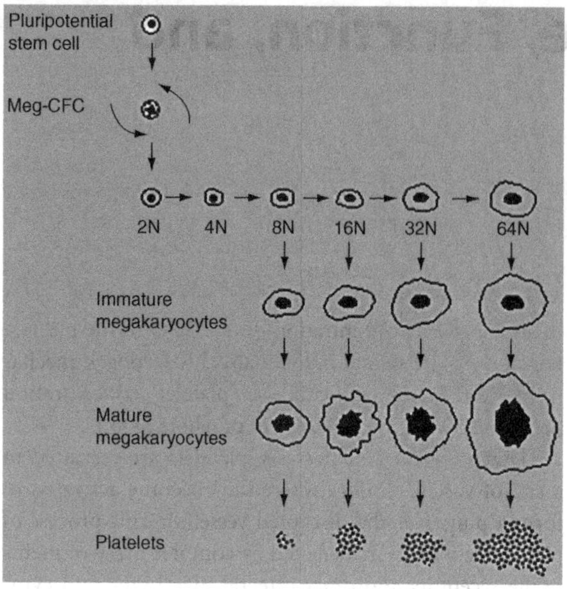

Figure 331.1
Thrombopoiesis. Illustration of the process of megakaryocytic differentiation and thrombopoiesis from the pluripotent bone marrow stem cell. The megakaryocyte first reaches a state of nuclear multiploidy and increases the size of the cytoplasm. Platelets are formed when hundreds of small cytoplasmic fragments are packaged in specialized phopholipid membranes surrounded by a central microtubular ring. Megakarocytic differentiation and thrombopoiesis are controlled by the hepatic production of the cytokine thrombopoietin

aggregate in the presence of fibrinogen. Like other coagulation assays, platelet aggregation and other tests of platelet function require careful interpretation and a firm grasp of their limitations.

Platelet Structure

Cytoskeleton

Normal circulating platelets are about 10 μm in diameter, and appear discoid in shape. The platelet plasma membrane consists of a complex arrangement of constituents including cholesterol, phospholipids, and integral membrane proteins. Many integral membrane proteins, including the adhesive receptors to fibrinogen and Von Willebrand factor, are anchored to an extensive platelet cytoskeleton composed chiefly of actin filaments. These actin filaments are arranged in a fine meshwork just below the plasma membrane and become less dense and more orthogonal in configuration deeper into the platelet cytoplasm. Just under the plasma membrane and surrounding the diameter of the platelet is a thick microtubule filament composed alpha and beta tubulin. ➋ *Figure 331.3* shows a circulating discoid platelet with the membrane peeled back and the cytoskeleton exposed. When platelets are activated to cover a vascular defect, the sub-plasma membrane microtubule ring contracts toward the center of the platelet as the actin cytoskeleton undergoes extensive rearrangement. This results in a dramatic shape change from the inactive, discoid platelet to a flattened platelet that looks somewhat like a "fried egg" spread out over an adhesive surface such a Von Willebrand factor, fibrinogen, or collagen.

The Plasma Membrane

Coincidental with the cytoskeletal changes that occur when platelets are activated to spread over a vascular defect, dramatic changes in structure of the activated platelet plasma membrane also occur and are critical to maintaining normal hemostasis. These events are summarized in ➋ *Fig. 331.4.* The overall effect of these plasma membrane changes is to form a phospholipid surface for the assembly of coagulation cascade components, particularly the *tenase* (FVIIIa/FIXa) and *prothrombinase* (FVa/FXa) complexes. These complexes require the "clottable" phospholipids (phophatidylserine and phosphatidylethanolamine) to achieve their maximal activity. In the resting or inactive state, circulating discoid platelets have an asymmetrical distribution of the phopholipid bilayer of the plasma membrane: Phophatidylcholine and phophatidylinositol, which do not support clotting ("non-clottable" phospholipids) are present predominantly on the outer plasma membrane. Phosphatidylserine and phosphatidylethanolamine, which efficiently support clotting, are present predominantly on the inner plasma membrane. This phopholipid membrane asymmetry is an energy-dependent process mediated, in part, by the integral membrane protein complex *aminophospholipid translocase.* Once platelets are activated to participate in hemostasis, the distribution of the membrane phospholipids is "scrambled" by another integral membrane protein called *scramblase.* The favorable clotting surface provided by phosphatidylserine and phosphatidylethanolamine translocates from the inner leaflet to the outer leaflet of the plasma membrane. In this activated phopholipid membrane configuration, the phospholipid-dependent

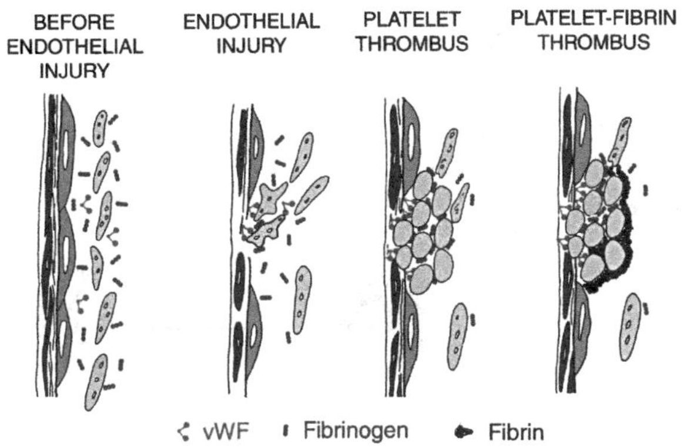

Figure 331.2
Primary and secondary phases of hemostasis. Formation of the platelet plug over a vascular defect is illustrated when Von Willebrand factor (*green*) binds to exposed sub-endothelial collagen and the platelet gpIB receptor. Once a layer of platelets cover the vascular defect, fibrinogen (*red*) further aggregates platelets on top of one another (through activation of platelet gpIIB-IIIA) to form a platelet plug. At the same time, tissue factor generated by injured endothelial cells associates with factor VIIa to start the extrinsic pathway of coagulation. With the platelet plug in place, the coagulation factors assemble on the activated platelet membrane surface to form a strong fibrin (*black*) covering that stabilizes and secures the platelet plug. The formation of the platelet plug by Von Willebrand factor and fibrinogen is referred to as the primary phase of hemostasis, and the production of fibrin by the plasma coagulation factors is referred to as the secondary phase of hemostasis

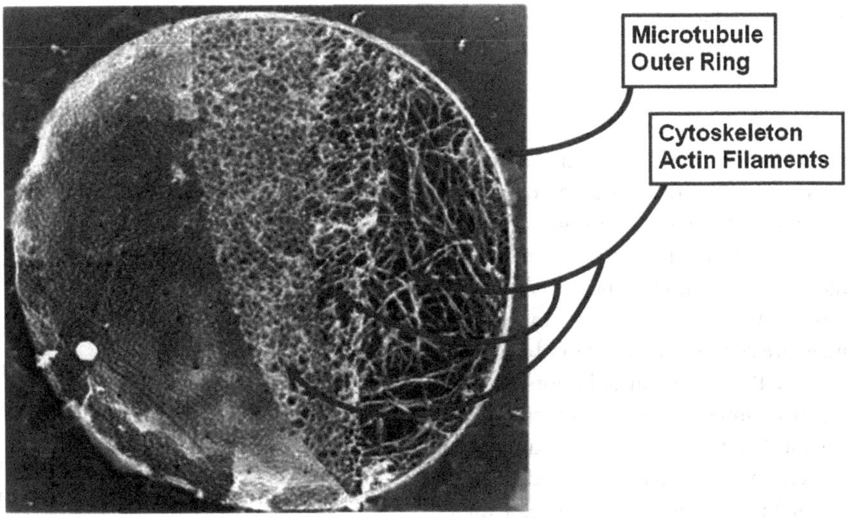

Figure 331.3
Platelet cytoskeleton. The cytoskeleton of the circulating discoid platelet is shown by electron micrograph. Immediately beneath the plasma membrane is a fine meshwork of filamentous actin which becomes more orthogonal and less dense deeper into the cytoplasm. An outer microtubule ring composed of a tubulin filament surrounds the platelet and contracts toward the center upon platelet activation and granular secretion

steps of the coagulation cascade are able to assemble on the platelet surface to generate a fibrin covering that anchors and protects the platelet plug. Accordingly, hemostasis is often divided into two phases: the primary phase in which platelets are localized to the wound by VWF and aggregated on top of the wound by fibrinogen, and a secondary phase in which the coagulation cascade (which is dependent on a "clottable"

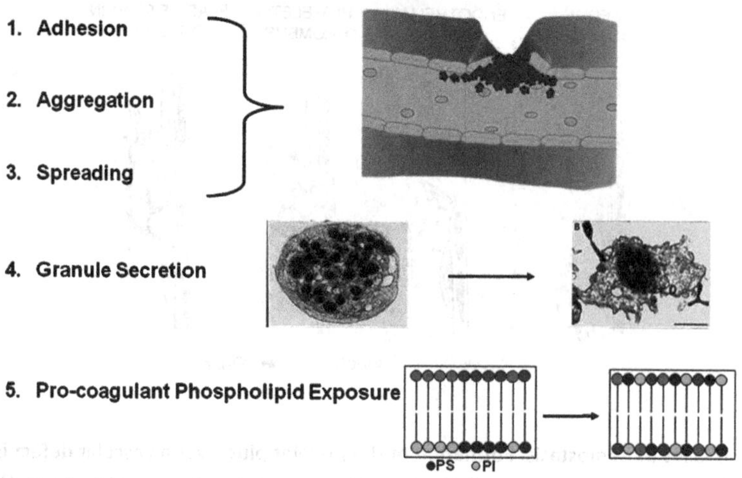

Figure 331.4
Multistep process of platelet activation. The process of platelet activation starts with platelet adhesion, aggregation, and spreading (Steps 1–3). Simultaneous central contraction of the microtubule ring with granule secretion as well as translocation of phophatidylserine [(PS) "clottable" phospholipid (Steps 4 and 5)] and "non-clottable" phosphatidylinositol (PI) are also illustrated

phospholipid surface provided by the localized, activated platelets) results in the activation of thrombin and the conversion of fibrinogen to fibrin.

Cytoplasmic Granules

Platelets also contain unique granules within their cytoplasm. These granules are of two distinct types: dense (or delta) granules and alpha granules. Dense granules are smaller than alpha granules and are composed mainly of calcium and magnesium ions, non-metabolic ATP and ADP, and the vasoconstrictive agent 5-hydroxytryptamine. Dense granules are composed chiefly of fibrinogen, Von Willebrand factor, P-selectin (an adhesion protein that is thought to play an important role in atherosclerosis), and platelet factor 4 (a homo-tetramer of uncertain function that is associated with heparin-induced thrombocytopenia). Both alpha and dense granules release their contents from the platelet cytosplasm after the platelet undergoes activation. During platelet activation, these granules merge with a specialized membranous system called the open canalicular system (OCS). The OCS is a complex membranous structure that is contiguous with the plasma membrane and serves as the pathway for transport of substances into the platelet and as conduits for the discharge of granule products secreted during the platelet release reaction (activation). Inherited deficiencies in platelet granule structure or function often result in mild to moderate bleeding disorders.

Adhesion Receptors: Von Willebrand Factor Receptor and Fibrinogen Receptor

Platelets express a number of important receptors on the plasma membrane surface that is essential for normal platelet function. These receptors can be grouped as adhesive, such as the fibrinogen and Von Willebrand factor receptors, or activating, such as the thrombin and collagen receptors. First the adhesive receptors will be discussed followed by the activating and other receptors. ➋ *Figure 331.5* shows a diagram of the major platelet receptors discussed below.

The Von Willebrand receptor is also known as platelet glycoprotein IB complex (gpIB). The complex is composed of two Ib-alpha, two Ib-beta, two gpV, and one gpIX polypeptides. This receptor complex is essential for localization of the platelet to the vascular defect and exposed sub-endothelium. Deficiencies of gpIB complex, known as Bernard–Soulier syndrome, have a severe lifelong bleeding disorder. A normal human platelet expresses about 25,000 gpIB receptor complexes. While gpIB is essential to localizing the platelet to the site of injury, it does not appear to have a major role in platelet activation. Accordingly, the gpIB-Von Willebrand factor interaction is critical but not sufficient for normal platelet function.

The other major adhesion receptor present on platelets is the glycoprotein IIB-IIIA complex (gpIIB-IIIA), also known as the fibrinogen receptor. This receptor complex, numbering about 50,000 copies per cell, is also

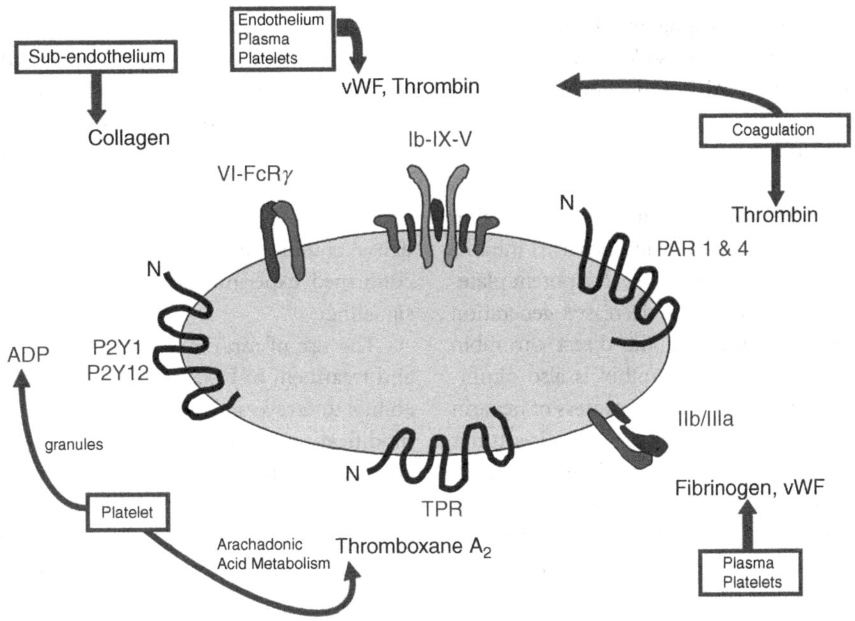

Figure 331.5
Platelet receptors. Representational view of platelet receptors is shown with their corresponding activating ligands. The most abundant receptors on the platelet surface are the adhesive receptors gpIIB-IIIA (50,000 copies/cell) and the gpIB complex (25,000 copies/cell). The other platelet receptors shown activate platelets by "priming" the gpIIB-IIIA receptor to bind fibrinogen

essential for normal platelet function. Accordingly, inherited deficiencies of gpIIB-IIIA, known as Glanzman's thrombasthenia, confers a lifelong bleeding disorder. The gpIIB-IIIA complex is a heterodimer, composed of one gpIIB and one gpIIIA polypeptide. The function of the gpIIB-IIIA complex is to aggregate platelets on top of the initial platelet plug. Once a thin layer of platelets is localized to the wound by the gpIB receptor complex and Von Willebrand factor, circulating fibrinogen binds to the platelet gpIIB-IIIA receptors, acting as a bridge between platelets. This aggregating step localizes more platelets to the site of injury and greatly strengthens the integrity of the platelet plug. Platelets that have not been sufficiently activated will not aggregate in the presence of fibrinogen. Accordingly, platelets must be "primed" by other platelet receptor agonists before they will aggregate. This platelet priming is sometimes referred to as inside-out signaling because it involves the release of intracellular calcium within the platelet cytoplasm in response to the priming step. The increase in intracellular calcium concentration causes a conformational change in the structure of the gpIIB-IIIA complex which allows tight binding with circulating fibrinogen. Thus, fibrinogen has two functions in normal hemostasis: It forms fibrin when digested by thrombin and it mediates platelet aggregation at the site of injury.

Nonadhesive Activating Receptors

There are several important activating receptors present on the platelet plasma membrane. These receptors "prime" the platelet by activating the gpIIB-IIIA receptor complex to bind fibrinogen, as discussed above. There are two major classes of receptor-activating agonists: weak and strong. For example, the thrombin receptor is a strong platelet agonist, while the epinephrine receptor is a relatively weak one. By weak or strong agonist, we mean the extent to which the agonist in question supports platelet aggregation through activation of the gpIIB-IIIA complex. What follows is a brief discussion about the major platelet-activating receptors and their corresponding agonists.

Thrombin is the most powerful physiologic platelet agonist known. Resting platelets exposed to physiologic concentrations of thrombin rapidly form aggregates in the presence of fibrinogen. Three distinct thrombin receptors have been characterized, two of which are present in human platelets. Thrombin receptors have thrombin recognition sequences and specific thrombin cleavage sites. When thrombin is present, the extracellular amino terminus of the receptor is cleaved by limited proteolysis. Cleavage of this amino terminus exposes a series of critical amino acid residues that results in activation of the receptor and intracellular signaling which activates the receptor. Thrombin receptors are also known as protease-activated receptors (PAR). PAR1 is the most numerous and potent thrombin receptor and is the major pathway by which platelets respond to thrombin. Human platelets also express PAR4, a relatively weak platelet agonist with unclear physiologic significance. Treatment with thrombin inhibitors (e.g., argatroban, hirudin, and heparin) inhibits platelet activation because thrombin is such a potent platelet agonist. Thus, in addition to the decreased generation of fibrin afforded by heparin and the direct thrombin inhibitors, platelet activation by thrombin is also diminished. This may account, in part, for the success of heparin in the treatment of acute arterial thromboembolic settings such as an evolving myocardial or cerebral infarction. Heparin's antiplatelet properties also contribute to its usefulness in an adjuvant therapy with thrombolytics (tPA and *urokinase*) and angioplasty procedures in similar clinical settings.

Platelets also contain two types of adenosine diphosphate (ADP) receptors: the P2Y1 and P2Y12 receptors. ADP is considered a relatively weak platelet agonist relative to thrombin in that treatment of platelets in solution with varying concentrations of ADP results in about 50% the amount of platelet aggregation than with thrombin. ADP is present in the platelet dense granules and is also secreted by endothelium and other cell types. After a layer of platelets is localized by VWF to the site of vascular injury, more platelets must aggregate on top of the base layer for normal hemostasis to proceed. Accordingly, the platelet must be "primed" by an agonist in order for the gpIIB-IIIA complex to recognize and bind fibrinogen (as discussed above). Thrombin plays such a role since it is a very strong platelet agonist and is being generated simultaneously through tissue factor exposure and the coagulation cascade. However, circulating thrombin inhibitors and binding of thrombin to the endothelium and other cell types limit the ability for thrombin to completely sustain platelet aggregation in the absence of ADP. Clinical evidence of the importance of the ADP pathway is demonstrated by the fact that rare inherited abnormalities of the P2Y12 receptor confer a moderate bleeding disorder similar to that of moderate type I or II Von Willebrand disease. The drug clopidogrel, currently used to treat coronary and peripheral artery diseases, is a P2Y12 inhibitor. The P2Y1 receptor is a much weaker agonist than even the P2Y12 receptor, and has not been shown to directly result in the activation of the gpIIIB-IIIA receptor.

The thromboxane receptor is also considered a moderately weak platelet agonist. Thromboxane (TX2) is a prostaglandin that is produced from membrane-derived arachadonic acid after platelet activation. The production of TX2, like many other prostaglandins, is dependent on the activity of the membrane-bound enzyme *cycloxegenase 1* (COX1). Inherited deficiencies in TX2 synthesis or the thromboxane receptor are rare. These patients have mild to moderate lifelong bleeding disorders. Interestingly, analysis of their platelet function shows a deficiency in dense granule secretion, an observation that has been confirmed experimentally by inhibiting TXA2 receptor signaling.

The use of aspirin (salicylic acid) for the prevention and treatment of heart disease and stroke is based on its ability to irreversibly inhibit platelet COX1 by covalent modification of a key serine residue (Ser 529) that blocks entry of the eicosanoid substrate to the active site of the enzyme. Non-aspirin anti-inflammatory drugs (such as ibuprofen and the majority of other NSAID class members) also inhibit platelet COX1, but unlike aspirin these drugs do not covalently modify the enzyme. Accordingly, the antiplatelet effect of the NSAID group is reversible and dependent on the half-life of the particular drug.

The major collagen receptor present on the platelet plasma membrane surface is glycoprotein VI or gpVI. Compared to thrombin, collagen is considered a moderately weak platelet activator. Accordingly, treatment of platelets with collagen in solution results in an aggregation response similar to that of ADP. Inherited defects of gpVI are rare and confer a mild to moderate bleeding disorder. The function of the collagen receptor is to activate the platelets to aggregate after they have been localized to the vascular sub-endothelium by VWF and the gpIB receptor complex. It is important to keep in mind that the platelet gpVI is not an adhesion receptor, although it does bind collagen. Adhesion of the platelets to collagen is primarily mediated by VWF and gpIB. Once localized to the collagen surface, the interaction between collagen and gpVI results in the activation of gpIIB-IIIA and aggregation to form a stable primary platelet plug over the vascular defect.

Platelets undergo a relatively weak aggregation response when exposed to epinephrine through activation of the alpha-2 adrenergic receptor. The activation of gpIIB-IIIA, and hence platelet aggregation in response to alpha-2-andrenergic receptor activation, is heavily dependent on the synthesis of TXA2 (thromboxane) and signaling through the TXA2 receptor. TXA2 is synthesized from arachadonic acid present in the plasma membrane as a result of intracellular signaling by the alpha-2-andrenergic receptor through the COX1 pathway. As a result of this TXA2-dependent aggregation in response to epinephrine, platelets that have been exposed to aspirin (or other NSAIDs that inhibit COX1 activity) do not aggregate normally in response to epinephrine. For this reason, epinephrine is often used as an agonist in clinical platelet aggregation studies.

Another weak platelet agonist is 5-hydroxytryptamine (serotonin), a constituent of the platelet dense granules. The corresponding receptor present on platelets is the 5HT2A isoform. Platelets do not synthesize serotonin but actively transport it into the dense granules by endocytosis in a process that is inhibited by selective serotonin uptake inhibitor drugs (SSRIs). With the widespread use of SSRI, there was concern that diminished activation of platelets by the decreased concentration of serotonin in the dense granules might cause bleeding due to platelet dysfunction. However, there does not appear to be an increased risk of bleeding or thrombosis associated with the use of SSRI medications.

Platelet Function

As mentioned in the introduction, platelet localization to site of a vascular injury is essential for normal hemostasis. Patients with platelet disorders or defects in the localization of platelets to the site of injury have mild to severe bleeding. On the other hand, activation of platelets near or on the site of a vascular atherosclerotic plaque (such as might occur in the setting of an acute myocardial infarction or stroke) is the leading cause of death in the modern industrialized world. Platelets are also important for normal wound healing and have been associated with the infectivity of malaria and other infections as well as the process of cancer metastasis. As a result of these observations, there is a great deal of interest in the physiology of platelet function. What follows is primarily a description of the role platelets play in normal hemostasis.

When a vessel is disrupted to cause bleeding, there is an almost instantaneous constriction of the lumen of the vessel near the injury site by reflex neurological pathways and the local release of vasoconstrictive substances. This vasoconstriction and the mechanical damage to the vessel wall and surrounding tissues results in a disruption of laminar blood flow and produces high shear forces at the site of injury. At the same time, the injured tissue exposes collagen, which is a main constituent of the basement membranes of almost every imaginable blood vessel. The high shear forces result in a conformational change in the structure of VWF from a globular to a linear configuration. In the linear configuration, the VWF is able to recognize and bind collagen and tether the platelet to the site via binding to gpIB, the VWF receptor complex. The exposed collagen also results in the activation of gpVI, the platelet collagen receptor. Signaling via gpVI results in the activation of the fibrinogen receptor, gpIIB-IIIA and platelets aggregate on top of the VWF bound platelets. Signaling through gpVI also results in the synthesis of TXA2 and release of ADP, epinephrine, and 5-hydroxytryptamine by the platelet dense granules. The effect of this "second wave" of platelet activation after localization by VWF and activation by collagen is to further strengthen the aggregation response. In fact, the activation of platelets to aggregate is a very redundant system such that defects in one component or another are unlikely to cause major bleeding [with the notable exception of disorders involving gpIIB-IIIA (Glanzman's thrombasthenia), gpIB (Bernard–Soulier disease), or the absence of VWF (type III Von Willebrand's disease)]. Tissue factor, which initiates the extrinsic pathway of coagulation when it binds factor VIIa, is also expressed by the injured endothelial cells and circulating monocytes which are localized to the site of the vascular injury. Tissue factor binding to circulating factor VIIa results in an initial burst of thrombin generation. Since thrombin is the most powerful physiologic activator of platelets to undergo aggregation, its production at the site of injury is critical to insure the adequate recruitment of platelets to form a platelet plug. Thrombin also activates fibrinogen to form a tough fibrin layer over the surface of the aggregated platelets. Accordingly, thrombin provides a key link between the primary phase of hemostasis, in which the platelets are localized and aggregated to the site of vascular injury, and the secondary phase of hemostasis, in which the coagulation proteins form fibrin.

Platelet function, as indicated in the preceding sections, involves more than plugging up a defect. The platelet membrane and cytoskeleton also undergo dramatic changes upon adhesion and activation. The platelet membrane changes its phopholipid distribution so that the high levels of "clottable" phophatidylserine and phosphatidylethanolamine appear on the outer leaflet of the plasma membrane. These membrane changes are essential to the localization of the clotting cascade protein complexes (*tenase* and *prothrombinase*, see above) and the efficient formation of thrombin and fibrin. The circulating discoid platelet also spreads and flattens over the vascular defect as a result of intracellular signaling pathways which rearrange the actin cytoskeleton filaments in an orthogonal configuration, with bundles of fibers composed of filamentous actin and myosin (stress fibers) arranged in a pattern connecting adjacent gpIIB-IIIA adhesion points (focal adhesions). The result is a firmly attached platelet plug covered by a thick fibrin meshwork.

Once the platelet forms a plug over the vascular defect that is anchored and covered with fibrin, clot retraction must then occur for normal wound healing to take place. The platelet-dependent process of clot retraction is poorly understood, but is an energy-dependent process in which the actin–myosin stress fibers contract in a manner similar to striated muscle. This filamentous contraction by the platelet brings the margins of the wound together and facilitates tissue repair with the recruitment of epithelium, fibroblast, and other cells. This process of clot retraction is distinct from thrombolysis, which involves the digestion of fibrin, though both processes overlap with respect to timing and their importance in normal wound healing.

Platelet Disorders

Platelet disorders are broadly grouped according to whether they are acquired or hereditary. Acquired platelet disorders will be covered first, followed by a brief discussion of selected hereditary disorders. ➲ *Table 331.1* summarizes the acquired and hereditary platelet disorders discussed below.

Acquired Platelet Disorders

Platelet function deficiencies can be acquired or hereditary. Most are acquired and due to drugs such as aspirin, which inhibits platelet function by interfering with COX1 activity (see above). Other mechanisms of drug-induced platelet dysfunction result from thrombocytopenia. Drug-induced thrombocytopenia is difficult to diagnose as many drugs are rare causes of thrombocytopenia that must be excluded by the largely empirical process of elimination of other causes. Severe thrombocytopenia soon after the start of a medication is the most straightforward presentation of drug-induced thrombocytopenia. For example, drugs such as the antibiotic vancomycin result in rapid immunologic clearance of platelets in some individuals. The mechanism of vancomycin-induced thrombocytopenia is due to antibody formation to the complex of vancomycin associated with the adhesive platelet receptor gpIIB-IIIA. Quinine may also cause an immune-mediated severe thrombocytopenia. In general, drug-induced immune thrombocytopenia resolves within a week or two of stopping the drug but may recur when the drug is reintroduced. Other drugs such as thiazide diuretics and some of the earlier NSAIDs which are not commonly used such as phenylbutazone and antineoplastic agents can cause amegakaryocytic thrombocytopenia. Treatment involves stopping the offending medication and supporting the patient with platelet transfusion as

◘ Table 331.1
Acquired and hereditary platelet disorders. Selected examples of common acquired and hereditary platelet disorders are shown with the primary mechanisms of platelet malfunction. See text for details

	Disorder	Mechanism of platelet dysfunction
Acquired	Drugs	Decrease production
		Immune clearance
	Liver disease	Decreased production
		Increased sequestration
		Membrane defects
	Vitamin B12 and folate Deficiencies	Decreased production
	Marrow stem cell disorders	Decreased production
		Structural defects
	ITP	Immune clearance
	Microangiopathic anemias	Platelet activation and consumption
Inherited	Membrane defects	Bernard–Soulier (gpIB)
		Glanzman's (gpIIB-IIIA)
	Storage pool disease	Alpha granule and dense granule
	Macrothrombocytopenia	May–Hegglin anomaly

necessary to prevent or treat bleeding. In the setting of acute myocardial infarction or after revascularization procedures, gpIIB-IIIA antagonists have proved very effective at reducing the rate of post-revascularization thrombosis. These antagonists are powerful antiplatelet agents that directly interfere with the binding of fibrinogen to gpIIB-IIIA, and hence stop platelet aggregation. These drugs are never administered outside the intensive care setting with close monitoring because of the high risk of bleeding. The gpIIB-IIIA antagonists are usually stopped within 24 h after the revascularization procedure. These drugs are available as an antibody (abciximab) or as small molecules (tirofiban, eptifibatide). The major side effect is thrombocytopenia and bleeding. The thrombocytopenia is characterized by the appearance of clumps of aggregated platelets on the peripheral smear together with a falling platelet count. The treatment is to stop the drug as soon as possible and consider administering platelet transfusions if there is bleeding or the platelet count is less than 50,000/μl.

Most drug-induced platelet disorders involve the occurrence of thrombocytopenia and bleeding with the notable exception being heparin-induced thrombocytopenia (HIT) or type II heparin-induced thrombocytopenia. In this case, the offending drug, unfractionated heparin, causes a platelet activation syndrome with a high risk of intravascular clotting. HIT usually develops within 4 days to 2 weeks of initiating unfractionated heparin with the onset of mild to moderate thrombocytopenia and often life-threatening venous and/or arterial thrombosis. The mechanism appears to be the formation of endogenous IgG antibodies to standard heparin in complex with platelet factor 4 (PF4). This antibody-heparin-PF4 complex activates platelets by associating with the FCR-gamma receptor present on the surface of the platelet plasma membrane. The FCR-gamma receptor is normally paired with the collagen receptor gpVI, where it functions as a moderately weak platelet agonist. However, when the FCR-gamma receptor is activated by the antibody-heparin-PF4 complex, the platelet aggregation response is similar to thrombin – the strongest physiological platelet agonist. Patients who develop thrombocytopenia within 2 weeks of starting unfractionated heparin demonstrate anti-PF4 antibodies in their serum and whose plasma confers brisk platelet aggregation in the presence of heparin are considered to have HIT. The treatment for HIT is to stop all heparin infusions of any kind. Furthermore, due to the risk of thrombosis in the setting of HIT, patients are treated with a non-heparin anticoagulant such as the direct thrombin inhibitors argatroban or hirudin until the platelet count returns to normal. If the patient with HIT has a thrombosis, heparin-free anticoagulation is maintained for at least 3 months.

There are many other causes of acquired thrombocytopenia which are often grouped according to whether the mechanism is due to decreased production, increased destruction, or sequestration. The most common cause of decreased platelet production (after drug toxicity) is liver disease. Hepatic dysfunction results in thrombocytopenia because of diminished thrombopoietin production by hepatocytes and synthetic membrane defects which shorten the circulating life of the platelet. Hypersplenism with increased platelet sequestration is also commonly associated with liver disease. Vitamin B12 and folate deficiencies are also important causes of thrombocytopenia due to poor platelet production. Finally, bone marrow stem cell disorders such as myelodysplasia, aplastic anemia, and acute and chronic leukemia adversely affect the production of megakaryocytes and the process of thrombopoiesis. Thrombocytopenia due to increased peripheral destruction is most commonly seen in immune disorders such as idiopathic thrombocytopenic purpura (ITP) and rheumatologic disorders.

ITP is an immune disorder that results in the clearance of platelets from the circulation by antibodies formed against platelet surface antigens. The most common target of the platelet autoantibodies is the gpIB receptor complexes; however, other platelet surface proteins and receptors have also been reported as targets. The mechanism behind the formation of these platelet autoantibodies is unclear. However, ITP is associated with low-grade lymphoproliferative disorders such as CLL as well as other immunological disorders such as AIDS. Interestingly, in children, ITP is almost always a self-limited disease, while in adults, the disease is almost always chronic or relapsing. While ITP can result in very low platelet counts, life-threatening spontaneous bleeding such as intracranial hemorrhage occurs in less than 1% of patients. Treatment of acute episodes of ITP in the adult or child usually includes immunosuppression agents. The first line of therapy is usually corticosteroids, which increases the platelet count to normal levels in about two thirds of patients. A favorable response to corticosteroids is associated with an increased chance of cure with splenectomy in adult patients. Patients who do not respond to corticosteroids are sometimes treated with the anti-CD20 monoclonal antibody rituximab. High-dose intravenous immune globulin and anti-Rh antibodies (Rho-D) can be used successfully to rapidly increase the platelet count within a day or two, but these medications usually result in short-lived remissions and are expensive. Because of the relatively low incidence of spontaneous bleeding in patients with ITP and the relatively high toxicity of the immunosuppressive drugs used to treat the disorder, patients are often left untreated if they maintain a platelet count of at least 30,000/μl. For patients with lower platelet counts or bleeding who have chronic ITP, thrombopoietin (TPO) is now available. There are two TPO preparations currently manufactured: one is taken orally on a daily basis and the other is given as a weekly subcutaneous injection. These TPO preparations have about a 90% response rate and are generally well tolerated. However, the thrombocytopenia returns when TPO is discontinued and long-term studies regarding the safety of these drugs is ongoing.

Other important platelet destructive or consumptive disorders are the microangiopathic hemolytic anemias, thrombocytopenic thrombotic purpura (TTP), disseminated intravascular coagulation (DIC), and the hemolytic-uremic syndrome (HUS). These disorders are characterized by microvascular thrombosis and thrombocytopenia due to systemic activation of platelets by ultra-large VWF (TTP and HUS) or by thrombin (DIC). These are life-threatening disorders with high mortality rates. Treatment of DIC and HUS involves addressing the underlying cause, which is often infection or malignancy. Successful treatment of TTP involves daily plasma exchange until the platelet count reaches normal levels. DIC and HUS do not respond to plasma exchange. About one third of patients diagnosed with TTP have a chronic relapsing form of the disease and must be treated with immunosuppression and plasma exchange at regular intervals. TTP treatment is best done at a major medical facility with the resources to perform plasma exchange and physicians with expertise in plasma exchange and blood banking.

Inherited Platelet Disorders

There are many rare familial platelet disorders that occur in isolated families. While these disorders are of scientific interest, they are rarely encountered by most physicians. Inherited disorders are grouped according to whether they involve membrane defects, disorders of granules, or macrothrombocytopenia.

The most important membrane defects are those which involve the adhesion receptors gpIB and gpIIB-IIIA, known as Bernard–Soulier syndrome and Glanzman's thrombasthenia. These disorders, like almost all inherited platelet disorders, are autosomal recessive in their inheritance pattern. Multiple genetic mutations in the genes coding for these disorders have been reported. Homozygous mutations result in severe, lifelong bleeding disorders. In the heterozygous state, these patients usually have mild bleeding disorders characterized by excessive post-traumatic bleeding. The diagnosis is usually suspected when the patient's platelets fail to aggregate in response to weak or strong agonists and confirmed by platelet flow cytometry using antibodies which recognize the corresponding surface receptors. Treatment for these disorders with platelet transfusions usually results in the development of allo-immunization or antibodies against the receptor. Recombinant factor VIIa has been used successfully to prevent perioperative and post-traumatic bleeding. Bone marrow stem cell transplantation would provide definitive treatment, but the mortality rate is unacceptably high with this therapy.

Platelet granule disorders, also known as platelet storage pool disease, encompass a range of disorders with variable reduction in the concentration and structure of dense granules, alpha granules, or both. These disorders are generally inherited in an autosomal-recessive pattern. The most common of these disorders is dense granule deficiency. These patients all have a mild to moderate bleeding disorder, characterized by bleeding when challenged by trauma or surgery. The formation and secretion of granules is a complex process involving many genes. Accordingly, the specific genetic mutations that cause platelet storage pool disease are largely undetermined. The diagnosis is made by analysis of platelet structure with electron microscopy or by flow cytometry using chemical probes that specifically recognize platelet granules. Treatment involves the appropriate use of DDAVP, antifibrinolytics such as epsilon aminocarproic acid or tranexamic acid, and platelet transfusions.

The macrothrobocytopenias are rare disorders that usually involve multiple inherited birth defects together with large platelets and thrombocytopenia. These patients generally have mild bleeding disorders, with most episodes of bleeding occurring after trauma or surgical procedures. The most common macrothrombocytopnenia is the May–Hegglin anomaly, a disorder that affects only leukocytes and platelets. The peripheral blood smear is often suggestive of this disorder because of the prevalent appearance of leukocyte cytoplasmic inclusion bodies and large platelets with mild thrombocytopenia.

Some specific genetic mutations have been found which account for a subset of May–Hegglin patients. These tests are available through specialized genetic laboratories.

Summary

Blood platelets have several important functions. They adhere to sites of vascular injury and spread over the defect, secrete their procoagulant granular contents, and serve as a "clottable" surface upon which coagulation can occur. Accordingly, platelets are essential for normal hemostasis, and patients with acquired or inherited defects in platelet function have mild to severe bleeding. The diagnosis and classification of platelet disorders is complex and often requires the assistance of specialized regional laboratories capable of ultrastructural analysis, DNA sequencing, and platelet function testing. Treatment for bleeding disorders in patients with platelet defects is variable, and may involve platelet transfusion, antifibrinolytic medications, recombinant factor VIIa, DDAVP, and cryoprecipitate.

References

Beardsley DS (2006) ITP in the 21st century. Hematology Am Soc Hematol Educ Program 402–407

Cohen I, Burk DL, White JG (1989) The effect of peptides and monoclonal antibodies that bind to platelet glycoprotein IIb-IIIa complex on the development of clot tension. Blood 73:1880–1887

Coughlin SR (2005) Protease-activated receptors in hemostasis, thrombosis and vascular biology. J Thromb Haemost 3(8):1800–1814

Du X (2007) Signaling and regulation of the platelet glycoprotein Ib-IX-V complex. Curr Opin Hematol 14(3):262–269

Gachet C (2008) P2 receptors, platelet function and pharmacological implications. Thromb Haemost 99(3):466–472

Handin RI (2005) Inherited platelet disorders. Hematology Am Soc Hematol Educ Program 396–402

Hartwig JH (2006) The platelet: form and function. Semin Hematol 3(Suppl 1):S94–S100

Kaushansky K (2008) Historical review: megakaryopoiesis and thrombopoiesis. Blood 111(3):981–986

Kuter DJ, Rummel M, Boccia R, Macik BG, Pabinger I, Selleslag D, Rodeghiero F, Chong BH, Wang X, Berger DP (2010) Romiplostim or standard of care in patients with immune thrombocytopenia. N Engl J Med 363(20):1889–1899

Li Z, Delaney MK, O'Brien KA, Du X (2010) Signaling during platelet adhesion and activation. Arterioscler Thromb Vasc Biol 30(12): 2341–2349

Mandava P, Thiagarajan P, Kent TA (2008) Glycoprotein IIb/IIIa antagonists in acute ischaemic stroke: current status and future directions. Drugs 68(8):1019–1028

Murugappan S, Shankar H, Kunapuli SP (2004) Platelet receptors for adenine nucleotides and thromboxane A2. Semin Thromb Hemost 30(4):411–418

Phillips DR, Charo IF, Parise LV, Fitzgerald LA (1998) The platelet membrane glycoprotein IIb-IIIa complex. Blood 71(4):831–843

Pozgajová M, Sachs UJ, Hein L, Nieswandt B (2006) Reduced thrombus stability in mice lacking the alpha2A-adrenergic receptor. Blood 108(2):510–514

Schlienger RG, Meier CR (2003) Effect of selective serotonin reuptake inhibitors on platelet activation: can they prevent acute myocardial infarction? Am J Cardiovasc Drugs 3(3):149–162

Von Drygalski A, Curtis BR, Bougie DW, McFarland JG, Ahl S, Limbu I, Baker KR, Aster RH (2007) Vancomycin-induced immune thrombocytopenia. N Engl J Med 356(9):904–910

Warkentin TE (2007) Heparin-induced thrombocytopenia. Hematol Oncol Clin North Am 21(4):589–607

Watson SP, Auger JM, McCarty OJ, Pearce AC (2005) GPVI and integrin alphaIIb beta3 signaling in platelets. J Thromb Haemost 3(8): 1752–1762

Wolfs JL, Comfurius P, Rasmussen JT, Keuren JF, Lindhout T, Zwaal RF, Bevers EM (2005) Activated scramblase and inhibited aminophospholipid translocase cause phosphatidylserine exposure in a distinct platelet fraction. Cell Mol Life Sci 62(13):1514–1525

332 The Phagocytic System

Hassan El Solh · Abdallah Al-Nasser · Saleh Al-Muhsen

Function and Morphology of the Phagocytic System

Phagocytes play a critical role in the initial response to infections with bacteria and fungi. They follow certain immune responses in order to combat and clear the infection. They adhere to the endothelial wall and subsequently migrate to the site of infection (chemotaxis). Once they ingest the pathogen (phagocytosis), they kill via different mechanisms including oxidative burst, proteases, and other toxic peptides. The phagocytes are also involved in the production of cytokines and other cellular mediators that participate in the inflammatory response. In addition, they contribute to the recognition of certain pathogens (opsonization or coating objects with certain proteins). Phagocytes originate within the bone marrow and move into the circulation (mobilization), and then exit to sites of inflammation (chemotaxis).

The phagocytic system consists of monocytes (mononuclear), neutrophils (polymorphonuclear), and eosinophils. Neutrophils and monocytes share many morphologic and functional characteristics. They originate from the same stem cell progenitors in the bone marrow. The proliferation and differentiation into mature leukocytes require stimulation by a variety of cytokines: interleukins and lineage-specific cytokines such as granulocyte-macrophage colony-stimulating factor (GM-CSF), granulocyte colony-stimulating factor (GCSF), and macrophage colony-stimulating factor (M-CSF). The neutrophils have nuclei with three to five segments and constitute the predominant type of phagocytes. Monocytes are characterized by their large size with lobulated nuclei and azurophilic granules. The eosinophils are distinguished by large red granules and are involved in the inflammatory and parasitic reactions.

Disorders of the Phagocytic System

The phagocytic disorders can be classified to abnormality in number, function, or both. Affected patients typically present with recurrent and severe bacterial and fungal infections in early childhood. Respiratory tract and skin dominate the affected organs. However, deep-seated abscesses and oral stomatitis are commonly encountered. In the last few decades, our knowledge of the phagocytic disorders has clearly been revolutionized by the discovery of the underlying molecular defects in many clinical phenotypes, largely through international collaborations. However, many remain to be identified. Nevertheless, addressing the details of all known phagocytic disorders is beyond the scope of this chapter and the most common disorders of the phagocytic system will only be discussed.

Abnormality in the Number of Phagocytes

Neutropenia

Neutropenia is defined as an absolute decrease in the number of circulating neutrophils in the peripheral blood. Neutropenia is considered severe if the absolute neutrophil count (ANC) is less than 0.5×10^9 cells/L, moderate if the ANC is $0.5–1.0 \times 10^9$ cells/L, and mild if the ANC is $1.0–1.5 \times 10^9$ cells/L. Neutropenia can be classified based on pathophysiology (disorders of production, maturation, or peripheral utilization) or on intrinsic defects in the myeloid progenitors as compared to extrinsic factors to the bone marrow, causing acquired neutropenia (➋ *Table 332.1*).

Congenital Neutropenia (CN)

Severe congenital Neutropenia (SCN) is a heterogeneous group of primary immune deficiency diseases conferring susceptibility to infections due to lack of neutrophils. It follows different mendelian inheritance, including autosomal dominant (AD), autosomal recessive (AR), and X-linked. There are some sporadic cases. Moreover, many syndromes are associated with severe neutropenia. SCN classically presents with persistent low neutrophil counts with typical myeloid maturation arrest at the level of promyelocytes in bone marrow studies. Recent discoveries have elucidated the underlying molecular defect of many SCN phenotypes.

Abdelaziz Y. Elzouki (ed.), *Textbook of Clinical Pediatrics*, DOI 10.1007/978-3-642-02202-9_332,

Table 332.1
Neutropenia in childhood

Congenital neutropenia (CN)
Non-syndromic CN
AD and sporadic SCN/ cyclic neutropenia due to mutations in ELA2
AR SCN due to mutations in HAX1
X-lined SCN due to mutations in WAS
SCN due to mutations in GFI1
CN associated with syndromic features
Reticular dysgenesis
Shwachman–Diamond–Oski syndrome
Chediak–Higashi Syndrome
Griscelli syndrome type 2
Hermansky–Pudlak syndrome type 2
p14 deficiency
Glycogen-storage disease
WHIM syndrome
Shwachman–Diamond Syndrome
Dykeratosis congenita
Neutropenia associated with T- and B-lymphocyte abnormalities
Acquired neutropenia
Bone marrow replacement
Infection
Ineffective granulopoiesis due to nutritional deficiencies
Neutropenia associated with metabolic diseases
Drug-induced neutropenia
Autoimmune neutropenia
Isoimmune neutropenia

Non-syndromic SCN

AD and Sporadic ELA2 Defect The most common form of SCN is caused by mutation in *ELA2*, the gene encoding neutrophil elastase. This disease presents as autosomal dominant or in a sporadic pattern. A subgroup of patients with the ELA2 mutation presents in an oscillatory cyclic pattern with a nadir every 3 weeks, giving rise to what is known as "Cyclic Neutropenia" with subsequent periodicity of clinical manifestations, including bacterial infections and stomatitis. Patients with cyclic neutropenia usually have a mild phenotype; however, death occurs in 10% due to overwhelming infections during the neutropenic nadir. Patients harboring the ELA2 mutation have a higher risk of myloid dysplasia and leukemia associated with somatic mutation in the granulocyte colony-stimulating factor receptor (GCSFR) gene.

AR: Kostmann Syndrome Although this is the classical autosomal recessive SCN that was described more than 50 years ago by Kostmann, the underlying molecular defect was only recently identified with a deficiency in HAX1, leading to increased apoptosis of myeloid cells. Patients might present with neurological abnormalities.

Other Rare Non-syndromic SCN These include X-linked neutropenia caused by mutation in *WAS*, the gene encoding Wiskott–Aldrich Syndrome protein and *GFI1*, a transcriptional repressor and splice control factor of the zinc-finger family of transcription factors with similar clinical presentation to common SCN.

Congenital Neutropenia Associated with Syndromic Features

Reticular Dysgenesis This is an autosomal recessive disease characterized by severe neutropenia and lymphopenia, resembling severe combined immune deficiency. The underlying molecular defect has been recently identified by mutations in the gene-encoding mitochondrial adenylate kinase 2. Patients usually die soon after birth with overwhelming infection in the early neonatal period unless offered hematopoietic stem cell transplantation. Bone marrow studies typically reveal arrest in myeloid differentiation at the promyelocytic stage, whereas erythrocytic and megakaryocytic maturation is generally normal.

Congenital Neutropenia with Hyperpigmentation Chediak–Higashi Syndrome (CHS) and Griscelli syndrome type 2 are associated with transient neutropenia and abnormal skin pigmentation. Hermansky–Pudlak syndrome type 2 (HPS2) and p14 deficiency are two other syndromes associated with abnormal pigmentation and neutropenia that is persistent. HPS2 consists primarily of hypopigmentation and prolonged bleeding times due to defective platelet granules. Patients with P14 deficiency may present with other features, including short stature, hypogammaglobulinemia and reduced numbers of B-cell subsets, and defective function of cytotoxic T cells. In contrast to the SCN, the bone marrow studies in all these four syndromes show normal maturation of the neutrophils. In CHS, GS2, and P14 deficiency, the abnormality is due to low levels of neutrophils and their impaired killing ability.

Congenital Neutropenia Associated with Glycogen-Storage Disease (GSD) Patents with GSD1b are not only characterized by abnormal glycogen storage, hypoglycemia, and lactic acidosis, but also demonstrate congenital neutropenia. This disease is caused by mutations in the glucose-6-phosphate translocase (G6PT, encoded by the gene SLC37A4), a transporter mediating translocation of G6P into the endoplasmic reticulum.

Another glucose metabolic disease was recently described, where, in addition to congenital neutropenia, patients may present with various congenital defects of the cardiovascular and/or urogenital system and increased visibility of superficial veins. It is caused by a defect in G6PC3.

WHIM Syndrome (Warts, Hypogammaglobulinemia, Immunodeficiency, Myelokathexis) WHIM is a rare autosomal dominant disease caused by mutation in the chemokine receptor gene *CXCR4*. It is characterized by multiple warts and hypogammaglobulinemia. Myelokathexis indicates dysregulated granulopoiesis which includes hypersegmentation and increased apoptosis. Severe infections are not typical because of the adequacy of neutrophils in the circulation during infection.

Shwachman–Diamond Syndrome This is a rare autosomal recessive disorder, characterized by exocrine pancreatic insufficiency, skeletal abnormalities, bone marrow dysfunction, and recurrent infections. Almost all patients suffer intermittent or cyclic neutropenia. Pancytopenia occurs in 25% of patients. Patients are at higher risk of bone marrow aplasia, myelodysplasia, and leukemia.

Dyskeratosis Congenita This is an X-linked recessive disorder characterized by nail dystrophy and skin hyperpigmentation. Some patients have marrow hypoplasia, and others (one third) have neutropenia.

Neutropenia Associated with T- and B-Lymphocyte Abnormalities Neutropenia has been described in severe combined immunodeficiency diseases, common variable immunodeficiency, agammaglobulinemia, and typically with hyper IgM syndrome, especially CD40 deficiency

Acquired Neutropenia

Bone Marrow Replacement

Neoplasms infiltrating the bone marrow induce neutropenia. Leukemia and lymphoma are the most common neoplasms that can cause neutropenia. Other disorders, such as osteopetrosis, myelofibrosis, and myelodysplastic syndrome, can result in severe neutropenia and pancytopenia.

Infection

Viral infection is the most common cause of transient neutropenia in children. Epstein–Barr virus, influenza A and B, measles, hepatitis A and B, respiratory syncytial virus, rubella, and varicella are noted to induce neutropenia. Other infections, such as typhoid, paratyphoid, tuberculosis, brucellosis, malaria, and rickettsial infections, can induce neutropenia through different mechanisms.

Ineffective Granulopoiesis due to Nutritional Deficiencies

Megalobalstic anemia secondary to nutritional deficiencies of folic acid or vitamin B12 has been associated with neutropenia.

Neutropenia Associated with Metabolic Diseases

Neutropenia can occur in children with metabolic disorders due to impairment of proliferation and differentiation of myeloid cells. These disorders include hyperglycinemia, propionic acidemia, methylmalonic acidemia, glycogen-storage disease type IB, and isovaleric acidemia.

Drug-Induced Neutropenia

The underlying cause of neutropenia associated with certain drugs is unclear. However, damage to the microenvironment of the bone marrow and/or immune-mediated destruction of neutrophils are the most likely mechanisms. The list of drugs reported to cause neutropenia includes antibiotics such as sulfonamides and penicillins; phenothiazines; antipyretics such as aspirin, acetaminophen, phenybutazone; anti-inflammatory agents such as penicillamine, levamisole, gold; and sedatives such as benzodiazepines and barbiturates.

Autoimmune Neutropenia

Patients may develop antineutrophil antibodies, causing rapid removal of neutrophils by the reticuloendothelial system. These patients may have recurrent infections and frequent hospitalizations. Therapy with corticosteroids has been shown to improve the neutrophil count in 50% of patients. High-dose intravenous immunoglobulin or splenectomy has been tried, but their efficacy is still unproven.

Isoimmune Neutropenia

Neutropenia occurring in the neonatal period can be due to neutrophil antibodies crossing the placenta from the mother after sensitization to the fetal neutrophil antigens. Usually, by the age of 7 weeks, the neutrophil count becomes normal.

Approach to Diagnosis and Therapy of Neutropenia

The diagnostic approach to neutropenia should focus through the history and physical examination on the following: duration, frequency, site, and severity of infection; family history; recent viral infection; medications; dysmorphic features; lymphadenopathy; and hepatosplenomegaly. Patients should have white blood cell counts and differentials twice per week for 6 weeks to evaluate the possibility of cyclic neutropenia. Patients with persistent neutropenia should undergo a bone marrow aspiration and biopsy for detecting malignant disorders and congenital etiologies. Antineutrophil antibody may be helpful to detect immune-mediated neutropenia. The Rebuck skin window test can assess neutrophil mobilization. The steroid mobilization test evaluates the storage pool size. Immunologic evaluation can detect immune deficiency disorders. Plasma and urine amino acid screening can be helpful in the diagnosis of metabolic diseases associated with neutropenia. Chromosomal studies can establish the diagnosis of Fanconi anemia. Exocrine pancreatic function tests can detect Shwachman syndrome.

In spite of improvement in antibiotic therapy and supportive care, infections and septicemia are still a major cause of morbidity and mortality. A patient with severe neutropenia presenting with a febrile illness has at least a 60% chance of having a bacterial infection. Accordingly, broad-spectrum antibiotics to cover gram-positive (especially Staphylococcus) and gram-negative organisms should be started immediately. Blood, urine, and, if indicated, throat and sputum cultures should be done, and the appropriate radiologic imaging should he performed. Patients should receive antibiotics for a few days (duration to be determined by the clinical course, results of cultures, and neutrophil levels). If the patient continues to be febrile for more than 5–7 days in spite of adequate antibiotic coverage, then antifungal therapy should be initiated empirically. Patients with proven bacterial or fungal sepsis may benefit from granulocyte transfusions if they are still neutropenic, especially for critically ill patients, although this still has not been studied in a randomized trial. Caution should be taken regarding transmission of infections such as hepatitis, toxoplasma, and cytomegalovirus. Also, there is a potential risk for pulmonary toxicity and transfusion-associated graft-versus-host disease. Patients with immune-mediated neutropenia may respond to steroid therapy. Cytokines, such as granulocyte colony stimulating factor (GCSF), have been instrumental in improving the outcome of many congenital neutropenia. In fact, before the GCSF era, most patients affected by the SCNs succumbed to severe sepsis. Since its introduction into the clinical practice, the morbidity and mortality of infection have decreased significantly. In spite of all this supportive therapy, the definite cure is only possible by hematopoietic stem cell transplantation in most SCNs.

Neutrophilia

When the ANC exceeds 7.5×10^9 cells/L, patients can be considered to have neutrophilia. Neutrophilia can occur as a result of any one or a combination of the following: increased production, enhanced release from marrow storage pool, decreased exit from the circulation, and reduced margination. ➲ *Table 332.2* lists possible etiologies of neutrophilia.

Eosinophilia

Allergic disorders are the most common cause of eosinophilia in the developed countries, and parasitic infections account for a large proportion of patients with esoinophilia in the developing countries. Other causes include tumors such as Hodgkin disease, and hypereosinophilic syndromes (eosinophilic leukemia and Löffler syndrome).

Basophilia

Hypersensitivity reactions are the most common cause of basophilia. Other disorders that are associated

Table 332.2
Causes of neutrophilia

Increased production
Infection
Chronic inflammation
Myeloproliferative disease
Leukemoid reactions
Tumors (nonhematologic)
Drug-induced neutrophilia (lithium)
Hemolytic anemia
Enhanced release from marrow storage pool and/or reduced margination stress
Exercise
Postsurgery
Postictal
Heat stroke
Steroids
Decreased exit from circulation
Splenectomy

with basophilia include ulcerative colitis, rheumatoid arthritis, chronic renal failure, tuberculosis, and myeloproliferative disorders.

Monocytosis

In malignant hematologic disorders such as preleukemia, juvenile chronic myeloid leukemia, and lymphoma are associated with monocytosis. Other causes include infections such as tuberculosis, bacterial endocarditis, and granulomatous diseases.

Disorders of the Phagocyte Morphology

Morphologic Variations in Neutrophils

These disorders affecting the morphology of neutrophils include nuclear as well as cytoplasmic abnormalities.

1. *Pelger–Huet Anomaly.* Neutrophils of patients with this anomaly have a limitation of segmentation of the nucleus to two lobes. The disorder is inherited as an autosomal dominant trait; however, it can he acquired in infections such as mycoplasma and malaria or in malignant diseases such as leukemia or lymphoma.
2. *Hereditary Hypersegmentation of Neurophils.* This is a benign condition characterized by hypersegmentation of the nucleus in the neutrophil into four to five lobes.
3. *Prevalence of Nuclear Appendages.* In women, nuclear appendages (female specific) are present in about 2–10% of neutrophils. An excessive number of appendages may be present in trisomy 13–15.
4. *Vacuolization.* Cytoplasmic vacuolization has been noted in neutrophils in association with infections and burns.
5. *Alder-Reilly Anomaly.* Prominent granules in neutrophils are present in Hurler syndrome. Other cells, such as monocytes and lymphocytes, may have similar granules.
6. *Chédiak–Higashi Syndrome.* The neutrophils and other leukocytes of patients with Chédiak–Higashi syndrome contain giant granules.
7. *Hermansky–Pudlak Syndrome.* This is an autosomal recessive disorder characterized by albinism and increased bleeding tendency due to platelet dysfunction. The macrophages in the bone marrow have ceroid-like pigment.
8. *May–Hegglin Anomaly.* This disorder is characterized by thrombocytopenia with giant platelets. There are pale blue inclusions present in neutrophils, eosinophils, monocytes, and basophils. It has an autosomal dominant inheritance.

Abnormality in the Function of Phagocytes

Abnormal function of phagocytes may occur at any step involved in the process of engulfment and destruction of foreign particles described at the beginning of this chapter (➋ *Fig. 332.1*).

Disorders of Adhesion

Leukocyte Adhesion Deficiency (LAD)

LAD is a heterogeneous group of disorders characterized by impairment of adhesion or chemotaxis of leukocytes to the site of infection. It is inherited as an autosomal recessive disorder. LAD-I is the most common and is caused by lack of glycoprotein molecules, the α subunits of the $\beta2$ integrin (CD18) shared by LFA-1 (CD11a), MAC-1 (CD11b), and P 150, 95 (CD11c).

Patients present with severe infections early in infancy without pus formation. They also have impaired wound healing manifesting early as delayed separation of the umbilical cord and omphalitis. Severe periodontitis, cellulitis, ulcerative skin lesions, and pneumonia are typical manifestation. Due to impaired trafficking of leukocytes, patients have an elevated peripheral neutrophil count. Flow cytometry using monoclonal antibodies to detect expression of the subunits of the $\beta2$ integrin can provide the diagnosis. The treatment of LAD should focus on the management of infections using appropriate antimicrobial therapy. Trimethoprim-sulfamethoxazole can be used for prophylaxis, and adequate oral hygiene is very important to prevent recurrent infections. Hematopoietic stem cell transplantation is the only modality which may provide definite cure in LAD.

LAD-II is caused by mutations in a GDP-fucose transporter. It was initially reported in two boys of Arab origin causing lack of expression of Sialyl Lewis^{X}, the ligand for E-selectin with subsequent impaired rolling of the leukocyte along the endothelium. In addition to the clinical manifestations of LAD-I, patients with this defect have short stature, facial dysmorphism, mental retardation, and Bombay blood-type phenotype due to generalized defect of fucose metabolism.

LAD-III is caused by a mutation of kindlin-3, which is involved in integrin signaling. Patients may have bleeding tendency due to impaired platelets adhesion.

A very rare clinical phenotype resembling LAD-I has been described with a mutation in Rac2 GTPase. It is

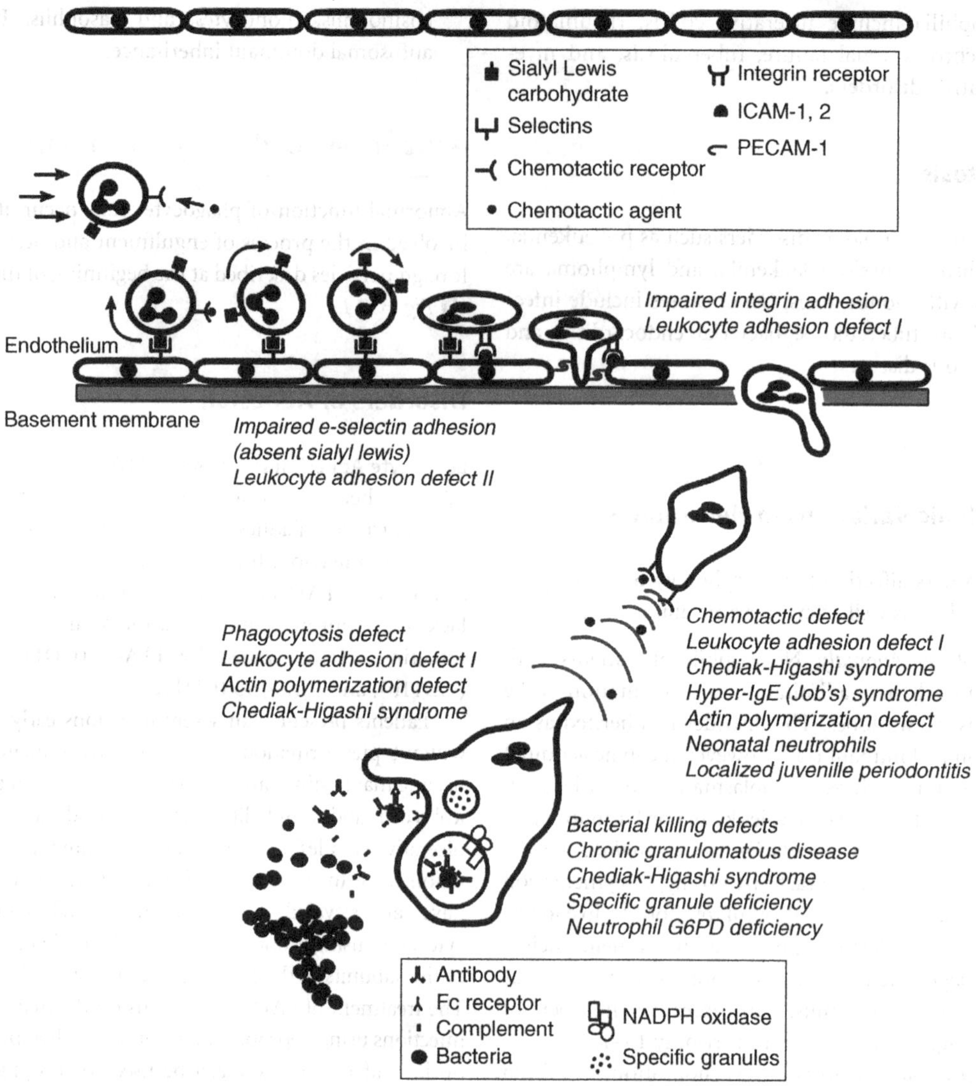

Figure 332.1

Steps in the response of circulating neutrophils to infection or inflammation (Reprinted with permission from Dinauer MC, Coates TD (2005) Disorders of phagocyte function and number. In Hoffman R, Benz J, Shattil S et al. (eds) Hematology: basic principles and practices. Elsevier Churchill Livingstone, Philadelphia, pp 787–830)

characterized by impaired neutrophil adhesion and motility, along with decreased neutrophil glucose-6-phosphate dehydrogenase (NADPH) oxidase activation and degranulation in response to chemoattractants.

Disorders of Chemotaxis

Patients with chemotactic disorders have recurrent bacterial (gram-positive and gram-negative) and fungal infections. The most common microorganism is Staphylococcus aureus. Several conditions are associated with defective chemotaxis, including inactivation of chemotactic factors (Hodgkin disease and cirrhosis of the liver); inhibitors of neutrophil responses (hyperimmunoglobulin E syndrome, localized juvenile periodontitis, rheumatoid arthritis, bone marrow transplantation, and drugs); deactivation of increased levels of chemotactic factors (Wiskott–Aldrich syndrome and bacterial sepsis); and phagocytic defects (neonatal neutrophilia, LAD,

Chédiak–Higashi syndrome, specific granule deficiency, and "lazy leukocyte" syndrome).

Hyperimmunoglobulin E (Job) Syndrome (HIGE)

HIGE a heterogeneous group of inherited disorders characterized by recurrent staphylococcal infections of the skin (cold abscesses) and lungs with subsequent formation of pneumatoceles. Candida infection is commonly encountered among HIGE patients. On the other hand, aspergillous frequently causes secondary pneumatocele infection. Chronic eczema and high levels of immunoglobulin E are consistent features of HIGE. AD and AR forms have been recently identified. The AD HIGE is caused by mutation in STAT-3 and is characterized by additional features, including defective shedding of primary teeth with double rows, scoliosis, easily bone fractures, joint hyperextensibility, coarse facial features, and aneurysms. In AR HIGE, patients might suffer viral infections but unlikely to present with skeletal or dental abnormalities. Vasculitis and autoimmunity are common in this phenotype. Mutations of the tyrosine kinase 2 gene (TYK2) have been identified as one of the causes of AR HIGE. Recently, a mutation in DOCK8 has been identified as a genetic cause of many AR HIGE patients. It is characterized by severe viral infection with HSV, extensive molluscum contagiosum, and several patients develop squamous-cell carcinomas. This phenotype is described as combined immunodeficiency with dysregulated IgE production. Patients with HIGE have variable defects in neutrophil chemotaxis. Treatment includes antibiotics for *S. aureus* infections and surgical drainage if indicated. Trimethoprim-sulfamethoxazole prophylaxis helps in decreasing the incidence of serious infections and improving the outcome. There is no definite treatment available for HIGE syndrome to date.

Neonatal Neutrophils

Neonatal neutrophils have defects in adhesion, chemotaxis, phagocytosis, and bactericidal activity, particularly in premature infants. The chemotactic deficiency is the most important one and has been attributed to abnormal regulation of cell adhesion molecules and decreased polymerization of F-actin in neutrophils after stimulation.

Disorders of Recognition

Complement (C3) deficiency is inherited as an autosomal recessive disorder, leading to recurrent infections due to absence of two major opsonins, C3b and C3bi.

Disorders of Ingestion

Neutrophilia in patients with LAD involves deficiency in ingestion of opsonized particles. Also, patients with deficiency of cytoskeleton-related 89-kDa protein or neutrophil actin polymerization have abnormal phagocytic function. Patients with paroxysmal nocturnal hemoglobinuria have deficiency of receptors (FcR III) that are important in the process of ingestion.

Disorders of Degranulation

Two main disorders belong to this category: Chédiak–Higashi syndrome and specific granule deficiency. Both are rare and inherited as autosomal recessive traits.

Chediak–Higashi Syndrome

CHS is a rare AR inherited disorder caused by mutation in *CHS1*, which encodes a large protein thought to regulate lysosomal and granule trafficking. It is characterized by partial oculocutaneous albinism, frequent and severe bacterial infections (*Staphylocuccs aureus*), and neuropathies (cranial and peripheral). Those who survive the recurrent infections develop diffuse lymphohistiocytic infiltration and pancytopenia "accelerated phase" and succumb to its complications. In addition to ineffective granulopoiesis, neutrophils have deficiency in chemotaxis and degranulation. Neutrophils from patients with Chédiak–Higashi syndrome have giant granules that appear to be a coalescence of azurophilic and specific granules. BM studies are often indicated as they are often more prominent in bone marrow neutrophils than in peripheral blood neutrophils. Management includes treatment of infections, such as prophylaxis with trimethoprim-sulfamethoxazole. If a suitable donor is available, hematopoietic stem cell transplantation can offer cure for this fatal disease.

Specific Granule Deficiency

Specific granule deficiency (SGD) is a rare disorder characterized by the absence of specific or secondary granules in developing neutrophils. It is caused by molecular defect involving the myeloid transcription factor C/EBPå. SGD neutrophils also demonstrate relatively severe chemotactic defect. Therefore, they present with severe infections of the skin, ears, lungs, and lymph nodes (*S. aureus*, *Proteus*, *Pseudomonas aeruginosa*, and *Candida*). The neutrophils lack or have empty specific granule vesicles (by electron microscopy) due to deficiency of certain proteins (defensins and lactoferrin). Treatment of SGD is supportive with prophylactic antibiotics, and prompt and prolonged treatment of infections.

Disorder of Signaling (Defect in IL-12/IFN-γ Axis)

The mononuclear phagocyte interaction with lymphocytes and monocytes through IL-12/IFN-γ axis is critical for the immune response against intracellular microorganisms, such as mycobacteria, salmonella, and listeria. The presence of pathogens as Mycobacterium triggers macrophages to produce IL-12. It binds to a specific receptor expressed by T and NK lymphocytes and induces secretion of IFN-γ that triggers macrophage microbicide on binding to the IFN-γ receptor. Defects of this crucial signaling pathway account for mendelian susceptibility to mycobacterial disease (MSMD). There are six MSMD-causing genes, including one X-linked gene (nuclear factor-kB–essential modulator [NEMO]) and five autosomal genes (IFN- γ receptor 1 [IFNGR1], IFN- γ receptor 2 [IFNGR2], signal transducer and activator of transcription 1 [STAT1], IL-12 p40 subunit [IL12P40], and IL-12 receptor b-subunit [IL12RB1]), producing heterogeneous clinical phenotypes of MSMD (➋ *Fig. 332.2*).

All forms of MSMD are characterized by increased susceptibility to environmental mycobacteria and to BCG vaccine strain. Salmonella, Listeria, and Histoplasma species infections can also be observed, especially in patients with IL12RB1 mutations.

Management of MSMD relies on aggressive therapy of infections, long-term prophylaxis. IFN-γ might be useful in patients with AD IFN- γ R1 deficiency, IL-12 p40 deficiency,

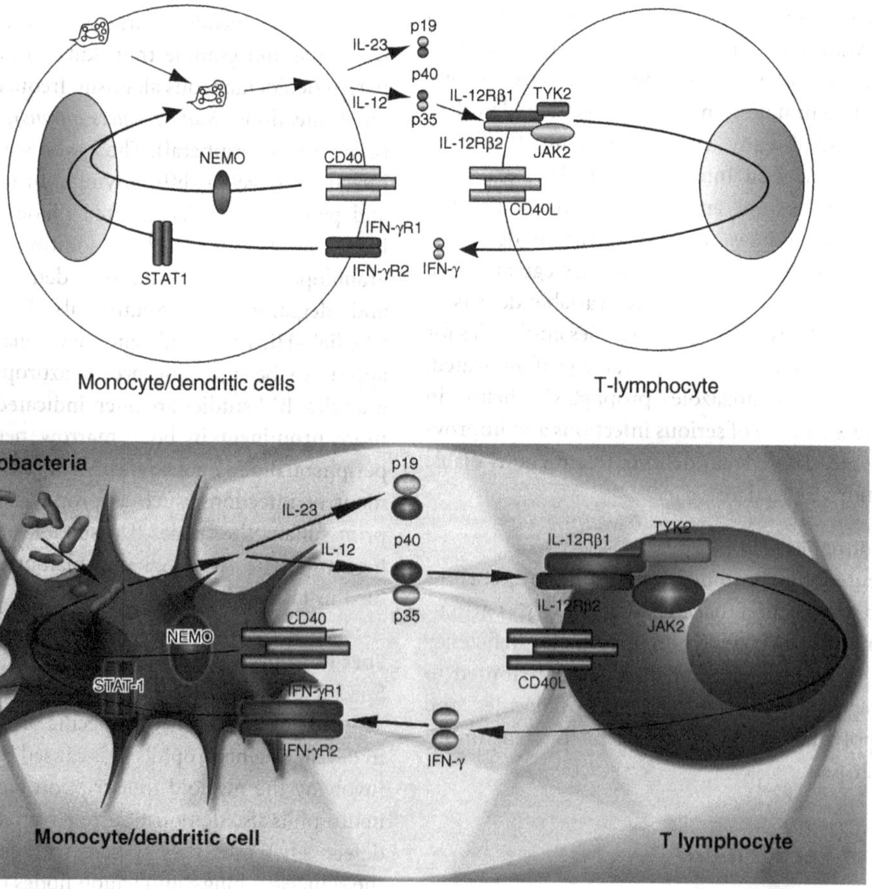

◘ Figure 332.2
MSMD-causing genes in the IL-12/23-IFN-g pathway. Schematic representation of host immune response against mycobacterial infection(Reprinted with permission from Al-Muhsen S, Casanova JL (2008). The genetic heterogeneity of mendelian susceptibility to mycobacterial diseases. J Allergy Clin Immunol 122(6):1043–1051)

or IL-12R defects. Bone marrow transplantation may provide cure for severe cases. However, the high mortality associated with graft rejection has limited this curative option.

Disorders of Intracellular Killing (Oxidative Metabolism)

Chronic Granulomatous Disease (CGD)

CGD is a heterogeneous group of inherited disorders caused by genetic defects in the components of the phagocyte's NADPH oxidase complex. Hence, the phagocytes are unable to generate the microbicidal reactive oxidant superoxide anion and its metabolites. As a result of the defect in this key host defense pathway, CGD patients suffer from recurrent life-threatening bacterial and fungal infections. Five genetic mutations involving the phagocytic oxidase system have been identified so far. The most common is an X-linked recessive defect in gP91phox, while three other AR defects were reported in P22phox, P47phox, and P67phox components of the NADPH oxidase system. A novel mutation in *NCF4*, the gene encoding P40phox, has also recently been reported in a boy who presented with granulomatous colitis, delineating the fourth AR form of CGD. International data indicate that X-linked is more common (65%); however, in highly inbred populations, the AR forms of the condition seem to be more frequent. Clinically, patients with CGD present with recurrent bacterial (*Staphylococcus aureus, Serratia marcescens, Salmonella*, and *Burkholdaria cepacia*) and fungal (*Aspergillus*) infections. In addition to susceptibility to infections, CGD patients are prone to develop noninfectious complications characterized by unregulated inflammation such as granulomatous colitis, chorioretinal lesions, and lupus-like disease. The diagnosis of CGD is based on a compatible clinical presentation and demonstration of a defective respiratory burst by nitroblue tetrazolium test which relies on the intracellular reduction of NBT by superoxide anion to a blue formozan precipitate that can be seen microscopically. More recently, a sensitive tool using flow cytometry to detect dihydrorhodamine 123 oxidative burst assay has been widely used in clinical practice. Genetic confirmation is the gold standard diagnostic test. Prenatal diagnosis can be done by percutaneous umbilical sampling or by puncture of placental vessels using fetoscopy. Treatment of patients with CGD includes appropriate management of infections (antibiotics and antifungal). Prophylaxis with trimethoprim-sulfamethoxazole and itraconazole antifungal prophylaxis have reduced the rate of serious infections substantially and hence improved the outcome. Introducing Interferon-γ prophylaxis was shown to be beneficial in reducing the frequency of serious infections. Hematopietic stem cell transplantation may provide definite cure for severe cases. CGD was formerly associated with a high mortality, but the current practice of prophylaxis with antimicrobials and IFN-γ, aggressive surgery, and early hematopoietic stem cell transplantation or gene therapy have improved the outcome substantially.

Glucose-6-Phosphate Dehydrogenase (G6PD) Deficiency

G6PD is an X-linked inherited disorder leading to a low concentration of NADPH. Patients have recurrent bacterial infections and hemolytic anemia. Diagnosis is made by testing neutrophil G6PD activity (<5% of normal) and erythrocyte G6PD levels. Treatment focuses mainly on appropriate management of infections.

Myeloperoxidase Deficiency (MPO)

MPO is the most common disorder of phagocyte function. It is inherited as autosomal recessive with variable expression. The defect results in diminished production of hydrochlorous acid (HOCI) required for killing of microorganisms (especially *Candida*). Usually patients are clinically asymptomatic but rarely may present with disseminated candidiasis. The deficiency may be acquired in acute myeloid leukemia. Diagnosis is made by testing neutrophils and monocytes for peroxidase (by histochemical analysis). Patients with MPO deficiency and diabetes are usually treated aggressively to prevent fungal infections. Otherwise, MPO does not require prophylactic antibiotics. Prognosis is usually excellent.

Glutathione Metabolism Disorders

Glutathione reductase deficiency and glutathione synthetase deficiency are uncommon and inherited as autosomal recessive traits. Diminished levels of these enzymes lead to toxic accumulation of hydrogen peroxidase due to decreased catabolism by glutathione. Patients may have hemolysis with oxidant stress and usually have a benign course (patients with glutathione synthetase deficiency may have metabolic acidosis, recurrent otitis media, and intermittent neutropenia).

References

Al-Muhsen SZ (2010) Gastrointestinal and hepatic manifestations of primary immune deficiency diseases. Saudi J Gastroenterol 16(2): 66–74

Al-Muhsen S, Casanova JL (2008) The genetic heterogeneity of mendelian susceptibility to mycobacterial diseases. J Allergy Clin Immunol 122(6):1043–1051

Al-Muhsen S, Al-Hemidan A, Al-Shehri A et al (2009) Ocular manifestations in chronic granulomatous disease in Saudi Arabia. J AAPOS 13(4):396–399

Al-Nasser AA, Harfi HA, Sahbah RJ et al (1993) Chediak-Higashi syndrome: report of five Saudi Arab children and review of the literature. Ann Saudi Med 13:321–327

Ambruso DR, Knall C, Abell AN et al (2000) Human neutrophil immunodeficiency syndrome is associated with an inhibitory Rac2 mutation. Proc Natl Acad Sci USA 97:4654–4659

Bainton DF (1980) The cells of inflammation: a general view. In: Weissman G (ed) The cell biology of inflammation, vol 2. Elsevier/North Holland, New York, pp 1–25

Beutler E (1994) G6PD deficiency. Blood 84:3613–3636

Bohn G et al (2007) A novel human primary immunodeficiency syndrome caused by deficiency of the endosomal adaptor protein p14. Nat Med 13(1):38–45

Boztug K et al (2009) A syndrome with congenital neutropenia and mutations in G6PC3. N Engl J Med 360(1):32–43

Burroughs L, Woolfrey A, Shimamura A (2009) Shwachman-Diamond syndrome: a review of the clinical presentation, molecular pathogenesis, diagnosis, and treatment. Hematol Oncol Clin North Am 23: 233–248

Casanova JL, Abel L (2007) Primary immunodeficiencies: a field in its infancy. Science 317:617–619

Cross AR, Noack D, Rae J et al (2000) Hematologically important mutations: the autosomal recessive forms of chronic granulomatous disease (first update). Blood Cells Mol Dis 26:561–565

Dinarello C, Mier J (1987) Lymphokines. N Engl J Med 317:940

Dinauer MC (2007) Disorders of neutrophil function: an overview. Meth Mol Biol 412:489–504

Dinauer MC, Coates TD (2005) Disorders of phagocyte function and number. In: Hoffman R, Benz J, Shattil S et al (eds) Hematology: basic principles and practices. Elsevier Churchill Livingstone, Philadelphia, pp 787–830

Donini M et al (2007) G-CSF treatment of severe congenital neutropenia reverses neutropenia but does not correct the underlying functional deficiency of the neutrophil in defending against microorganisms. Blood 109(11):4716–4723

Engelhardt KR, McGhee S, Winkler S et al (2009) Large deletions and point mutations involving the dedicator of cytokinesis 8 (DOCK8) in the autosomal-recessive form of hyper-IgE syndrome. J Allergy Clin Immunol 124(6):1289–1302.e4

Etzioni A (2010) Defects in the leukocyte adhesion cascade. Clin Rev Allergy Immunol 38(1):54–60

Etzioni A, Alon R (2004) Leukocyte adhesion deficiency III: a group of integrin activation defects in hematopoietic lineage cells. Curr Opin Allergy Clin Immunol 4:485–490

Gallin JI (1992) Disorders of phagocytic cells. In: Gallin JI, Goldstein IM, Syndrome R (eds) Inflammation: basic principles and clinical correlates, 2nd edn. Raven Press, New York, p 859

Germeshausen M, Grudzien M, Zeidler C, Abdollahpour H, Yetgin S, Rezaei N et al (2008) Novel HAX1 mutations in patients with severe congenital neutropenia reveal isoform-dependent genotype-phenotype associations. Blood 111:4954–4957

Gombart AF, Koeffler HP (2002) Neutrophil specific granule deficiency and mutations in the gene encoding transcription factor C/EBP (epsilon). Curr Opin Hematol 9:36–42

Gorlin RJ et al (2000) WHIM syndrome, an autosomal dominant disorder: clinical, hematological, and molecular studies. Am J Med Genet 91(5):368–376

Grimbacher B, Holland SM, Gallin JI et al (1999) Hyper-IgE syndrome with recurrent infections – an autosomal dominant multisystem disorder N. Engl J Med 340:692–702

Grimbacher B, Holland SM, Puck JM (2005) Hyper-IgE syndromes. Immunol Rev 203:244–250

Hernandez PA et al (2003) Mutations in the chemokine receptor gene CXCR4 are associated with WHIM syndrome, a combined immunodeficiency disease. Nat Genet 34(1):70–74

Heyworth PG, Curnutte JT, Rae J et al (2001) Hematologically important mutations: X-linked chronic granulomatous disease (second update). Blood Cells Mol Dis 27:16–26

Heyworth PG, Cross AR, Curnutte JT (2003) Chronic granulomatous disease. Curr Opin Immunol 15:578–584

Holland SM (2010) Chronic granulomatous disease. Clin Rev Allergy Immunol 38(1):3–10

Horwitz M et al (1999) Mutations in ELA2, encoding neutrophil elastase, define a 21-day biological clock in cyclic haematopoiesis. Nat Genet 23(4):433–436

Horwitz MS et al (2007) Neutrophil elastase in cyclic and severe congenital neutropenia. Blood 109(5):1817–1824

Hutchinson R, Boxer LA (1990) Disorders of granulocyte and monocyte production. In: Benz EJ, Cohen HJ, Furie B et al (eds) Hematology: basic principles and practice. Churchill Livingstone, New York, pp 193–204

Jung J et al (2006) Identification of a homozygous deletion in the AP3B1 gene causing Hermansky-Pudlak syndrome, type 2. Blood 108(1): 362–369

Klein C, Welte K (2010) Genetic insights into congenital neutropenia. Clin Rev Allergy Immunol 38(1):68–74

Klein C, Phillipe N, Le Deist F et al (1994) Griscelli C. Partial albinism with immunodeficiency (Griscelli syndrome). J Pediatr 125:886–895

Lekstrom-Himes JA, Gallin JI (2000) Immunodeficiency diseases caused by defects in phagocytes. N Engl J Med 343(23):1703–1714

Malech HL, Galin JI (1987) Current concepts. Immunology: neutrophils in human diseases. N Engl J Med 317:687

Matute JD, Arias AA, Wright NA et al (2009) A new genetic subgroup of chronic granulomatous disease with autosomal recessive mutations in p40phox and selective defects in neutrophil NADPH oxidase activity. Blood 114:3309–3315

Melis D et al (2005) Genotype/phenotype correlation in glycogen storage disease type 1b: a multicentre study and review of the literature. Eur J Pediatr 164(8):501–508

Minegishi Y, Saito M, Morio T, Watanabe K, Agematsu K, Tsuchiya S et al (2006) Human tyrosine kinase 2 deficiency reveals its requisite roles in multiple cytokine signals involved in innate and acquired immunity. Immunity 25:745–755

Minegishi Y, Saito M, Tsuchiya S, Tsuge I, Takada H, Hara T et al (2007) Dominantnegative mutations in the DNA-binding domain of STAT3 cause hyper-IgE syndrome. Nature 448:1058–1062

Nauseef WM (1998) Insights into myeloperoxidase biosynthesis from its inherited deficiency. J Mol Med 76:661–668

Notarangelo LD (2010) Primary immunodeficiencies. J Allergy Clin Immunol 125(2 Suppl 2):S182–S194

Notarangelo LD, Fischer A, Geha RS, Casanova JL et al (2009) Primary immunodeficiencies: 2009 update: from the International Union of Immunological Societies Expert Committee on Primary Immunodeficiencies. J Allergy Clin Immunol 124(6):1161–1178. Erratum in: J Allergy Clin Immunol, 2010, 125(3):771–773

Pannicke U et al (2009a) Reticular dysgenesis (aleukocytosis) is caused by mutations in the gene encoding mitochondrial adenylate kinase 2. Nat Genet 41(1):101–105

Pannicke U, Hönig M, Hess I, Friesen C et al (2009b) Reticular dysgenesis (aleukocytosis) is caused by mutations in the gene encoding mitochondrial adenylate kinase 2. Nat Genet 41(1):101–105. Epub 30 Nov 2008

Pizzo PA (2004) Fever and neutropenia. In: Kliegman R, Greenbaum L (eds) Patricia lye practical strategies in pediatric diagnosis and therapy, 2nd edn. Elsevier, Philadelphia, pp 1071–1084

Rosenberg PS et al (2006) The incidence of leukemia and mortality from sepsis in patients with severe congenital neutropenia receiving long-term G-CSF therapy. Blood 107(12):4628–4635

Rosenzweig SD, Holland SM (2004) Phagocyte immunodeficiencies and their infections. J Allergy Clin Immunol 113(4):620–626

Schäffer AA, Klein C (2007) Genetic heterogeneity in severe congenital neutropenia: how many aberrant pathways can kill a neutrophil? Curr Opin Allergy Clin Immunol 7(6):481–494

Smith OP, Hann IM, Chessels JM, Reeves BR, Milla P (1996) Haematological abnormalities in Shwachman-Diamond syndrome. Br J Haematol 94:279–284

Svensson L, Howarth K, McDowall A et al (2009) Leukocyte adhesion deficiency-III is caused by mutations in KINDLIN3 affecting integrin activation. Nat Med 15:306–312

Tassone L, Notarangelo LD, Bonomi V, Savoldi G, Sensi A, Soresina A et al (2009) Clinical and genetic diagnosis of warts, hypogammaglobulinemia, infections, myelokathexis (WHIM) syndrome in 10 patients. J Allergy Clin Immunol 123(1170–3):e1–e3

Ward DM, Shiflett SL, Kaplan J (2002) Chediak-Higashi syndrome: a clinical and molecular view of a rare lysosomal storage disorder. Curr Mol Med 2:469–477

Wei ML (2006) Hermansky-Pudlak syndrome: a disease of protein trafficking and organelle function. Pigment Cell Res 19(1):19–42

Winkelstein JA, Marino MC, Johnston RB Jr, Boyle J, Curnutte J, Gallin JI et al (2000) Chronic granulomatous disease. Report on a national registry of 368 patients. Med Baltim 79:155–169

Yang Kuender D, Quie Paul G, Hill Harry R (2007) Phagocytic system. In: Hans Ochs, Smith CI, Jennifer Puck (eds) Primary immunodeficiency diseases: a molecular and genetic approach, 2nd edn. Oxford University press, Philadelphia, pp 103–120

Zhang Q, Davis JC, Lamborn IT, Freeman AF et al (2009) Combined immunodeficiency associated with DOCK8 mutations. N Engl J Med 361(21):2046–2055. Epub 23 Sept 2009

333 Bone Marrow Failure Disorders

Hassan El Solh · Abdallah Al-Nasser · Peter Kurre

The term "bone marrow failure syndromes" (BMF) captures a heterogeneous group of disorders that result in an effective mismatch between blood and immune cell production in the bone marrow and peripheral demand. Most often clinical symptoms of cytopenia bring children to medical attention and prompt laboratory evaluation. However, in children, given the compensatory capacity of their cardiovascular system, relatively greater baseline incidence of infections and their general propensity for minor trauma, they often present relatively late in the process. The clinical presentation is further compounded by the frequently insidious nature of onset and can be masked by disease specific symptoms in other organs. For example, children with cytopenia following infection may undergo evaluation for predominant fevers and skin findings. Indeed, with some regularity the diagnosis is unsuspected and even incidental during evaluation for more common childhood problems, especially infections, recurrent bleeding, or failure to thrive. On rare occasions, patients will be referred because siblings or family members have been diagnosed with a specific BMF disorder. Notwithstanding specific symptoms, the hemogram often reveals a variable degree and combination of multi- or single lineage count decrements.

Etiologic considerations are broad, covering specific acquired and multi-system heritable genetic disorders. Medical history and physical evaluation can provide critical clues to guide differential diagnosis and tailor choice of ancillary studies. However, in the absence of acute blood loss or evidence of immune mediated destruction, further evaluation will almost always require a bone marrow evaluation and, where available, more specialized biochemical and genetic testing. Setting appropriate expectations with patient, family, and other providers, the often extensive evaluation may not always establish a definitive diagnosis, but is crucial in making appropriate treatment recommendations and excluding heritable etiologies that require family counseling.

General Considerations

Definitive hematopoiesis during human development follows a carefully orchestrated series of in utero developmental phases. Beginning in the aorta-gonadomesonephros region of the early fetus, production of blood and immune cells passes through a placental phase with subsequent expansion in the fetal liver before ultimately moving to the bone marrow at 22 weeks of gestation. Trabecular bone provides the scaffold structure that supports the stromal, hematopoietic, osteoblastic, as well as endothelial cellular components and extracellular matrix that comprise the hematopoietic microenvironment. It is widely believed that hematopoiesis and immunopoiesis are hierarchically organized in a system of successive steps of differentiation and progressive restriction with functional specializations of cells. All mature cells in the blood stream are derived from rare hematopoietic stem cells residing in the bone marrow microenvironment and capable of asymmetric division. Cell fate decisions determine self-renewal and differentiation activity and match blood and immune cell production to physiologic needs. Driving the process of amplification and specification is a network of endocrine and paracrine signaling molecules and their cognate cellular receptors. Hematopoietically active cytokines, interleukins, adhesion molecules, and growth factors are responsible for maintaining cells in quiescence and providing hierarchically specific cues to initiate proliferation and cell type specific coordinated expansion. For example, during adjustment to lower partial oxygen pressures at high elevations, hypoxia signaling in the kidney will result in erythropoietin secretion and selective activation of red blood cell progenitors in the bone marrow to increase production of oxygen carrier capacity. Similarly, pathophysiologic events such as infection or bleeding can trigger massive increases in production and mobilization of leukocytes or platelets. Expansion of virus specific T-cells on the other hand provides an instructive model for interleukin-2 and its role during induced clonal proliferation of immune cells in response to a very specific viral agent. The often remarkably advanced and tightly controlled signaling effects reflect the combined diversity of ligands and receptors.

Differential Diagnosis

Children presenting with signs of single or multilineage cytopenias offer a broad differential diagnosis. Patient age,

Abdelaziz Y. Elzouki (ed.), *Textbook of Clinical Pediatrics*, DOI 10.1007/978-3-642-02202-9_333,

physical findings, and specific circumstances can help guide the work up and narrow relevant diagnoses. Principally, infections, environmental exposures, nutritional deficiencies, immune dysregulation, malignant, or benign infiltrative bone marrow processes must be considered.

Evaluation

Physical examination and thorough patient and family history are cornerstones in the diagnosis of BMF, often providing critical clues to tailor additional investigations. The relatively greater proportion of children in whom marrow aplasia is merely the presenting manifestation of an underlying heritable condition emphasizes their critical importance. The distinction between acquired and inherited etiologies in children is crucial, not only for proper treatment and to avoid unnecessary toxicities, but also to initiate family counseling. In some conditions, such as Fanconi Anemia, characteristic physical stigmata are obvious in only a minority of patients and their absence should never lead the clinician to dismiss the diagnosis. In other instances, such as thrombocytopenia with absent radii, abnormalities on physical exam are obvious and the diagnosis more straightforward. Several ancillary studies are useful to ascertain the diagnosis and begin to delineate more specific etiologies:

Quantitative cytopenic abnormalities of individual or all hematopoietic lineages in the peripheral blood often lead to symptomatic presentation, prompt further work up and lead to specialty referral. The complete hemogram provides a wealth of information about the patient's hematological status and may help narrow the differential diagnoses to be pursued. Normal range values for blood cell counts and indices should be interpreted with consideration of age, gender, and laboratory reference standards. Separately, a blood smear for microscopic evaluation and reticulocyte stains should be included to assess cell morphology and bone marrow red cell compensatory activity, respectively.

The bone marrow evaluation is a key for the classification of cytopenias and provides an opportunity for several separate tests. Ideally, the decalcified Giemsa stained bone marrow biopsy captures the architecture, cellular composition, and extracellular matrix of hematopoietic tissue. Additional, more specific histochemical stains can help answer questions of iron stores, infection, malignant (e.g., leukemia) or nonmalignant (e.g., glycogen storage disease) displacement of hematopoietic cells. However, the hallmark finding in bone marrow failure is the adipose replacement and proportional decrease of hematopoietic elements inappropriate for age. Reduced cellularity (defined as <30% averaged for multiple fields of view) and variable peripheral cytopenias are defining diagnostic features of bone marrow failure, regardless of etiology. A bone marrow aspirate is usually obtained to evaluate size and morphology (dysplasia, nuclear bridging), but also cytogenetic analysis for karyotype abnormalities. Depending on circumstance, immunophenotyping, or fluorescence in situ hybridization (FISH) studies may be desired to delineate aplastic anemia (AA) from hypoplastic myelodysplastic syndrome (MDS) or lymphomatous invasion. Incidental diagnosis of fatty marrow replacement has been reported in patients who underwent magnetic resonance imaging for unrelated causes, but radiologic evaluation, other than for specific symptoms, has no routine role in the diagnostic algorithm. Additionally indicated diagnostic tests are discussed in the context of specific diagnoses below.

Acquired Aplastic Anemia (AAA)

Pathophysiologically AA is widely considered to reflect immune destruction of stem cells with the resulting progressive depletion of mature blood and immune cells. The degree of peripheral blood neutropenia, reticulocytopenia, thrombocytopenia, and the proportion of hematopoietic elements in the bone marrow are usually used to grade severity. Values of $<500 \times 10^9$/l for neutrophils, <1% reticulocytes, $<20{,}000 \times 10^9$ platelets, and <30% cellularity define severe disease, often associated with a transfusion requirement for red blood cells and platelets. Most practitioners will consider therapeutic intervention only in such cases, whereas moderately severe disease may progress or resolve in up to 30% of cases without intervention. The incidence ranges from two to six cases per million without ethnic or gender predilections, but with notable regional differences between western and eastern hemisphere.

Etiology

Paul Ehrlich's initial description associated with pregnancy in a young woman is now considered exceedingly rare. But, notwithstanding its shared pathophysiology, the most common finding will be idiopathic bone marrow failure without a known cause even though several specific etiologies and common associations that alter treatment decision making must be considered in children.

Infections

A wide range of infections has been associated with prolonged cytopenias. Especially in children, these can be asymptomatic and are often transient. However, congenital or postnatal infection with parvovirus (*B19* strain), human immunodeficiency virus (HIV-1, or rarely -2), Epstein Barr Virus (EBV), or Cytomegalovirus (CMV) may result in sustained low blood counts. Failure to eradicate these infections may also provide clues to underlying immunodeficiencies. Hypocellular cytopenias have long been appreciated as sequelae of, or rarely concurrent with, A, B, or C viral hepatitis. Regionally different incidences for AA range from 2% to 5% of children with hepatitis and a slightly higher percentage in patients who received orthotopic liver grafts. Clinically heterogeneous, even patients with substantial and life-threatening liver failure, organ function recovers and does not necessarily affect treatment, complications, response to therapy, or ultimate prognosis. Serological or pathogen-specific nucleic acid based laboratory evidence will help distinguish past from active infection and can be helpful guiding successful treatment.

Drugs

When it was in more widespread medical use, chloramphenicol was linked to aplastic anemia. Case reports also implicate more commonly used drugs, including sulfonamides, carbamazepines, cimetidine and quinacrine, and others. Mechanistic insight into this etiology is missing and no specific test will be helpful in ascertaining this etiology.

Chemicals and Toxins

Environmental exposure to aerosolized benzene in particular is an established cause of marrow dysfunction and occasionally myelodysplasia. But, while patients and caregivers often focus on this etiology, it is in fact very rare in industrialized western society. A particularly informative recent study suggests that environmental exposure to pesticides and other agents including organophosphates may be a problem in other parts of the world. An extensive exposure and occupational history is important in making the diagnosis.

Etiologies such as ionizing radiation or graft versus host disease (GVHD) are well-established causes of marrow aplasia and pancytopenia, but the context dependence makes their diagnosis more straightforward.

Paroxysmal Nocturnal Hemoglobinuria (PNH)

PNH is a clonal stem cell disorder resulting from somatic mutations in PIG-A gene and the production of blood cells defective for glycosylphosphatidyl-inositol (GPI) anchorage of several cell surface proteins. Clinically PNH is characterized by periodic lysis of red blood cells with resulting intravascular hemolysis. However, considerable overlap exists in the clinical presentation and diagnostic findings of patients with idiopathic AA and those with PNH. Indeed, commonalities between the two entities have been interpreted to indicate an immune pathophysiology for PNH, as well. Care should be exercised to distinguish the two from each other, and the existence of coagulation abnormalities and symptoms of thrombosis may be considered defining features of classic PNH. Accordingly, the demonstration of clonal deficiencies of select cell surface proteins in red blood cell or leukocyte lineages should not be automatically considered diagnostic of PNH since positive tests have been found in many patients with marrow failure. Historically, testing relied on sucrose lysis, with more recent flow-cytometry based assays greatly increasing sensitivity and quantitation. A prognostic role for PNH clones and the value of sequential analyses in guiding treatment has been suggested.

Complicating matters further, PNH has been well documented as a potential late complication after treatment with immunosuppressive agents.

Myelodysplasia (MDS)

Primary, non-treatment related myelodysplasia is a rare form of bone marrow dysfunction in childhood that may progress to acute myeloid leukemia. Cytopenias bringing the patients to medical attention and the diagnosis of a hypocellular bone marrow overlap with those of AA. Importantly, many patients present evidence not only of morphologic dysplasia on examination of smears, but also hallmark chromosomal aberrations. Accordingly, all patients with bone marrow failure undergoing a marrow aspiration procedure should have a cytogenetic analysis for karyotypic abnormalities. Numeric and gross structural abnormalities will be readily apparent. Depending on availabilities of laboratory facilities for further testing, additional studies for characteristic abnormalities such as loss of chromosome 7 or gains in chromosome 8 using FISH are indicated. Myelodysplasia and leukemia can be the initial presenting sign of cancer prone genetic disorders, including Fanconi Anemia and Shwachman–Diamond Syndrome. This, along with the generally infrequent occurrence of myelodysplasia in children, implies the need to test these children for genetic disorders, especially in the very young.

Laboratory Findings

The backbone of the diagnostic work up is a complete peripheral blood count with indices, reticulocyte count and leukocyte differential. A blood film may hold additional valuable information on cell shape, morphology, and size. The bone marrow aspirate and biopsy should be evaluated for morphology and cellular composition and cellularity. Cytogenetic testing to exclude cases of myelodysplasia is important. When available, flowcytometric immunophenotyping to exclude leukemic involvement is helpful. Additional studies helpful in confirming the diagnoses and considering differential etiology include peripheral blood chromosome breakage testing to exclude Fanconi Anemia. Immunologic evaluation may include determination of immunoglobulin subclasses, lymphocyte subsets, the presence, and compositions of PI negative clones. Underlying viral infections should be excluded, especially HIV, hepatitis, and parvovirus. Radiological imaging has no routine role in the diagnostic work up of AA.

Therapy

Supportive Care is the backbone of treatment of patients with AA. Because most will present with cytopenias, diagnosis and treatment of infections as well as the need for transfusions are principal concerns in newly presenting patients. Neutropenic patients frequently come to medical attention with recurrent febrile episodes, oral mucosal ulcers, and fevers of unexplained origin. Symptom-guided diagnostics are indicated, although frequently unrevealing, and appropriate broad-spectrum antibiotics should be considered under these circumstances, especially in patients with indwelling central venous catheters. The role of empiric antibiotic coverage in patients is more controversial, although many practitioners consider antifungal coverage and prophylaxis against *pneumocystis carini* important. Children have profound cardiovascular reserve and the signs and symptoms of anemia routinely occur late with hemoglobin values often <6 g/dl. The transfusion of chronically adjusted patients requires judicious and slow correction, often over the course of several days. Normal hemoglobin values are not the goal, rather, improving oxygen delivery to tissues to relieve immediate symptoms of fatigue and exertion with post-transfusion target range between 8 and 10 g/dl. Because, patients are often neutropenic and lymphopenic, they should be considered immunocompromised even before receiving treatment. Therefore, to avoid transfusion associated immune reactions and minimize transmission of pathogens, transfusions of whole blood, red blood cells, or platelets should be prepared to eliminate viable lymphocytes (γ-irradiation) and filtered to remove trace leukocyte carriers of cytomegalovirus whenever possible. Long-term complications of transfusions include blood group and human leukocyte antigen (HLA) sensitization. They may accelerate transfusion requirements and sensitize the patient to transfusion associated immune reactions. HLA matching of platelets or family directed donation is often technically feasible, but should be strenuously avoided so as to not increase the risk of subsequent rejection in any patient who is considered for a stem cell transplant procedure in the future. The hemoglobin contained in red blood cells is complexed with iron, and transfusion of blood in patients unable to mobilize stores during red blood cell production in the bone marrow can lead to iron deposition and end organ dysfunction in liver, heart, and pancreas. Therefore, transfusion of blood products should always be judicious to minimize side effects. White blood cells and especially granulocytes are rarely transfused in cases of severe invasive infections.

Hematopoietic growth factors in the treatment of AA produce no sustained responses by themselves, but may have a role in the context of immunosuppressive therapy. Whether long-term use of G-CSF contributes to clonal evolution of myelodysplasia or acute myeloblastic leukemia is controversial. Androgenic steroids can temporarily improve hematopoietic output and are widely used in some parts of the world, but their side effects make long-term use problematic.

The treatment algorithm for idiopathic severe AA is subject to patient specific considerations and available resources and can therefore be regionally different. However, because the pathophysiology of AA is widely agreed to be an immune elimination of bone marrow stem cells, suppression or replacement of immune function are the principal considerations. Based on risk-benefit ratio and local resources, stem cell transplantation from an HLA matched sibling is the primary modality, followed by a variety of immunosuppressive strategies. Transplantation of stem cells from an unrelated donor is a potentially curative option for patients who fail immune suppression.

Immunosuppression Therapy (IST)

The incidental observation of sustained endogenous recovery following graft failure in AA patients undergoing transplantation provides powerful evidence for the immunological basis of AA. Based on a landmark randomized trial, the modern backbone of AA treatment is a course of rabbit or horse derived anti-lymphocyte or anti-thymocyte globulin (ATG). The combination with calcineurin inhibitor cyclosporine in particular has proved effective in inducing partial or complete remission in a majority of patients. Response to treatment is notoriously slow, but white blood cell count recovery can be hastened by addition of granulocyte colony stimulating factor. Responses may be drug dependent and the disease may recur, but immunosuppression can present a viable functional cure allowing independence from transfusions and high survival rates in children. Re-treatment with a second course of ATG will provide remission in about half the patients, without gains after switching between globulin preparations. Survival after IST is improved for younger patients with less severe disease who respond to treatment early, whereas clonal evolution to myelodysplasia or leukemia is frequently fatal. In aggregate, between 15% and 20% of long-term survivors develop late clonal disease (MDS, AML, and PNH).

Corticosteroids have not been effective in producing sustained remissions whereas cyclopshophamide can be successful, but immunosuppression is profound and complications can be severe.

Bone Marrow Transplantation

Transplantation of bone marrow stem cells is the only curative treatment of AA. Resources and donor availability permitting, transplantation of hematopoietic stem cells from an HLA matched related sibling donor is the treatment of choice. Improvements in supportive care and transfusion practices result in long-term survival rates in children exceeding 90%. Conditioning with ATG and high dose cyclopshophamide combined with adequate stem cell dose leads to stable donor chimerism with acceptable toxicities and effective prophylaxis against graft versus host disease. Unlike patients with malignancy, those with AA do not benefit from GVHD and the use of peripheral blood stem cell grafts worsens outcomes. Endocrine late effects on growth, thyroid, and gonadal functions are less frequent than following high dose radiation conditioning, but secondary malignancies have been seen.

Inherited Bone Marrow Failure Disorders

Fanconi Anemia (FA, OMIM: 227650)

A heritable multi-system disorder with great phenotypic diversity, Fanconi Anemia comprises a combination of physical anomalies, progressive bone marrow failure, and propensity to develop cancer. Mutations in at least 12 genes are the basis for predominantly autosomal inheritance, except for one rare form inherited in autosomal dominant fashion. Remarkably, most of the affected proteins functionally cooperate in a molecular pathway involved in genome damage repair. The phenotypic presentation of these subgroups, referred to as complementation groups, show considerable overlap, although some groups seem to follow a more severe and rapidly progressive course. Historically, radii and thenar abnormalities, microcephaly, as well as short stature have been considered characteristic physical findings, prompting a diagnostic work up. However, more recent studies of presymptomatic siblings and routine screening for excessive chromosomal breakage of children with any form of marrow failure reveal that over one third of patients ultimately diagnosed with FA do not have obvious findings on physical exam. Therefore, specific screening for chromosome breakage must be considered in any child with marrow failure, whether single or multilineage. FA is a multi-system disorder and many patients suffer from endocrine dysfunction with thyroid and growth hormone imbalance, glucose homeostasis, and reproductive function. Patients should be followed at routine intervals.

Bone marrow failure in FA is characteristically progressive and slow. Children commonly present with symptoms of cytopenias and are often followed for years before definitive intervention. Guidelines for transfusion and infection apply as in any form of aplastic anemia. Temporary responses to androgenic steroids and use of granulocyte colony stimulating factor have been described. The only curative treatment remains transplantation of hematopoietic stem cells from and unaffected HLA matched individual, preferably a matched family member who has tested negative for FA. However, caution must be exercised in selecting conditioning regimens, as patients will suffer excessive mucosal toxicities from chemotherapeutic regimen and especially higher doses of radiation used in AA. Low doses of cyclopshophamide combined with ATG produce rapid and reliable engraftment of unmanipulated marrow grafts. An alternative approach intended to reduce rates of GVHD has been to deplete the graft of T-cells. Especially in the unrelated donor setting, where graft failure, frequently severe GVHD, and invasive infections compromise outcomes, this can be of benefit. The risk of FA patients developing myelodysplasia or leukemia is several hundred folds in excess of those in the general population. While the successful replacement of blood and immune system in FA presents a cure for the bone marrow manifestations of the disease, other organ systems remain at risk. Most notably, the risk for epithelial cancers of the head/neck region and the female genital tract is high. As follows from observations on conditioning regimen toxicity, selecting chemotherapeutic agents, or radiation doses, effective at eradicating cancer cells, while limiting toxicity is a challenge that applies to treatment of any cancer in children with FA. Early detection is of key importance and screening for head-neck and gynecological cancers are recommended where available. The lifespan for children with FA has greatly improved with an improved understanding of disease biology, supportive care, and advances in modifying conventional treatment regimens. However, genetic counseling remains important.

Dyskeratosis Congenita (DC, OMIM: 127550)

Children with congenital dyskeratosis show characteristic reticular skin changes, dysplastic nails, oral leukoplakia, and progressive bone marrow failure. Presentation and severity are heterogeneous and can vary among individuals within affected families. Longitudinal studies reveal an increased risk of solid tumors, MDS, leukemias, and pulmonary fibrosis. Classic dyskeratosis is thought to be a severe form in a spectrum of disorders of telomere biology. Rare forms of DC can present with significant neurologic and cognitive dysfunction. Most patients come to medical attention with macrocytic anemia. Evaluation of bone marrow and peripheral blood smear in conjunction with clinical findings is the key to establishing the diagnosis. More recently the diagnosis of shortened telomeres in multiple leukocyte subsets has been proposed as a sensitive and specific assay, though limited in availability. This test can be useful for screening children fulfilling clinical criteria. Subsequent mutation sequencing can be confirmatory for patients and helpful for family carrier screening. Depending on which genes harbor mutations, inheritance mode can be autosomal dominant, recessive (*TERC, TERT, TINF, NHP2 NOP10*) or even x-linked (*DKC1*). Treatment is symptomatic as in other BMF syndromes, relying on transfusion support and aggressive treatment of infections. Androgens, growth factors, erythropoietin, and G-CSF have been used with variable success, but the risk of complications including virilization and rare reports of splenic rupture, respectively, should be carefully weighed. In patients with symptomatic bone marrow failure who have an available HLA matched and non-affected sibling donor, transplantation of hematopoietic stem cells is the recommended treatment. Pulmonary and hepatic cirrhosis can complicate transplantation suggesting that non-myeloablative conditioning strategies result in improved long-term outcomes.

Shwachman–Diamond Syndrome (SDS, OMIM 260400)

The combination of exocrine pancreatic insufficiency, marrow failure and metaphyseal dysostoses comprise the principal findings in Shwachman–Diamond Syndrome. The overwhelming majority of cases reflect mutations in the Shwachman–Bodian–Diamond gene on chromosome 7. The gene product has prominent functions in mitotic spindle formation and ribosome biogenesis. Patients most commonly present with chronic or intermittent neutropenia, but other cell lines are also frequently affected, reflecting the underlying quantitative and qualitative stem cell abnormalities. Additionally, immune function can be abnormal in SDS patients with variable cellular defects of neutrophil polarization and migration, B, T, and NK cell number. Like patients with other bone marrow failure syndromes, SDS patients are at greatly increased risk for developing MDS and myeloid leukemia. These often go hand in hand with cytogenetic abnormalities, such as loss of chromosome 7. Notwithstanding, cytogenetic abnormalities also occur without over signs of dysplasia and can wax and wane, putting their clinical significance in question. Compromised exocrine pancreatic function results in steatorrhea and reduced absorption of fat-soluble vitamins. Failure to thrive and growth failure are frequent presenting signs. Imaging studies will reveal a small pancreas. Liver abnormalities are also common. Pathologic correlates in liver and pancreas are fatty replacements. Remarkably, symptoms may vary over time with many patients recovering sufficient pancreatic function in later years. Specific testing for fecal elastase or serum pancreatic trypsinogen with a negative sweat chloride test to exclude cystic fibrosis will help establish the diagnosis. Metaphyseal dysostosis of the long bones are found in roughly half the patients, although they are frequently asymptomatic. Rarely, rib cage anomalies can result in respiratory compromise. Structural cardiac anomalies have been described in several patients and cardiovascular complications can manifest after high dose therapy in the context of transplantation.

Treatment is predominantly symptom based and should include supplemental vitamins, antibiotics to treat infections, and transfusions when needed. Routine follow up by hematologist, gastroenterologist, endocrinologist, and genetic counselor are recommended. Stem cell transplantation can be curative for hematological manifestations and has been performed successfully using matched related and non-affected, as well as unrelated donors. Different conditioning strategies have been used depending in part on donor availability and whether patients progressed to MDS and AML. The ideal timing in patients with asymptomatic cytopenias is a matter of discussion and institutional preference.

Reticular Dysgenesis (OMIM 267500)

This is a severe form of inherited immunodeficiency and an exceedingly rare disorder of leukocyte and immune function manifesting in infancy. Patients will present with agranulocytosis, lymphopenia, thymic hypoplasia and absent immune function. Recent evidence suggests that a defect in mitochondrial metabolism may be causative. Overwhelming infections are frequent causes of death, but stem cell transplantation is potentially curative.

Congenital Amegakaryocytic Thrombocytopenia (CAMT, OMIM: 604498)

CAMT is a hypomegakaryocytopenic thrombocytopenia commonly diagnosed during infancy with an inherent propensity to progress to AA. Thrombocytopenia in these patients can be severe, with potentially life-threatening bleeding requiring transfusion of platelets. Additional congenital anomalies can be seen, mostly involving heart, kidney, or neuromotor function. The differential diagnosis should include TAR (below) and the Wiskott–Aldrich Syndrome as well as neonatal alloimmune thrombocytopenia. The diagnosis is often established on clinical grounds with bone marrow confirmation and where available genetic testing. The molecular defect rests on mutations in the thrombopoietin (TPO) receptor, c-MPL, coinciding with high levels of the cytokine in patients. The role of TPO in stem cell pool maintenance and differentiation is consistent with the frequent evolution to AA in patients. Cytokine and steroid treatment can have transient benefit, but transfusion is the main therapeutic recourse to treat symptoms. The definitive treatment and only known cure is the transplantation of stem cells from unaffected HLA matched donors. It is unclear if patients with CAMT suffer an increased risk of malignancy.

Pure Red Cell Aplasia

Diamond Blackfan Anemia (DBA, OMIM;105650)

DBA is the principal cause of inherited erythroid specific bone marrow failure. Care should be taken to distinguish it from acquired causes of red cell aplasia, namely Pearson Syndrome; transient erythroblastopenia of childhood (TEC); and secondary immune or malignancy associated forms. The incidence in the population is 5–7 cases per million without gender or ethnic predilection. DBA is inherited in autosomal dominant mode in 45%, but de novo mutations are frequent. More than 90% of patients are diagnosed within the first year of life based on anemia, either related to symptoms or in the work up of the cephalic, thumb, cardiac or urogenital malformations seen in up to 50% of DBA patients. Short stature is diagnosed in 30%. At the extremes of the spectrum, some carriers are clinically silent while other patients present with nonclassical DBA picture indistinguishable from AA. There is no significant correlation between patient presentation, disease severity, clinical response to treatment and genotype. A macrocytic normochromic anemia with reticulocytopenia is found most often in the context of a normal bone marrow cellularity with dramatically reduced (<5%) erythroid precursors resulting from increased apoptosis in the erythroid precursors. In distinction to TEC, the anemia tends to be macrocytic and red cell adenosine deaminase (ADA) is elevated in 85% of individuals. Haploinsufficiency in one of at least seven responsible genes identified to date results in ribosomal dysfunction. But, while mutation sequencing in patients can therefore be useful, where available, for confirmation, family or prenatal screening, these genes account for only 43% of DBA patients. Erythropoietic failure in DBA is characteristically responsive to steroids, the mainstay of treatment. Up to 80% of patients respond to steroids, with about half each experiencing sustained responses and drug-dependent erythropoiesis versus relapse to transfusion dependence, respectively. Up to 20% will remit over time. However, related to potentially severe and debilitating effects steroids can have on immune function, neuromotor and musculoskeletal development, many practitioners favor transfusion for infants. In general, hemoglobin levels between 8 and 9 g/dl permit musculoskeletal growth without undue suppression of hematopoiesis and excessive transfusional iron loading. Surveillance bone densitometry measurements may be indicated where available to detect developing osteoporosis early. As in cases of multilineage bone marrow failure, or hemoglobinopathies, the only curative treatment for DBA is transplantation. The indication for transplantation is often predicated on development of side effects of steroids treatment and transfusion associated iron overload. Outcomes for patients less than 10 years of age with available HLA matched sibling donors is up to 90% survival, while results in older patients and following unrelated donor transplantation are significantly worse. Anecdotal reports indicate occasional response to cyclosporine, metoclopramide and leucine in steroid resistant patients. Finally, it must be noted that patients with DBA, as with other BMF syndromes suffer an excessive risk for cancer at a generally earlier onset than the general population. Reports show predominant leukemia, MDS, lymphoma, and sporadic breast cancer or melanoma.

Transient Erythroblastopenia of Childhood (TEC)

Often the principal competing diagnostic consideration, TEC is an acquired, self-limiting disorder of erythropoiesis in children 1–4 years old and rarely in infants younger than 6 months. A normochromic and normocytic anemia with reticulocytopenia can last up to several months. A bone marrow evaluation is usually not indicated, only revealing erythroblastopenia while mostly normal red cell ADA levels are potentially useful in distinguishing DBA in the acute setting. A viral etiology has been suggested and there may be overlap with herpes, or parvovirus B19 infections. Close follow up and supportive care including transfusions for symptomatic patients may be required. The prognosis for complete recovery is excellent and treatment is not usually indicated, although empiric use of IVIG has been proposed for persistence.

Congenital Dyserythropoetic Anemia (CDA, type I–III)

CDA comprises a group of rare inherited disorders defined by ineffective erythropoiesis. CDA I (OMIM: 224120) presents with congenital macrocytic anemia and occasionally intrauterine hydrops. Infants tend to show signs of hepatomegaly and jaundice. However, some patients are not diagnosed until well into child and even adulthood. A moderate anemia is lifelong with jaundice and splenomegaly that may be delayed in onset. Additionally, some patients come to attention with dyskeratotic skin pigment changes and limb anomalies, specifically syndactily and metatarsal bone duplication. Autosomal recessive inheritance based on mutations in *CDAN1* has been reported in Bedouin populations. CDA is diagnosed based on evidence of ineffective erythropoiesis with high reticulocyte counts and low serum haptoglobin. Elevated indirect bilirubin is evidence of intramedullary and extramedullary hemolysis. The bone marrow exam shows characteristic erythroid hyperplasia with double nucleated erythroblasts and prominent ultrastructural abnormalities. Chromatin bridging occurs in over 50% and occasionally increased non-ringed sideroblasts and peripheral elliptocytosis are seen. It is important to exclude megaloblastic anemias, MDS, and myeloid leukemia, subtype M6. The administration of interferon alpha 2a can increase hemoglobin values.

Hemochromatosis is a frequent long-term complication, secondary to transfusion and increased intestinal absorptions. Patients requiring transfusions need to be monitored for iron load and end organ functions. Surveillance evaluation of hemoglobin, bilirubin, and ferritin is recommended. Similarly, where available, gall bladder ultrasound to evaluate for cholelithiasis and T2 MRI to determine cardiac as well as hepatic iron load is helpful. Chelation therapy may be indicated.

CDA type II (OMIM: 224100) is a more frequent and potentially more severe anemia characteristically associated with expression of an antigen that reacts with a naturally occurring cold reacting IgM antibody and abnormal glycoprotein band 3. Bone marrow evaluation shows multinuclearity in >50% of erythroblasts. Splenectomy has been found to be helpful in reducing bilirubin and improve anemia. Those benefits are sustained, but do not alter iron absorption. Malformations are less common.

CDA type III (OMIM: 105600) is a very rare form running a mild course with autosomal dominant inheritance. Diagnostically, it is distinguished by giant multinucleated erythroblasts and occasional monoclonal gammopathy.

Thrombocytopenia with Absent Radii (TAR, OMIM: 274000)

The characteristic association of an absent radial bone and isolated thrombocytopenia makes this rare syndrome straightforward to diagnose. The majority of patients are diagnosed with associated bleeding during the neonatal period and many have additional orthopedic anomalies of other long bones. Bleeding can be severe, frequently gastrointestinal and occasionally intracranial. Thrombocytopenia typically resolves with time, but transfusions may be required. Not all patients recover normal platelet counts and resolution often takes until school age. No specific genetic test is indicated and a bone marrow is not required. The inheritance pattern is unknown.

Neutropenia Syndromes

Bone marrow failure with predominant neutropenia, including *ELANE* related congenital and cyclic neutropenia, is discussed elsewhere in this book.

Unclassified Bone Marrow Dysfunction

Not all bone marrow failure syndromes can be classified. This often causes considerable anguish and uncertainty among patients, parents, and practitioners. While symptomatic treatment is unaffected and should follow the standard of care for transfusions and in treating infections, clinical judgment has to be exercised to determine appropriate surveillance of blood counts and bone marrow status. As research into bone marrow failure has seen a recent resurgence, new genetic abnormalities and testing will become available.

References

Bacigalupo A et al (1995) Antilymphocyte globulin, cyclosporin, and granulocyte colony-stimulating factor in patients with acquired severe aplastic anemia (SAA): a pilot study of the EBMT SAA Working Party. Blood 85:1348–1353

Ballmaier M et al (2001) c-mpl mutations are the cause of congenital amegakaryocytic thrombocytopenia. Blood 97:139–146

Bernheim M, Monnet P, Germain D (1963) Congenital hypoplastic amegakaryocytic thrombopenia. (Study of 3 new cases and review of the literature). Pédiatrie 18:367–385

Blank U, Karlsson G, Karlsson S (2008) Signaling pathways governing stem-cell fate. Blood 111:492–503

Bottiger LE, Westerholm B (1972) Aplastic anaemia. 3. Aplastic anaemia and infectious hepatitis. Acta Med Scand 192:323–326

Champlin R, Ho W, Gale RP (1983) Antithymocyte globulin treatment in patients with aplastic anemia: a prospective randomized trial. N Engl J Med 308:113–118

de la Fuente J, Dokal I (2007) Dyskeratosis congenita: advances in the understanding of the telomerase defect and the role of stem cell transplantation. Pediatr Transplant 11:584–594

Doherty L et al (2010) Ribosomal protein genes RPS10 and RPS26 are commonly mutated in Diamond-Blackfan anemia. Am J Hum Genet 86:222–228

Drachtman RA, Alter BP (1992) Dyskeratosis congenita: clinical and genetic heterogeneity. Report of a new case and review of the literature. Am J Pediatr Hematol Oncol 14:297–304

Dror Y, Squire J, Durie P, Freedman MH (1998) Malignant myeloid transformation with isochromosome 7q in Shwachman-Diamond syndrome. Leukemia 12:1591–1595

Dunn DE et al (1999) Paroxysmal nocturnal hemoglobinuria cells in patients with bone marrow failure syndromes. Ann Intern Med 131:401–408

Ehrlich P (1888) Ueber einen Fall von Anaemie mit Bemerkungen ueber regenerative Veraenderungen des Knochenmarks. Charite Annalen 13:300–309

Frickhofen N, Kaltwasser JP (1988) Immunosuppressive treatment of aplastic anemia: a prospective, randomized multicenter trial evaluating antilymphocyte globulin (ALG) versus ALG and cyclosporin A. Blut 56:191–192

Fuhrer M et al (1998) Relapse and clonal disease in children with aplastic anemia (AA) after immunosuppressive therapy (IST): the SAA 94 experience. German/Austrian pediatric aplastic anemia working group. Klin Pädiatr 210:173–179

Fuhrer M et al (2005) Immunosuppressive therapy for aplastic anemia in children: a more severe disease predicts better survival. Blood 106:2102–2104

Goldenberg NA, Graham DK, Liang X, Hays T (2004) Successful treatment of severe aplastic anemia in children using standardized immunosuppressive therapy with antithymocyte globulin and cyclosporine A. Pediatr Blood Cancer 43:718–722

Gonzalez-Casas R, Garcia-Buey L, Jones EA, Gisbert JP, Moreno-Otero R (2009) Systematic review: hepatitis-associated aplastic anaemia–a syndrome associated with abnormal immunological function. Aliment Pharmacol Ther 30:436–443

Guiguet M, Baumelou E, Mary JY (1995) A case-control study of aplastic anaemia: occupational exposures. The French cooperative group for epidemiological study of aplastic anaemia. Int J Epidemiol 24:993–999

Hedberg VA, Lipton JM (1988) Thrombocytopenia with absent radii. A review of 100 cases. Am J Pediatr Hematol Oncol 10:51–64

Heimpel H et al (2006) Congenital dyserythropoietic anemia type I (CDA I): molecular genetics, clinical appearance, and prognosis based on long-term observation. Blood 107:334–340

Heiss NS et al (1998) X-linked dyskeratosis congenita is caused by mutations in a highly conserved gene with putative nucleolar functions. Nat Genet 19:32–38

Hibbs JR et al (1992) Aplastic anemia and viral hepatitis. Non-A, Non-B, Non-C? JAMA 267:2051–2054

Howard SC et al (2004) Natural history of moderate aplastic anemia in children. Pediatr Blood Cancer 43:545

Issaragrisil S et al (2006) The epidemiology of aplastic anemia in Thailand. Blood 107:1299–1307

Kahl C et al (2005) Cyclophosphamide and antithymocyte globulin as a conditioning regimen for allogeneic marrow transplantation in patients with aplastic anaemia: a long-term follow-up. Br J Haematol 130:747–751

Kaito K et al (1998) Long-term administration of G-CSF for aplastic anaemia is closely related to the early evolution of monosomy 7 MDS in adults. Br J Haematol 103:297–303

Kaufman DW et al (1996) Drugs in the aetiology of agranulocytosis and aplastic anaemia. Eur J Haematol Suppl 60:23–30

Kirwan M, Dokal I (2009) Dyskeratosis congenita, stem cells and telomeres. Biochim Biophys Acta 1792:371–379

Kumar M, Alter BP (1998) Hematopoietic growth factors for the treatment of aplastic anemia. Curr Opin Hematol 5:226–234

Kurtzman G, Frickhofen N, Kimball J, Jenkins DW, Nienhuis AW, Young NS (1989) Pure red-cell aplasia of 10 years' duration due to persistent parvovirus B19 infection and its cure with immunoglobulin therapy. N Engl J Med 321:519–523

Lavabre-Bertrand T et al (2004) Long-term alpha interferon treatment is effective on anaemia and significantly reduces iron overload in congenital dyserythropoiesis type I. Eur J Haematol 73:380–383

Lessard J, Faubert A, Sauvageau G (2004) Genetic programs regulating HSC specification, maintenance and expansion. Oncogene 23:7199–7209

Lipton JM, Atsidaftos E, Zyskind I, Vlachos A (2006) Improving clinical care and elucidating the pathophysiology of Diamond Blackfan anemia: an update from the Diamond Blackfan anemia registry. Pediatr Blood Cancer 46:558–564

Maciejewski JP, Risitano A, Kook H, Zeng W, Chen G, Young NS (2002) Immune pathophysiology of aplastic anemia. Int J Hematol 76(Suppl 1):207–214

Mathe G et al (1970) Bone marrow graft in man after conditioning by antilymphocytic serum. Br Med J 2:131–136

Muir KR et al (2003) The role of occupational and environmental exposures in the aetiology of acquired severe aplastic anaemia: a case control investigation. Br J Haematol 123:906–914

Mukhina GL, Buckley JT, Barber JP, Jones RJ, Brodsky RA (2001) Multilineage glycosylphosphatidylinositol anchor-deficient haematopoiesis in untreated aplastic anaemia. Br J Haematol 115:476–482

Orfali KA, Ohene-Abuakwa Y, Ball SE (2004) Diamond Blackfan anaemia in the UK: clinical and genetic heterogeneity. Br J Haematol 125:243–252

Pannicke U et al (2009) Reticular dysgenesis (aleukocytosis) is caused by mutations in the gene encoding mitochondrial adenylate kinase 2. Nat Genet 41:101–105

Pongtanakul B, Das PK, Charpentier K, Dror Y (2008) Outcome of children with aplastic anemia treated with immunosuppressive therapy. Pediatr Blood Cancer 50:52–57

Schrezenmeier H et al (2007) Worse outcome and more chronic GVHD with peripheral blood progenitor cells than bone marrow in HLA-matched sibling donor transplants for young patients with severe acquired aplastic anemia. Blood 110:1397–1400

Shalev H, Kapelushnik J, Moser A, Dgany O, Krasnov T, Tamary H (2004) A comprehensive study of the neonatal manifestations of congenital dyserythropoietic anemia type I. J Pediatr Hematol Oncol 26:746–748

Shwachman H, Diamond LK, Oski FA, Khaw KT (1964) The syndrome of pancreatic insufficiency and bone marrow dysfunction. J Pediatr 65:645–663

Socie G et al (1993) Malignant tumors occurring after treatment of aplastic anemia. European bone marrow transplantation-severe aplastic anaemia working party. N Engl J Med 329:1152–1157

Socie G, Rosenfeld S, Frickhofen N, Gluckman E, Tichelli A (2000) Late clonal diseases of treated aplastic anemia. Semin Hematol 37:91–101

Tichelli A, Gratwohl A, Nissen C, Speck B (1994) Late clonal complications in severe aplastic anemia. Leuk Lymphoma 12: 167–175

Tiu R, Maciejewski J (2006) Immune pathogenesis of paroxysmal nocturnal hemoglobinuria. Int J Hematol 84:113–117

van der Schoot CE, Huizinga TW, van 't Veer-Korthof ET, Wijmans R, Pinkster J, von dem Borne AE (1990) Deficiency of glycosyl-phosphatidylinositol-linked membrane glycoproteins of leukocytes in paroxysmal nocturnal hemoglobinuria, description of a new diagnostic cytofluorometric assay. Blood 76:1853–1859

Vlachos A et al (2008) Diagnosing and treating diamond blackfan anaemia: results of an international clinical consensus conference. Br J Haematol 142:859–876

Weissman IL (2000) Stem cells: units of development, units of regeneration, and units in evolution. Cell 100:157–168

West BC, DeVault GA Jr, Clement JC, Williams DM (1988) Aplastic anemia associated with parenteral chloramphenicol: review of 10 cases, including the second case of possible increased risk with cimetidine. Rev Infect Dis 10:1048–1051

Willig TN et al (1999) Identification of new prognosis factors from the clinical and epidemiologic analysis of a registry of 229 Diamond-Blackfan anemia patients. DBA group of Societe d'Hematologie et d'Immunologie Pediatrique (SHIP), Gesellshaft fur Padiatrische Onkologie und Hamatologie (GPOH), and the European Society for Pediatric Hematology and Immunology (ESPHI). Pediatr Res 46:553–561

Wilson A, Trumpp A (2006) Bone-marrow haematopoietic-stem-cell niches. Nat Rev Immunol 6:93–106

Young NS, Kaufman DW (2008) The epidemiology of acquired aplastic anemia. Haematologica 93:489–492

334 Developmental Hemostasis

Rowena C. Punzalan · Veronica H. Flood

The Hemostatic System in the Neonate

In neonates, the coagulation system is dynamic and its development continues after birth. This phenomenon is more evident in premature neonates. ➤ *Figure 334.1* shows the prenatal development of components of the hemostatic system. Establishing reference ranges is complicated, as multiple reference ranges are needed, blood samples are difficult to obtain, and the amount of blood obtained is limited. In addition, more subjects are needed because of greater variability. Therefore, interpretation of coagulation test results in infants should take into account the age-dependent normal values.

Overall, in newborns, there is enhanced primary hemostasis, but decreased thrombin generation; in turn, there is reduced ability for anticoagulation and a hypofibrinolytic state. In the healthy newborn, all of these factors balance out and, therefore, do not lead to increased bleeding or thrombosis. In sick and preterm neonates, there are many acquired disturbances that can predispose to either bleeding or thrombosis.

Primary Hemostasis

Platelets can be found in the peripheral circulation at 11 weeks of gestation and have generally reached adult levels by 18 weeks of gestation (➤ *Fig. 334.1*). Platelet function in neonates is slightly different than that seen in adults, with most studies indicating decreased responsiveness to the agonists ADP, collagen, epinephrine, and thrombin. Ristocetin-induced platelet aggregation is increased, likely secondary to higher von Willebrand factor levels in the neonate. Activation of platelets may occur in the neonate during childbirth. Neonates are not, however, at high risk of bleeding from platelet dysfunction despite these physiologic changes.

Coagulation

Neonates have overall decreased thrombin generation. Levels of the vitamin K–dependent factors (II, VII, IX, and X) and factor XI are significantly decreased compared to values in adults; the levels of fibrinogen and factors V and VIII are similar to adult values (➤ *Table 334.1*). In healthy neonates, the prothrombin time (PT) is prolonged up to 2s above the adult reference ranges, while the activated partial thromboplastin time (aPTT) is $\geq$20 s or more above adult values. Von Willebrand factor is increased and ultra large molecular weight multimers are present at birth, which may explain the shorter bleeding time. Progressive maturation of the coagulation system occurs unless a coincident problem is present, with adult levels achieved by 6 months of age for some clotting factors but not until adolescence for others. Premature neonates are somewhat more likely than term neonates to have achieved adult levels by age 6 months. In otherwise well infants, the decreased coagulant factor levels are not associated with clinical bleeding.

Anticoagulation and Fibrinolysis

Both anticoagulation and fibrinolysis are thought to be downregulated in newborns. Plasma concentrations of naturally occurring anticoagulant proteins (antithrombin, protein C, and protein S) are significantly lower at birth than during later childhood and adulthood. Plasminogen and plasmin generation are reduced and plasmin inhibitors are increased. These observed decreases in anticoagulant and fibrinolytic factors usually do not cause thrombosis in otherwise healthy newborns. Being a sick neonate is a known risk factor for thrombosis, but the contribution of these decreased levels to this risk is unknown. All these differences need to be taken into account when interpreting lab values and managing anticoagulation in neonates.

Hemorrhagic Disorders in the Neonate

Most hemorrhagic disorders in the neonate are acquired. Thrombocytopenia likely contributes to most of these, but often coexists with other coagulation disturbances. Several inherited coagulation problems can also manifest in this age group.

Abdelaziz Y. Elzouki (ed.), *Textbook of Clinical Pediatrics*, DOI 10.1007/978-3-642-02202-9_334,

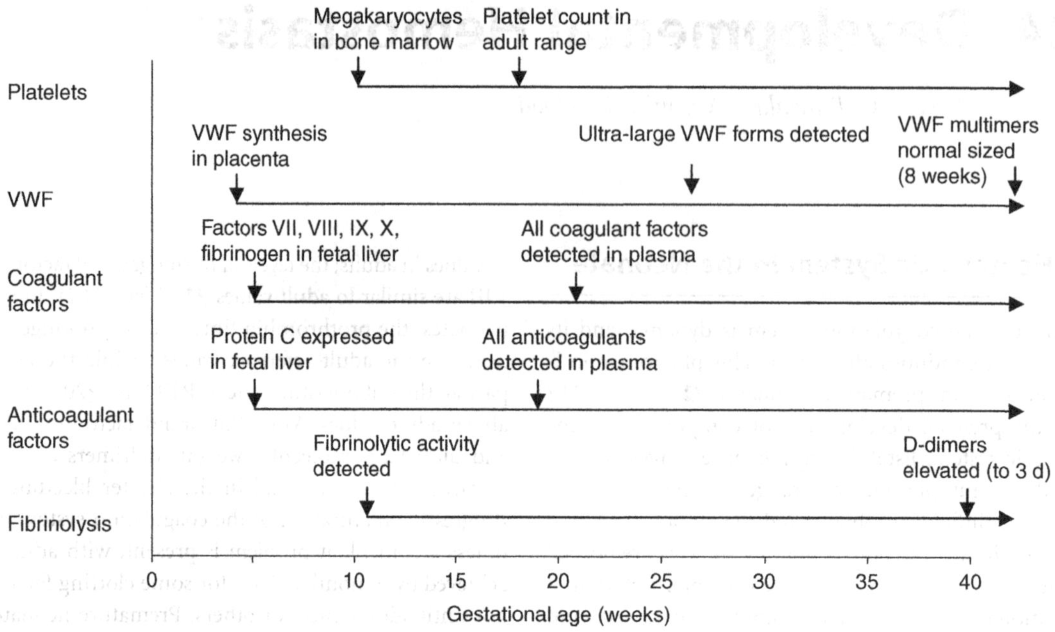

Figure 334.1

Fetal development of the hemostatic system. *VWF* von Willebrand factor (Cited from Manco-Johnson MJ (2005) Development of hemostasis in the fetus. Thromb Res 115:55–63; Cantor A (2009) Developmental hemostasis: Relevance to newborns and infants. In: Orkin SA, Fisher DE, Look AT, Lux SE, Ginsburg D, Nathan DG (eds) Nathan and Oski's hematology of infancy and childhood. Saunders Elsevier, Philadelphia)

Evaluation of the Bleeding Neonate

The most important consideration in the initial evaluation of the bleeding neonate is the clinical setting in which the bleeding occurs. Bleeding in an otherwise healthy neonate is more suggestive of an inherited coagulation disorder or immune-mediated thrombocytopenia. In a sick or premature neonate, abnormal bleeding is usually from acquired causes and often is multifactorial, including medications. Sepsis or surgery can cause a consumptive coagulopathy or disseminated intravascular coagulation (DIC). Protein loss (from chest or peritoneal drainage) can involve coagulation factors, but this is usually balanced by loss of anticoagulant factors as well. Maternal factors, including drugs (anticoagulants, antiepileptics, and antituberculosis drugs) and illness (preeclampsia) should always be considered. Complications during delivery can cause activation of the coagulation system and DIC. As discussed below, vitamin K deficiency may cause significant bleeding in the neonatal period. Finally, family history should be investigated, although not all affected infants will have a family history of bleeding disorders.

The bleeding manifestation is another very important consideration, especially in the presentation of an inherited bleeding disorder. Congenital coagulation disorders may present with oozing from the umbilical cord stump, scalp bleeding, cephalohematomas, bleeding from IV puncture sites, bleeding with circumcision, mucocutaneous bleeding, and bleeding with invasive procedures (➋ *Table 334.2*). Sometimes, anemia may be the only manifestation of increased bleeding, so for unexplained anemia a source of bleeding should always be sought. Although not uncommon in premature infants, intracranial hemorrhage (ICH) in a term or late preterm infant without significant trauma should prompt an investigation for a bleeding disorder. In 349 newborns with hemophilia, bleeding consisted of ICH, more commonly subdural (27%) and increased bleeding with circumcision (30%) and heel stick (16%).

Laboratory Testing in Neonates

In the laboratory evaluation of a neonate with abnormal bleeding, it is important to consider sampling problems.

Table 334.1
Reference values for coagulation tests in healthy infants [mean (range of 95% of the population)][a]

Test or level	30–36 Weeks gestation infant	Term infant	1 Month–1 year	Children 1–5 years	Adults
Screening tests					
PT (s)	13 (10.6–16.2)	15.6 (14.4–16.4)	13.1 (12.1–14.6)	13.3 (12.1–14.5)	13 (11.5–14.5)
aPTT (s)	53.6 (27.5–79.4)	38.7 (34.3–44.8)	39.3 (35.1–46.3)	37.7 (33.6–43.8)	33.2 (28.6–38.2)
Platelet function screen					
Collagen/epinephrine closure time (s)		81 (61–108)		109 (92–126)	106 (82–142)
Collagen/ADP closure time (s)		56 (48–65)		89 (69–109)	85 (67–111)
Bleeding time (min)	3.4 (1.7–5.2)	1.8 (1.2–2.4)		6 (2.5–10)	4 (1–7)
Coagulant factors					
Fibrinogen (g/L)	243 (150–373)	2.8 (1.92–3.74)	2.42 (0.82–3.83)	2.82 (1.62–4.01)	3.1 (1.9–4.3)
Factor II (%)	45 (20–77)	54 (41–69)	90 (62–103)	89 (70–109)	110 (78–138)
Factor V (%)	88 (41–144)	81 (64–103)	113 (94–141)	97 (67–127)	118 (78–152)
Factor VII (%)	67 (21–113)	70 (52–88)	128 (83–160)	111 (72–150)	129 (61–199)
Factor VIII (%)	111 (50–213)	182 (105–329)	94 (54–145)	110 (36–185)	160 (52–290)
Factor IX (%)	35 (19–65)	48 (35–56)	71 (43–121)	85 (44–127)	130 (59–254)
Factor X (%)	41 (11–71)	55 (46–67)	95 (77–122)	98 (72–125)	124 (96–171)
Factor XI (%)	30 (8–52)	30 (7–41)	89 (62–125)	113 (65–162)	112 (67–196)
Factor XII (%)	38 (10–66)	58 (43–80)	79 (20–132)	85 (36–136)	115 (35–207)
VWF (%)	136 (78–210)	153 (86–220)	107 (62–152)		92 (59–125)
Anticoagulants and fibrinolytics					
Antithrombin (%)	38 (14–62)	76 (58–90)	109 (72–134)	116 (101–131)	96 (66–124)
Protein C (%)	28 (12–44)	32 (24–40)	77 (28–124)	94 (50–134)	103 (54–166)
Protein S (%)	26 (14–38)	36 (28–47)	102 (29–162)	101 (67–136)	75 (54–103)
Plasminogen (U/mL)	1.7 (1.12–2.48)	1.95 (1.25–2.65)	3.01 (2.21–3.01)[b]		3.36 (2.84–4.24)
tPA (ng/mL)	8.48 (3–16.7)	9.6 (5–18.9)	2.8 (1–6.0)[b]		4.9 (1.4–8.4)
α_2AP (U/mL)	0.78 (0.4–1.16)	0.85 (0.55–1.15)	1.11 (0.83–1.39)[b]		1.02 (0.63–1.35)
PAI (U/mL)	5.4 (0–12.2)	6.4 (2–15.1)	8.1 (6–13)[b]		3.6 (0–11)

PT prothrombin time, *aPTT* activated partial thromboplastin time, *VWF* von Willebrand factor, *tPA* tissue plasminogen activator, *α_2AP* α_2 antiplasmin-1, *PAI* plasminogen activator inhibitor

[a]Adapted from Monagle P, Barnes C, Ignjatovic V, Furmedge J, Newall F, Chan A, De Rosa L, Hamilton S, Ragg P, Robinson S, Auldist A, Crock C, Roy N, Rowlands S (2006) Developmental haemostasis. impact for clinical haemostasis laboratories. Thromb Haemost 95:362–372; Andrew M, Paes B, Milner R, Johnston M, Mitchell L, Tollefsen DM, Powers P (1987) Development of the human coagulation system in the full-term infant. Blood 70:165– 172; Carcao MD, Blanchette VS, Dean JA, He L, Kern MA, Stain AM, Sparling CR, Stephens D, Ryan G, Freedman J, Rand ML (1998) The platelet function analyzer (PFA-100): A novel in-vitro system for evaluation of primary haemostasis in children. Br J Haematol 101:70–73; Lippi G, Manzato F, Franchini M, Brocco G, Florenziani G, Guidi G (2001) Establishment of reference values for the PFA-100 platelet function analyzer in pediatrics. Clin Exp Med 1:69–70; Del Vecchio A, Latini G, Henry E, Christensen RD (2008) Template bleeding times of 240 neonates born at 24 to 41 weeks gestation. J Perinatol 28:427–431

[b]Value at 180 days

In newborns, there is often a volume limit to the amount of blood that can be collected, so the appropriate tubes that will yield the correct anticoagulant-to-blood sample ratio should be used. This is particularly important in neonates with polycythemia, which can cause spurious prolongation of the PT and aPTT. Activation of coagulation of the blood sample may occur more often in neonates because of the often difficult blood draws. Sample contamination, for instance, with heparin from central line sites of blood draw, may be more common in neonates

Table 334.2

Clinical presentation and treatment of rare congenital coagulation disorders

Factor deficiency	Clinical presentation	Treatment
Fibrinogen[a]	Umbilical stump bleeding, circumcision bleeding, soft tissue bleeding; infrequent ICH	Cryoprecipitate, FFP, fibrinogen concentrate
Factor II	Mucosal bleeding; surgical or trauma bleeding; rare joint bleed, ICH	FFP, PCC Aminocaproic acid
Factor V	Factor level does not predict severity of bleed, but homozygotes usually have spontaneous bleeding; mucous membrane bleed; ICH, subdural bleed; umbilical stump bleed; GI bleed; surgery/trauma bleed	FFP rFVIIa, FEIBA, platelets for those with inhibitors
Factor VII[a]	ICH, GI bleeding, soft tissue bleeding in very young; epistaxis, bruising, gum bleeding, postoperative bleeding; menorrhagia	rFVIIa PCC, FFP
Factor X[a]	ICH, umbilical stump bleed, GI bleed, bleed from needle punctures; menorrhagia, easy bruising, epistaxis, hematoma, hemarthrosis	PCC, FFP Factor X concentrate (Switzerland)
Factor XI	Circumcision bleeding, subdural hemorrhage; surgical (especially mucosal surgery) bleeding	FFP Factor XI concentrate
Factor XIII[a]	Umbilical stump bleed (80%); ICH (20–25%); delayed wound healing, abnormal scar, mucosal bleed, recurrent soft tissue bleed	Cryoprecipitate, FFP Factor XIII concentrate
Alpha2 antiplasmin-1	Umbilical stump bleed	Tranexamic acid Aminocaproic acid (no data in neonates)

Source: Modified from Saxonhouse MA, Manco-Johnson MJ (2009) The evaluation and management of neonatal coagulation disorders. Semin Perinatol 33:52–65

ICH intracranial hemorrhage, *FFP* fresh frozen plasma, *PCC* prothrombin complex concentrate

[a]Disorders most likely to present in the neonatal period

because of the smaller blood volumes. As above, age-appropriate reference ranges should always be used when interpreting results (*Table 334.1*). However, even those values should be interpreted with care, as there can be overlap of the abnormal and normal values. A striking example of this is the values for aPTT, which can be physiologically prolonged in neonates, but may be "normal" in the presence of hemophilia.

Evaluation of hemostasis in neonates is similar to that performed in older children. A complete blood count is essential to determine platelet number. Review of the peripheral blood smear is useful to evaluate platelet size and granularity. PT and aPTT provide a general screen of clotting factors. Fibrinogen levels may also be useful to detect consumption or decreased fibrinogen production. The platelet function analyzer (PFA), although intended to provide an assessment of platelet function, has suboptimal sensitivity and specificity for diagnosis of both von Willebrand disease and platelet function defects. Some studies have shown shorter PFA closure times in term infants, but no data exists for premature infants and a normal range is not well established for neonates. Platelet aggregation studies will demonstrate platelet function, but the amount of blood required and need for a specialty laboratory restrict the general application of this test. *Table 334.3* details the laboratory studies useful in workup of neonatal hemostasis.

Congenital Deficiency of Coagulant Factors

The most common congenital disorders of coagulation are deficiencies of factors VIII and IX (hemophilia A and B, respectively). These, along with congenital disorders of primary hemostasis (von Willebrand disease, platelet function defects), are discussed in a previous chapter.

Clinically significant congenital deficiencies of fibrinogen, prothrombin, and factors V, combined V/VIII, VII, X, XI, and XIII, combined vitamin K–dependent factors (prothrombin and factors VII, IX, X), and the contact

Table 334.3
Evaluation of neonatal hemostasis

Screening tests	Diagnostic tests
CBC	Factor VIII
PT	Factor IX
aPTT	Factor XIII
Fibrinogen	Von Willebrand factor (antigen, activity)
d-Dimer	Platelet glycoprotein expression
Platelet function analysis	Platelet aggregation

factors are rare and usually inherited as autosomal-recessive traits. Those most likely to present in the neonatal period include deficiencies of factors VII, X, and XIII, and deficiency or dysfunction of fibrinogen (*Table 334.2*). Of note, recent studies show that deficiencies in factor XII, prekallikrein, and high-molecular-weight kininogen may prolong the aPTT but do not cause abnormal bleeding. Patients with congenital coagulant factor deficiencies are usually treated episodically for acute bleeding or surgery. The mainstay of treatment is coagulation factor replacement. Generally, neonates with single-factor deficiencies are treated with either recombinant or plasma-derived concentrates for the specific factor whenever available, which allows the administration of adequate and precise doses in relatively small volumes. These products have also been treated to minimize the risk of viral disease transmission. Recombinant factor VIIa (rFVIIa) is used both as bypassing agent in the treatment of hemophilia with inhibitors and replacement therapy for bleeding or surgery for patients with factor VII deficiency. Cryoprecipitated antihemophilic factor is used as a source most frequently of fibrinogen and rarely of factor XIII. However, purified factor XIII concentrate and a virus-inactivated fibrinogen concentrate are available. A factor XI concentrate is available in Europe. Prothrombin complex concentrates or plasma may be used for the treatment and prophylaxis of bleeding in patients with deficiency of prothrombin, factor VII and X, and the vitamin K–dependent factors. There is no factor V concentrate available.

Acquired Coagulant Factor Deficiency

Common acquired disorders include liver disease, DIC, and hemorrhagic disease of the newborn.

Liver Disease in the Neonate

Liver disease in neonates may lead to disorders of coagulation. Since the liver is the site of synthesis for the majority of coagulation factors, hepatic dysfunction will lead to a decrease in procoagulant factors as well as some anticoagulant factors. The PT and PTT will be prolonged, and fibrinogen should be low. Bleeding, particularly mucosal bleeding, is common. Treatment consists of coagulation factor replacement via plasma infusions and cryoprecipitate. Fresh frozen plasma at a dose of 10–20 mL/kg should increase clotting factors by approximately 1% per mL given per kilogram of body weight. Evaluation and treatment for the underlying cause of liver disease will be required.

Disseminated Intravascular Coagulation

Prolonged PT and PTT may also represent consumption of coagulation factors due to DIC. Sepsis is the most common cause in neonates, particularly those in intensive care units. Infants with DIC may present with either bleeding or thrombosis. Congenital protein C or protein S deficiency should be suspected in the setting of purpura fulminans, although infection may also cause this presentation. D-dimers are usually elevated in DIC, but these elevations are usually non-specific. Treatment is aimed at eradicating the underlying cause. Administration of plasma, cryoprecipitate, or platelets may be required, but should be reserved for those infants who are actually symptomatic. Heparin anticoagulation in DIC is occasionally used in patients with evidence of thrombosis, but there is a paucity of evidence to support its effectiveness.

Previously, treatment of patients with coagulopathy due to synthetic or consumptive processes was restricted to replacement with fresh frozen plasma to replete all coagulation factors, and/or cryoprecipitate to replete fibrinogen, factor VIII, and von Willebrand factor. Recently, rFVIIa has become available and has been widely used in this setting, although it is not generally recommended due to the potential risk of thrombosis.

Hemorrhagic Disease of the Newborn

Vitamin K is a cofactor in γ-carboxylation of procoagulant factors II, VII, IX, and X, as well as anticoagulant factors such as protein C and S. Vitamin K levels are decreased in the newborn as compared to adults. Therefore, those clotting factors that depend on vitamin K–mediated posttranslational modification will be decreased in the newborn period. Deficiency of vitamin K leads to a relative decrease in procoagulant factors, which may lead to clinically significant bleeding. Such bleeding, originally termed hemorrhagic disease of the newborn, is now referred to as vitamin K–dependent bleeding, or VKDB.

Early VKDB presents within the first day of life with severe bleeding, often intracranial hemorrhage or GI bleeds. Early VKDB may be due to maternal medications such as anticonvulsants leading to chronically low vitamin K levels throughout pregnancy. Classic VKDB presents in the first week of life in infants with inadequate intake. The incidence is approximately 1 in 10,000 births without prophylaxis. Late VKDB presents within 6 months of birth in breast-fed infants or infants with malabsorption disorders such as cystic fibrosis or celiac disease. Usual sites of bleeding include the skin and GI tract, although intracranial hemorrhage is unfortunately not an uncommon presenting feature.

Supplementation with vitamin K is recommended for newborn infants to increase levels of the vitamin K–dependent proteins and prevent bleeding in the neonatal period. A great deal of debate has occurred regarding the relative merits of IM versus oral vitamin K, particularly due to the concern for an increased risk of leukemia which had been reported in an earlier British study. Subsequent studies, however, have failed to show a link between IM vitamin K and cancer. Some countries, however, recommend the use of oral vitamin K preferentially. If vitamin K is administered orally, it is important to recognize that multiple doses are required to prevent late VKDB. IM vitamin K at a dose of 0.5–1 mg is recommended for all neonates. In the event that an oral regimen is chosen, typical dosing is 1–2 mg on day of life 1, then again around 1 week and around 4 weeks of age. Alternate regimens prescribe 2 mg of oral vitamin K weekly until the infant is 3 months of age.

Diagnosis of VKDB is made on the basis of a prolonged PT and prolonged PTT, with a greater prolongation in the PT as compared to the PTT. Vitamin K–dependent clotting factors will be low, with normal levels of nonvitamin K–dependent clotting factors such as factor V and factor VIII. Treatment should not wait for confirmation of the diagnosis, but rather vitamin K should be administered as soon as the diagnosis is suspected. If severe bleeding, such as intracranial hemorrhage or GI bleeding, is present, emergent treatment may be required. Fresh frozen plasma is usually readily available, but other treatment options include prothrombin complex concentrates or rFVIIa.

Neonatal Thrombocytopenia and Other Platelet Defects

Quantitative platelet disorders in neonates may be due to decreased production or increased destruction (*Table 334.4*). Decreased production is typically secondary to inherited platelet disorders. Congenital amegakaryocytic thrombocytopenia, a disorder where megakaryocytes are absent or significantly reduced, presents with petechiae or bruising. Thrombocytopenia-absent radii (TAR) syndrome is, as the name implies,

Table 334.4
Differential diagnosis of neonatal thrombocytopenia

Immune-mediated	Inherited quantitative defects	Qualitative defects	Acquired thrombocytopenias
Neonatal alloimmune thrombocytopenia	Congenital amegakaryocytic thrombocytopenia	Drugs: aspirin, indomethacin	Sepsis
Maternal ITP	TAR syndrome	Diet	DIC
Neonatal ITP	Wiskott–Aldrich syndrome	Maternal alcohol use	Necrotizing enterocolitis
Drug-dependent antibodies	Jacobsen syndrome	Maternal tobacco use	Kasabach–Merritt syndrome
	X-linked macrothrombocytopenia	Maternal diabetes	Perinatal asphyxiation
	Bernard–Soulier syndrome	Nitric oxide	
	Velocardiofacial syndrome	ECMO	
	MYH-9 disorders		

ITP immune-mediated thrombocytopenic purpura, *ECMO* extracorporeal membrane oxygenation a syndrome where thrombocytopenia is associated with skeletal abnormalities including radial hypoplasia. The diagnosis is generally not difficult due to the characteristic limb appearance. Wiskott–Aldrich syndrome is an X-linked thrombocytopenia which also manifests with eczema and immune deficiency. Platelets are characteristically small. Neonates may present with bloody diarrhea, but infection due to the immune deficiency is also a serious risk.

There are several disorders that lead to decreased platelet production and large platelets. Jacobsen syndrome, otherwise known as Paris–Trousseau syndrome, involves macrothrombocytopenia as well as mental retardation, facial dysmorphogenesis, and cardiac abnormalities. The defect has been localized to a deletion of part of chromosome 11. X-linked macrothrombocytopenia is due to mutations in GATA-1 and may also present with anemia. Bernard–Soulier syndrome is a defect in glycoprotein (GP) Ib or associated proteins GPIX or GPV. Platelets are large and characterized by defective aggregation in response to ristocetin, which induces VWF binding to platelet GPIb. Platelet aggregation with other agonists, however, is normal in Bernard–Soulier syndrome. Velocardiofacial syndrome, a gene deletion syndrome involving chromosome 22q11.2, may manifest with macrothrombocytopenia similar to that seen in Bernard–Soulier syndrome due to deletion of the GPIbα gene in this region. Macrothrombocytopenia may also be caused by a defect in MYH-9, the myosin heavy chain, which has now been found to be the underlying problem in a number of platelet disorders, including Epstein syndrome, Fechtner syndrome, May–Hegglin anomaly, and Sebastian syndrome.

Qualitative platelet disorders are generally due to medications or other treatments the neonate is receiving. Maternal medications, diet, alcohol, or tobacco use may also induce temporary platelet dysfunction. Maternal diabetes may actually lead to platelet hyperreactivity with increased platelet aggregation, although the clinical significance of this finding is unclear. Aspirin and nonsteroidal anti-inflammatory drugs (NSAIDs) lead to platelet dysfunction, either permanently with the use of aspirin or temporarily with the use of other NSAIDs. Indomethacin is frequently used to induce closure of a patent ductus arteriosus in premature infants, and may contribute to qualitative platelet dysfunction in newborns. Nitric oxide also interferes with platelet adhesion by inhibition of platelet aggregation in response to ADP. Extracorporeal membrane oxygenation (ECMO) is associated with bleeding complications, primarily due to the need for anticoagulation and depletion of clotting factors, but is also associated with platelet dysfunction due to chronic activation.

Neonatal Alloimmune Thrombocytopenia

Platelet destruction may occur through immune-mediated or nonimmune mechanisms. The most common cause of immune-mediated thrombocytopenia in neonates is neonatal alloimmune thrombocytopenia (NAIT). NAIT is quite common, with an incidence of around 1:1,000. In NAIT, the father's platelets have an antigen not present on maternal platelets. When the infant inherits this antigen, the mother recognizes it as foreign and makes antibodies, which cross the placenta and lead to thrombocytopenia in the fetus. Thrombocytopenia may be severe. NAIT carries a high risk of intracranial hemorrhage, up to 20% of affected neonates. Diagnosis is made by testing the reactivity of maternal serum against the father's platelets. The most frequent antigen responsible for NAIT is HPA-1a, or Pl^{A1}, although other antigens may also cause NAIT. Treatment involves infusion of platelets lacking the causative antigen. Until a suitable donor is found, washed maternal platelets may be used, as these are typically the most readily available. Some blood banks stock HPA-1a negative platelets for use in such cases. While waiting for suitable platelets to become available, random donor platelets may be used, as infants may still respond. In addition, IVIG may be used for NAIT, typically at a dose of 1 g/kg. Head ultrasound is recommended to evaluate any infant at risk of intracranial hemorrhage.

Maternal autoimmune thrombocytopenia may lead to temporary thrombocytopenia in the neonate due to IgG antibodies crossing the placenta in mothers affected with immune-mediated thrombocytopenic purpura (ITP) or systemic lupus erythematosus (SLE). Passive antibodies are more common with true ITP in neonates due to an endogenous antibody, a rare occurrence except in the setting of immune dysfunction. Drug-dependent antibodies may also cause immune-mediated thrombocytopenia less commonly in this age group. Thrombocytopenia due to acquired antibodies will resolve within the first several months of life.

Nonimmune Thrombocytopenia

Destruction may also be nonimmune-mediated. Thrombocytopenia is common in the NICU setting, present in anywhere from 6% to 22% of infants. The most common cause in sick neonates is sepsis, which commonly presents with thrombocytopenia and may also present with DIC. Both bacterial and viral infections may be the cause. Some infections may also lead to decreased production. Premature infants may also experience thrombocytopenia related to necrotizing enterocolitis, respiratory distress syndrome, and persistent pulmonary hypertension. Perinatal asphyxiation has been associated with thrombocytopenia. Vascular malformations such as Kasabach–Merritt syndrome lead to consumption of platelets (and coagulation factors). Affected infants may present with systemic bleeding due to the severe thrombocytopenia.

Treatment of decreased platelet function or decreased platelet number due to a production defect consists of administration of platelets, generally at a dose of 10–15 mL/kg. Unless there is a treatable underlying cause, platelet support may need to be continued for some time. The precise threshold for transfusion is not entirely clear. Most physicians consider a platelet count less than 50,000 to signify an increased risk of bleeding. A survey of neonatologists showed that most transfused a bleeding neonate with a platelet count of <50,000, but most used a platelet count of <20,000 as the threshold for prophylactic transfusions. Transfusion thresholds of 30,000 as compared to 50,000 in one study did not demonstrate a difference in risk of hemorrhage.

Thrombotic Disorders in the Neonate

Like the neonate, the study of thrombosis in infants and children is rapidly evolving. During childhood, the greatest risk of thromboembolism is in the neonatal period. The greatest incidence reported, from the Canadian childhood thrombosis registry, is 2.4 per 1,000 admissions to the neonatal intensive care unit. As in hemostasis, the delicate balance between coagulation and anticoagulation proteins may be disturbed by a number of acquired conditions, which then can predispose to thromboembolism. Most infants who develop abnormal clots have comorbid conditions that predispose to thrombosis. However, given that not all sick neonates develop clots and that thrombosis sometimes occur in newborns who are otherwise healthy, genetic factors may also play a role. Virchow's triad, the intersection between the vasculature, blood flow, and blood clotting proteins, applies to neonatal thrombosis as well (➲ *Table 334.5*).

Table 334.5
Virchow's triad in the neonate

Abnormal vessel wall	Inflammation
	Intravascular catheters damage endothelium
	Thrombosed chorionic vessels embolize to fetal vessels
	Local thrombi from patent ductus arteriosus
Stasis of blood flow	Large catheters in small veins
	Increased blood viscosity, polycythemia
	Poor deformability of newborn red cells
Altered constituents of blood	Shock/consumption
	Sepsis/inflammation
	Extracorporeal membrane oxygenation (ECMO)
	Congenital disorders

Source: Modified from Thornburg C, Pipe S (2006) Neonatal thromboembolic emergencies. Semin Fetal Neonatal Med 11:198–206

Thrombophilia is the term used to describe a range of defects in coagulation, fibrinolysis, endothelial cells, and primary hemostasis that can predispose to thrombosis. Most of these conditions are inherited, but some, like antiphospholipid syndrome, may be acquired (➲ *Table 334.6*). In the neonate, antiphospholipid antibodies are most likely maternal.

Deficiency of Anticoagulant Proteins

Of the congenital anticoagulant factor deficiencies, homozygous protein C and protein S deficiency are the most clinically significant. Purpura fulminans is characterized by acute onset of microvascular thrombosis followed by perivascular hemorrhage. Although purpura fulminans can be associated with acquired factors (like DIC and meningococcal infections), if it occurs in the newborn period, inherited protein C (and less commonly protein S) deficiency needs to be ruled out. Protein C concentrate (nonactivated) may be used for the management of both acquired and congenital protein C deficiency. A plasma transfusion would be needed to replace protein S.

Also, aside from the physiologically low anticoagulant protein levels in neonates, many acquired conditions can affect these levels. Congenital heart disease, hepatic dysfunction, and nephrotic syndrome have all been associated with decreased anticoagulant protein levels in the plasma. Antithrombin deficiency in the newborn is most commonly acquired, in association with cardiopulmonary bypass or ECMO, which can cause activation of the coagulation system and consumption of coagulant and anticoagulant proteins because of the interaction with the

Table 334.6
Prothrombotic risk factors

Inherited thrombophilia	Acquired conditions
Factor V Leiden mutation	Central venous line
Prothrombin G20210A mutation	Cancer
Hyperhomocysteinemia	Congenital heart disease
Increased lipoprotein (a) levels	Hyperalimentation
Protein C deficiency	Infection
Protein S deficiency	Nephrotic syndrome
Antithrombin deficiency	Liver failure
Dysfibrinogenemia	Antiphospholipid syndrome
Increased fibrinogen, factor VIII (probably inherited)	ECMO
	Polycythemia
	Perinatal complications
	Sepsis

Source: Modified from Thornburg C, Pipe S (2006) Neonatal thromboembolic emergencies. Semin Fetal Neonatal Med 11:198–206; Andrew (1994); deVeber (2001)

biomaterials in the circuit, as well as a systemic inflammatory reaction; this deficiency is usually manifested by difficulty in obtaining therapeutic heparin effect. A purified antithrombin concentrate is available. However, because thrombosis in neonates is likely multifactorial, in the absence of an actual thrombus, it is unclear whether factor replacement would be of benefit in these situations.

Thrombotic Manifestations in the Neonate

Thrombotic manifestations in neonates include ischemic perinatal stroke (IPS), cerebral sinus venous thrombosis (CSVT), venous systemic thrombosis, renal vein thrombosis, portal vein thrombosis, and arterial systemic thrombosis.

The clinical presentation of IPS is often subtle and nonspecific, including seizures, poor feeding, and lethargy. Often diagnosis is delayed until hemiparesis is evident, sometimes months later. The etiology of IPS remains unclear. In a recent meta-analysis, it was found that genetic prothrombotic risk factors significantly contributed to the risk of stroke in children; as other risk factors were also present in many instances, the significance of this is unclear. IPS does not seem to independently increase the risk of recurrent thromboembolic disease. Given that the diagnosis of IPS is frequently delayed, the prognosis generally better than in older children and adults, and the risk of bleeding is high, anticoagulation or aspirin therapy is not generally recommended for neonates with initial IPS unless there is an embolic source.

In the Canadian pediatric stroke registry, the incidence of CSVT was 0.67 per 100,000 children per year, and neonates were the most commonly affected group. Risk factors include head and neck disorders, dehydration, perinatal complications, and bacterial sepsis; of note, prothrombotic disorders were found in 20% of neonates with CSVT. In pediatric CSVT, in contrast to adults, non-anticoagulation resulted in increased thrombus propagation, while anticoagulation (with heparin, low-molecular-weight heparin, or warfarin) did not increase the risk of fatal bleeding or bad outcome, with neonates having the best outcome. Evidence-based practice guidelines for anticoagulation in children recommend, but not strongly, anticoagulation for neonatal CSVT for 6 weeks to 3 months.

The incidence of venous thromboembolism in children varies among registries, but the association with acquired risk factors is consistent with the presence of a central venous line (CVL), the most common association. These thrombi are often asymptomatic or associated only with CVL dysfunction. Other risk factors in neonates include congenital heart disease, sepsis, and hyperalimentation. Despite the risk of thrombosis associated with CVL in children, prophylactic anticoagulation has not been proven effective at prevention.

Renal vein thrombosis (RVT) comprises up to 33–58% of neonatal thrombotic events according to registry data. In a recent meta-analysis, 7% occurred in utero and 67% occurred in the first day of life; most children were born >36 weeks age of gestation (73%). Features at presentation included macroscopic hematuria (55%), thrombocytopenia (47%), and a palpable mass (42%). Associated conditions included perinatal asphyxia (29%), maternal diabetes (8%), and dehydration (1.5%). The thrombus extended into the inferior vena cava in 44%, and there was adrenal hemorrhage in 14%. Fifty-three percent of those tested had at least one thrombophilia. Anticoagulation or thrombolytic therapy does not seem to change the long-term outcome in children with RVT. Evidence-based guidelines recommend observation for unilateral RVT and anticoagulation or fibrinolytic therapy for bilateral RVT, depending on the renal dysfunction.

Portal vein thrombosis (PVT) can be associated with umbilical vein catheterization and omphalitis. Diagnosis is by ultrasound, and it is often found incidentally. Treatment with anticoagulation and catheter removal is usually indicated as portal hypertension can develop over time.

Arterial systemic thrombosis in neonates is usually iatrogenic, associated with catheterization. Spontaneous arterial thrombosis is uncommon in neonates, usually involves the aorta, and can have a mortality rate of up to 33%. For extensive arterial thrombosis, thrombolysis or surgical thrombectomy should be performed; for less extensive thrombosis, anticoagulation may be considered.

Testing for Thrombophilia

Although older guidelines recommend testing for genetic thrombophilia for all neonates with thrombosis, more recent studies have questioned the utility of such testing given that the ability of such testing to improve clinical outcome even in adults is unclear. This lack of evidence is even more apparent in children, such that the effect of thrombophilia on duration of anticoagulation is not addressed in the most recent evidence-based practice guidelines. Clearly, neonates with purpura fulminans and, possibly, those with very extensive unexplained thrombi, should be tested, as replacement therapy may be necessary.

Treatment of Neonatal Thrombosis

Although heparin and low-molecular-weight heparin have been used safely in neonates with thrombosis, efficacy has not been clearly established, except possibly in CSVT. There are no randomized control trials, and current evidence supports anticoagulation for neonates with thrombi only weakly. Consultation with a hematologist is recommended. When needed, low-molecular-weight heparin and heparin are given at higher doses per kilogram body weight than those in adults because of the increased volume of distribution in infants. Initial check of the low-molecular-weight heparin level and periodic monitoring of aPTT and heparin level are recommended.

References

Ahlsten G, Ewald U, Kindahl H, Tuvemo T (1985) Aggregation of and thromboxane B2 synthesis in platelets from newborn infants of smoking and non-smoking mothers. Prostaglandins Leukot Med 19:167–176

American Academy of Pediatrics Committee on Fetus and Newborn (2003) Controversies concerning vitamin K and the newborn. American Academy of Pediatrics Committee on fetus and newborn. Pediatrics 112:191–192

Andrew M, Kelton J (1984) Neonatal thrombocytopenia. Clin Perinatol 11:359–391

Andrew M, Paes B, Milner R, Johnston M, Mitchell L, Tollefsen DM, Powers P (1987) Development of the human coagulation system in the full-term infant. Blood 70:165–172

Andrew M, Paes B, Milner R, Johnston M, Mitchell L, Tollefsen DM, Castle V, Powers P (1988) Development of the human coagulation system in the healthy premature infant. Blood 72:1651–1657

Andrew M, Vegh P, Johnston M, Bowker J, Ofosu F, Mitchell L (1992) Maturation of the hemostatic system during childhood. Blood 80:1998–2005

Andrew M, David M, Adams M, Ali K, Anderson R, Barnard D, Bernstein M, Brisson L, Cairney B, De Sai D (1994) Venous thromboembolic complications (VTE) in children: First analyses of the Canadian registry of VTE. Blood 83:1251–1257

Ballmaier M, Germeshausen M (2009) Advances in the understanding of congenital amegakaryocytic thrombocytopenia. Br J Haematol 146:3–16

Bleyer WA, Hakami N, Shepard TH (1971) The development of hemostasis in the human fetus and newborn infant. J Pediatr 79:838–853

Bolton-Maggs PH, Perry DJ, Chalmers EA, Parapia LA, Wilde JT, Williams MD, Collins PW, Kitchen S, Dolan G, Mumford AD (2004) The rare coagulation disorders–review with guidelines for management from the united kingdom haemophilia centre doctors' organisation. Haemophilia 10:593–628

Bosticardo M, Marangoni F, Aiuti A, Villa A, Grazia Roncarolo M (2009) Recent advances in understanding the pathophysiology of Wiskott-Aldrich syndrome. Blood 113:6288–6295

Budarf ML, Konkle BA, Ludlow LB, Michaud D, Li M, Yamashiro DJ, McDonald-McGinn D, Zackai EH, Driscoll DA (1995) Identification of a patient with Bernard-Soulier syndrome and a deletion in the DiGeorge/velo-cardio-facial chromosomal region in 22q11.2. Hum Mol Genet 4:763–766

Calhoun DA, Christensen RD, Edstrom CS, Juul SE, Ohls RK, Schibler KR, Sola MC, Sullivan SE (2000) Consistent approaches to procedures and practices in neonatal hematology. Clin Perinatol 27:733–753

Cantor A (2009) Developmental hemostasis: Relevance to newborns and infants. In: Orkin SA, Fisher DE, Look AT, Lux SE, Ginsburg D, Nathan DG (eds) Nathan and Oski's hematology of infancy and childhood. Saunders Elsevier, Philadelphia

Carcao MD, Blanchette VS, Dean JA, He L, Kern MA, Stain AM, Sparling CR, Stephens D, Ryan G, Freedman J, Rand ML (1998) The platelet function analyzer (PFA-100): A novel in-vitro system for evaluation of primary haemostasis in children. Br J Haematol 101:70–73

Castle V, Andrew M, Kelton J, Giron D, Johnston M, Carter C (1986) Frequency and mechanism of neonatal thrombocytopenia. J Pediatr 108:749–755

Castle V, Coates G, Mitchell LG, O'Brodovich H, Andrew M (1988) The effect of hypoxia on platelet survival and site of sequestration in the newborn rabbit. Thromb Haemost 59:45–48

Chalmers EA (2006) Epidemiology of venous thromboembolism in neonates and children. Thromb Res 118:3–12

Chang TT (2008) Transfusion therapy in critically ill children. Pediatr Neonatol 49:5–12

Citak A, Emre S, Sairin A, Bilge I, Nayir A (2000) Hemostatic problems and thromboembolic complications in nephrotic children. Pediatr Nephrol 14:138–142

Cochran JB, Losek JD (2007) Acute liver failure in children. Pediatr Emerg Care 23:129–135

Cornelissen M, von Kries R, Loughnan P, Schubiger G (1997) Prevention of vitamin K deficiency bleeding: Efficacy of different multiple oral dose schedules of vitamin K. Eur J Pediatr 156:126–130

Del Vecchio A, Latini G, Henry E, Christensen RD (2008) Template bleeding times of 240 neonates born at 24 to 41 weeks gestation. J Perinatol 28:427–431

deVeber G, Roach ES, Riela AR, Wiznitzer M (2000) Stroke in children: Recognition, treatment, and future directions. Semin Pediatr Neurol 7:309–317

deVeber G, Andrew M, Adams C, Bjornson B, Booth F, Buckley DJ, Camfield CS, David M, Humphreys P, Langevin P, MacDonald EA, Gillett J, Meaney B, Shevell M, Sinclair DB, Yager J, Canadian Pediatric Ischemic Stroke Study Group (2001) Cerebral sinovenous thrombosis in children. N Engl J Med 345:417–423

Dickneite G, Pragst I, Joch C, Bergman GE (2009) Animal model and clinical evidence indicating low thrombogenic potential of fibrinogen concentrate (haemocomplettan P). Blood Coagul Fibrinolysis 20:535–540

Dong F, Li S, Pujol-Moix N, Luban NL, Shin SW, Seo JH, Ruiz-Saez A, Demeter J, Langdon S, Kelley MJ (2005) Genotype-phenotype correlation in MYH9-related thrombocytopenia. Br J Haematol 130:620–627

Dreyfus M, Kaplan C, Verdy E, Schlegel N, Durand-Zaleski I, Tchernia G (1997) Frequency of immune thrombocytopenia in newborns: A prospective study. immune thrombocytopenia working group. Blood 89:4402–4406

Ekelund H, Finnstrom O, Gunnarskog J, Kallen B, Larsson Y (1993) Administration of vitamin K to newborn infants and childhood cancer. BMJ Clin Res Ed 307:89–91

Flood VH, Galderisi FC, Lowas SR, Kendrick A, Boshkov LK (2008) Hemorrhagic disease of the newborn despite vitamin K prophylaxis at birth. Pediatr Blood Cancer 50:1075–1077

Goldenberg NA, Manco-Johnson MJ (2006) Pediatric hemostasis and use of plasma components. Best Practice & Research. Clin Haematol 19:143–155

Golding J, Greenwood R, Birmingham K, Mott M (1992) Childhood cancer, intramuscular vitamin K, and pethidine given during labour. BMJ Clin Res Ed 305:341–346

Greenhalgh KL, Howell RT, Bottani A, Ancliff PJ, Brunner HG, Verschuuren-Bemelmans CC, Vernon E, Brown KW, Newbury-Ecob RA (2002) Thrombocytopenia-absent radius syndrome: A clinical genetic study. J Med Genet 39:876–881

Greenway A, Massicotte MP, Monagle P (2004) Neonatal thrombosis and its treatment. Blood Rev 18:75–84

Gruenwald CE, Manlhiot C, Crawford-Lean L, Foreman C, Brandao LR, McCrindle BW, Holtby H, Richards R, Moriarty H, Van Arsdell G, Chan AK (2010) Management and monitoring of anticoagulation for children undergoing cardiopulmonary bypass in cardiac surgery. J Extra-Corpor Technol 42:9–19

Hubbard D, Tobias JD (2006) Intracerebral hemorrhage due to hemorrhagic disease of the newborn and failure to administer vitamin K at birth. South Med J 99:1216–1220

Israels SJ, Rand ML, Michelson AD (2003) Neonatal platelet function. Semin Thromb Hemost 29:363–372

Jaggers J, Lawson JH (2006) Coagulopathy and inflammation in neonatal heart surgery: Mechanisms and strategies. Ann Thorac Surg 81: S2360–S2366

Kaapa P, Knip M, Viinikka L, Ylikorkala O (1986) Increased platelet thromboxane B2 production in newborn infants of diabetic mothers. Prostaglandins Leukot Med 21:299–304

Kaplan C, Morel-Kopp MC, Clemenceau S, Daffos F, Forestier F, Tchernia G (1992) Fetal and neonatal alloimmune thrombocytopenia: Current trends in diagnosis and therapy. Transfus Med Oxf Engl 2:265–271

Kelton JG, Blanchette VS, Wilson WE, Powers P, Pai KR, Effer SB, Barr RD (1980) Neonatal thrombocytopenia due to passive immunization: Prenatal diagnosis and distinction between maternal platelet alloantibodies and autoantibodies. N Engl J Med 302:1401–1403

Kenet G, Lutkhoff LK, Albisetti M, Bernard T, Bonduel M, Brandao L, Chabrier S, Chan A, de Veber G, Fiedler B, Fullerton HJ, Goldenberg NA, Grabowski E, Gunther G, Heller C, Holzhauer S, Iorio A, Journeycake J, Junker R, Kirkham FJ, Kurnik K, Lynch JK, Male C, Manco-Johnson M, Mesters R, Monagle P, van Ommen CH, Raffini L, Rostasy K, Simioni P, Strater RD, Young G, Nowak-Gottl U (2010) Impact of thrombophilia on risk of arterial ischemic stroke or cerebral sinovenous thrombosis in neonates and children: A systematic review and meta-analysis of observational studies. Circulation 121:1838–1847

Key NS, Negrier C (2007) Coagulation factor concentrates: Past, present, and future. Lancet 370:439–448

Klebanoff MA, Read JS, Mills JL, Shiono PH (1993) The risk of childhood cancer after neonatal exposure to vitamin K. N Engl J Med 329:905–908

Koepke JA, Rodgers JL, Ollivier MJ (1975) Pre-instrumental variables in coagulation testing. Am J Clin Pathol 64:591–596

Kulkarni R, Lusher J (2001) Perinatal management of newborns with haemophilia. Br J Haematol 112:264–274

Kurnik K, Kosch A, Strater R, Schobess R, Heller C, Nowak-Gottl U, Childhood Stroke Study G (2003) Recurrent thromboembolism in infants and children suffering from symptomatic neonatal arterial stroke: A prospective follow-up study. Stroke 34:2887–2892

Larsen EC, Zinkham WH, Eggleston JC, Zitelli BJ (1987) Kasabach-Merritt syndrome: Therapeutic considerations. Pediatrics 79: 971–980

Lau KK, Stoffman JM, Williams S, McCusker P, Brandao L, Patel S, Chan AK, Thrombosis CP, Hemostasis N (2007) Neonatal renal vein thrombosis: Review of the English-language literature between 1992 and 2006. Pediatrics 120:e1278–e1284

Levi M, Toh CH, Thachil J, Watson HG (2009) Guidelines for the diagnosis and management of disseminated intravascular coagulation. British Committee for Standards in Haematology. Br J Haematol 145:24–33

Lippi G, Manzato F, Franchini M, Brocco G, Florenziani G, Guidi G (2001) Establishment of reference values for the PFA-100 platelet function analyzer in pediatrics. Clin Exp Med 1:69–70

Lippi G, Franchini M, Montagnana M, Guidi GC (2007) Coagulation testing in pediatric patients: The young are not just miniature adults. Semin Thromb Hemost 33:816–820

Lopez JA, Andrews RK, Afshar-Kharghan V, Berndt MC (1998) Bernard-Soulier syndrome. Blood 91:4397–4418

Manco-Johnson MJ (2005) Development of hemostasis in the fetus. Thromb Res 115:55–63

Manco-Johnson MJ, Grabowski EF, Hellgreen M, Kemahli AS, Massicotte MP, Muntean W, Peters M, Nowak-Gottl U (2002) Laboratory testing for thrombophilia in pediatric patients. on behalf of the subcommittee for perinatal and pediatric thrombosis of the scientific and standardization committee of the international society of thrombosis and haemostasis (ISTH). Thromb Haemost 88: 155–156

Marlar RA, Neumann A (1990) Neonatal purpura fulminans due to homozygous protein C or protein S deficiencies. Semin Thromb Hemost 16:299–309

Mathew P, Young G (2006) Recombinant factor VIIa in paediatric bleeding disorders–a 2006 review. Haemoph Off J World Fed Hemoph 12:457–472

Mattina T, Perrotta CS, Grossfeld P (2009) Jacobsen syndrome. Orphanet J Rare Dis 4:9

Messinger Y, Sheaffer JW, Mrozek J, Smith CM, Sinaiko AR (2006) Renal outcome of neonatal renal venous thrombosis: Review of 28 patients and effectiveness of fibrinolytics and heparin in 10 patients. Pediatrics 118:e1478–e1484

Middeldorp S, van Hylckama Vlieg A (2008) Does thrombophilia testing help in the clinical management of patients? Br J Haematol 143:321–335

Moharir MD, Shroff M, Stephens D, Pontigon AM, Chan A, MacGregor D, Mikulis D, Adams M, de Veber G (2010) Anticoagulants in pediatric cerebral sinovenous thrombosis: A safety and outcome study. Ann Neurol 67:590–599

Monagle P, Adams M, Mahoney M, Ali K, Barnard D, Bernstein M, Brisson L, David M, Desai S, Scully MF, Halton J, Israels S, Jardine L, Leaker M, McCusker P, Silva M, Wu J, Anderson R, Andrew M, Massicotte MP (2000) Outcome of pediatric thromboembolic disease: A report from the Canadian childhood thrombophilia registry. Pediatr Res 47:763–766

Monagle P, Barnes C, Ignjatovic V, Furmedge J, Newall F, Chan A, De Rosa L, Hamilton S, Ragg P, Robinson S, Auldist A, Crock C, Roy N, Rowlands S (2006) Developmental haemostasis. impact for clinical haemostasis laboratories. Thromb Haemost 95:362–372

Monagle P, Chalmers E, Chan A, DeVeber G, Kirkham F, Massicotte P, Michelson AD, College A, American College of Chest, P (2008) Antithrombotic therapy in neonates and children: American college of chest physicians evidence-based clinical practice guidelines (8th edn). Chest 133:887S–968S

Morris JL, Rosen DA, Rosen KR (2003) Nonsteroidal anti-inflammatory agents in neonates. Paediatr Drugs 5:385–405

Muller F, Renne T (2008) Novel roles for factor XII-driven plasma contact activation system. Curr Opin Hematol 15:516–521

Murray NA, Howarth LJ, McCloy MP, Letsky EA, Roberts IA (2002) Platelet transfusion in the management of severe thrombocytopenia in neonatal intensive care unit patients. Transfus Med Oxf Engl 12:35–41

Nichols KE, Crispino JD, Poncz M, White JG, Orkin SH, Maris JM, Weiss MJ (2000) Familial dyserythropoietic anaemia and thrombocytopenia due to an inherited mutation in GATA1. Nat Genet 24:266–270

Nurden P, Nurden AT (2008) Congenital disorders associated with platelet dysfunctions. Thromb Haemost 99:253–263

Odegard KC, McGowan FX Jr, Zurakowski D, DiNardo JA, Castro RA, del Nido PJ, Laussen PC (2002) Coagulation factor abnormalities in patients with single-ventricle physiology immediately prior to the fontan procedure. Ann Thorac Surg 73:1770–1777

Odegard KC, Zurakowski D, Hornykewycz S, DiNardo JA, Castro RA, Neufeld EJ, Laussen PC (2007) Evaluation of the coagulation system in children with two-ventricle congenital heart disease. Ann Thorac Surg 83:1797–1803

Odegard KC, Zurakowski D, DiNardo JA, Castro RA, McGowan FX Jr, Neufeld EJ, Laussen PC (2009) Prospective longitudinal study of coagulation profiles in children with hypoplastic left heart syndrome from stage I through Fontan completion. J Thorac Cardiovasc Surg 137:934–941

Oliver WC (2009) Anticoagulation and coagulation management for ECMO. Semin Cardiothorac Vasc Anesth 13:154–175

Puetz J, Darling G, Brabec P, Blatny J, Mathew P (2009) Thrombotic events in neonates receiving recombinant factor VIIa or fresh frozen plasma. Pediatr Blood Cancer 53:1074–1078

Quiroga T, Goycoolea M, Munoz B, Morales M, Aranda E, Panes O, Pereira J, Mezzano D (2004) Template bleeding time and PFA-100 have low sensitivity to screen patients with hereditary mucocutaneous hemorrhages: Comparative study in 148 patients. J Thromb Haemost JTH 2:892–898

Raffini L, Thornburg C (2009) Testing children for inherited thrombophilia: More questions than answers. Br J Haematol 147:277–288

Roberts I, Stanworth S, Murray NA (2008) Thrombocytopenia in the neonate. Blood Rev 22:173–186

Roseff SD, Luban NL, Manno CS (2002) Guidelines for assessing appropriateness of pediatric transfusion. Transfusion 42:1398–1413

Rothenberger S (2002) Neonatal alloimmune thrombocytopenia. Ther Apher Off J Int Soc Apher Jpn Soc Apher 6:32–35

Saracco P, Parodi E, Fabris C, Cecinati V, Molinari AC, Giordano P (2009) Management and investigation of neonatal thromboembolic events: Genetic and acquired risk factors. Thromb Res 123:805–809

Saxonhouse MA, Manco-Johnson MJ (2009) The evaluation and management of neonatal coagulation disorders. Semin Perinatol 33:52–65

Saxonhouse MA, Sola MC (2004) Platelet function in term and preterm neonates. Clin Perinatol 31:15–28

Shapiro AD, Jacobson LJ, Armon ME, Manco-Johnson MJ, Hulac P, Lane PA, Hathaway WE (1986) Vitamin K deficiency in the newborn infant: Prevalence and perinatal risk factors. J Pediatr 109:675–680

Shearer MJ (2009) Vitamin K deficiency bleeding (VKDB) in early infancy. Blood Rev 23:49–59

Strauss RG, Levy GJ, Sotelo-Avila C, Albanese MA, Hume H, Schloz L, Blazina J, Werner A, Barrasso C, Blanchette V (1993) National survey of neonatal transfusion practices: II. Blood component therapy. Pediatrics 91:530–536

Suarez CR, Gonzalez J, Menendez C, Fareed J, Fresco R, Walenga J (1988) Neonatal and maternal platelets: Activation at time of birth. Am J Hematol 29:18–21

Sutor AH (1995) Vitamin K deficiency bleeding in infants and children. Semin Thromb Hemost 21:317–329

Sutor AH, von Kries R, Cornelissen EA, McNinch AW, Andrew M (1999) Vitamin K deficiency bleeding (VKDB) in infancy. ISTH Pediatric/Perinatal Subcommittee. International society on thrombosis and haemostasis. Thromb Haemost 81:456–461

Suttie JW (1993) Synthesis of vitamin K-dependent proteins. FASEB J Off Publ Fed Am Soc Exp Biol 7:445–452

Thornburg C, Pipe S (2006) Neonatal thromboembolic emergencies. Semin Fetal Neonatal Med 11:198–206

Ts'ao CH, Green D, Schultz K (1976) Function and ultrastructure of platelets of neonates: Enhanced ristocetin aggregation of neonatal platelets. Br J Haematol 32:225–233

Tsai HM, Sarode R, Downes KA (2002) Ultralarge von Willebrand factor multimers and normal ADAMTS13 activity in the umbilical cord blood. Thromb Res 108:121–125

Tunnacliffe A, Jones C, Le Paslier D, Todd R, Cherif D, Birdsall M, Devenish L, Yousry C, Cotter FE, James MR (1999) Localization of Jacobsen syndrome breakpoints on a 40-mb physical map of distal chromosome 11q. Genome Res 9:44–52

van Ommen CH, Heijboer H, Buller HR, Hirasing RA, Heijmans HS, Peters M (2001) Venous thromboembolism in childhood:

A prospective two-year registry in the Netherlands. J Pediatr 139:676–681
Van Winckel M, De Bruyne R, Van De Velde S, Van Biervliet S (2009) Vitamin K, an update for the paediatrician. Eur J Pediatr 168:127–134
Varela AF, Runge A, Ignarro LJ, Chaudhuri G (1992) Nitric oxide and prostacyclin inhibit fetal platelet aggregation: A response similar to that observed in adults. Am J Obstet Gynecol 167:1599–1604
Veldman A, Fischer D, Nold MF, Wong FY (2010) Disseminated intravascular coagulation in term and preterm neonates. Semin Thromb Hemost 36:419–428
von Kries R, Hachmeister A, Gobel U (2003) Oral mixed micellar vitamin K for prevention of late vitamin K deficiency bleeding. Archives of disease in childhood. Fetal Neonatal Ed 88:F109–F112
Whaun JM, Smith GR, Sochor VA (1980) Effect of prenatal drug administration on maternal and neonatal platelet aggregation and PF4 release. Haemostasis 9:226–237
Williams MD, Chalmers EA, Gibson BE, Haemostasis and Thrombosis Task Force, British Committee for Standards in Haematology (2002) The investigation and management of neonatal haemostasis and thrombosis. Br J Haematol 119:295–309

335 Bleeding Disorders

Hassan M. Yaish · Eugenia Chang

Familial bleeding disorders affecting males have been described in religious and historical texts for thousands of years. Hemophilia A (classic hemophilia) and B (Christmas Disease) are clinically indistinguishable and discussed together in this chapter. Some of most famous individuals affected with hemophilia have been the descendents of Queen Victoria of England and the Empress of the Indies, including Czar Alexis. The downfall of the Russian aristocracy is partially attributed to the poor health of Czar Alexis and the royal family's dependence upon their physician, Rasputin, for advice. Analysis of Czar Alexis' DNA revealed a substitution in exon 4 of the factor IX gene. Schonlein termed the disease hemophilia in the 1820s. In the early twentieth century, experiments by several investigators determined that the plasma and, more specifically, the "globulin fraction" of blood plasma could correct the clotting defect of the blood of affected patients in vivo and in vitro, leading to identification of coagulation factors VIII and IX in the 1940s and eventually to the characterization and sequencing of factor VIII and IX in the 1980s. Since the 1980s, rapid progress has been made in high purity factor replacement and prophylactic therapy for these populations and has opened the door to the potential for gene therapy.

Classification

The incidence of hemophilia is 1:6,000 live male births with no racial predilection. Eighty to eighty-five percent of patients have factor VIII deficiency (hemophilia A) and 10–15% of patients with factor IX deficiency (hemophilia B), 2–3% with factor XI deficiency (hemophilia C). Severity is determined by the patient's baseline level of factor VIII or IX. factor levels are expressed as % activity, with 1 ml of normal plasma containing 100% activity and expressed as units/dL. In both hemophilia A and B, severe patients have levels of <1%, moderate with levels of 1–5% and mild with levels of >5%. Plasma factor levels correlate with frequency and severity of bleeding episodes.

Diagnosis

Hemophilia is suspected in a bleeding male patient with a prolonged aPTT on screening tests. However, some patients with mild factor VIII and IX deficiencies may have a normal aPTT. A hemophilia patient typically has a normal PT, platelet count, and bleeding time/PFA testing. Mixing studies exclude inhibitors and confirm the presence of a factor deficiency. Definitive diagnosis is based in direct assays of plasma factor VIII and IX activity levels.

The diagnosis of hemophilia is suspected based upon family history in two third of patients. One third of patients have a new mutation. Although severe patients tend to present within the first year of life, mild or moderate patients may not present until after injury or surgery in adulthood. Because inheritance is X-linked, almost all patients are male, with very rare homozygous female patients. Female carriers are variably affected and are more commonly detected by screening and treated as necessary.

Factor IX is a vitamin K-dependent factor, with low, normal neonatal levels, reaching the level of adult normals at 4–6 months of age. Factor VIII levels in newborns are similar to adult normals. Patients with mild factor VIII deficiency should also have von Willebrand factor (VWF) levels measured to differentiate mild von Willebrand disease from mild hemophilia A. The normal range of activity is 50–150%, with a typical ratio of factor VIII:VWF of 1:1. Overall, hemophilia A affected individuals and carriers have decreased levels of factor VIII, but normal plasma levels of the carrier, VWF, thus resulting in a factor VIII:VWF ratio of less than 1:1. On the other hand, patient with von Willebrands disease have decreased levels of both with a relative decrease in VWF. In the case of factor IX deficiency, carriers may have decreased levels of Factor IX activity as well. There are rare families with mutations in hormone-dependent promoters (factor IX Leyden) that have bleeding symptoms that improve with age.

Abdelaziz Y. Elzouki (ed.), *Textbook of Clinical Pediatrics*, DOI 10.1007/978-3-642-02202-9_335,

Prenatal Diagnosis and Carrier Detection

Since description and sequencing of the Factor VIII and IX molecules, more than 2,000 different mutations of factor VIII and factor IX have been described. Utilizing this data has allowed earlier and more accurate detection of affected patients and carriers. The genes for factor VIII and factor IX are both located on the X chromosome at q28 and q27.1, respectively. The factor VIII gene is 186 kb with 26 exons. The factor IX gene is considerably smaller at 34 kb and 8 exons. Both genes have a number of normal allelic variants that can be associated with ethnicity.

In the case of hemophilia A, 45% of severe cases are due to "inversions" of the factor VIII gene at intron 22, which result from intrachromosomal recombination. Nearly all spontaneous mutations are due to an inversion of intron 22. Point or small mutations resulting in truncated proteins and inversions of intron 1 and the inverted repeat 5′ end of the factor VIII gene cause the remaining cases of severe factor VIII deficiency. Missense mutations comprise of nearly all patients with moderate or mild hemophilia A.

In the case of Hemophilia B, there is also a high spontaneous rate of mutation, but there is no single common mutation. While most patients with mild or moderate disease have missense point mutations, patients with severe disease have a variety of large mutations, frame shift splice junction, nonsense or missense mutations. This heterogeneity makes the screening of carriers of factor IX deficiency more complex than that of factor VIII deficiency.

Carriers for Hemophilia A and B can be detected by direct gene mutation analysis, linkage studies, or by measurement of reduced plasma factor VIII or IX activity. Only two third of carriers are detected by reduced plasma factor activity, with the remainder having normal plasma levels.

Prenatal and antenatal screening is available to those families in whom the mutation is known or linkage analysis has been performed. While helpful for the expectant families, the infant's factor levels are not essential to make delivery room recommendations, discussed later in this chapter. Genetic counseling is recommended for all known carriers to discuss testing options and optimal delivery room management of potentially affected males.

Preimplantation diagnosis can be performed using molecular techniques or preimplantation sex screening by biopsying the embryo at the cleavage stage or biopsy of the polar body of the oocyte. Prenatal diagnosis can be performed as early as 10–12 weeks gestation using chorionic villus sampling or at 15 weeks' gestation using amniocentesis. If DNA markers are not known, fetal blood sampling for the purpose of measuring factor VIII activity can be done at 20 weeks gestation. Unfortunately, measuring fetal factor IX levels are not helpful in detecting factor IX deficiency because of the physiologically low factor IX levels in the normal fetus and newborn.

Presentation and Clinical Manifestation

Patients with both hemophilia A and B present in a similar manner. These patients have decreased thrombin formation resulting in friable and delayed clot formation. They commonly present with bleeding following minor or no trauma. Bleeding is frequently prolonged or recurrent. Thirty percent of patients present with bleeding with circumcision, 1–2% present with intracranial hemorrhage. Other bleeding manifestations include deep muscle and joint hemorrhage, bruising, hematomas, posttraumatic bleeding, postsurgical bleeding, oozing after dental procedures or oral injury, epistaxis, gastrointestinal, renal, and retroperitoneal bleeding. The most disabling long-term sequellae are related to repeated joint and muscular hemorrhages. Many patients treated prior to 1985 also have acquired HIV and/or slowly progressive liver disease from hepatitis C. These associated diseases and the cost of hemophilia treatment add social and economic difficulties to the psychological and physical challenges that this population faces.

In the severe patient (70% of A and 50% of B), bleeding in the neonatal period and muscular bleeding associated with immunization is common. Once the child begins to walk, both spontaneous and posttraumatic joint and muscle bleeds are seen. Moderate hemophiliacs (15% of hemophilia A and 30% of B) more commonly present with posttraumatic bleeding. Mild patients (15% of hemophilia A and 20% of B) frequently are not diagnosed until they have prolonged or severe posttraumatic or postsurgical bleeding.

Hemarthrosis is the hallmark of hemophilia, accounting for 90% of serious bleeding episodes. Knees, elbows, and other large joints are involved in 80% of the bleeding episodes. Bleeds can be spontaneous or following minimal trauma. Patients describe an "aura" of warmth or tingling sensation hours before the joint bleed is evident. While mild bleeds can resolve in several hours, severe bleeds can cause significant joint swelling, lasting for weeks. Once several bleeds occur in a joint, the synovium, which normally makes lubricating fluid for the joint, begins to proliferate and becomes hypertrophied, friable, leading to increased risk of repeated bleeding, cartilaginous damage, and eventual severe arthropathy. There are validated radiologic and joint examination scoring systems to assist in quantification and follow-up of joint outcomes in hemophilia (➋ *Tables 335.1* and ➋ *335.2*).

Repeated bleeding episodes eventually cause loss of joint space, bone cysts, crippling arthritis, and eventual fusion of the joint. Chronic synovitis can be treated with surgical or radiosynovectomy, while end-stage arthropathy is frequently treated with joint fusion or replacement.

Deep muscle bleeding is another common manifestation of hemophilia. Of particular interest is bleeding within the retroperitoneal muscles. Large bleeds can occur in the iliopsoas muscles, causing lower quadrant abdominal pain that can mimic appedicitis or referred pain to the groin or hip, easily confused with hip

Table 335.1
Orthopedic joint scoring system (Gilbert score)

	Score[a]			
	0	1	2	3
Chronic Pain	No pain	Mild pain	Moderate pain partial or occasional interference with occupation or ADL	Severe pain
	No functional deficit	Does not interfere with occupation or activities of daily living (ADL)	Use of non-narcotic medications	Interferes with occupation or ADL
	No analgesic use (except with acute hemarthrosis)	May require non-narcotic analgesic	May require occasional narcotic medications	Requires frequent use of non-narcotic and narcotic medications
Axial deformity				
Elbow	None	≤10° varus or valgus	>10° varus or valgus	–
Knee	No deformity (0–7° valgus)	8–15° valgus or 0–5° varus	>15° valgus or >5° varus	–
Ankle	No deformity	≤10° valgus or ≤5° varus	>10° valgus or >5° varus	–
Contracture Flexion	<15° fixed flexion contracture (FFC)	–	≥15° FFC	–
Equinus	<15°	–	≥15°	–
Joint physical findings				
Instability range of motion[b]	None	Slight (noted on examination but does not interfere with function or require bracing)	Severe (creates a function deficit or requires bracing)	–
Pronation and supination[b]	0–10%	11–33%	33–100%	–
Chronic swelling	None		Present	–
Atrophy	None/minimal (<1 cm)	Present	–	–
Crepitus on motion	None	Present	–	–

[a]Sum of the elbows, knees, and ankles = joint score; maximum possible score = 90
[b]Expressed as percentage loss of full range of motion.
Source: Adapted from Pipe SW, Valentino LA (2007) Hemophilia 13(suppl 4):1–16

Table 335.2
Radiologic joint score (Pettersson score)

Type of change	Finding	Score[a]
Osteoporosis	Absent	0
	Present	1
Enlarged epiphysis	Absent	0
	Present	1
Irregular subchondral surface	Absent	0
	Partially involved	1
	Totally involved	2
Narrowing of joint space	Absent	0
	Present; joint space >1 mm	1
	Present; joint space <1mm	2
Subchondral cyst formation	Absent	0
	1 Cyst	1
	>1 Cyst	2
Erosion of joint margins	Absent	0
	Present	1
Gross incongruence of articulating bone ends	Absent	0
	Slight	1
Joint deformity	Absent	0
	Slight	1
	Pronounced	2

[a]Maximum possible joint score = 13; maximum possible total joint score (Sum of elbows, knees, and ankles) =78.
Source: Adapted from Gilbert MS (1993) Semin Hematol 30:3–6

hemarthrosis. The patient with an iliopsoas bleed will hold his leg flexed and inwardly rotated. Non-contrast CT scan of the abdomen and pelvis or ultrasound can confirm the diagnosis. Large muscle bleeds of the extremities can lead to a compartment syndrome, where the hematoma can compromise the neurovascular integrity of the limb, requiring surgical fasciotomy to save the limb.

Gross hematuria is another characteristic manifestation of hemophilia. These episodes are typically spontaneous and painless. Severe pain should raise the suspicion of urinary tract obstruction due to blood clot. Treatment is controversial, but most practitioners treat with hydration, corticosteroids, and factor replacement. Antifibrinolytics are contraindicated.

Intracranial hemorrhages and bleeds around the airway are among the most life-threatening complications of hemophilia and account for 25% of hemorrhagic deaths in hemophilia.

Treatment for Hemophilia

Treatment is focused on prevention of injury, local control of bleeding, and replacement therapy. The surroundings of the infant should be cleared of objects that may cause injury. Once the child starts walking, close supervision and guidance are essential to prevent trauma. As the child becomes older, sports, such as swimming, should be encouraged and contact sports should be avoided. Participation in physical activity and physiotherapy improves strength and mobility, decreases bleeding, and prevents the development of hemophilic muscle atrophy.

Local control of a bleeding episode is a helpful adjunct to replacement therapy. RICE is a frequently used mnemonic by the National Hemophilia Foundation to teach essentials of local control: Rest, Ice, Compression, and Elevation. Topical therapies to stop an active bleeding can also be useful to reduce usage of factor replacement therapy.

Replacement Therapy

The earliest attempts to treat hemophiliacs by providing them with blood obtained from normal individuals were undertaken by a British physician 100 years before the relationship between effective blood transfusion and the temporary replacement of a missing blood coagulation factor was understood and appreciated. For many years, blood transfusion was the only effective mode of therapy until fresh frozen plasma (FFP) was developed. FFP was more practical to administer and provided more factor per volume than whole blood. Cryoprecipitate was introduced later and became the treatment of choice until lyophilized factor concentrates were available in the 1970s. Development of factor concentrates has enabled patients with hemophilia to undergo orthopedic and dental treatment, followed by home infusion therapy with factor concentrates. Life expectancy for patients with hemophilia without inhibitor increased from 11 years in 1921 to 71.2 years after 2000, now approaching the life expectancy of a normal male.

One of the great tragedies of the hemophilia population was the HIV epidemic. Between 1979 and 1985, 55% of treated hemophiliacs were infected with HIV-1 virus and 60–95% with hepatitis C, due to exposure to factor replacement products. Each lot of these factor concentrates is manufactured from more than 2,000 blood donors. In response to the HIV epidemic, the 1980s brought numerous methods of factor purification including monoclonal antibody purification of factors, viral inactivation with heat and solvent detergent treatment methods, as well as recombinant factor VIII and factor IX products.

Several types of purified factor VIII concentrates are currently available. Lower-purity, plasma-derived, VIII concentrate products containing VWF and VIII can be used to treat hemophilia A, but this has been largely replaced by high purity factor concentrates. Since the late 1980s, monoclonal antibody purified products that are virally inactivated with a combination of pasteurization, dry heat treatment, and solvent detergent methods have been available (Monarc-P(no longer available)®, Hemophil M®). Over the last 20 years, recombinant factor VIII products have been widely used. Purity in these products has progressively improved over the three generations of recombinant factor products. First-generation products include human albumin in the final product (Recombinate®), second-generation products (Helixate FS®, Kogenate FS®) only contain human or animal albumen in the cell culture medium, and third-generation products contain no human or animal albumin in their production (Advate®). Since deleting the B domain of the factor VIII molecule does not alter its activity but increases yields of the recombinant protein, several B domain–deleted second- and third-generation products have also been used (Refacto(no longer available), Xyntha®).

Much of the emphasis of newer factor VIII products has been on purity and safety, but currently commercially available products contain essentially the same factor VIII molecule. Future factor VIII products may have more favorable properties that improve its ease of use.

For patients with factor IX deficiency, previously, only low purity prothrombin complex concentrates (PCC) were available. These products contain factors II, variably activated VII, IX, and X. These products have been largely replaced by plasma-derived, monoclonal antibody–purified factor IX concentrates (Mononine®, AlphaNine SD®) and third-generation recombinant factor IX products (Benefix®).

Despite the number of factor concentrate products available, the fundamentals of factor replacement therapy have remained the same: prompt and adequate therapy to achieve a hemostatic level for the type of bleeding being treated. One milliliter of normal plasma contains 1u of clotting activity of all coagulation factors, including factor VIII and IX (➋ *Table 335.3*). Since plasma volume is 45 mL/kg of body weight and has 100% activity for both factor VIII

Table 335.3
Guidelines for factor replacement therapy for hemophilia A and B

Type of bleed	Goal hemostatic level	Factor VIII dose	Factor IX dose
Soft tissue, muscle, joint	40–80%	20–40 u/kg daily	40–80 u/kg
Oral mucosa	50%	25 u/kg	50 u/kg
Epistaxis, GI, GU	100% initially then 30% until healing	50 u/kg initially then 15 u/kg	100 u/kg initially then 30 u/kg
CNS, trauma, surgery or life threatening	100% initially then 50–100% until wound healing	50 u/kg initially then 25–50 u/kg until wound healing	100 u/kg initially then 50–100 u/kg until wound healing

and IX, in a normal individual, infusion of 45 u/kg would be expected to raise the factor level from 0–100% of normal. In the case of factor VIII, 1 U factor VIII/kg will raise the level 2%, with a half-life of 8–12 h. Because of the increased rate of diffusion of the smaller factor IX molecule to the extravascular space, 1U factor IX/kg will raise the factor level by 1%, with a half-life of 18–24 h.

Home Infusion/Self Therapy Program

Virtually, all patients with reliable family support and adequate vascular access are candidates for home infusion therapy. Most families can be trained when the patient is 3–8 years of age to perform home infusion therapy. Families with even younger patients can be trained, if a permanent indwelling vascular access device (portacath) or arteriovenous fistula is placed. Refer to Sangostino for a review of vascular access issues in patients with hemophilia.

This has opened the door to routine prophylactic treatment that permits these patients to participate in most physical activities.

Infusion Schedules

Many older and mild/moderate hemophilia patients treat themselves "on demand" (episodic factor replacement for bleeding episodes or trauma). Mild or moderate hemophiliacs will frequently infuse prior to higher risk physical activity, such as downhill skiing. However, the mainstay of treatment for a severe hemophiliac is routine scheduled prophylactic infusion therapy. Joint outcomes in severe hemophiliacs that are treated "on demand" are poor, prompting clinical trials that have demonstrated improved long-term joint outcomes in patients that receive routine prophylactic infusions. Many patients that are treated on demand will begin secondary prophylaxis after repeated bleeding episodes in order to decrease symptoms in a target joint (a joint with recurrent bleeding).

In essence, severe hemophiliacs can be converted to a moderate phenotype with routine infusions of factor VIII (25–40 units/kg) one to four times per week or factor IX (50 units/kg) one to two times per week. A study by Collins et al., elegantly demonstrated that decreasing the time with factor VIII levels of <1% in patients with hemophilia A by infusing with factor VIII replacement therapy at least three times per week correlated with decreased total bleeding episodes and hemarthrosis. Studies performed in patients with factor IX deficiency also demonstrated the efficacy of prophylactic infusions (15–50 units/kg) in preventing bleeding episodes. With the advent of routine prophylaxis, many severe hemophiliacs lead a life full of activities much like their healthy peers without daily fear of life-threatening hemorrhage.

Ancillary Pharmacologic Therapies

Desmopressin: Desmopressin or 1-deamino-8-D-argnine vasopressin (DDAVP) stimulates a transient, fourfold increase in factor VIII levels by releasing factor VIII stored in endothelial cells and platelets. This is an effective alternative therapy for patients with mild hemophilia A. Administration of 0.3 mcg/kg of DDAVP in 30–50 mL of saline IV over 15–30 min results in peak factor VIII level at 30–60 min. A concentrated nasal spray (Stimate®) administers 150 mcg/spray and can be self-administered in the home. 150 mcg is sufficient for a child <50 kg, 300 mcg is indicated for a >50 kg person, with the nasal spray peak levels are attained at 60–90 min. Fluids should be restricted in patients receiving DDAVP because of the risk of hyponatremia. Tachyphylaxis (temporary cessation of response) can occur with repeated doses of DDAVP, even if given no more frequently than daily. Transient facial flushing, hyponatremia, hypertension, and headache can occur after administration.

Antifibrinolytic therapy: Another effective method of controlling bleeding in the hemophilia patient is the use of antifibrinolytics to stabilize and protect the friable clot. Clots in the oropharynx are particularly sensitive to degradation due to the high levels of fibrinolytic enzymes in saliva. Two agents are available, ϵ-aminocaproic acid (EACA, Amicar®) and tranexamic acid (Cyclokapron®). Both can be administered intravenously or orally. Generally these agents are administered in patients with oronasopharyngeal bleeding, for 2–5 days to permit healing of the mucosa. The greatest risk with these agents is thrombosis. Administration with prothrombin complex concentrates or with urinary tract bleeding is relatively contraindicated due to the risk of thrombosis and urinary tract obstruction, respectively.

Topical therapy: There are three categories of topical treatments: sealants, matrix dressings, and other topical therapies. Sealants include Tisseel VH®, topical thrombin, and cyanoacrylate. The matrix dressings promote fibrin formation. Finally, other materials such as zeolite and hydrophilic polymers that form artificial scabs can be used to assist with hemostasis.

Future therapeutic strategies: Due to improved understanding of the factor VIIa, VIII, and IX molecules, one future avenue of treatment would be to improve the stability, potency, and half-life of the molecules and facilitate alternative delivery systems such as oral and intrapulmonary routes. Current clinical trials include agents with extended half-lives, improving the convenience of prophylactic factor infusion. Even more attractive is the potential to cure disease using gene therapy or hepatocyte transfer. While a number of these approaches utilizing adenoviral, adeno-associated viral, and retroviral vectors have been tried in clinical trials, thus far these approaches have not resulted in sufficient long-term factor VIII or IX protein levels and have been limited by immunologic response.

Delivery Room Management of Potential Hemophilia Patients

The risk of intracranial hemorrhage in hemophilia patients delivered vaginally is 4% compared to 0.5% in patients delivered by cesarean section. The risk is tripled in deliveries assisted by forceps or vacuum extraction which is contraindicated when delivering a potential hemophilia patient. Fetal scalp electrodes also increase the risk of bleeding in affected infants and should be avoided. After delivery, umbilical cord blood specimens can be sent to determine if the infant is affected and requires additional care or observation. Ideally, a 4.5 mL specimen should be drawn from a double clamped 10 in. section of cord, drawn from the umbilical vein, and placed into a citrated syringe or tube after discarding the initial 1–2 mL. This method decreases the risk of hemorrhage in the affected infant due to difficult venopuncture. Routine factor infusion after delivery is not indicated, but a high index of suspicion for bleeding and low threshold for prompt intervention with factor replacement therapy for bleeding episodes is essential.

Management of Carriers

There is great variability to symptomatology of carriers for factor VIII and IX deficiency. Ten percent of carriers of factor VIII and IX deficiency are symptomatic with levels of less than 35% and 30%, respectively. Patients with depressed factor VIII and IX levels of <50% (50 IU/dL) may require factor replacement therapy for severe bleeding episodes, delivery, or surgery. Factor VIII levels increase during pregnancy and should be evaluated in the event of unusual bleeding and during the last trimester to determine if intervention is necessary. Factor VIII levels also rise in response to inflammation, estrogen therapy, and aerobic exercise. Carriers with blood type O also have factor VIII levels that are 25% lower than those with blood group A, B, or AB. Factor IX levels do not increase during pregnancy, so a postpubertal baseline level should be adequate to determine the necessity of treatment for delivery.

Management of Hemophiliac Patients with Inhibitors to Factor VIII or IX

Ten to fifteen percent of patients with severe hemophilia A, 3% of patients with severe hemophilia B, and 2.7–13% of mild/moderate hemophilia A eventually become refractory to factor replacement therapy due to the development of immunoglobulin G (IgG) antibodies to factor VIII or IX. The risk factors for inhibitor development include genotype, major histocompatibility class II alleles, polymorphisms in immune response genes (IL10, TNFa, CTLA4), reason for first treatment (surgery vs routine infusion), >5 days of initial exposure, and some suggestion that initial continuous infusion may increase the risk. There are two preferred methods of evaluating inhibitors: the Nijmegen assay and the Bethesda assay. The Nijmegen assay is a modification of the Bethesda assay that has improved specificity and inter-laboratory reliability, but the Bethesda assay continues to be more widely used. Both assays quantify inhibitors to the A2 domain better than for inhibitors to the C2 domain. The unit utilized to measure the titer of inhibitor is the Bethesda unit (BU). This is defined as the amount of inhibitor present in 1 ml of the patient's plasma that neutralizes 50% of the factor VIII or IX in 1 ml of normal plasma. Patients with inhibitors to factor VIII and IX are divided into low titer (<5 BU), high titer (5–30 BU), and very high titer patients (>30 BU) for purposes of treatment recommendations. Patients with low-titer inhibitors that do not increase in response to factor replacement therapy are known as low responders (25% of hemophilia A inhibitor patients), whereas those that have rapidly increasing titers with repeated exposure to factor replacement are high responders (75% of hemophilia A inhibitor patients). Typically, the inhibitor titer begins to rise 2–3 days after reexposure to replacement therapy and reaches a peak at 7–21 days, decreasing slowly if there are no further exposures to factor replacement. The highest risk of development of inhibitors is in the first 50 days of exposure to factor replacement therapy, with only rare patients developing inhibitors after 150 exposure days. Once formed, high-titer inhibitors in high responders tend to persist and low-titer inhibitors in low responders tend to disappear without recurrence.

Treatment of these patients is challenging and complex. Low-titer, low-responder patients can generally be treated with higher and more frequent doses of factor replacement therapy. Some treating physicians will change from a recombinant factor to a plasma-derived factor in inhibitor patients. For patients with high titer inhibitors or high responders, plasmapheresis can reduce titers temporarily to permit emergent treatment of a life-threatening hemorrhage with factor replacement.

There are other options for the treatment of hemophilia A in the presence of inhibitors. Porcine factor VIII (Hyate:C) at a dose of 100–150 u/kg can be used to treat acute bleeds, but is associated with allergic reactions and hematologic side effects. It may cause an amnestic response to both human and porcine factor VIII. Once anti-porcine inhibitor titers rise to 15–20 BU, the product becomes less effective.

Bypass therapy with prothrombin complex concentrates (PCC, Proplex® at 100 u/kg) and activated prothrombin complex concentrates (aPCC, FEIBA® at 50–75 u/kg) is effective for treatment of acute bleeds in inhibitor patients with both hemophilia A and B, but is not used for prophylaxis because of the risks of thrombosis and amnesis associated with their use. Both of these products contain Vitamin K–dependent factors, including activated factor II, VII, IX, X, explaining their ability to bypass factor VIII and IX with the activated factor X and VII.

There is now 20 years of experience administering recombinant activated factor VII (NovoSeven®). It is highly effective in hemophilia A and B patients with inhibitors. Dosing is variable and can range from (35–300 mcg/kg). Its use is limited by its short half-life (2.7 h in adults and 1.3 h in children) and its cost. In the subset of hemophilia B patients with inhibitors and anaphylaxis associated with factor IX administration, it is currently the only treatment option for acute bleeds, as they can develop proteinuria due to immune complex formation with repeated factor IX exposure. There is in vitro evidence that demonstrates a synergistic effect between the use of aPCC with recombinant VIIa, but clinical trials are needed, given the potential risk of thrombosis with concurrent use.

The best solution for hemophilia patients with inhibitors is to eradicate them with immune tolerance therapy. When successful, this permits the use of factor replacement products, frequently at normal dosing. Induction of immune tolerance is possible in 60–80% of hemophilia A patients. The success rate in hemophilia B patients with inhibitors appears to be significantly lower. The process of immune tolerance is time consuming and expensive. There are several methods currently being utilized including high dose factor replacement therapy (frequently by continuous infusion), cyclophosphamide, corticosteroids, and intravenous immunoglobulins. There are promising preliminary findings with the use of cyclosporin, mycophenylate mofetil, and rituximab therapy.

Comprehensive Hemophilia Clinic

Because of the complexity of the ongoing care of these patients, most patients in the USA are managed in a federally funded network of comprehensive hemophilia clinics. These clinics have a staff experienced in the complex medical and psychosocial needs of this population. Comprehensive clinics usually include hemophilia physicians, nurses, orthopedists, infectious disease specialists, dentists, social workers, genetic counselors, nutritionists, and physical therapists.

Factor XI Deficiency (Hemophilia C)

Hemophilia C comprises only 2–3% of hemophilia. The gene is 23 kb and located on the long arm of chromosome 4. It is autosomal recessive and most symptomatic patients have factor XI levels of 1–10% of normal. Symptoms are most typically post surgical, posttraumatic, epistaxis, menorrhagia, and hematuria. Spontaneous bleeding is rare. Bleeding tendency and factor levels do not always correlate, likely due to coinheritance of additional hemostatic defects, VWF levels, reduced thrombin-activatable fibrinolysis inhibitor levels (TAFI), and abnormalities in platelet associated factor XI. Over half of the reported cases are in the Jewish population with a gene frequency of 1:8 of Ashkenazi Jews. The half-life of factor XI is 45–55 h. Treatment is FFP or solvent detergent pooled plasma. In France, a plasma-derived factor XI concentrate (Hemoleven) is available as well. DDAVP and antifibrinolytic therapy can be an effective adjunct. Rare patients with abnormalities in platelet-associated factor XI may require platelet transfusion as well.

Factor Deficiencies Associated with Laboratory Abnormalities but No Bleeding Tendency

Factor XII deficiency, prekallikrein (Fletcher factor), and HMW kininogen (Fitzgerald factor) deficiency can all result in impressive prolongation of the aPTT but are not associated with bleeding tendency. In patients with a prolonged aPTT and absence of bleeding, this diagnosis is suggested with a mixing study demonstrating factor deficiency but normal factor VIII, IX, and XI levels. The diagnosis can be confirmed with factor assays.

von Willebrand disease

General

von Willebrand disease (VWD) is the most common congenital bleeding disorder, with an incidence of over 1% in the general population. VWD was initially described by Eric A. von Willebrand in 1926 in a family with a bleeding disorder affecting both males and females and distinctive from hemophilia. Many patients have symptoms and laboratory findings that can be confused with hemophilia A (➲ *Table 335.4*). Mucocutaneous bleeding is more common than joint bleeding. The disease is caused by qualitatively abnormal and quantitatively decreased levels of von Willebrand factor (VWF). VWF is a carrier protein for factor VIII, complexed together in a 1:1 ratio. The gene for VWF is located on chromosome 12. Among the three main clinical subtypes of VWD, a significant overlap between normal individuals and patients with type 1 VWD, makes the diagnosis very challenging.

Physiologic Regulation of von WF Synthesis and Release

VWF is a multimeric glycoprotein consisting of dimeric subunits. The multimers are classified as low, intermediate, and high depending upon their molecular weight. The protein is synthesized by both the megakaryocyte and the endothelial cell. VWF produced by the endothelial cell is high molecular weight (HMW) and stored in Weibel–Palade bodies. VWF produced in the megakaryocytes is LMW and stored in the alpha granules of the platelets. Secretion is facilitated by two pathways, constitutive from the platelets and regulated from endothelial cells in response to vascular endothelial damage and other endothelial cell stimulation. Levels vary according to inflammation, exercise, vasopressin, pregnancy, and blood group type, with blood type O individuals having significantly lower levels of VWF.

Function of von Willebrand Factor

VWF serves two key roles in normal hemostatis: it is a cofactor for platelet adhesion and the carrier protein for factor VIII procoagulant. In platelet adhesion, VWF promotes the attachment of platelets to the areas of vessel injury. To optimize the availability of VWF at the site of injury, a highly active form of the protein (HMW multimers) is stored in the α granules of the platelets

Table 335.4
Differences between von Willebrand disease and hemophilia

	von Willebrand disease	Hemophilia A
Symptoms	Mucous membrane bleeds and bruising (epistaxis, menorrhagia)	Joint and muscle bleeds
Sexual distribution	Males and females	Males
Incidence	1/100 or more	1/6,000 males
Abnormal protein	von Willebrand factor	Factor VIII
Function	Platelet adhesion and carrier to factor VIII	Clotting cofactor
Site of synthesis	Endothelial cells and megakaryocytes	Liver
Gene location	Chromosome 12	X chromosome
BT	Often prolonged	Normal
PTT	Prolonged or normal	Prolonged
Factor VIII	Low normal or decreased	Decreased or absent
VWF:Ag	Decreased or absent	Normal or increased
VWF:Rcof	Decreased or abnormal	Normal or increased

BT bleeding time, *PTT* partial thromboplastin time, *VWF:Ag* von Willebrand factor antigen, *VWF:Rcof* von Willebrand factor/ristocetin cofactor activity and the endothelial cells. When such cells sense tissue injury (e.g., by contact with thrombin), they instantly mobilize the stored protein. Each HMW multimeric unit has a binding site for (a) the receptor glycoprotein (GP) Ib on nonactivated platelets, (b) the integrin-type receptors (GPIIb/IIIa on activated platelets), and (c) fibrillar collagen and heparin-like molecules. Each multimeric unit can also facilitate factor VIII binding onto platelet surface templates to mediate the coagulation process. The result is bridging of the platelets and vascular endothelium (adhesion) to GPIb as well as the platelets with other platelets (aggregation) via GPIIb/IIIa, resulting in the formation of the platelet plug. Adhesive proteins such as fibrinogen also react with the GPIIb/IIIa on the surface of the activated platelets and contribute to platelet aggregation and platelet plug formation in primary hemostasis.

LMW and intermediate-molecular-weight (IMW) multimers have fewer platelet binding sites and serve as carriers for factor VIII, unlike the HMW multimers, which are rich in platelet bridging sites. In secondary hemostasis, which facilitates fibrin clot formation, VWF, a carrier of factor VIII, will deliver this important component to the site of adherent platelets, resulting in clot formation. VWF also stabilizes factor VIII, protecting it from premature activation by activated factor X or inactivation by protein C, and preventing it from binding to phospholipids and activated circulating platelets. Unbound factor VIII is an unstable molecule that decays rapidly in the circulation. This probably explains, at least in part, the low factor VIII activity (factor VIII:C) in some types of VWD, such as type 2N.

Genetics of von Willebrand Disease

Typically, VWD is a heterozygous autosomally inherited disorder with depressed levels of VWF or function. Patients with severe disease are usually homozygotes or double heterozygotes, with an autosomal recessive pattern of inheritance (➋ *Table 335.5*).

Classification of VWD

There are three types of von Willebrand Disease and a group of individuals that are classified as “low von Willebrand factor” (➋ *Table 335.6*).

Type I: The most common subtype of VWD is type I, accounting for 80% of affected individuals. These patients have a heterozygous or partial deficiency of structurally normal VWF. There is an overrepresentation of individuals with the blood group O due to the lower levels in this population. Ten percent of patients have the Y1584C missense mutation. Most other known mutations are also missense mutations. A distinct variant of type I VWD is type 1 Vicenza, characterized by a markedly decreased half-life. Adding to the mystery of VWD, there are affected patients that do not have detectable mutations in the VWF gene and do not demonstrate linkage, suggesting that there may be other genetic interactions that modify level of VWF:Rcof. These patients range from those with mild bleeding disorder to those who are asymptomatic. The diagnosis can be challenging because of the many factors affecting circulating VWF levels. Because these patients have present but reduced levels of VWF and factor VIII in the platelets and endothelial cells, they respond to DDAVP.

Low VWF: There is considerable controversy in the diagnosis of individuals with VWF 30–50IU/dL. 2.5% of the general population has a VWF level in this range. Many of the individuals with levels in this range do not demonstrate typical inheritance for VWD or abnormalities in the VWF gene. Linkage to VWF gene abnormalities was only present in 51% of these individuals. These individuals have a mild bleeding tendency, occasionally can require treatment for bleeding, and may have some protective effect against thrombosis. This group of individuals is currently classified as having low von Willebrand factor, a risk factor for bleeding.

Type 2: 15–20% of patients belong to this type. These patients have both qualitative and quantitative abnormalities in VWF. These variants can have decreased numbers of HMW and IMW VWF multimers with variable bleeding tendency. Inheritance is can be dominant or recessive. There are a number of subgroups of this type. All of these subtypes have missense mutations that impair functional domains of the VWF molecule responsible for binding to GP1b, factor VIII, or multimerization.

Type 2a: This is the most common type 2 variant. This subtype has a lack or relative decrease of high and intermediate weight multimers of VWF. Mutations are in the A2 domain. Sixty percent of cases are either R1597W or Q or Y, or S1506L. These mutations affect the multimerization of VWF. There are two groups of these patients: group I that have impaired secretion of HMW multimers due to abnormal transport and group II that have mutations with a greater susceptibility to in vivo proteolysis.

Type 2b: This subtype also has a lack of high molecular weight multimers, with the exception of the New York/ Malmo variant. Mutations are in the A1 domain. Ninety percent of cases are due to R1306W, R1308C, V1316M,

Table 335.5

Main characteristics of von Willebrand disease types

Type of VWD	Laboratory	Multimers	Mutations associated	Comments
Type 1	Concurrent reduction of FVIII:C and VWF in plasma; VWF:RCo/VWF: Ag ≥ 0.6	All multimers present; some minor abnormalities may be evident using sensitive methods	Missense mutations scattered over the entire gene. Possible dominant-negative effect. Y1584C in about 10%. Single null allele not associated with bleeding.	Usually co-dominant or dominant-negative. Ideal candidates for desmopressin. Short VWF half-life in VWD Vicenza (R1205H) and other rare mutations.
Type 2A	Usually VWF:RCo/VWF: Ag < 0.6	Lack or relative decrease of the high molecular weight (HMW) and of intermediate multimers	Mutations in A2 domain; R1597W or Q or Y and S1506L represent about 60% of cases.	Usually co-dominant. Two mechanisms demonstrated by expression experiments. Group I: impaired secretion of HMW multimers, due to defective intracellular transport. Group II: normal synthesis and secretion of a VWF with greater susceptibility to in vivo proteolysis. Patients of the latter group may respond to desmopressin.[27]
Type 2B	Usually VWF:RCo/VWF: Ag < 0.6; RIPA occurs at low ristocetin concentration	Lack of HMW multimers; a normal pattern is present in New York/Malmö variant	Mutations in A1 domain; 90% of cases are due to R1306W, R1308C, V1316M, and R1341Q.[51] P1266L associated with gene conversion and New York/Malmö phenotype.[12]	Usually co-dominant. Enhanced affinity of abnormal VWF for platelet GpIb receptor. Thrombocytopenia after desmopressin and sometimes during pregnancy or stress situations; thrombocytopenia may aggravate bleeding risk conferred by the abnormal VWF.
Type 2M	Usually VWF:RCo/VWF: Ag < 0.6;	Large multimers present; inner abnormalities may be evident (e.g., "smeary pattern")	A few heterogeneous mutations recurrent (e.g., R1315C, G1324S/A, R1374C/H).	Usually co-dominant. Some overlap with Type 2A may occur. Desmopressin may be useful in selected cases.
Type 2N	VWF may be normal or only slightly reduced; FVIII:C/VWF:Ag < 0.5; defective FVIII-VWF binding	All multimers present	Mutations in NH2-terminus; R854Q largely the most frequent mutation.	Usually recessive. Bleeding only for homozygosity or compound heterozygosity. Heterozygosity for R854Q in up to 2% of population in Northern Europe. Desmopressin may be useful for the majority of minor bleedings
Type 3	Virtual absence of VWF; markedly reduced FVIII:C (<5 IU/dL)	Lack of multimers	Mutations scattered over the entire gene, but some (e.g., 2,430delC exon 18[a] or Arg2535stop) are particularly recurrent in North Europe. High prevalence of null mutations (stop codons, frameshift, gene deletions).	Recessive. Desmopressin does not work since cellular storage is devoid of VWF

[a]Mutation responsible for VWD in the original family described by E von Willebrand.

Source: Adapted from Rodeghiero et al. (2009) Hematology 2009:113–123

Table 335.6
Laboratory findings and inheritance in von Willebrand disease variants

	Type 1	Type 2A	Type 2B	Type 2M	Type 2N	Type 3
Test	P	R	R	P	N	P
BT						
VIII:C	R	R/N	R/N	R/N	R	R
VWF:Ag	R	R/N	R/N	N	N	R
VWF:Rcof	R	R	R	R	N	R
RIPA	N/R	R	I	R	R	R
Multimer	N	Abn	Abn	N	N	Usually absent
Inheritance	AD	AD	AD	AD	AD	AR
Frequency	70–80%	10–12%	3–5%	0–1%	0–1%	1–3%

BT bleeding time, *VIII:C* factor VIII procoagulant, *VWF:Ag* von Willebrand factor antigen, *VWF:Rcof* von Willebrand factor/ristocetin cofactor activity, *RIPA*, ristocetin-induced platelet aggregation, *P* prolonged, *R* reduced, *N* normal, *I* increased, *Abn* abnormal, *AD* autosomal dominant, *AR* autosomal recessive

and R1341Q. The New York/Malmo phenotype has the P1266L mutation. These mutations are associated with an increased affinity for the platelet Gp1b receptor leading to increased thrombocytopenia after desmopressin, pregnancy, or stress.

Type 2M: This subtype is characterized by the presence of large multimers, but have decreased function of the VWF, resulting in a VWF:Rcof/VWF:Ag of <0.6. Mutations are heterogeneous and there is some overlap with type 2a.

Type 2N (Normandy): This subtype is characterized by mutations in the NH2 terminus leading to impaired binding and subsequent rapid decay of factor VIII. The most frequent mutation is R854Q. Up to 2% of the Northern European population is heterozygous for this mutation. Bleeding is only seen in individuals that are homozygous or double heterozygotes. These patients mimic hemophilia A patients.

Type 3: These patients inherit disease in an autosomal recessive manner. They are severely affected with virtual absence of VWF and markedly reduced FVIII:C. The mutations associated with this subtype are scattered over the entire gene, many of which are null mutations. This subtype has an increased risk of inhibitor development with exposure to VWF. DDAVP does not work in this population.

Platelet-type Pseudo VWD: This disorder is actually a mutation in the platelet GP1b gene resulting in increased affinity for the VWF. This disease clinically resembles type 2B. There are reduced levels of HMW multimers in these individuals because of the adsorption of VWF by the platelets.

Acquired VWD: Some autoimmune and lymphoproliferative diseases and less frequently solid tumors, such as Wilms tumor, congenital heart disease, hypothyroidism, or liver diseases are occasionally associated with a hemorrhagic diathesis resembling congenital VWD, but characterized by the presence of antibodies to VWF. Some pharmacologic agents have also been implicated in the development of acquired VWD, such as dextran, valproate, and ciprofloxacin. A prolonged infusion of factor VIII preparations devoid of VWF (recombinant preparations) has resulted in a similar syndrome due to binding of all available VWF by the excessive factor VIII, resulting in complete consumption of VWF, leaving behind a large amount of unbound factor VIII that is then rapidly cleared from the circulation.

Clinical Presentation and Diagnosis

The clinical manifestations of VWD are frequently mild and might go unnoticed until the patient is subjected to physical or surgical trauma. Many patients do not recognize their symptoms as abnormal and go undiagnosed. The most frequent symptoms are easy bruising and mucous membrane bleeding, such as epistaxis, menorrhagia, dental, and gastrointestinal bleeding. Deep muscle bleeds and hemarthrosis are uncommon, with the exception of individuals with type 3 VWD. Differentiating between normal individuals and those with mild VWD requires a combination of family history, characterization of bleeding symptoms, and careful laboratory evaluation.

Given the variation of VWF levels within a single individual, diagnosis may require repeating assays numerous times. In the adult literature bleeding scores distinguish between affected individuals and normal with low levels. Unfortunately, bleeding scores have not proven to be consistent in children, given their limited past bleeding history.

Laboratory Diagnosis of VWD

Laboratory diagnosis of VWD can be difficult because of the overlap between normal and affected individuals. In the most characteristic cases, aPTT is prolonged, bleeding time is prolonged, but PT, platelet counts, and platelet morphology is normal. Unfortunately normal screening tests are relatively insensitive and a number of patients will require specific testing for VWD. In patients with suspected VWD, it is important to exclude bleeding disorders that present with similar symptoms such as primary disorders of platelet function and number.

The bleeding time is abnormal in the presence of qualitative or quantitative platelet abnormalities, or abnormalities of connective tissues. It is variably prolonged in VWD and is occasionally normal in mild forms of disease. Ingestion of medications such as aspirin and nonsteroidal anti-inflammatory drugs can inhibit platelet function, resulting in a prolonged bleeding time, so it is not sufficient for diagnosis of VWD. Because of inherent variability in the Ivy bleeding time, many centers have replaced its use with automated platelet functional analyzers such as PFA-100™. The analyzers use either collagen/epinephrine or collagen/ADP to stimulate platelet adherence to block a small aperture, and this appears to be more reproducible than the Ivy bleeding time.

Initial evaluation includes measurement of VWF antigen (VWF:Ag), VWF activity by evaluating the ability to bind to platelet GP1b in the presence of ristocetin (VWF: Rco), factor VIII activity (VWF:VIIIc) and ABO blood type. The diagnosis of VWD is complex and may require serial evaluations of suspected patients and/or performing platelet aggregations. It is particularly difficult to diagnose individuals on hormone replacement therapy or during acute infections, as both of these factors increase the circulating VWF. Menstruating female patients have variation in their VWF levels during the menstrual cycle, with lowest levels day 1–4 and highest levels on day 9–10 of the menstrual cycle. Diagnosis of VWD is confirmed with a VWF:Rcof of <30%. Depending upon the subtype, the individuals may have a normal or decreased VWF:Ag. When the VWF:Rcof is 30–50%, individuals with a family history, abnormal multimeric analysis, or detectable VWF mutation have VWD. Other individuals are classified as low VWF and have a bleeding tendency, likely due to factors outside of the VWF gene that modulate activity or levels of VWF. Additional tests are performed in patients with confirmed VWD to classify their disease and determine therapeutic options (➋ *Table 335.7*).

Table 335.7
Phenotypic analysis of VWD

Test	Type	Measurement
VWF:Ag[a]	Initial	Antigen; quantity of protein
VWF:Rco[a]	Initial	Ristocetin cofactor activity; ability to bind platelet Gplb in the presence of ristocetin
FVIII:C[a]	Initial	FVIII coagulant activity
VWF:A[c]	Initial	Monoclonal antibody binding to a functional epitope of the A1 loop: immunoassay of Gplb binding
RIPA	Subtyping	Ability to aggregate platelets at varying doses of ristocetin. Aggregation at low doses of ~0.5 mg/ml indicates 2B VWD
VWF:FVIIIB[a]	Subtyping	FVIII binding capacity. Reduced values indicate 2N VWD
VWF:CB[a]	Subtyping	Collagen binding capacity. Reduced values correlate with reduction in HMW multimers
VWFpp[b]	Subtyping	Quantity of propeptide. Elevated VWFpp/VWF:Ag ratio indicates enhanced clearance rate from plasma
Multimer profile	Subtyping	Aberrant profiles can indicate reduction in dimerisation/multimerisation HMW multimer loss enhanced or reduced ADAMTS13 cleavage enhanced clearance and mutations that replace/ introduce cysteine residues affecting disulphide bonding

[a]Abbreviations recommended for VWF and its activities
[b]Abbreviations approved at ISTH-SSC on VWF 2009
Source: Goodeve AC (2010) Blood Reviews 24:123–134

Treatment of VWD

The goals of treatment of VWD are to prevent spontaneous bleeding, hasten hemostasis, or prevent postoperative bleeding. This can be achieved by administration of several different treatments. The first is DDAVP, to stimulate the release of VWF and factor VIII from tissue storage sites. The next is plasma-derived factor VIII concentrates rich in VWF. Currently not available in the USA are purified VWF and recombinant VWF.

Desmopressin: This agent is the first line of therapy for individuals with low von Willebrand, VWD types 1, 2a. Some patients with 2B, 2M, and 2N can also be treated with DDAVP. Pretesting is indicated for patients to determine response and to evaluate for degree of resultant thrombocytopenia in type 2b patients. Desmopressin is available for intravenous and intranasal administration. Dosing is identical to that for mild hemophilia. The intravenous dosing is 0.3 mcg/kg over 20–30 min in normal saline. The intranasal dosing is one puff (150 mcg) for patients <50 kg and two puffs (300 mcg) for those over 50 kg, similar to that of hemophilia A.

Plasma-derived products: Intermediate purity factor VIII/VWF virally inactivated factor VIII products are the treatment of choice for individuals with type 3 and most type 2B patients. Dosing is dependent upon the product and can be dosed in VWF:Rcof or factor VIII units. Products currently licensed in the USA for the treatment of VWD include Alphanate®, Humate-P®, and Wilate®. Koate-DVI is not currently licensed for use in VWD, but contains both factor VIII and VWF. Each of these products contains a different ratio of VWF:factor VIII. Dosing and products are not interchangeable. Only in emergent, life-threatening bleeding should cryoprecipitate (1 unit/5kg) be administered.

Purified VWF products: There are purified VWF products that are currently in clinical development. Initial studies of purified, plasma-derived products were limited by the need to either coinfuse factor VIII or allow 24 h for native factor VIII to bind to the VWF. A recombinant VWF product coexpressed with recombinant factor VIII is currently under development as well.

Recombinant factor VIII products: Most types of VWD cannot be treated with recombinant factor VIII products. The exception to this is severe type 3 patients. These patients are at increased risk for development of VWF inhibitors and are occasionally treated with recombinant factor VIII products.

Ancillary therapy: The antifibrinolytic agents described for the treatment of mucous membrane bleed in hemophilia, namely, EACA (Amicar®) or Tranexamic acid (Cyklocapron®), are also recommended in the management of mucous membrane bleeding in VWD.

References

Bajaj SP, Thompson AR (2006) Molecular and structural biology of factor IX. Chapter 7. In: Colman RW et al (eds) Hemostasis and thrombosis: basic principles and clinical practice, 5th edn. Lippincott-Raven, Philadelphia, pp 131–150

Bray GL, Luban NL (1987) Hemophilia presenting with intracranial hemorrhage. A approach to the infant with intracranial bleeding and coagulopathy. Am J Dis Child 141:1215–1217

Castaman G, Tosetto A, Goodeve A, Federici AB, Lethagen S, Budde U, Batlle J, Meyer D, Mazurier C, Goudemand J, Eikenboom J, Schneppenheim R, Ingerslev J, Habart D, Hill F, Peake I, Rodeghiero F (2010) The impact of bleeding history, von Willebrand factor and PFA-100(®) on the diagnosis of type 1 von Willebrand disease: results from the European study MCMDM-1VWD. Br J Haematol 151(3):245–251, Epub 25 Aug 2010

Collins PW, Blanchette VS, Fischer K, Björkman S, Oh M, Fritsch S, Schroth P, Spotts G, Astermark J, Ewenstein B, rAHF-PFM Study Group (2009) Break-through bleeding in relation to predicted factor VIII levels in patients receiving prophylactic treatment for severe hemophilia A. J Thromb Haemost 7(3):413–420

Coppola A, Di Minno MN, Santagostino E (2010) Optimizing management of immune tolerance induction in patients with severe haemophilia A and inhibitors: towards evidence-based approaches. Br J Haematol 150(5):515–528. Epub 22 June 2010

Darby SC, Keeling DM, Spooner RJ et al (2004) The incidence of factor VIII and factor IX inhibitors in the hemophilia population of the UK and their effect on subsequent mortality, 1977–99. J Thromb Haemost 2:1047–1054

DiMichele D (2007) Inhibitor development in haemophilia B: an orphan disease in need of attention. Br J Haematol 138(3):305–315

d'Oiron R, Pipe SW, Jacquemin M (2008) Mild/moderate haemophilia A: new insights into molecular mechanisms and inhibitor development. Haemophilia 14(Suppl 3):138–146

Fischer K, Van der Born JG, Molho P, Negrier C, Mauser Bunschoten EP, Roosendaal G, de Kleijn P, Grobbee DE, Van den Berg HM (2002) Prophylactic versus on demand treatment strategies for severe hemophilia: comparison of costs and long term outcome. Haemophilia 8:745–752

Gilbert MS (1993) Prophylaxis: musculoskeletal evaluation. Semin Hematol 3(Suppl 2):3–6

Gitschier J, Wood WI, Goralka TM, Wion KL, Chen EY, Eaton DH, Vehar GA, Capon DJ, Lawn RM (1984) Characterization of the human factor VIII gene. Nature 312(5992):326–330

Gomis M, Querol F, Gallach JE, González LM, Aznar JA (2009) Exercise and sport in the treatment of haemophilic patients: a systematic review. Haemophilia 15(1):43–54. Epub 21 Aug 2008

Goodeve AC (2010) The genetic basis of von Willebrand disease. Blood Rev 24(3):123–134. Epub 20 Apr 2010

Goodnight SH, Hathaway WE (eds) (2001) Disorders of hemostasis and thrombosis: a clinical guide, 2nd edn. McGraw-Hill, Lancaster, pp 115–161

Goralka TM et al (1984) Characterization of the human factor VIII gene. Nature 312:326–330

Hathaway W, Corrigan J (1991) Report of scientific and standardization subcommittee on neonatal hemostasis. Normal coagulation data for fetuses and newborn infants. Thromb Haemost 65(3):323–325

Hay CRN, Ludlam CA, Colvin BT et al (1998) Factor VIII inhibitors in mild and moderate severity haemophilia A. Thromb Haemost 79:762–766

Hopff f uber die Hemophilie oder die Erbiche. CW Becker, Wurzburg (1828)

Kaufman RJ, Antonarakis SE, Fay PJ (2006) Factor VIII and hemophilia A. In: Colman RW et al (eds) Hemostasis and thrombosis: basic principles and clinical practice, 5th edn. Lippincott-Raven, Philadelphia, pp 151–175

Kempton CL, White GC 2nd (2009) How we treat a hemophilia A patient with inhibitors. Blood 113(1):11–17

Kessler CM, Gill JC, White GC 2nd, Shapiro A, Arkin S, Roth DA, Meng X, Lusher JM (2005) B-domain deleted recombinant factor VIII preparations are bioequivalent to a monoclonal antibody purified plasma-derived factor VIII concentrate: a randomized, three-way crossover study. Haemophilia 11(2):84–91

Klintman J, Astermark J, Berntorp E (2010) Combination of FVIII and bypassing agent potentiates in vitro thrombin production in haemophilia A inhibitor plasma. Br J Haematol 151(4):381–386. Epub 1 Oct 2010

Kouides PA (2006) Aspects of the laboratory identification of von Willebrand disease in women. Semin Thromb Hemost 32(5):480–484

Kreuz W, Escuriola-Ettingshausen C, Funk M, Schmidt H, Kornhuber B (1998) When should prophylactic treatment in patients with hemophilia A and B start? – The German experience. Haemophilia 4:413–417

Kulkarni R (2004) Alternative and topical approaches to treating the massively bleeding patient. Clin Adv Hematol Oncol 2(7):428–431

Kurachi S, Huo JS, Ameri A, Zhang K, Yoshizawa AC, Kurachi K (2009) An age-related homeostasis mechanism is essential for spontaneous amelioration of hemophilia B Leyden. Proc Natl Acad Sci U S A 106(19):7921–7926. Epub 28 Apr 2009

Lannoy N, Hermans C (2010) The 'Royal Disease' haemophilia A or B? A Haemotologic mystery is finally solved. Haemophilia 16(6):843–847

Lavery S (2009) Preimplantation genetic diagnosis of haemophilia. Br J Haematol 144(3):303–307. Epub 22 Nov 2008

Ljung R, Petrini P, Nilsson IM (1990) Diagnostic symptoms of severe and moderate hemophilia A and B. A survey of 140 cases. Acta Paediatr Scand 79:196–200

Lofqvist T, Nilsson IM, Berntorp E, Pettersson H (1997) Haemophilia prophylaxis in young patients. J Intern Med 241:395–400

Manco-Johnson MJ, Abshire TC, Shapiro AD, Riske B, Hacker MR, Kilcoyne R, Ingram JD, Manco-Johnson ML, Funk S, Jacobson L, Valentino LA, Hoots WK, Buchanan GR, DiMichele D, Recht M, Brown D, Leissinger C, Bleak S, Cohen A, Mathew P, Matsunaga A, Medeiros D, Nugent D, Thomas GA, Thompson AA, McRedmond K, Soucie JM, Austin H, Evatt BL (2007) Prophylaxis versus episodic treatment to prevent joint disease in boys with severe hemophilia. N Engl J Med 357(6):535–544

Mauser Bunschoten EP, van Houwelingen JC, Sjamsoedin Visser EJ, van Dijken PJ, Kok AJ, Sixma JJ (1988) Bleeding symptoms in carriers of hemophilia A and B. Thromb Haemost 59(3):349–352

Metjian AD, Wang C, Sood SL, Cuker A, Peterson SM, Soucie JM, Konkle BA, HTCN Study Investigators (2009) Bleeding symptoms and laboratory correlation in patients with severe von Willebrand disease. Haemophilia 15(4):918–925. Epub 7 Apr 2009

Monahan PE, Liesner R, Sullivan ST, Ramirez ME, Kelly P, Roth DA (2010) Safety and efficacy of investigator-prescribed BeneFIX prophylaxis in children less than 6 years of age with severe haemophilia B. Haemophilia 16(3):460–468. Epub 4 Jan 2010

Oldenburg J, Pavlova A (2006) Genetic risk factors for inhibitors to factors VIII and IX. Haemophilia 12(Suppl 6):15–22

Orkin SH, Nathan DG, Ginsburg D, Look AT, Fisher DE, Lux SE (2009) Hematology of infancy and childhood, 7th edn. Saunders Elsevier, Philadelphia, pp 1487–1524

Patek AJ, Taylor FHL (1937) Hemophilia. II some properties of substances obtained from human plasma effective in acceleration coagulation of hemophiliac blood. J Clin Invest 16:113–124

Pergantou H, Matsinos G, Papdopoulos A, Platokouki H, Aronis S (2006) Comparative study of validity of clinical, xray, and magnetic resonance imaging scores in evaluation and management of haemophlic arthropathy in children. Haemophilia 12:241–247

Pipe S (2009) Visions in haemophilia care. Thromb Res 124(Suppl 2): S2–S5

Pipe SW, High KA, Ohashi K, Ural AU, Lillicrap D (2008) Progress in the molecular biology of inherited bleeding disorders. Haemophilia 14(Suppl 3):130–137

Plug I, Mauser-Bunschoten EP, Bröcker-Vriends AH, van Amstel HK, van der Bom JG, van Diemen-Homan JE, Willemse J, Rosendaal FR (2006a) Bleeding in carriers of hemophilia. Blood 108(1):52–56. Epub 21 Mar 2006

Plug I, Van Der Bom JG, Peters M, Mauser-Bunschoten EP, De Goede-Bolder A, Heijnen L, Smit C, Willemse J, Rosendaal FR (2006b) Mortality and causes of death in patients with hemophilia, 1992–2001: a prospective cohort study. J Thromb Haemost 4(3):510–516

Puetz J (2010) Optimal use of recombinant factor VIIa in the control of bleeding episodes in hemophilic patients. Drug Des Devel Ther 4:127–37

Ramgen O (1962) A clinical and medico-social study of haemophilia in Sweden. Acta Med Scand Suppl 379:111–190

Rodeghiero F, Castaman G, Tosetto A (2009) Optimizing treatment of von Willebrand disease by using phenotypic and molecular data. Hematology Am Soc Hematol Educ Prog 2009(1):113–123

Rosner F (1969) Hemophilia in the Talmud and rabbinic writings. Ann Intern Med 70:833–837

Sadler JE (2009) Low von Willebrand factor: sometimes a risk factor and sometimes a disease. Hematology Am Soc Hematol Educ Program 2009:106–112

Santagostino E, Mancuso ME (2008) Barriers to primary prophylaxis in haemophilic children: the issue of the venous access. Blood Transfus 6(Suppl 2):S12–S16

Schneider T (1976) Circumcision and "uncircumcision". S Afr Med J 50:556–558

Sharathkumar AA, Pipe SW (2008) Bleeding disorders. Pediatr Rev 29(4):121–129

Stobart K, Iorio A, Wu JK (2006) Clotting factor concentrates given to prevent bleeding and bleeding-related complications in people with hemophilia A or B. Cochrane Database Syst Rev 2:CD003429

Thompson AR (2003) Structure and function of the factor VIII gene and protein. Semin Thromb Hemost 29:11–22

Toole JJ, Knopf JL, Wozney JM et al (1984) Molecular cloning of tha cDNA encoding human antihemophilic factor. Nature 312:342–347

Verbruggen B, van Heerde WL, Laros-van Gorkom BA (2009) Improvements in factor VIII inhibitor detection: from Bethesda to Nijmegen. Semin Thromb Hemost 35(8):752–759. Epub 18 Feb 2010

Yoshitake S, Schach BG, Foster DC et al (1985) Nucleotide sequence of the gene for human factor IX (antihemophilic factor B). Biochemistry 24:3736–3750

336 Introduction to Hemostasis and Bleeding Disorders Other Than Hemophilia

Hassan M. Yaish · Eugenia Chang

► *Gone are the days of simply saying, "Pass the fresh frozen plasma; if something is missing, it is bound to be there."*

Hemostasis is defined as arrest of blood flow within or outside blood vessel. Thrombosis, on the other hand, indicates "the formation and propagation of blood clot in a vessel."

Thrombotic events were described by Virchow in 1856; he believed at the time that elements leading to the formation of thromboembolism in the veins are related to alterations in blood flow, blood vessels, and constitution of the blood. Even though such facts were individually known and have been described by others earlier, they were put together and came to be known as "Virchow's Triad."

What is currently known about the pathophysiology of thrombus formation is very similar to the description provided by Virchow. Slowing of blood flow by any means, damaging the endothelium of the blood vessels, or alteration in procoagulants or inhibitors component of the blood are the main activities leading to thrombotic events.

In the physiologic state, hemostasis is a balance between closely coordinated groups of plasma factors designed to keep the blood in a fluid state and yet capable of forming efficient clotting when blood vessels are damaged. These factors are categorized as *procoagulants* (clot promoting) *anticoagulant* proteins (clotting inhibitors), and *fibrinolytic* proteins (clot lysing). They interact with physiologic surfaces such as the platelets, vascular endothelium, and subendothelial matrix, all of which are known to promote the function of the various clotting factors.

The physiology of the hemostatic system in infancy and childhood is profoundly different from that in adults. It is a dynamic and constantly maturing system with multiple reference ranges that reflect both gestational and postnatal age. After the age of 6 months, however, adult reference ranges are usually used in children, with the exception of Protein C (PC), which remains lower until adolescence.

Physiology of Hemostasis

As a result of injury to the blood vessel endothelium, several events take place simultaneously, as the affected vessel constricts (vascular phase) and the homostatic process proceeds through four well-coordinated functional phases:

1. The *initiation* phase of "platelets plug formation," or the primary hemostatic phase
2. The *propagation* phase by the activated clotting factors leading to fibrin clot formation (the secondary or plasma phase)
3. The *termination* phase by the coagulation inhibitors
4. The *fibrinolytic* phase leading to clot lyses by the fibrinolytic system

Initiation Phase

In the *initiation* phase, the functional response of activated platelets at the site of injury includes four different phases:

1. *Adhesion* which involves the deposition of platelets on the damaged endothelium with the exposed collagen acting as strong platelets activator and the Von Willebrand's factor as adhesive to bridge the platelets to the endothelium
2. *Aggregation* which is the formation of platelets clump by platelet–platelet interaction utilizing fibrinogen as another adhesive protein in the plasma
3. *Release reaction* which is the secretion of various platelets chemicals and proteins (ADP, Thromboxane A2) from storage sites to aid in the process of plug formation (➋ *Fig. 336.1*)
4. *Procoagulant activity* (PF3) which contributes to thrombin generation

Abdelaziz Y. Elzouki (ed.), *Textbook of Clinical Pediatrics*, DOI 10.1007/978-3-642-02202-9_336,

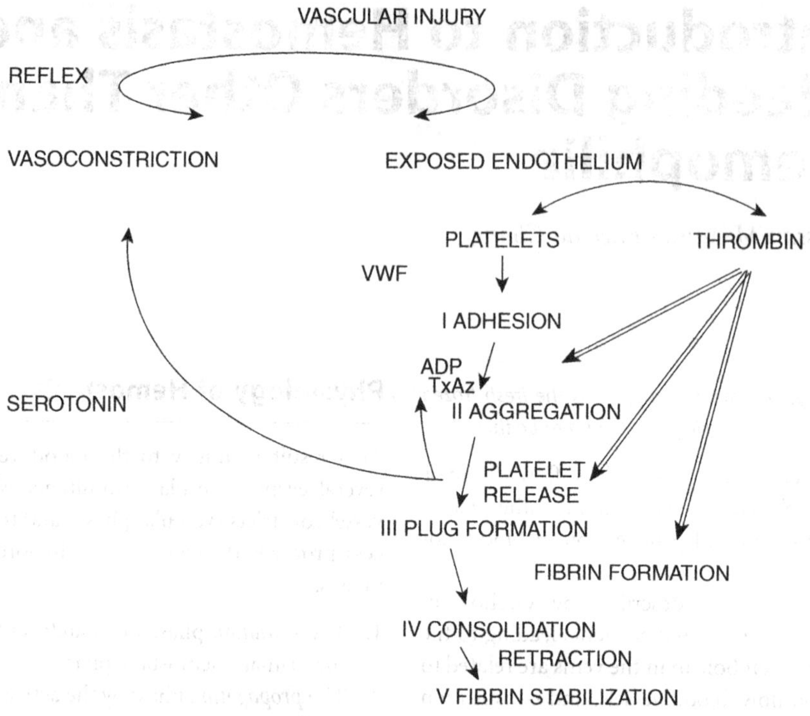

Figure 336.1
The formation of platelet plug (primary hemostatic mechanism)

Propagation Phase

Propagation phase results from a sequential activation of a series of zymogens (proenzymes) to active enzymes resulting in significant stepwise response amplification. This process represents the coagulation cascade which proceeds in three phases through one of two pathways, the *intrinsic* and the *extrinsic* pathways which were initially thought to be distinct and independent pathways. At the present time, however, it is known that they are closely interrelated and the extrinsic pathway is not actually intrinsic, since the tissue factor itself is now known to be present in the circulation and is the main element in the initiation of coagulation and not the intrinsic system as it was believed earlier. The formation of *multiple component macromolecular complexes* such as the intrinsic and extrinsic Tenases (X-ase) and the prothrombinase (*Fig. 336.2*), the first to activate FX and the second to activate FII in the process of thrombin generation), support the function of the various enzymes involved in the process of coagulation. Such complexes amplify the response in the various reactions significantly. For example, thrombin is generated from prothrombin through the prothrombinase complex 300,000 times more efficient than when produced from Prothrombin and Xa alone. The role of the platelets in providing surfaces for the various reactions and the role of its procoagulant function are very essential in the coagulation process. Patients with thrombocytopenia however do not exhibit the major bleeding manifestations that patients with clotting factors deficiencies show, unless the platelets counts are profoundly low. This suggests that small numbers of normal platelets is adequate for the clotting process.

The two traditional coagulation pathways are capable of producing *thromboplastin* in the initial phase, for the purpose of activating FX which activates FII into thrombin, which in turn carries out the last step of the coagulation cascade converting fibrinogen into fibrin to enforce and strengthen the platelet plug.

In the *intrinsic pathway* is activated by the exposure of the blood to the negatively charged surfaces (such as the Kaolin in vitro for measuring the aPTT). The *extrinsic pathway* on the other hand is activated by the Tissue factor (TF) exposure, or tissue factor–like material such as thromboplastin used in the in vitro process of measuring prothrombin time (PT). Activation of FX is the end result of both pathways that activates FII to FIIa or thrombin which in turn activates the soluble plasma fibrinogen to insoluble fibrin clot by splitting it into four small peptides

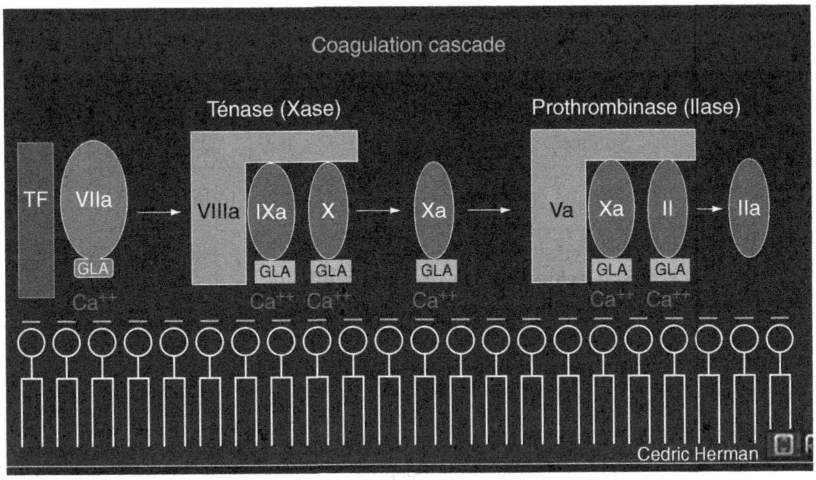

Figure 336.2
Macromolecular complexes for activation of FX (Tenase) and FII (II ase)

(two fibrinopeptide A and two fibrinopeptide B molecules). These fibrin monomers then polymerize spontaneously to form fibrin. Another one of the many functions of thrombin is activation of FXIII (fibrin stabilizing agent) to FXIIIa which in turn causes covalent bonding of the fibrin strands resulting in stable clot (➔ *Fig. 336.3*).

It is now known that the exposure of TF at the wound site and its interaction with FVIIa is the primary physiologic event in initiating the clotting process. Only a small amount of thrombin is generated in this reaction which is capable of priming the clotting cascade, activating platelets and components of the intrinsic pathway (FVIII, FIX, FXI) which will be responsible for the amplification and the bulk generation of thrombin in the propagation phase. This interpretation of the clotting process is supported by the fact that deficiencies in FXII, HK, and PK (members of the contact factors) do not cause any bleeding disorder. Deficiency of FXI (contact factor), however, may be associated with mild bleeding symptoms. It is clear now that the classical classification of the clotting pathways into intrinsic and extrinsic (even though useful for interpretation of the clotting tests) is not physiologically accurate as was indicated earlier. The term "extrinsic" was initially introduced to indicate that TF is present only in tissues extrinsic to circulation. It is known now that TF is present in the circulation. Furthermore, the separation of the two pathways is also theoretical, since they clearly interact together. Finally, the major role of thrombin in sustaining the clotting process through a feedback mechanism is recognized (➔ *Fig. 336.3*).

Termination Phase

The two main circulating enzymatic inhibitors are involved in this process, the antithrombin (AT), (previously antithrombin III), and the tissue factor pathway inhibitor (TFPI). In addition a clotting-initiated inhibitory process, the protein C pathway (PC), and other platelets and vascular modulators such as prostacyclin, thromboxane A2, and nitric oxide (NO) are also involved in the termination phase (➔ *Fig. 336.4*). In the newborn and young infants, AT, PC, and PS are deficient which explain in part the high incidence of thrombotic events in this age group. Thrombin which is known to be a major procoagulant now plays a different role in the termination phase. Once it is bound to thrombomodulin and AT, it creates a conformational change which activates PC, forming another multiple macromolecular complex, of inhibitory nature, and no longer activates platelets or cleaves fibrinogen (➔ *Fig. 336.5*). FVa and FVIIIa are cleaved by this complex, thus Tenase and Prothrombinase are inhibited. TFPI, an enzymatic inhibitor which circulates in the plasma (20%) and on endothelial surfaces (80%), inhibits FXa, directly and could form complex with such factor to inhibit TF/FVIIa. The level of this inhibitor increases significantly in plasma after parenteral administration of heparin, a phenomena that explains the effective anticoagulation effect of LMW heparin despite its weak antithrombin activity. The role of prostacyclin and thromboxane A2 in the termination phase is mainly by blocking platelet activation which is discussed under the topic of Platelets.

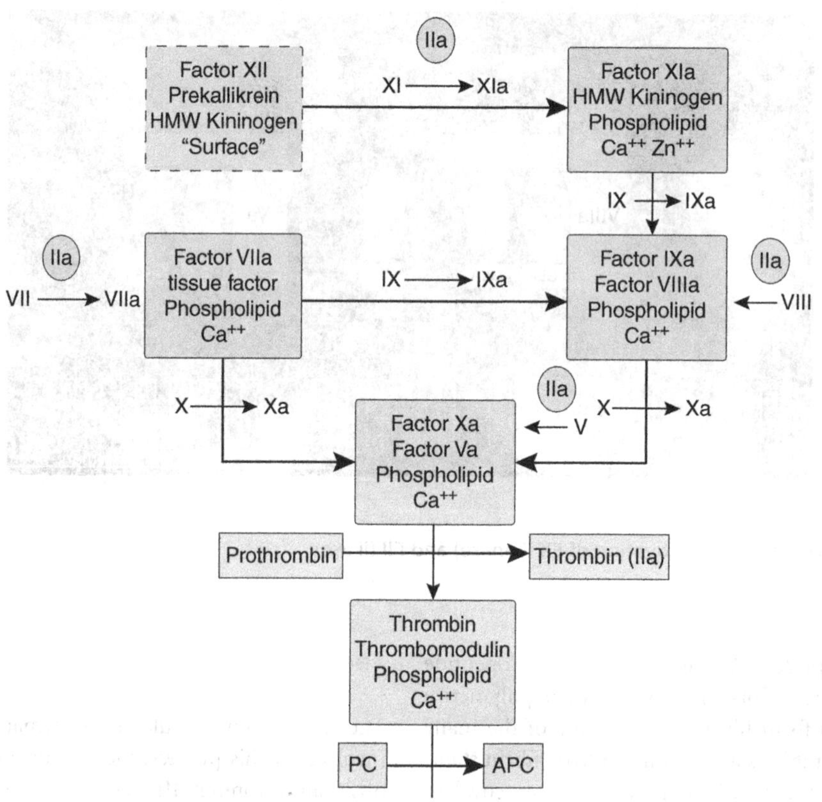

■ Figure 336.3

The revised coagulation cascade showing the role of TF in initiating the clotting system The interaction between the intrinsic and the extrinsic pathways. And the feed back mechanism of the Thrombin (IIa) in mediating various reactions

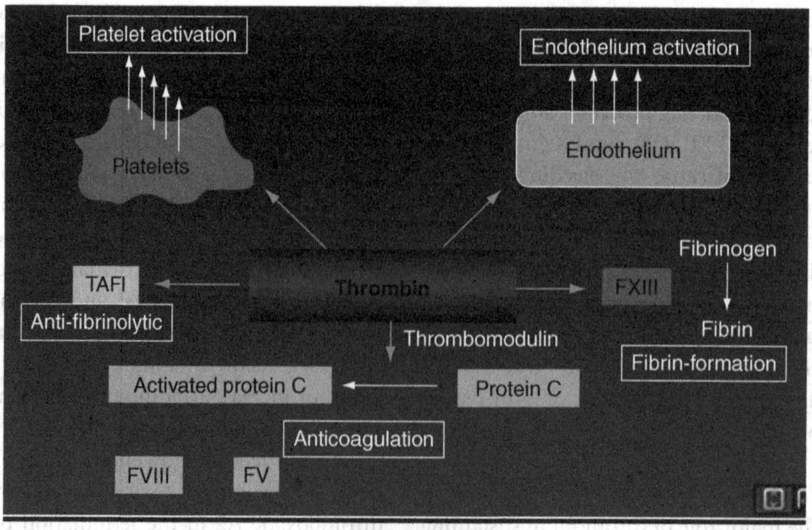

■ Figure 336.4

Thrombin multiple thrombotic and antithrombotic functions

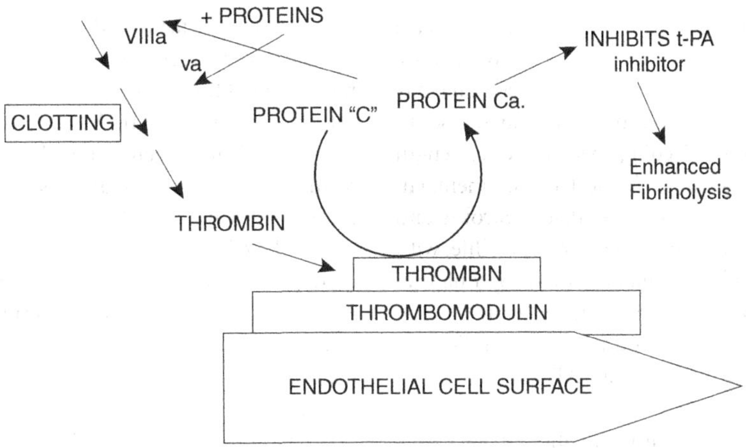

Figure 336.5
Protein C/protein S pathway

Clot Termination and Fibrinolysis

The residual clot in this stage lyses by the activation of plasminogen to plasmin, a process mediated by the intravascular activator tPA. Urokinase on the other hand is the major activator of plasminogen in the extravascular compartment. Plasmin cleaves fibrin, fibrinogen, and other proteins and clotting factors. It cleaves the polymerized fibrin strands at multiple sites resulting in the production of fibrin degradation products (FDP), one of such products is the D-Dimers which represent monomers that have been cross-linked by FXIIIa. Plasmin activator inhibitor (PAI) and alpha-2 anti-plasmin are inhibitors of the fibrinolytic process, the first is an anti-tPA and the second inhibits plasmin. They prevent the process of over fibrinolysis and if deficient, some thrombotic disorders may develop.

Evaluation of the Patient with a Suspected Hemostatic Defect

History and Physical Examination

It is said that the medical history in the patient with suspected bleeding or thrombotic disorder, when done effectively, is the most sensitive "test" for such disorders. The history and the physical examination should focus on (a) whether the suspected defect is hereditary or acquired, and (b) whether it is related to a primary or secondary hemostatic mechanism defect. The first is usually determined by the finding of documented bleeding disorders in family members or manifestations highly suggestive of such disorders. The second requires determination of the site and the nature of the bleeding manifestations. Mucous membrane bleeds (epistaxis, menorrhagia, hematuria, or gastrointestinal bleeds), petechiae of the skin, and multiple small ecchymoses are all characteristic of the defect in the primary hemostatic mechanism in patients with quantitative or qualitative platelet disorders or blood vessel abnormalities. Patients with a defective secondary hemostatic mechanism (coagulation system) usually present with joint and deep muscle bleeds, hematomas, and large spreading ecchymotic lesions. A combination of both manifestations may be encountered in the occasional patient with severe von Willebrand disease (VWD). It is also important to evaluate the severity and duration of the bleed, whether it was spontaneous or induced, and what was required to control it.

Previous surgical procedures should be reviewed. Tooth extraction, tonsillectomy, and circumcision are of particular value, even though the absence of bleed after this last procedure does not exclude a coagulation defect. The age of onset of the bleeding or thrombotic episode may give a clue to the diagnosis. A history of poor wound healing or delayed umbilical cord stump separation may suggest factor XIII deficiency. Epistaxis, a frequent manifestation of coagulation defect in the child, should be evaluated carefully. Several other conditions are known to cause epistaxis and should be considered. Epistaxis in the teenager has more significance than in the younger child. Epistaxis episodes occurring in clusters during a respiratory infection or in certain seasons are less likely to represent a coagulation problem, unlike epistaxis that causes anemia or requires cautery. Drug history is also significant in both determining the cause of the bleed and interpreting an abnormal coagulation test (e.g., bleeding time (BT) or platelet function tests after NSAID drugs ingestion). Evaluation of the adolescent with menorrhagia also requires certain skills in determining the significance of the symptom. Young women going into menarche may not know what is normal. It is important in such cases to quantitate the amount of bleeding (pads per day), length of bleeding in days, and timing of cycle. Chronic anemia in such patients may indicate a clotting defect. Strokes and thrombosis are most common at the extremes of life, with preterm infants and elderly adults each having a natural predisposition to thrombosis. The occurrence of stroke in a child beyond the neonatal period is often an indication of inherited thrombophilia such as AT, protein C, or protein S deficiency.

In addition to the previously mentioned elements, physical examination should include looking for loose skin (hyperelasticity) and hyperflexibility of the joints. Telangiectasia should also be sought on skin and mucous membranes. Both conditions may give clues to the presence of a systemic disease known to be associated with a hemostatic defect.

Laboratory Evaluation

The laboratory evaluation of children of all ages presenting with bleeding complications should include a prothrombin time (PT), activated partial thromboplastin time (aPTT), BT (or PFA if indicated), thrombin time (TT), and fibrinogen level. One should remember, however, that the laboratory evaluation is not conclusive in many hemorrhagic conditions and may even be in the normal range in the presence of a bleeding disorder that requires a completely different set of tests. For this reason, the importance of a careful history and good physical examination in directing the clinician to an appropriate laboratory evaluation cannot be overemphasized. It is also important to know the normal values for each of the tests performed in relation to the patient's age, since many of the coagulation factors do not reach adult values until the child is 6 months of age or older.

Prothrombin Time

This test measures phase II of coagulation or, more precisely, the function of the extrinsic pathway. The test is performed by adding exogenous thromboplastin (tissue factor) and calcium to the patient's plasma. Thromboplastin complexes with factor VIIa to activate the extrinsic pathway clotting system. The test is most sensitive to deficiencies of factors at the initiation of the extrinsic pathway, such as factor VII and factor X. It is less sensitive to deficiencies of prothrombin itself. The normal values range from 11.5 to 14 S. This test does not measure the activities of factors XII, XI, IX, VIII, or XIII. Since the thrombopalstin reagent differs by the lab and the manufacturer, and so the instruments used in different laboratories to measure the PT, one expects the sensitivity of the test to the effect of Wafarin (for which the test is usually used) to vary as well. For this reason, the INR (International Normalized Ratio), a derivative of the PT was introduced to correct this deficiency and to standardize the test. The INR is calculated by dividing the patient's PT by the control PT (the midpoint of the normal range for that lab) multiplied by the ISI (International Sensitivity Index); this value is provided by the manufacturer based on the sensitivity of their reagent to the effect of Warfarin. If the reagent is less sensitive, the ISI will have a greater value. The INR should not be utilized for evaluation of liver functions, since it is calibrated with plasma from individuals on Warfarin and thus its sensitivity to factor deficiencies related to liver disease cannot be predicted.

Activated Partial Thromboplastin Time

This test measures the time required for the clotting of plasma that has been activated by incubation with an inert activator (kaolin, celite, etc.) when calcium and platelets (or lipid substitute for platelets) are added. In this process, thromboplastin is formed internally (intrinsic system) by activation of the clotting factors. Unlike in the PT testing procedure, thromboplastin is not added in this test, therefore, it is described as "partial." The test therefore measures the function of the intrinsic pathway, and it is most sensitive to deficiencies of factors at the initiation of the intrinsic pathway, such as factor XII, Fletcher factor (prekallikrein), and Fitzgerald factor (HMW kininogen). These three factors, when deficient, give the longest partial thromboplastin times (PTTs), despite the fact that they are not associated with any bleeding disorder. The sensitivity of the PTT reagents is variable, and the normal value should be established for each of the PTT reagents in each laboratory. The variation of sensitivity can be appreciated when a PTT is found to be normal with factor IX as low as 10–13% or prolonged in patients with a factor VIII level of 60% (normal range). The optimal PTT, however, should be prolonged when factor VIII or factor IX is below 30–40% of normal (➋ *Table 336.1*).

The PTT measures factors XII, XI, IX, and VIII. It does not measure factors VII or XIII. In both the PT and the PTT, a prolonged value may indicate a relevant factor

Table 336.1
The clotting factors

Factors	Common name	Biologic half-life(h)	Plasma level
I	Fibrinogen	90	200–400
II	Prothrombin	60	50–150
III	Total thromboplastin	?	0
IV	Calcium		
V	Labile factor	12–36	50–150
VI	Activated labile factor	Part of V	
VII	Stable factor	6–8	50–150
VIII	Antihemophilic factor	8–12	50–150
IX	Christmas factor	12–24	50–150
VWF	Von Willebrand factor	8–12	50–150
X	Stuart factor	32–58	50–150
XI	Plasma thromboplastin antecedent	48–72	50–150
XII	Hageman factor	48–52	50–150
XIII	Fibrin-stabilizing factor	72–120	50–150
High-molecular-weight kininogen	Fitzgerald factor	136	
Prekallikrein	Fletcher factor		

deficiency or the presence of an inhibitor. To determine which condition is present, an inhibitor mix is performed where equal amounts of the patient's and normal plasmas are mixed and a PTT is performed. A normal PTT indicates a factor deficiency, while lack of correction indicates the presence of inhibitor; a low inhibitor titer could be misdiagnosed as deficiency since the mixing study could correct a weak titer, which usually neutralizes the factor activity present in the normal plasma. Should a bleeding tendency exist in addition to the prolonged PTT, then the inhibitor is probably directed against factor VIII, IX, or XI. If no bleeding manifestations are present, the inhibitor is probably of the "lupus anticoagulant" type.

Heparin Anti-Xa

The heparin anti-Xa test is listed here not as a diagnostic test for patients with bleeding disorders, but for the sake of comparison with aPTT test when used for monitoring of anticoagulation therapy with heparin. This test is becoming available in almost all centers, and has gained grounds in replacing aPTT for monitoring UH therapy, in addition to monitoring the treatment with LMW heparin. The many shortcomings of aPTT for monitoring UH treatment make this test a very attractive alternative. It is basically the same test used to derive the therapeutic range for aPTT each time a new reagent is used. It is an ideal test for patients with heparin resistance, and for monitoring UH therapy in the newborn whose base line aPTT is already prolonged. The test is not affected by tube under fill, elevated FVIII or FI due to inflammation, or factors deficiency except for AT.

Bleeding Time

The bleeding time is currently underutilized or unavailable in many laboratories for various reasons, even though a quick, relatively not expensive, and noninvasive test to replace it is not available. The most commonly used method for measuring the BT is the modified Ivy method. An incision is made on the volar surface of the forearm using a standardized template that controls the depth and the length of the incision while a blood pressure cuff is applied to the arm and inflated to 20–40 mmHg. At 30-s intervals, drops of blood are blotted from the margin of the incision. Normally, blood flow stops at 4–8 min. Despite all efforts to standardize this test, a high degree of variability continues to exist. Therefore, it is usually advantageous, whenever possible, to have a technologist in the laboratory to perform this test at all times. This test is not perfect, and it has a high degree of variability and poor sensitivity, yet for lack of alternative tests, it continues to be the best screening test available for assessing the vascular and platelet phases of hemostasis. Bleeding times are prolonged in the presence of thrombocytopenia, thrombocytopathy, connective tissue diseases (Ehlers-Danlos syndrome), and some cases of VWD.

Thrombin Time

This test evaluates phase III of the coagulation cascade. It measures the time required for plasma to clot after the addition of thrombin (factor IIa), which converts fibrinogen to fibrin. The normal TT is 15–20 s. It is prolonged by heparin, fibrin split products, uremia, decreased fibrinogen, or dysfibrinogenemia. In the presence of heparin, the TT can be performed by adding snake venom (reptilase) instead of thrombin, since this agent is not usually affected by heparin. Other coagulation tests are more specific for certain hemostatic processes. Euglobulin clot lysis time (ELT), for instance, is a crude test designed to measure the fibrinolytic activity. It is performed by using acetic acid to precipitate a euglobulin fraction of the plasma. This fraction is then clotted with thrombin or calcium. The time required for the clot to lyse is then measured (usually 2–4 h). A long ELT may be related to a low plasminogen level, reduced activator, or an extremely increased level of fibrinogen. A short ELT, however, indicates increased activators and/or reduced fibrinogen. Plasminogen, plasminogen activators, and inhibitor assays, as well as assays for fibrin degradation products (FDPs) are other tests for the assessment of the fibrinolytic system.

The marked differences in the various clotting factor levels between newborns and older children and adults make it necessary to discuss the neonatal coagulation system separately. ➋ *Table 336.2* shows reference values for coagulation tests in the healthy full-term infant during the first 6 months of life compared to adult values. The striking differences at this stage in life include a prolonged PT, mostly related to the low level of vitamin K–dependent factors; a prolonged PTT, attributed to low levels of the four contact factors (XI, XII, prekallikrein, and HMW kininogen); a BT that is slightly short; and a prolonged TT, which is probably related to the presence of the "fetal" type of fibrinogen at this age. Factors V and VIII, Von Willebrand Factor (VWF), and fibrinogen are not decreased at birth and might actually be elevated. The inhibitors levels are either elevated or low; AT, protein C, and protein S are all low at birth; and other inhibitors are usually higher than adult levels. As for fibrinolysis in the newborn, plasminogen and α_2-antiplasmin are decreased while tissue plasminogen activator (tPA) and PAI are twice the adult values (➋ *Table 336.3*).

Platelet Counts

The platelet component of hemostasis is less difficult to evaluate. Both its quantitative and qualitative aspects can be measured. Thrombocytopenia in infants and children, including premature babies, is defined as it is in adults: a platelet count of less than 150×10^9/L. There is a linear relationship between platelet counts and the BT – the

Table 336.2

Normal coagulation values in the healthy full-term infant during the first 6 months of life[a]

Test	Day 1	Day 5	Day 30	Day 90	Day 180	Adult
PT (s)	13.0(10.1–15.9)[b]	12.4(10.0–15.3)[b]	11.8(10.0–14.3)[b]	11.9(10.0–14.2)[b]	12.3(10.7–13.9)[b]	12.4(10.8–13.9)
INR	1.00(0.53–1.62)	0.89(0.53–1.48)	0.79(0.53–1.26)	0.81(0.53–1.26)	0.88(0.61–1.17)	0.89(0.64–1.17)
APTT (s)	42.9(31.3–54.3)	42.6(25.4–59.8)	40.4(32.0–55.2)	37.1(29.0–50.1)[b]	35.5(28.1–42.9)[b]	33.5(26.6–40.3)
TCT (s)	23.5(19.0–28.3)[b]	23.1(18.0–29.2)	24.3(19.4–29.2)	25.1(20.5–29.7)[b]	25.5(19.8–31.2)[b]	25.0(19.7–30.3)
Fibrinogen (g/L)	2.83(1.67–3.99)[b]	3.12(1.62–4.62)[b]	2.70(1.62–3.78)[b]	2.43(1.50–3.79)[b]	2.51(1.50–3.87)[b]	2.78(1.56–4.00)
II	0.48(0.26–0.70)	0.63(0.33–0.93)	0.68(0.34–1.02)	0.75(0.45–1.05)	0.88(0.60–1.12)	1.08(0.70–1.46)
V	0.72(0.34–1.08)	0.95(0.45–1.45)	0.98(0.62–1.34)	0.90(0.48–1.32)	0.91(0.55–1.27)	1.06(0.62–1.50)
VII	0.66(0.28–1.04)	0.89(0.35–1.43)	0.90(0.42–1.38)	0.91(0.39–1.43)	0.87(0.47–1.27)	1.05(0.67–1.43)
VIII	1.00(0.50–1.78)[b]	0.88(0.50–1.54)[b]	0.91(0.50–1.57)[b]	0.79(0.50–1.25)[b]	0.73(0.50–1.09)	0.99(0.50–1.49)
vWf	1.53(0.50–2.87)	1.40(0.50–2.54)	1.28(0.50–2.46)	1.18(0.50–2.06)	1.07(0.50–1.97)	0.92(0.50–1.58)
IX	0.53(0.15–0.91)	0.53(0.15–0.91)	0.51(0.21–0.81)	0.67(0.21–1.13)	0.86(0.36–1.36)	1.09(0.55–1.63)
X	0.40(0.12–0.68)	0.49(0.19–0.79)	0.59(0.31–0.87)	0.71(0.35–1.07)	0.78(0.38–1.18)	1.06(0.70–1.52)
XI	0.38(0.10–0.66)	0.55(0.23–0.87)	0.53(0.27–0.79)	0.69(0.41–0.97)	0.86(0.49–1.34)	0.97(0.67–1.27)
XII	0.53(0.13–0.93)	0.47(0.11–0.83)	0.49(0.17–0.81)	0.67(0.25–1.09)	0.77(0.39–1.15)	1.08(0.52–1.64)
PK	0.37(0.18–0.69)	0.48(0.20–0.76)	0.57(0.23–0.91)	0.73(0.41–1.05)	0.86(0.56–1.16)	1.12(0.62–1.62)
HK	0.54(0.06–1.02)	0.74(0.16–1.32)	0.77(0.33–1.21)	0.82(0.30–1.46)[b]	0.82(0.36–1.28)[b]	0.92(0.50–1.36)
XIIIa	0.79(0.27–1.31)	0.94(0.44–1.44)[b]	0.93(0.39–1.47)[b]	1.04(0.36–1.72)[b]	1.04(0.46–1.62)[b]	1.05(0.55–1.55)
XIIIb	0.76(0.30–1.22)	1.06(0.32–1.80)	1.11(0.39–1.73)[b]	1.16(0.48–1.84)[b]	1.10(0.50–1.70)[b]	0.97(0.57–1.37)

[a]Values are expressed as means followed by lower and upper normals in 95% of the population
[b]Values similar to those in adults

Table 336.3
Hemostatic mechanisms of the newborn compared to older children and adults

Hemostatic mechanism	Typical values versus adults
Coagulation Factors	
Fibrinogen	Normal limit
Factors II, VII, IX, X	Very low
Factors VIII, VWF	Normal to increased
Factors XI, XII, high-molecular-weight kininogen	Slightly low–low normal
Prekallikrein	
Factors V and XIII	Low normal
Inhibitors	
Antithrombin III	Low
Proteins C and S	Low
Heparin cofactor II	Low
α_2-Macroglobulin	High
α_1-Antitrypsin	Normal
Fibrinolytic components	
Plasminogen	Low
Plasminogen activators	High
Plasminogen activator inhibitors	Normal/high
Plasmin inhibitors	Low

lower the platelet count, the more prolonged the BT. The etiology of thrombocytopenia, however, plays a role in this relation. Patients whose thrombocytopenia is due to lack of marrow production of platelets, as in aplastic anemia or leukemia, may reveal prolonged BTs at a platelet count of 80,000/μL or lower. In consumptive thrombocytopenias (e.g., idiopathic thrombocytopenic purpura), however, the BT will remain normal until the platelet count drops below 30,000–40,000/μL. If the BT is disproportionate to the platelet count, a qualitative platelet defect, VWD, or a vascular defect should be suspected. Ingestion of anti-inflammatory agents, including aspirin, may prolong the BT; therefore, such testing should be delayed for a minimum of 1 week after the drug ingestion.

Platelet Function Tests

These studies delineate the functional abnormalities of the platelet. One test is based on the increase in light transmittance of a platelet suspension when a platelet activator is added to the suspension. This increase in light transmittance is recorded on a chart for interpretation. Various disorders of platelet function have specific aggregation pattern. Release of platelet-specific proteins (platelet factor 4 and platelet factor 3) is one of the other studies that may be performed to delineate platelet participation in the secondary hemostatic mechanism.

Platelet Function Analyzer-100

(PFA-100) is a relatively new, rapid, and simple in vitro test for the evaluation of platelet function. Some clinicians hoped that the test will be able to replace the vanishing bleeding time (BT), and decrease the need for the traditional, more complicated, and demanding platelet aggregation testing with various agonists. The test is based on simulating the in vivo hemostatic plug formation and is initiated by aspiration of a citrated whole blood sample at high shear rate through a 150 μm aperture in a membrane coated with collagen and epinephrine (CEPI) or collagen and ADP (CADP). Mediated by VWF, platelets adhere to the collagen on the membrane causing them to aggregate in and around the aperture which results in closure of the aperture and arrest of blood flow. The time in seconds needed to reach this point is called "the closure time." Several pre-analytic variables were found to interfere with the test results including: a low level of VWF in the plasma, the high concentration of the citrate in the specimen, an O blood group, low platelet counts or low hematocrit, as well as ingestion of drugs which may affect platelet function such as NSAIDs. All could prolong the closure time giving the impression of a platelet function defect. PFA-100 is now commonly used in clinical practice for the purpose of screening for platelet defects. In our experience, the test is frequently abnormal in many patients with VWD especially those with significantly low VWF.

Congenital Coagulation Disorders

Phase I Disorders: The Hemophilias

The hemophilias are the most common severe inherited bleeding disorders of children and adults. Probably originally named hemorrhaphilia, the disorder was referred to as hemophilia by Schönlein in the early 1800s. Its sex-linked inheritance was recognized 50 years before the Mendelian principles of genetics were introduced. Legg further distinguished hemophilia from other known bleeding disorders on the basis of clinical symptoms, i.e., a congenital tendency to bleed into joints and muscles. It was not until 1920 that the etiology of hemophilia was attributed to a defect in blood clotting rather than gout or tuberculosis. In the 1940s and 1950s, coagulation factors VIII and IX were identified: the first as the deficient factor in hemophilia A (classic hemophilia) and the second as the deficient protein in hemophilia B (Christmas disease). In the 1970s, factor VIII was isolated from its carrier protein in the plasma, VWF, which has helped to distinguish two previously confused bleeding disorders, hemophilia A and VWD. Since both hemophilia A and B are indistinguishable clinically, they are discussed together in the chapter on bleeding disorders in hemophilia. VWD will also be discussed in that chapter. Hemophilia C, a significantly less common type of hemophilia resulting from deficiency of factor XI, is discussed separately.

Disorders of the Second Phase of Coagulation

The factors that might be involved in this phase are factor II (prothrombin), factor V, factor VII, and factor X. All are produced in the liver, and, with the exception of factor V, they all require vitamin K for their synthesis. Together with factor IX (which is also vitamin K dependent), they are called the "prothrombin complex factors." Vitamin K is needed for the Y-carboxylation of glutamic acid residues, which converts the inactive precursors into active forms. These precursors are described as protein induced by vitamin K absence (PIVKA). The precursor protein for factor II, for instance, is called PIVKA-II.

Factor II (Prothrombin) Deficiency

Quick reported the first case of prothrombin deficiency and, fewer than 100 cases were reported so far. The condition is of autosomal recessive inheritance and could be homozygous, heterozygous, or compound heterozygous. In the first and the third conditions, the activity level may range from <1% to 20% based on the variants reported. This level is about 50% in the heterozygous. The antigen however is usually normal in almost all cases, suggesting a dysprothrombinemia. Heterozygous are usually asymptomatic while homozygous patients present with easy bruising, epistaxis, menorrhagia, and, rarely, joint bleeds. The PT is usually prolonged in the presence of normal TT, and the diagnosis is confirmed by measuring the functional level of the factor. FFP was the treatment of choice for significant bleed (half-life of FII is 3 days). Prothrombin complex concentrates (PCCs) could be used in severe cases after the prothrombin content of that particular brand is checked.

Factor V Deficiency: Owren's Disease

This is a very rare condition with an incidence of one in a million. It is inherited as autosomal recessive and in the severe form (<1% level) is associated with umbilical stump bleed, easy bruising, epistaxis, and menorrhagia. Facor V was previously known as the labile factor since it is not stable in the plasma. Unlike FVIII and IX deficiency, spontaneous Joint bleeds are very unusual. The severity is frequently attributed to the deficient FV in the platelets. Both PT and PTT are prolonged, with normal TCT. FFP (less than 2–3 months old) is the treatment of choice for significant bleed (half-life is 36 h), with local and antifibrinolytic agents for the mild bleed. Platelet transfusion could be considered in the very rare situation of severe nonresponding bleed.

Factor VII Deficiency

The incidence of this deficiency is about 1:500,000. It has a similar mode of inheritance (AR) like the other factors described earlier. The level does not correlate well with the bleeding manifestations in many cases due to the fact that it depends on the reagent used in measuring the factor level. Human tissue factor gives more accurate values which correlate more with the clinical symptoms. This could explain why some patients with <1% level have no bleeding manifestations while others manifest severe disease with hemophilia A and B–like symptoms including hemarthrosis and ICH. The PT is prolonged with normal PTT and TCT. A level of 5–10% is adequate for hemostasis in mild bleed and 15–25% for surgery. Since half-life of FVII is very short (3–4 h), FFP is not practical for treatment. PCCs or recombinant VIIa are usually used.

Factor X Deficiency

This is another rare inherited coagulation factor deficiency with an incidence of 1:500,000. Bleeding manifestations seem to correlate well with the level of the factor. They range from mild to very severe with hemophilia-like symptoms including severe hemarthrosis. Both PT and PTT are prolonged, and so the Russell's viper venum time (measures direct activation of FX). Patients with amyloidosis may have an associated FX deficiency which is difficult to manage due to the shortened half-life in this disease. FFP and PCCs products are used for treatment of bleeds in FX deficiency. A level of 10–15% is usually adequate. Since half-life is about 40 h, the patients could be managed with FFP.

Factor XI Deficiency (Hemophilia C)

In the individual homozygous for factor XII deficiency, a marked prolongation of the PTT is usually encountered without any evidence of bleeding tendency. Similar findings are encountered with deficiencies of two other contact factors. The prekallikrien (Fletcher) factor and the HMW kininogen (Fitzgerald) factor both result in prolonged PTTs without any bleeding tendency.

Factor XII Deficiency (Hageman Factor)

The deficiency of factor XII is not associated with bleeding and does not require any treatment. The PTT is usually very long in the homozygous (>100 s). Adults with FXII deficiency were reported to have tendency for thrombosis, spontaneous abortion, myocardial infarction, and pulmonary embolism.

Factor XIII Deficiency (Fibrin Stabilizing Factor)

Since this deficiency was first described in 1960, 200 proved cases were reported. The condition is extremely rare and estimated at one in several millions. The protein is present in the plasma as well as the platelets (50% of body total FXIII activity). The condition could be suspected in a bleeder when all coagulation tests are normal. The bleeding manifestations start very early in life with umbilical stump hemorrhage in 80% of the cases. Poor wound healing, bleeding after circumcision, and gum bleed during teething. Females develop recurrent spontaneous abortions, and males develop oligospermia and infertility. ICH could occur in as many as 30% of the cases and is the leading cause of death in this deficiency. The diagnosis is made by clot solubility in urea or by factor level measurement. Only low level of this factor is needed for hemostasis (5%), and since half-life is 9–10 days, prophylactic therapy to prevent intracranial bleed is effective. FFP or cryoprecipitate every 4–6 weeks or, FXIII concentrate by IV infusion every 5–6 weeks will be adequate.

Disorders of the Third Phase of Coagulation

The inherited disorders of fibrinogen (α-fibrinogenemia, hypofibrinogenemia, and dysfibrinogenemia) may present in the homozygous newborn with a clinical picture of delayed umbilical cord bleeds (similar to factor XIII deficiency). Heterozygous newborns are usually asymptomatic except after major challenge. Cryoprecipitate provides effective therapy. Each bag contains 200–250 mg of fibrinogen; 100-mg/kg infusions provide adequate hemostatic levels. Frequent infusions are not necessary since the half-life of fibrinogen is 3–5 days. In dysfibrinogenemia, the fibrinogen level is usually normal despite bleeding manifestations and prolonged TT. This disorder is usually inherited as an autosomal dominant trait.

Aquired Coagulation Disorders

Vitamin K Deficiency

Neonatal vitamin K deficiency (hemorrhagic disease of the newborn) is discussed somewhere else in this text; therefore, only postnatal vitamin K deficiency is presented here. Late manifestations of vitamin K deficiency are reported more frequently in breast-fed infants (low vitamin K in breast milk) and infants with chronic diarrhea, fat malabsorption (celiac disease, systic fibrosis), biliary atresia, hepatitis, and α_1-antitrypsin deficiency. Infants and children on chronic broad-spectrum antibiotics are also susceptible to vitamin K–deficiency hemorrhagic complications. Prophylactic oral administration of water-soluble vitamin K to such infants is indicated (2–3 mg/day for children and 5–10 mg/day for adolescents and adults). In advanced liver disease, the production of the precursor proteins is defective, so vitamin K supplementation is not expected to be of any value. Prolonged PTs and PTTs are the only abnormal coagulation findings. Factor assays may delineate the nature of the problem.

Liver Disease and Liver Transplant

As many as 85% of children with significant liver disease manifest coagulation abnormalities that are directly proportional to the severity of the liver condition. About 15% of such patients manifest significant clinical hemorrhagic disorders. Decreased synthesis of clotting proteins is the major contributing factor, even though other factors, such as poor clearance of the products of hemostasis, activation of the clotting and fibrinolytic systems, and loss of clotting factors into ascitic fluid, may also be involved. Fulminant liver disease in both newborns and older children may result from viral hepatitis, hypoxia, and shock. Treatment involves replacement therapy. FFP contains all the coagulation factors except fibrinogen, which is provided by cryoprecipitate. Lethal hepatic disorders have been treated with liver transplant since the mid-1980s. Survival rates for such children are on the order of 80%. Two major causes of morbidity and mortality in such patients are intraoperative bleeding and postoperative vascular thrombotic events in the transplanted vessels (portal vein and hepatic artery). This second complication is significantly more common in infants less than 1 year of age (20–25%) than in adults (3–5%).

The incidence is also related to the quality of the graft. Damaged blood vessels for instance increase the rate of thrombotic complications. The clinical features and precipitating factors for coagulopathy in liver transplant vary according to the stage of the procedure. In the preimplant stage for instance, the coagulopathy reflects the underlying liver disease, as well as the effect of clotting factors dilution due to frequent blood product replacement. In the a hepatic stage, the lack of clotting factors synthesis as well as lack of clearance of activated products are the main reasons for the profound coagulopathy, fibrinolysis, and possible DIC encountered in this stage. A very high level of tPA is generated within minutes after the donor liver is placed. In the reimplantation stage, factors and inhibitors of coagulation are gradually restored, fibrinolysis begins to resolve, fibrinogen and plasminogen levels increase while FDPs gradually decrease.

Disseminated Intravascular Coagulation (Consumptive Coagulopathy)

DIC is not a disorder in itself but a process that is secondary to a large variety of underlying conditions. The name indicates the presence of diffuse fibrin deposits scattered in the microvasculature. Both hemorrhagic and thrombotic complications are usually encountered. The first are the result of reduced clotting factors, which were consumed in the circulation, in addition to active fibrinolysis, which also contributes to the bleeding process. The thrombotic complications are the result of increased clotting triggered by various precipitating factors. Underlying disease processes may occur at all ages or be unique to a certain age group. Unique to newborns are adverse events affecting the fetoplacental unit that result in asphyxia and shock, which cause release of tissue thromboplastin that triggers the intravascular clotting process. Other pathologic disorders related to prematurity, such as respiratory distress syndrome, congenital viral infection, hypothermia, and meconium aspiration, may all initiate disseminated intravascular coagulation (DIC). The recent improvements in the care of neonates, together with a better understanding of the DIC process, have significantly changed both the classic clinical picture and the outcome of the affected newborns.

The diagnosis of DIC is based on compatible clinical features in conjunction with abnormal screening tests (PT, aPTT), low levels of certain coagulation factors (fibrinogen, factor V, factor VIII) and inhibitors (AT, heparin cofactor II, protein C), elevated fibrinogen/fibrin split products (FDPs), thrombocytopenia, and fragmented red blood cells (➋ *Table 336.4*). Milder forms of DIC are diagnosed by tests that measure the subtle effects of small amounts of thrombin or plasmin. These include fibrin monomers, thrombin–AT complexes, FDPs, and *D*-dimer. Positive tests alone, however, cannot confirm the process of DIC.

The cornerstone of the management of DIC is the treatment of the underlying disease and its complications. The decision to treat the secondary hemostatic complications has been an issue of debate for some time. Currently, however, the old argument that replacement therapy with plasma products may "fuel the fire" is believed to be theoretical and not true. If the patient is symptomatic

Table 336.4
Laboratory findings in children with three acquired coagulation defects

Test	Disseminated intravascular coagulation	Vitamin K deficiency	Liver disease
Partial thromboplastin time	P	P	P
Prothrombin time	P	P	P
Thrombin time	P	N	P
Platelet counts	L	N	N/L
Fibrin split products	+	N	±
Fibrinogen	L	N	L
Factor VIII	L	N	N
Factor V	L	N	L

P prolonged, *L* low, *N* normal, *N/L* normal or low, + increased due to hemostatic abnormalities, replacement therapy with FFP, exchange transfusion, cryoprecipitate, or platelet transfusion should be initiated. A reasonable therapeutic approach is to maintain a normal PTT, platelets of 50×10^9/L, and fibrinogen of 1.0 g/L. Treatment with anticoagulants such as heparin has also been an issue of controversy. The current recommendation is to restrict heparin therapy to infants with purpura fulminans, usually secondary to meningococcemia. This disorder is characterized by small and large vessel thrombi leading to organ and limb damage. Heparin is probably not indicated in children with skin necrosis only. Heparin is given either as intermittent intravenous administrations in a dose of 75–100 IU/kg every 4 h or as continuous infusion with 50–70 IU/kg as a bolus followed by 1525 IU/kg/h. This therapy should be closely monitored with serial measurements of the anti-Xa or aPTT. In children with evidence of organ or limb necrosis, anticoagulant therapy with heparin may be helpful.

Fibrinolysis

Fibrinolysis is the process responsible for the removal and degradation of the fibrin clot, whether the clot is formed physiologically, as a result of inflammation, tissue repair, or hemostasis, or precipitated by a pathologic process, such as deep vein thrombosis, pulmonary embolism, or DIC. In the first situation, the clot plays a temporary role and must be removed when normal tissue structure and function are restored. In pathologic circumstances, however, the fibrinolytic system, for some reason, fails to dissolve the fibrin clot. Similar to the other coagulation and thrombosis processes, the fibrinolytic system action is coordinated through the interaction of activators, zymogens, enzymes, and inhibitors to provide local activation at sites of fibrin deposition. Activation of the fibrinolytic system can also be achieved by intrinsic or extrinsic pathways. In intrinsic pathway, the activated contact factors (XIIa, XIa, prekallikrein) are known to activate plasminogen to plasmin while the intrinsic coagulation system is being activated. In the extrinsic system (activators are not in the plasma), however, two serine proteases tissue activators have been identified: the first is tPA and the second is urokinase-type plasminogen activator. Both have been produced by recombinant DNA and are available for therapeutic purposes.

Plasminogen is the precursor of the active fibrinolytic enzyme plasmin. It is produced by the liver and present in the plasma as a single-chain molecule. When activated to a two-chain plasmin molecule, a smaller molecule cleaved by plasmin with an amino-terminal lysine is produced (lys-plasminogen). This molecule has higher affinity for binding to fibrin and greater reactivity with plasminogen activators, through sites known as lysine-binding sites. Lysine analogs such as EACA are capable of binding to these sites on plasminogen, thus competing with the lysine-like sites on fibrin, resulting in inhibition of fibrinolysis by rendering the fibrin protected from binding with plasmin or plasminogen. The physiologic fibrinolytic inhibitor α_2-antiplasmin is also mediated in part by binding to the same sites of plasminogen. Plasmin is capable of hydrolyzing proteins other than fibrin and fibrinogen; factor V, factor VIII, complement components, adrenocorticotropic hormone, growth hormone, and glucagon are some examples. Together with other fibrinolytic system inhibitors such as PAI, α_2-antiplasmin plays an important role in the regulation of fibrinolysis.

Once the clot is physiologically formed, fibrinolysis is instantly stimulated. Plasminogen, activated by tPA and single-chain urokinase plasminogen activator (SCU-PA), binds to fibrin while fast-acting inhibitors such as α_2-antiplasmin and PAI-1 go into action. Both are more efficient when their substrates (plasmin for the first and tPA for the second) are free in the plasma rather than bound to other proteins. This allows plasminogen activation on the fibrin while avoiding its effect systemically. When therapeutic quantities of tPA are infused, however, virtually all the plasminogen in the plasma is converted to plasmin, overcoming the neutralizing capacity of antiplasmin and leading eventually to fibrinogenolysis (the lytic state).

References

Andrew M, Shmidt B (1994) Hemorrhagic and thrombotic complications in children. In: Colman RW, Hirsh J, Marder VJ et al (eds) Hemostasis and thrombosis: basic principles and clinical practice. Lippincott, Philadelphia, pp 989–1022

Baur KA, Rosenberg RD (1991) Role of antithrombin III as a regulator of in vivo coagulation. Semin Hematol 28:10

Binette TM, Taylor FB Jr, Peer G et al (2007) Thrombin – thrombomodulin connects coagulation and fibrinolysis: more than an invetro phenomenon. Blood 110:3168

Brass LF (2003) Thrombin and platelet activation. Chest 124:185

Furie B, Furie BC (2008) Mechanism of thrombus formation. N Engl J Med 359:938

Grabowski EF, Corrigan JJ Jr (1995) Hemostasis: general consideration. In: Miller DR, Baehner RL (eds) Blood diseases of infancy and childhood. Mosby, St. Louis, pp 849–865

Mann, KG, Brummel- Ziedins, K (2009) Blood coagulation. In: Nathan DG, and Oski (eds) Hematology of infancy and childhood, 7th edn. pp 1399–1418

Osterud B, Rapaport SI (1977) Activation of factor IX by the reaction product of tissue factor and factor VII: additional pathway for

initiating blood coagulation. Proc Natl Acad Sci USA 74:5260–5264
Porte RJ, Knot EA, Bontembo FA et al (1998) Hemostasis in liver transplantation. Gastroenterol 97:488
Rapaport SI, Rao LV (1995) The tissue factor pathway: how it has become "Prima ballerina". Thromb Haemost 74:7
Santoro SA, Eby CS (2000) Laboratory evaluation of hemostatic disorders. In: Hoffman R, Benz EJ Jr, Shattil SJ et al (eds) Hematology: basic principles and practice. Churchill Livingstone, New York, pp 1841–1850
Sixma JJ, Wester J (1977) The thrombostatic plug. Semin Hematol 14:265

337 Pediatric Venous Thromboembolism

Brian R. Branchford · Neil A. Goldenberg

The incidence of pediatric venous thromboembolism (VTE) is increasing and has become a significant cause of morbidity and mortality in infants and children. It is therefore crucial for the primary care pediatrician and subspecialist alike to appreciate the epidemiology, etiologies, presentations, diagnostic evaluation, management, and outcomes of VTE in neonates and older children.

The objectives of this narrative review are to: (1) briefly consider physiologic mechanisms of hemostasis; (2) discuss epidemiology, etiology, and clinical presentation of VTE in children; and (3) present diagnostic measures and treatment options.

Background: Brief review of physiologic mechanisms of hemostasis.

Coagulation is not, in itself, a pathologic condition. Indeed, coagulation and fibrinolysis dynamically interact in the normal physiological state, and it is only when coagulation is insufficiently inhibited or fibrinolysis is excessively inhibited that pathologic thrombosis results. Understanding these processes in normal physiology will facilitate a comprehension of pathologic thrombosis.

Hemostasis is defined as the process by which blood flow from within a vessel is arrested. It is helpful to conceive of hemostasis in two major phases – primary and secondary – that interact in dynamic fashion. Primary hemostasis is triggered when blood vessel damage (i.e., endothelial injury) exposes subendothelial tissue factor (TF) and collagen to flowing blood. Von Willebrand factor and fibrinogen then mediate platelet adhesion and aggregation, resulting in the formation of a platelet plug. Additionally, platelet activation results in surface exposure of phospholipid, forming the scaffold for the plasma clotting reactions of secondary hemostasis. In secondary hemostasis, coagulation activation is initiated as exposed subendothelial TF combines with small amounts of circulating activated factor VII, forming a complex that directly activates factor X (Xa). This is known as the TF pathway (formerly called the extrinsic pathway) of the coagulation cascade. Subsequently, through the common pathway, Xa combines with activated factor V (Va) as the prothrombinase complex, converting prothrombin to thrombin. This process of thrombin generation via the TF pathway is described as thrombin initiation. Thrombin generation is greatly upregulated (described as thrombin propagation) when thrombin activates factor XI, which in turn activates factors VIII (VIIIa) and IX (IXa) through the "contact pathway" (historically known as the "intrinsic pathway") of the coagulation cascade. VIIIa and XIa form a "tenase" complex, converting factor X to Xa, ultimately generating thrombin through the common pathway. The thrombin propagation phase of secondary hemostasis is also mediated by thrombin-induced activation of factors VIII and V. Thrombin is important in the conversion of soluble fibrinogen to insoluble fibrin, forming polymers (fibrils) that are cross-linked by factor XIII to form a hemostatic clot that, in the venous system, is rich in fibrin and interspersed with platelets. Thrombin also serves to activate platelets, thereby fueling further platelet plug and clot formation.

Principal regulators of coagulation activation include the native anticoagulants (antithrombin, protein C, and protein S), thrombomodulin, and tissue factor pathway inhibitor. Antithrombin (formerly known as antithrombin III) is the primary inhibitor of circulating thrombin. Protein C inhibits activation of factors V and VIII. Protein S and thrombomodulin serves as cofactors for protein C.

The coagulation system is in dynamic balance with the fibrinolytic system. In the fibrinolytic system, clot-bound plasminogen is converted by tissue plasminogen activator to plasmin, which cleaves fibrin into monomers and dimers. This process mediates clot lysis, and the fibrin monomers and dimers produced also inhibit further fibrin polymerization.

Further discussion of genetic and acquired thrombophilia traits is beyond the scope of this review, but details can be found in several other texts.

Epidemiology

Historically, the incidence of VTE in children has been perceived to be low. Review of data from multiple recent patient registries revealed an estimated cumulative incidence of 0.07 per 10,000 individuals (5.3 per 10,000 hospitalizations) for extremity deep venous thrombosis (DVT) and/or pulmonary embolism (PE) among non-neonatal Canadian children, and an incidence rate of 0.14

Abdelaziz Y. Elzouki (ed.), *Textbook of Clinical Pediatrics*, DOI 10.1007/978-3-642-02202-9_337,

per 10,000 Dutch children per year for VTE in general. An evaluation of the National Hospital Discharge Survey and census data for VTE in the United States from 1979 to 2001 disclosed an overall incidence rate of 0.49 per 10,000 individuals per year. During a recent 7-year period of study the annual rate of pediatric VTE increased by 70%, from 34 to 58 cases per 10,000 hospital admissions.

A bimodal age distribution of the incidence rate for childhood VTE is noted, with peak rates in neonates and adolescents. The Dutch registry, for example, indicated a VTE incidence rate of 14.5 per 10,000 per year in the neonatal period, approximately 100 times greater than the overall rate in childhood, while the VTE-specific incidence rate in the United States among adolescents 15–17 years of age was determined to be 1.1 per 10,000 per year, a rate nearly threefold that observed overall in childhood.

Most recently, an analysis of the Pediatric Health Information System (PHIS) database from 2001 to 2007 revealed that approximately 1 in 200 hospitalized children are diagnosed with VTE. This figure likely includes both patients who developed VTE in hospital as well as those children admitted for VTE that developed outside the hospital.

Etiology

Virchow's triad consists of venous stasis, endothelial damage, and the hypercoagulable state. This group of clinical situations encapsulates the primary risk factors responsible for pathogenesis of VTE. In children, greater than 90% of VTE are risk-associated (as compared to approximately 60% in adults), with risk factors in children often disclosed from more than one component of this triad. Of the clinical prothrombotic risk factors, one of the most common is an indwelling central venous catheter. Over 50% of cases of DVT in children and over 80% of cases in newborns occur in association with central venous catheters. The presence of an indwelling central venous catheter, underlying malignancy or disorder for which bone marrow transplantation was undertaken, and congenital cardiac disease and its corrective surgery were all highly prevalent in the Canadian pediatric thrombosis registry, whereas underlying infectious illness and the presence of an indwelling central venous catheter were identified as pervasive clinical risk factors in a recent cohort study analysis from the United States. A recent review of the Pediatric Health Information System revealed that a majority (63%) of children with VTE had >1 coexisting chronic complex medical condition and that pediatric malignancy was the medical comorbid condition associated most strongly with recurrent VTE.

As noted above, thrombophilia may be caused by any alteration in hemostatic balance that increases thrombin production, enhances platelet activation/aggregation, mediates endothelial activation/damage, or inhibits fibrinolysis. Regarding the hypercoagulable state, blood-based risk factors for VTE in children include both inherited and acquired thrombophilic conditions. Potent thrombophilic conditions (e.g., severe anticoagulant deficiencies, antiphospholipid antibodies) in children are frequently acquired, rather than congenital. By contrast, the common congenital thrombophilia traits (e.g., heterozygosity for the factor V Leiden or prothrombin G20210A polymorphisms) tend to be more mild.

Common examples of acquired thrombophilia in children include: increased factor VIII activity with significant infection and inflammatory states; anticoagulant deficiencies due to consumption in bacterial sepsis and disseminated intravascular coagulopathy (DIC) or to the production of inhibitory antibodies in acute viral infection; and para-infectious development of antiphospholipid antibodies (APA). In order to provide an appreciation of the magnitude of VTE risk increase associated with several congenital/genetically influenced thrombophilia traits, population-based VTE risk estimates derived from the adult literature are shown in *Table 337.1*. As seen in the Table, the addition of standard-dose estrogen oral contraceptive pill to an underlying heterozygous factor V Leiden (in large part by virtue of a "double-hit" to the protein C pathway) would be expected to increase the risk for VTE from a baseline risk of 15 per 10,000 US females aged 15–17 years per year to a risk of over 500 per 10,000, or 5%, per year.

Table 337.1
VTE risk estimates for selected thrombophilia traits and conditions

Trait/condition	VTE risk estimate (× baseline)
Hyperhomocysteinemia	2.5
Prothrombin 20210 mutation, heterozygous	2–3
Oral contraceptive pill (OCP; standard-dose estrogen)	4
Factor V Leiden mutation, heterozygous	2–7
OCP+Factor V Leiden mutation, heterozygous	35
Factor V Leiden mutation, homozygous	80

Clinical Presentation

The degree of clinical suspicion for acute VTE in children should be primarily influenced by the following characteristics: (1) clinical signs and symptoms; (2) personal history of VTE; (3) clinical prothrombotic risk factors; (4) family history of early (e.g., before age 50 years) VTE or other vascular events; and (5) known thrombophilia traits/risk factors. In many cases, information from this last category is not available at the time of clinical presentation with possible VTE.

The signs and symptoms of VTE vary based upon anatomic location.

Limb Deep Venous Thrombosis

The classic manifestation of acute limb DVT is painful unilateral extremity swelling. The presence of Homan's sign (pain upon manual calf compression or with forced dorsiflexion of the foot while the knee is flexed) or the presence of a palpable cord in the popliteal fossa may suggest lower extremity DVT; however, these physical findings are both insensitive and nonspecific. In upper extremity DVT with extension into, and occlusion of, the superior vena cava (SVC), signs and symptoms may include swelling and/or erythema of neck and face, visualization of superficial collateral vessels in the chest, bilateral periorbital edema, and headache.

Pulmonary Embolism

Pulmonary embolism usually presents with sudden- or progressive-onset dyspnea and/or pleuritic chest pain, and is occasionally accompanied with hypoxemia (particularly in settings of extensive or proximal PA involvement). Associated right heart failure (cor pulmonale) may manifest with hepatomegaly, visible superficial collateral vessels in the abdomen, and/or peripheral edema. Proximal PE and especially saddle embolus can present with cyanosis or sudden cardiopulmonary collapse. In many cases, however, PE may be asymptomatic or subtle in children, especially when involving limited segmental or subsegmental branches of the pulmonary arteries. At the same time, the most peripheral PE near the pleura frequently causes pleuritic reactions (pleuritis) and/or effusions that are quite symptomatic. In one retrospective series, only 50% of affected children had clinical symptoms attributable to PE.

Cerebral Sinovenous Thrombosis

Signs and symptoms of acute cerebral sinovenous thrombosis (CSVT) may include severe and persistent headache, blurred vision, neurologic signs (e.g., cranial nerve palsy, papilledema), or seizures. Although not signs and symptoms of the CSVT per se, one must also be attentive to the constellation of findings in otitic hydrocephalus and Gradenigo's syndrome (the triad of suppurative otitis media, pain in the distribution of the trigeminal nerve, and abducens nerve palsy), in which otitis media is complicated by mastoiditis and petrositis, with development of thrombus in the adjacent sigmoid or lateral sinus. Mastoid tenderness, fever, and findings (or recent history) of otitis media should therefore prompt suspicion for this disorder.

Renal Vein Thrombosis

Renal vein thrombosis (RVT) is classically associated with hematuria and thrombocytopenia, sometimes accompanied by anemia and hypertension. Bilateral involvement is sometimes associated with uremia and/or oliguria. RVT is most common during the neonatal period and may be noted on physical exam as a flank mass. RVT in older children is often associated with nephrotic syndrome (a risk factor for VTE in general), and may therefore present with peripheral and/or periorbital edema.

Portal Vein Thrombosis and Hepatic Vein Thrombosis

Portal vein thrombosis (PVT) characteristically presents with splenomegaly, and is associated with thrombocytopenia and, often, anemia; gastrointestinal bleeding at presentation typically signals the presence of gastroesophageal varices due to portal hypertension.

Hepatic vein thrombosis without PVT is typically asymptomatic, and usually found incidentally upon abdominal imaging.

Intracardiac Deep Venous Thrombosis

Isolated intracardiac thrombosis in association with cardiac surgery or central venous catheter placement is most often asymptomatic. Thrombocytopenia, described for RVT above, can also be seen with intracardiac (e.g., right atrial) thrombus.

Internal Jugular DVT and Lemierre's Syndrome

Internal jugular vein thrombosis may manifest with neck pain or swelling. Lemierre's syndrome (classically caused by Fusobacterium, but occasionally identified with other potentially causative organisms) is associated with fever, trismus, and a palpable thrombus in the lateral triangle of the neck.

Diagnosis

Radiologic Evaluation

The importance of radiologic imaging lies in its dual ability to confirm the clinical diagnosis of VTE as well as define both the extent and occlusiveness of thrombosis. The gold-standard for diagnosis of venous thrombosis is conventional venography, but the utility of this modality is limited by its invasive nature and the associated risks.

Currently, when DVT of an extremity is suspected, compression ultrasonography with Doppler color flow imaging is typically used for confirmation. When the thrombus may involve or extend into deep pelvic or abdominal veins, computed tomography venography (CTV) or magnetic resonance venography (MRV) is often required.

If involvement of the central thoracic vasculature (e.g., right atrial thrombosis, SVC thrombosis) is suspected, echocardiogram may be used in addition to CT or MRI. In the case of asymptomatic non-occlusive extremity DVT disclosed by ultrasound, CTV, MRV with gadolinium contrast, or conventional venography may be necessary for diagnostic confirmation. To establish a diagnosis of DVT of the jugular venous system (such as in suspected cases of Lemierre's syndrome), compression ultrasound with Doppler imaging is typically used.

PE in children is commonly evaluated with spiral CT angiography or by ventilation-perfusion scan. The latter, however, is generally suboptimal in cases involving other potentially confounding lung pathologies or at centers without sufficient expertice with this modality. CSVT is typically diagnosed by MRV or CTV. This diagnosis occasionally is made in the course of head imaging (e.g., plain CT or MRI) for another cause. RVT is most often diagnosed clinically in neonates and is supported by Doppler ultrasound findings of intrarenal vascular resistive indices; however, in some cases a discrete thrombus may be suggested by Doppler ultrasound (especially when extending into the inferior vena cava) or may be further disclosed via MRV. When RVT occurs in older children, Doppler ultrasound or CTV is often diagnostic. Similarly, portal vein thrombosis is typically visualized by Doppler ultrasound or CTV.

In some cases, new-onset venous thrombosis is being evaluated in patients with anatomic abnormalities of the venous system, including extensive collateral venous circulation due to a prior VTE episode, May-Thurner anomaly (left iliac vein is compressed by right iliac artery, causing increased risk of DVT due to compressive stasis), or atretic IVC with azygous continuation. For these patients, more sensitive methods such as CTV or MRV are often required to define the vascular anatomy as well as the presence, extent, and occlusiveness of thrombosis. Conventional venography may also be required.

Disadvantages of MRV include its expense, and necessity of sedation in young, developmentally delayed, or anxious children. Additionally, its use during acute VTE evaluation requires availability of MR-trained technologists. However, MRV offers a significant advantage over CTV by providing diagnostic sensitivity at least as great as CTV (particularly when gadolinium enhancement is used for scenarios in which non-occlusive thrombus must be distinguished from flow artifact), without significant radiation exposure.

Laboratory Evaluation

A thorough diagnostic laboratory evaluation in the setting of pediatric acute VTE should include a complete blood count, DIC panel, comprehensive thrombophilia evaluation (see Etiology, above), and beta-HCG testing in postmenarchal females. Additional laboratory studies may also be necessary depending upon associated medical conditions and possible VTE involvement of specific organ systems. ➋ *Table 337.2* summarizes a panel of thrombophilia traits and markers that each have been identified as risk factors for VTE in pediatric studies, and as such have been recommended by the Scientific and Standardization Committee Subcommittee on Perinatal and Pediatric Haemostasis of the International Society on Thrombosis and Haemostasis for the diagnostic laboratory evaluation of acute VTE in children. This comprehensive panel includes tests of anticoagulant deficiency (e.g., protein C, protein S, antithrombin), procoagulant excess (e.g., factor VIII), mediators of hypercoagulablity and/or endothelial damage (e.g., APA, lipoprotein(a), homocysteine), and markers of coagulation activation (e.g., D-dimer).

Significant debate currently surrounds the issue of comprehensive laboratory testing for thrombophilia traits

Table 337.2
Thrombophilic conditions and markers tested during comprehensive diagnostic laboratory evaluation of acute VTE in children

Condition/marker	Testing method(s)
Genetic	
Factor V Leiden polymorphism	PCR
Prothrombin 20210 polymorphism	PCR
Elevated plasma lipoprotein(a) concentration[a]	ELISA
Acquired or genetic	
Antithrombin deficiency	Chromogenic (functional) assay
Protein C deficiency	Chromogenic (functional) assay
Protein S deficiency	ELISA for free (i.e., functionally active) protein S antigen
Elevated plasma factor VIII activity[b]	One-stage clotting assay (aPTT-based)
Hyperhomocysteinemia	Mass spectroscopy
Antiphospholipid antibodies	ELISA for anticardiolipin and anti-beta-2-glycoprotein-I IgG and IgM; clotting assay (dilute Russell Viper Venom time or aPTT-based phospholipid neutralization method for lupus anticoagulant)
Disseminated intravascular coagulation	Includes platelet count, fibrinogen by clotting method (Clauss), and D-dimer by semiquantitative or quantitative immunoassay (e.g., latex agglutination)
Activated protein C resistance	Clotting assay (aPTT-based)

[a]Although designated here as genetic, lipoprotein(a) may also be elevated as part of the acute phase response
[b]Noted as worthy of consideration in original International Society on Thrombosis and Haemostasis recommendations; this has since been shown to be a prognostic marker in pediatric thrombosis. Additional testing involving the fibrinolytic system and systemic inflammatory response is also noted as worthy of consideration

in children with, or at heightened risk of, VTE. Many of the current guidelines are based upon consensus expert opinion or low-grade clinical evidence. Indeed, given the low incidence of VTE in the general pediatric population, widespread, unselected thrombophilia screening would neither be ethical nor cost-effective.

A comprehensive thrombophilia assessment is likely to have greatest clinical utility among individuals with a personal or close family history of a thrombotic event before the age of 55 years. A recent analysis of comprehensive laboratory evaluation in 56 children with positive family history of early VTE, but negative personal history of the same, advocated a risk-stratified approach to laboratory-based thrombophilia evaluation in these asymptomatic children that would target individuals with familial early VTE. Particularly in children and young adults, populations in which the incidence of VTE is low, efforts to identify individuals with clinical risk factors for VTE who have meaningful underlying thrombophilia may provide a rational approach to VTE prevention by targeting a subpopulation at heightened risk, in which comprehensive laboratory testing would be more beneficial.

Conventional Therapy

Table 337.3 provides a summary of conventional antithrombotic agents and corresponding target anticoagulant levels, based upon recent pediatric recommendations for both initial (i.e., acute phase) and extended (i.e., subacute phase) treatment. Conventional anticoagulants attenuate hypercoagulability, decreasing the risk of thrombus progression and embolism, while relying principally upon intrinsic fibrinolytic mechanisms to dissolve the thrombus. The most commonly employed conventional anticoagulants in children include heparins (either unfractionated [UFH] or low molecular weight heparin [LMWH] varieties) and warfarin. Heparins work by enhancing the activity of antithrombin, as discussed above. Warfarin acts through antagonism of vitamin K, thus interfering with gamma-carboxylation of the vitamin K-dependent procoagulant factors II, VII, IX, and X, as well as intrinsic anticoagulant proteins C and S.

Initial anticoagulant therapy for the acute phase of VTE in children involves UFH or LMWH. Two LMWH agents commonly employed in the United States (based upon labeling for adult VTE) are enoxaparin and

Table 337.3

Recommended intensities and durations of conventional antithrombotic therapies in children, by etiology and treatment agent (adapted from current consensus-based recommendations)

Episode	Agents and target anticoagulant activities				Duration of therapy, by etiology
	Initial treatment		Extended treatment		
First	UFH	03–0.7 anti-Xa U/mL	Warfarin	INR 2.0–3.0	Resolved risk factor: 3–6 months
	LMWH	0.5–1.0 anti-Xa U/mL	LMWH	0.5–1.0 anti-Xa U/mL	No known clinical risk factor: 6–12 months
					Chronic clinical risk factor: for duration of risk factor (often with prophylactic dosing, after initial 3–6 months of therapeutic dosing)
					Potent congenital thrombophilia: indefinite
Recurrent	UFH	0.3–0.7 anti-Xa U/mL	Warfarin	INR 2.0–3.0	Resolved risk factor: 3–6 months
	LMWH	0.5–1.0 anti-Xa U/mL	LMWH	0.5–1.0 anti-Xa U/mL	No known clinical risk factor: indefinite
					Chronic clinical risk factor: for duration of risk factor (often with prophylactic dosing, after initial 3–6 months of therapeutic dosing)
					Potent congenital thrombophilia: indefinite

dalteparin. In recent years, LMWH has become increasingly popular as the first-line agent for initial anticoagulant therapy in children given the relative ease of subcutaneous administration, the decreased need for blood monitoring of anticoagulant efficacy, and a decreased risk of the development of heparin-induced thrombocytopenia (HIT). LMWH is not ideal in all situations, however. UFH has a much shorter half-life than LMWH, and is therefore preferred in circumstances of heightened bleeding risk, upcoming surgery/invasive procedure, or labile acute clinical status, since the anticoagulant effect rapidly dissipates following cessation of the drug. Additionally, because LMWH is partly eliminated through the renal system, UFH (which is largely heptically eliminated) is more appropriate for acute VTE therapy in the setting of significantly impaired renal function.

Common initial dosing for UFH in non-neonatal children begins with an IV loading dose of 50–75 U/kg followed by a continuous IV infusion of 15–20 U/kg/h. Due to lower antithrombin levels in full-term neonates, a maintenance dose of up to 50 U/kg/h may be required for these patients, especially if the clinical condition is complicated by antithrombin consumption. The starting dose for enoxaparin in non-neonatal children commonly ranges between 1.0 and 1.375 mg/kg subcutaneously on an every-12-h schedule and does not require a bolus dose. In full-term neonates, a dose of 1.5 mg/kg is typically necessary. For dalteparin, on the other hand, initial maintenance dosing of 1.0–1.5 mg/kg (100–150 anti-Xa U/kg) appears appropriate based upon available pediatric data.

Anti-factor Xa activity levels can be used to follow either type of heparin therapy, whether UFH or LMWH. Anti-Xa level should be obtained 6–8 h after initiation of UFH infusion or 4 h following any one of the first few doses of LMWH. For UFH, the therapeutic range is 0.3–0.7 anti-Xa activity U/mL, while for LMWH the therapeutic range is 0.5–1.0 U/mL. When the anti-Xa assay is not available, the activated partial thromboplastin time (aPTT) may be used (with a goal aPTT of approximately 1.5–2 times the upper limit of age-appropriate normal values); however, this approach is especially suboptimal in the pediatric age group, in which transient antiphospholipid antibodies are common and may alter the clotting endpoint. Notably, one study of pediatric heparin monitoring demonstrated inaccuracy of aPTT approximately 30% of the time. When dosed by weight in childhood, LMWH does not require frequent monitoring, but anti-Xa activity should be evaluated with changes in renal function, weight shifts >10% of baseline, or in clinical situations where bleeding side effect is of particular concern. In addition, there are cases of acute VTE in which acquired antithrombin deficiency is related to consumption in acute infection or inflammation. In these instances, the anti-Xa activity may rise as antithrombin levels normalize with resolution of the acute illness, warranting follow-up evaluation of anti-Xa in the subacute period.

Controversy exists regarding length of therapy during both the acute and subacute phases of anticoagulation for VTE in children. Due to lack of pediatric data, the recommended duration of heparinization of 5–10 days during the initial therapy for acute VTE has been extrapolated from adult data. UFH treatment is rarely maintained beyond the acute period, given the risk of osteoporosis with extended administration and the inconvenience of continuous intravenous administration. Although adult data suggest efficacy of subcutaneous administration of unfractionated heparin for acute VTE, this has only been evaluated for the acute therapy period prior to extended therapy with warfarin, and the appropriateness of such an approach in children has not been established.

Extended anticoagulant therapy (i.e., subacute phase) for VTE in children may employ LMWH or warfarin. For warfarin anticoagulation, warfarin is often started during the acute phase. As above, however, severe congenital PC deficiencies can present as VTE in early childhood and are associated with warfarin skin necrosis. Warfarinization should, therefore, be initiated only after therapeutic anticoagulation is achieved with a heparin agent. Due to the relatively short half-life of PC, warfarin's interference with its activation can result in a transient hypercoagulable state. It is therefore also important to use LMWH or UFH as a "bridge" until warfarin reaches effective levels.

A common starting dose for warfarin in children is 0.1 mg/kg orally once daily. Warfarin is monitored by international normalized ratio (INR), derived from the measured prothrombin time. The therapeutic INR range for warfarin anticoagulation in VTE is 2.0–3.0. Recent adult data do not agree with the historical evidence for maintaining a higher INR (2.5–3.5) in the presence of APA; however, pediatric data are lacking with regard to both optimal dose intensity and duration in children with APA syndrome. The INR is typically checked after the first 5 days of initiation of (or dosing change in) warfarin therapy, and weekly thereafter until stable. As levels become more stable, less frequent monitoring is often feasible. The INR should also be evaluated at the time of any bleeding manifestations or increased bruising. Warfarin must be discontinued at least 5 days prior to invasive procedures, with an INR obtained prior to the procedure to ensure resolution of anticoagulant effect. In some situations, an anticoagulant transition, or "bridge," to LMWH can be performed, to minimize the time off anticoagulation perioperatively.

As mentioned above, clear recommendations for long-term duration of anticoagulant therapy are not available, and depend heavily on clinical situation, as well as provider preference. For initial VTE in children in the absence of potent chronic thrombophilia (e.g., APA syndrome, homozygous anticoagulant deficiency, homozygous factor V Leiden or prothrombin 20210), the recommended duration of anticoagulant therapy is 3–6 months in the presence of an underlying reversible risk factor (e.g., postoperative VTE) and 6–12 months when idiopathic. In the case of chronic risk factors (systemic lupus erythematosus), the initial 3–6 months consist of therapeutic dosing, followed by prophylactic dosing for the duration of the risk factor's presence. Recurrent VTE is treated for 3–6 months in the presence of an underlying reversible risk factor, and indefinitely when idiopathic. As above in the case of chronic risk factors (systemic lupus erythematosus), the initial 3–6 months of therapy for recurrent VTE consist of therapeutic dosing, followed by prophylactic dosing for the duration of the risk factor's presence. In the setting of APA syndrome or potent congenital thrombophilia, the treatment duration for first-episode VTE is often indefinite. Some evidence suggests that children with SLE and persistence of the lupus anticoagulant (LA) have a 16- to 25-fold greater risk of TEs than children with SLE and no LA. However, in children with primary (i.e., idiopathic) or secondary (i.e., associated with SLE or other underlying chronic inflammatory condition) APA syndrome, it is possible that the autoimmune disease will become quiescent in later years, such that the benefit of continued therapeutic anticoagulation as secondary VTE prophylaxis may be reevaluated. Some experts have recommended consideration of low-dose anticoagulation as secondary VTE prophylaxis following a conventional 3- to 6-month course of therapeutic anticoagulation for VTE in children with SLE who have APA syndrome. Such low-dose, or prophylactic, anticoagulation might, for example, consist of enoxaparin 1.0–1.5 mg/kg subcutaneously once daily, enoxaparin 0.5 mg/kg subcutaneously twice daily, or daily warfarin with a goal INR of 1.5. However, further study to optimize the intensity and duration of therapy/secondary prophylaxis for VTE in children with APA syndrome is urgently needed, especially given the recent evidence in adult VTE that secondary prophylaxis with low-dose warfarin not only may offer little risk reduction beyond no anticoagulation, but also is associated with bleeding complications despite a reduced warfarin dose.

A multicenter randomized trial is underway to determine whether a shorter duration of anticoagulant therapy (i.e., 6 weeks) is appropriate for pediatric VTE associated with identifiable reversible risk factors and no potent genetic thrombophilia state.

Novel/Emerging Therapies and New/Alternative Anticoagulants

Direct Thrombin Inhibitors

Direct thrombin inhibitors inhibit thrombin directly via its active site or by binding to its target on fibrin. This class includes intravenously administered drugs such as bivalirudin and argatroban, as well as oral alternatives such as dabigatran.

The intravenous direct thrombin inhibitors are indicated for the treatment of heparin-induced thrombocytopenia (HIT), particularly when associated with acute thrombosis (HITT), and are also used in patients with a history of HIT.

Dabigatran is an oral direct thrombin inhibitor, which has been approved in Europe and Canada since 2008 for venous thromboembolism (VTE) prophylaxis in the setting of orthopedic surgery, and was recently approved in the US for stroke prevention in adults with atrial fibrillation. A recent meta-analysis of the three phase-3 studies, RE-MODEL, RE-MOBILIZE, and RE-NOVATE, supported the individual trials' conclusions of noninferiority to enoxaparin. Results of the RE-COVER study which compared dabigatran with warfarin for the treatment of acute VTE in 2,539 patients were recently reported and showed equivalent rates of recurrent VTE without significantly different major bleeding episodes in patients treated with dabigatran versus those who received warfarin.

Xa Inhibitors

Factor Xa inhibitors, including fondaparinux, inhibit the activation of factor X, thereby indirectly inhibiting thrombin. Fondaparinux is an entirely synthetic pentasaccharide that is structurally related to the antithrombin-binding site of heparin. In contrast to heparin, which interacts with many plasma components, the pentasaccharide selectively binds to antithrombin, causing it to rapidly inhibit factor Xa, a key enzyme in the coagulation pathway.

Rivaroxaban, an oral factor Xa inhibitor, is already approved for VTE prophylaxis following hip and knee replacement in Europe and Canada, and appears near to approval in the United States. The RECORD series of clinical trials compared rivaroxaban to subcutaneous enoxaparin for the prevention of venous thromboembolism after orthopedic surgery and illustrated both efficacy and safety. Another Factor Xa inhibitor, apixaban, is currently in trials for VTE treatment and post-orthopedic surgery prophylaxis.

Intravenous direct thrombin inhibitors are routinely monitored by aPTT, with the therapeutic goal ranging from a 1.5- to 3.0-fold aPTT prolongation. A variety of factor Xa inhibitors and oral direct thrombin inhibitors are undergoing preclinical development or evaluation in adult clinical trials.

Both the factor Xa inhibitors and the direct thrombin inhibitors are also being evaluated for their efficacy in stroke prevention in the setting of atrial fibrillation. Though these new agents may allow for similar efficacy and safety as warfarin for long-term oral anticoagulation therapy or prevention, significant cost may be prohibitive. Also, despite the inconvenience of frequent lab monitoring of warfarin, it is an effective means of evaluating compliance. An effective antidote or reversal agent for these drugs (such as protamine sulfate might be used for overdose of unfractionated heparin or LMWH) is not currently available. Therefore, optimal safety information regarding dosing regimens is of vital importance. It is hoped that head-to-head trials of these new anticoagulants will provide useful information regarding the challenges that will arise in optimal therapeutic selection.

Thrombolytic Modalities

Systemic TPA

One treatment approach that is becoming more common in children with hemodynamically significant PE or extensive limb-threatening VTE is the use of thrombolysis. The conventional anticoagulants discussed above act by attenuating clot progression while intrinsic fibrinolysis occurs physiologically. Thrombolytics, on the other hand, promote fibrinolysis directly. Tissue-type plasminogen activator (TPA) is an intrinsic activator of the fibrinolytic system, and can be administered in its recombinant form by various routes (e.g., systemic bolus, systemic short-duration infusion, systemic low-dose continuous infusion, local catheter-directed infusion with or without interventional mechanical thrombectomy/thrombolysis). A recent cohort study analysis of children with acute lower extremity DVT, who had an a priori high risk of poor post-thrombotic outcomes by virtue of completely veno-occlusive thrombus and plasma FVIII activity >150 U/dL or D-dimer concentration >500 ng/mL, revealed that a thrombolysis regimen followed by standard anticoagulation may substantially reduce the risk of post-thrombotic syndrome when compared to standard anticoagulation alone. However, bleeding risk must be carefully assessed prior to the use of this approach.

Percutaneous Mechanical/ Pharmacomechanical Thrombolysis (PMT/PPMT)

Percutaneous mechanical/pharmacomechanical thrombolysis (PMT/PPMT), using a combination of intravenous mechanical clot disruption and local TPA infusion, is a therapeutic option that is gaining popularity. This procedure may be followed by catheter-directed thrombolytic infusion (CDTI), a practice in which TPA is administered locally over a period of 1–2 days following the procedure.

One recent prospective cohort study evaluated 16 children who suffered from completely occlusive proximal limb DVT in association with acute elevation of FVIII and D-dimer who elected to undergo PMT/PPMT within 60 days of symptom onset. PMT/PPMT was successfully conducted in 15 cases and CDTI was employed adjunctively in 11 of these for the purpose of providing local therapy only, thereby reducing the risks of systemic thrombolysis (including systemic bleeding risks involving critical sites such as the central nervous system). There were no peri-procedural major bleeding events, but one symptomatic pulmonary embolism occurred. Clot lysis was achieved in 94% of cases. There were five acute local recurrences within 1 week (all of which were successfully re-lysed). Despite acute local re-thrombosis in 40%, 83% of these were successfully re-lysed, and late recurrent DVT occurred in 31% overall. These data suggest that PMT with/without adjunctive CDTI can be used safely in adolescents with DVT known to be at high a priori risk for PTS. Although signs and/or symptoms of PTS were still observed in some patients even when PMT was performed within 10 days of symptom onset, the rate of functionally significant PTS occurred in only 25% of these high-risk patients.

At the time of this writing, the existing literature contains no randomized control trials of PMT, in children or adults. Indeed, prospective data on this lytic intervention for DVT are limited to two adult studies, which were actually focused more upon CDTI, and PMT was reported in just a few cases in each study. Retrospective studies, on the other hand, are somewhat more numerous. Eight retrospective studies exist, totaling approximately 200 adult DVT patients treated by PMT with/without adjunctive CDTI. However, published experience with a regimen of PMT followed by adjunctive CDTI as described above is limited to three retrospective adult studies.

Regarding the safety of PMT with/without CDTI, only six cases of acute major bleeding and zero cases of acute symptomatic PE were reported among the nine retrospective studies, out of a total of 279 patients. Acute thrombolysis rates were high across the eight retrospective studies, suggesting potential efficacy. However, long-term patency was only reported by Lin and colleagues, who determined a rate of 65%. No cases of acute recurrent DVT were reported among a cumulative total of 62 subjects in the retrospective studies wherein this outcome was assessed. These findings identify PMT with adjunctive CDTI as a therapeutic option worthy of further prospective study as an effective and potentially safer (decreased systemic bleeding risks involving critical sites such as the central nervous system) alternative to systemic thrombolysis in children with occlusive proximal limb DVT who have adverse prognostic biomarkers at acute presentation.

Other Antithrombotic Agents

Various other antithrombotic products await further clinical trials to demonstrate efficacy. For example, as mentioned above, protein C concentrate can be useful as an adjunct to standard heparin therapy for VTE or purpura fulminans due to microvascular thrombosis in severe congenital protein C deficiency or in children with sepsis, particularly in meningococcemia. In addition, various case series have suggested a role for antithrombin replacement in VTE prevention in children and young adults with congenital severe antithrombin deficiency, for the prevention of L-asparaginase-associated VTE in pediatric acute lymphoblastic leukemia (ALL), and as combination therapy with defibrotide in the prevention and treatment of hepatic sinusoidal obstruction syndrome (formerly termed veno-occlusive disease) in children undergoing hematopoietic stem cell transplantation. The potential benefit for VTE risk reduction using a regimen of antithrombin replacement combined with daily prophylactic LMWH during induction and consolidation phases of therapy in ALL has now also been suggested by a historically controlled cohort study of the BFM 2000 protocol experience in Europe. As noted above, antithrombin replacement may also be worthy of consideration in patients receiving heparin therapy for acute VTE in whom significant antithrombin deficiency prevents the achievement of therapeutic anti-Xa levels (i.e., heparin "resistance"). This may be the case in nephrotic syndrome-associated VTE. Additionally, neonates with clinical conditions complicated by antithrombin consumption as described above are particularly predisposed to such heparin "resistance," due to a physiologic relative deficiency of this key intrinsic thrombin inhibitor.

Another complementary therapy to consider in children of appropriate size with persistent prothrombotic risk factor(s) who suffer from recurrent VTE (especially PE) is the placement of temporary vena caval filters. However, recommended use of these devices in pediatric VTE is generally restricted to the setting of inability or contraindication to anticoagulate (typically transient). The impact of non-retrievable devices upon the vena cava of the developing child has not been well studied, and experience with surgical removal of non-retrievable vena caval filters is quite limited. Consequently, the use of non-retrievable vena caval filters in pediatrics should be undertaken with caution.

Outcomes

Both acute and long-term complications of VTEs, and their associated therapy, must be considered. Short-term adverse outcomes of the thrombotic event itself may include post-thrombotic hemorrhage (in the brain, testis, or adrenal gland), early recurrent VTE (including DVT and PE), SVC syndrome in upper extremity DVT, acute renal insufficiency in RVT, catheter-related sepsis or malfunction (sometimes necessitating surgical replacement) in CRT, severe acute venous insufficiency leading to venous infarction with limb gangrene in rare cases of occlusive DVT involving the extremities, and/or death from hemodynamic instability in extensive intracardiac thrombosis or proximal PE. Additionally, one must consider the major hemorrhagic complications of antithrombotic interventions.

Given the long-term risks of recurrence, disease sequelae, and functional impairment, VTE must also be considered as a chronic disorder in children. Long-term adverse outcomes in pediatric VTE have recently been reviewed, and include: recurrent VTE, chronic hypertension and renal insufficiency in RVT, variceal hemorrhage in portal vein thrombosis, chronic SVC syndrome involving occlusion in upper extremity VTE, and development of the post-thrombotic syndrome (PTS): a condition of chronic venous insufficiency following DVT.

Mortality

While VTE-specific mortality in children is quite low, ranging from 0% to 2%, a considerably higher all-cause mortality reflects the severity of underlying conditions (e.g., sepsis, cancer, congenital cardiac disease) in pediatric VTE. Neonate-specific outcomes data in pediatric non-RVT VTE reflect an all-cause mortality of 12–18%, including one series of premature infants with CRT treated with enoxaparin.

Recurrent Venous Thromboembolism

Registry and cohort study data in all types of pediatric VTE indicate that children appear to have a lower risk of recurrent thromboembolism than adults (cumulative incidences at 1–2 years of 6–11% versus 12–22%, respectively). However, the risk of PTS in children with DVT of the limbs appears to be at least as great as that in adults (cumulative incidences at 1–2 years of 33–70% versus 29%, respectively). Additionally, it should be noted that a German cohort study of children with spontaneous VTE (i.e., VTE in the absence of identified clinical risk factors) revealed that the cumulative incidence of recurrent VTE at a median follow-up time of 7 years was 21%. These findings suggest that, in this subgroup of pediatric VTE, the risk for recurrent events is long-lived.

Major Bleeding

With regard to major bleeding complications occurring during the anticoagulation period, frequencies in children range from 0% to 9% in recent studies.

Post-thrombotic Syndrome

The manifestations of PTS (as described above) may include edema, visibly dilated superficial collateral veins, venous stasis dermatitis, and (in the most severe cases) venous stasis ulcers. A recent systematic review of 19 studies totaling 977 patients with upper and lower extremity DVT, revealed a PTS frequency of 26%. The pathophysiology of PTS is thought to derive from venous valvular reflux and/or persistent thrombotic veno-occlusion following DVT, both of which ultimately result in venous hypertension.

Outcomes by Thrombus Type/Location

A clot's location has been found to be quite important with regard to long-term sequelae. Specifically, outcomes of VTE in children may differ among particular anatomic sites. In a Canadian study of CRT in children from 1990 to 1996, VTE-specific mortality was 4% among all children, and was 20% among those children in whom CRT was complicated by PE. No major bleeding episodes were observed. At a median follow-up of 2 years, the cumulative incidence of symptomatic recurrent VTE was 6.5%, and PTS developed in 9% of children. In other series of RVT (primarily among neonates), VTE-related death has been quite uncommon, and the cumulative incidence of recurrent VTE has ranged from 0% to 4%. The cumulative incidence of chronic hypertension in RVT in these studies was reported at 22–33%. For CSVT, the pediatric literature reflects a VTE-specific mortality ranging from 4% to 20%, with a cumulative incidence of recurrent VTE of 8% for neonatal CSVT cases and 17% for CSVT occurring in older children. Long-term neurologic sequelae were noted in 17–26% of neonatal CSVT cases and the cumulative incidence of such sequelae in childhood (i.e., non-neonatal) CSVT has ranged widely between 8% and 47%. It should be noted that both the proportion of children anticoagulated, and the duration of therapy, in the aforementioned pediatric series of RVT and CSVT varied considerably across studies. With regard to portal vein thrombosis, few pediatric series reporting outcomes have been published; however, it appears that the risk of developing recurrent gastrovariceal bleeding in this population is substantial, occurring in many cases even after surgical interventions have been undertaken to reduce portal hypertension. For PE in childhood, long-term outcomes such as chronic pulmonary hypertension and pulmonary function have yet to be established, but remain important to evaluate.

Residual thrombus burden is an additional outcome of interest, but of unclear prognostic significance. A correlation has been shown between D-dimer levels and residual thrombosis at time of anticoagulant treatment discontinuation and the risk of recurrence. Additionally, some evidence indicates that persistent thrombosis is associated with the development of venous valvular insufficiency, an important risk factor for (albeit an imperfect correlate of) the development of PTS. The prevalence of residual thrombosis despite adequate anticoagulation in neonatal VTE has ranged from 12% in a small series of premature newborns with CRT to 62% in full-term neonatal VTE survivors. Among primarily older children, the prevalences of persistent thrombosis have ranged broadly from 37% to 68% in the few longitudinal studies that have employed systematic radiological evaluation of thrombus evolution.

Prognostic Factors and Predictors of Outcome

It has been reported that thrombophilia and markers of coagulation activation are common in pediatric VTE, while potent genetic thrombophilia states are less frequently encountered; nevertheless, the latter are more likely to present in the pediatric age than in older adulthood.

Part of the difficulty with treating childhood VTE is lack of knowledge regarding the natural course of the disease in this population. The ability to predict clinically relevant long-term outcomes of VTE at diagnosis and during the acute/subacute phases of treatment is essential to establishing a future risk-stratified approach to antithrombotic management in children.

As VTE becomes increasingly recognized in children, discussion regarding the appropriate laboratory evaluation for thrombophilia continues. Comprehensive thrombophilia evaluation is recommended in children with VTE. In the future, validated global assays of overall coagulative and fibrinolytic capacities may provide an initial diagnostic evaluation tool to direct more specific testing, and could perhaps be prognostically important.

Previous studies have defined the strong associations of homozygous anticoagulant deficiencies and APA syndrome with recurrent VTE. Over the past several years, the presence of multiple thrombophilia traits has been identified as prognostic for recurrent VTE, and the radiologic finding of complete veno-occlusion at diagnosis of DVT has been associated with an increased risk of persistent thrombosis (which in turn has been associated with the development of venous valvular insufficiency, as noted above). A recent meta-analysis of searches of electronic databases from 1970 to 2007 evaluated the impact of certain thrombophilia traits on recurrence of VTE, reported as odds ratios (OR), which ranged from 2.63 for the factor II variant to 9.44 for antithrombin deficiency. Significant association was found for all inherited thrombophilia traits except factor V Leiden (OR 0.64) and elevated lipoprotein(a) (OR 0.81).

In addition, plasma FVIII activity >150 U/dL and D-dimer concentration >500 ng/mL at the time of diagnosis of VTE in children, as well as following 3–6 months of standard anticoagulation have been shown to predict a composite adverse thrombotic outcome, characterized by persistent thrombosis, recurrent VTE, and/or the development of PTS, adding to evidence for the prognostic utility of these markers in adult VTE.

The finding that evaluation of thrombophilic states in children with VTE may be useful in predicting these pediatric thrombotic outcomes provides optimism that a risk-stratified approach to intensity and duration of antithrombotic therapy may soon be established.

References

Agnelli G, Becattini C (2008) Treatment of DVT: how long is enough and how do you predict recurrence. J Thromb Thrombolysis 25(1):37–44

Andrew M, David M, Adams M et al (1994a) Venous thromboembolic complications (VTE) in children: first analyses of the Canadian registry of VTE. Blood 83:1251–1257

Andrew M, Marzinotto V, Massicotte P et al (1994b) Heparin therapy in pediatric patients: a prospective cohort study. Pediatr Res 35:78–83

Bauer KA et al (2001) Fondaparinux compared with enoxaparin for the prevention of venous thromboembolism after elective major knee surgery. N Engl J Med 345:1305–1310

Berube C, Mitchell L, Silverman E et al (1998) The relationship of antiphospholipid antibodies to thromboembolic events in pediatric patients with systemic lupus erythematosus: a cross-sectional study. Pediatr Res 44:351–356

Bick RL (2003) Prothrombin G20210A mutation, antithrombin, heparin cofactor II, protein C, and protein S defects. Hematol Oncol Clin North Am 17:9–36

Bjarnason H, Kruse JR, Asinger DA, Nazarian GK, Dietz CA Jr, Caldwell MD, Key NS, Hirsch AT, Hunter DW (1997) Iliofemoral deep venous thrombosis: safety and efficacy outcome during 5 years of catheter-directed thrombolytic therapy. J Vasc Interv Radiol 8: 405–418

Buck JR, Connor RH, Cook WW et al (1981) Pulmonary embolism in children. J Pediatr Surg 16:385–391

Bush RL, Lin PH, Bates JT, Mureebe L et al (2004) Pharmacomechanical thrombectomy for treatment of symptomatic lower extremity deep venous thrombosis: safety and feasibility study. J Vasc Surg 40:965–970

Cahn MD, Rohrer MJ, Martella MB, Cutler BS (2001) Long-term follow-up of Greenfield inferior vena cava filter placement in children. J Vasc Surg 34:820–825

Calhoun M, Ross C, Pounder E et al (2010) High prevalence of thrombophilic traits in children with family history of thromboembolism. J Pediatr 157(3):485–489

Cynamon J, Stein EG, Dym RJ et al (2006) A new method for aggressive management of deep vein thrombosis: retrospective study of the power pulse technique. J Vasc Interv Radiol 17:1043–1049

David M, Andrew M (1993) Venous thromboembolic complications in children. J Pediatr 123:337–346

De Graaf J et al (1988) Gradenigo syndrome: a rare complication of otitis media. Clin Neurol Neurosurg 90(3):237–239

de Kleijn ED, de Groot R, Hack CE et al (2003) Activation of protein C following infusion of protein C concentrate in children with severe meningococcal sepsis and purpura fulminans: a randomized, double-blinded, placebo-controlled, dose-finding study. Crit Care Med 31:1839–1847

De Schryver ELLM, Blom I, Braun KPJ et al (2004) Long-term prognosis of cerebral venous sinus thrombosis in childhood. Dev Med Child Neurol 46:514–519

deVeber GA, MacGregor D, Curtis R et al (2000) Neurologic outcome in survivors of childhood arterial ischemic stroke and sinovenous thrombosis. J Child Neurol 15:316–324

deVeber G, Andrew M, Adams C et al (2001) Cerebral sinovenous thrombosis in children. N Engl J Med 345:417–423

Dreyfus M, Magny JF, Bridey F et al (1991) Treatment of homozygous protein C deficiency and neonatal purpura fulminans with a purified protein C concentrate. N Engl J Med 325:1565–1568

Dreyfus M, Masterson M, David M et al (1995) Replacement therapy with a monoclonal antibody purified protein C concentrate in newborns with severe congenital protein C deficiency. Semin Thromb Hemost 21:371–381

Eichinger S, Minar E, Bialonczyk C et al (2003) D-dimer levels and risk of recurrent venous thromboembolism. J Am Med Assoc 290: 1071–1074

Eriksson BI, Dahl OE, Rosencher N et al (2007a) Oral dabigatran etexilate vs. subcutaneous enoxaparin for the prevention of venous thromboembolism after total knee replacement; the RE-MODEL randomized trial. J Thromb Haemost 5:2178–2185

Eriksson BL, Dahl OE, Rosencher N, RE-NOVATE Study Group et al (2007b) Dabigatran etexilate versus enoxaparin for prevention of venous thromboembolism after total hip replacement: a randomized, double-blind, non-inferiority trial. Lancet 370:949–956

Eriksson BI, Borris LC, Friedman RJ et al (2008) Rivaroxaban versus enoxaparin for thromboprophylaxis after hip arthroplasty. N Engl J Med 358:2765–2775

Ettingshausen CE, Veldmann A, Beeg T et al (1999) Replacement therapy with protein C concentrate in infants and adolescents with meningococcal sepsis and purpura fulminans. Semin Thromb Hemost 25:537–541

Gandini R, Maspes F, Sodani G et al (1999) Percutaneous ilio-caval thrombectomy with the Amplatz device: preliminary results. Eur Radiol 9:951–958

Ginsburg JS (2009) Oral thrombin inhibitor dabigatran etexilate vs North American enoxaparin regimen for prevention of venous thromboembolism after knee arthroplasty surgery: the RE-MOBILIZE writing committee. J Arthroplasty 24(1):1–9

Goldenberg NA (2005) Long-term outcomes of venous thrombosis in children. Curr Opin Hematol 12:370–376

Goldenberg NA, Knapp-Clevenger R, Manco-Johnson MJ et al (2004) Elevated plasma factor VIII and D-dimer levels as predictors of poor outcomes of thrombosis in children. N Engl J Med 351:1081–1088

Goldenberg NA, Knapp-Clevenger R, Hays T, Mando-Johnson M (2005) Lemierre's and Lemierre's-like syndromes in children: survival and thromboembolic outcomes. Pediatrics 116:543–548

Goldenberg NA, Knapp-Clevenger R, Durham JD, Manco-Johnson MJ (2007) A thrombolytic regimen for high-risk deep venous thrombosis may substantially reduce the risk of post-thrombotic syndrome in children. Blood 110:45–53

Goldenberg NA et al (2008) Thrombophilia states and markers of coagulation activation in the prediction of pediatric venous thromboembolic outcomes: a comparative analysis with respect to adult evidence. Hematol Am Soc Hematol Educ Program 2008(1):236–244

Goldenberg NA et al (2010a) The "parallel-cohort RCT": novel design aspects and application in the Kids-DOTT trial of pediatric venous thromboembolism. Contemp Clin Trials 31(1):131–133

Goldenberg NA, Branchford BR, Wang M et al (2011) Percutaneous mechanical and pharmacomechanical thrombolysis for occlusive deep venous thrombosis of the proximal limb in adolescents: findings from an institution-based prospective inception cohort study of pediatric venous thromboembolism JVIR (in press)

Goldenberg NA et al (2010). Post thrombotic syndrome in children: a systematic review of frequency of occurrence, validity of outcome measures, and prognostic factors. Haematologica (in press)

Goodnight S, Hathaway W (2001) Disorders of hemostasis and thrombosis: a clinical guide, 2nd edn. McGraw-Hill, New York

Gurakan F, Eren M, Kocak N et al (2004) Extrahepatic portal vein thrombosis in children: etiology and long-term follow-up. J Clin Gastroenterol 38:368–372

Haussmann U, Fischer J, Eber S et al (2006) Hepatic veno-occlusive disease in pediatric stem cell transplantation: impact of pre-emptive antithrombin III replacement and combined antithrombin III/defibrotide therapy. Haematologica 91:795–800

Hoyer PF, Gonda S, Barthels M (1986) Thromboembolic complications in children with nephritic syndrome. Risk and incidence. Acta Paediatr Scand 75:804–810

Hull RD, Raskob GE, Rosenbloom D et al (1990) Heparin for 5 days as compared with 10 days in the initial treatment of proximal venous thrombosis. N Engl J Med 322:1260–1264

Jackson LSM, Xiu-Jie W, Dudrick SJ et al (2005) Catheter-directed thrombolysis and/or thrombectomy with selective endovascular stenting as alternatives to systemic anticoagulation for treatment of acute deep vein thrombosis. Am J Surg 190:864–868

Kahn SR, Dsmarais S, Ducruet T et al (2006) Comparison of the Villalta and Ginsberg clinical scales to diagnose the post-thrombotic syndrome: correlation with patient-reported disease burden and venous valvular reflux. J Thromb Haemost 4:907–908

Kearon C, Ginsberg JS, Kovacs MJ et al (2003) Comparison of low-intensity warfarin therapy with conventional-intensity warfarin therapy for long-term prevention of recurrent venous thromboembolism. N Engl J Med 349:631–639

Kearon C, Ginsberg JS, Julina JA et al (2006) Comparison of fixed-dose weight-adjusted UFH and low-molecular-weight heparin for acute treatment of venous thromboembolism. J Am Med Assoc 296:935–942

Keidan I, Lotan D, Gazit G et al (1994) Early neonatal renal venous thrombosis: long-term outcome. Acta Pediatr 83:1225–1227

Kenet G, Waldman D, Lubetsky A et al (2004) Paediatric cerebral sinus vein thrombosis. Thromb Haemost 92:713–718

Konkle BA, Bauer KA, Weinstein R et al (2003) Use of recombinant human antithrombin in patients with congenital antithrombin deficiency undergoing surgical procedures. Transfusion 43:390–394

Kosch A, Kuwertz-Broking E, Heller C et al (2004) Renal venous thrombosis in neonates: prothrombotic risk factors and long-term follow-up. Blood 104:1356–1360

Kovacs MJ (2004) Long-term low-dose warfarin use is effective in the prevention of recurrent venous thromboembolism. J Thromb Haemost 2:1041–1043

Kuhle S, Massicotte P, Chan A et al (2004) A case series of 72 neonates with renal vein thrombosis: data from the 1-800-NO-CLOTS registry. Thromb Haemost 92:929–933

Kyrle PA, Minar E, Hirschl M et al (2000) High plasma levels of factor VIII and the risk of recurrent venous thromboembolism. N Engl J Med 343:457–462

Lassen MR, Ageno W, Borris LC et al (2008) Rivaroxaban versus enoxaparin for thromboprophylaxis after total knee arthroplasty. N Engl J Med 358:2776–2786

Lewy PR, Jao W (1974) Nephrotic syndrome in association with renal vein thrombosis in infancy. J Pediatr 85:359–365

Lin PH, Zhou W, Dardik A, Mussa F et al (2006) Catheter-direct thrombolysis versus pharmacomechanical thrombectomy for treatment of symptomatic lower extremity deep venous thrombosis. Am J Surg 192:782–788

Manco-Johnson M (2006) How I treat venous thrombosis in children. Blood 107:21–29

Manco-Johnson MJ, Grabowski EF, Hellgreen M et al (2002) Laboratory testing for thrombophilia in pediatric patients. On behalf of the subcommittee for perinatal and pediatric thrombosis of the scientific and standardization committee of the International Society on Thrombosis and Haemostasis (ISTH). Thromb Haemost 88:155–156

Mann K, Brummel-Ziedins K (2009) Blood coagulation. In: Orkin S et al (eds) Nathan and Oski's hematology of infancy and childhood, 7th edn. Elsevier, Philadelphia

Massicotte MP, Dix D, Monagle P et al (1998) Central venous catheter related thrombosis in children: analysis of the Canadian Registry of venous thromboembolic complications. J Pediatr 133:770–776

Massicotte P, Julian JA, Gent M et al (2003) An open label randomized controlled trial of low molecular weight heparin compared to heparin and coumadin for the treatment of venous thromboembolic events in children: the REVIVE trial. Thromb Res 109:85–92

Meissner MH, Manzo RA, Bergelin RO et al (1993) Deep venous insufficiency: the relationship between lysis and subsequent reflux. J Vasc Surg 18:596–605

Meister B, Kropshofer G, Klein-Franke A et al (2008) Comparison of low-molecular-weight heparin and antithrombin versus antithrombin alone for the prevention of thrombosis in children with acute lymphoblastic leukemia. Pediatr Blood Cancer 50(2):298–303

Michaels LA, Gurian M, Hagyi T et al (2004) Low molecular weight heparin in the treatment of venous and arterial thromboses in the premature infant. Pediatrics 114:703–707

Mitchell L, Andrew M, Hanna K et al (2003) Trend to efficacy and safety using antithrombin concentrate in prevention of thrombosis in children receiving L-asparaginase for acute lymphoblastic leukemia. Results of the PARKAA study. Thromb Haemost 90:235–244

Mocan H, Beattie TJ, Murphy AV et al (1991) Renal venous thrombosis in infancy: long-term follow-up. Pediatr Nephrol 5:45–49

Monagle P, Andew M (2003) Nathan and Oski's hematology of infancy and childhood, 6th edn. Elsivier, Philadelphia

Monagle P, Adams M, Mahoney M et al (2000) Outcome of pediatric thromboembolic disease: a report from the Canadian childhood thrombophilia registry. Pediatr Res 47:763–766

Monagle P, Chan A, Massicotte P, Chalmers E, Michelson AD (2004) Antithrombotic therapy in children: the seventh ACCP conference on antithrombotic and thrombotic therapy. Chest 126 (Suppl 3):645S–687S

Muller FM, Ehrenthal W, Hafner G, Schranz D (1996) Purpura fulminans in severe congenital protein C deficiency: monitoring of treatment with protein C concentrate. Eur J Pediatr 155:20–25

Newman P, Newman D (2009) Platelets and the vessel wall. In: Orkin S et al (eds) Nathan and Oski's hematology of infancy and childhood, 7th edn. Elsevier, Philadelphia

Nohe N, Flemmer A, Rumler R et al (1999) The low molecular weight heparin dalteparin for prophylaxis and therapy of thrombosis in childhood: a report on 48 cases. Eur J Pediatr 158:S134–S139

Nowak-Göttl U, Junker R, Kruez W et al (2001) Risk of recurrent venous thrombosis in children with combined prothrombotic risk factors. Blood 97:858–862

Nuss R, Hays T, Manco-Johnson M (1994) Efficacy and safety of heparin anticoagulation for neonatal renal vein thrombosis. Am J Hematol Oncol 16:127–131

Oren H, Devecioglu O, Ertem M et al (2004) Analysis of pediatric thrombotic patients in Turkey. Pediatr Hematol Oncol 21:573–583

Palareti G, Legnani C, Cosmi B et al (2002) Risk of venous thromboembolism recurrence: high negative predictive value of D-dimer performed after oral anticoagulation is stopped. Thromb Haemost 87:7–12

Parikh S, Motarjeme A, McNamara T et al (2008) Ultrasound-accelerated thrombolysis for the treatment of deep vein thrombosis: initial clinical experience. J Vasc Interv Radiol 19:521–528

Pipe S, Goldenberg N (2009) Acquired diseases of hemostasis. In: Orkin S et al (eds) Nathan and Oski's hematology of infancy and childhood, 7th edn. Elsevier, Philadelphia

Prandoni P, Lensing AWA, Cogo A et al (1996) The long-term clinical course of acute deep venous thrombosis. Ann Intern Med 125:1–7

Protack CD, Bakken AM, Patel N et al (2007) Long-term outcomes of catheter directed thrombolysis for lower extremity deep venous thrombosis without prophylactic inferior vena cava filter placement. J Vasc Surg 45:992–997

Raffini L et al (2009) Dramatic increase in venous thromboembolism in children's hospitals in the United States from 2001 to 2007. Pediatrics 124(4):1001–1008

Revel-Vilk S, Sharathkumar A, Massicotte P et al (2004) Natural history of arterial and venous thrombosis in children treated with low molecular weight heparin: a longitudinal study by ultrasound. J Thromb Haemost 2:42–46

Rivard GE, David M, Farrell C, Schwarz HP (1995) Treatment of purpura fulminans in meningococcemia with protein C concentrate. J Pediatr 126(4):646–652

Schmidt B, Andrew M (1995) Neonatal thrombosis: report of a prospective Canadian and international registry. Pediatrics 96:939–943

Schulmna S et al (2009) Dabigatran versus warfarin in the treatment of acute venous thromboembolism. N Engl J Med 24(361):2342–2352

Shi H-J, Huang Y-H, Shen T et al (2009) Percutaneous mechanical thrombectomy combined with catheter-directed thrombolysis in the treatment of symptomatic lower extremity deep venous thrombosis. Eur J Radiol 71:350–355

Stein PD, Kayali R, Olson RE et al (1994) Incidence of venous thromboembolism in infants and children: data from the National Hospital Discharge Survey. J Pediatr 145:563–565

van Ommen C, Monagle P, Peters M et al (1999) Pulmonary embolism in childhood. In: van Beek E, Oudkerk M, ten Cate JW (eds) Pulmonary embolism: epidemiology, diagnosis, and treatment. Blackwell, Oxford

van Ommen CH, Heijboer H, Buller HR et al (2001) Venous thromboembolism in childhood: a prospective two-year registry in the Netherlands. J Pediatr 139:676–681

van Ommen CH, Heijboer H, van den Dool EJ et al (2003) Pediatric venous thromboembolic disease in one single center: congenital prothrombotic disorders and the clinical outcome. J Thromb Haemost 1:2516–2522

Verhaeghe R, Stockx L, Lacroix H, Vermylen J, Baert AL (1997) Catheter-directed lysis of iliofemoral vein thrombosis with use of rt-PA. Eur Radiol 7:996–1001

Vukovich T, Auberger K, Weil J et al (1988) Replacement therapy for a homozygous protein C deficiency state using a concentrate of human protein C and S. Br J Haematol 70:435–440

Young G et al (2008) Impact of inherited thrombophilia on venous thromboembolism in children: a systematic review and meta-analysis of observational studies. Circulation 118(13):1373–1382

Zaunschirm A, Muntean W (1986) Correction of hemostatic imbalances induced by L-asparaginase therapy in children with acute lymphoblastic leukemia. Pediatr Hematol Oncol 3:19–25

Pediatric Oncology

H. Stacy Nicholson

338 Incidence, Epidemiology and Survival

H. Stacy Nicholson

Introduction

Compared to cancer during adulthood, childhood cancer is rare. In the USA, the incidence of cancer between ages 0–19 is 16.7 per 100,000 (15.2 per 100,000 for ages 0–14). The most common malignancy is acute lymphoblastic leukemia (ALL) with 3.5 per 100,000 followed by central nervous system (CNS) tumors at 2.9 per 100,000. Over the past three decades, survival has improved for most pediatric cancers. In the USA, 81.4% of children and adolescents diagnosed with cancer between the ages of 0 and 19 between 1999 and 2006 survived for more than 5 years. The incidence rates and chances of surviving at least 5 years for the major childhood cancers are shown in ➔ *Table 338.1.*

Cancer in Developing Nations

Childhood cancer incidence and mortality differs in high- vs. low-income nations, and these differences should be further studied in order to better understand etiology, in particular. While cancer survival rates for children are similar in all high-income nations to what is seen in the USA, most of the world's children live in middle- and low-income nations. In developing nations, the proportion of children relative to the total population is greater, and access to health care is often lower. As the treatment for infectious diseases and other more common diseases in children has improved, the impact of childhood cancer in developing counties has increased. We shouldn't accept that survival rates will always remain lower in developing nations. "Twinning" countries – creating partnerships between developed and developing countries in order to improve the treatment of childhood cancer – is an approach that holds great promise for bringing the benefits of effective anticancer therapy to more of the world's children.

Etiology

In most cases of childhood cancer, the cause is unknown. Environmental factors do not play a large causal role in childhood cancer in contrast to many adult malignancies. Cancer in childhood or adolescence differs significantly from adult malignancies. Adult cancers are primarily carcinomas, while children get leukemia, brain tumors, embryonic cancers, and sarcomas. Thus, in children, the etiology is more likely to be genetic, rather than environmental. There are exceptions – benzene can lead to leukemia, and radiation can lead to brain tumors and other solid malignancies. Also, in Sub-Saharan Africa, the Epstein–Barr virus (EBV) is known to cause Burkitt lymphoma, and EBV is also associated with lymphoproliferative diseases in transplant survivors. Human Papilloma Virus (HPV) is associated with cervical, penile, and some head and neck cancers – while these tumors do not often affect children and adolescents, the prevention of these cancers is becoming possible with the advent of

Table 338.1
Incidence and survival of major childhood cancers in the United States (diagnosed before age 20)

Cancer	Incidence (per 100,000)	5 year relative survival (%)
Bone	0.8	70.1
Brain	3.0	74.8
Hodgkin's lymphoma	1.4	96.1
Acute lympoblastic leukemia (ALL)	3.2	85.9
Acute myeloid leukemia	0.8	56.5
Neuroblastoma	1.0	71.7
Non-Hodgkin lymphoma	1.2	84.1
Soft tissue sarcoma	1.1	76.3
Wilms' tumor	0.6	92.1
OVERALL	16.7	81.4

Incidence rates are per 100,000 and are age-adjusted to the 2000 US standard population. 2007 data given. Survival data are for children diagnosed at ages 0–19 between 1999 and 2006

Abdelaziz Y. Elzouki (ed.), *Textbook of Clinical Pediatrics*, DOI 10.1007/978-3-642-02202-9_338,

vaccines against HPV. HIV is associated with Kaposi's sarcoma and non-Hodgkin's lymphoma, and Hepatitis B and other viruses may be causal in some liver tumors.

Secondary cancers occur in a small proportion of cancer survivors due to therapies such as chemotherapy and radiotherapy and, in some, a genetic predisposition to cancer. Secondary cancers are discussed in the chapter ➋ on late complications of therapy.

The incidence of cancer in children who are genetically predisposed to cancer is higher. This predisposition may be due to genetic factors that have either been inherited or develop spontaneously. Some of the more common-known cancer predisposition syndromes are outlined in ➋ *Table 338.2.* Rarely, the same cancer may occur in multiple members of a family. Bilateral cancers in paired organs, such as bilateral retinoblastoma or bilateral Wilms tumor, is evidence for a genetic predisposition as are positive family histories. Familial cancers have been most commonly reported in retinoblastoma, childhood leukemia, and Wilms tumor. Mathematical modeling of the earlier

Table 338.2
Cancer predisposition syndromes in children

Condition	Tumors	Genetic defect	Comments
Hereditary retinoblastoma (RB)	Retinoblastoma; osteosarcoma	RB1	80% with bilateral RB will have a negative family history
Down syndrome	Acute lymphoblastic leukemia; acute megakaryoblastic leukemia; JMML	Trisomy 21	Contribution of trisomy to tumorigenesis is not known
Li Fraumeni syndrome	Sarcomas; breast cancer; brain tumors; leukemia	p53	Family history key
Fanconi anemia	Acute leukemia Head and neck carcinomas Cervical carcinoma	Multiple Fanconi	Chromosomal breakage syndrome
Bloom syndrome	Acute leukemias		
Ataxia telangiectasia	Lymphoma Leukemia Gastric carcinoma	ATM (11q22–q23)	Truncal ataxia; oculocutaneous telangiectasias
Neurofibromatosis type I	Neurofibromas; optic nerve gliomas; astrocytomas; pheochromocytoma; AML; myelodysplasia; myeloproliferative syndromes;	NF1 gene (17q11.2)	Variable severity of NF1; very large gene
Neurofibromatosis type II	Vestibular schwanomas; meningiomas;	NF2 (19)	Most often diagnosed in adulthood
Tuberous sclerosis	Subependymal giant cell astrocytomas (SEGA); renal angiomyolipomas	TSC1 (9q34) TSC2 (16p13.3)	Variable intelligence; seizures
Gorlin syndrome	Medulloblastoma Basal cell carcinomas	PTCH	
Turcot syndrome	Colon cancer and CNS tumors (medulloblastoma, high-grade astrocytomas)	APC gene; hereditary nonpolyposis colon cancer (HNPCC)	Family history of colon cancer, particularly at a young age.
WAGR	Wilms tumor	WT1 (11p13)	Wilms tumor, aniridia, genitourinary abnormalities; mental retardation
Beckwith Wiedeman syndrome (BWS)	Wilms tumor Hepatoblastoma Adrenocortical carcinoma	11p15	Screening for liver, adrenal and kidney tumors key during childhood

age at onset of bilateral retinoblastoma led to Knudsen's two-hit model of cancer etiology. Furthermore, children with an underlying cancer predisposition syndrome have an increased risk of a second cancer. Thus, updating the family history for cancer in all first- and second-degree relatives should occur at diagnosis and periodically throughout treatment and follow-up as new cancers occurring in adult relatives may be informative. Finally, children with immunodeficiencies have an increased risk of lymphoma and lymphoproliferative diseases.

Cancer During Infancy

During the first year of life, the types of cancers that occur differ from what is seen in later childhood. While leukemia remains the most common cancer during infancy, its incidence is less than half of what occurs at age 2, and acute myelogenous leukemia (AML) is more common relative to *all* than in older children. As in other ages, brain and other Central Nervous System (CNS) tumors are the most common solid malignancy, and neuroblastoma is also common. Neuroblastoma is the most common cancer in the first month of life.

Adolescent and Young (Aya) Adult Cancers

In the USA, older adolescents (15 years and older) and young adults (up to 40 years) have not seen the same degree of improvement in survival compared to children and older adults. This is likely due to differing tumor biology, impaired access to care, and insufficient supportive care infrastructure. Efforts to improve outcomes in the AYA population are being studied.

References

Ahmedin J, Siegel R, Xu J, Ward E (2010) Cancer statistics, 2010. CA Cancer J Clin 60:277–300

American Society of Clinical Oncology (2003) Policy statement update: Genetic testing for cancer susceptibility. J Clin Oncol 21:2397–2406

DeBaun M, Tucker MA (1998) Risk of cancer during the first 4 years of life in children from the Beckwith-Wiedemann Syndrome Registry. J Pediatr 132:398–400

Eiler ME, Frohnmayer D, Frohnmayer L et al (eds) (2008) Fanconi anemia: Guidelines for diagnosis and management, 3rd edn. Fanconi Anemia Research Fund, Inc., Eugene, OR

Eng C, Li FP, Abramson DH et al (1993) Mortality from second tumors among long-term survivors of retinoblastoma. J Natl Cancer Inst 85:1121–1129

German J, Ellis N (2002) Bloom syndrome. In: Vogelstein B, Kingler RW (eds) The genetic basis of human cancer, 2nd edn. McGraw-Hill, Inc; NY, New York, pp 267–288

Howard SC, Metzger ML, Wilimas JA et al (2008) Childhood cancer epidemiology in low-income countries. Cancer 112:461–472

Kinzler KW, Volgelstein B (1993) Cancer. A gene for neurofibromatosis 2. Nature 363:495–496

Knudsen AG Jr (1971) Mutation and cancer: Statistical study of retinoblastoma. Proc Natl Acad Sci USA 68:820–823

Li FP, Fraumeni JF Jr (1969) Rhabdomyosarcoma in children: Epidemiologic study and identification of a familial cancer syndrome. J Natl Cancer Inst 43:1365–1373

Lo Muzio L (2008) Nevoid basal cell carcinoma syndrome (Gorlin syndrome). Orphanet J Rare Dis 3:32

Malkin D (2004) Predictive genetic testing for childhood cancer: Taking the road less traveled by. J Pediatr Hematol Oncol 26:546–548

Malkin D, Li FP, Strong LC et al (1990) Germ line p53 mutations in a familial syndrome of breast cancer, sarcoma and other neoplasms. Science 250:1233–1238

Masera G (2009) Bridging the childhood cancer mortality gap between economically developed and low-income countries. J Pediatr Hematol Oncol 31:720–712

Matsui I, Tanimura M, Kobayashi N et al (1991) Neurofibromatosis type I and childhood cancer. Cancer 72:2746–2754

Mori T, Nagase H, Horii A et al (1994) Germ-line and somatic mutations of the APC gene in patients with Turcot syndrome and analysis of APC gene in brain tumors. Genes Chromosom Cancer 9:168–172

Narod SA, Stiller C, Lenoir GM (1991) An estimate of the heritable fraction of childhood cancer. Br J Cancer 63:993–999

Orem J, Otieno MW, Remick SC (2004) AIDS-associated cancer in developing nations. Curr Opin Oncol 16:468–476

Ribeiro PC, Piu CH (2005) Saving the children – improving childhood cancer treatment in developing countries. NEJM 352:2158–2160

Ross JA, Spector LG, Robison LL, Olshan AF (2005) Epidemiology of leukemia in children with Down syndrome. Pediatr Blood Cancer 44:8–12

www.seer.cancer.gov.

339 Evaluation of Abdominal Masses and Enlarged Lymph Nodes in Children

Gregory Blaschke · H. Stacy Nicholson

Abdominal Masses

Childhood tumors that commonly present with an abdominal mass include neuroblastoma, Wilms' tumor, hepatoblastoma, rhabdomyosarcoma, lymphoma, and ovarian tumors. Prompt investigation of suspected abdominal masses leads to more effective and more cost effective treatment.

Often, abdominal masses are discovered by parents or by physicians during health maintenance visits. In order to maximize the chances of discovering abdominal masses, a careful history and physical exam should be part of each health maintenance visit during childhood. In addition to allowing the parents to describe any concerns, including the following items in a review of systems will be helpful in uncovering abdominal masses:

- Abdominal pain
- Hematuria
- Irritability
- Weight loss
- Vomiting
- Changes in bowel habits

The physical examination should include careful palpation of the entire abdomen, and this may be done in any position that ensures cooperation and a successful exam. The history and physical can yield clues as to the diagnosis. Hematuria suggests Wilms' tumor or a rhabdomyosarcoma of the genitourinary system. Hypertension may accompany neuroblastoma, and symptoms of intestinal obstruction suggest a Burkitt's lymphoma of the bowel wall.

Any suspected abdominal mass should be promptly evaluated, and an abdominal ultrasound (US) is useful as the initial imaging modality as it is typically readily available and spares the child from radiation exposure that accompanies computerized tomography (CT).

Once an abdominal mass is confirmed, surgical consultation is warranted. The history, exam, and imaging often suggest a likely diagnosis; based on this presumed diagnosis, any indicated staging tests may be done before surgery. This will assist the surgeon in surgical planning, and a preoperative chest CT eliminates confusion regarding whether findings represent postoperative atelectasis or metastatic disease.

Enlarged Lymph Nodes

Enlarged lymph nodes are a common finding in healthy children, and few such nodes represent malignancy. Lymph nodes are most often enlarged in response to an infection, and one generally sees resolution with successful treatment of the underlying cause. Pyomyositis is more common in many tropical parts of the world. Common infectious causes include staph aureus, tuberculosis, or sarcoidosis. Preceding trauma may be in the history and drainage is part of treatment. Nontender, firm nodes in unusual locations or ones that continue to increase after 2 weeks or fail to regress in 4–6 weeks should lead to biopsy. Tender adenitis may require a trial of antibiotics.

Table 339.1
Typical differences between benign and malignant causes of enlarged lymph nodes

Characteristic	Benign adenopathy	Malignancy
Onset	Rapid and associated with other signs and symptoms of infection, such as fever.	Progresses slowly over time. May be the only symptom present.
Size	Usually <3 cm	Can be small or large; will generally increase in size over time and may become confluent
Consistency	Soft, warm	Firm, rubbery, or hard
Tenderness	Usually present	Usually absent

Abdelaziz Y. Elzouki (ed.), *Textbook of Clinical Pediatrics*, DOI 10.1007/978-3-642-02202-9_339,

Fluctuant adenopathy may require cautious surgical involvement or drainage, and usually excision to avoid chronic drainage tracks depending on infectious etiology. However, enlarged nodes may be the initial manifestation of leukemia (particularly T-cell acute lymphoblastic leukemia (ALL)), Hodgkin Disease, non-Hodgkin lymphoma, or histiocytosis. Rarely, an enlarged node may represent regional or metastatic spread from an undiagnosed solid tumor. Adenopathy associated with malignancy does not resolve and typically progresses over time. ➲ *Table 339.1* lists clinical features that typically accompany both benign and malignant adenopathy.

References

Brodeur AE, Brodeur GM (1991) Abdominal masses in children: neuroblastoma, wilms tumor, and other considerations. Pediatr Rev 12: 196–206

Chandler JC, Gauderer MW (2004) The neonate with an abdominal mass. Pediatr Clin North Am 51(4):979–997, ix

Golden CB, Feusner JH (2002) Malignant abdominal masses in children: quick guide to evaluation and diagnosis. Pediatr Clin North Am 49:1368–1392

Hoffer FA (2005) Magnetic resonance imaging of abdominal masses in the pediatric patient. Semin Ultrasound CT MRI 26:212–223

Irish MS, Pearl RH, Caty MG, Glick PL (1998) The approach to common abdominal diagnosis in infants and children. Pediatr Clin North Am 45:729–772

Kaste SC, McCarville MB (2008) Imaging pediatric abdominal tumors. Semin Roentgenol 43(1):50–59

Olson OE (2008) Imaging of abdominal tumors: CT or MRI? Pediatr Radiol 38(Suppl 3):S452–S458

Pearl RH, Irish MS, Caty MG, Glick PL (1998) The approach to common abdominal diagnoses in infants and children. Part II. Pediatr Clin North Am 45:1287–1326

Restrepo R, Oneto J, Lopez K, Kukreja K (2009) Head and neck lymph nodes in children: the spectrum from normal to abnormal. Pediatr Radiol 39(8):836–846

Vural S, Baskin D, Dogan O et al (2010) Diagnosis in childhood abdominal Burkitt's lymphoma. Ann Surg Oncol 17:2476–2479

Wang J, Pei G, Yan J et al (2010) Unexplained cervical lymphadenopathy in children: Prredictive factors for malignancy. J Pediatr Surg 45(4): 784–788

Wolf AD, Lavine JE (2000) Hepatomegaly in neonates and children. Pediatr Rev 21:303–310

340 Principles of Diagnosis

Gregory Blaschke · H. Stacy Nicholson

Introduction

When a child is suspected of having a malignancy, there is an urgent need to obtain the correct specific histopathological diagnosis and to fully document the stage (degree of spread). A precise diagnosis and correct staging informs both the prognosis and determines the correct treatment plan. Thus, ensuring that all tissues are handled correctly and that all required staging tests are obtained is crucial. In general, a histopathological diagnosis, either from tumor excision, biopsy, or needle aspiration, must be obtained. Exceptions to this rule include sites where biopsies pose excessive risk (such as brainstem tumors) and some oncologic emergencies, such as when a child with a mediastinal mass presents with severe respiratory and/or circulatory compromise. Each cancer has a distinct panel of diagnostic studies needed for proper staging, and these are discussed in each disease entity. Guiding general principles are the topic of this chapter.

When a primary care physician diagnoses or strongly suspects a childhood malignancy, prompt referral to a center with pediatric oncologists, pediatric surgeons, advanced imaging resources, and pathological resources is indicated.

Diagnostic Studies

Blood, Bone Marrow, and Spinal Fluid

A complete blood count (CBC) is generally performed whenever leukemia or a solid tumor is suspected. Children with leukemia will usually have blasts on the blood smear; however, cytopenias in one or more cell lines may be the only evidence for leukemia. Similarly, solid tumors with metastatic spread to the bone marrow may lead to cytopenias on the CBC.

Serum chemistries should be obtained to ensure adequate hepatic, renal, and other organ function prior to initiating therapy. LDH should be measured if lymphoma is suspected, and uric acid must be measured in leukemias and lymphomas in order to minimize the risk of tumor lysis syndrome with the initiation of therapy. When applicable, serum tumor markers should be obtained. Tumor markers are discussed with each disease entity.

Bone marrow aspiration is required to establish the diagnosis of leukemia and in staging solid tumors that can metastasize to marrow. In addition to standard morphology, cytogenetic studies and flow cytometry need to be obtained. In leukemia, chromosomal number (ploidy), some chromosomal translocations and cell surface markers have prognostic and treatment implications. Bone marrow biopsies are also important in the staffing workup for lymphomas and for some solid tumors.

Performing a lumbar puncture for cerebrospinal fluid (CSF) cytology is indicated in some brain tumors (medulloblastoma, ependymoma, primitive neuroectodermal tumors (PNET)), in leukemia and lymphoma, and in parameningeal rhabdomyosarcomas.

Radiological Studies

Chest X-rays (CXR) are frequently obtained in children with newly diagnosed cancer, and an urgent CXR should be obtained in children with leukemia or lymphoma to check for a mediastinal mass (➲ *Fig. 340.1*). A CXR is typically obtained in children with a solid tumor, but computerized tomography (CT) of the chest should also be done, making a CXR less important. Abdominal ultrasound may be useful as a screening tool, but the degree of information obtained from CT scans or magnetic resonance imaging (MRI) has made these modalities the gold standard. MRI is the imaging modality of choice in CNS tumors, while CT scans are typically better in evaluating bone. Nuclear medicine scans are used to evaluate for bony metastases and are used in staging and following patients with lymphoma.

Tissue Diagnosis

Proper treatment is only possible following a correct pathological diagnosis. Biopsies can be obtained via surgery or by a needle biopsy. Consultation with the pathologist prior to the procedure can be helpful, particularly when a needle biopsy is planned, in order to ensure that enough tissue is available to establish the diagnosis and perform all required studies. Frozen-section examination of the tumor

Abdelaziz Y. Elzouki (ed.), *Textbook of Clinical Pediatrics*, DOI 10.1007/978-3-642-02202-9_340,

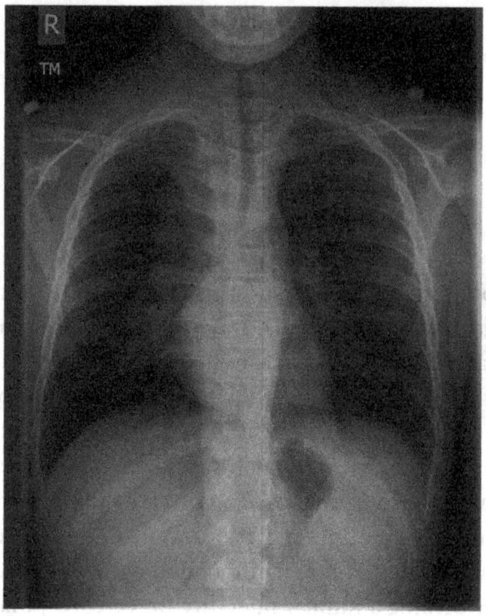

a

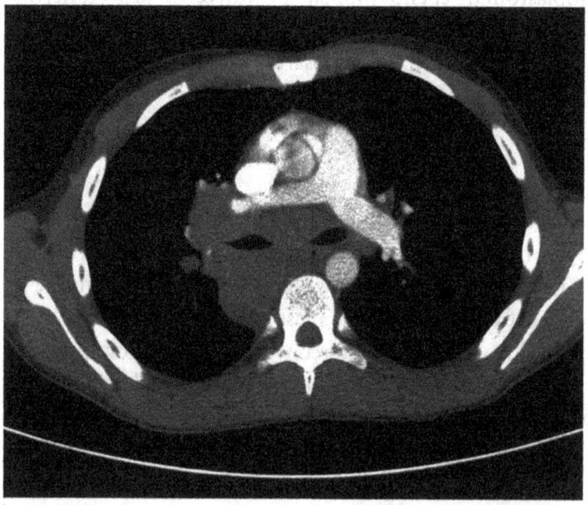

b

Figure 340.1
(a) CXR of 18-year-old male with respiratory distress showing anterior mediastinal mass. (b) Chest CT with intravenous contrast showing mediastinal mass with compression of both main-stem bronchi.Images courtesy of Katharine Hopkins, MD

during surgery can ensure that the tumor has indeed been biopsied and guide the surgeon in making clinical decisions. In some tumors, evaluating the margins of the excised mass for active tumor must be done to assist in determining prognosis and assigning treatment. Providing the pathologist with fresh tissue may be required for cytogenetics, molecular studies and flow cytometry. Such studies are becoming more important with molecular staging of tumors and leukemias. Again, preoperative consultation with the pathologist can ensure that the proper studies are performed.

Family- and Community-Centered Care

While the primary care provider may not make the definitive diagnosis, it is always helpful to collaboratively "break the news" regarding the concern for cancer to the family as part of referral process. Indeed, the desires and abilities in the context of the family and community will often determine the initial referral location. Definitive care may require additional referral to alternative sites that specialize in specific treatments or cancers. Many family, community, and multidisciplinary partners can assist in informing the family and assisting with the process of referral.

References

Dixon-Woods M, Findlay M, Young B et al (2001) Parent's accounts of obtaining a diagnosis of childhood cancer. Lancet 357:670–674

Fernbach DJ (1985) The role of the family physician in the care of the child with cancer. CA Cancer J Clin 35:258–270

Franzius C, Juergens KU (2009) PET/CT in paediatric oncology: indications and pitfalls. Pediatr Radiol 39(Suppl 3):446–9

Golden CB, Feusner JH (2002) Malignant abdominal masses in children: quick guide to evaluation and diagnosis. Pediatr Clin North Am 49:1368–1392

Hoffer FA (2005) Magnetic resonance imaging of abdominal masses in the pediatric patient. Seminars Ultrasound CT MRI 26:212–223

Irish MS, Pearl RH, Caty MG, Glick PL (1998) The approach to common abdominal diagnosis in infants and children. Pediatr Clin North Am 45:729–72

Pearl RH, Irish MS, Caty MG, Glick PL (1998) The approach to common abdominal diagnoses in infants and children. Part II. Pediatr Clin North Am 45:1287–326

Raab CP, Gartner JC Jr (2009) Diagnosis of childhood cancer. Primary Care; Clinics Office Practice 36:671–84

341 Principles of Cancer Chemotherapy in Children

H. Stacy Nicholson

Introduction

Children and adolescents with cancer are best treated at a referral center with adequate resources to assemble a team consisting of pediatric oncologists, radiation oncologists, and surgeons, as well as nursing staff and others who support the children and families. The pediatric oncologist typically leads the team, and most pediatric cancers are treated with chemotherapy, either alone or in combination with surgery and radiation.

Chemotherapy simply means using medicines to treat cancer, and there are a few key principles and definitions that broadly apply, regardless of diagnosis. Using chemotherapy in solid tumors following surgery, even without evidence of metastatic disease, is defined as adjuvant chemotherapy. Chemotherapy administered before the definitive surgical procedure is referred to as neoadjuvant chemotherapy. One of the most important advances in the use of chemotherapy was the recognition that combination chemotherapy, using two or more drugs with differing mechanisms of action, would help overcome drug resistance. Dose intensity, the amount of chemotherapy delivered over a specified interval of time, is another key principle of associated with improved efficacy and survival.

Chemotherapy dosing is typically based on the body surface area (BSA), which more closely correlates to the patient's volume than weight. In infants (less than 12 months) or children weighing less than 12 kg, BSA-based dosing often results in an overdose, so weight-based dosing is used. During the first month of life, in particular, drug clearance may be slow due to immature liver and renal function.

Protocol-driven therapy is the standard of care in children with cancer, and randomized phase III clinical trials have resulted in steady improvements in survival. When available, such trials are usually offered to families at diagnosis.

Major Classes of Chemotherapy

Most chemotherapy agents interfere in the process of cell replication. The most commonly used chemotherapy drugs in children are listed in ➲ *Table 341.1.*

Alkylating Agents

Alkylating agents are used against most pediatric cancers. These highly reactive compounds form covalent bonds by attaching an alkyl group to DNA, creating DNA-DNA and DNA-protein crosslinks. Alkylating agents include mechlorethamine (nitrogen mustard), cyclophosphamide, ifosfamide, thiotepa, the nitrosoureas, melphalan, and busulfan. Cyclophosphamide and ifosfamide are prodrugs, requiring activation by hepatic metabolism. Their dose-limiting toxicity is hematological toxicity, and all can cause nausea and vomiting and mucositis. Cyclophosphamide and ifosfamide can cause hemorrhagic cystitis, which can be prevented by the concomitant use of mesna.

There are related drugs that also covalently bond to DNA. The platinators cisplatin and carboplatin bind a platinum group to DNA and dacarbazine, procarbazine and temozolomide covalently bind methyl groups to DNA.

Antimetabolites

Antimetabolites are structural analogues of the building blocks or cofactors used in the synthesis of DNA and/or RNA. These agents are active against many childhood cancers and are critical in the treatment for childhood acute lymphoblastic leukemia (ALL). Methotrexate, a folate analogue, can be given by multiple routes: oral (PO), intravenous (IV), intramuscular (IM), or

Abdelaziz Y. Elzouki (ed.), *Textbook of Clinical Pediatrics*, DOI 10.1007/978-3-642-02202-9_341,

Table 341.1
Chemotherapy agents most commonly used in children and adolescents

Drug	Mode of administration	Precautions	Major toxicity	Major use in pediatric oncology
Alkylating agents				
Nitrogen mustard (NM)	IV	Avoid extravasation	Myelosuppression N/V	Hodgkin disease (HD)
Cyclophosphamide (cytoxan, CTX)	IV, PO	Brisk diuresis, use mesna with high doses	Hemorrhagic cystitis, myelosuppression, infertility N/V	Leukemias Lymphomas Sarcomas Neuroblastoma
Ifosfamide	IV	Brisk diuresis, mesna must be used	Hemorrhagic cystitis, myelosuppression, infertility N/V	Sarcomas Germ cell tumors
Cisplatin (CDDP)	IV	Brisk diuresis	Renal dysfunction Hearing loss Severe N/V	Medulloblastoma Neuroblastoma Germ cell tumors Osteosarcoma
Carboplatin	IV		Myelosuppression Hearing loss N/V Allergic reactions	Brain tumors Germ cell tumors Neuroblastoma Sarcomas
Plant products				
Vincristine	IV	Avoid extravasation	Peripheral neuropathy	Leukemia Lymphoma Rhabdomyosarcoma Wilms
Vinblastine	IV	Avoid extravasation	Myelosuppression	HD Germ cell tumors
Etoposide (VP-16)	IV, PO	Avoid rapid infusion	Myelosuppression	ALL, AML, NHL, Neuroblastoma Sarcomas Brain tumors
Antimetabolites				
Methotrexate	PO, IV, IT	Adjust dose if renal function is poor; do not use if patient has effusions	Myelosuppression, mucositis	ALL Non-Hodgkin Lymphoma (NHL) Osteosarcoma
6-Mercaptopurine	PO	Adjust dose with hepatic dysfunction	Myelosuppression, hepatic dysfunction	ALL
6-Thioguanine	PO	Adjust dose with hepatic dysfunction	Myelosuppression, hepatic dysfunction	ALL AML
Cytosine arabinoside (Ara C)	IV, IT		Myelosuppression, mucositis	ALL AML

Table 341.1 (Continued)

Drug	Mode of administration	Precautions	Major toxicity	Major use in pediatric oncology
Antitumor antibiotics				
Doxorubicin (adriamycin)	IV	Avoid extravasation	Cardiomyopathy	ALL
		Cumulative dose cannot exceed 550 mg/m^2	Myelosuppression	AML
			Mucositis	Most solid tumors
Daunomycin	IV	Avoid extravasation	Cardiomyopathy	ALL
		Cumulative dose cannot exceed 550 mg/m^2	Myelosuppression	AML
			Mucositis	
Bleomycin	IV	Cumulative dose cannot exceed 250 mg/m^2	Pulmonary fibrosis	HD
				Germ cell tumors
Dactinomycin (actinomycin D)	IV	High dose associated with severe hepatic damage	Myelosuppression	Wilms
			N/V	Sarcomas
			Veno-occlusive disease (VOD)	
			Mucositis	
Miscellaneous				
L-Asparaginase	IM	Allergic reaction (can be delayed)	Myelosuppression	ALL
			Anaphylaxis	
			Coagulation issues	
			Pancreatitis	
			Hyperglycemia	
Prednisone	PO		Hyperglycemia	ALL
			Weight gain	NHL
			Hypertension	HD

ALL Acute lymphoblastic leukemia, *AML* acute myelogenous leukemia, *HD* Hodgkin disease, *NHL* non-Hodgkin disease, *N/V* nausea and vomiting

intrathecal (IT). Dosing varies widely, including high-dose therapy with leucovorin rescue. The thiopurines, mercaptopurine and thioguanine, are oral agents active in ALL, during the maintenance phase. Failure to comply with maintenance therapy is associated with relapse, especially in adolescents. Cytarabine, a pyrimidine analog, is active against lymphoid malignancies and can be given IT.

Anthracyclines

The anthracyclines doxorubicin and daunomycin are effective against most childhood cancers, although their poor penetration of the blood-brain barrier limits their use against central nervous system tumors. Anthracyclines have several mechanisms of action, including becoming intercalated into DNA and inhibition of topoisomerase II, a key DNA repair enzyme. Monitoring cardiac function and limiting the cumulative dose is important, as these drugs are associated with cardiomyopathy as a late complication.

Tyrosine Kinase Inhibitors

The use of imatinib mesylate in chronic myelogenous leukemia (CML) has transformed the treatment of CML and is the first broad application of rationally designed therapy. Imatinib inhibits the action of the abnormal tyrosine kinase that is the *BCR-ABL* fusion protein. Imatinib is similarly effective in pediatric CML, and trials are ongoing in pediatric ALL with the Philadelphia chromosome. Such drugs will be increasingly important in the coming decades.

Other Agents

The vinca alkaloids vincristine and vinblastine bind to tubulin and interfere with the microtubular spindles involved in mitosis. Vincristine is more widely used, and has neurotoxicity (pain and/or weakness) as its dose-limiting toxicity. Etoposide is a topoisomerase II inhibitor active in both solid tumors and leukemia, and asparaginase is an enzyme that deletes asparagine, an essential amino acid in lymphoblasts.

Steroids, including prednisone and dexamethasone, are active against lymphoid malignancies. These medications induce apoptosis, in both malignant and normal lymphoid cells.

References

Adamson PC, Balis FM, Berg S, Blaney SM (2006) General principles of chemotherapy. In: Pizzo PA, Poplack DG (eds) Principles and practice of pediatric oncology. Lippincott Williams & Wilkins, Philadelphia, pp 290–365

Berg SL, Grisell DL, DeLaney TF, Balis FM (1991) Principles of treatment of pediatric solid tumors. Pediatr Clin N Am 38:249–267

Cheung N-KV, Heller G (1991) Chemotherapy dose intensity correlates strongly with response, median survival, and median progression-free survival in metastatic neuroblastoma. J Clin Oncol 9:1050–1058

Druker BJ, Talpaz M, Resta DJ et al (2001) Efficacy and safety of a specific inhibitor of the BCR-ABL tyrosine kinase in chronic myeloid leukemia. N Engl J Med 344:1031–1037

Druker BJ, Guilhot F, O'Brien SG et al (2006) Five-year follow-up of patients receiving imatinib for chronic myeloid leukemia. N Engl J Med 355:2408–2417

DeVita VT (1983) The relationship between tumor mass and resistance to chemotherapy. Cancer 51:1209–1220

Eilber FC, Rosen G, Eckardt J et al (2001) Treatment-induced pathologic necrosis: A predictor of local recurrence and survival in patients receiving neoadjuvant therapy for high-grade extremity soft tissue sarcoma. J Clin Oncol 19:3203–3209

Esteller M, Garcia-Foncillas J, Andion E et al (2000) Inactivation of the DNA-repair gene *MGMT* and the clinical response of gliomas to alkylating agents. N Engl J Med 343:1350–1354

Goldie JH, Coldman AJ (1979) A mathematical model for relating the drug sensitivity of tumors to their spontaneous mutation rate. Cancer Treat Rep 63:1727–1733

Goldie JH, Coldman AJ (1986) Theoretical considerations regarding the early use of adjuvant chemotherapy. Recent Results Cancer Res 103:30–35

Martin DS (1981) The scientific basis for adjuvant chemotherapy. Cancer Treat Rev 8:169–189

Morgan E, Baum E, Breslow N et al (1988) Chemotherapy-related toxicity in infants treated according to the Second National Wilms' Tumor Study. J Clin Oncol 6:51–55

Pinkel D (1958) The use of body surface area as a criterion of drug dosage in cancer chemotherapy. Cancer Res 18:853–856

Smith MA, Ungerleider RS, Horowitz ME, Simon R (1991) Influence of doxorubicin dose intensity on response and outcome for patients with osteogenic sarcoma and Ewing's sarcoma. J Natl Cancer Inst 83:1460–1470

Trimble EL, Ungerleider RS, Abrams JA et al (1993) Neoadjuvant therapy in cancer treatment. Cancer 72:3515–3524

342 Pediatric Radiation Therapy

Carol Marquez

Treating children with radiation therapy presents unique challenges. Fortunately, in the last 20 years, many improvements have occurred that address and mitigate these challenges. Those improvements have been in the field of radiation oncology, in the development and results of pediatric clinical trials, and in the care and management of children in designated children's hospitals. Taken together, they represent a significant advance on the prognosis of pediatric malignancies and on the quality of life of the pediatric patients.

Improvements in Radiation Therapy

There have been significant advances in the planning and delivery of radiation therapy in the last two decades. In the early 1990s, treatment planning became based on CT images versus plain x-ray images. This switch allowed for a 3D rendering of the tumor and normal structures and for a "beams' eye view (BEV)" perspective of those relationships (see ➋ *Fig. 342.1*). The linear accelerator is designed to deliver dose from a wide variety of table positions and gantry positions. Only by having a BEV can the radiation oncologist visualize the tumor and normal tissue in oblique and noncoplanar angles. With this perspective, the radiation oncologist is able to design a treatment field that may spare more normal tissues. Having the CT information about normal structures also allowed for more accurate information about the dose delivered to those structures. With the development of the multileaf collimator (see ➋ *Fig. 342.2*), a device that is part of the linear accelerator that allows for precise, rapid, computer-controlled shaping of the beam of radiation, a treatment planning technique called intensity modulated radiation therapy (IMRT) was possible. The multileaf collimator shapes the beam while the dose is being delivered, thereby varying the intensity of the radiation and the subsequent dose within each beam of radiation that is used. This modulation of the dose produces a heterogeneous dose distribution within the treatment field. With IMRT, doses to nearby critical structures can be significantly reduced, especially in those tumors that wrap around critical normal structures, such as the spinal cord or parotid gland, where a concave dose distribution is desirable. IMRT is very useful in pediatric tumors that arise near these critical structures such as rhabdomyosarcoma or Ewing's sarcoma.

Given the rapid fall off of the dose outside of the target volume in IMRT plans, it is necessary to verify the accuracy of the patient's position immediately prior to treatment delivery. This need required the development of image-guided radiation therapy (IGRT). With IGRT, imaging of the patient is performed on the treatment table and the images are compared to the images obtained at the time of treatment simulation to verify that the patient is in the same position so that the dose is delivered accurately. The imaging modalities that may be used for IGRT include ultrasound, orthogonal films, or a CT that is part of the treatment machine (cone beam CT) (see ➋ *Fig. 342.3*). This process of verifying treatment position means that the patient and the target volume are within millimeter accuracy on a daily basis. This level of accuracy provides less variability in day-to-day setup. This decrease in variability and increase in accuracy in turn allows for a decrease in the additional margin placed around the tumor that has been historically necessary. The potential downside for the patient especially in the pediatric population is the increased exposure to x-rays when kV x-rays or cone beam CT is used as the modality for IGRT.

Stereotactic radiosurgery (SRS) is a technique of delivering a high single dose of radiation to a small volume (<2 cm) with high precision using stereotactic guidance often with rigid immobilization such as a frame or a relocatable mask. Multiple intersecting beams are used so that a high dose is given at the point of intersection (the "isocenter") and a lower dose is given to the surrounding brain because multiple beams are used. This technique is ideally suited for intracranial well-circumscribed spherical targets such as brain metastasis but is also indicated in the treatment of primary tumors such as acoustic neuromas, meningiomas or pituitary adenomas, and in the benign conditions of arteriovenous malformations or trigeminal neuralgia. In the pediatric population, SRS has been used for the treatment of astrocytomas, recurrent medulloblastomas, and recurrent ependymomas. Radiosurgery is helpful in the setting of recurrent disease because the

Abdelaziz Y. Elzouki (ed.), *Textbook of Clinical Pediatrics*, DOI 10.1007/978-3-642-02202-9_342,

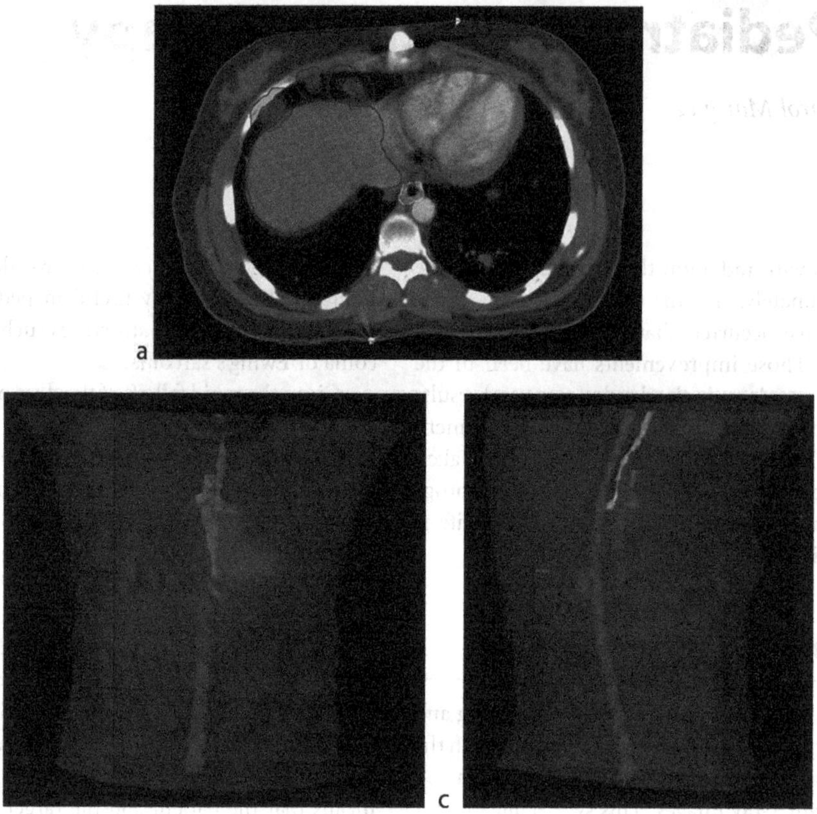

Figure 342.1
(a) CT for treatment planning with metastatic lung lesions contoured in *red*; (b) Beam's eye view (BEV) of tumor volume and relationship to lung, liver in AP view; and (c) BEV of tumor volume and relationship to spinal cord in oblique view

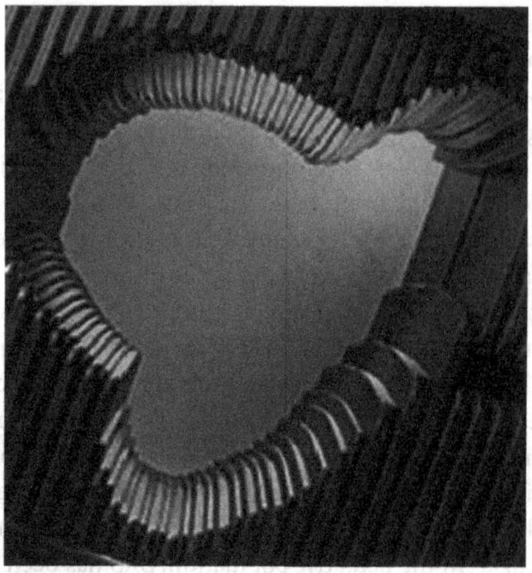

Figure 342.2
Multileaf collimator with computer-controlled leaves that shape the radiation beam to conform to the target volume

amount of dose given beyond the target is very limited which is important in patients who have previously received a larger field of radiation. There are several technologies that are available to perform SRS and they include gamma knife, cyberknife, and a linear accelerator.

In the last 10 years, the principles of SRS have been applied to extracranial targets such as small primary lung tumors or liver tumors, so-called stereotactic body radiotherapy (SBRT). In SBRT, the treatment is delivered over 2–5 fractions usually separated by several days. Each fraction delivers a dose of 4–20 Gy, which is determined by the volume being treated, the disease being treated, and the location of the target volume with respect to nearby critical structures. With SBRT, the use of IGRT is mandatory because of the high dose being given and the few numbers of fractions delivered. In pediatric patients, SBRT has shown promising results in lung metastases from Ewing's sarcoma but the results are otherwise limited in the pediatric setting.

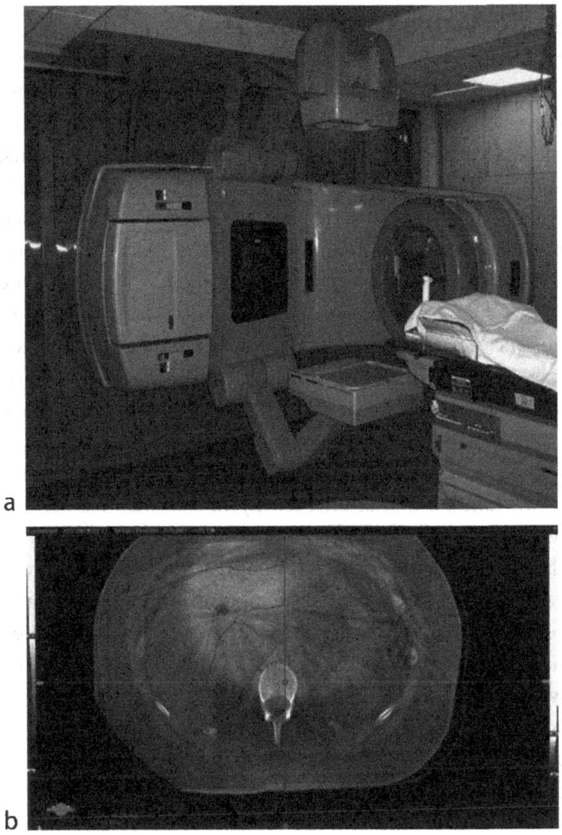

Figure 342.3
(a) Linear accelerator with cone beam CT, arms that are perpendicular to the head of the machine. This device generates kV photons and, when rotated completely around the patient, a CT is generated; (b) CT image generated by the cone beam CT

One of the more promising innovative technologies for the treatment of pediatric malignancies is proton beam therapy. Protons are a particle form of radiation, not photons or x-rays which are produced in therapeutic linear accelerators. The pattern of protons' dose deposition is unique where the dose is deposited at a finite range or depth. When protons reach this depth, they deposit all of their radiation, something called the Bragg peak (see *Fig. 342.4*). This pattern of dose deposition results in a lower entrance and exit dose. Having this Bragg peak means that, if there is a critical structure near a target volume, then proton radiation therapy has the potential to deliver a lower dose to that critical structure. This difference in dose distribution may mean a lower total dose to the entire body as in the craniospinal irradiation for medulloblastoma or to a nearby critical structure in a patient with rhabdomyosarcoma. The limitation on proton radiation therapy is the cost of building and running a facility which has results in a limited number of facilities. Protons have a physical dose distribution advantage over x-rays or photons but no biologic advantage. The next technology that has both a spatial dose distribution and biologic effect advantage is carbon ions. There are very few of these facilities (none in the USA) and little experience in pediatric patients in part due to the concern of lack of long-term follow-up with its use and the potential for increased long-term toxicity given its unique biologic properties.

While technologic improvements have significantly improved the care of pediatric patients, parallel improvements in combined modality therapy have allowed for the reduction of treatment volume, dose reduction, and careful selection of patients for radiation therapy. As stated previously, the use of IMRT and IGRT have provided improved conformity of dose and accuracy of delivery so that normal tissue margins may be reduced. Improvements in imaging of low and intermediate brain tumors and the ability to fuse those images with the treatment planning CT may allow for treatment volume reduction, a critical endpoint in brain tumors. This concept is the study of children's oncology group (COG) protocol ACNS 0221 where patients with low-grade gliodmas who have progressive non-resectable disease are given radiation therapy and the margin of normal brain is reduced from the traditional 2 cm to 0.8–1 cm. This reduction in the volume of normal brain that is within the target volume of radiation may result in a significant improvement in the long-term functional outcome of these patients who have an excellent prognosis. Volume reduction is also achieved through the use of pre-radiation chemotherapy. In Hodgkin's lymphoma when radiation is given with chemotherapy, it is delivered only to the involved field and not to a traditional mantle or subtotal nodal field. This modification allows for (in some patients) a significant reduction in the amount of lung, heart, and, in females, breast tissue that is included in the radiation therapy field.

Dose reduction is another important means of reducing the long-term toxicity of radiation therapy. An excellent example of this concept is medulloblastoma where in patients with standard risk disease who receive chemotherapy, a dose of 23.4 Gy is given to the craniospinal axis as opposed to 36 Gy for those who do not or who have high-risk disease. This dose reduction provides a decrease in overall toxicity while maintaining excellent cure rates, progression-free survival of 79% at 5 years. A further dose reduction is currently being investigated in COG ACNS 0331. In this study, patients with standard risk disease who are less than 7 years old are randomized to

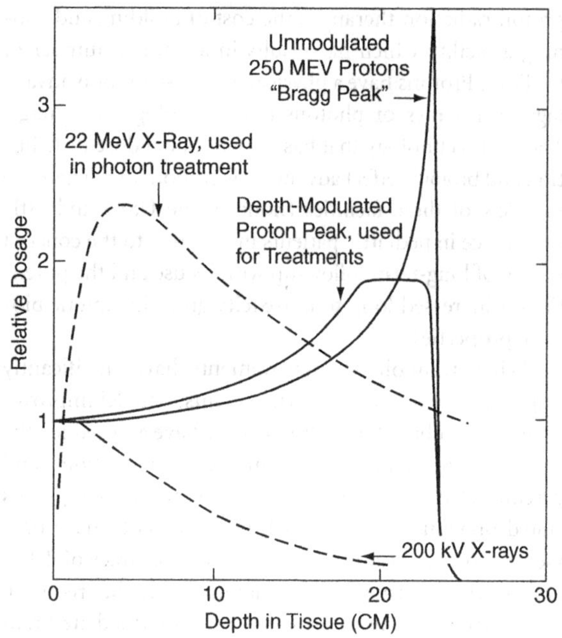

Figure 342.4
Bragg peak for protons demonstrating decrease in both entrance and exit dose when compared to x-rays (photons) of low (200 kV) or high (22 MeV) energy

either 18 Gy or 23.4 Gy for the craniospinal portion of their treatment. In addition, all of the patients regardless of age are randomized to either have the entire posterior fossa boosted to 55.8 Gy or to only the tumor bed plus 2 cm margin. This approach has been piloted at other institutions with success. This age cutoff of 7 years is chosen for the randomization because the deleterious impact of radiation is more evident in younger children.

Patient selection or eliminating radiation therapy altogether in certain groups of patients is probably the most important method of reducing its toxicity. Over the last 20 years, the use of radiation therapy has been stopped in patients with Stage 1, Group I rhabdomyosarcoma, several groups of patients with acute lymphoblastic leukemia (ALL) for prophylactic cranial irradiation, and for Stage I Wilm's tumor with favorable histology. There is a current COG protocol AREN 0533 that investigates the elimination of whole-lung irradiation in patients with Stage IV Wilm's disease, favorable histology with spread to the lungs. For those patients who have a complete response to chemotherapy based on CT performed at 6 weeks and no loss of heterozygosity at 1p16q, no whole-lung irradiation will be given. If successful, this elimination of radiation therapy in this group of patients will decrease both their pulmonary and cardiac toxicity.

Importance of Clinical Trials

One of the most notable contrasts between the management of pediatric and adult oncology patients is the increased enrollment in clinical trials in pediatric patients. It is widely believed that this participation in clinical trials is one of the major factors contributing to the continued success in managing childhood cancers. There are several advantages to a strong clinical trial group such as the COG. These advantages include the ability to ask and answer therapeutic questions reliably, several of which have been outlined above. Another advantage is the relative standardization of care, where a randomized clinical trial clearly outlines what the standard arm is and how it should be followed. A final advantage that is especially important for radiation therapy in the era of emerging technologies is that quality assurance is required prior to the use of any emerging technology. This quality assurance review is performed at a national center, quality assurance review center (QARC) prior to any patient being treated using a technique such as IMRT, SRS, or image fusion, when the patient is being treated on a cooperative group study or a pharmaceutical industry study. In addition, treatment plans are reviewed at a central location and feedback is given to the investigator so that, if necessary, modifications can be made. This same process of central review of treatment fields and plans has also been instituted in the German Hodgkin Study Group (GHSG) with a resultant improvement in the quality of radiation delivered on those studies.

Receiving Care in a Children's Hospital

The care of an ill child requires an array of specialized services. By having a hospital that focuses only on the care of pediatric patients, all of those specialized services can be brought together and together they are improved. In treating a child with cancer, the modalities of surgery, chemotherapy, and radiation therapy all are often part of the treatment regimen. Having these groups of physicians working closely together in multidisciplinary teams allows for improved communication and collaboration. In radiation therapy, young patients often need to be sedated for their daily treatments so it is essential to have pediatric sedation services that are available, reliable, and safe. Also, in most radiation therapy departments, pediatric patients will be the minority of patients treated. Yet it is important that the staff have a comfort level in working with patients and, importantly, their families. For those departments who rarely treat a child, this comfort can be hard to achieve and both the child and the family find the treatment difficult.

As more children are cured of their cancer, there will be more survivors who will need to transition to care as adolescents and young adults and who may experience the long-term toxicity of radiation therapy. Unfortunately, the effects of radiation therapy may continue to be seen many years after treatment is complete. Issues regarding growth, fertility, and the occurrence of second malignant neoplasms (SMNs) are of particular importance. This area of interest, adolescent and young adult (AYA), is growing and new research and programs are being developed specifically for it. Again, the issues facing these survivors require a multidisciplinary team.

References

Combs SE, Kulozik AE (2009) Carbon ion radiotherapy for pediatric patients and young adults treated for tumors of the skull base. Cancer 115(6):1348–1355

Ding GX, Coffey C (2009) Radiation dose from kilovoltage cone beam computed tomorgraphy in an image-guided radiaotherapy procedure. Int J Radiat Oncol Biol Phys 73(2):610–617

Ernst-Stecken A, Lambrecht U (2006) Hypofractionated stereotactic radiotherapy for primary and secondary intrapulmonary tumors: first results of a phase I/II study. Strahlenther Onkolgie 182:696–702

Fogliata A, Nicolini G (2007) On the performances of different IMRT treatment planning systems for selected paediatric cases. Radiat Oncol 2:7

Hodgson DC, Goumnerova GL (2001) Radiosurgery in the management of pediatric brain tumors. Int J Radiat Oncol Biol Phys 50:929–935

Kano H, Niranjan A (2009a) Outcome predictors for intracranial ependymoma radiosurgery. Neurosurgery 64(2):287–288

Kano H, Niranjan A (2009b) Stereotactic radiosurgery for pilocytic astrocytomas part 2: outcomes in pediatric patients. J Neurooncol 95(2):219–229

Kozak KR, Adams J (2009) A dosimetric comparison of proton and intensity-modulated photon radiotherapy for pediatric parameningeal rhabdomyosarcomas. Int J Radiat Oncol Biol Phys 74(1):179–186

Merchant TE, Hua C (2008) Proton versus photon radiotherapy for common pediatric brain tumors: comparison of models of dose characteristics and their relationship to cognitive. Pediatr Blood Cancer 51(1):110–117

Merchant TE, Kun L (2008) Multi-institution prospective trial of reduced-dose craniospinal irradiation (23.4 Gy) followed by conformal posterior fossa (36 Gy) and primary site irradiation (55.8 Gy) and dose-intensive chemotherapy for average-risk medulloblastoma. Int J Radiat Oncol Biol Phys 70(3):782–787

O'Brien MM, Donaldson S (2010) Second malignant neoplasms in survivors of pediatric Hodgkin's lymphoma treated with low-dose radiation and chemotherapy. J Clin Oncol 28(7):1232–1239

Sterzing F, Stoiber E (2009) Intensity modulated radiotherapy (IMRT) in the treatment of children and adolescents – a single instiution's experience and a review of the literature. Radiat Oncol 4:37

Yuh GE, Loredo L (2004) Reducing toxicity from craniospinal irradiation: using proton beams to treat medulloblastoma in young children. Cancer 10:386–390

343 Hematopoietic Stem Cell Transplantation

Hassan El Solh · Abdallah Al-Nasser · Eneida R. Nemecek

Hematopoietic Stem Cell Transplantation (HSCT) can cure many malignant and nonmalignant childhood diseases. As new indications for HSCT arise, and donor and stem cell sources expand, the number of bone marrow transplants performed is increasing. This modality, once only available in limited institutions, is now used worldwide. Many pediatric care providers encounter patients in their practice who will or have undergone HSCT, thus it is important for pediatricians to understand the basics of this therapeutic modality, its potential benefits, and acute and long-term risks.

Stem Cell Sources

The main goal of HSCT is to infuse hematopoietic progenitor cells in a host to totally or partially replace host defective cells affected by cancer or other disorders. Bone marrow is the most direct source for hematopoetic progenitor cells, but they can also be obtained from peripheral blood and placental (cord) blood.

Marrow is obtained from donors through a procedure referred to as *bone marrow harvest.* A harvest is performed in an operating room under general anesthesia, and involves directly extracting bone marrow, usually from the posterior iliac crests using bone marrow aspirate needles. The extracted marrow product is filtered to remove debris and collected in a bag mixed with anticoagulant. The amount of marrow volume removed is limited by the weight of the donor (maximum of 15 ml/kg) recipient and usually does not exceed 20 ml/kg of the intended recipient weight. Bone marrow can be harvested from donors of any age. The procedure is usually performed as outpatient procedure or may involve a short overnight hospital stay. The harvest procedure is well tolerated by the donor. The most common side effect is mild to moderate pain at the aspiration sites usually lasting a few days. Blood transfusion to a donor is rarely needed but may be indicated when the donor is substantially smaller than the recipient. The incidence of significant complications for donors has been reported to be very low.

A second source of hematopoietic progenitors is *peripheral blood stem cells.* The donor receives subcutaneous injections of granulocyte colony-stimulating factor for several days to mobilize the stem cells from the bone marrow to the peripheral blood, after which the cells are collected by apheresis. For this procedure, the donor has two venous catheters placed and is connected to an apheresis machine, which separates and collects the stem cells and returns other blood components back to the patient. Some donors, particularly those of small size, require central venous catheters for this procedure and may need transfusions or red cell priming of the apheresis machine to undergo this procedure, making it a less appealing approach to obtain cells from young children donors. Umbilical *cord blood* is a rich source of hematopoietic progenitors. After delivering the baby and clamping of the cord, placental blood can be collected using sterile technique by direct venipuncture of the cord vessels. Cord blood collection poses no risk to the mother or newborn. The collected cord blood can then be cryopreserved and stored until used.

Donor Selection

Hematopoietic cells can be obtained from the recipient, also referred to as *autologous*, or from another donor (*allogeneic*). When the donor is an identical twin sibling, it is referred to as *syngeneic.*

An Autologous transplant is traditionally used to "rescue" patients after high-dose chemotherapy for lymphoma or other solid tumors. Allogeneic transplant is used for treatment of patients with malignancies considered at high risk for relapse with conventional chemotherapy and for some patients with nonmalignant disorders.

An allogeneic donor may be a sibling, a parent, another relative, or unrelated. The selection of an allogeneic donor is determined primarily by compatibility of the human leukocyte antigen (HLA) system. Improvement in the understanding of the genetics of the HLA system has played a major role in advancing the field of transplantation. The HLA system contains a set of tightly linked genes

Abdelaziz Y. Elzouki (ed.), *Textbook of Clinical Pediatrics*, DOI 10.1007/978-3-642-02202-9_343,

located on chromosome 6. These genes are inherited as one group from each parent, called a haplotype. The overall chance that two siblings inherit the same set of maternal and paternal haplotypes is 25%. Due to heterogeneity in HLA types, in addition to other contributing factors such as the trend towards reduced family size in developed countries, there is only a 30% chance of finding an HLA-identical sibling for a given patient. The chance of a parent or other relatives fully matching a child is very small, but they may serve as partially matched or haploidentical ("half-matched") donors. This latter type of donor is sometimes the only choice available for patients with ethnicities poorly represented in the donor registries. Approximately 45% of all allogeneic transplants performed worldwide are from adult unrelated donors. These individuals join donor registries voluntarily where their HLA typing data become available to search coordinators looking for a match for a potential recipient anywhere in the world. This process is conducted with a great degree of confidentiality to protect the identity and safety of both donor and recipient. Unrelated donors are ideally matched at 8 of 8 HLA loci, or in some cases partially mismatched at one or 2 HLA loci.

Indications for HSCT in Childhood Diseases

The list of diseases for which marrow transplantation is clinically used continues to grow and includes a wide variety of malignant and nonmalignant disorders (*Table 343.1*). The choice of donor and stem cell source are influenced by the type of disease being treated and time constraints.

Table 343.1
Indications for HSCT in children

Allogeneic	Autologous
Malignant disorders	Ewing sarcoma
Acute lymphoblastic leukemia	Recurrent germ cell tumors
Acute myeloid leukemia	Malignant Brain tumors
Chronic myeloid leukemia	Recurrent Lymphoma
Juvenile myelomonocytic leukemia /Juvenile chronic myeloid leukemia	High-risk Neuroblastoma
Myelodysplastic syndrome	
Lymphoma relapsed after autologous transplantation	
Nonmalignant disorders	
Severe aplastic anemia	
Bone Marrow Failure syndromes	
Hemoglobinopathies (Thalassemia major, Sickle cell disease)	
Primary (congenital) immunodeficiency diseases	
Hemophagocytic lymphohistiocytosis	
Inborn errors of metabolism (Mucopolysaccharidosis, Sphingolipidosis, Malignant osteopetrosis, Adrenoleukodystrophy)	

Allogeneic HSCT

Allogeneic BMT has been proven to be an effective treatment for hematologic malignancies, bone marrow failure syndromes, primary immunodeficiency disorders and inborn errors of metabolism. According to reports from the Center for International Blood and Marrow Transplant Research (CIBMTR), the most common source of allogeneic stem cells for children is bone marrow (52%) followed by peripheral blood stem cells (28%) and cord blood (20%).

In malignancies the primary goal is to eradicate all malignant cells, usually by administering high doses of chemotherapy agents and/or total body irradiation, and infusing the normal blood cells of the donor. The donor cells repopulate the host bone marrow space and may also mediate an immunological response against the cancer cells, referred to as the "graft-versus-leukemia" or "graft-versus-tumor" effect. Many patients with hematologic malignancies not cured with conventional chemotherapy treatment have benefited from allogeneic HSCT. The 3-year probability of survival for patients with acute leukemia younger than 20 years ranges between 70% for those with disease in first remission and 37% for those with more advanced disease at the time of transplant. Acute myeloid leukemia in first or greater remission and acute lymphoblastic leukemia in second or greater remission are the most common indications for allogeneic HSCT In children. Chronic myeloid leukemia (CML), juvenile myelomonocytic leukemia, and myelodysplastic syndrome, are rare malignant hematologic disorders in children treated with allogeneic stem cell transplantation. The number of transplants for adult CML has significantly decreased since the development of oral tyrosine kinase inhibitors such as imatinib mesylate, and is reserved primarily for patients not responding to treatment with these biological modifiers. For children with CML, the emphasis is still on transplantation.

The indications for allogeneic HSCT for nonmalignant diseases are varied. The goal of HSCT in the nonmalignant setting is to fully or partially replace defective cells of the host with normal cells from a healthy donor. Severe aplastic anemia and bone marrow failure syndromes where one or more of the hematopoietic cell lines are defective such as Diamond-Blackfan anemia, congenital neutropenia and Fanconi anemia have been cured with HSCT. The long-term survival of children undergoing allogeneic HSCT for severe aplastic anemia is 70–80%. Inherited hemoglobinopathies such as sickle cell anemia and thalassemias can also be cured by allogeneic BMT. Around 70% of patients with severe combined immunodeficiency have long-term survival with full immunoreconstitution within 6 months after HLA-matched allogeneic transplant. Similarly, many other primary immundeficiencies can be corrected with HSCT. Inborn errors of metablism such as malignant osteopetrosis and lysosomal storage diseases have been reported to be cured by allogeneic HSCT. However, there is still a paucity of data from prospective clinical trials for these disorders.

Autologous HSCT

Autologous HSCT in children is used in the setting of malignant disorders, usually solid tumors or recurrent lymphomas, to facilitate blood count recovery after administration of high doses of chemotherapy agents. One of the most common indications for autologous HSCT in children is high-risk neuroblastoma. Randomized clinical trials have shown a modest clinical advantage of consolidative therapy with autologous HSCT over conventional chemotherapy, with long-term survival of 50% for patients with disease in complete or good partial remission prior to transplant. Patients with recurrent chemoresponsive Hodgkin or non-Hodgkin lymphoma may also benefit from consolidation with autologous BMT, with long-term survival ranging between 40% and 50% depending on the type of lymphoma and disease burden at the time of transplantation. Other less common indications for autologous BMT include brain tumors and other neoplasms such as germ cell tumors and Ewing sarcoma.

The Transplant Process

Prior to transplant, both patient and allogeneic HSCT donor must undergo extensive multidisciplinary evaluations. This typically includes a comprehensive history and physical exam, laboratory evaluations such as complete blood counts, serum chemistries, and infectious serology testing. The recipient also undergoes testing to confirm disease status, general health status, and organ functions (echocardiogram, electrocardiogram, pulmonary function testing, creatinine clearance, etc.). Assessment of family support and psychosocial needs is also an integral part of the pre-transplant assessment. Once the patient and donor receive medical clearance, the recipient starts the transplant preparative regimen, also referred to as conditioning regimen.

The intensity of the conditioning regimen depends on the disease being treated, type of donor used, and the general health status of the recipient and its predicted ability to tolerate such therapy. Conditioning starts usually about 1 week before the infusion of stem cells. More intense myeloablative regimens are used to treat malignant disorders. Regimens of reduced or minimal intensity may be used to treat patients with nonmalignant disorders and those with malignancies who due to poor health status are deemed unable to tolerate full myeloablative regimens. After conditioning, the patient receives the hematopoietic cells on “day zero.”

During the acute phase of transplant, the patient has profound pancytopenia and immunosuppression and may also experience acute side effects from the conditioning therapy. Patients remain isolated in the hospital for about 3–4 weeks until the new donor cells engraft and they are free of major complications from the transplant process. Patients are usually followed by the transplant team until at least 3 months post transplant, after which they return to the care of their primary care or oncology providers.

Early Complications of HSCT

The early complications are related to infections, toxicities related to the preparative regimen, graft-versus-host disease (GVHD), and graft rejection.

The most common cause of morbidity and mortality during the early phase of transplant is infections. Risk factors for infections include immunosuppression, indwelling venous catheters, GVHD, and coexisting toxicities such as mucositis. Various measures have been taken to isolate the transplant patient from possible infections. Protection measures include hand washing, wearing a mask, minimizing nonessential contacts, and using hospital rooms equipped with high-energy particulate air (HEPA) filters, when available. Infections prophylaxis has significantly improved the outcome of HSCT by reducing the number of infectious complications. Patients should be aggressively monitored and promptly treated for symptoms or signs of systemic infections. The absence of neutropenia does not necessarily mean that the patient is not immunosuppressed. The ability to fight infections is also affected by absence of cellular and humoral responses, and by the multiple medications used to suppress the immune system to prevent GVHD. Infections can be caused by bacterial, fungal, or viral pathogens and can present in any form, from localized to overwhelming sepsis. Empirical broad-spectrum antibiotics should be started during the neutropenic period and continued until neutrophil engraftment is achieved. Patients should receive Pneumocystis prophyalxis, antifungal prophylaxis to cover for Candida species and molds, and antiviral prophylaxis with acyclovir until off immunosuppressive therapy. Cytomegalovirus (CMV) infection or reactivation has decreased significantly with the use of CMV-negative blood products CMV-serosurveillance and preemptive antiviral prophylaxis with ganciclovir or foscarnet. Other viruses such as adenovirus, respiratory syncytial virus, and parainfluenza and influenza virus continue to be causes of major morbidity and infectious mortality in transplant patients. Prevention of infections and, when available, prompt institution of antiviral therapy are the recommended management for these viral pathogens.

Regimen-related toxicities are the second most common cause of death during the first 100 days post transplant. Any organ can be affected during transplant. The most common organ toxicity is mucositis of the oropharyngeal region. Diarrhea and enteritis may also occur in a high percentage of patients, particularly those receiving myeloablative therapy. Some other manifestations of toxicity include noninfectious pneumonitis, veno-occlusive disease of the liver, hemorrhagic cystitis, acute renal insufficiency or failure, and cardiac dysfunction. Veno-occlusive disease of the liver presents as weight gain, fluid retention, hyperbilirubinemia, and right upper quadrant (hepatic) tenderness. Although most toxicities are reversible and respond to supportive medical management, some can be irreversible or fatal. The average incidence of severe/fatal regimen-related toxicities in children is about 15%, ranging from 0 to 50% depending on predisposing factors. Some factors associated with an increased risk for toxicity are age (infants are at higher risk), intense pre-transplant treatment, and use of myeloablative regimens. Aggressive and prompt institution of supportive care and/or intensive care is key to prevent irreversible injury or death from toxicities in transplant patients.

Graft-Versus-Host Disease

As the new allogeneic donor cells establish within their new environment, they can recognize host antigens as foreign and generate an immune response. This response, known as graft-versus-host disease (GVHD), ranges from subclinical to a severe reaction with multiple manifestations.

Acute GVHD typically presents in the first 3 months post transplant. The organs most commonly affected are skin (rash, erythema, bullae formation), gut (anorexia, nausea/vomiting, watery or bloody diarrhea, abdominal cramps), or liver (elevation of hepatic enzymes with hyperbilirubinemia and liver dysfunction). Since acute immune reactions between the donor and host are expected events in the transplant setting, immunosuppressive medications are given prophylactically before and during the first 3 months post transplant. GVHD prophylaxis usually consists of combinations of two or more drugs that act by reducing the number and function of T-cells. The most common combinations are calcineurin inhibitors (cyclopsporine or tacrolimus) with methotrexate, mycophenolate mofetil, anti-thymocyte, or alemtuzumab globulin. Drugs are used at therapeutic doses early during transplant, and then slowly tapered over 3–6 months if there is no evidence of GVHD. Despite prophylaxis, the incidence of acute GVHD ranges from 25% in matched sibling transplants to 70% in unrelated donor transplants. Acute GVHD is graded depending on the extent and areas of disease involvement.

Chronic GVHD usually occurs after the first 3 months post transplant, although in some patients clinical signs and symptoms have been described at an earlier time after transplant. Skin manifestations of chronic GVHD include desquamation, scleroderma-like changes, pigmentation, and lichenoid changes. Chronic GVHD of the liver is characterized by hyperbilirubinemia and elevation of the hepatic enzymes. Patients with chronic GVHD of the intestine may have abdominal pain, diarrhea, malabsorption, wasting syndrome, and, in the late phases, strictures of the gastrointestinal tract. Lungs acan be affected by chronic GVHD, manifesting as obstructive lung disease or bronchiolitis obliterans. Involvement of the eyes is also common, with keratoconjunctivitis sicca, blurred vision, and photophobia. Oral manifestations include ulcers, leukoplakia, dry mouth, dysphagia, and sensitivity to certain foods. Joints can be affected by serositis or scleroderma. Thrombocytopenia may occur in chronic GVHD, and it is usually one of the poor prognostic factors of the disease.

There are several alternatives for therapy of GVHD. The goal in the treatment of GVHD is to provide therapy that is sufficient to ameliorate the signs and symptoms without excessively compromising the immune system of the host, a challenging task. Drugs and therapies are added/tapered in response to changes in clinical status until the desired effect is observed. Systemic steroids (prednisone, methylprednisolone) are the first line of therapy. About 50% of patients with acute GVHD respond to steroid therapy, but many require extended therapy with steroids or other agents. Prolonged use of steroids is associated with many side effects including weight gain, myalgia, arthralgia, hyperglycemia, hypertension, increased risk for infections, osteopenia, avascular necrosis of the bones typically the hip, and mood changes, among others. Second line therapies for patients not responding to steroids include monoclonal antibodies against T-cells or cytokines (anti-thymocyte globulin, alemtuzumab, daclizumab, etanercept), macrolide antibiotics (sirolimus or rapamycin), and antimetabolites (pentostatin). Localized skin disease can sometimes be treated with topical therapies (tacrolimus or steroid creams) or with ultraviolet light therapy (psoralens and ultraviolet light absorber, PUVA). Extracorporeal photopheresis (ECP) is a new technique that applies the PUVA concept to systemic GVHD, currently reserved for patients resistant to other modalities. This technique consists of removing a fraction of the lymphocytes of the patient by apheresis, exposing the cell fraction ex vivo to PUVA, and returning the treated cells to the patient. Through complex mechanisms, this procedure generates an immunomodulatory effect and increases immune tolerance of the donor T-cells toward the host.

Long-Term Complications of HSCT

With an increasing number of long-term survivors of HSCT and extended observation periods, long-term sequelae are becoming of significant importance and primary concern for all physicians who care for HSCT patients. After engraftment of stem cells and recovery of blood counts, it takes approximately 1 year after HSCT to recover a fully functional immune system; until then, cellular and humoral responses are impaired. Many patients, especially those with GVHD, have hypogammaglobulinemia and require intravenous gammaglobulin replacement. Patients are at risk for reactivation of dormant viruses (Herpes and Varicella) during the first year post transplant. After transplant, most children lose titers to previously administered immunizations. Most cannot mount adequate responses to immunizations for the first year post transplant. After a year post transplant, most children need to be re-immunized for childhood diseases. Live virus vaccines are not given until 2 years post transplant because of the potential risk of acquiring primary viral infections or complications from the vaccine.

As more patients survive the intense transplant process, the incidence of other long-term sequelae increases as well. Risk factors for the development of late effects include younger age at time of transplant, use of radiation in the conditioning regimen, and presence of chronic GVHD. The most frequent late sequelae of transplant are endocrine deficiencies. Manifestations include growth hormone deficiency and growth failure, hypogonadism and infertility, hypothyroidism, adrenal insufficiency, and diabetes. Endocrine problems are much more common in patients receiving TBI and/or cranial radiation. Chronic organ dysfunction may also occur. Lung problems include obstructive or restrictive disease and bronchiolitis obliterans; an inflammatory disease of unknown etiology that is almost always associated with chronic GVHD. Other late effects include cataracts, dental problems, cardiotoxicity, chronic renal insufficiency, learning disabilities, psychosocial adjustment problems, and secondary malignancies.

Monitoring of late effects and guidance significantly improve the quality of life of transplant patients. In addition to routine care by their primary providers, many transplant centers patients offer comprehensive long-term follow-up evaluations. Patients and their primary health care providers are informed of the results of these evaluations, and recommendations are given to address existing problems.

Transplant is a life-changing experience for patients and their families. Although most of the physical effects of transplant resolve within the first years post transplant, patients and families take years to recover from the psychosocial impact of this process. Hence the involvement of support staff such as social workers, child life specialists and counseling, early and through the transplant is extremely important. Despite the many complications associated with HSCT, most patients and their families report good quality of life post transplant. The pediatrician is an important part of the transplant process by facilitating prompt referral to the transplant center and, once the transplant is completed and the patient has returned back to their care, by providing adequate surveillance for side effects and late effects of bone marrow transplantation.

References

American Academy of Pediatrics Section on Hematology/Oncology, American Academy of Pediatrics Section on Allergy/Immunology, Lubin BH, Shearer WT (2007) Cord blood banking for potential future transplantation. Pediatrics 119(1):165–170

Bach FH, van Rood JJ (1976a) The major histocompatibility complex – genetics and biology (Part I). N Engl J Med 295(15):806–813

Bach FH, van Rood JJ (1976b) The major histocompatibility complex – genetics and biology (Part III). N Engl J Med 295(17):927–936

Balduzzi A, Valsecchi MG, Silvestri D, Locatelli F, Manfredini L, Busca A, Iori AP, Messina C, Prete A, Andolina M, Porta F, Favre C, Ceppi S, Giorgiani G, Lanino E, Rovelli A, Fagioli F, De Fusco C, Rondelli R, Uderzo C, for the Associazione Italiana Ematologia Oncologia Pediatrica-BMT Group (2002) Transplant-related toxicity and mortality: an AIEOP prospective study in 636 pediatric patients transplanted for acute leukemia. Bone Marrow Transplant 29(2):93–100

Buckner CD, Clift RA, Sanders JE, Stewart P, Bensinger WI, Doney KC, Sullivan KM, Witherspoon RP, Deeg HJ, Appelbaum FR et al (1984) Marrow harvesting from normal donors. Blood 64(3):630–634

Center for International Blood and Marrow Transplant Research, National Marrow Donor Program, European Blood and Marrow Transplant Group, American Society of Blood and Marrow Transplantation, Canadian Blood and Marrow Transplant Group, Infectious Disease Society of America, Society for Healthcare Epidemiology of America, Association of Medical Microbiology and Infectious Diseases Canada, Centers for Disease Control and Prevention (2009) Guidelines for preventing infectious complications among hematopoietic cell transplant recipients: a global perspective. Bone Marrow Transplant 44(8):453–558

Cohen A, Békássy AN, Gaiero A, Faraci M, Zecca S, Tichelli A, Dini G, EBMT Paediatric and Late Effects Working Parties (2008) Endocrinological late complications after hematopoietic SCT in children. Bone Marrow Transplant 41(Suppl 2):S43–S48

Faraci M, Békássy AN, De Fazio V, Tichelli A, Dini G, EBMT Paediatric and Late Effects Working Parties (2008) Non-endocrine late complications in children after allogeneic haematopoietic SCT. Bone Marrow Transplant 41(Suppl 2):S49–S57

Filipovich AH, Weisdorf D, Pavletic S, Socie G, Wingard JR, Lee SJ, Martin P, Chien J, Przepiorka D, Couriel D, Cowen EW, Dinndorf P, Farrell A, Hartzman R, Henslee-Downey J, Jacobsohn D, McDonald G, Mittleman B, Rizzo JD, Robinson M, Schubert M, Schultz K, Shulman H, Turner M, Vogelsang G, Flowers ME (2005) National Institutes of Health consensus development project on criteria for clinical trials in chronic graft-versus-host disease: I. Diagnosis and staging working group report. Biol Blood Marrow Transplant 11(12):945–956

Gaziev J, Lucarelli G (2003) Stem cell transplantation for hemoglobinopathies. Curr Opin Pediatr 15(1):24–31

Gross TG, Hale GA, He W, Camitta BM, Sanders JE, Cairo MS, Hayashi RJ, Termuhlen AM, Zhang MJ, Davies SM, Eapen M (2010) Hematopoietic stem cell transplantation for refractory or recurrent non-Hodgkin lymphoma in children and adolescents. Biol Blood Marrow Transplant 16(2):223–230

Lasky LC, Bostrom B, Smith J, Moss TJ, Ramsay NK (1989) Clinical collection and use of peripheral blood stem cells in pediatric patients. Transplantation 47(4):613–616

Ljungman P, Bregni M, Brune M, Cornelissen J, de Witte T, Dini G, Einsele H, Gaspar HB, Gratwohl A, Passweg J, Peters C, Rocha V, Saccardi R, Schouten H, Sureda A, Tichelli A, Velardi A, Niederwieser D, European Group for Blood and Marrow Transplantation (2010) Allogeneic and autologous transplantation for haematological diseases, solid tumours and immune disorders: current practice in Europe 2009. Bone Marrow Transplant 45(2):219–234

Martins da Cunha A, Gin N, Padmos A et al (1993) Allogeneic bone marrow transplantation for infantile osteopetrosis: Saudi Arabian experience. Blood 82(suppl 1):667

Mackall C, Fry T, Gress R, Peggs K, Storek J, Toubert A et al (2009) Background to hematopoietic cell transplantation, including post transplant immune recovery. Bone Marrow Transplant 44(8):457–462

MacMillan ML, Davies SM, Nelson GO, Chitphakdithai P, Confer DL, King RJ, Kernan NA (2008) Twenty years of unrelated donor bone marrow transplantation for pediatric acute leukemia facilitated by the National Marrow Donor Program. Biol Blood Marrow Transplant 14(9 Suppl):16–22

Mehta P, Locatelli F, Stary J, Smith FO (2010) Bone marrow transplantation for inherited bone marrow failure syndromes. Pediatr Clin North Am 57(1):147–170

Meyers JD, Reed EC, Shepp DH, Thornquist M, Dandliker PS, Vicary CA, Flournoy N, Kirk LE, Kersey JH, Thomas ED et al (1988) Acyclovir for prevention of cytomegalovirus infection and disease after allogeneic marrow transplantation. N Engl J Med 318(2):70–75

Pasquini MC, Wang Z (2009a) Current use and outcome of hematopoietic stem cell transplantation: Part I CIBMTR summary slides, 2009. CIBMTR Newsletter [serial online] 15(1):7–11

Pasquini MC, Wang Z (2009b) Current use and outcome of hematopoietic stem cell transplantation: Part II-CIBMTR Summary Slides, 2009. CIBMTR Newsletter [serial online] 15(2):7–11

Prasad VK, Kurtzberg J (2010) Transplant outcomes in mucopolysaccharidoses. Semin Hematol 47(1):59–69

Pulsipher MA, Nagler A, Iannone R, Nelson RM (2006) Weighing the risks of G-CSF administration, leukopheresis, and standard marrow harvest: ethical and safety considerations for normal pediatric hematopoietic cell donors. Pediatr Blood Cancer 46(4):422–433

Sanders JE, Buckner CD, Leonard JM, Sullivan KM, Witherspoon RP, Deeg HJ, Storb R, Thomas ED (1983) Late effects on gonadal function of cyclophosphamide, total-body irradiation, and marrow transplantation. Transplantation 36(3):252–255

Sanders JE (2008) Growth and development after hematopoietic cell transplant in children. Bone Marrow Transplant 41(2):223–227

Szabolcs P, Cavazzana-Calvo M, Fischer A, Veys P (2010) Bone marrow transplantation for primary immunodeficiency diseases. Pediatr Clin North Am 57(1):207–237

Walters MC, Storb R, Patience M, Leisenring W, Taylor T, Sanders JE, Buchanan GE, Rogers ZR, Dinndorf P, Davies SC, Roberts IA, Dickerhoff R, Yeager AM, Hsu L, Kurtzberg J, Ohene-Frempong K, Bunin N, Bernaudin F, Wong WY, Scott JP, Margolis D, Vichinsky E, Wall DA, Wayne AS, Pegelow C, Redding-Lallinger R, Wiley J, Klemperer M, Mentzer WC, Smith FO, Sullivan KM (2000) Impact of bone marrow transplantation for symptomatic sickle cell disease: an interim report. Multicenter investigation of bone marrow transplantation for sickle cell disease. Blood 95(6):1918–1924

Woods WG, Ramsay NKC, Kersey JH (1986) Long term follow-up of individuals undergoing allogeneic bone marrow transplantation for acute lymphoblastic leukemia. J Clin Oncol 4:1015–1016

344 Supportive Care of the Child with Cancer

H. Stacy Nicholson

Introduction

Curing a child with cancer requires prompt and accurate diagnosis and staging, and safe delivery of risk-adjusted therapy. In addition, supportive treatments that decrease side effects, increase patient safety, and support health and healing are also important and ensure improved health and quality of life during anticancer therapy. Supportive care can also be life saving.

Venous Access

Most chemotherapy drugs are administered by the intravenous (IV) route. Repeated IV infusions and blood tests are the norm. IV chemotherapy can be delivered via a peripheral vein or via an indwelling central venous catheter. Using peripheral IVs risk extravasations of medications into surrounding soft tissues, and some chemotherapy agents (particularly the vinca alkaloids and anthracyclines) can cause tissue destruction. The surgical implantation of indwelling central venous catheters facilitates both chemotherapy delivery and blood tests. There are two main types of devices: those that end with an external catheter and those that end in a reservoir under the skin.

Procedures and Sedation

There are several routine procedures associated with childhood cancer. Bone marrow aspirations (BMA) are performed to diagnose and monitor leukemia and are required for staging some solid tumors. Marrow fluid is aspirated using a specially designed needle, and the site most commonly used is the posterior superior iliac spine. During a BMA, children are under deep sedation, delivered by an anesthesiologist or other highly trained provider, or are more lightly sedated (conscious sedation) with the concomitant use of locally injected analgesia. Conscious sedation, often using the combination of an opiate and a benzodiazepine, can be delivered by the practitioner performing the BMA and his or her team. Bone marrow biopsies should always be done with the patient under deep sedation or general anesthesia.

Lumbar punctures (LP) generally require less sedation than BMAs, but local analgesia is important. Preventing pain during procedures will improve comfort and increase compliance with care. In older children, using distraction or other non-medicinal techniques can be very effective for LPs and IV placement.

Pain Control

Pain in children with cancer may be caused by the cancer itself (at diagnosis, relapse, or during the terminal phase of illness), procedures (see above), surgical procedures, or as a side effect of therapy, such as mucositis (mouth sores). Using a pain scale so that the child can effectively communicate his or her pain can be helpful in monitoring the effectiveness of the analgesia. Depending upon severity, pain medications will range from acetaminophen to opiates. When opiates are used for more than a few days, children may develop tachyphylaxis, requiring an increasing amount of medication to achieve the same results. If prolonged use of opiates is required, long-acting formulations may be used to deliver a baseline level of analgesia combined with short acting opiates for breakthrough pain.

Antiemetics

Many chemotherapy drugs and radiation cause nausea and vomiting. Fortunately, the past two decades have brought new antiemetic medications that are highly effective. Drugs used to control nausea in children undergoing chemotherapy include 5-HT_3 receptor inhibitors (ondansetron, granisetron, and dolasetron), steroids (dexamethasone), phenothiazines, and/or metoclopramide. Although expensive, 5-HT_3 receptor inhibitors have become the agents of choice as they are highly effective in most patients and

Abdelaziz Y. Elzouki (ed.), *Textbook of Clinical Pediatrics*, DOI 10.1007/978-3-642-02202-9_344,

have a low risk of side effects. Children whose nausea cannot be controlled with a single medication may require combination therapy.

Transfusion Therapy

Children with cancer often experience cytopenias, either from disease (in leukemia or solid tumors metastatic to bone marrow) or as a side effect of therapy. Myelosuppression is the most common dose-limiting side effect of chemotherapy. Packed red cells and platelets are most commonly used blood components. Indications for transfusion based on blood count results will vary by institution, but symptoms that warrant red cell transfusions include tachycardia, orthostatic hypotension, and fatigue. The transfusion of prophylactic platelets is supported by some, but many centers only use platelets when children experience bleeding. White cell transfusions are sometime done in neutropenic patients with persistent sepsis; however, white cell transfusions are controversial. All blood products should be irradiated prior to transfusion to prevent graft-versus-host disease, and leukodepletion by filtration can decrease cytomegalovirus (CMV) transmission.

Nutrition

Children are often malnourished at diagnosis, and children need good nutrition to heal following radiation and chemotherapy treatments. Nutritional status should be assessed in all patients and support offered if needed. The oral route is preferred when possible, and success can be enhanced by enriching the calorie content and ensuring effective pain management for mucositis. Appetite stimulants can help in some children. If a patient cannot take sufficient calories by mouth, the use of a nasogastric (NG) tube or gastrostomy tube (G-tube) to facilitate delivery of enteral nutrition may be effective. If enteral nutrition cannot be tolerated, total parenteral nutrition (TPN) can be delivered by a central venous catheter.

Oncologic Emergencies

There are several unique emergencies that occur in children with cancer, including mediastinal masses with respiratory compromise and spinal cord compression. Similarly, anticancer therapy can cause serious side effects that require immediate attention, such as serious life-threatening infections.

Superior Vena Cava Syndrome

The anterior mediastinum in children is rich in lymphoid tissue, and these structures are in close proximity with the trachea and both main-stem bronchi, the heart, and major blood vessels, including the superior vena cava (SVC). Some lymphomas or leukemias are accompanies by rapid lymph node growth. In the anterior mediastinum, such growth can lead to a mass that compresses the SVC, leading to facial plethora, cyanosis, and petechiae. Impairment of venous drainage from the brain may result in somnolence and confusion. Airway compression may lead to severe respiratory compromise and is the greatest concern in these patients. Sedation should be avoided and therapy with steroids and/or radiation needs to be administered as a life-saving measure, even if the ability to make a histopathological diagnosis is compromised.

Spinal Cord Compression

Masses that involve or invade the spinal canal can present with spinal cord compression (SCC), either at diagnosis or at relapse. Symptoms include back pain, weakness, inability to walk, sensory changes, or changes in bowel or bladder function. In children, SCC occurs most commonly in children with sarcomas, neuroblastomas, or brain tumors. The time from symptom onset to treatment is inversely related to the chances of the patient recovering lost function. Thus, treatment decisions must be made promptly and immediately initiated. Treatment can include surgical decompression, steroids, or external beam radiation.

Fever and Neutropenia

Infections are the most common complications of anticancer therapy and can be life threatening. Parents must be educated about the risk of infections so that the child is immediately brought to medical attention immediately upon developing a fever. Upon arrival at the clinic or emergency department, the child should be promptly evaluated with a detailed history and thorough physical examination, blood count, and blood cultures. The physical examination should especially focus on seeking specific sites of infection, and extra attention should be given to the oral cavity, sinuses, lungs, abdomen, perianal region, and any tunneled catheters. If neutropenic (absolute neutrophil count (ANC) $<500/mm^3$ or $<1{,}000/mm^3$ and likely to be decreasing), broad-spectrum antibiotics should be administered, the child should be admitted to the hospital for further antibiotics and monitoring. Antibiotics will continue until the child is no longer neutropenic. Any signs of septic shock should be promptly addressed with fluid resuscitation and consultation with a pediatric critical care unit.

Infections

Throughout therapy, children with cancer are immunosuppressed and susceptible to infection from bacteria, viruses, and fungi. Serious bacterial infections are more likely when children are neutropenic, and prolonged neutropenia increases the risk of invasive fungal disease. The likelihood of a specific organism varies by institution and may change over time, so knowing which bacteria typically cause sepsis in a given population and hospital will inform the antibiotic choice. Empiric antibiotics for fever and neutropenia should include coverage for gram-negative organisms, including Pseudomonas species and for gram-positive organisms such as Staph aureus and coagulase negative Staphylococcus. If fever persists for 5–7 days, empiric antifungal therapy is indicated. Typical antimicrobial choices are listed in *Table 344.1*.

In addition to bacteremia, immunocompromised hosts are susceptible to other bacterial infections, including sinusitis, pneumonia, perianal cellulitis, typhlitis, and other areas of cellulitis. Invasive fungal disease can include candidal esophagitis, fungal sinusitis, and invasive fungal pneumonia, either with candida or mucor. Mucor has a poor prognosis and must include aggressive surgical management in addition to antifungal medical therapy.

Viral infections that are dangerous in immunocompromised hosts include varicella zoster, herpes simplex, Epstein–Barr virus, and cytomegalovirus (CMV). Disseminated varicella is particularly problematic, with a high degree of lethality from encephalitis, pneumonia, or hepatic failure. Following a Varicella exposure, prophylaxis with varicella immune globulin within 72 h can prevent or ameliorate illness, and if varicella occurs, hospitalization and treatment with acyclovir is indicated. Varicella vaccine, although a live attenuated vaccine, is safe and effective in immunocompromised hosts. Zoster also requires treatment but is less likely than primary Varicella to disseminate.

Immunization with live-attenuated viruses (measles, mumps, rubella, polio (Sabin)) should not be given before the child completes chemotherapy and immune mechanisms are restored. Killed virus vaccines, such as those against diphtheria, tetanus, pertussis, and polio (Salk only), can be used safely in children receiving chemotherapy (*Table 344.2*).

Table 344.1
Common infectious complications in immmunocompromised hosts and treatment

Indication	Treatment of choice	Comments
Fever and neutropenia (F&N)	Third-generation cephalosporin (ceftazadime)	Alternatively, use three-drug combination, including:
		• Anti-pseudomonas penicillin (ticarcillin, piperacillin)
		• Anti-staphylococcal penicillin (oxacillin, nafcillin)
		• Aminoglycoside (gentamycin)
		If a specific site of infection is identified, it should be treated in addition to empiric coverage
Persistent F&N (5–7 days)	Amphotericin B	Alternatively, use may fluconazole
		Lipid encapsulated formulations of amphotericin may be less toxic
Pneumocystis jiroveci	1. TMP/SMX	Must be used as prophylaxis – 2 consecutive days per week
	2. Pentamadine	Used at therapeutic doses for treatment
Varicella	Acyclovir	Use high-dose therapy with sufficient fluids. Monitor renal function closely

Pneumocystis jirovecii (previously known as *P.carinii*) is a yeast-like fungus that causes opportunistic pneumonia in immunocompromised hosts. This pneumonia is universally fatal if not treated but can be easily and effectively prevented with prophylactic trimethoprim-sulfamethoxazole (TMP/SMX) given on 2 successive days each week. In patients with contraindications to TMP/SMX, a monthly infusion of pentamadine is used as prophylaxis. At therapeutic doses, these medications are also used for treatment.

There are additional and unique infectious risks associated with bone marrow transplantation (BMT). These are discussed in the chapter on BMT.

Table 344.2
Antibiotic usage in immunocompromised hosts

Drug	Dose	Organisms	Comments
Antibiotics			
Ceftazadime	100 mg/kg/day divided every 8 h	Pseudomonas	Third-generation cephalosporin
			Most common antibiotic for empiric coverage of fever and neutropenia (F&N)
Cefepime	100 mg/kg/day divided every 8 h	Pseudomonas, gram negative, gram positive	Can be used in setting of resistance to ceftazadime
Imipenem	50 mg/kg/day divided every 6 h	Pseudomonas, gram negative, gram positive	Excellent anaerobic coverage
Aztreonam	100–150 mg/kg/day divided every 6 h	Gram negative	No gram-positive coverage
Vancomycin	25–40 mg/kg/day divided every 6–12 h	Gram positive	Use only when clinically indicated
			Monitor levels and renal function
Antifungals			
Amphotericin B	0.5 mg/kg daily (empiric)	Candida	Monitor renal function closely
	1–1.5 mg/kg daily (therapeutic)	Aspergillus	Sodium loading prior to infusion protective for kidneys
Fluconazole	3–12 mg/kg/day	Candida	Use high doses in life-threatening conditions
Acyclovir	1500 mg/m^2 divided every 8 h	Varicella Zoster (VZV)	May use half this dose for HSV
		Herpes simplex (HSV)	Adequate hydration with high doses will limit nephrotoxicity
Anti-pneumocystis agents			
Trimethoprim – sulfamethoxazole	20 mg/kg/day divided every 12 h	Pneumocistis jiroveci	Monitor for bone marrow suppression
Pentamadine	4 mg/kg/day	Pneumocistis jiroveci	Use in TMP/SMX contraindication or treatment failure

Psychosocial Support

Providing psychosocial support to patients and their families is an important aspect of care in pediatric oncology. Helping them deal with accepting the diagnosis, ensuring compliance with therapy, and adjusting to being a cancer survivor are all important aspects of support. Practical supportive measures may include assisting families with housing for those who must travel to get care and helping ensure access to prescription medications. Supporting the child during procedures with medical play and distractions can help diminish the pain experienced with these procedures.

Support for the medical, nursing, and other staff is also important as there can be an emotional toll in dealing with children who have cancer.

Rehabilitation

Maximizing function and quality of life in children undergoing anticancer therapy may require rehabilitation services. Children with central nervous system (CNS) tumors may require intensive rehabilitation, including physical therapy, occupational therapy, and speech therapy following tumor resection, and this should be done in a way that does not interfere with the timely initiation of adjuvant therapies. Children with CNS tumors and others who receive cranial radiation may have learning difficulties after therapy and may benefit from cognitive remediation and accommodations from their teachers. Children with bone and other extremity sarcomas may also need physical therapy to adjust to amputation or following a limb-sparing surgical procedure.

Unique Aspects in Developing Countries

In developing countries, children often present with higher-stage disease, and they are more likely to be malnourished and impoverished. Medical resources may also be decreased compared to developed nations. Knowing the usual differences for a given country or region will help physicians design local standards of care.

References

Barbi E, Gerarduzzi T, Marchetti R et al (2003) Deep sedation with propofol by nonanesthesiologists: a prospective pediatric experience. Arch Pediatr Adolesc Med 157:1097–1103

Boogard W, van der Sande JJ (1993) Diagnosis and treatment of spinal cord compression in malignant disease. Cancer Treat Rev 19:129

Ellenby MS, Tegtmeyer K, Lai S, Braner DAV (2006) Videos in clinical medicine: lumbar puncture. N Engl J Med 355:e12

Malempati S, Joshi S, Lai S et al (2009) Videos in clinical medicine: bone marrow aspiration and biopsy. N Engl J Med 361:e28

Michon J (2002) Incidence of anemia in pediatric cancer patients in Europe: results of a large international survey. Med Pediatr Oncol 39:448–450

Pinkerton CR, Williams D, Wootton C et al (1990) 5-HT3 antagonist ondansetron–an effective outpatient antiemetic in cancer treatment. Arch Dis Child 65:822–825

Pisciotto PT, Benson K, Hume H, Glassman AB, Oberman H, Popovsky M, Hines D, Anderson K (1995) Prophylactic versus therapeutic platelet transfusion practices in hematology and/or oncology patients. Transfusion 35:498–502

Pollock ES (1993) Emergency department presentation of childhood malignancies. Hematol Oncol Emerg 11:517–529

Ricketts RR (2001) Clinical management of anterior mediastinal tumors in children. Semin Pediatr Surg 10:161–168

Saxonhouse M (2004) Platelet transfusions in the infant and child. In: Hillyer C, Strauss R, Luban NLC (eds) Handbook of pediatric transfusion medicine. Academic, San Diego, pp 253–270

Schiff D (2003) Spinal cord compression. Neurol Clin 21:67–86

Schiffer CA (2001) (2001) Platelet transfusion for patients with cancer: clinical practice guidelines of the American Society of Clinical Oncology. J Clin Oncol 19(5):1519–1538

Walco GA, Cassidy RC, Schechter NL (1994) Pain, hurt, and harm – The ethics of pain control in infants and children. N Engl J Med 331:541–544

Walker SM (2008) Pain in children: recent advances and ongoing challenges. Br J Anaesth 101:101–110

Walsh TJ, Roilides E, Groll AH et al (2006) Infectious complications in pediatric cancer patients. In: Pizzo PA, Poplack DG (eds) Principles and practice of pediatric oncology, 5th edn. Lippincott Williams & Wilkins, Philadelphia, pp 1269–1329

Wong EC, Perez-Albuerne E, Moscow JA, Luban NL (2005) Transfusion management strategies: a survey of practicing pediatric hematology/oncology specialists. Pediatr Blood Cancer 44:119–127

345 Childhood Leukemia

Hassan El Solh · Abdallah Al-Nasser · Asim Belgaumi

Definition/Classification

Leukemias are a group of malignant diseases with a unifying origin from hematopoietic cells. They result from clonal proliferation of a malignantly transformed cell of hematopoietic lineage with differentiation arrest. The type of leukemia is determined by the normal counterpart of the malignant clone and also by the stage of differentiation at the time of arrest. As such, leukemias can be lymphoid or myeloid; and even within these broad categories further sub-classifications can be made based on the particular cell involved. The most common subtype of leukemia seen in children is acute lymphoblastic leukemia (ALL).

Although by far the majority of leukemias originates from and involves the bone marrow, this in itself is not a requisite and in rare cases a diagnosis of leukemia can be made without bone marrow involvement by conventional diagnostic methods.

Etiology

The precise etiology of leukemia in humans is not known. There are, however, several factors which may play a presumed role in the pathogenesis of human leukemia, including genetic predisposition, viral infection, congenital immune deficiency diseases, ionizing radiation, and certain toxic chemicals that can facilitate its development. Leukemia-associated genetic changes have been identified in umbilical cord blood samples, indicating a prenatal initiation of at least common childhood acute lymphoblastic leukemia. However, such prenatal cytogenetic changes are probably only predisposing factors and require post natal events, such as viral infections, to fully realize the leukemic phenotype. Constitutional chromosomal abnormalities are associated with childhood leukemia. Children with trisomy 21 (Down syndrome) are approximately 15-times more likely to develop leukemia, particularly acute myeloid leukemia, than normal children. Congenital syndromes that result in DNA instability, such as Fanconi anemia, Bloom syndrome and ataxia telangiectasia, also result in an increased predisposition to leukemogenesis. Although environmental factors, such as ionizing radiation or toxic chemicals, have the potential to produce leukemias, these are rarely associated with childhood leukemia in practice.

Epidemiology

Leukemias are the most common malignancy in children, constituting about 30% of all pediatric cancers. The average annual incidence of childhood leukemias from developed countries is about three to four cases per 100,000 children. The incidence reported from Saudi Arabia is somewhat lower, between two and three cases per 100,000 children. The data from India report an incidence that varies considerably from 1.5 to 5.6 per 100,000 children, with the lower incidence in the rural areas and the highest in the urban centers. Whether development and urbanization contribute to leukemogenesis or, as is more likely, case acquisition is better in the cities is as yet undetermined. Within the pediatric age group the incidence is highest between 1 and 4 year of age and corresponds to the peak incidence for common childhood ALL.

Acute lymphoblastic leukemia (ALL) accounts for 70–75% of all leukemias seen in this age group. Precursor B-cell ALL constitutes the majority of cases seen, with T-ALL accounting for about 15–20% in most reports. The proportion of T-ALL seems to be higher and significantly variable (20–60%) in less developed rural populations, which may be related to environmental factors. Acute myeloid leukemia (AML) accounts for about 25% of all cases. Chronic myeloid leukemia (CML) and juvenile myelomonocytic leukemia (JMML) are rare and together account for 5% of all childhood leukemias. The peak incidence of ALL occurs at approximately 3–4 years of age. The incidence of AML remains stable from birth to age 10 years and increases slightly during the teen ages.

Pathogenesis

Like all malignant disorders, leukemia is a clonal disease, originating from a single cell. Genetic mutations within this

Abdelaziz Y. Elzouki (ed.), *Textbook of Clinical Pediatrics*, DOI 10.1007/978-3-642-02202-9_345,

cell provide an evolutionary "survival advantage." Such "advantageous" mutations also result in a predisposition for further genetic mutation which, as they accumulate, result in the development of a malignant phenotype, the leukemic cell. There is clear evidence that the initiating steps in a significant proportion of childhood leukemia begins in utero. This is certainly true for infantile leukemia harboring the *MLL* gene, and has also been noted in a significant proportion of post-infancy childhood ALL and AML. What is also evident is that the leukemic predisposition induced by the in utero genetic changes requires a postnatal "second-hit." Current evidence seems to indicate an aberrant immune response to common infectious exposures which may be one of the intervening events leading to phenotypic leukemia. The pre-leukemic latent phase often lasts 2–4 years but may be as long as 14 years. The monoclonal and intrauterine origin of leukemia is most evident in the concordance of acute leukemia in monozygotic twins, which is estimated to be as high as 25%. The risk is higher in infancy and diminishes with age.

Clinical Manifestations

Presenting signs and symptoms of leukemia are usually nonspecific and are usually a manifestation of the underlying anemia, thrombocytopenia, and neutropenia. Pallor, fatigue, petechiae, purpura, bleeding, and fever are often present. Bone pain particularly affecting the long bones is common. In addition, joint effusions and arthralgias may be present due to leukemic infiltration of the peri-articular bone. Evidence for leukemic infiltration of organs, such as hepatomegaly, splenomegaly, and lymphadenopathy, may be evident on physical examination. Chloromas or granulocytic sarcomas are discrete tumors seen in patients with AML. Central nervous system (CNS) involvement can manifest as seizures, cranial nerve palsy, and/or symptoms and signs of increased intracranial pressure.

Laboratory abnormalities most often reflect the underlying failure of production of normal blood elements. Although white blood cell counts are often increased in patients with leukemia, many patients, in fact, have reduced white blood cells (WBC) counts. Thrombocytopenia and anemia are seen almost universally. Electrolyte abnormalities may also be seen, particularly if there is ongoing tumor lysis syndrome (TLS). In such cases elevated serum potassium, phosphate and uric acid, and hypocalcemia may be seen even prior to initiation of chemotherapy. Leukemic infiltration of the kidneys may result in renal dysfunction with elevation of serum creatinine. Disseminated intravascular coagulopathy (DIC) may occur in any type of leukemia, but this is more common in the acute promyelocytic leukemia.

Differential diagnosis includes nonmalignant conditions like juvenile rheumatoid arthritis, infectious mononucleosis, aplastic anemia, and idiopathic (immune) thrombocytopenic purpura. In infants any infection may result in a marked elevation of WBC counts and a leukoerythroblastic picture, mimicking leukemia.

Diagnosis

Childhood leukemias are systemic diseases that may affect any organ of the body, causing manifestations that may mimic other diseases. Children with leukemia are usually referred to a tertiary care center, where comprehensive programs for treatment of such diseases are available.

Although leukemic blast cells may be present in the peripheral blood, the definitive diagnosis is usually established upon examination of bone marrow aspirate specimens. Most patients have anemia and thrombocytopenia at diagnosis. Leukocyte counts may be elevated, normal, or low. Blast cells may be present in the peripheral blood. Bone marrow aspirate should be done in order to more completely characterize the leukemic cells. On occasion, when the peripheral white blood cell count is elevated the diagnosis can be completed without performing a bone marrow aspirate. The characterization of the leukemic blasts is done by morphologic assessment utilizing special stains, immuno phenotyping, cytogenetic and molecular studies. Establishment of the immune phenotype by flow-cytometric analysis is now considered the cornerstone of leukemia diagnosis. This is essential in defining the cell-type of origin, and helps in determining the treatment strategy that would be used.

Cytogenetic and molecular genetic studies have now become extremely important in determining the prognosis and in risk stratification of therapy. In ALL, genetic abnormalities within the leukemic cell have been shown to confer either a good-risk or a poor-risk genotype. This obviously would determine treatment intensity and outcome. This is probably even more evident in AML, where cytogenetic abnormalities now form the basis for AML subtype categorization, according to the current World Health Organization (WHO) Classification.

Other diagnostic studies include evaluation of the cerebrospinal fluid (CSF), and testicular-evaluation in boys. In patients with T-cell ALL, chest X-ray may show a mediastinal mass.

Treatment

General Concepts in the Initial Management of Childhood Leukemias

Chemotherapy remains the mainstay of therapy for children with leukemias. Over the years the use of radiation therapy, particularly cranial radiation therapy, has lost some of its value, and now indications for radiation therapy are limited. Bone marrow transplantation is used for a limited number of higher risk leukemia patients and does contribute toward achieving a higher cure rate. These treatment strategies are different for the different types of leukemias encountered and are outlined in more detail below.

Supportive measures are critical in stabilizing the patients prior to initiation of therapy. Hydration and correction of electrolyte disturbances are essential. As all patients with leukemia are at risk of tumor lysis syndrome (TLS) and the resultant renal compromise due to hyperuricemia, they all should be well hydrated to maintain a brisk urine output. Although urine alkalinization has been a component of TLS prevention for many years, it is now evident that alkalinization does not add to the beneficial effect of a high urine flow, and is no longer recommended.

Even with normal or high WBC counts, newly diagnosed patients with leukemia should be considered as immunocompromised. Any evidence or even suspicion of infection should be treated aggressively with broad spectrum intravenous antibiotics. While blood product transfusion for anemia or thrombocytopenia is indicated, this should be undertaken judiciously, particularly in patients with markedly elevated WBC count. Hyperleukocytosis, particularly in patients with AML, may result in hyperviscosity and resultant obstruction of small vasculature. Red blood cell transfusions may aggravate the signs and symptoms of hyperviscosity. Adequate hydration is usually sufficient in preventing hyperviscosity, although some patients with very high WBC counts may need leukapheresis in order to induce rapid reductions in the WBC counts. Such patients with high WBC counts and those with massive organomegaly have a large tumor load and with initiation of therapy remain at a high risk for TLS. The best treatment for TLS is its prevention with good hydration and the use of agents such as allopurinol and urate oxidase to decrease uric acid levels.

Good nutritional support, including total parenteral nutrition (TPN) when needed for critically ill patients, should be provided. Psychosocial support of the patient and the family including education about the disease and its therapy is of extreme importance to enable the treating team to deliver therapy.

Acute Lymphoblastic Leukemia

Childhood ALL is a heterogeneous group of leukemias, all sharing a common characteristic of lymphoid origin. This is reflected in the cellular differentiation markers and the morphology. Broadly, ALL can be divided into B-cell and T-cell types; however, the true nomenclature for these should be precursor B-cell and precursor T-cell lymphoblastic leukemias. Mature B-cell ALL, which was previously also categorized morphologically as the FAB L3 subtype, is now no longer included within this group of diseases and is reclassified as Burkitt leukemia/lymphoma. Distinct subtypes of precursor B-ALL with recurrent genetic lesions are now identified.

Central Nervous System (CNS) leukemia is diagnosed by the presence of lymphoblasts in the cerebrospinal fluid (CSF) as detected by centrifugation. For diagnosis of leukemic involvement of the testis, fine-needle aspiration or open biopsy is required to determine the presence of lymphoblasts. In the bone marrow, the lymphoblasts can be characterized by morphologic, biochemical markers, immunologic, and cytogenetic.

Morphology

Morphologic features of the leukemic lymphoblasts are best determined on examination of a bone marrow aspirate specimen. Most often the bone marrow is diffusedly infiltrated with the monomorphic leukemic lymphoblasts, with marked reduction in the normal marrow elements. Occasionally the numbers of lymphoblasts in the bone marrow may be less, making a distinction between ALL and bone marrow involvement of a lymphoblastic lymphoma difficult. An arbitrary cut off of 25% has been used to make this distinction. The lymphoblasts vary in size from small to medium sized cells. The cytoplasm is often scanty, but can be of a moderate amount and occasionally (10% of cases) may have coarse azurophilic granules. Generally, the nuclear cytoplasm (N/C) ratio is high and the nuclei often have prominent nucleoli.

The FAB classification of lymphoblastic leukemias, which is based primarily on the morphological characteristics, is no longer considered to be of clinical significance and is not used any more.

Biochemical Characterization

With current available diagnostic tools, cytochemistry seldom contributes to the diagnosis of ALL. Lymphoblasts are universally negative for myeloperoxidase, Sudan black, and esterase stains. Periodic acid-Schiff (PAS) reaction is positive in most cases and is present in a coarse granular distribution. Terminal deoxynucleotidyl transferase (TdT) is found in the majority of patients with ALL.

Immuno Phenotype

Immuno phenotyping is the mainstay of ALL diagnosis and is used to characterize the leukemic cell. The leukemic transformation and clonal expansion can occur at different stages of maturation in the process of lymphoid differentiation and this is reflected in the expression pattern of cellular proteins in the malignant cells. Although most immunophenotyping is conducted using flowcytometry, immunohistochemical staining can also be used. The basic principle involves the use of monoclonal antibodies (moAbs) directed at surface and cytoplasmic proteins of the malignant cells. These moAbs are then identified by using fluorescent or chromogenic tags. Expression of lineage-specific markers such as CD19, cytoplasmic CD79a and cytoplasmic CD22 for B-cells, and cytoplasmic CD3 surface CD2 and CD7 for T-cells is indicative. However no individual marker is enough on its own to finalize the diagnosis and most often a pattern of expression is utilized. Some markers have been shown to have a prognostic association, such as CD10 which is commonly seen in patients with B-cell precursor ALL and is indicative of a more favorable prognosis.

Precursor B-ALL constitutes approximately 80–85% of all ALL, while 15–20% of ALL cases are T-cell ALL. This distinction is also of clinical importance as there are differences in disease presentation and response to therapy. T-ALL tends to occur in older children as compared to B-lineage ALL and generally presents with a higher WBC count. T-ALL is also associated with thymic infiltration presenting as a mediastinal mass. Patients with T-ALL require more intensive therapy, in spite of which they have a somewhat worse outcome than B-lineage ALL.

Not all ALL cases adhere to a specific lineage. Although occasional aberrant myeloid marker positivity is seen in ALL, this does not necessarily result in a diagnosis of mixed phenotype acute leukemia (MPAL). Clear guidelines are now available for the diagnosis of MPAL and require the expression of lineage specific markers of more than one cellular lineage. These MPAL tend to confer a worse prognosis, but may be amenable to therapy which includes agents effective against both lymphoid and myeloid leukemias.

Cytogenetic Studies

With the advances in cell culture methodology and improved chromosomal banding techniques, cytogenetic analysis has contributed significantly to the understanding of the biology and treatment of ALL. More recently the availability of molecular tools, such as polymerase chain reaction (PCR) and fluorescence in situ hybridization (FISH), has made it easier to identify genetic lesions. These techniques have also allowed the identification of cryptic translocations that are not evident on routine chromosomal banding. Certain recurrent cytogenetic abnormalities have been identified in ALL that have clinical and prognostic importance and these are now categorized separately.

Numerical abnormalities, with duplications and deletions of whole chromosomes, are seen quite frequently in leukemic blasts. These are non-random with extra copies of chromosomes 21, X, 14, and 4 encountered most often. Children with more than 52 chromosomes in their leukemia cells (hyperdiploid >52) tend to have a significantly better prognosis. This is determined either by routine karyotyping, or by the DNA index (the ratio of the average number of chromosomes in the lymphoblasts/normal diploid number 46) which can be determined by flowcytometry or FISH. Patients with DNA index >1.16 have a good prognosis. Extremes of chromosome numbers, near haploid or near tetraploid, confer an extremely poor prognosis. Recent studies have identified that trisomies of specific chromosomes (chromosomes 4, 10, and 17) rather than the total chromosome number may in fact be more important in determining the prognosis.

Specific structural chromosomal abnormalities also occur in ALL and several are considered clinically significant enough to warrant separate categorization. Precursor B-ALL with the Philadelphia chromosome (t(9:22); *BCR-ABL1* translocation) and those with rearrangements of the *MLL* gene at the 11q23 locus have a poor prognosis. *MLL* gene rearrangements occur due to translocations between chromosome 11 at the q23 locus and several variable partner chromosomes (t(v;11q23)); however, chromosome 4 is the most common. These translocations characterize the leukemias seen in infancy and are related to the poor prognosis of these patients. Translocation (12;21) (p13;q22) (*TEL-AML1 or ETV6-RUNX1*) is a cryptic translocation that is found in 20–25% of precursor B-ALL and is now considered the most common cytogenetic abnormality in ALL. Patients with this translocation have good prognosis. Other encountered translocations include t(1:19) and t(9;11).

Although several translocations are also encountered in patients with T-ALL, none are clearly identified as having a prognostic or clinical impact.

Prognostic Factors

Age at diagnosis and initial WBC count are the most significant clinical prognostic factors identified. In fact, patients with a WBC count<50 × 10^9/L and age between 1 and 10 years are considered to have an especially good risk. Infancy (age <1 year) is universally recognized as a poor prognostic factor, particularly due to its association with *MLL* gene rearrangements. Older patients (≥10 years of age) have a relatively poor prognosis which may be related to a higher proportion of patients with the T-cell phenotype and the absence of good-risk cytogenetic features. Cytogenetic abnormalities, as outlined above, have prognostic significance. Several studies reported that girls have a better prognosis than boys, although with recent treatment protocols this difference is less evident. Immune phenotype also appears to correlate with prognosis, with T-ALL being associated with a worse outcome than precursor B-ALL. Patients with T-ALL tend also to present with higher WBC counts and have more extramedullary involvement, particularly CNS involvement.

Leukemic infiltration of extramedullary sanctuary sites, such as the CNS and testicles, confers a worse outcome. This is especially significant for patients with CNS involvement who tend to have a higher risk of relapse, including bone marrow recurrences. The best outcome is seen in younger, non-infant, patients with B-ALL who have either the t(12;21) or hyperdiploidy with trisomies of chromosomes 4, 10, and 17.

Treatment

Treatment of ALL is primarily chemotherapy based and is risk-stratified. Risk stratification implies the use of higher intensity of therapy for those patients who are at a greater risk for relapse, and less intense therapy for those who at lower risk for relapse in order to avoid treatment-related toxicity. Risk stratification is based on the prognostic features available at diagnosis as outlined above, and also on response to therapy. Early response to therapy is determined by peripheral blood and bone marrow evaluation following 1 and 2 weeks of induction therapy.

Although different ALL treatment protocols utilize somewhat differing chemotherapeutic agents, certain universally applied features are present. Treatment for ALL is composed of well defined phases of therapy. The initial phase is induction, which usually utilizes three or four drugs (vincristine, prednisone, L-asparaginase, and daunomycin). This phase of therapy is aimed at rapid reduction of leukemic infiltrates and results in a 2–4 log reduction in the lymphoblasts burden.This phase is followed by the consolidation phase which further reduces systemic leukemic infiltrates. Therapy during the consolidation phase is also aimed at prevention of relapse in the CNS. The preventive therapy involves administration of intrathecal chemotherapy. Post consolidation the patients are placed on a prolonged continuation therapy phase which primarily includes antimetabolite (mercaptopurine and methotrexate) chemotherapy. This continuation phase is interspersed with either one or two intensification phases which are reminiscent of induction and consolidation. Total duration of therapy is usually between 2 and 3 years.

Radiation therapy was a standard component of ALL treatment; however, over the past 2 decades the need and indications for radiation therapy have been severely restricted. Currently, craniospinal radiation therapy is still required for patients diagnosed with CNS leukemia and testicular radiation therapy is administered to those boys with testicular leukemia. Clinical trials exploring further reductions in these indications are underway. These restrictions are desirable due to concerns that radiotherapy contributes to the long-term neurotoxicity.

Hematopoietic Stem Cell Transplantation (HSCT) is not required for the majority of patients with ALL. However, certain categories of patients with very high risk features, such as those with *BCR-ABLX* translocation or with *MLL* gene rearrangements, do benefit from BMT in first remission.

Outcome and Prognosis

Bone marrow relapse is the principal form of treatment failure in patients with ALL. Other sites of relapse include the CNS and, in boys, the testicles.

Prognosis of patients with ALL has improved significantly in recent years. Currently, approximately 70–80% of children with ALL achieve prolonged disease-free survival (>5 years after finishing therapy) and are considered cured. In patients with low risk features, this figure has reached 90%.

Acute Myelogenous Leukemia

The transformation event in AML could theoretically occur in any cell along the pathway from pluripotent stem cell to committed hematopoietic cells. Although derived from cells of the myeloid lineage, AML is a heterogeneous group that can originate from and be reminiscent of any hematopoietic cell lineage, including erythroid and megakaryocytic.

Morphology

As with ALL, the morphologic classification, according to the FAB system, has lost its reliability and is no longer used. Lineage assignment and prognosis is now better determined by immunophenotype and genetic characteristics. Due to the various cell lineages involved and the fact that AML may occur at any phase of myeloid differentiation, no unifying morphologic characteristics can be enumerated for AML myeloblasts. These myeloblasts are described according to the presumed cells of origin (myeloid, monocytic, megakaryocytic, and erythroid) and the degree of cellular differentiation/maturation. In general, myeloblasts are larger in size than lymphoblasts and have more copious cytoplasm. Granularity is often encountered and Auer rods are considered diagnostic of myeloid malignancy. Myeloperoxidase detection by cytochemistry or flowcytometry conclusively assigns myeloid lineage to the leukemic cells; this however is not positive in all AML subtypes.

Immuno Phenotype

As with ALL, immuno phenotyping is the mainstay of AML diagnosis and subtype assignment. Often a relatively large panel of moAbs is applied, and the patterns of expression are used to reach a diagnosis. Certain markers are seen more consistently, with at least one of the following markers, CD33, CDI3, CD15, CD11b, CD 14, and CD34, being expressed in more than 90% of AML cases.

Cytogenetic Studies

Genetic alterations form the basis of AML subclassification and prognostic risk assignment. Certain recurrent genetic abnormalities are frequently seen in AML cells. These structural changes are associated with specific subtypes of AML and have prognostic implications. Translocation (8;21)(q22;q22)/*RUNX1-RUNX1T1* is the most commonly occurring translocation in de novo AML. This is found mostly in myeloid leukemia with maturation (prior FAB M2 subtype). Related genetic abnormalities include inv(16)(p13.1q22) (p13.1;q22)/*CBFB-MYH11* or the t(16;16), which is often associated with the myelomonocytic subtype of AML. This translocation and t(8;21) involve the genes for the subunits of the heterodimeric DNA binding transcriptional regulator, the Core Binding Factor (CBF), which has been shown to be essential for the normal development of all hematopoietic lineages. The presence of either of these translocations confers a more chemo-sensitive phenotype and results in better disease free survivals. Interestingly, the *RUNX1* gene is also involved in the t(12;21)/*RUNX1-ETV6* translocation in ALL which also results in improved prognosis.

AML with the t(15:17)(q22;q12)/*PML-RARA* translocation is uniquely associated with a more mature myeloid cell type (Acute promyelocytic leukemia; prior FAB M3 subtype). This AML also has a better outcome, which is primarily associated with the use of *all-trans* retinoic acid (ATRA) as a component of treatment. As in ALL the *MLL* gene rearrangements involving translocations of the chromosome 11q23 are often seen and can involve numerous translocation partner genes. These translocations are more often seen in the younger age group and tend to confer a worse overall outcome, except for t(9;11)(p22;q23)/*MLLT3-MLL* which has an intermediate prognosis. In addition to their presence in *de novo* AML, *MLL* gene rearrangements are frequently seen in cases of treatment-related AML, particularly those associated with prior topoisomerase II inhibitor therapy. Numeric changes in certain chromosomes or loss/gain of major chromosomal segments are often seen in AML associated with myelodysplasia. Most commonly associated changes include −7/del(7q), −5/del(5q), and trisomy 8.

Several other gene mutations, in addition to the structural chromosomal abnormalities, are seen in AML. These include mutations in genes such as *FLT3, NPM, WT1, and KIT.* These mutations have varying effects on prognosis.

Prognostic Factors

Prognostic risk stratification in AML is determined more by the primary cell of origin and the cytogenetic aberration than by specific clinical features. As mentioned above, t(8;21) and inv(16)/t(16:16) have a favorable outcome, as does APL with t(15;17). Myelodysplastic syndrome (MDS) associated cytogenetic abnormalities such as −7, del(5q) and +8 are associated with a significantly poor outcome, which is probably related to the association with MDS rather than the effect of any particular genetic abnormality. *MLL* gene rearrangements in *de novo* AML is not necessarily associated with a poor outcome, but confers a particularly bad prognosis in patients with outcome and treatment-related AML (t-AML).

Certain AML subtypes generally are known to have a worse outcome. These include acute megakaryocytic leukemia and erythroleukemia. Interestingly, megakaryocytic leukemia in children with Down's syndrome (DS), 4 years of age, has a particularly good outcome to chemotherapy.

Treatment

The treatment strategy for AML requires therapy to be intensive, multi-agent, and sequential. Although clear phases of therapy are well not defined, as in all treatment, the first two cycles of chemotherapy are generally considered to constitute the remission induction phase. Cytosine arabinoside and anthracyclines are considered to be the effective agents for remission induction. Often other chemotherapy agents, such as thioguanine or etoposide, are included in the induction regime. With current treatment approximately 85% of AML patients are expected to achieve remission following first line induction therapy.

Post remission induction therapy includes either two or three further cycles of multi-agent chemotherapy, or allogeneic hematopoietic stem cell transplantation (HSCT). Most often HSCT is timed to follow either second or third cycle of chemotherapy, depending on the timing of achievement of remission. Indication for HSCT has evolved over the last decade, and not all patients now need transplantation. Patients within the lower risk group, with good-risk cytogenetic changes, can be treated effectively with chemotherapy alone. Most physicians would now offer HSCT to patients with intermediate risk status only if there is a matched related donor. Patients in the poorest risk group, those with MDS-related AML, t-AML, or non DS megakaryocytic leukemia, continue to be candidates for HSCT even from alternative donor sources. Autologous SCT is no longer considered an option for treatment of pediatric AML.

Special consideration must be given to t(15;17) positive APL. In addition to the anthracycline and cytosine arabinoside these patients are induced with ATRA. Pharmacological doses of ATRA act by overcoming the effect of the retinoic acid receptor α (RARA) mutation and inducing cellular differentiation, maturation, and apoptosis. Due to the good outcome with chemotherapy, HSCT is not indicated in APL. Post remission therapy now includes a maintenance phase using antimetabolites (mercaptopurine and methotrexate) with pulses of ATRA.

Prognosis

With current intensive therapy around 50–60% of children with AML are expected to survive long term. This survival is dependent on risk stratification, with over 70% survival for the low risk AML patients and around 30% for those with high risk AML.

Chronic Myeloid Leukemia

Chronic Myeloid Leukemia (CML) is rare in the pediatric age group, accounting for less than 5% of all leukemias. It is a myeloproliferative neoplastic disease that originates in an abnormal pluripotent hematopoietic stem cell. CML is characterized by the presence of the *BCR-ABL* translocation (t(9;22)(q34;q11.2)). This translocation results in the abnormally small chromosome 22, known as the Philadelphia chromosome. Although the initial presentation primarily includes neutrophilic leukocytosis, all myeloid lineages are involved. In fact, some lymphoid and endothelial cells may also harbor the *BCR-AB*[1] translocation.

Patients most often present in the chronic phase with marked hyperleukocytosis, and massive hepatosplenomegaly. As opposed to the acute leukemias, even with very high WBC counts, the platelet count is not reduced and may be elevated. Generalized lymphadenopathy may present and occasionally there is leukemic blast infiltration of skin or other soft tissues. The natural history of CML is triphasic, with the initial presentation usually in the chronic phase; untreated CML progresses on to accelerated and blastic phases. Rarely, patients with CML will present in the later phases, which most often is myeloid in origin and resembles AML. In some cases blastic transformation can be lymphoid and patients may present with disease indistinguishable clinically from ALL.

The *BCR-ABL* translocation driven abnormal Eyrosine kinase activity that defines CML has been the target also resulted in the development of the treatment approach to this disease. Treatment of CML is now based upon the use of tyrosine kinase inhibitors (TKI) that target the abnormally enhanced tyrosine kinase activity of the chimeric BCR-ABL protein. Imatinib mesylate was the first such TKI to be developed and remains the standard agent for fist line therapy. Imatinib mesylate monotherapy has resulted in not only complete cytogenetic remissions, but also in reductions in the leukemic clone to levels less than 1 in 10^5 cells. However, it is still unclear if TKI therapy can achieve durable cures and current treatment approaches recommend indefinite continuation of the TKI therapy.

Allogeneic HSCT remains the only proven curative therapeutic option for patients with CML. However, with the advent of TKI therapy the status of HSCT has become controversial. While transplant has become significantly uncommon in the treatment of chronic phase CML in adult patients, many pediatric oncologists still opt for transplantation for their patients. The need for possible lifelong TKI therapy has to be balanced against the potential toxic morbidity and mortality associated with HSCT. Many pediatric oncologists will now recommend HSCT if a matched related donor is available, and continue with TKI therapy for all other patients. Patients with advanced phase CML need to be treated more aggressively and HSCT remains the unequivocal treatment of choice.

Juvenile Myelomonocytic Leukemia (JMML)

Juvenile myelomonocytic leukemia (JMML) is a clonal proliferative hematopoietic disorder which occurs in infancy or early childhood. It primarily results in monocytosis andgranulocytosis and is distinguished from CML by the absence of the *BCR-ABL* fusion gene. It is quite rare and comprises only 2–3% of all childhood leukemias. Diagnostic criteria for JMML include not only the absence of *BCR-ABL*[1], but also require peripheral blood monocytosis and less than 20% blasts in the blood marrow. Other features that may be seen are elevated hemoglobin F, immature granulocytes in the peripheral blood, elevated WBC count to more than 10×10^9/L, and clonal chromosomal abnormalities including monosomy 7.

While chemotherapy and differentiation agents, such as cis-retinoic acid, have been used for cytoreduction, curative therapy is only achievable with HSCT. Without transplantation most children die of organ dysfunction due to leukemic infiltration at a median survival of less than 1 year.

References

Al-Eid HS, Arteh SO (2004) Cancer incidence report, Saudi Arabia. Saudi Cancer Registry, Ministry of Health of Kingdom of Saudi Arabia, Saudi Arabia

Al-Seraihy A, Owaidah TM, Ayas M, El-Solh H, Al-Mahr M, Al-Ahmari A, Belgaumi AF (2009) Clinical characteristics and outcome of biphenotypic acute leukemia in children. Haematologica 94(12): 1682–1690, Epub 27 Aug 2009

Arber DA, Brunning RD, Le Beau MM, Falini B, Vardiman JW, Porwit A, Thiele J, Bloomfield CD (2008) Acute myeloid leukemia with recurrent genetic abnormalities. In: Swerdlow SH, Campo E, Harris NL, Jaffe ES, Pileri SA, Stein H, Thiele J, Vardiman JW (eds) WHO classification of tumours of haematopoietic and lymphoid tissues, 4th edn. International Agency for Research on Cancer, Lyons

Arora RS, Eden TOB, Kapoor G (2009) Epidemiology of childhood cancer in India. Indian J Cancer 46(4):264–273

Baumann I, Bennett JM, Niemeyer CM, Thiele J, Shannon K (2008) Juvenile myelomonocytic leukemia. In: Swerdlow SH, Campo E, Harris NL, Jaffe ES, Pileri SA, Stein H, Thiele J, Vardiman JW (eds) WHO classification of tumours of haematopoietic and lymphoid tissues, 4th edn. International Agency for Research on Cancer, Lyons

Belgaumi AF, Al-Shehri A, Ayas M, Al-Mahr M, Al-Seraihy A, Al-Ahmari A, El-Solh H (2010) Clinical characteristics and treatment outcome of pediatric patients with chronic myeloid leukemia. Haematologica 95(7):1211–1215, Epub 21 Apr 2010

Borowitz MJ, Chan JKC (2008) Precursor lymphoid neoplasms. In: Swerdlow SH, Campo E, Harris NL, Jaffe ES, Pileri SA, Stein H, Thiele J, Vardiman JW (eds) WHO classification of tumours of haematopoietic and lymphoid tissues, 4th edn. International Agency for Research on Cancer, Lyons

Burke MJ, Willert J, Desai S, Kadota R (2009) The treatment of pediatric Philadelphia positive (Ph+) leukemias in the Imatinib era. Pediatr Blood Cancer 53(6):992–995

Castro-Malaspina H, Schaison G, Passe S, Pasquier A, Berger R, Bayle-Weisgerber C, Miller D, Seligmann M, Bernard J (1984) Subacute and chronic myelomonocytic leukemia in children (juvenile CML). Clinical and hematologic observations, and identification of prognostic factors. Cancer 54(4):675–686

Coiffier B, Altman A, Pui CH, Younes A, Cairo MS (2008) Guidelines for the management of pediatric and adult tumor lysis syndrome: an evidence-based review. J Clin Oncol 26(16):2767–2778

Gaynon PS, Angiolillo AL, Carroll WL, Nachman JB, Trigg ME, Sather HN, Hunger SP, Devidas M, Children's Oncology Group (2010) Long-term results of the children's cancer group studies for childhood acute lymphoblastic leukemia 1983–2002: a Children's Oncology Group Report. Leukemia 24(2):285–297, Epub 17 Dec 2009

Greaves MF (2002) Childhood leukemia. BMJ 324(7332):283–287

Greaves MF, Maia AT, Wiemels JL, Ford AM (2003) Leukemia in twins: lessons in natural history. Blood 102(7):2321–2333, Epub 5 June 2003

Gregory J, Feusner J (2009) Acute promyelocytic leukemia in childhood. Curr Oncol Rep 11(6):439–445

Harris MB, Shuster JJ, Carroll A et al (1992) Trisomy of leukemic cell chromosomes 4 and 10 identifies children with B-progenitor cell acute lymphoblastic leukemia with a very low risk of treatment failure: a Pediatric Oncology Group study. Blood 79:3316–3324

Harrison CJ, Hills RK, Moorman AV, Grimwade DJ, Hann I, Webb DK, Wheatley K, de Graaf SS, van den Berg E, Burnett AK, Gibson BE (2010) Cytogenetics of childhood acute myeloid leukemia: United Kingdom Medical Research Council Treatment trials AML 10 and 12. J Clin Oncol 28(16):2674–2681, Epub 3 May 2010

Hasle H, Baumann I, Bergsträsser E, Fenu S, Fischer A, Kardos G, Kerndrup G, Locatelli F, Rogge T, Schultz KR, Starý J, Trebo M, van den Heuvel-Eibrink MM, Harbott J, Nöllke P, Niemeyer CM, European Working Group on childhood MDS (2004) The International Prognostic Scoring System (IPSS) for childhood myelodysplastic syndrome (MDS) and juvenile myelomonocytic leukemia (JMML). Leukemia 18(12):2008–2014

Inaba H, Fan Y, Pounds S, Geiger TL, Rubnitz JE, Ribeiro RC, Pui CH, Razzouk BI (2008) Clinical and biologic features and treatment outcome of children with newly diagnosed acute myeloid leukemia and hyperleukocytosis. Cancer 113(3):522–529

Kang HJ, Shin HY, Choi HS, Ahn HS (2004) Novel regimen for the treatment of juvenile myelomonocytic leukemia (JMML). Leuk Res 28:167–170

Kaspers GJ, Zwaan CM (2007) Pediatric acute myeloid leukemia: towards high-quality cure of all patients. Haematologica 92(11):1519–1532

Lowe EJ, Pui CH, Hancock ML, Geiger TL, Khan RB, Sandlund JT (2005) Early complications in children with acute lymphoblastic leukemia presenting with hyperleukocytosis. Pediatr Blood Cancer 45(1):10–15

Millot F, Traore P, Guilhot J, Nelken B, Leblanc T, Leverger G, Plantaz D, Bertrand Y, Bordigoni P, Guilhot F (2005) Clinical and biological features at diagnosis in 40 children with chronic myeloid leukemia. Pediatrics 116(1):140–143

Mori H, Colman SM, Xiao Z, Ford AM, Healy LE, Donaldson C, Hows JM, Navarrete C, Greaves M (2002) Chromosome translocations and covert leukemic clones are generated during normal fetal development. Proc Natl Acad Sci USA 99(12):8242–8247, Epub 4 June 2002

Möricke A, Zimmermann M, Reiter A, Henze G, Schrauder A, Gadner H, Ludwig WD, Ritter J, Harbott J, Mann G, Klingebiel T, Zintl F, Niemeyer C, Kremens B, Niggli F, Niethammer D, Welte K, Stanulla M, Odenwald E, Riehm H, Schrappe M (2010) Long-term results of five consecutive trials in childhood acute lymphoblastic leukemia performed by the ALL-BFM study group from 1981 to 2000. Leukemia 24(2):265–284, Epub 10 Dec 2009

Niemeyer CM, Kratz CP (2008) Paediatric myelodysplastic syndromes and juvenile myelomonocytic leukaemia: molecular classification and treatment options. Br J Haematol 140(6):610–624

Ortega JJ, Madero L, Martín G, Verdeguer A, García P, Parody R, Fuster J, Molines A, Novo A, Debén G, Rodríguez A, Conde E, de la Serna J, Allegue MJ, Capote FJ, González JD, Bolufer P, González M, Sanz MA, PETHEMA Group (2005) Treatment with all-trans retinoic acid and anthracycline monochemotherapy for children with acute promyelocytic leukemia: a multicenter study by the PETHEMA Group. J Clin Oncol 23(30):7632–7640

Paulsson K, Johansson B (2009) High hyperdiploid childhood acute lymphoblastic leukemia. Genes Chromosom Cancer 48(8):637–660

Pui CH, Relling MV, Downing JR (2004) Acute lymphoblastic leukemia. N Engl J Med 350:1535–1548

Pui CH, Pei D, Sandlund JT, Ribeiro RC, Rubnitz JE, Raimondi SC, Onciu M, Campana D, Kun LE, Jeha S, Cheng C, Howard SC, Metzger ML, Bhojwani D, Downing JR, Evans WE, Relling MV (2010) Long-term results of St Jude Total Therapy Studies 11, 12, 13A, 13B, and 14 for childhood acute lymphoblastic leukemia. Leukemia 24(2):371–382, Epub 10 Dec 2009

Rubnitz JE (2008) Childhood acute myeloid leukemia. Curr Treat Options Oncol 9(1):95–105, Epub 28 May 2008

Stiller CA, Kroll ME, Boyle PJ, Feng Z (2008) Population mixing, socioeconomic status and incidence of childhood acute lymphoblastic leukaemia in England and Wales: analysis by census ward. Br J Cancer 98(5):1006–1011, Epub 5 Feb 2008

Surveillance Epidemiology and End Results (2010) SEER Cancer Statistics Review 1975–2007. Available from http://www.seer.cancer.gov/csr/1975_2007/index.html. Accessed 6 Jul 2010

Suttorp M (2008) Innovative approaches of targeted therapy for CML of childhood in combination with paediatric haematopoietic SCT. Bone Marrow Transplant 42:S40–S46

Webb DK, Harrison G, Stevens RF, Gibson BG, Hann IM, Wheatley K, MRC Childhood Leukemia Working Party (2001) Relationships between age at diagnosis, clinical features, and outcome of therapy in children treated in the Medical Research Council AML 10 and 12 trials for acute myeloid leukemia. Blood 98(6):1714–1720

Wiemels JL, Cazzaniga G, Daniotti M, Eden OB, Addison GM, Masera G, Saha V, Biondi A, Greaves MF (1999) Prenatal origin of acute lymphoblastic leukaemia in children. Lancet 354(9189):1499–1503

346 Non-Hodgkin Lymphoma

H. Stacy Nicholson

Introduction

Non-Hodgkin lymphoma (NHL) is the term applied to all solid lymphoid neoplasms other than Hodgkin disease (HD). Some are closely related to acute lymphoblastic leukemia (ALL) and are treated similarly. The incidence of NHL in children below 15 years of age in the USA is 7.4 per 100,000. NHL is much more common than HD in the first decade of life, and children with immunodeficiencies have a greater risk of NHL. NHL is the third most common childhood cancer, following leukemia and brain tumors.

Histological Subtypes

NHL is a group of diverse lymphoid malignancies. Improved understanding of tumor immunology, cytogenetics, and molecular biology has improved both the classification and treatment strategies for NHL. Each major subtype NHL needs to be understood separately. Major subtypes of NHL include Burkitt Lymphoma (BL), lymphoblastic lymphoma (LL), diffuse large B-Cell lymphoma, and anaplastic large-cell lymphoma.

Burkitt lymphoma is a fast-growing B-cell malignancy with a high proliferation rate. The pathology generally shows sheets of homogeneous cells with a classical "starry sky" appearance. Cell surface antigens include CD19, CD20, CD79a, and CD10, and surface immunoglobulin. Most BLs have characteristic translocations, including t(8;14), t(2;8) or t(8;22); these translocations fuse an immunoglobulin component gene with an oncogene.

Lymphoblastic lymphoma (LL) is closely related to ALL and can be either of B or T-cell origin. Cell surface antigens, cytogenetic abnormalities, and molecular biology of LL are identical to the corresponding cell origin ALL.

Diffuse large B-cell Lymphoma accounts for about one-third of all childhood NHLs. Cells express a number of B-cell antigens, including CD19, CD20, CD22, and Cd79a.

Clinical Features

NHL often presents with either persistent, progressive adenopathy, or as a medical emergency, including respiratory distress from a mediastinal mass or intestinal obstruction due to a mass arising from a Peyer's patch in the small intestine (most commonly terminal ileum). Most NHLs have a high rate of growth, and prompt referral to a childhood cancer center is important. Clinical features differ by type of NHL.

There are at least two main types of Burkitt lymphoma. In developed countries, BL often primarily involves the intestine and presents as an abdominal mass with or without intestinal obstruction. African BL is often associated with the Epstein–Barr Virus (EBV) and presents as a large facial mass.

Lymphoblastic lymphoma often presents with a mediastinal mass and may have malignant effusions, often leading to respiratory distress or failure. LL can be of either B- or T-cell origin, and clinical features are similar to ALL of the same lineage. For example, both T-cell ALL and T-cell LL are likely to present with a mediastinal mass and are more likely to involve the central nervous system (CNS).

Diffuse large B-cell lymphomas can present in a large variety of ways, but typically with sizable adenopathy, including mediastinal masses. This subtype is often disseminated and is the subtype most associated with immunodeficiencies.

Laboratory Features

Unless the bone marrow is involved, the complete blood count is usually normal. Similarly, unless there is hepatic involvement or renal failure from the acute tumor lysis syndrome (ATLS), blood chemistries are often normal. Lactate dehydrogenase (LDH) is usually markedly elevated. Uric acid, electrolytes, and renal function must be following closely at diagnosis and during the first few days of treatment, to prevent or treat ATLS.

Diagnostic Studies and Staging

Diagnosis depends upon a biopsy, and pathological tests should include cytogenetics and flow cytometry.

Abdelaziz Y. Elzouki (ed.), *Textbook of Clinical Pediatrics*, DOI 10.1007/978-3-642-02202-9_346,

Table 346.1
St. Jude (Murphy) staging system for non-Hodgkin lymphoma (NHL)

Stage	Description
I	• A single extranodal tumor or single nodal group, exclusive of the mediastinum or abdomen
II	• A single extranodal tumor with regional node involvement
	• Two or more nodal groups, on the same side of the diaphragm
	• Two extranodal tumors with or without regional node involvement on the same side of the diaphragm
	• Primary GI tract tumor (usually ileocecal) with or without regional node involvement
III	• Two extranodal tumors involving both sides of the diaphragm
	• Two or more nodal groups, involving both sides of the diaphragm
	• All primary intrathoracic tumors (mediastinal, pleural)
	• All extensive primary intra-abdominal tumors
	• All paraspinal or epidural tumors
IV	• Any of the above stages, with bone marrow or central nervous system involvement

In children with an effusion, malignant cells from an aspirate will usually yield the diagnosis. Performing the staging workup rapidly is important, given the urgent need to start therapy. Computerized tomography (CT) of the neck, chest, abdomen, and pelvis should be done, including the Waldeyer Ring, and bone marrow and cerebrospinal fluid should be tested in all NHL patients. A modification of the Murphy staging system is used in NHL (see *Table 346.1*), supplemented by a risk stratification schema for B-cell lymphomas (*Table 346.2*).

Treatment

Treatment differs by subtype, but all are treated with chemotherapy. Beyond establishing the diagnosis, there is little role for surgery in the treatment of NHL. Patients with intestinal obstruction need an emergency laparotomy with tumor resection. Radiotherapy is not part of standard therapies for NHL but may be used for palliation in patients with recurrent disease.

Chemotherapy is the mainstay of NHL therapy and has many similarities to treatment strategies used in ALL.

Table 346.2
Risk stratification of B-cell lymphomas

Stratum	Description
A	• Resected stage I and abdominal stage II
B	• Multiple extraabdominal sites, nonresected stage I, II, III
	• Stage IV may be in this group if less than 25% of bone marrow or cells in CSF are malignant
C	• Intra-abdominal stage IV
	• Bone marrow involvement with greater than 25% of cells being malignant

This system is used in addition to the Murphy staging system

CHOP (cyclophosphamide, doxorubicin, vincristine and prednisone) is the most commonly used combination chemotherapy and is effective in Burkitt lymphoma, diffuse large B-cell lymphoma and anaplastic large-cell lymphoma. In addition, COPAD (cyclophosphamide, doxorubicin, vincristine, and prednisone), COPADM (cyclophosphamide, doxorubicin, vincristine, prednisone, and high-dose methotrexate), and COMP (cyclophosphamide, vincristine, methotrexate, and prednisone) are used in BL. COPAD and COPADM are also used in large B-cell lymphoma. These are all dose-intensive combinations with significant toxicities and need to be administered in a pediatric oncology referral center. Lymphoblastic lymphomas are treated very similarly to ALL, and treatment may include CHOP with an ALL-Type maintenance using oral mercaptopurine and methotrexate. Monoclonal antibodies directed at cell surface markers have activity in NHL and are being studied in combination with chemotherapy.

Prognosis

Most types and stages of NHL have an excellent prognosis. Low stage BL has a 90–95% survival rate, and large B-cell lymphoma and anaplastic large-cell lymphoma have 90% survival rates. Even with advanced stages, most children have at least a 70% chance of survival. However, recurrent NHL can be quite difficult to treat.

References

Al-Samawi AS, Aulaqi SM, Al-Thobhani AK (2009) Childhood lymphomas in Yemen. Saudi Med J 30:1192–1196

Bangerter M, Brudler O, Heinrich B, Griesshamnuer M (2007) Fine needle aspiration cytology and flow cytometry in the diagnosis and subclassification of non-Hodgkin's lymphoma based on the World Health Organization classification. Acta Cytolgica 51:390–398

De Moerloose B, Suciu S, Bertrand Y et al (2010) Improved outcome with pulses of vincristine and corticosteroids in continuation therapy of children with average risk acute lymphoblastic leukemia (ALL) and lymphoblastic non-Hodgkin lymphoma (NHL): report of the EORTC randomized phase 3 trial 58951. Blood 116:36–44

Emoti CE, Enosolease ME (2008) The effect of accessibility to drugs on outcome of therapy in patients with malignant lymphoma. Niger Postgrad Med J 15:10–14

Filipovich AH, Mathur A, Kamat D et al (1994) Lymphoproliferative disorders and other tumors complicating immunodeficiencies. Immunodeficiency 5:91–112

Fridrik MA, Hausmaninger H, Lang A et al (2010) Dose-dense therapy improves survival in aggressive non-Hodgkin's lymphoma. Ann Hematol 89(3):273–282

Gross TG, Termuhlen AM (2007) Pediatric non-Hodgkin's lymphoma. Curr Oncol Rep 9:459–465

Hochberg J, Waxman IM, Kelly KM et al (2009) Adolescent non-Hodgkin lymphoma and Hodgkin lymphoma: state of the science. Br J Haematol 144:24–40

Li B, Shi YK, He XH et al (2008) Primary non-Hodgkin lymphomas in the small and large intestine: clinicopathological characteristics and management of 40 patients. Int J Hematol 87:375–381

Meinhardt A, Burkhardt B, Zimmermann M et al (2010) Phase II window study on rituximab in newly diagnosed pediatric mature B-cell non-Hodgkin's lymphoma and Burkitt leukemia. J Clin Oncol 28:3115–3121

Murphy SB (1980) Classification, staging and end results of treatment of childhood non-Hodgkin's lymphomas: dissimilarities from lymphomas in adults. Semin Oncol 7:332–339

Mwanda WO, Orem J, Fu P et al (2009) Dose-modified oral chemotherapy in the treatment of AIDS-related non-Hodgkin's lymphoma in East Africa. J Clin Oncol 27:3480–3488

Okur FV, Krance R (2010) Stem cell transplantation in childhood non-Hodgkin's lymphomas. Curr Hematol Malig Rep 5:192–199

Reiter A (2007) Diagnosis and treatment of childhood non-Hodgkin lymphoma. Hematology 285–296

Salzburg J, Burkhardt B, Zimmermann M et al (2007) Prevalence, clinical pattern, and outcome of CNS involvement in childhood and adolescent non-Hodgkin's lymphoma differ by non-Hodgkin's lymphoma subtype: a Berlin-Frankfurt-Munster Group Report. J Clin Oncol 25:2915–2922

Sandlund JT (2007) Should adolescents with NHL be treated as old children or young adults? Hematology 297–303

Sant M, Allemani C, De Angelis R et al (2008) Influence of morphology on survival for non-Hodgkin lymphoma in Europe and the United States. Eur J Cancer 44:579–587

Shabbat S, Aharoni J, Sarid L et al (2009) Rituximab as monotherapy and in addition to reduced CHOP in children with primary immunodeficiency and non-Hodgkin lymphoma. Pediatr Blood Cancer 52:664–666

Tai E, Pollack LA, Townsend J et al (2010) Differences in non-Hodgkin lymphoma survival between young adults and children. Arch Pediatr Adolesc Med 164:218–224

Wayne AS, Reaman GH, Helman LJ (2008) Progress in the curative treatment of childhood hematologic malignancies. J Natl Cancer Inst 100:1271–1273

347 Hodgkin Disease

H. Stacy Nicholson

Introduction

Hodgkin disease (HD) is a B-cell lymphoid malignancy that occurs in 2 per 100,000 children before the age of 15 years in the USA. In the USA and other developed nations, HD is primarily a disease of adolescence and young adults with a second peak in older adulthood (>50 years). In the developing world, the age distribution is shifted toward younger children.

Pathology

HD is diagnosed from a lymph node biopsy and requires the demonstration of the classic Reed–Sternberg (RS) cells in a background of lymphocytes, histiocytes, eosinophils, and plasma cells. The RS cell is the malignant cell of HD and is of B-cell lineage. There are four histopathological subtypes of HD: lymphocyte predominance (LP), nodular sclerosis (NS), mixed cellularity (MC), and lymphocyte depletion (LD). NS is the most common subtype in the USA and Western Europe, and MC is the most common in the developing world. Subtype is related to prognosis – LP rarely disseminates and has a good prognosis, while LD is likely to disseminate and has a poor prognosis (➋ *Fig. 347.1*).

Clinical Features

HD usually presents as painless progressive adenopathy which ultimately will coalesce into a large mass. Most commonly, HD starts above the diaphragm and involves cervical, axillary, or intrathoracic nodes. In one-third of patients, the initial site is below the diaphragm and can include the inguinal and/or intraabdominal nodes. HD can spread to other organs, including spleen, liver, and bone marrow.

Some patients with HD have a classic constellation of symptoms, including fever, night sweats, and weight loss – these are called "B" symptoms and are important in staging newly diagnosed patients. Severe pruritis can also be a presenting symptom.

Diagnostic Studies and Staging

Following histopathological diagnosis, the staging workup in HD requires that all major nodal groups on both side of the diaphragm be imaged. The most common imaging modality is computerized tomography (CT), which should include the neck (including the Waldeyer ring), chest, abdomen, and pelvis. Nuclear scintography (gallium or PET) may be useful, but staging laparatomy and lymphangiograms are no longer routinely used. Bone marrow aspirates and biopsies are done in all but those with stages IA or IIA HD, and bone scans are needed only if symptoms suggest bony involvement.

The Ann Arbor staging system is the accepted standard (➋ *Table 347.1*). Based on the number and site of involved lymph node chains, patients are stratified into four main stages, I–IV. Furthermore, patients are classified as having either A or B disease based on the absence or presence, respectively, of the classic triad of constitutional symptoms (fever, weight loss, night sweats.) Untreated, HD will predictably progress to a higher stage, although stage at diagnosis usually reflects the underlying tumor biology.

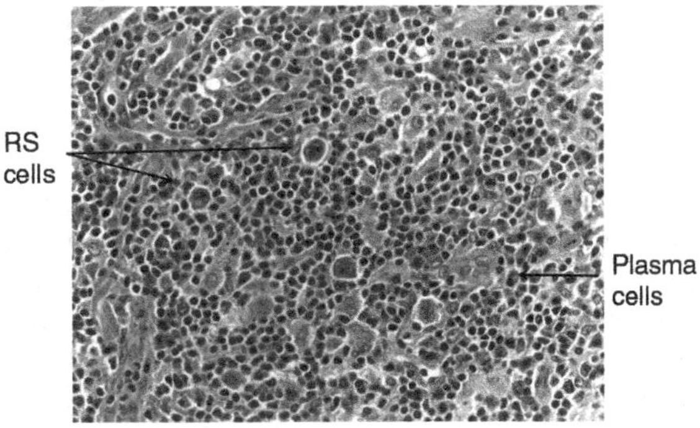

Figure 347.1
Nodular sclerosing Hodgkin disease: Hematoxalin-eosin stain – 20×: Reed–Sternberg cells with binuclear and mononuclear forms in the background of fibrosis, admixed with eosinophils, plasma cells, and small lymphocytes (Courtesy of Guang Fan, MD, PhD)

Abdelaziz Y. Elzouki (ed.), *Textbook of Clinical Pediatrics*, DOI 10.1007/978-3-642-02202-9_347,

Table 347.1
Ann Arbor staging of Hodgkin disease

Stage	
I	Disease is limited to one lymphatic region or one extra nodal site, excluding liver or bone marrow.
II	Disease involves two or more lymphatic regions on one side of the diaphragm
III	Disease involves lymphatic regions on both sides of the diaphragm (may involve spleen).
IV	Disease involves lymph nodes in any pattern. In addition, liver, bone marrow, lungs, CNS, or other organs are involved.

Treatment

Treatment is based on stage and may involve chemotherapy, radiation, or both. Generally, the role of surgery is limited to establishing the diagnosis. Treatment has evolved over the past few decades, resulting in excellent survival. Chemotherapy is now used in all but very low-stage patients, and radiation is being used more sparingly. With the realization that women who received chest radiation for HD during adolescence have a high risk of breast cancer, treatment strategies for males vs. females have diverged, with radiation being used less in females.

Radiotherapy

Radiation is an effective treatment for HD and has been used since the 1940s and is used without chemotherapy for low-risk patients with low-stage disease. Dosage varies by stage and site but generally does not exceed 40 Gy.

Chemotherapy

MOPP (mechlorethamine, vincristine (Oncovine®), procarbazine, and prednisone) chemotherapy was one of the first combinations of chemotherapy demonstrated to be effective in cancer. MOPP and variations of MOPP are still used in the treatment of HD. However, MOPP has significant long-term toxicities, including infertility and secondary malignancies. A second combination, ABVD (Adriamycin, bleomycin, vinblastine, and dacarbazine) is also effective. Combination therapy for HD continues to evolve, with combinations that use both MOPP and ABVD, and modifications of MOPP, most commonly with cyclophosphamide being substituted for mechlorethamine (COPP).

Prognosis

With stage-appropriate therapy, most children and adolescents with HD will become long-term survivors, and patients with low-stage disease have survival rates in excess of 90%. Even with stage IV disease, most become long-term survivors. However, HD is one of the few childhood malignancies where a relapse can occur more than 5 years after diagnosis. Thus, close follow-up is required through the first decade and lifelong follow-up is advised to monitor for late effects of therapy. Following relapse, some children have been cured using high-dose chemotherapy and autologous bone marrow transplantation.

References

Armitage JO (2010) Early-stage Hodgkin's lymphoma. N Engl J Med 363:653–662

Bartlett NL, Rosenberg SA, Hoppe RT et al (1995) Brief chemotherapy, Stanford V, and adjuvant radiotherapy for bulky or advanced-stage Hodgkin's disease: A preliminary report. J Clin Oncol 13: 1080–1088

Bhatia S, Robison LL, Oberlin O et al (1996) Breast cancer and other second neoplasms after childhood Hodgkin's disease. N Engl J Med 334:745–751

Bonadonna G, Zucali R, Monfardini S et al (1975) Combination chemotherapy of Hodgkin's disease with adriamycin, bleomycin, vinblastine, and imidazole carboxamide versus MOPP. Cancer 36:252–259

Canellos GP, Anderson JR, Propert KJ et al (1992) Chemotherapy of advanced Hodgkin's disease with MOPP, ABVD, or MOPP alternating with ABVD. N Engl J Med 327:1478–1484

Devita VT Jr, Serpick AA, Carbone PP (1970) Combination chemotherapy in the treatment of advanced Hodgkin's disease. Ann Intern Med 73:881–895

Diehl V, Sieber M, Ru¨ffer U et al (1997) BEACOPP: an intensified chemotherapy regimen in advanced Hodgkin's disease. The German Hodgkin's lymphoma study group. Ann Oncol 8:143–148

Ferme C, Eghbali H, Meerwaldt JH et al (2007) Chemotherapy plus involved-field radiation in early-stage Hodgkin's disease. N Engl J Med 357:1916–1927

Gurney JG, Young JL Jr, Roffers SD, et al. Soft Tissue Sarcomas. In: Ries LAG, Smith MA, Gurney JG, et al (eds). Cancer incidence and survival among children and adolescents: United States SEER Program 1975–1995. NIH Pub. No. 99–4649. National Cancer Institute, SEER Program, 111, Bethesda, MD

Henderson TO, Amsterdam A, Bhatia S et al (2010) Systematic review: surveillance for breast cancer in women treated with chest radiation for childhood, adolescent, or young adult cancer. Ann Int Med 152:444–455, W144-54

Horning SJ, Hoppe RT, Breslin S et al (2002) Stanford V and radiotherapy for locally extensive and advanced Hodgkin's disease: mature results of a prospective clinical trial. J Clin Oncol 20:630–637

Kaplan HS, Rosenberg SA (1966) The treatment of Hodgkin's disease. Med Clin North Am 50:1591–1610

Rosenberg SA, Kaplan HS (1966) Evidence for an orderly progression in the spread of Hodgkin's disease. Cancer Res 26:1225–1231

Seam P, Janik JE, Longo DL, DeVita VT (2009) Role of chemotherapy in Hodgkin's lymphoma. Cancer J 15:150–154

Straus DJ, Portlock CS, Qin J et al (2004) Results of a prospective randomized clinical trial of doxorubicin, bleomycin, vinblastine, and dacarbazine (ABVD) followed by radiation therapy (RT) versus ABVD alone for stages I, II, and IIIA nonbulky Hodgkin disease. Blood 104:3483–3489

Tucker MA, Coleman CN, Cox RS et al (1988) Risk of second cancers after treatment for Hodgkin's disease. N Engl J Med 318:76–81

348 The Histiocytoses

Suman Malempati · H. Stacy Nicholson

Introduction

The histiocytoses of childhood are a diverse and relatively uncommon group of disorders. Despite considerable heterogeneity in clinical manifestations, these diseases have in common the proliferation of cells of the mononuclear phagocyte system. The World Health Organization (WHO) has utilized a general classification scheme that is based on both clinical presentation as well as histologic features (➋ *Table 348.1*). According to this scheme, Class I defines Langerhans cell histiocytosis, Class II includes histiocytoses of mononuclear phagocytes other than Langerhans cells, and Class III denotes malignant histiocytic disorders.

Class I Histiocytosis

Langerhans Cell Histiocytosis (LCH) is characterized by a non-malignant clonal proliferation of a specific-type of dendritic cell, known as the Langerhans cell. Until the 1980s, LCH was known as Histiocytosis X, as the cell of origin was undetermined. Histiocytosis X, which was coined in 1953, was a term used to unify several related clinical syndromes, including Hand-Schuller-Christian syndrome, Letterer-Siwe disease, eosinophilic granuloma, and Hashimoto-Pritzker syndrome into one clinical entity. Despite the wide variation in clinical manifestations, the central role of the Langerhans Cell unites these disorders.

Epidemiology

It is difficult to obtain an exact incidence rate of LCH due to heterogeneity of clinical manifestations of the disease and possible underrecognition of this condition. The annual pediatric incidence of LCH has been estimated to be 2–6 cases per million children. LCH tends to occur in young children with a peak incidence between 1 and 4 years of age. Young children with LCH have a higher frequency of more severe disease, and most cases with multisystem involvement occur before the age of 2 years. Older children and adults are more likely to have disease limited to bony sites. There appears to be a higher incidence of cancer in patients with LCH, although a causal association has never been demonstrated.

Pathogenesis

LCH is characterized by a clonal proliferation of Langerhans cells. Langerhans cells are antigen-presenting cells of monocyte lineage that are normally found in the skin and other organs. The typical LCH lesion contains histiocytes including Langerhans cells, lymphocytes, eosinophils, and sometimes neutrophils and plasma cells. While the disease is thought to be immunologically mediated and result from disordered immune regulation, an exact cause of the disease has not been elucidated. Evidence suggests that the abnormal proliferation of histiocytes, though clonal, is reactive rather than malignant.

Clinical Manifestations

The manifestations of LCH range from an idolent localized lesion to widely disseminated aggressive disease. The most commonly affected system is the skeleton, with bone lesions present in 80% of cases. In the past, eosinophilic granuloma was the term used to describe LCH involving single or multiple bone sites without visceral involvement. A unifocal bone lesion is the most common manifestation of the disease and comprises approximately 30% of cases. Bone lesions are often painless and are usually accompanied by a soft-tissue mass. The skull is the most common site. Skull lesions may be associated with other head and/or neck manifestations such as chronic otitis media, mastoiditis, "floating teeth" with mandible involvement, and cervical lymphadenopathy. Patients with base of skull lesions are also at risk for intracranial complications – most commonly diabetes insipidus (DI). Involvement of the spine can result in vertebral collapse, and there can be risk of spinal cord impingement. Extremity lesions may be painful or painless and can sometimes lead to pathologic fracture.

Abdelaziz Y. Elzouki (ed.), *Textbook of Clinical Pediatrics*, DOI 10.1007/978-3-642-02202-9_348,

Skin is the next most commonly involved organ, and skin rash is often part of disseminated disease. The rash associated with LCH is characterized by a crusting vesiculopustular exanthem with a similar appearance to seborrheic dermatitis. It frequently occurs on the scalp and postauricular region, but can also be seen on the trunk and inguinal region. A syndrome associated with skin-only involvement of LCH in the neonate is known as congenital self-healing histiocytosis or Hashimoto-Pritzker syndrome. As the name suggests, the lesions typically resolve by 3–4 months of age without treatment.

Disseminated LCH usually occurs in children less than 1–2 years of age and can be life-threatening. The organs most commonly involved include the liver, spleen, lymph nodes, and bone marrow. Pulmonary involvement is rare in children, but can occur with disseminated disease. This is in contrast to primary pulmonary LCH that occurs in adults without other systemic involvement. Pulmonary LCH in adults is often associated with smoking tobacco.

Central nervous system involvement of LCH is common and can lead to devastating consequences. DI results from infiltration of LCH cells into the hypothalamus or pituitary stalk and occurs in up to 20% of patients with LCH. DI often occurs after other manifestations of the disease and is typically seen in patients with multisystem disease and those with skull bone involvement. Cranial nerve palsies and lesions in the cerebellum resulting in ataxia can also occur.

Diagnostic Evaluation

The diagnostic evaluation of patients with suspected LCH should begin with a thorough history and physical examination. Evaluation of patients with skull bone lesions and suspected LCH should include appraisal of CNS symptoms as well as symptoms of polyuria and polydypsia. Physical examination must include assessment for skin rash, lymphadenopathy, hepatosplenomegaly, and cranial nerve deficits. Imaging is necessary to characterize any suspected bone lesions. The classic radiologic findings are "punched out" lesions on plain x-rays (*Figs. 348.1* and *348.2*). Lesions are typically well demarcated, and reactive sclerosis is unusual at diagnosis. Other evaluations are helpful to determine extent of disease. A complete bone survey is necessary to evaluate for occult bone lesions in any patient diagnosed with LCH. Cytopenias see on a peripheral complete blood count may indicate bone marrow involvement. Bone marrow aspirates and biopsies should also be performed if cytopenias are present. A brain MRI is important to evaluate for intracranial lesions in patients who have skull bone involvement. Guidelines for diagnostic evaluation for patients with suspected LCH are shown in *Table 348.2.*

While clinical and radiographic features may suggest a diagnosis of LCH, pathologic evaluation of involved tissue is necessary for definitive diagnosis. On light microscopy, LCH lesions will show mixed population of cells that includes large histiocytes with few cytoplasmic vacuoles (Langerhans cells) along with an abundance of eosinophils

Table 348.1
Classification of histiocytic disorders

Class I	Class II	Class III
Langerhans cell histiocytosis	*Non-langerhans histiocytoses*	*Malignant histiocytoses*
• Eosinophilic Granuloma	• HLH – Familial HLH – Secondary HLH	• *Acute Monocytic Leukemia*
• Hand-Schuller Christian		• *Malignant Histiocytosis*
• Letterer-Siwe		• *Histiocytic Sarcoma*
• Hashimoto-Pritzker	• Rosai-Dorfman	
	• Juvenile Xanthogranuloma	

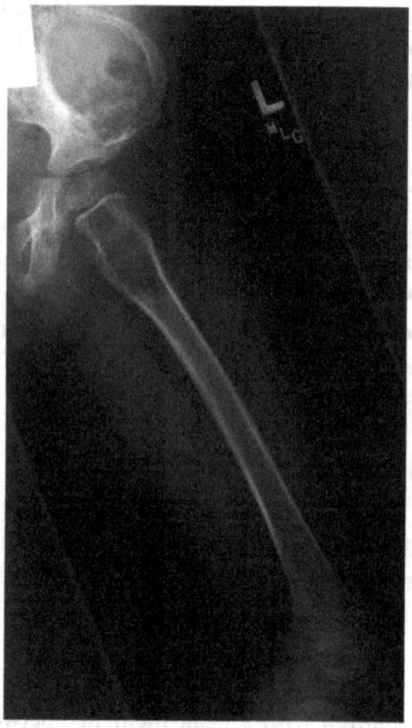

Figure 348.1
Lateral radiograph showing a large lytic lesion in the neck and intertrochanteric region of the femur

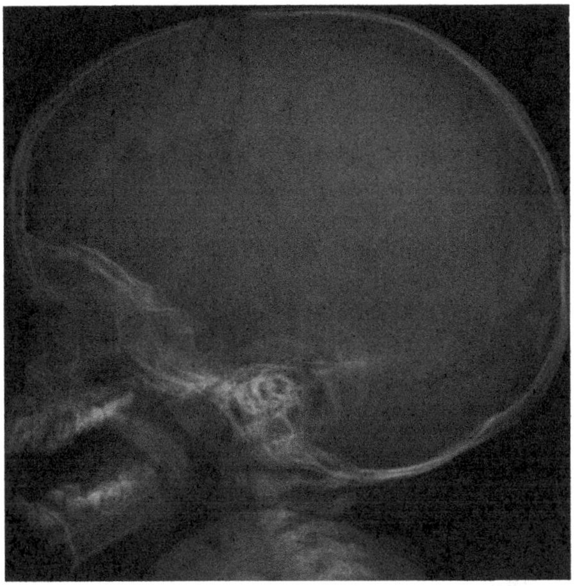

Figure 348.2
Radiograph of the skull showing a large geographic lytic lesion in the right fronto-parietal bone with 2 smaller lesions nearby

Table 348.2
Diagnostic evaluation for suspected LCH

• History
– Neurologic symptoms
– Polyuria/polydypsia
• Physical exam
– Bone lesions/masses
– Skin rash
– Lymphadenopathy
– Liver and Spleen Size
– Neurologic Exam/Cranial Nerves
• Laboratory tests:
– CBC
– Serum chemistries, LFTs
– Urine and serum osmolarity
• Imaging tests:
– Complete skeletal survey
– Brain MRI (if skull bone lesions present)
• Tissue diagnosis:
– Biopsy of involved lesion or organ
– Bone marrow aspirates/biopsies (if multisystem disease or cytopenias present)

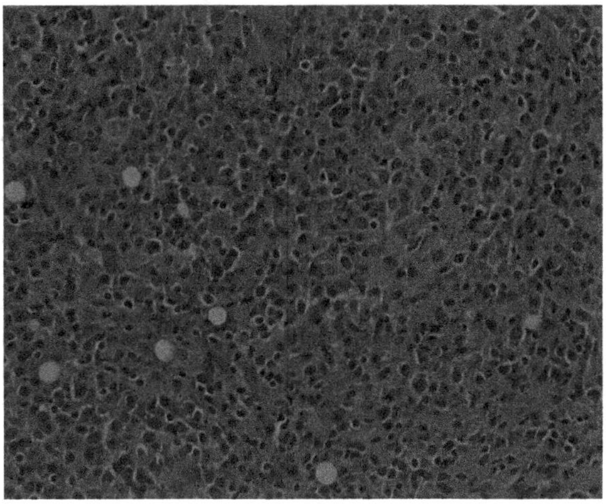

Figure 348.3
Light microscopy of LCH lesion

and lymphocytes (*Fig. 348.3*). Immunohistochemical staining shows positivity for CD1a antigen and S-100 protein. More recently staining for CD207 also known as Langerin has been used. Presence of the typical light microscopic findings along with positivity for CD1a or CD207 is diagnostic of LCH. Demonstration of rod-shaped organelles known as Birbeck granules by electron microscopy is also diagnostic.

Treatment and Prognosis

The appropriate management of patients with LCH depends on the location and extent of disease. The goal of treatment should be control of disease and prevention of long-term consequences rather than complete ablation. Patients with single-system disease may require minimal to no treatment as the natural history can include spontaneous resolution. Solitary bone lesions may be treated with curettage alone. Aggressive surgical resection is not necessary. Low-dose radiation therapy may also be used to treat bone lesions that are in locations that cause risk for permanent damage to underlying structures. Patients with skin-only disease may not need to be treated or can be treated with topical corticosteroids. The prognosis for patients with single-system disease is excellent.

Patients with multisystem disease and organ dysfunction have a significant risk of death and require systemic treatment. Chemotherapy has been used effectively to induce disease regression. Effective agents against LCH include prednisone, vinblastine, mercaptopurine, methotrexate, and more recently, 2-chlorodeoxyadenosine

(2-CDA). Combinations of these agents have been evaluated in multinational randomized clinical trials by the Histiocyte Society. Allogeneic hematopoeitic stem cell transplant has also been used for patients with refractory, progressive LCH.

While the prognosis for most patients with LCH is very good, the risk of late sequelae is high. Long-term complications of LCH occur in up to 30–50% of survivors of LCH. These permanent sequelae include diabetes insipidus and other endocrinopathies, neurologic and developmental abnormalities, orthopedic problems, and hearing impairment. Whether systemic therapy may decrease the frequency of these complications is debatable.

Class II Histiocytosis

The Class II histiocytoses are a heterogeneous group of disorders that are characterized by a proliferation of phagocytic cells. These disorders are thought to be reactive processes which result in infiltration of normal cells of monocyte/macrophage lineage. The major disease in this category is hemophagocytic lymphohistiocytosis (HLH), which has both familial and secondary forms. Other benign disorders in this category include sinus histiocytosis with massive lymphadenopathy (Rosai-Dorfman Disease) and juvenile xanthogranuloma.

Epidemiology

The primary familial form of HLH typically manifests in infancy or early childhood. There are multiple genetic abnormalities that can lead to the clinical manifestations of HLH syndrome. The disease is typically inherited in an autosomal recessive pattern, although there is often no family history. Familial HLH is rare with an estimated incidence of 1 in 50,000 live births. Among familial cases, the most common genetic abnormalities found involve mutations of the *perforin* gene, which are found in about one-third of patients with HLH.

Secondary HLH results from an abnormal immune response to an infection or other process. The incidence of secondary HLH is unclear as the disease is likely underdiagnosed. It is possible that the condition is now being recognized and diagnosed more frequently. Infection-associated secondary HLH has been reported after viral, bacterial, fungal, and parasitic infections. HLH is a known complication of EBV infection, particularly in patients with x-linked lymphoproliferative disease. It occurs more frequently in children with underlying immunodeficiency.

Clinical Manifestations

The most common clinical features of HLH are prolonged fever, hepatosplenomegaly, and cytopenias. Patients also often present with rash, lymphadenopathy, and coagulopathy. The Histiocyte Society has developed a set of diagnostic criteria for HLH based on clinical signs and specific laboratory abnormalities (➋ *Table 348.3*). These diagnostic guidelines are valid for both familial and secondary HLH. While HLH is a non-malignant disorder, patients are often critically ill at presentation and the disease is often fatal without treatment. Most of the signs and symptoms and HLH are non-specific and the condition can be difficult to distinguish from sepsis or hepatitis. Patients can also have CNS involvement which may manifest as seizures or ataxia.

Diagnostic Evaluation

The presenting signs and symptoms of HLH are non-specific and establishing a definitive diagnosis can be difficult. Physical exam should include evaluation for organomegaly and lymphadenopathy. The splenomegaly is often profound and out of proportion to what would be expected from an underlying bacterial of viral infection. Laboratory evaluation should include a complete blood count, coagulation profile, serum ferritin, and serum triglycerides. Biopsy of bone marrow, lymph nodes, spleen, or liver may show a lymphohistiocytic infiltrate with

Table 348.3
Diagnostic criteria for HLH

Detection of a characteristic genetic abnormality (i.e., perforin or MUNC 13-4 mutations) OR Presence of at least 5 of 8 criteria listed below:
• Fever (persistent daily)
• Splenomegaly
• Cytopenia of at least 2 cell lines
– Hemoglobin < 9 g/dL
– Platelets $< 100{,}000/\mu L$
– Neutrophils $< 1{,}000/\mu L$
• Hypertriglyceridemia and/or hypofibrinogenemia
• Hemophagocytosis in bone marrow, spleen, or lymph nodes without evidence of malignancy
• Elevated serum ferritin (> 500 μg/L)
• Elevated soluble IL-receptor alpha (CD25)
• Low or absent NK-cell function

hemophagocytosis. However, hemophagocytosis is not always identified and is not required for the diagnosis of HLH. Specialized tests that include measurement of soluble interleukin-2 receptor and NK-cell activity may need to be sent to a reference laboratory. A definitive diagnosis of familial HLH can be made by detection of one of the characteristic genetic mutations, which are present in approximately 50% of cases.

Treatment and Prognosis

Initial therapy for HLH consists of chemotherapy with immunosuppressive agents. The Histiocyte Society's HLH-2004 protocol treats patients with a combination of etoposide, cyclosporin A, and dexamethasone. Hematopoietic stem cell transplant is commonly used and is the treatment of choice for patients with familial HLH.

Without treatment HLH is usually rapidly fatal. Survival rates with stem cell transplant for familial HLH are better than 50%.

Other Class II Histiocytoses

Sinus histiocytosis with massive lymphadenopathy, also known as Rosai-Dorfman disease, is a benign, reactive process characterized by enlargement of cervical lymph nodes associated with systemic symptoms. Patients with this condition often have fevers, night sweats, and weight loss. The disease usually resolves spontaneously, but may require treatment due to life-threatening airway obstruction. Effective treatments include corticosteroids, chemotherapy, and radiation.

Juvenile xanthogranuloma is benign histiocytic process that occurs in infants and young children. Lesions are usually confined to the skin, but multisystem involvement can occur. Solitary cutaneous lesions almost always regress spontaneously. Treatment with chemotherapy as has been used for LCH is effective for systemic disease.

Class III Histiocytoses

The Class III Histiocytoses consist of malignant disorders of mononuclear phagocyte lineage, including acute monocytic leukemia, malignant histiocytosis, and histiocytic sarcoma. Acute monocytic leukemia is considered a subtype of acute myelogenous leukemia (M5) and is discussed in more detail in ➲ Chap. 345, "Childhood Leukemias". True malignant histiocytosis is a very rare systemic disease. The clinical manifestations may be very similar to HLH. Fever, lymphadenopathy, hepatosplenomegaly, and skin lesions are common signs. It is now recognized that many malignancies previously diagnosed as malignant histiocytosis actually represent anaplastic large cell lymphoma (see ➲ Chap. 346, "Non-Hodgkin Lymphoma"). Systemic chemotherapy can be effective in the treatment of the malignant histiocytoses.

References

Alston RD, Tatevossian RG et al (2006) Incidence and survival of childhood Langerhans cell histiocytosis in Northwest England from 1954 to 1998. Pediatr Blood Cancer 48(5):555–560

Broadbent V, Gadner H et al (1989) Histiocytosis syndromes in children: II. Approach to the clinical and laboratory evaluation of children with Langerhans cell histiocytosis. Clinical writing group of the histiocyte society. Med Pediatr Oncol 17(6):492–495

Bucsky P, Favara B et al (1994) Malignant histiocytosis and large cell anaplastic (Ki-1) lymphoma in childhood: guidelines for differential diagnosis – report of the histiocyte Society. Med Pediatr Oncol 22(3):200–203

Favara BE, Jaffe R (1994) The histopathology of langerhans cell histiocytosis. Br J Cancer Suppl 23:S17–S23

Favara BE, Feller AC et al (1997) Contemporary classification of histiocytic disorders. The WHO committee on histiocytic/reticulum cell proliferations. Reclassification working group of the histiocyte society. Med Pediatr Oncol 29(3):157–166

Filipovich AH (2005) Life-threatening hemophagocytic syndromes: current outcomes with hematopoietic stem cell transplantation. Pediatr Transplant 9(Suppl 7):87–91

Filipovich A, McClain K et al (2010) Histiocytic disorders: recent insights into pathophysiology and practical guidelines. Biol Blood Marrow Transplant 16(Suppl 1):S82–S89

Gadner H, Heitger A et al (1994) Treatment strategy for disseminated Langerhans cell histiocytosis. DAL HX-83 Study Group. Med Pediatr Oncol 23(2):72–80

Grois N, Tsunematsu Y et al (1994) Central nervous system disease in langerhans cell histiocytosis. Br J Cancer Suppl 23:S24–S28

Grois N, Potschger U et al (2006) Risk factors for diabetes insipidus in langerhans cell histiocytosis. Pediatr Blood Cancer 46(2):228–233

Hamre M, Hedberg J et al (1997) Langerhans cell histiocytosis: an exploratory epidemiologic study of 177 cases. Med Pediatr Oncol 28(2):92–97

Harris NL, Jaffe ES et al (1999) World Health Organization classification of neoplastic diseases of the hematopoietic and lymphoid tissues: report of the Clinical Advisory Committee meeting-Airlie House, Virginia, November 1997. J Clin Oncol 17(12):3835–3849

Haupt R, Nanduri V et al (2004) Permanent consequences in langerhans cell histiocytosis patients: a pilot study from the histiocyte society-late effects study group. Pediatr Blood Cancer 42(5):438–444

Henter JI, Arico M et al (1997) HLH-94: a treatment protocol for hemophagocytic lymphohistiocytosis. HLH study Group of the Histiocyte Society. Med Pediatr Oncol 28(5):342–347

Henter JI, Horne A et al (2007) HLH-2004: diagnostic and therapeutic guidelines for hemophagocytic lymphohistiocytosis. Pediatr Blood Cancer 48(2):124–131

Howarth DM, Gilchrist GS et al (1999) Langerhans cell histiocytosis: diagnosis, natural history, management, and outcome. Cancer 85(10):2278–2290

Jubran RF, Marachelian A et al (2005) Predictors of outcome in children with langerhans cell histiocytosis. Pediatr Blood Cancer 45(1):37–42

Kanitakis J, Zambruno G et al (1988) Congenital self-healing histiocytosis (Hashimoto-Pritzker). An ultrastructural and immunohistochemical study. Cancer 61(3):508–516

Komp DM (1987) Historical perspectives of langerhans cell histiocytosis. Hematol Oncol Clin North Am 1(1):9–21

Ladisch S, Jaffe ES (2006) The histiocytoses. In: Pizzo PA, Poplack DG (eds) Principles and practice of pediatric oncology. Lippincott Williams & Wilkins, Philadelphia, pp 768–785

Ladisch S, Gadner H et al (1994) LCH-I: a randomized trial of etoposide vs. vinblastine in disseminated langerhans cell histiocytosis. The histiocyte society. Med Pediatr Oncol 23(2):107–110

Lichtenstein L (1953) Histiocytosis X; integration of eosinophilic granuloma of bone, Letterer-Siwe disease, and Schuller-Christian disease as related manifestations of a single nosologic entity. AMA Arch Pathol 56(1):84–102

Malempati S, Nicholson HS (2009) Langerhans cell histiocytosis. In: Greer JP, Foerster J, Rodgers GM et al (eds) Wintrobe's clinical hematology. Lippincott Williams & Wilkins, Philadelphia, pp 1572–1581

Mittheisz E, Seidl R et al (2007) Central nervous system-related permanent consequences in patients with langerhans cell histiocytosis. Pediatr Blood Cancer 48(1):50–56

Stine KC, Saylors RL et al (1997) 2-Chlorodeoxyadenosine (2-CDA) for the treatment of refractory or recurrent langerhans cell histiocytosis (LCH) in pediatric patients. Med Pediatr Oncol 29(4):288–292

Weitzman S, Jaffe R (2005) Uncommon histiocytic disorders: the non-Langerhans cell histiocytoses. Pediatr Blood Cancer 45(3):256–264

Willman CL, Busque L et al (1994) Langerhans'-cell histiocytosis (histiocytosis X)–a clonal proliferative disease. N Engl J Med 331(3):154–160

349 Central Nervous System Tumors in Children

Rebecca Loret de Mola · Kellie J. Nazemi

Introduction

Brain tumors are the most common solid tumor in children and are the second most common malignancy of childhood. The incidence of brain tumors peaks in the first decade and then again in later adulthood. Supratentorial tumors predominate during the first 2 years of life and then again in adolescence and young adulthood. Throughout the rest of the first decade, infratentorial tumors are more common. Tumors with embryonal histology such as medulloblastoma, supratentorial primitive neuroectodermal tumor (PNET), atypical teratoid rhabdoid tumor (AT/RT), and pineoblastoma occur more frequently in children than adults, and medulloblastoma is the most common type of malignant brain tumor in children. Gliomas can be benign or malignant and can occur anywhere along the neuroaxis.

Cancer arises from mutations that occur in genes that regulate cell growth and death. These mutations can occur in the entire germline or only within the somatic cells of the tumor itself. A small fraction of children with brain tumors have germline mutations, either inherited or de novo, which predisposes them to develop central nervous system (CNS) tumors. Several inherited syndromes, such as neurofibromatosis and tuberous sclerosis, are associated with an increased risk of CNS tumors. There is also an increased incidence of CNS tumors with previous exposure to ionizing radiation. However, in the majority of cases, the cause of a brain or spinal cord tumor in a child is unknown and is likely multifactorial.

CNS tumors and their treatment can cause significant physical, neurocognitive, psychological, and neuroendocrine morbidity. Long-term morbidity often exceeds that of other childhood malignancies, and mortality is the highest of all pediatric cancers.

Signs and Symptoms of Central Nervous System Tumors

The presentation of brain tumors can generally be classified into two categories: increased intracranial pressure (ICP) and localizing signs/symptoms. CNS tumors often cause increased ICP by causing obstruction of CSF pathways. Signs and symptoms of increased ICP can be vague and generalized or can be more severe and life threatening. The classic presentation is early morning headaches relieved with vomiting, and a late finding is mental status decline. The early signs of increased ICP can be similar to other common childhood complaints, so many children with brain tumors have been initially treated for more common childhood illnesses, such as viral gastroenteritis or influenza.

Nearly two-thirds of patients with newly diagnosed pediatric brain tumors have a history of chronic or frequent headaches. In elementary school children, the prevalence of headache is approximately 40–50% and up to 60–80% in adolescents. Typically, headaches associated with a brain tumor worsen over time. Clear indicators that something serious is occurring are headaches that awaken a child from sleep, headaches associated with vomiting, or headaches in addition to an objective neurologic finding. The location of the headache is not typically helpful, but a constant occipital headache and neck pain with hyperextension is an ominous sign of tonsillar herniation. The structures of the posterior fossa and the back of the head are both innervated by branches of the upper cervical roots, so a complaint of worsening occipital headache may be a sign of an infratentorial tumor causing increased ICP. This scenario warrants urgent neuroimaging and referral to a neurosurgeon in the setting of an Emergency Department.

A study conducted by the Childhood Brain Tumor Consortium showed that more than 98% of newly diagnosed brain tumor patients who complained of a headache at presentation also had at least one objective neurologic finding. These included mental status changes, abnormal eye movements, optic disc distortion, asymmetric motor or sensory examination, coordination problems, or abnormal deep tendon reflexes. Therefore, it is very important to do a complete neurologic examination on any child presenting with a headache.

In infants and young children, the signs and symptoms of a brain tumor can be more subtle. Increased ICP can be

Abdelaziz Y. Elzouki (ed.), *Textbook of Clinical Pediatrics*, DOI 10.1007/978-3-642-02202-9_349,

demonstrated by macrocephaly, irritability, poor feeding, and lethargy. In very young children, cranial sutures can separate due to increased ICP even after closure of the fontanelles. Head circumference should be measured and plotted for all children up to at least 3 years of age. This should be done at every routine primary care visit, as well as any visit for headaches or other unexplained symptoms in a younger child. A late and ominous sign of increased ICP in very young children is the "setting sun sign" of the eyes which is caused by pressure on the nerves that control eye movement. The eyes are forced downward and pupillary responses are typically sluggish.

Localizing signs of CNS tumors may include seizures, cranial nerve dysfunction, endocrine dysfunction, cerebellar dysfunction (ataxia or dysmetria), bowel or bladder dysfunction, abnormal or asymmetric strength, abnormal sensation, or asymmetric deep tendon reflexes. Declining school performance or personality/behavioral changes are other common complaints, but are less easily classified as localizing signs. Lesions of the pineal region are associated with Parinaud's Ophthalmoplegia. This is a triad including severely impaired upward gaze, dilated pupils that react to accommodation but not to light, and a specific form of nystagmus called convergence retraction nystagmus. The latter is more easily recognized by an ophthalmologist, but is best recognized when the patient attempts to look up.

Tumors confined to the optic nerve produce monocular vision loss. Chiasmatic tumors present with complex visual field loss as well as loss of acuity. In infants, these tumors may present with unilateral or bilateral nystagmus with head nodding and head tilt, also known as spasmus nutans. Those that are located more posteriorly in the optic tract present with hemianopsia. Optic pathway tumors are very common in patients with Neurofibromatosis Type I. These patients must be screened by annual ophthalmologic examination, but MRI is only recommended if there is abnormality or change in their vision or visual fields because treatment is only indicated when there is evidence of vision change.

Tumors located in the hypothalamus in infants may present with the diencephalic syndrome, which is characterized by failure to thrive, emaciation, paradoxical euphoric mood, and increased appetite.

Diagnosis of Central Nervous System Tumors

Magnetic Resonance Imaging (MRI) of the brain and/or spine is the best diagnostic study to order when a CNS tumor is suspected. It offers the best diagnostic sensitivity and does not expose the patient to radiation. Although CT scanning does cause radiation exposure, it is sometimes needed for initial urgent evaluation of patients with increased ICP. MRI "quick brain" is a newer technique that may offer the information needed in an urgent situation, without the radiation exposure associated with CT scanning. Indications for neuroimaging with MRI in the child that has a headache include, but are not limited to: association with seizures, association with recumbent position or vomiting, occipital location, exacerbation with straining, presence of other ominous signs such as Cushing's Triad (bradycardia, hypertension, irregular respirations), altered mental status, presence of objective neurologic findings, optic disc distortion or papilledema, asymmetry on physical examination, coordination problems, and macrocephaly in infants and toddlers.

Seizures due to non-oncologic causes are more common than seizures due to brain tumors, so they do not always warrant urgent neuroimaging. However, unless the presentation is clearly consistent with a simple febrile seizure or absence seizure, MRI of the brain is recommended because of the severe consequences that could arise if a brain tumor is not recognized. Any patient with an EEG showing focal abnormalities should be further evaluated with MRI. All simple and complex partial seizures and most unexplained generalized seizures should prompt imaging. Seizure features associated with an increased risk of a brain tumor include a change in preexisting seizure features, status epilepticus as first presentation of a seizure, resistance of seizures to medical control, and prolonged postictal focal symptoms or deficits.

Once a CNS tumor is identified, neurosurgical intervention is often indicated, for diagnostic and treatment purposes. Initial care may require urgent treatment of hydrocephalus. Ultimately, histologic examination of the tumor by a neuropathologist will guide further treatment planning in most cases. There are several scenarios in which neurosurgical intervention may not be appropriate, so it is important that newly diagnosed pediatric brain tumor patients are evaluated at a center that has specialists in pediatric neurosurgery and pediatric neuro-oncology.

Common Types of Pediatric CNS Tumors

Embryonal Tumors: Medulloblastoma, sPNET, AT/RT

Medulloblastoma is an embryonal neuroepithelial tumor and is the most common malignant brain tumor in childhood. It accounts for 20% of all primary pediatric brain tumors and 40% of posterior fossa tumors. There is a peak incidence in the first decade of life around ages 5–7 and there is a male predominance of 2:1. Medulloblastoma has the greatest propensity of the CNS tumors to metastasize outside of the neuroaxis at a rate of about 4–7%. The most common sites of metastasis are bone, bone marrow, liver, lung, and lymph nodes.

Research continues on the genetic and biologic properties of medulloblastoma, and the most common chromosomal abnormality is isochromosome 17q. Trisomy 7 is the second most common abnormality. Several prognostic features have been identified and influence treatment recommendations. In general, age less than 3 years, residual tumor bulk of $>1.5\ cm^2$ after surgical resection, and presence of metastasis either within or outside of the CNS have been associated with high-risk disease and a worse prognosis. There are newer histopathologic markers of high-risk disease as well.

Supratentorial primitive neuroectodermal tumor (sPNET) has been called cerebral medulloblastoma in the past but recent molecular evidence indicates that this tumor is different from medulloblastoma, though the two are often discussed together. sPNET is a rare type of CNS tumor accounting for only 2–3% of all CNS tumors. It is more common during the first decade and 90% occur in the cerebral hemispheres. Males and females are affected equally. This tumor also has a propensity to metastasize with up to 30% with CSF seeding in some series. It can also metastasize outside of the neuroaxis and has been reported in the bone and lung. Treatment for sPNET has historically been based on treatment for medulloblastoma; however, the overall outcome of these patients is significantly worse than those with medulloblastoma, suggesting inherent biologic differences.

Pineoblastoma is a primitive undifferentiated tumor that is distinguished from medulloblastoma and sPNET by its location. It occurs most frequently in the first decade of life and there is an equal incidence among males and females. These tumors can spread within the CNS; however, seeding outside of the CNS is rare.

Therapy for medulloblastoma, sPNET, and pineoblastoma consists of maximal safe surgical resection, crainospinal radiation with focal boost to the local tumor site, and systemic chemotherapy. Ongoing research is aimed at further delineating clinical and biologic prognostic factors as well as optimization of therapy for these patients.

Historically, atypical teratoid rhabdoid tumor (AT/RT) was probably mistaken for medulloblastoma or sPNET. But further research identified distinct histologic and cytogenetic features that distinguish it from other tumor types. Deletion of chromosome 22 and alterations of the hSNF5/INI-1 gene have been described. Lack of INI-1 expression has been shown to be a characteristic feature of AT/RT, and the immunohistochemical stain is now used routinely by neuropathologists.

AT/RT is a rare tumor that occurs more commonly in young children with a median age of 24 months. About 60% of these tumors are supratentorial and there is a male predominance of 2:1. It is known to metastasize and leptomeningeal spread at diagnosis has been reported to occur in 20–25% of patients. These tumors tend to be very aggressive, with formerly reported median event-free survival reported of 10 months and median survival about 17 months from diagnosis. In spite of the historically poor prognosis and aggressive nature of this disease, a more recent treatment regimen has been reported by Chi et al. showing promising results for many patients. In general, these patients are treated with maximal surgical resection, radiation, and systemic chemotherapy.

Ependymoma

Ependymomas account for approximately 9% of all primary CNS tumors in children. These tumors are generally located within or adjacent to the ependymal lining of the ventricular system or the central canal of the spinal cord. Ninety percent are intracranial, and of these, 60% are located in the posterior fossa. The remaining 10% are located in the spinal cord and these tend to occur in adolescents. The highest incidence of these tumors is in the first 7 years of life and there is a slight predominance in males. Typically, ependymomas are locally invasive, although the reported incidence of systemic metastasis is approximately 7%. The single most important prognostic factor in ependymoma treatment is the degree of surgical resection. Survival rates are higher (about 70%) following a gross total resection compared with 0–50% survival following less than a complete resection. It has also been found that ependymomas of the spinal cord are associated with the best outcome. Children less than age three have had historically poorer outcomes, though the reasons for this are unclear. These patients are more likely to have tumors located in the posterior fossa and gross total resection is often more difficult in this location because of its characteristic wrapping around the brainstem and cranial nerves. Due to their age, these children often receive delayed radiation therapy which may also impact their overall survival. Focal radiation therapy increases survival rates in most scenarios. Chemotherapy has not been shown to improve overall survival for patients with completely or incompletely resected ependymomas.

Low-Grade Gliomas

Low-grade gliomas are a diverse tumor group that includes grade I (pilocytic) astrocytoma, grade II (fibrillary or diffuse) astrocytoma low-grade oligodendroglioma, low-grade ganglioglioma, pleiomorphic xanthoastrocytoma (PXA), and a variety of low-grade mixed glial tumors such as oligoastrocytoma. In general, they are slow-growing tumors with insidious onset of symptoms and relatively benign histologic appearance. Long-term outcomes are most dependent on the ability to achieve complete surgical resection. The average age at diagnosis is between 6 and 9 years and boys are affected more than girls. Dissemination outside of the CNS is very rare and reported in only about 5% of cases.

Most supratentorial and cerebellar low-grade gliomas are astrocytomas. Classic cerebellar pilocytic astrocytomas are the most common type of low-grade glioma and account for 80–85% of low-grade tumors in the cerebellum. Diffuse or fibrillary astrocytomas account for approximately 15% of cerebellar astrocytomas and are more likely to undergo anaplastic transformation compared to the pilocytic variant, though this malignant transformation is observed less in the pediatric population than it is in adults. Prognostic factors for low-grade gliomas are inconsistent in the literature. Complete surgical resection is thought to be very important for long-term disease-free survival in most series, and these tumors tend to be amenable to repeat surgical resection.

The standard of care for this group of tumors is complete surgical resection when possible. When complete resection is accomplished for pilocytic astrocytomas, cure rates are as high as 90–100%. If there is residual disease after initial resection or if there is tumor recurrence, repeat resection should be attempted if it can be done safely and it is felt that a complete resection can be achieved. Adjuvant therapy, such as radiation or chemotherapy, is often used for progressive or symptomatic residual tumors that cannot be completely resected. Radiation is known to be effective in delaying time to further progression, but it has not been shown to significantly affect overall survival in patients with unresectable tumors. Chemotherapy is often used in preadolescent children to avoid radiation in this young population. There are multiple outpatient chemotherapy regimens that offer a modest rate of disease stabilization or partial response. Complete regression of these tumors is rare with chemotherapy and ultimately, many patients experience progression of their disease and require multiple treatment regimens over a period of many years.

Brainstem Glioma

Brainstem gliomas are a heterogenous group of tumors with distinct subtypes. They are subdivided into non-diffuse brainstem tumors and diffuse intrinsic pontine gliomas (DIPG). Non-diffuse tumors of the brainstem account for 20% of all brainstem gliomas and include focal midbrain, dorsally exophytic, and cervicomedullary tumors. The non-diffuse brainstem tumors tend to be slow-growing, low-grade tumors with a more favorable prognosis and treatment response than DIPG. The majority of DIPG arise from the pons and can infiltrate into surrounding structures making them extremely difficult to treat and contributing to their overall dismal prognosis. Brainstem tumors make up 10–20% of all CNS tumors in children less than 15 years of age and the majority occur in children less than 10 years old with a median age of 6–7 years at diagnosis. Ninety percent are of glial origin and there is an equal incidence among males and females. Overall, the 5 year survival for all types of brainstem tumors is between 20% and 30%.

Brainstem gliomas are classified by their location rather than histology. The current standard of care does not include biopsy when radiographic features are classic for a DIPG, but historically most have been found to be diffuse astrocytoma (grades II, III, or IV). The majority of non-diffuse brainstem gliomas are low-grade astrocytomas.

Surgical treatment of non-diffuse brainstem gliomas is dependent on the degree of infiltration into normal structures, and often due to their location, surgical resection is not possible. However, if possible, debulking of dorsally exophytic, tegmental and non-tectal midbrain tumors, and cervicomedullary tumors should be considered. Radiation therapy is the conventional treatment for brainstem gliomas. The role of chemotherapy in the treatment of non-diffuse brainstem gliomas remains unknown and trials are ongoing, but the outpatient regimens of low-grade gliomas are sometimes used.

Diffuse intrinsic pontine gliomas have a universally poor prognosis and treatment of these lesions has historically been directed toward symptom relief rather than cure. The conventional treatment has been radiation therapy and several studies have investigated the use of hyperfractionated external beam radiotherapy (HFRT) versus standard radiotherapy. However no statistically significant difference in progression-free or overall survival was found between patients treated with HFRT vs. standard radiation therapy. The role of chemotherapy in DIPG is not currently known, and there is little evidence to suggest that the use of chemotherapy has a significant impact on the overall outcome of these patients. If left untreated, the median survival of DIPG patients is 20 weeks. Radiation is thought to increase this median survival by approximately 2–3 months. Due to the overall dismal prognosis of DIPG, any treatment that could provide even a modest improvement in survival would have a large impact in the outcomes of these patients. Clinical trials are ongoing.

Germ Cell Tumors

Two-thirds of germ cell tumors are located in the region of the pineal gland and the remaining one-third are in the suprasellar region. They account for 40–65% of tumors in the pineal region, and are more common in the second decade of life with a peak incidence between 10 and 14 years of age. There is a male-to-female predominance of at least 2:1.

These tumors are a spectrum of embryonal neoplasms and teratomas thought to arise from totipotent germ cells. Sixty percent of these tumors are germinoma, 30% teratomas or mixed nonmalignant histology, and 10% malignant histology such as choriocarcinoma, endodermal sinus tumor (yolk sac tumor), and embryonal carcinoma. Collectively, immature teratomas, mixed germ cell tumors, endodermal sinus tumor, choriocarcinoma, and embryonal carcinomas are referred to as non-germinomatous germ cell tumors (NGGCT). Leptomeningeal spread occurs in approximately 10% of cases and in the highly malignant subgroups, systemic metastases can occur to the lungs, bone, and lymph nodes. Evaluation of the spine with MRI is important in the work up of these tumors due to their propensity to seed the CNS.

The histology of these tumors is prognostically significant. Germinomas are highly curable with 5 year survival rates as high as 95%. However, NGGCT generally have much poorer survival rates ranging from 20% to 75%. Disseminated disease and young age have also been associated with a worse prognosis; however, in younger patients this may be due to the fact that they often have disseminated disease at diagnosis and cannot safely receive crainospinal radiation which may be important in some cases.

Patients with NGGCT often have one or two associated tumor markers present in the serum or cerebrospinal fluid, alpha fetoprotein (AFP), and beta human chorionic gonadotropin (beta-hCG). If so, up-front surgical resection and even biopsy are not indicated. The presence of a pineal and/or suprasellar mass and elevated tumor markers is pathognomonic for NGGCT. Neoadjuvant chemotherapy has become the standard of care for NGGCT because of the high-risk nature of surgical manipulation in the pineal region. Germinomas can also have slightly elevated tumor markers, but the levels are modest compared to the more malignant germ cell tumors. Because the treatment for germinoma differs from that of NGGCT, it is generally recommended that tumor biopsies be obtained when there is not a significant elevation in at least one of the tumor markers.

Due to the location of these tumors, complete surgical resection is often not possible without causing significant morbidity. Surgery is no longer the up-front treatment approach for this group of tumors. Germinomas are extremely radiation sensitive and surgery can often be avoided using chemotherapy and radiation alone. NGGCT are also treated initially with chemotherapy, and definitive therapy is radiation. Surgical resection is often used in germ cell tumors when there is residual tumor following initial chemotherapy. The histology of the residual tumor is often a benign or mature form of germ cell tumor. These tumors are also known to have a propensity for CSF seeding, but there is great debate about the extent of radiation needed to optimize therapy in patients who do not have documented dissemination at the time of diagnosis. Focal radiation at the site of the initial tumor is standard, but debate resides in whether ventricular volume radiation or craniospinal radiation is most appropriate in these patients. Chemotherapy regimens are platinum based, and in combination with other chemotherapy agents and radiation therapy are capable of producing response rates of 48–90% depending on the tumor type. It is important to note that mature teratomas have a unique treatment approach among germ cell tumors. They are not thought to be sensitive to radiation or chemotherapy, and are therefore treated with maximal surgical resection alone.

Supratentorial High-Grade Gliomas

Supratentorial high-grade gliomas account for 7–11% of all pediatric CNS tumors. Sixty-six percent occur within the cerebral hemispheres, 20% are in deep midline structures of the cerebrum midline, and 15% are located in the posterior fossa or brainstem. The median age at diagnosis is 9 years and the male-to-female ratio is 1:1. The most common malignant glial neoplasms are high-grade astrocytomas such as anaplastic astrocytoma (grade III) and glioblastoma multiforme (grade IV), but this broad category can also include anaplastic oligodendroglioma, anaplastic ganglioglioma, high-grade pleomorphic xanthoastrocytoma (PXA), and high-grade mixed glial tumors such as anaplastic oligoastrocytoma. These lesions tend to be clinically aggressive, locally and regionally invasive, and can rarely disseminate to the lung, lymph nodes, bone, and liver.

The most important prognostic factor in these patients is the extent of surgical resection. As a group, those who have had a near-complete or complete resection experience significantly longer progression-free survival than those with incomplete resections. Disease site has also been shown to be prognostic of outcome. Patients with tumor in deep midline structures have poorer survival rates compared to those with hemispheric lesions, presumably due to the inability to safely resect tumors in the deep midline structures.

Radiation therapy is considered a standard component of therapy for these patients. It is rarely curative, but when used in combination with chemotherapy has been shown to provide a small improvement in survival. Many different combination regimens have been studied in both the adult and pediatric populations with little to no improvement in prolonging time to progression. Regimens using myeloablative chemotherapy with peripheral stem cell rescue have a high up-front morbidity/mortality and have not shown improvement in outcomes for these patients. Multiple phase I and II trials are underway in the adult and pediatric populations in an effort to identify effective therapeutic agents.

Choroid Plexus Tumors

Tumors of the choroid plexus account for approximately 1–4% of brain tumors in children. These are tumors of young children and the median age at diagnosis is 10–32 months, with males and females being equally affected. Eighty-five percent arise in the lateral ventricles, 10–15% in the fourth ventricle, and 5–10% in the third ventricle. These tumors are classified as either choroid plexus papilloma (CPP) or choroid plexus carcinoma (CPC). CPP are more common, accounting for 80–90% of choroid plexus tumors, are typically very slow growing, and are treated with surgical resection only. CPC accounts for 10–20% of choroid plexus tumors and behave more aggressively because they are less differentiated and more anaplastic. Leptomeningeal spread can be seen in CPC and in atypical CPP, a form of papilloma with some anaplastic features.

The degree of surgical resection and tumor histology are the important prognostic factors in these tumors. With complete resection of a CPP, long-term survival is almost 100%. In CPC, outcomes tend to be less favorable due to local invasion and propensity of this tumor to disseminate throughout the CNS. However, studies of CPC treatment have shown that complete resection does appear to affect long-term survival and this should therefore be the surgical goal. Ventriculoperitoneal shunting may be required following tumor resection because of persistent hydrocephalus, which can occur in up to 60% of patients postoperatively. Radiation therapy is frequently used postoperatively in patients with CPC if there is evidence of residual disease and/or leptomeningeal dissemination, but its use must be carefully considered in this young patient population and can often be delayed by using chemotherapy. It has been difficult to clearly define the role of chemotherapy in CPC because it is so rare and therefore difficult to establish clinical trials with enough power to answer questions about efficacy. Treatment protocols for malignant brain tumors in children under the age of 3 years are often used.

Optic Pathway Gliomas

Optic pathway tumors arise in the optic nerves, optic chiasm, or optic tracts. They account for 5% of pediatric CNS tumors. Seventy-five percent occur in the first decade of life and males and females are equally affected. The incidence of optic pathway tumors is increased in patients with Neurofibromatosis Type I (NF-1) with up to 28% of patients with NF-1 being affected in some reports. Involvement of the optic chiasm appears to be more common in patients without NF-1 and unilateral or bilateral optic nerve involvement is more commonly seen in patients with NF-1. Histologically these tumors are typically low-grade pilocytic or fibrillary astrocytomas and malignant degeneration is very rare. Tumor growth tends to be slow, though there can be local spread of disease into surrounding brain parenchyma, and vision decline can sometimes occur in the absence of radiographic increase in tumor size. Serial ophthalmologic evaluation is at least as important, if not more important, than the routine imaging that is done after diagnosis of an optic pathway tumor.

Three prognostic variables have been shown to have an impact on outcome in optic pathway tumors. Tumors involving the chiasm and hypothalamus tend to have a worse prognosis, as do those that occur in children younger than 3–5 years of age. Optic gliomas in the setting of NF-1 tend to have a more indolent course and can even regress without any treatment. For this reason, optic gliomas in NF-1 patients are monitored with serial MRIs and ophthalmologic exams including visual fields. When a decline in vision is documented, chemotherapy should be initiated to prevent any further impact on vision. Regimens including alkylating agents should be avoided in NF-1 patients because of the increased risk of second malignancies.

Biopsy of these tumors can cause vision impairment, so biopsy of these lesions must be considered very carefully. Because these tumors are so common in patients with NF-1, this diagnosis can be made based on radiographic appearance of an optic pathway tumor alone. For patients who do not have NF-1, biopsy is often recommended in order to define the histological type and further direct therapy. In cases in which a unilateral tumor has already caused severe vision changes, then surgical resection could be considered. Radiation therapy has been shown to be effective in stabilizing or improving existing disease, and it has been shown to improve vision in some patients and can also prevent further vision loss. Toxicity from radiation therapy should be taken into consideration as up to 50% of prepubertal patients will experience endocrine toxicity due to radiation of the adjacent hypothalamic-pituitary axis. In preadolescent children, delaying radiation therapy by using chemotherapy may help avoid or decrease the endocrinologic sequelae that can occur after radiation to this region. Chemotherapy is also used for patients with NF-1 who require treatment for an optic pathway tumor, in order to avoid radiation altogether in this patient population, if at all possible. The risk of second malignancy associated with radiation, such as glioblastoma multiforme or sarcomas, is likely higher in patients with NF-1. All patients with optic pathway tumors should undergo serial ophthalmologic exams regardless of the treatment or observation approach.

Craniopharyngioma

Craniopharyngiomas account for 6–9% of all childhood primary CNS tumors. There is a bimodal age distribution with a peak at age 8–10 years and again in older adults (50–74 years). This tumor is rarely seen in children less than age 2. There is an equal predominance among males and females. These tumors are generally suprasellar in location. Histologically, they are benign, but they often become functionally malignant due to the location and impairment of the hypothalamic-pituitary axis.

The extent of tumor resection is an important prognostic factor in craniopharyngioma. Those with complete resection have significantly better survival rates compared to those with incomplete resection. Tumor size has also been shown to be of prognostic significance; however, this may be secondary to degree of resectability. Patients with pure cystic lesions appear to have better survival than those with solid or mixed solid and cystic tumors, and children less than 5 years of age seem to have a worse prognosis compared to older children.

Surgical resection is the mainstay of treatment for craniopharyngioma. Approximately 90% of children with craniopharyngioma will have neuroendocrine deficits at the time of presentation, and 50–90% will have visual field defects. Tumor resection may exacerbate neuroendocrine deficits and their management needs to be optimized prior to surgery. Preoperative stress dosing of steroids followed by a postoperative taper are important in the management of these patients. Due to the location of these tumors, significant morbidity can be encountered if a radical complete resection is attempted. Debate continues in the neurosurgical literature regarding radical resection of these tumors versus less radical surgery and postoperative radiation therapy. Approximately 50–75% of patients will have recurrence of their disease after a partial resection; however, cure rates improve to 60–85% if radiation therapy is given postoperatively. Chemotherapy has no established role in the treatment of craniopharyngioma.

Late Effects of Childhood CNS Tumors

The 5 year overall survival of a child with a brain tumor has improved to 60% over the past several decades. However, despite successful treatment for a brain tumor, many children will experience significant long-term side effects either directly because of their tumor or as sequelae from treatment. These patients may experience physical, cognitive, neurologic, and endocrinologic side effects that may diminish their overall quality of life.

Radiation therapy alone is responsible for several adverse side effects including endocrine dysfunction, neuropsychological deficits, radiation necrosis, vasculopathy such as stroke or Moya Moya disease, and an increased risk of a secondary tumor. Radiation effects are inversely related to age at treatment; those who are treated at a younger age experience a higher degree of sequelae from their treatment. Full brain irradiation to children less than 3 years of age has been associated with severe intellectual deficits and significant impairment diminishing the likelihood that they will be independent, functioning adults. For this reason, full cranial radiation therapy should be avoided in children less than 3 years of age.

Growth failure is also a common side effect seen in patients who undergo radiation therapy. Radiation therapy impairs the secretion of growth hormone, decreases the growth of the spinal cord and vertebral column in those undergoing spinal radiation, and can induce precocious puberty which prematurely fuses bony epiphyses. The concomitant use of chemotherapy further exacerbates the severity of growth failure experienced in these patients. Due to the concern of stimulating tumor recurrence, the use of growth hormone replacement remains controversial and is generally not recommended until many years after disease control or stabilization.

Secondary to the use of platinum agents in the treatment of many pediatric brain tumors, sensorineural hearing loss is a frequent complication among survivors. Radiation therapy can also exacerbate these deficits.

Management of survivors of childhood brain tumors should include a multidisciplinary team consisting of pediatric oncologists, endocrinologists, neurosurgeons, radiation oncologists, neuroradiologists, nurses, nurse practioners, neuropsychologists, psychologists, physical and occupational therapists, speech therapists, school teachers, and social workers. The child should be seen at least yearly for both physical and neuropsychological exams for at least the first 5 years after therapy is completed. Surveillance for recurrence of disease is also an important part of the long-term management of these patients. Recurrence or progression can occur several months to years after therapy has been completed.

A childhood diagnosis of a brain tumor or spinal cord tumor is a major challenge in the lives of patients and their families. Treatment of these types of cancers requires a highly specialized team to treat not only the acute disease process, but also to manage the long-term physical and emotional effects these tumors and their therapies have. Therapies for CNS tumors of childhood have improved over the past several decades, but there is still much work to be done. Further research is mandatory to better understand these tumors biologically, improve therapeutic approaches, and ultimately, improve survival and quality of life for these patients.

References

Albright AL, Price RA, Guthkelch AN (1985) Diencephalic gliomas of children. A clinicopathologic study. Contemp Neurosurg 55:2789–2793

Anonymous (1991) The epidemiology of headache among children with brain tumor. Headache in children with brain tumors. The childhood brain tumor consortium. J Neurooncol 10:31–46

Barkovich AJ, Krischer J, Kun LE et al (1990) Brain stem gliomas: a classification system based on magnetic resonance imaging. Pediatr Neurosurg 16:73–83

Becker LE, Yates AJ (1986) Astroctyic tumors in children. In: Finegold M (ed) Pathology of neoplasia in children and adolescents. WB Saunders, Philadelphia, p 373

Berger C, Thiesse P, Lellouch-Tubiana A et al (1998) Choroid plexus carcinomas in childhood: clinical features and prognostic factors. Neurosurgery 42:470–475

Biegel JA, Tan L, Zhang F et al (2002) Alterations of the hSNF5/INI1 gene in central nervous system atypical teratoid/rhaboid tumors and renal and extrarenal rhabdoid tumors. Clin Cancer Res 8: 3461–3467

Blaney SM, Kun LE, Hunter J et al (2006) Tumors of the central nervous system. In: Pizzo PA, Poplack DG (eds) Principles and practice of pediatric oncology., pp 786–864

Bleyer WA (1999) Epidemiologic impact of children with brain tumors. Childs Nerv Syst 15:758–763

Bouffet E, Perilongo G, Canete A et al (1998) Intracranial ependymomas in children: a critical review of prognostic factors and a plea for cooperation. Med Pediatr Oncol 30:319–329

Bruno LA, Rorke LB, Norris DG (1981) Primitive neuroectodermal tumors of infancy and childhood. In: Humphrey GB, Dehner LP, Grindey GB (eds) Pediatric oncology. Nijhoff, Boston, pp 265–267

Bunin GR, Surawicz TS, Witman PA et al (1998) The descriptive epidemiology of craniopharyngioma. J Neurosurg 89:547–551

Campbell JW, Pollack IF, Martinez AJ et al (1996) High-grade astrocytomas in children: radiologically complete resection is associated with an excellent long-term prognosis. Neurosurgery 38:258–264

Chan MY, Foong AP, Heisey BM et al (1998) Potential prognostic factors of relapse-free survival in childhood optic pathway glioma: a multivariate analysis. Pediatr Neurosurg 29:23–28

Chi SN, Zimmerman MA, Yao X, Cohen KJ et al (2009) Intensive multimodality treatment for children with newly diagnosed CNS atypical teratoid rhabdoid tumor. J Clin Oncol 27:385–389

Chow E, Reardon DA, Shah AB et al (1999) Pediatric choroid plexus neoplasms. Int J Radiat Oncol Biol Phys 44:249–254

Civitello LA, Packer RJ, Rorke LB et al (1988) Leptomenigeal dissemination of low-grade gliomas in childhood. Neurology 38:562–566

Eberhart CG, Cohen KJ, Tihan T et al (2003) Medulloblastomas with systemic metastases: evaluation of tumor histopathology and clinical behavior in 23 patients. J Pediatr Hematol Oncol 25:198–203

Evans AE, Jenkin RD, Sposto R et al (1990) The treatment of medulloblastoma. Results of a prospective randomized trial of radiation therapy with and without CCNU, vincristine, and prednisone. J Neurosurg 72:572–582

Finlay JL, Boyett JM, Yates AJ et al (1995) Randomized phase III trial in childhood high-grade astrocytoma comparing vincristine, loustine, and prednisone with the eight-drugs-in-1-day regimen. Childrens Cancer Group. J Clin Oncol 13:112–123

Fisher PG, Breiter SN, Carson BS et al (2000) A clinicopathologic reappraisal of brain stem tumor classification. Identification of pilocytic astrocytoma and fibrillary astrocytoma as distinct entities. Cancer 89:1569–1576

Fouladi M, Wallace D, Langston JW et al (2003) Survival and functional outcome of children with hypothalamic/chiasmatic tumors. Cancer 15:1084–1092

Gaffney CC, Sloane JP, Bradley NJ et al (1985) Primitive neuroectodermal tumours of the cerebrum. Pathology and treatment. J Neurooncol 3:23–33

Gajjar A, Sanford FA, Heideman R et al (1997) Low-grade astrocytoma: a decade of experience at St. Jude Children's Research Hospital. J Clin Oncol 15:2792–2799

Greenberg ML (1999) Chemotherapy of choroid plexus carcinoma. Childs Nerv Syst 15:571–577

Griffin CA, Hawkins AL, Packer RJ et al (1988) Chromosome abnormalities in pediatric brain tumors. Cancer Res 48:175–180

Gupta N, Banerjee A, Haas-Kogan D (2004) Pediatric CNS tumors. Springer, Berlin

Gurney JG, Kadan-Lottick N (2001) Brain and other central nervous system tumors: rate, trends, and epidemiology. Curr Opin Oncol 13:160–166

Gurney JG, Smith MA, Bunin GR (1999) Cancer incidence and survival among children and adolescents. United States SEER program 1975–1999. NIH Pub No 99–4649. National Cancer Institute, SEER Program, Bethesda, pp 51–63

Healey EA, Barnes PD, Kupsky WJ et al (1991) The prognostic significance of postoperative residual tumor in ependymoma. Neurosurgery 28:666–671

Heideman RL, Kuttesch J Jr, Gajjar AJ et al (1997) Supratentorial malignant gliomas in childhood: a single institution perspective. Cancer 80:497–504

Hirsch JF, Sainte RC, Pierre-Kahn A et al (1989) Benign astrocytic and oligodendrocytic tumors of the cerebral hemispheres in children. J Neurosurg 70:568–572

Hirtz D, Ashwal S, Berg A et al (2000) Practice parameter: evaluating a first nonfebrile seizure in children: report of the quality standards subcommittee of the American Academy of Neurology, The Child Neurology Society, and The American Epilepsy Society. Neurology 55:616–623

Horn B, Heeideman R, Geyer R et al (1999) A multi-institutional retrospective study of intracranial ependymoma in children: identification of risk factors. J Pediatr Hematol Oncol 21:203–211

Housepian EM, Chi TL (1993) Neurofibromatosis and optic pathways gliomas. J Neurooncol 15:51–55

Hukin J, Epstein F, Lefton D et al (1998) Treatment of intracranial ependymoma by surgery alone. Pediatr Neurosurg 29:40–45

Janss AJ, Grundy R, Cnaan A et al (1995) Optic pathway and hypothalamic/chiasmatic gliomas in children younger than age 5 years with a 6-year follow up. Cancer 75:1051–1059

Jemal A, Clegg LX, Ward E et al (2004) Annual report to the nation on the status of cancer 1975–2001, with a special feature regarding survival. Cancer 101:3–27

Jenkin D, Berry M, Chan H et al (1990) Pineal region germinomas in childhood treatment considerations. Int Radiat Oncol Biol Phys 18:541–545

Judkins AR, Mauger J, Ht A et al (2004) Immunohistochemical analysis of hSNF5/INI1 in pediatric CNS neoplasms. Am J Surg Pathol 28: 644–650

Kleihues P, Berger PC, Scheithauer B, O'Fallon J et al (1988) Grading of astrocytomas. A simple and reproducible method. Cancer 62: 2152–2165

Kun LE, Kovnar EH, Sanford RA (1998) Ependymomas in children. Pediatr Neurosci 14:57–63

Legler JM, Ries LA, Smith MA et al (1999) Cancer surveillance series [corrected]: brain and other central nervous system cancers: recent trends in incidence and mortality. J Natl Cancer Inst 91: 1382–1390

Lesniak MS, Klem JM, Weingart J et al (2003) Surgical outcome following resection f contrast-enhanced pediatric brainstem gliomas. Pediatr Neurosurg 39:314–322

Lewis DW (2007) Headaches in children and adolescents. Curr Probl Pediatr Adolesc Health Care 37:207–246

Lewis DW, Packer RJ, Raney B et al (1986) Incidence, presentation, and outcome of spinal cord disease in children with systemic cancer. Pediatrics 78:438–443

Marchese MJ, Chang CH (1990) Malignant astrocytic gliomas in children. Cancer 65:2771–2778

Mason WP, Grovas A, Halpern S et al (1998) Intensive chemotherapy and bone marrow rescue for young children with newly diagnosed malignant brain tumors. J Clin Oncol 16:210–221

Matsutani M, Sano K, Takakura K et al (1997) Primary intracranial germ cell tumors: a clinical analysis of 153 histologically verified cases. J Neurosurg 86:446–455

McNeil DE, Cote TR, Clegg L et al (2002) Incidence and trends in pediatric malignancies medulloblastoma/primitive neuroectodermal tumor: a SEER update: surveillance epidemiology and end results. Med Pediatr Oncol 39:190–194

Nazemi KJ, Malempati S (2009) Emergency department presentation of childhood cancer. Emerg Med Clin N Am 27:477–495

Packer RJ (2005) Progress and challenges in childhood brain tumors. J Neurooncol 75:239–242

Packer RJ, Cohen BH, Cooney K (2000) Intracranial germ cell tumors. Oncologist 5:312–320

Pencale P, Sainte-Rose C, Lellouch-Tubiana A et al (1998) Papillomas and carcinomas of the choroid plexus in children. J Neurosurg 88: 521–528

Pierre-Kahn A, Hirsch JF, Vinchon M et al (1993) Surgical management of brain-stem tumors in children: results and statistical analysis of 75 cases. J Neurosurg 79:845–852

Pollack IF (1994) Brain tumors in children. N Engl J Med 331:1500–1507

Pollack IF, Hurtt M, Pang D et al (1994) Dissemination of low grade intracranial astrocytomas in children. Cancer 73:2869–2878

Pollack IF, Gerszten PC, Martinez AJ et al (1995a) Intracranial ependymomas of childhood: long-term outcome and prognostic factors. Neurosurgery 37:655–666

Pollack IF, Claassen D, al Shboul Q et al (1995b) Low-grade gliomas of the cerebral hemispheres in children: an analysis of 71 cases. J Neurosurg 82:536–547

Pollack IF, Shultz B, Mulvihill JJ (1996) The management of brainstem gliomas in patients with neurofibromatosis 1. Neurology 46:1652–1660

Richmond IL, Wara WM, Wilson CB (1980) Role of radiation therapy in the management of craniopharyngiomas in children. Neurosurgery 6:513–517

Rickert CH, Paulus W (2001) Epidemiology of central nervous system tumors in childhood and adolescence based on the new WHO classification. Childs Nerv Syst 17:503–511

Robertson PL, Zeltzer PM, Boyett JM et al (1998) Survival and prognostic factors following radiation therapy and chemotherapy for ependymomas in children: a report of the Children's Cancer Group. J Neurosurg 88:695–703

Ron E, Modan B, Boice JD Jr et al (1988) Tumors of the brain and nervous system after radiotherapy in childhood. N Engl J Med 319:1033–1039

Rorke LB, Packer RJ, Biegel JA (1996) Central nervous system atypical teratoid/rhaboid tumors of infancy and childhood: definition of an entity. J Neurosurg 85:56–65

Rousseau P, Habrand JL, Sarrazin D et al (1994) Treatment of intracranial ependymomas of children: review of a 15-year experience. Int J Radiat Oncol Biol Phys 28:381–386

Smith MA, Freidlin B, Ries LA et al (1998) Trends in reported incidence of primary malignant brain tumors in children in the United States. J Natl Cancer Inst 90:1269–1277

Smoots DW, Geyer JR, Lieberman DM et al (1998) Prediciting disease progression in childhood cerebellar astrocytoma. Childs Nerv Syst 14:636–648

Tarbell NJ, Loeffler JS, Silver B et al (1991) The change in patterns of relapse in medulloblastoma. Cancer 68:1600–1604

Wallner KE, Gonzales MF, Edwards MS et al (1988) Treatment results of juvenile pilocytic astrocytoma. J Neurosurg 69:171–176

Wilne SH, Ferris RC, Nathwani A et al (2006) The presenting features of brain tumors: a review of 200 cases. Arch Dis Child 91:502–506

Wilne S, Collier J, Kennedy C et al (2007) Presentation of childhood CNS tumors: a systematic review and meta-analysis. Lancet Oncol 8:685–695

Wisoff JH, Boyett JM, Berger MS et al (1998) Current neurosurgical management and the impact of the extent of resection in the treatment of malignant gliomas of childhood: a report of the Children's Cancer Group trial no. CCG-945. J Neurosurg 38: 258–264

Yang HJ, Nam DH, Wang KC et al (1999) Supratentorial primitive neuroectodermal tumor in children: clinical features, treatment outcome and prognostic factors. Childs Nerv Syst 15:377–383

350 Neuroblastoma and Other Sympathetic Nervous System Tumors

Stephen S. Roberts

Definition

Tumors of the sympathetic nervous system in children consist of neuroblastoma and its variants, ganglioneuroblastoma, and ganglioneuroma, as well as pheochromocytoma/paraganglioma. Pheochromocytomas and paragangliomas are very rare in children, with an incidence of less than 0.3 cases per million per year. They are called pheochromocytomas when arising from the adrenal gland and paragangliomas when extra-adrenal and can occur anywhere from the neck to the pelvis. The majority of these tumors are benign (~90%) and present because of systemic symptoms such as hypertension due to catecholamine secretion. Because these tumors are quite rare and usually benign, we will confine the remainder of this discussion to neuroblastoma only.

Few tumors exhibit such diversity of behavior and outcome as neuroblastoma. This varies from spontaneous regression and differentiation, often without therapy, to aggressive, treatment-resistant disease that is frequently fatal despite intensive multimodality therapy.

Etiology

The etiology of neuroblastoma is unknown. Although several studies have investigated potential links between environmental factors, maternal drug exposures, and parental occupations and increased risk of neuroblastoma, to date, no consistent and definitive associations have been identified. Neuroblastoma has been positively associated with various congenital anomalies, especially urogenital and cardiac abnormalities, and in patients with congenital central hypoventilation syndrome (CCHS) and Hirschsprung's disease. Presumably this represents disordered development in shared neurodevelopmental pathways but the exact cause and relationship remains unknown.

Epidemiology

Neuroblastoma is the most common extracranial solid tumor of childhood and the most common cancer of infancy, accounting for 8–10% of all childhood cancers. In industrialized countries, the prevalence is roughly 1 case per 7,000 births, with an incidence of approximately 8–10 per million per year. This incidence appears to be similar throughout the developed world. Rates in developing countries are less clear; several reports have suggested that rates are lower, particularly in sub-Saharan Africa. However, it is unknown if this represents true lower incidence or underreporting. There is a very slight increase in incidence among boys versus girls (1.1:1).

Because neuroblastomas generally produce and secrete catecholamines whose metabolites (vanillylmandelic acid, VMA and homovanillic acid, HVA) are detectable in the urine, there have been several attempts at mass screenings of infants. These screenings were conducted in Japan, Germany, and Montreal, Canada in the 1980s and 1990s with the hope of detecting neuroblastoma at an earlier stage. Unfortunately, while these screening efforts did lead to an increased detection of low-stage neuroblastoma in infants, they did not lower the prevalence or the mortality rates of those children over 1 year of age with higher stage disease. Therefore, at this time, routine screening of infants for neuroblastoma is not recommended. It is possible that in the future, screening may be recommended for children with identifiable predisposition syndromes.

Pathogenesis

Neuroblastoma serves as a model disease where detailed genetic analyses have enabled biology-based risk stratification and treatment. There are multiple genetic changes that have been identified in NB, several of which are strongly correlated with disease outcome and are an integral part of our understanding of the development and treatment of this disease. Recently, several different groups

Abdelaziz Y. Elzouki (ed.), *Textbook of Clinical Pediatrics*, DOI 10.1007/978-3-642-02202-9_350,

reported germline mutations in the anaplastic lymphoma kinase (ALK) and PHOX2B genes in a small subset of neuroblastoma patients with familial predisposition. Mutations in these genes strongly predispose to development of neuroblastoma. However, the vast majority of children with NB do not have heritable risk factors predisposing them to the development of the disease. Instead, acquired somatic changes in neural crest stem cells appear to be the underlying cause leading to NB development.

Most neuroblastomas contain genomic level aberrations, including amplifications, translocations, and whole chromosome losses and gains. Many of these changes are nonrandom and have prognostic significance. Detailed analysis of these recurrent changes has led Maris et al. to propose a model for neuroblastoma development and progression. This model proposes that all neuroblastomas arise from a common precursor but that different types of genomic changes lead to two distinct subtypes of NB with very different clinical behaviors. Further, their model suggests that neuroblastomas that are biologically unfavorable do not evolve from favorable tumors but are distinct subtypes from the beginning. The first type of NB is characterized by loss and gain of whole chromosomes and few or no segmental chromosome abnormalities. These NBs are generally hyperdiploid, lack genetic changes associated with biologically unfavorable disease, and are most common in young children under 18 months of age. The prognosis for these tumors is generally excellent, with many undergoing spontaneous differentiation and/or apoptosis. In contrast, the second type of NB is characterized by recurrent segmental chromosome abnormalities. Nonrandom alterations of numerous chromosomes have been identified, including deletions of 1p36 and 11q and unbalanced gain of chromosome 17q. However, the most important genomic alteration is amplification of the MYCN oncogene, which tends to portend a particularly grim prognosis. MYCN amplification is associated with advanced disease, older age (>18 months), and poor outcome. The overall prevalence of MYCN amplification is approximately 20% and is essentially always present at the time of diagnosis, strongly suggesting it is an inherent feature of a subset of aggressive neuroblastomas and not an acquired late event. Thus, determination of MYCN amplification status is a standard part of neuroblastoma characterization at diagnosis due to its clear biological importance.

Pathology

Neuroblastoma is classically defined as a small, round, blue-cell tumor of childhood. Other malignancies in this group include non-Hodgkin lymphomas, Ewing sarcoma family tumors, and soft tissue sarcomas such as rhabdomyosarcoma. There are three histopathological subtypes: neuroblastoma, ganglioneuroblastoma, and ganglioneuroma. These three types represent a spectrum of differentiation from malignant to benign. Typically, the cells are small and uniform in size, with dark nuclei and little cytoplasm. Nearly all neuroblastoma form neuropil, collections of primitive neurites, and the Homer-Wright pseudorosette, a classic finding, is a ring of neuroblasts surrounding a core of eosinophilic neuropil. These pseudorosettes, however, are found in a minority of tumors. Ganglioneuromas represent a fully mature, benign collection of ganglion cells, Schwann cells, and neuropil. Ganglioneuroblastomas represent the spectrum of differentiation between malignant neuroblastoma and mature, benign ganglioneuromas.

Histopathology has been used to prognostically classify neuroblastomas; the most common system was developed by Shimada et al., and utilizes patient age, Schwannian cell stroma, mitosis-karyorrhexis index, and differentiation state to classify tumors as favorable or unfavorable. This system was recently modified with the goal of making it more reproducible around the world and is now known as the International Neuroblastoma Pathology Classification (INPC) system.

Clinical Manifestations

The clinical manifestations depend on the primary site of the tumor as well as any metastases that may be present. Approximately 65% of primary tumors arise in the abdomen; most of the remainder are thoracic or cervical in origin. No primary tumor is found in about 1% of patients. Most children with NB are diagnosed by age 5 and nearly all occur before age 10. Neuroblastoma is often disseminated at diagnosis, with spread most commonly involving locoregional lymph nodes as well as bone, bone marrow, liver, and skin. Lung and central nervous system metastases are rare.

Abdominal neuroblastoma may present with abdominal pain or fullness but is often asymptomatic and discovered incidentally, frequently by a caregiver. Thoracic neuroblastoma is frequently discovered incidentally on chest radiographs obtained for other reasons. Rarely, large thoracic tumors can cause mechanical obstruction and lead to compression of the superior vena cava and/or trachea (superior vena cava and superior mediastinal syndromes, respectively). High-level thoracic lesions and cervical neuroblastomas can cause Horner Syndrome (unilateral ptosis, myosis, and anhydrosis). Any paraspinal neuroblastoma may extend through the neural foramina of the vertebral bodies and cause nerve root or spinal cord compression. This may lead to symptoms such as weakness, paralysis, bowel and/or bladder dysfunction, and radicular pain. Bone marrow involvement may lead to anemia and bleeding, while widespread cortical bone metastases are frequently seen and cause pain, limp, and significant irritability in younger patients.

Neuroblastoma is classically associated with several distinct presentations. Tumor infiltration of the periorbital bones causing proptosis and periorbital ecchymoses is a frequent manifestation of disseminated disease (➋ *Fig. 350.1*). Likewise, infants less than 1 year of age will frequently present with multiple bluish, painless, subcutaneous nodular lesions. These are generally associated with stage 4S disease, spontaneous regression, and an excellent prognosis.

Two distinct paraneoplastic syndromes have been associated with neuroblastoma. The first, opsoclonus-myoclonus syndrome, is found in 2–4% of patients with neuroblastoma and is characterized by rapid, jerking eye movements, myoclonus, and ataxia. Thought to be an immune-mediated cross reaction between antibodies against the tumor and elements of the normal nervous system, these children tend to have low-stage disease and an excellent prognosis. Unfortunately, as many as 80% will have long-term neurologic sequelae, including significant cognitive deficits. The other paraneoplastic syndrome is intractable secretory diarrhea, hypokalemia, and dehydration caused by tumor secretion of vasoactive intestinal peptide, known as VIP syndrome. These tumors are usually ganglioneuroblastomas or ganglioneuromas and removal of the primary tumor generally leads to resolution of the diarrhea and excellent long-term survival.

Systemic manifestations such as hypertension, tachycardia, and flushing are rarely seen with neuroblastoma, as opposed to pheochromocytomas, because they do not secrete epinephrine.

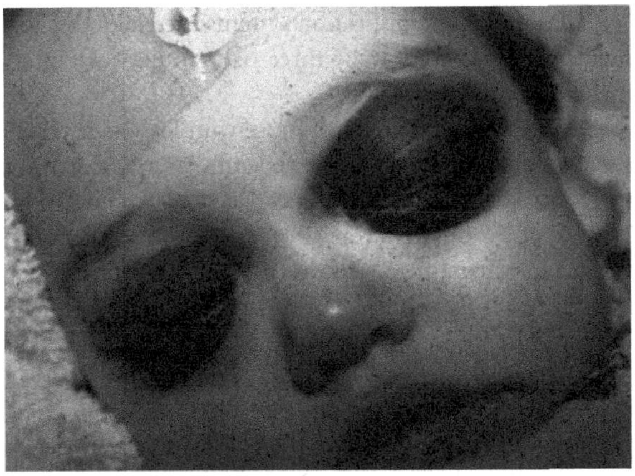

Figure 350.1
Periorbital ecchymoses in a child with high-risk neuroblastoma

Diagnosis

All patients suspected to have neuroblastoma require a comprehensive evaluation to ensure accurate staging and risk stratification. The diagnosis of neuroblastoma is made by either pathologic identification of neuroblasts from tumor biopsy or unequivocal presence of neuroblastoma in a bone marrow aspirate along with the presence of elevated serum or urine catecholamine levels. Whenever feasible, every effort should be made to perform a tumor biopsy, especially in young children under 18 months of age, as the biological information obtained is critical in proper determination of risk category and subsequent therapy planning.

A thorough physical exam should include evaluation of any masses, palpation for presence of hepatomegaly, neurological evaluation for weakness or paralysis, and examination of lymph nodes, skin, and skull for evidence of metastases. The imaging modality of choice for delineation of the primary tumor is CT scan. In general, most patients should receive a CT of the chest, abdomen, and pelvis, with evaluation of the head, neck, and spine if clinically indicated. All patients should have bilateral bone marrow aspirates and biopsies to evaluate for the presence of marrow disease. Likewise, evaluation of the bony skeleton should be performed. This has classically been done with plain radiography and Technetium-99 scintigraphy. More recently, radiolabeled metaiodobenzylguanidine (MIBG) scans, using either ^{123}I- or ^{131}I-MIBG, have become increasingly important in evaluating NB. ^{123}I-MIBG is more sensitive and specific than a Tc-99 bone scan or ^{131}I-MIBG. Whenever possible, both Tc-99 and ^{123}I-MIBG scanning should be performed at diagnosis as approximately 10% of tumors are not MIBG avid. Positron emission tomography is generally less sensitive than MIBG scanning and does not currently play a role in routine diagnostic imaging of neuroblastoma.

Tissue samples obtained should be evaluated for the presence of specific cytogenetic abnormalities, DNA ploidy, and the presence of MYCN amplification. Standard cytogenetic testing or specific fluorescent in situ hybridization techniques are routinely used. This information is critical for subsequent risk stratification, with all major cooperative groups worldwide incorporating this information in their schema.

Differential Diagnosis

The differential diagnosis includes ganglioneuroma, which occurs in the same sites as its malignant counterpart. Intrathoracic neurofibromatosis tumors can mimic neuroblastomas radiologically, but they tend to be more nodular in outline, and grow along the course of the intercostal nerves, which results in characteristic indentations along the inferior costal margin. Tumors arising in the retroperitoneum may be confused with Wilms' tumor; the latter, however, tend to feel smooth to palpation in contrast to the nodular feel of a neuroblastoma and generally lack the characteristic intratumoral calcifications seen in imaging studies of neuroblastomas. Cervical neuroblastomas may be confused with cervical adenitis or lymphomas. Lack of tenderness upon palpation of the mass is a key finding allowing differentiation between NB and infectious etiologies. Additionally, neuroblastomas may present with weakness or paralysis of the lower extremities due to tumor extension through the neural foramina causing spinal cord compression. A thorough history, physical exam, and imaging studies are needed to differentiate NB from other primary neurologic causes of weakness and paralysis. Since NB frequently metastasizes to bone marrow, its presenting symptoms can mimic leukemia with pallor, fatigue, recurrent fevers, and bruising and petechiae being common; bone marrow aspiration will distinguish between these entities.

Pathologically, neuroblastoma must be distinguished from the other small round blue-cell tumors of childhood mentioned above. This can be done by identification of neuropil and pseudorosettes and more specifically by immunohistochemical staining for neural markers such as neurofilament proteins, synaptophysin, and neuron-specific enolase (NSE).

Treatment

Treatment is determined by risk group stratification. Currently, all of the major cooperative groups use similar risk group classification schemes that include disease stage, patient age (less than 12–18 months versus greater than 12–18 months) at diagnosis, and MYCN amplification status. DNA ploidy, additional cytogenetic analyses, and histopathology are incorporated with some variability. Stage of disease is a key component of risk group assignment.

Table 350.1
International neuroblastoma staging system

Stage 1	Localized tumor confined to the area of origin; complete gross excision, with or without microscopic residual disease; identifiable ipsilateral and contralateral lymph nodes negative microscopically
Stage 2A	Unilateral tumor with incomplete gross excision; identifiable ipsilateral and contralateral lymph nodes negative microscopically
Stage 2B	Unilateral tumor with complete or incomplete gross excision; positive ipsilateral regional lymph nodes; identifiable contralateral lymph nodes negative microscopically
Stage 3	Tumor infiltrating across the midline with or without regional lymph node involvement, or midline tumor with bilateral regional lymph node involvement
Stage 4	Dissemination of tumor to distant lymph nodes, bone, bone marrow, liver, and/or other organs (except as defined in stage 4S)
Stage 4S	Localized primary tumor as defined for stage 1 or 2 with dissemination limited to liver, skin, and/or less than 10% of bone marrow; limited to infants less than 1 year of age

Currently, the international neuroblastoma staging system (INSS) is used around the world as the primary staging system (➲ *Table 350.1*). Recently, an international consensus group developed a newer staging and risk stratification system called the international neuroblastoma risk group (INRG) staging and classification systems. These will likely be the future international standards.

All of the risk stratification systems used allow assignment into one of generally three risk groups: low, intermediate, and high risk.

Low-risk patients include those with low-stage (INSS stage 1 or 2) disease, and are generally of a younger age (<18 months) and do not have MYCN amplification. Treatment for this group involves surgical resection only. Importantly, complete resection is not necessary in these low-risk patients and therefore aggressive and potentially morbid surgeries should be avoided. Chemotherapy and radiation therapy are rarely needed and should be reserved for the patient that experiences disease recurrence. Some patients with low-risk disease (INSS stage 4S and incidentally found perinatal tumors) are successfully managed through observation only with no active intervention.

Treatment of intermediate risk patients is somewhat more complex and includes local control surgery followed by moderately intensive chemotherapy, with the precise regimen varying by cooperative group. Radiation therapy is reserved for those intermediate risk patients with residual disease that has not responded to chemotherapy.

High-risk neuroblastoma is treated with aggressive, multimodality therapy including surgery, radiotherapy, chemotherapy, and biological/immunotherapy. The current standard therapy for high-risk patients in North America, Europe, and Japan includes intensive induction chemotherapy followed by surgery, radiation therapy, and autologous stem cell supported myeloablative therapy. This is then followed by a period of biological/immunotherapy targeting remaining minimal residual disease that uses 13-*cis* retinoic acid as a differentiating agent. Additionally, the Children's Oncology Group recently reported that the addition of immunotherapy directed at the neuroblastoma tumor antigen GD2 significantly improved survival in these patients, and future therapies will likely include some form of immune-based treatment.

Prognosis

Prognosis varies greatly by risk group. Currently, with observation and/or surgical resection alone, patients with low-risk disease have survival rates in excess of 95% in the developed world. Intermediate risk patients also do very well with moderate chemotherapy and have survival rates of over 90%. Prognosis for high-risk disease, however, remains poor. Historically, 5-year event-free survival rates have been less than 20%. Using the current intensive, multimodality therapy regimens, survival rates have increased to 40–50%. While this is an improvement over historical rates, there is room for substantial improvement. Additionally, significant long-term side effects of intensive therapy remain a large issue for those high-risk patients that are cured of their disease.

Prevention

Currently, there is no known preventive strategy for neuroblastoma.

References

Attiyeh EF, London WB, Mosse YP et al (2005) Chromosome 1p and 11q deletions and outcome in neuroblastoma. N Engl J Med 353(21):2243–2253

Azizkhan RG, Shaw A, Chandler JG (1985) Surgical complications of neuroblastoma resection. Surgery 97(5):514–517

Bagatell R, Beck-Popovic M, London WB et al (2009) Significance of MYCN amplification in international neuroblastoma staging system stage 1 and 2 neuroblastoma: a report from the International Neuroblastoma Risk Group database. J Clin Oncol 27(3):365–370

Brodeur GM (2003) Neuroblastoma: biological insights into a clinical enigma. Nat Rev Cancer 3(3):203–216

Brodeur GM, Hogarty MD, Mosse YP et al (2011) Neuroblastoma. In: Pizzo PA, Poplack DG (eds) Principles and practice of pediatric oncology, 6th edn. Lippincott Williams & Wilkins, Philadelphia

Brodeur GM, Pritchard J, Berthold F et al (1993) Revisions of the international criteria for neuroblastoma diagnosis, staging, and response to treatment. J Clin Oncol 11(8):1466–1477

Brodeur GM, Nakagawara A (1992) Molecular basis of clinical heterogeneity in neuroblastoma. Am J Pediatr Hematol Oncol 14(2):111–116

Brodeur GM, Seeger RC, Barrett A et al (1988) International criteria for diagnosis, staging, and response to treatment in patients with neuroblastoma. J Clin Oncol 6(12):1874–1881

Brodeur GM, Seeger RC, Schwab M et al (1984) Amplification of N-myc in untreated human neuroblastomas correlates with advanced disease stage. Science 224(4653):1121–1124

Cheung NK, Kushner BH, Yeh SD et al (1998) 3F8 monoclonal antibody treatment of patients with stage 4 neuroblastoma: a phase II study. Int J Oncol 12(6):1299–1306

Cohn SL, Pearson AD, London WB et al (2009) The International Neuroblastoma Risk Group (INRG) classification system: an INRG task force report. J Clin Oncol 27(2):289–297

El Shafie M, Samuel D, Klippel CH et al (1983) Intractable diarrhea in children with VIP-secreting ganglioneuroblastomas. J Pediatr Surg 18(1):34–36

Evans AE, Silber JH, Shpilsky A et al (1996) Successful management of low-stage neuroblastoma without adjuvant therapies: a comparison of two decades, 1972 through 1981 and 1982 through 1992, in a single institution. J Clin Oncol 14(9):2504–2510

George RE, Sanda T, Hanna M et al (2008) Activating mutations in ALK provide a therapeutic target in neuroblastoma. Nature 455(7215):975–978

Haas-Kogan DA, Swift PS, Selch M et al (2003) Impact of radiotherapy for high-risk neuroblastoma: a children's cancer group study. Int J Radiat Oncol Biol Phys 56(1):28–39

Ho PT, Estroff JA, Kozakewich H et al (1993) Prenatal detection of neuroblastoma: a ten-year experience from the Dana-Farber Cancer Institute and Children's Hospital. Pediatrics 92(3):358–364

Janoueix-Lerosey I, Schleiermacher G, Michels E et al (2009) Overall genomic pattern is a predictor of outcome in neuroblastoma. J Clin Oncol 27(7):1026–1033

Kaatsch P (2010) Epidemiology of childhood cancer. Cancer Treat Rev 36(4):277–285

Kushner BH, Cheung NK (1996) Allelic loss of chromosome 1p in neuroblastoma. N Engl J Med 334(24):1608–1609

Kushner BH, Cheung NK, LaQuaglia MP et al (1996a) International neuroblastoma staging system stage 1 neuroblastoma: a prospective study and literature review. J Clin Oncol 14(7):2174–2180

Kushner BH, Cheung NK, LaQuaglia MP et al (1996b) Survival from locally invasive or widespread neuroblastoma without cytotoxic therapy. J Clin Oncol 14(2):373–381

Kushner BH, Kramer K, LaQuaglia MP et al (2003) Neuroblastoma in adolescents and adults: the Memorial Sloan-Kettering experience. Med Pediatr Oncol 41(6):508–515

La Quaglia MP, Kushner BH, Su W et al (2004) The impact of gross total resection on local control and survival in high-risk neuroblastoma. J Pediatr Surg 39(3):412–417. Discussion 412–417

Look AT, Hayes FA, Nitschke R et al (1984) Cellular DNA content as a predictor of response to chemotherapy in infants with unresectable neuroblastoma. N Engl J Med 311(4):231–235

Look AT, Hayes FA, Shuster JJ et al (1991) Clinical relevance of tumor cell ploidy and N-myc gene amplification in childhood neuroblastoma: a pediatric oncology group study. J Clin Oncol 9(4):581–591

Maris JM (2005) The biologic basis for neuroblastoma heterogeneity and risk stratification. Curr Opin Pediatr 17(1):7–13

Maris JM (2010) Recent advances in neuroblastoma. N Engl J Med 362(23):2202–2211

Maris JM, Weiss MJ, Guo C et al (2000) Loss of heterozygosity at 1p36 independently predicts for disease progression but not decreased overall survival probability in neuroblastoma patients: a children's cancer group study. J Clin Oncol 18(9):1888–1899

Matthay KK, Edeline V, Lumbroso J et al (2003) Correlation of early metastatic response by 123I-metaiodobenzylguanidine scintigraphy with overall response and event-free survival in stage IV neuroblastoma. J Clin Oncol 21(13):2486–2491

Matthay KK, Villablanca JG, Seeger RC et al (1999) Treatment of high-risk neuroblastoma with intensive chemotherapy, radiotherapy, autologous bone marrow transplantation, and 13-cis-retinoic acid. Children's Cancer Group. N Engl J Med 341(16):1165–1173

Menegaux F, Olshan AF, Reitnauer PJ et al (2005) Positive association between congenital anomalies and risk of neuroblastoma. Pediatr Blood Cancer 45(5):649–655

Monclair T, Brodeur GM, Ambros PF et al (2009) The International Neuroblastoma Risk Group (INRG) staging system: an INRG task force report. J Clin Oncol 27(2):298–303

Mosse YP, Greshock J, Margolin A et al (2005) High-resolution detection and mapping of genomic DNA alterations in neuroblastoma. Genes Chromosomes Cancer 43(4):390–403

Mosse YP, Laudenslager M, Longo L et al (2008) Identification of ALK as a major familial neuroblastoma predisposition gene. Nature 455(7215):930–935

Mueller S, Matthay KK (2009) Neuroblastoma: biology and staging. Curr Oncol Rep 11(6):431–438

Olshan AF, De Roos AJ, Teschke K et al (1999) Neuroblastoma and parental occupation. Cancer causes control 10(6):539–549

Plantaz D, Mohapatra G, Matthay KK et al (1997) Gain of chromosome 17 is the most frequent abnormality detected in neuroblastoma by comparative genomic hybridization. Am J Pathol 150(1):81–89

Rudnick E, Khakoo Y, Antunes NL et al (2001) Opsoclonus-myoclonus-ataxia syndrome in neuroblastoma: clinical outcome and antineuronal antibodies-a report from the Children's Cancer Group Study. Med Pediatr Oncol 36(6):612–622

Sabbah RS, Ayas M, Laban MA (2001) Tumors of the sympathetic nervous system. In: Elzouki AY, Harfi HA, Nazer HM (eds) Textbook of clinical pediatrics, 1st edn. Lippincott Williams & Wilkins, Philadelphia

Seeger RC, Brodeur GM, Sather H et al (1985) Association of multiple copies of the N-myc oncogene with rapid progression of neuroblastomas. N Engl J Med 313(18):1111–1116

Shimada H, Ambros IM, Dehner LP et al (1999a) Terminology and morphologic criteria of neuroblastic tumors: recommendations by the International Neuroblastoma Pathology Committee. Cancer 86(2):349–363

Shimada H, Ambros IM, Dehner LP et al (1999b) The International Neuroblastoma Pathology Classification (the Shimada system). Cancer 86(2):364–372

Shimada H, Chatten J, Newton WA Jr et al (1984) Histopathologic prognostic factors in neuroblastic tumors: definition of subtypes of ganglioneuroblastoma and an age-linked classification of neuroblastomas. J Natl Cancer Inst 73(2):405–416

Shulkin BL, Shapiro B (1998) Current concepts on the diagnostic use of MIBG in children. J Nucl Med 39(4):679–688

Stiller CA, Parkin DM (1992) International variations in the incidence of neuroblastoma. Int J Cancer 52(4):538–543

Trochet D, Bourdeaut F, Janoueix-Lerosey I et al (2004) Germline mutations of the paired-like homeobox 2B (PHOX2B) gene in neuroblastoma. Am J Hum Genet 74(4):761–764

Villablanca JG, Khan AA, Avramis VI et al (1995) Phase I trial of 13-cis-retinoic acid in children with neuroblastoma following bone marrow transplantation. J Clin Oncol 13(4):894–901

White PS, Thompson PM, Seifried BA et al (2001) Detailed molecular analysis of 1p36 in neuroblastoma. Med Pediatr Oncol 36(1):37–41

Woods WG, Gao RN, Shuster JJ et al (2002) Screening of infants and mortality due to neuroblastoma. N Engl J Med 346(14): 1041–1046

Yu AL, Gilman AL, Ozkaynak MF et al (2010) Anti-GD2 antibody with GM-CSF, interleukin-2, and isotretinoin for neuroblastoma. N Engl J Med 363(14):1324–1334

351 Wilms' Tumor and Other Primary Renal Neoplasms

Susan J. Lindemulder

Definition/Classification

Wilms' tumor is the most common primary tumor of the kidney in children. There are several other tumor types including clear cell sarcoma of the kidney, rhabdoid tumor of the kidney, congenital mesoblastic nephroma, and renal cell carcinoma that also arise from the kidney, but they are much less common. The development of modern treatment regimens using a combination of surgery, chemotherapy, and radiation therapy has greatly improved the cure rate for Wilms' tumor.

Epidemiology

Wilms' tumor is typically diagnosed in children younger than 15 years and approximately 500 new cases are diagnosed per year in the United States. The prevalence worldwide is approximately 1 in 10,000 children under the age of 15 years. Globally, the incidence is substantially lower in Asian populations. Although various studies have explored environmental risk factors, it is likely that genetics play a larger role than the environment.

Wilms' tumor most often occurs in previously healthy children; however, there is a higher incidence of Wilms' tumor in children with certain recognized syndromes which are associated with other congenital malformations. These syndromes can typically be grouped into either overgrowth syndromes or non-overgrowth syndromes. The overgrowth syndromes are characterized by malformations such as macroglossia, nephromegaly, and hemihypertrophy, and include: Beckwith–Wiedemann syndrome, isolated hemihypertrophy, Perlman syndrome, Sotos syndrome, and Simpson-Golabi-Behemel syndrome. The non-overgrowth syndromes are characterized by various other malformations and include: isolated aniridia, trisomy 18, WAGR syndrome, Blooms syndrome, Alagille syndrome, Denys–Drash syndrome, and Frasier syndrome. The phenotypic characteristics of these syndromes are summarized in ➋ *Table 351.1*.

Pathogenesis

Multiple genes have been identified as playing a role in the development of Wilms' tumor. The first gene identified and the most studied is WT1 which was discovered through the study of patients with WAGR syndrome. WT1 is located on chromosome 11p13 in a region which also contains the gene responsible for aniridia. The gene is a tumor suppressor gene which codes for a transcription factor responsible for regulating other transcription factors important in cell growth and differentiation. A second gene important to the development of Wilms' tumor was discovered through the study of BWS patients. The WT2 gene is located on chromosome 11p15, and Wilms' tumor develops when there is loss of heterozygosity. The loss of heterozygosity is thought to upregulate an oncogene, resulting in tumor formation.

There is a recognized familial predisposition for Wilms' tumor which is rare and only accounts for a small percentage of new cases. Two genes have been identified as playing a role in familial Wilms' tumor, FWT1 located on chromosome 17q and FWT2 located on chromosome 19q.

Other chromosomal abnormalities are seen with increased incidence in studies of Wilms' tumor samples. Loss of heterozygosity in chromosome 16q and 11p have been suggested to be associated with poor prognosis unrelated to stage of disease. The role of p53 in the development of Wilms' tumor is also under investigation, although Wilms' tumor is not commonly seen in the Li Fraumeni syndrome.

Pathology

Three cell types are commonly seen in the histology of Wilms' tumor: blastemal, stromal, and epithelial. These three cell types reflect stages of normal renal development. A single specimen does not need to include all three cell types to be diagnostic for Wilms' tumor. Histology is further classified as

Abdelaziz Y. Elzouki (ed.), *Textbook of Clinical Pediatrics*, DOI 10.1007/978-3-642-02202-9_351,

Table 351.1
Characteristics of syndromes associated with Wilms' tumor

Syndrome	Phenotypic characteristics
Overgrowth syndromes	
Beckwith–Wiedemann syndrome	Macrosomia, macroglossia, visceromegaly, embryonal tumors, omphalocele, neonatal hypoglycemia, ear creases/pits, adrenocortical cytomegaly, renal abnormalities
Isolated hemihyperplasia	Asymmetric growth without other abnormalities
Perlman syndrome	Polyhydramnios, neonatal macrosomia, visceromegaly, nephromegaly, distinctive facial appearance, renal dysplasia
Sotos syndrome	Typical facial appearance, tall stature, learning disability, behavioral problems, congenital cardiac anomalies, neonatal jaundice, renal anomalies, scoliosis, seizures
Simpson-Golabi-Behemel syndrome	Macrosomia, distinctive craniofacial features, mental retardation, skeletal anomalies, hand anomalies
Non-overgrowth syndromes	
Isolated aniridia	Panocular abnormalities
Trisomy 18	Prominent occiput, short eye fissures with droopy eyelids, micrognathia, external ear variations, rocker-bottom feet, redundant skin on back of neck, congenital heart defects, hand anomalies
WAGR syndrome	Wilms' tumor, aniridia, genitourinary anomalies, mental retardation
Blooms syndrome	Small body size, immunodeficiency, sun-sensitive facial erythema
Alagille syndrome	Bile duct paucity, congenital cardiomyopahty, facial dysmorphy, vertebral defects, ocular abnormalities, renal anomalies
Denys–Drash syndrome	Ambiguous genitalia, congenital nephropathy leading to renal failure
Frasier syndrome	Complete gonadal dysgenesis and nephritic syndrome

"favorable" or "unfavorable" based on the absence or presence of anaplastic nuclear changes. Anaplasia is characterized by multipolar mitotic figures and marked nuclear enlargement. Nephrogenic rests can also be found within areas of the kidney not affected by Wilms' tumor and increase the risk for developing tumor in the remaining kidney.

Clear cell sarcoma of the kidney is the second most common renal cancer in children and has a poorer prognosis than Wilms' tumor. It requires more aggressive treatment and has a wider range of metastatic spread (lungs, bone, brain, soft tissues). Clear cell sarcoma was named for the classic pale-stained tumor cells that are seen in cords and nests separated by vascular septa.

Rhabdoid tumor of the kidney is highly aggressive and occurs more commonly in children less than 2 years. Patients often present with widely metastatic disease, and the majority die within 1 year. Cells in rhabdoid tumors have nuclei with a large single nucleolus, giving the appearance of an "owl's eye."

Congenital mesoblastic nephroma occurs in infants with a median age of 2 months. There are three histological types: the classic type, the cellular type, and the mixed type. The cellular type is the most common and shares histologic features with infantile fibrosarcoma and also has the chromosomal translocation t(12;15) which is seen in infantile fibrosarcoma. Congenital mesoblastic nephromas tend to grow into the hilar areas and perirenal soft tissues, and they require radical surgical excision for cure.

Renal cell carcinoma is the most common primary cancer of the kidney in adults but it is rare in children. The histologic features are papillary, clear cell, and mixed. The papillary subtype is the most common in children. Renal cell carcinoma is difficult to treat, and survival is often limited to weeks or months after diagnosis.

Clinical Manifestations: Symptoms, Signs

The most common clinical presentation of renal masses in children is painless abdominal swelling or mass noted by the parents. At diagnosis, abdominal pain or hematuria are often also present. Hypertension is diagnosed in a significant percentage of patients during the initial work-up of a renal mass.

On physical exam, a large mass can be palpated, and it is noted to arise from the flank. It often will not move with respiration. Signs of venous obstruction can be noted if tumor thrombus has invaded the renal vein or inferior vena cava. Given the link between Wilms' tumor and various syndromes, physical examination should include assessment for the stigmata of these syndromes including: aniridia, facial dysmorphism, hemihypertrophy, macroglosia, genitourinary abnormalities, cryptorchidism, and pseudohermaphroditism.

Diagnosis

The diagnostic work-up for a renal mass includes laboratory evaluation, radiology studies, and pathologic analysis of tissue. A complete blood count, liver, and renal function testing should be done to evaluate organ function. A urinalysis should be done to evaluate for hematuria.

Imaging studies are very important in the diagnosis of a renal mass as, in some cases, treatment is initiated based on the characteristic imaging of these tumors. Commonly, an abdominal ultrasound is the first study completed and shows whether the mass is solid or cystic in character, the size of the mass, involvement of other organs and, if Doppler measurement is done, the presence of tumor thrombus in the inferior vena cava. These are all vital aspects in considering initial surgical management. Computed tomography (CT) scan with contract enhancement is often also done to further evaluate the extent of the mass and further define involvement in the other kidney. The typical appearance of a Wilms' tumor on CT is a well-defined mass pushing other structures out of the way but not invading them. The remaining normal kidney is often seen appearing like a "claw" on one aspect of the mass. This can often distinguish Wilms' tumor from neuroblastoma arising from the adrenal gland as neuroblastoma often has an ill-defined margin and almost always invades the surrounding structures. Abdominal MRI may be useful to characterize nephrogenic rests in the other kidney. Chest x-ray is done to evaluate for presence of pulmonary metastases, and CT of the chest can be done to evaluate for masses which may not be seen on chest x-ray.

Other radiologic studies may be indicated based on the diagnosis. Clear cell sarcoma and renal cell carcinoma can spread to the bones, and therefore a bone scan and skeletal survey should be done for patients with clear cell sarcoma and bone scan for those with renal cell carcinoma. Clear cell sarcoma, rhabdoid tumor, and renal cell carcinoma can also spread to the brain, and a MRI or CT with contrast should be done to assess for metastases.

Once all diagnostic studies have been completed to confirm the diagnosis, the patient is staged to determine the appropriate treatment. The staging characteristics for Wilms' tumor are documented in ➋ *Table 351.2.*

Differential Diagnosis

The differential diagnosis includes both benign and malignant etiologies. Primary renal cancers would include Wilms' tumor, congenital mesoblastic nephroma, clear cell sarcoma of the kidney, rhabdoid tumor of the kidney, and renal cell carcinoma. Neuroblastoma is a childhood cancer often arising from the adrenal gland which is also included in the differential diagnosis. Benign etiologies include polycystic kidney disease, renal abscess, and hydronephrosis.

Treatment

Surgery is required for all patients with Wilms' tumor and other renal tumors. The objective of surgery is to remove the entire tumor without rupturing the tumor capsule. This almost always requires a nephrectomy. In addition, the surgeon can visually examine the abdomen for other suspicious lesions in the lymph nodes and other structures and biopsy as needed. There are two approaches to the timing of surgery. North American practice is to attempt pretreatment resection whenever possible to facilitate careful examination of histologic characteristics before treatment related changes occur. The approach outside of North America has been resection after delivery of some chemotherapy to lessen the risk of intraoperative rupture and facilitate an easier surgical procedure. The results with combined modality therapy are very good with both surgical approaches.

Table 351.2
Staging for Wilms' tumor

Stage	Characteristics
I	• Tumor limited to the kidney and completely resected • Renal capsule intact (no previous biopsy) • No involvement of renal sinus vessels or evidence of tumor beyond the margin of resection
II	• Tumor extends beyond the kidney but is completely resected (margins negative) • One of the following: penetration of renal capsule, invasion of renal sinus vessels
III	• Gross or microscopic tumor remaining • Tumor spillage before or during surgery • Lymph nodes within the abdomen or pelvis involved by tumor • Extension of tumor thrombus within the vena cava • Previous biopsy
IV	• Hematogenous spread or lymph node metastases outside of the abdomen
V	• Bilateral tumor at diagnosis

The surgical approach to bilateral disease is different with a goal to salvage as much renal function as possible. Therefore, patients undergo an initial biopsy and staging of both kidneys with exploration for suspicious lymph nodes or other lesions. Then, preoperative chemotherapy is given to allow for response before surgery is undertaken to remove the tumors and maximize the amount of kidney remaining.

Radiation to the flank is indicated for Stage III tumors. The recommended dose is 10.5 Gy of radiation to the affected flank. Whole abdomen radiation is only indicated for patients who have ascites positive for tumor cells or tumor rupture. Whole lung irradiation at a dose of 12 Gy is recommended for patients presenting with lung metastases seen on diagnostic chest x-ray. Irradiation of other involved metastatic sites, including the brain, liver, bone, and lymph nodes, is also indicated for patients who have metastatic involvement. In patients with anaplasia, clear cell sarcoma or rhabdoid tumor, radiation is recommended for the flank and all involved sites of disease.

For favorable histology Wilms' tumor the treatment regimen involves combined chemotherapy treatment with Vincristine and Dactinomycin for Stage I and II disease with the addition of Doxorubicin for Stage III and IV disease. Cyclophosphamide or cyclophosphamide and etoposide have been studied for patients with stage IV disease, anaplasia, or clear cell sarcoma. The prognosis for rhabdoid tumor and renal cell carcinoma remain poor and no optimal chemotherapy regimen has been determined. The benefit of chemotherapy in the treatment of congenital mesoblastic nephroma is under investigation.

Prognosis

Overall, all stages of Wilms' tumor are highly curable. Specific prognostic considerations are based on tumor size, patient age, histology, lymph node mestastases, and local features. The most important prognostic feature is the presence of anaplasia. Although the outcomes of patients with Stage I disease do not vary significantly according to anaplasia, for all other stages, the presence of anaplasia confers a worsened prognosis. Patients younger than 2 years of age appear to have a much better prognosis than older children.

The prognosis for clear cell sarcoma of the kidney has improved with the addition of chemotherapy agents. Congential mesoblastic nephroma has an excellent prognosis often with surgery alone. The prognosis for rhabdoid tumor of the kidney and renal cell carcinoma remains very poor in children.

Prevention

Screening ultrasound is recommended every 3 months until the age of 8 years for children with recognized syndromes which carry a predisposition for Wilms' tumor.

References

Alessandri JL, Cuillier F, Ramful D et al (2008) Perlman syndrome: report, prenatal findings and review. Am J Med Genet 146A(19): 2532–2537

Auber F, Jeanpierre C, Denamur E et al (2009) Management of Wilms tumours in Drash and Frasier syndromes. Pediatr Blood Cancer 52(1):55–59

Bourdeaut F, Guiochon-Mantel A, Fabre M et al (2008) Alagille syndrome and nephroblastoms: unusual coincidence of two rare disorders. Pediatr Blood Cancer 50(4):908–911

D'Angio GJ (2007) The National Wilms Tumor Study: a 40 year perspective. Lifetime Data Anal 13(4):463–470

Davidoff AM (2009) Wilms' tumor. Curr Opin Pediatr 21(3):357–364

Dome JS, Perlman EJ, Ritchey ML et al (2006) Renal tumors. In: Pizzo PA, Poplack DG (eds) Principles and practice of pediatric oncology, 5th edn. Lippincott Williams and Wilkins, Philadelphia

Green DM (2007) Controversies in the management of Wilms tumour-immediate nephrectomy or delayed nephrectomy? Eur J Cancer 43(17):2453–2456

Hartkamp J, Roberts SG (2008) The role of the Wilms' tumour-suppressor protein WT1 in apoptosis. Biochem Soc Trans 36(Pt 4):629–631

Jain D, Hui P, McNamara J et al (2001) Bloom syndrome in sibs: first reports of hepatocellular carcinoma and Wilms tumor with documented anaplasia and nephrogenic rests. Pediatr Dev Pathol 4(6):585–589

James A, Culver K, Golabi M (2006) Simpson-Golabi-Behemel syndrome. In: Pagon RA, Bird TC, Dolan CR et al (eds) GeneReviews. University of Washington, Seattle

Lee H, Khan R, O'Keefe M (2008) Aniridia: current pathology and management. Acta Ophthalmol 86(7):708–715

Morrison AA, Viney RL, Ladomery MR (2008) The post-transcriptional roles of WT1, a multifunctional zinc-finger protein. Biochim Biophys Acta 1785(1):55–62

Mueller RF (1994) The Denys-Drash syndrome. J Med Genet 31(6): 471–476

Rao A, Rothman J, Nichols KE (2008) Genetic testing and tumor surveillance for children with cancer predisposition syndromes. Curr Opin Pediatr 20(1):1–7

Shaw J (2008) Trisomy 18: a case study. Neonatal Netw 27(1):33–41

Tan TY, Amor DJ (2006) Tumour surveillance in Beckwith-Wiedemann syndrome and hemihyperplasia: a critical review of the evidence and suggested guidelines for local practice. J Paediatr Child Health 42(9):486–490

Tatton-Brown K, Rahman N (2007) Sotos syndrome. Eur J Hum Genet 15(3):264–267

Van den Heuvel-Eibrink MM, Grundy P, Graf N et al (2008) Characteristics and survival of 750 children diagnosed with a renal tumor in the first 7 months of life: a collaborative study by the SIOP/GPOH/SFOP, NWTSG, and UKCCSG Wilms Tumor Study Groups. Pediatr Blood Cancer 50(6):1130–1134

Vujanic GM, Sandstedt B (2010) The pathology of Wilms' tumour (nephroblastoma): the International Society of Paediatric Oncology approach. J Clin Pathol 63(2):102–109

Zhuge Y, Cheung MC, Yang R et al (2010) Pediatric non-Wilms renal tumors: subtypes, survival, and prognostic indicators. J Surg Res [epub April 21]

352 Hepatic Tumors

H. Stacy Nicholson · Suman Malempati

Introduction

Primary liver tumors are rare in children, and in the USA, occur at a rate of 1.8 per million before the age of 15 years. In infants and children less than 5 years of age, hepatoblastoma (HB) accounts for nearly all liver tumors, and hepatocellular carcinoma (HCC) becomes more common in older children; HCC is the primary hepatic tumor in adolescents. In areas where Hepatitis B is prevalent, the incidence of primary liver tumors in children is higher, and the relative proportion of tumors that are HCC is higher. Benign primary liver tumors also occur and include hemangiomas and hamartomas. The liver is also a common site for metastases of other childhood malignancies, including neuroblastoma. This chapter focuses on the malignant hepatic tumors.

Pathology

Diagnosis is made by histopathological examination of the resected tumor or biopsy. HB is further divided into pure fetal, embryonal, or mixed fetal-embryonal histology. Alpha-fetoprotein (AFP), the predominant protein in serum before birth, is produced by embryonic hepatocytes and remains present for the first few months of life; thus, one must take care in interpreting AFP levels in infants. Serum AFP is elevated in 40% of children with HCC and in nearly all patients with HB. AFP should be measured at diagnosis in all patients, and if elevated, should be followed during treatment and follow-up. Normal or low AFP levels at the diagnosis of HB is associated with worse prognosis.

Clinical Features

Hepatoblastoma most commonly occurs in infants and very young children. Patients typically present with an abdominal mass, most often noted by a parent or physician. However, children with advanced disease may also present with abdominal pain, malaise, and weight loss. Jaundice is rare, and when present, suggests a primary hepatobiliary tumor, such as rhabdomyosarcoma.

Diagnostic Studies and Staging

Ultrasound is often used as the initial imaging modality in a child with an abdominal mass; however, computerized tomography (CT) or magnetic resonance imaging (MRI) of the abdomen is needed to define the extent of the mass and its relationship to hepatic landmarks. The importance of this imaging cannot be overemphasized, as surgical planning will be dependent upon this information. Abdominal radiographs are rarely helpful. All patients should be evaluated for metastases with a chest X-ray (CXR) and CT of the lungs.

Treatment

Once the imaging studies indicate a primary hepatic tumor, a team approach to treatment planning, involving the pediatric surgeon and pediatric oncologist, ensures that a coordinated plan for surgery and chemotherapy is in place. Radiotherapy is of limited use and is typically limited to a few children with unresectable disease or following recurrence.

Surgery

For patients with HB and HCC, complete resection is necessary for cure. Patients who undergo primary complete resection of HB have an excellent prognosis with a 90% long-term survival rate. However, only one-third to one-half of liver tumors in children can be safely resected at initial diagnosis. For children with hepatoblastoma, chemotherapy can induce significant tumor shrinkage, which may allow a tumor becoming resectable in up to two-thirds of patients. Chemotherapy is less effective for HCC. In children without metastatic disease but whose primary tumor remains unresectable, liver transplantation can be curative. Finally, in some patients, surgical excision of pulmonary metastases has improved survival.

Abdelaziz Y. Elzouki (ed.), *Textbook of Clinical Pediatrics*, DOI 10.1007/978-3-642-02202-9_352,

Chemotherapy

Cisplatin-based chemotherapy has greatly improved the survival of children with HB, and the use of combination chemotherapy is recommended for most children with HB or HCC, including those who have had a complete resection. In addition, chemotherapy may make a previously unresectable tumor amenable to surgery. Chemotherapy is not necessary for children with resectable pure fetal histology HB, as complete surgical resection alone is curative. Agents with the most activity against HB include doxorubicin, cisplatin, 5-fluorouracil, and vincristine, which are commonly used in combination. While similar approaches are used in both HB and HCC, HCC is much less chemosensitive.

Prognosis

Prognosis is related to the extent of disease at diagnosis, the histologic subtype, and whether the tumor can be surgically excised. Multi-modality therapy has resulted in long-term survival rates in excess of 75%.

References

Czauderna P, Otte JB et al (2005) Guidelines for surgical treatment of hepatoblastoma in the modern era–recommendations from the Childhood Liver Tumour Strategy Group of the International Society of Paediatric Oncology (SIOPEL). Eur J Cancer 41:1031–1036

Haas JE, Muczynski KA et al (1989) Histopathology and prognosis in childhood hepatoblastoma and hepatocarcinoma. Cancer 64: 1082–1095

http//seer.cancer.gov

Li J, Thompson TD et al (2008) Cancer incidence among children and adolescents in the United States, 2001–2003. Pediatrics 121: e1470–e1477

Perilongo G, Shafford E et al (2004) Risk-adapted treatment for childhood hepatoblastoma. Final report of the second study of the International Society of Paediatric Oncology–SIOPEL 2. Eur J Cancer 40:411–421

Wolf AD, Lavine JE (2000) Hepatomegaly in neonates and children. Pediatr Rev 21:303–310

353 Soft Tissue Sarcomas

Suman Malempati · H. Stacy Nicholson

Introduction

As a group, soft tissue sarcomas are the most common solid tumor in children outside the central nervous system (CNS). In general, these tumors arise from the primitive embryonic mesenchyme, and include neoplasms of muscle, connective tissue, supportive tissue, and vascular tissue. Tumors may arise anywhere in the body where these tissues occur, but are most commonly seen in the extremities, head and neck regions, and genitourinary tract. Rhabdomyosarcoma is the most common soft tissue sarcoma in children and is the primary focus of this chapter.

Rhabdomyosarcoma

The cause of rhabdomyosarcoma is unknown; however, improved understanding of its biology may lead to an improved understanding of its etiology and to new treatments. The annual incidence in the USA in children less than 20 years of age is 4.3 cases per million. Rhabdomyosarcoma occurs in all ages, from birth to adulthood, but there are two distinct age peaks. Two-third of cases of rhabdomyosarcoma are diagnosed in children less than 6 years of age, but a second peak occurs in adolescents between the ages of 14 and 18 years. Adolescents with rhabdomyosarcoma are more likely to have tumors of the extremities. Rhabdomyosarcoma is slightly more common in males, and compared to Caucasians, rates are lower in African-Americans and in Asian populations. Rhabdomyosarcoma occurs more frequently in certain familial cancer predisposition syndromes, including Li–Fraumeni, neurofibromatosis type 1, and Gardner syndrome.

Histologic Types and Histopathology

Rhabdomyosarcoma is one of the "small round blue cell" tumors of childhood, and requires a skilled pathologist to confirm the diagnosis. The primary histopathological subtypes are embryonal (including botryoid), alveolar, and pleomorphic histologies. Alveolar rhabdomyosarcoma is associated with a specific chromosomal translocation, t(2;13), resulting in Pax3-FOXO fusion transcription factor that drives pathogenesis. Alveolar rhabdomyosarcoma more commonly occurs in extremity sites in adolescents and young adults and is associated with a worse prognosis. Pleomorphic rhabdomyosarcoma typically occurs in adults and can be very difficult to treat.

Clinical Features

Although rhabdomyosarcoma is a tumor of primitive skeletal muscle cells, it can occur in sites in the body that do not normally contain skeletal muscle. Common sites of involvement are the head and neck region (orbit, nasopharynx, sinuses, and superficial face), the genitourinary tract (bladder, vagina, and testis), extremities, and the trunk including retroperitoneum. Adolescents with rhabdomyosarcoma are more likely to have tumors of the extremities.

Signs and symptoms depend upon the site of the primary tumor. Head and neck tumors may present with pain, proptosis, orbital swelling, nasal obstruction, sinusitis, epistaxis, dysphasia, or hoarseness. Acquired denasalized speech, asymptomatic serous otitis media, persistent earache or aural discharge or unexplained facial palsy should raise the suspicion about such tumors. Approximately 25% of head and neck rhabdomyosarcoma in children occur in the orbit, and 50% occur in parameningeal regions.

Hematuria or urinary retention may be the presenting symptoms of tumors arising in the bladder or prostate, which are common sites in young children. Vaginal rhabdomyosarcoma, often called botryoides, due to the characteristic grapelike cluster of tumor may present with bloody mucoid discharge in young girls before a mass is seen. Paratesticular tumors are usually painless and can be mistaken for hydroceles. Patients with rhabdomyosarcoma of the extremities typically present with a painless mass.

Abdelaziz Y. Elzouki (ed.), *Textbook of Clinical Pediatrics*, DOI 10.1007/978-3-642-02202-9_353,

Diagnostic Studies and Staging

Diagnosis is made by histopathological examination of a tumor or biopsy, and all patients need to be evaluated for metastases. Rhabdomyosarcoma may involve regional lymph nodes, and distant spread most often involves the lungs, bone, and bone marrow. Imaging of the primary site may involve X-rays, computerized tomography (CT), and/or magnetic resonance imaging (MRI). To evaluate for metastases, CT scanning of the chest, abdomen and pelvis, bone scan, and bone marrow biopsies are typically done. Imaging of regional lymph nodes is important and lymph node sampling may be necessary for complete staging. For parameningeal tumors, a lumbar puncture should be performed to evaluate CSF cytology. Correct staging is important in assigning treatment and in counseling the patients and families about prognosis.

Treatment

Treatment needs to be assigned based on site, histology, and extent of metastatic spread. The clinical grouping system developed by the Intergroup Rhabdomyosarcoma Study (*Table 353.1*) is used to assign treatment, which generally includes surgery and chemotherapy, with or without radiotherapy.

Table 353.1
Intergroup rhabdomyosarcoma study clinical grouping system

Group	
I	Localized disease, completely resected. Regional nodes not involved. No metastases. (a) Confined to the muscle or organ of origin. (b) Infiltration outside the muscle or organ of origin – continuous with primary tumor.
II	(a) Grossly resected tumor with microscopic residual disease. No lymph node involvement; no metastases. (b) Regional disease, completely resected. Lymph nodes can be positive or negative; no metastases. (c) Regional disease with completely resected involved lymph nodes, with microscopic residual disease; no metastases.
III	Incomplete resection or biopsy. Gross residual disease is present.
IV	Metastatic disease present at onset.

Surgery

When the primary tumor can be surgically removed with negative margins, that is the preferred initial approach. However, tumors at many sites, including most head and neck tumors, cannot be completely excised and are simply biopsied. The initial surgical approach is key in assigning patients to the appropriate clinical group (*Table 353.1*).

Radiotherapy

External beam radiation is used in combination with surgery and chemotherapy in most patients with rhabdomyosarcoma. However, if the initial surgery results in a complete resection with negative margins, radiation may not be needed. Conversely, if only a biopsy is performed at diagnosis, radiation is often part of the treatment plan, even if a second surgery results in a complete resection. Doses are typically between 3,600 to 5,000 cGy.

Chemotherapy

The use of combination chemotherapy with vincristine, actinomycin-D, and cyclophosphamide (VAC) has improved the survival rates for children with rhabdomyosarcoma and has been the standard since the 1970s. VAC chemotherapy is typically given every 3 weeks and the duration of therapy depends upon clinical group and histology. Patients with embryonal histology occurring in "favorable" sites may be treated with vincristine and actinomycin-D alone. There are other active chemotherapy drugs in rhabdomyosarcoma, but addition of these agents has generally not improved survival compared to VAC. As more is understood about the biology of rhabdomyosarcoma, targeted therapy will increasingly be studied and may be added to combination therapy with surgery, chemotherapy, and radiation.

Prognosis

Prognosis varies by histology, clinical group, and, increasingly, molecular characterization. Patients with Group I disease have a 5-year survival rate that exceeds 90%. At the other end of the spectrum, those with Group IV disease (distant metastases) have a 5-year survival rate of approximately 25%. Favorable sites include orbital and paratesticular tumors, and masses in the trunk and extremities typically have a worse prognosis.

Other Soft Tissue Sarcomas

Other soft tissue sarcomas that occur in children include synovial sarcoma, malignant peripheral nerve sheath tumor, undifferentiated sarcoma, fibrosarcoma, liposarcoma, leiomyosarcoma, and others. These tumors typically arise in the extremities and trunk, and, unlike rhabdomyosarcoma, are unusual in the head and neck. Non-rhabdomyosarcomatous soft tissue sarcoma (NRSTS) usually presents as a painless mass. NRSTS can occur as secondary malignancies within a field of prior radiation in patients previously treated for cancer. While the surgical approach is similar to that used for rhabdomyosarcoma, these tumors are typically less susceptible to chemotherapy in particular. These tumors also vary in degree of aggressiveness and propensity to spread. The rarity of these tumors has impaired the ability to conduct robust clinical trials, and surgeons and oncologists must collaborate closely in determining the best treatment approach for each patient.

References

Arndt CA, Crist WM (1999) Common musculoskeletal tumors of childhood and adolescence. N Engl J Med 341(5):342–352

Dagher R, Helman L (1999) Rhabdomyosarcoma: an overview. Oncologist 4(1):34–44

Gurney JG, Young JL Jr, Roffers SD et al (1999) Soft tissue sarcomas. In: Ries LAG, Smith MA, Gurney JG et al (eds) Cancer incidence and survival among children and adolescents: United States SEER Program 1975–1995, NIH Pub. No. 99-4649. National Cancer Institute, SEER Program, 111, Bethesda

Raney RB, Anderson JR et al (2001) Rhabdomyosarcoma and undifferentiated sarcoma in the first two decades of life: a selective review of intergroup rhabdomyosarcoma study group experience and rationale for Intergroup Rhabdomyosarcoma Study V. J Pediatr Hematol Oncol 23(4):215–220

Stiller CA, Parkin DM (1994) International variations in the incidence of childhood soft tissue sarcomas. Paediatr Perinat Epidemiol 8: 107–119

Stiller CA, McKinney PA, Bunch KJ et al (1991) Childhood cancer and ethnig groups in Britain: a United Kingdom Children's Cancer Group (UKCCSG) study. Br J Cancer 64:543–548

354 Primary Malignant Tumors of Bone

Suman Malempati

Introduction

As a group, malignant bone tumors account for 5% of all cancers in children (age 0–19 years) in the USA. The vast majority of bone cancers that occur in the pediatric population are osteosarcoma and Ewing sarcoma. Both of these are aggressive high-grade malignancies that are diagnosed most frequently in the second decade of life. Chondrosarcoma can occur in children, but is much less common. There are a variety of nonmalignant conditions from which bone malignancies must be distinguished.

Epidemiology

Osteosarcoma is the most common malignant tumor of bone with an annual incidence rate of approximately five cases per million children in the USA. The incidence of osteosarcoma is similar in many Western European countries, but tends to be lower in Asian and many African countries. The annual incidence of Ewing sarcoma is approximately 3/million children in the USA, and is almost exclusively diagnosed in Caucasians. Ewing sarcoma very rarely occurs in persons of African or Asian descent. There is a slight male predominance of both osteosarcoma and Ewing sarcoma. Chondrosarcoma is diagnosed much less frequently with an annual incidence rate of 0.3–0.4/million children.

The peak incidence of malignant bone tumors is during the second decade of life. Both osteosarcoma and Ewing sarcoma are most commonly diagnosed around the time of the adolescent growth spurt. The average age of onset for Ewing sarcoma is younger than for osteosarcoma. In contrast to osteosarcoma, which very rarely occurs before the age of 8, Ewing sarcoma may be diagnosed in younger children and infants. Both Ewing sarcoma and osteosarcoma also occur in young adults in the 3rd and 4th decades of life. Osteosarcoma diagnosed in older adults is typically associated with previous radiation exposure.

Pathogenesis

The cause of bone malignancies is unknown in most cases. However, a variety of genetic and environmental factors predispose patients to the development of osteosarcoma (➲ *Table 354.1*). Hereditary retinoblastoma with germline mutations of loss of the Rb tumor suppressor gene, germline p53 mutations (Li-Fraumeni syndrome), and Rothmund–Thompson syndrome are all associated with a very high risk of osteosarcoma. In addition, children with Paget's disease of bone and osteogenesis imperfecta, and those who have been exposed to ionizing radiation have a higher incidence of osteosarcoma.

In contrast, Ewing sarcoma is not typically associated with radiation exposure or cancer predisposition syndromes. The pathogenesis of Ewing sarcoma is related to chimeric proteins that are the result of recurrent translocations involving the *ews* gene at 22q12 locus and members of the *ets* family of transcription factors. It is now known that the EWS-ETS fusion proteins play an essential role in the tumorigenesis of Ewing sarcoma.

Clinical Manifestations

The most common presenting symptom in patients diagnosed with bone tumors is pain with or without swelling at the involved site. Initially, the pain is often intermittent, but becomes more constant and more severe over time. There is often a history of trauma at the onset of symptoms, but there is no evidence that trauma is causative. The trauma likely draws the patient's and caregiver's attention to the affected site. Patients eventually diagnosed with bone tumors are often initially treated with rest, ice and anti-inflammatory medication for presumed injury. It is common for there to be delay of several months from onset of symptoms to diagnosis of a bone tumor. A malignant bone tumor should be suspected with any "pathologic fracture" that occurs in an unusual site or after seemingly minor trauma. Systemic symptoms such

Abdelaziz Y. Elzouki (ed.), *Textbook of Clinical Pediatrics*, DOI 10.1007/978-3-642-02202-9_354,

Table 354.1
Conditions associated with increased risk of osteosarcoma

• Hereditary retinoblastoma
• Li-Fraumeni syndrome
• Rothmund–Thompson syndrome
• Bloom syndrome
• Werner syndrome
• Paget disease
• Enchondromatosis
• Osteogenesis imperfecta

Table 354.2
Conditions that mimic malignant bone tumors

Infections
• Osteomyelitis
Benign lesions
• Osteoid osteoma
• Chondroblastoma
• Osteochondroma
• Aneurysmal bone cyst
• Langerhans cell histiocytosis (Eosinophilic granuloma)
Other malignancies
• Lymphoma
• Metastatic small round blue cell tumor

as fever and weight loss may be seen, particularly with Ewing sarcoma.

Osteosarcoma typically arises at the metaphyses of long bones, with almost one-half of primary tumors occurring around the knee joint (distal femur or proximal tibia). The proximal humerus is the next most common site. In contrast, Ewing sarcoma more commonly occurs in flat bones. When long bones are affected with Ewing sarcoma, the diaphyses are usually the involved sites rather than the metaphyses. The bones of the pelvis are the most frequently involved sites of Ewing sarcoma, accounting for approximately 25% of cases.

Diagnostic Evaluation

The initial evaluation of patients with suspected bone tumors should include a thorough history and physical examination. Signs and symptoms may be nonspecific. *Table 354.2* lists a variety of conditions that mimic

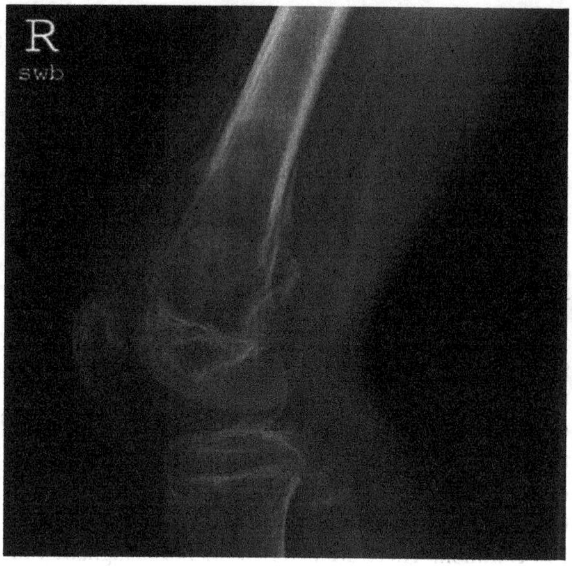

Figure 354.1
Lateral radiograph of the knee showing "Codman's triangle" resulting from elevation of periosteum from underlying bone

malignant bone tumors. A history of fever, weight loss, and/or night sweats should alert the physician to the possibility of cancer, although patients with bone tumors often have no symptoms other than pain. Suspected bone tumors must be distinguished from injuries. Injury-associated pain usually gets better with rest, whereas pain due to a malignant bone tumor does not remit and progressively worsens over time. Pain that is severe enough to wake a child or adolescent from sleep deserves further evaluation. Physical exam reveals tenderness at the involved site. There is also often a soft-tissue mass associated with primary tumors of bone.

The initial radiographic evaluation should be a plain radiograph of the involved bone. Plain x-ray will show a destructive lesion in the involved bone with disruption of the cortex. A classic radiographic finding in osteosarcoma and Ewing sarcoma, known as "Codman triangle," results from elevation and detachment of periosteum from bone along with subperiosteal new bone formation (*Fig. 354.1*). A "sunburst" periosteal reaction is often seen in osteosarcoma due to a rapidly growing mass (*Fig. 354.2*).

In order to better determine the extent of bone involvement of a suspected bone tumor, either magnetic resonance imaging (MRI) or computed tomography (CT) is necessary. In regard to surgical planning, MRI is more accurate and useful for evaluating intraosseus tumor

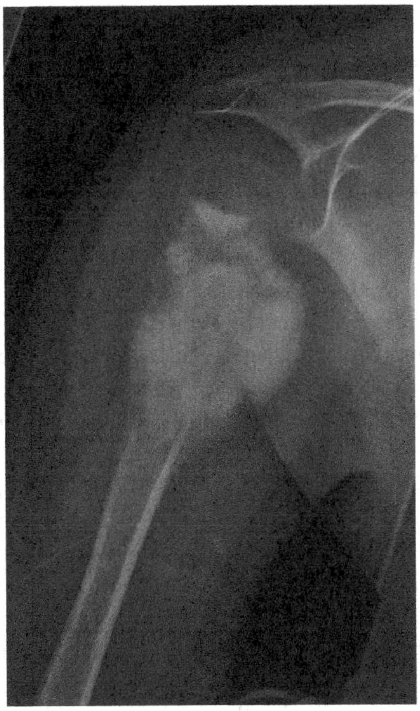

Figure 354.2
Radiograph showing the classic "Sunburst" pattern of periosteal reaction in a patient with osteosarcoma of the proximal humerus

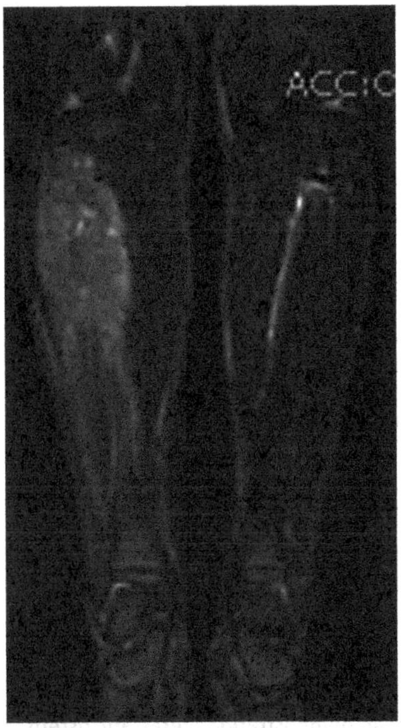

Figure 354.3
T1-weighted MRI image of Ewing sarcoma of the fibula with large soft-tissue component

extent, joint involvement, subcutaneous fat planes, and association with neurovascular structures (➋ *Fig. 354.3*).

Evaluation for distant metastases is critical. Approximately 20–25% of patients with Ewing sarcoma and osteosarcoma have detectable metastases at diagnosis. The most common site of metastases is the lungs. While plain radiographs of the chest can often detect metastatic lesions, chest CT scan is considerably more sensitive (➋ *Fig. 354.4*). Radionuclide bone scan (technetium-99m) is also standard in the USA for detection of bone metastases, which occur in approximately 10% of patients with newly diagnosed malignant bone tumors. In addition, approximately 10% of patients with Ewing sarcoma will have detectable metastases to bone marrow. Therefore, bone marrow biopsies from bilateral posterior iliac crests are critical.

While presenting signs and symptoms, location and pattern of the lesion, and characteristic findings on imaging may suggest the presence of a malignant bone tumor, definitive diagnosis requires biopsy and histologic assessment. The approach to the biopsy is critical as the biopsy tract will also need to be resected at the time of surgical resection. Biopsy without consideration of planning for the definitive local control surgery can hinder the ability to perform a future limb-salvage procedure in the patient.

Histologic evaluation of conventional osteosarcoma reveals a high-grade malignant lesion with large spindle-shaped cells, irregular nuclei, and mitotic figures intermixed with a stroma containing areas of osteoid. Conventional high-grade osteosarcoma is often further characterized as osteoblastic, chondroblastic, or fibroblastic based on the pattern of differentiation. This distinction, however, is clinically meaningless. Other variants that are similar to conventional osteosarcoma include telangiectatic, small cell, and periosteal osteosarcoma. An additional variant, parosteal osteosarcoma, is similar to periosteal in that it arises from the cortex of bone, but does not invade into the medullary cavity. Parosteal osteosarcoma tends to behave more indolently than conventional osteosarcoma and does not metastasize.

Ewing sarcoma is one of the "small round blue cell tumors" of childhood. It can be distinguished from rhabdomyosarcoma, neuroblastoma, and lymphoma based on the pattern of histochemical staining. The pattern of staining shows some evidence of neural differentiation with typical expression of CD99, S-100, and neuron-specific enolase.

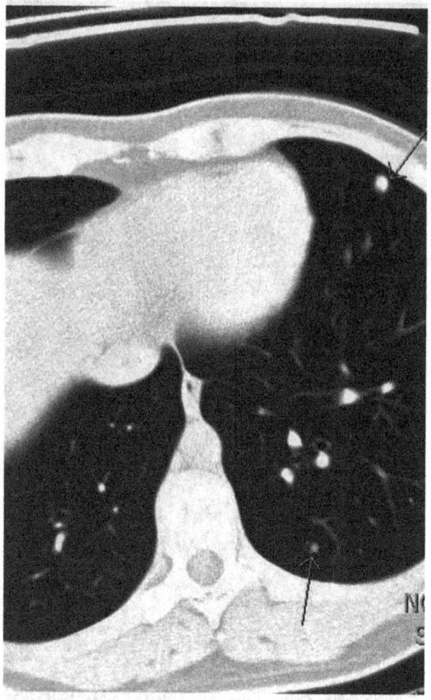

Figure 354.4
Chest CT scan demonstrating metastatic osteosarcoma

Fluorescent in situ hybridization or chromosome analysis of tumor cells is critical to assess for rearrangements of the *ews* gene on chromosome 22, which can be detected in more than 95% of cases of Ewing sarcoma. The most common rearrangement is the characteristic t(11;22)(q24;q12) reciprocal translocation, which results in the chimeric EWS-FLI1 transcription factor. Presence of this translocation is pathognomic for Ewing sarcoma.

Treatment and Prognosis

Treatment of malignant bone tumors involves both systemic and local therapy. Significant improvements have been made in both systemic therapies as well local control techniques over the past few decades. Currently, at least two-thirds of patients with Ewing sarcoma and osteosarcoma without detectable metastatic disease can be cured. A comparison of clinical features, treatment, and prognosis between Ewing sarcoma and osteosarcoma is shown in *Table 354.3*.

Osteosarcoma

Since the 1970s, chemotherapy has been a vital component to the treatment of patients with osteosarcoma. Prior to the use of chemotherapy, survival rate with surgical resection alone was less than 20%. Most patients died from metastatic disease to lungs. Neo-adjuvant chemotherapy is now standard. Chemotherapy given before surgical resection allows for early initiation of systemic control as well as the histologic assessment of tumor necrosis in response to chemotherapy. Degree of tumor necrosis after initial chemotherapy has been shown to be prognostic, as patients with 10% or greater viable tumor at the time of definitive surgery have a significantly higher risk of recurrence.

Chemotherapeutic agents that are most active against osteosarcoma are doxorubicin, cisplatin, methotrexate, and ifosfamide. Standard therapy in North America and Europe involve combinations of these agents before and after definitive surgery. While chemotherapy has improved prognosis, complete surgical resection of all tumor with clear margins remains essential for cure. Amputation has been a traditional approach and remains effective. However, improved surgical techniques and neo-adjuvant chemotherapy allow a higher proportion of patients to undergo limb-sparing procedures (*Fig. 354.5*). Radiation therapy is not considered a viable option for local control as osteosarcoma tumors are relatively radioresistant. However, for tumors that not resectable (such as primary tumors of the pelvis), radiation therapy can be effective as palliation.

Patients who present with metastatic disease have a poor prognosis. Less than 20% of patients with metastatic disease will be long-term survivors. Along with standard chemotherapy, local control to all metastatic sites, including pulmonary metastatecomy, is critical to offer any chance of long-term cure.

Patients diagnosed with parosteal osteosarcoma have a much more favorable prognosis with complete surgical resection alone. These tumors can recur locally without complete resection with wide margins, but metastatic spread is not typically seen. These patients can be treated without chemotherapy.

Ewing Sarcoma

Current treatment for Ewing sarcoma involves multimodal therapy. Neo-adjuvant chemotherapy is now standard. For patients with localized disease, the addition of Ifosfamide and Etoposide to Vincristine, Doxorubicin, and Cyclophosphamide has been shown to improve survival. Dose intensity is critical and a recent study has shown that delivering the agents on a compressed every 2 week schedule is more effective at preventing disease recurrence.

Table 354.3
Comparison of osteosarcoma and Ewing sarcoma

	Osteosarcoma	Ewing sarcoma
Annual incidence rate (age 0–19 in Western countries)	~5/million	~3/million
Race	All races	Caucasian (rare in persons of African or Asian descent)
Primary tumor site	Metaphyses of long bones	Flat bones
		Diaphyses of long bones
		Extraskeletal
Radiographic signs	"Sunburst"	"Onion-skinning"
	Sclerotic destruction	Lytic lesion
Treatment	Chemotherapy	Chemotherapy
	Surgery	Surgery
		Radiation
Prognosis (long-term survival)		
Localized	~65%	~75%
Metastatic	<20%	~20–30%

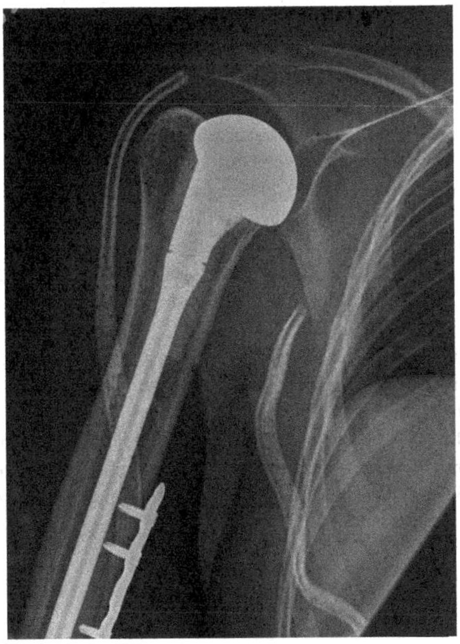

Figure 354.5
Radiograph demonstrating limb salvage surgery with reconstruction using a composite allograft/metal prosthesis

As with osteosarcoma, local control is also critical. In general, complete surgical resection with clear margins is considered the most effective means of local control. However, Ewing sarcoma is much more radiosensitive than osteosarcoma. Therefore, radiation therapy may be an effective means of local control if the alternative would be a mutilating operative surgery. Prognosis depends on site of primary tumor and presence of metastatic disease. Up to 75% of patients with localized extremity tumors can be cured. Patients with centrally located tumors (such as in the pelvis) and those with metastatic disease have poorer outcomes.

Chondrosarcoma

The only known curative therapy for chondrosarcoma is surgical resection. Chemotherapy has no proven benefit in regard to preventing recurrence if complete surgical resection is achieved. Prognosis is poor for patients in whom surgical resection cannot be achieved. Chemotherapy and radiation therapy may be used to slow tumor progression, but neither modality has been shown to affect long-term outcome.

Summary and Future Directions

As malignant tumors of bone are relatively uncommon in children, diagnosis can be difficult. Both Ewing sarcoma and osteosarcoma most commonly occur in adolescents during the second decade of life. While there is a higher incidence of osteosarcoma in some familial cancer predisposition syndromes and after radiation exposure, the etiology of most cases of bone tumors is unknown. Bone malignancy should be suspected for persistent pain, swelling, and palpable mass as well as if a pathologic fracture occurs. The outlook for patients with malignant bone tumors has improved considerably with multimodal therapy. Future advances in treatment will likely include better risk stratification of patients based on tumor biology, improved local control techniques (both surgical and radiation therapy), and the incorporation of molecular targeted therapies into current treatment plans.

References

Arndt CA, Crist WM (1999) Common musculoskeletal tumors of childhood and adolescence. N Engl J Med 341(5):342–352

Bernstein M, Kovar H et al (2006) Ewing sarcoma family of tumors: Ewing sarcoma of bone and soft tissue and the peipheral primitive neuroectodermal tumors. In: Pizzo PA, Poplack DG (eds) Principles and practice of pediatric oncology. Lippincott Williams and Wilkins, Philadelphia

Dunst J, Schuck A (2004) Role of radiotherapy in Ewing tumors. Pediatr Blood Cancer 42(5):465–470

Eyre R, Feltbower RG et al (2009a) Epidemiology of bone tumours in children and young adults. Pediatr Blood Cancer 53(6):941–952

Eyre R, Feltbower RG et al (2009b) Incidence and survival of childhood bone cancer in northern England and the West Midlands, 1981–2002. Br J Cancer 100(1):188–193

Ferrari S, Palmerini E (2007) Adjuvant and neoadjuvant combination chemotherapy for osteogenic sarcoma. Curr Opin Oncol 19(4): 341–346

Fuchs N, Bielack SS et al (1998) Long-term results of the co-operative German-Austrian-Swiss osteosarcoma study group's protocol COSS-86 of intensive multidrug chemotherapy and surgery for osteosarcoma of the limbs. Ann Oncol 9(8):893–899

Gorlick R, Anderson P et al (2003) Biology of childhood osteogenic sarcoma and potential targets for therapeutic development: meeting summary. Clin Cancer Res 9(15):5442–5453

Grier HE (1997) The Ewing family of tumors. Ewing's sarcoma and primitive neuroectodermal tumors. Pediatr Clin North Am 44(4):991–1004

Grier HE, Krailo MD et al (2003) Addition of ifosfamide and etoposide to standard chemotherapy for Ewing's sarcoma and primitive neuroectodermal tumor of bone. N Engl J Med 348(8):694–701

Grimer RJ, Carter SR et al (1999) Osteosarcoma of the pelvis. J Bone Joint Surg Br 81(5):796–802

Han I, Oh JH et al (2008) Clinical outcome of parosteal osteosarcoma. J Surg Oncol 97(2):146–149

Kim HJ, Chalmers PN et al (2010) Pediatric osteogenic sarcoma. Curr Opin Pediatr 22(1):61–66

Klein MJ, Siegal GP (2006) Osteosarcoma: anatomic and histologic variants. Am J Clin Pathol 125(4):555–581

Li J, Thompson TD et al (2008) Cancer incidence among children and adolescents in the United States, 2001–2003. Pediatrics 121(6): e1470–e1477

Link MP, Gebhardt MC et al (2006) Osteosarcoma. In: Pizzo PA, Poplack DG (eds) Principles and practice of pediatric oncology. Lippincott Williams and Wilkins, Philadelphia

Mahajan A, Woo SY et al (2008) Multimodality treatment of osteosarcoma: radiation in a high-risk cohort. Pediatr Blood Cancer 50(5):976–982

Mialou V, Philip T et al (2005) Metastatic osteosarcoma at diagnosis: prognostic factors and long-term outcome – the French pediatric experience. Cancer 104(5):1100–1109

Nagarajan R, Neglia JP et al (2002) Limb salvage and amputation in survivors of pediatric lower-extremity bone tumors: what are the long-term implications? J Clin Oncol 20(22):4493–4501

Provisor AJ, Ettinger LJ et al (1997) Treatment of nonmetastatic osteosarcoma of the extremity with preoperative and postoperative chemotherapy: a report from the Children's Cancer Group. J Clin Oncol 15(1):76–84

Rodriguez-Galindo C, Spunt SL et al (2003) Treatment of Ewing sarcoma family of tumors: current status and outlook for the future. Med Pediatr Oncol 40(5):276–287

Stiller CA, Bielack SS et al (2006) Bone tumours in European children and adolescents, 1978–1997. Report from the Automated Childhood Cancer Information System project. Eur J Cancer 42(13):2124–2135

van den Berg H, Dirksen U et al (2008) Ewing tumors in infants. Pediatr Blood Cancer 50(4):761–764

Wittig JC, Bickels J et al (2002) Osteosarcoma: a multidisciplinary approach to diagnosis and treatment. Am Fam Physician 65(6):1123–1132

Womer RB, Daller RT et al (2000) Granulocyte colony stimulating factor permits dose intensification by interval compression in the treatment of Ewing's sarcomas and soft tissue sarcomas in children. Eur J Cancer 36(1):87–94

355 Retinoblastoma

H. Stacy Nicholson

Retinoblastoma (RB) is a highly malignant tumor of the retina, occurring in infants and young children. Many cases are probably congenital, and RB occurs in 1 of 18,000 live births in the USA. RB can be either genetic or sporadic. Familial RB occurs at an earlier age and is often bilateral. It can be inherited from a parent, usually in an autosomal dominant fashion, or can develop from spontaneous mutations. An estimated 15% of unilateral RB is genetic, with the remainder being sporadic. The RB1 gene is located at 13q14.

Histology

Retinoblastoma is one of the embryonal neoplasms of childhood. Often the histological examination shows sheets of malignant cells, similar to other small round blue cell tumors. The degree of retinal differentiation varies.

Clinical Features

The most common presentation is of leukocoria, or of a "white reflex." Sometimes, the child may present with a "squint." Untreated, RB will cause complete loss of vision, globe destruction, and direct extension into the orbit, orbital bones, and central nervous system. Metastases can occur in lymph nodes, bone, and bone marrow (➔ *Figs.355.1* and ➔ *355.2*).

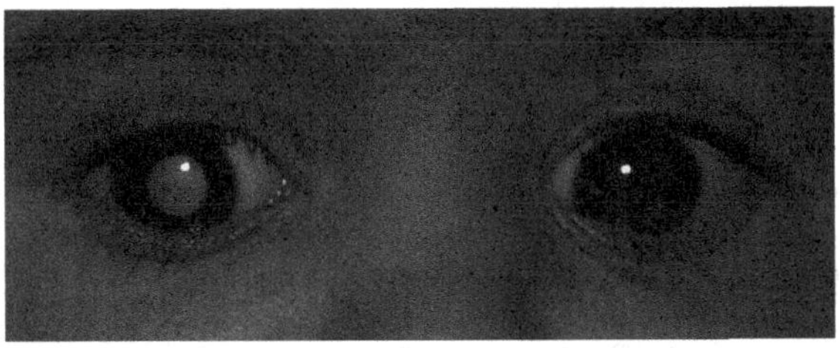

◘ Figure 355.1
Leukocoria in a 3-year-old girl with newly diagnosed unilateral retinoblastoma (Courtesy of Tim Stout, MD, PhD)

Diagnostic Studies and Staging

The diagnosis is initially established by an examination of the retina under anesthesia by an ophthalmologist. Biopsy is not done, in order to prevent seeding of the orbit. To assess the degree of tumor, orbital ultrasound or computerized tomography (CT) may be used. In patients with suspected optic nerve invasion or extensive choroidal invasion, a magnetic resonance image (MRI) of the orbits and brain should be obtained, as well as cerebrospinal fluid (CSF) for cytology. The MRI should show whether the pineal gland also is involved – this is known as "trilateral" retinoblastoma. Bone scan and bone marrow aspirates should be performed if distant metastases are suspected clinically.

Treatment

Treatment needs to be individualized and may involve surgery, cryotherapy and photocoagulation, radiation, and/or chemotherapy. Close collaboration between the pediatric ophthalmologist and pediatric oncologist in creating an individualized treatment plan is needed.

Surgery and Other Local Therapies

For advanced RB, enucleation is the treatment of choice. This includes tumors with invasion of the optic nerve, choroid or obits, as well as anterior chamber invasion. In small tumors that are away from the macula, cryotherapy, thermotherapy, and/or photocoagulation can be used as a means of saving the globe.

Radiotherapy

Retinoblastoma is radiosensitive and external beam radiation is used in children with advanced disease. Brachytherapy can also be delivered using "plaque radiotherapy."

Abdelaziz Y. Elzouki (ed.), *Textbook of Clinical Pediatrics*, DOI 10.1007/978-3-642-02202-9_355,

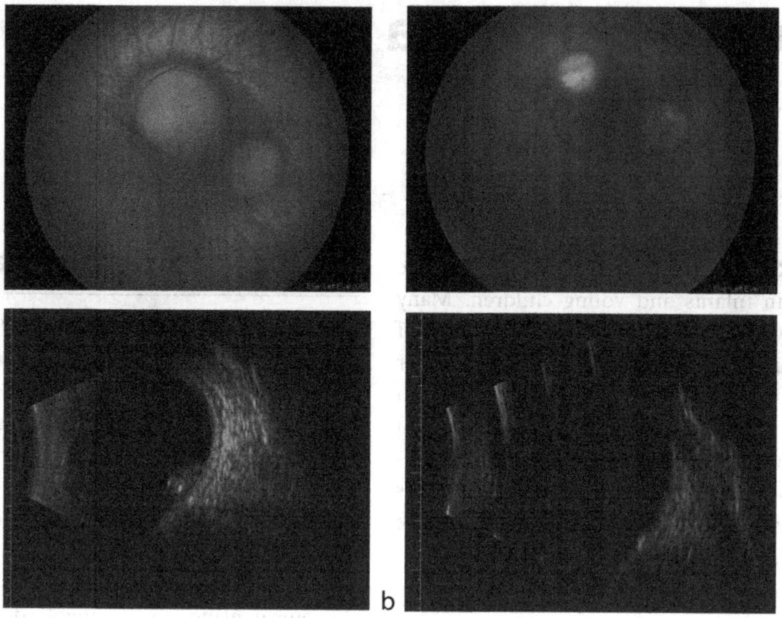

Figure 355.2
Unilateral retinoblastoma in a 6-month-old boy. The upper panels show the retina and the lower panel shows the ultrasound: (a) is at presentation and (b) shows the results following treatment with laser combined with chemotherapy (etoposide, vincristine, and carboplatin) (Courtesy of Tim Stout, MD, PhD)

Radiation carries a substantial risk of secondary cancers, especially in children with bilateral or other forms of genetic RB.

Chemotherapy

Chemotherapy is used in all patients with metastatic disease. Furthermore, chemotherapy is increasingly being used to shrink tumors so that they are amenable to local globe-sparing therapy. Agents that are active in RB include carboplatin, vincristine, etoposide, teniposide, cyclophosphamide, and doxorubicin.

Prognosis

In early stage unilateral disease, the prognosis is excellent, with more than 90% of children surviving. Most of these will have intact vision. Follow-up examinations of the retina under anesthesia to ensure that disease does not develop in the contralateral eye should be done until age 3. Patients with metastatic disease at diagnosis have a poor prognosis.

References

Canturk S, Qaddoumi I, Khetan V et al (2010) Survival of retinoblastoma in less-developed countries impact of socioeconomic and health-related indicators. Br J Ophthal 94:1432–1436

Cohen VM, Kingston J, Hungerford JL (2009) The success of primary chemotherapy for group D heritable retinoblastoma. Br J Ophthal 93:887–890

Dimaras H, Rushlow D, Halliday W et al (2010) Using RB1 mutations to assess minimal residual disease in metastatic retinoblastoma. Transl Res 156:91–97

Dimaras H, Heon E, Budning A et al (2009) Retinoblastoma CSF metastasis cured by multimodality chemotherapy without radiation. Ophthal Genet 30:121–126

Du W, Searle JS (2009) The rb pathway and cancer therapeutics. Curr Drug Targets 10:581–589

Gallie B (2009) Canadian guidelines for retinoblastoma care. Can J Ophthal 44:639–642

Lin P, O'Brien JM (2009) Frontiers in the management of retinoblastoma. Am J Ophthal 148:192–198

Maki JL, Marr BP, Abramson DH (2009) Diagnosis of retinoblastoma: how good are referring physicians? Ophthal Genet 30:199–205

Mallipatna AC, Sutherland JE, Gallie BL (2009) Management and outcome of unilateral retinoblastoma. J AAPOS 13:546–550

Marees T, van Leeuwen FE, de Boer MR (2009) Cancer mortality in long-term survivors of retinoblastoma. Eur J Cancer 45:3245–3253

Mehta M, Sethi S, Pushker N et al (2010) Typical and atypical presentations of retinoblastoma. J Pediatr Ophthalmol Strabismus 47:320

Phan IT, Stout T (2010) Retinoblastoma presenting as strabismus and leukocoria. J Pediatr 157:858

Rodjan F, de Graaf P, Moll AC et al (2010) Brain abnormalities on MR imaging in patients with retinoblastoma. Am J Neuroradiol 31:1385–1389

Sastre X, Chantada GL, Doz F et al (2009) Proceedings of the consensus meetings from the International Retinoblastoma Staging Working Group on the pathology guidelines for the examination of enucleated eyes and evaluation of prognostic risk factors in retinoblastoma. Arch Pathol Lab Med 133:1199–1202

Shields CL, Shields JA (2010) Retinoblastoma management: advances in enucleation, intravenous chemoreduction, and intra-arterial chemotherapy. Cur Opin Ophthal 21:203–212

Shin JY, Kim JH, Yu YS et al (2010) Eye-preserving therapy in retinoblastoma: prolonged primary chemotherapy alone or combined with local therapy. Korean J Ophthalmol 24:219–224

Wright KD, Qaddoumi I, Patay Z et al (2010) Successful treatment of early detected trilateral retinoblastoma using standard infant brain tumor therapy. Pediatr Blood Cancer 55:570–572

356 Germ Cell Tumors

Suman Malempati · H. Stacy Nicholson

Introduction

Germ cell tumors in children develop from the primordial germ cells, and arise in either the gonads or in sites associated with the normal migration of germ cells during embryogenesis. When these tumors occur outside the gonads, presumably they arise from germ cells that did not migrate properly. Germ cell tumors in children are rare, occurring at a rate of 10.7 per million children less than 19 years of age. When combined, these tumors represent 2–4% of all childhood malignancies in the USA. Extragonadal germ cell tumors typically occur in the pelvis, retroperitoneum, mediastinum, and in the central nervous system (CNS). CNS germ cell tumors are covered in the CNS tumor ➋ Chap. 349, "Central Nervous System Tumors in Children".

Pathology

The category of germ cell tumors is comprised of a variety of histologic subtypes. However, regardless of site, there are common pathological features that all germ cell tumors share. As the name suggests, germ cell tumors arise from primordial germ cells that undergo embryonal or extraembryonic differentiation. Histologic subtypes include benign and mature teratomas, yolk sac tumor, choriocarcinoma, and germinomas (also known as dysgerminomas or seminomas) among others. All of the different subtypes can be components of a mixed malignant germ cell tumor. Benign teratomas commonly occur soon after birth, yolk sac tumors typically occur between the ages of 1 and 5 years, and dysgerminomas and malignant teratomas occur predominately in adolescents. Teratomas have well-differentiated tissues from all three germ layers – endoderm, ectoderm, and mesoderm – and can be either cystic or solid. Many germ cell tumors may produce tumor markers that can be used in establishing the diagnosis and in monitoring for therapeutic response and disease recurrence. Tumors with a trophoblastic element (such as choriocarcinoma) may produce beta-human chorionic gonadotrophin (β-hCG) and those with a yolk sac element may produce alpha-fetoprotein (AFP).

Treatment Issues Common to All Sites

Complete surgical resection is the goal for all tumors and is often curative in benign teratomas and low-stage malignant germ cell tumors. However, as germ cell tumors are typically chemosensitive, surgeons should avoid an operative approach that would be disfiguring or compromise fertility. For a given patient, treatment is guided by both site and histology.

Testicular Germ Cell Tumors

Although most testicular tumors in children (75%) are germ cell tumors, one must also consider the possibility of a paratesticular rhabdomyosarcoma or leukemic infiltration when evaluating a new patient with a testicular mass. Typically, a testicular germ cell tumor will present as a rapidly growing, nontender, scrotal mass. While most testicular germ cell tumors in children are localized, a metastatic workup should be performed, including computerized tomography (CT) of the chest, abdomen, and pelvis, and a bone scintigraphy. Following surgery, a scrotal ultrasound within a month should be performed, and AFP should be followed in those with elevated levels at diagnosis.

For those without metastatic disease, treatment requires orchiectomy with a high excision of the cord via an inguinal approach. Retroperitoneal node dissection is not indicated and chemotherapy is not necessary. Patients with metastatic disease respond well to chemotherapy consisting of cisplatin, bleomycin, and etoposide (PEB) or cisplatin, bleomycin, and vinblastine (PVB). The prognosis is generally excellent with up to 90% survival even in patients with metastatic disease.

Ovarian Germ Cell Tumors

Ovarian germ cell tumors typically occur in early adolescence, and most ovarian tumors in children are of germ cell origin. Patients present with either abdominal pain or a mass, and other causes, such as ovarian torsion, should be considered. Ultrasound of the abdomen is usually

Abdelaziz Y. Elzouki (ed.), *Textbook of Clinical Pediatrics*, DOI 10.1007/978-3-642-02202-9_356,

the initial study obtained. Additional studies should include measurement of serum levels of AFP and β-hCG and CT scan of the chest, abdomen, and pelvis, and bone scintigraphy. There are four main histological subtypes: mature (benign) teratoma, immature (malignant) teratoma, dysgerminoma, and yolk sac tumors. Treatment may include surgery, with or without chemotherapy, depending upon the tumor type and extent of disease. Standard chemotherapy is the same as for testicular germ cell tumors and the prognosis is excellent.

Sacrococcygeal Tumors

Although rare (one per 40,000 live births), sacrococcygeal teratomas are among the most common tumors in the newborn. Females are more often affected than males (4:1), and the presentation is typically a large mass between the coccyx and rectum. Complete excision, including the coccyx, is usually curative. Most of these are benign teratomas, but a small percentage may have malignant components. Close follow-up after surgery is necessary because of a small risk of recurrent tumor with malignant elements. Serial measurements of the serum AFP level are recommended as persistently elevated AFP for age may be a marker of previously unrecognized malignant elements.

Mediastinal Tumors

Thoracic germ cell tumors typically occur in the anterior mediastinum in adolescent males and occur at a higher frequency in those with Klinefelter syndrome (47, XXY). Histology can be mixed and often includes yolk sac tumor, germinoma, choriocarcinoma, and teratoma. Tumor markers including AFP and β-hCG are often elevated in serum. Treatment usually includes surgery and chemotherapy, and if a complete resection can be accomplished, this improves survival. Rarely, these tumors are sometimes associated with hematological malignancies or can contain foci of sarcomatous elements.

References

Dehner LP (1983) Gonadal and extragonadal germ cell neoplasia of childhood. Hum Pathol 14:493–511

http//seer.cancer.gov

Li J, Thompson TD et al (2008) Cancer incidence among children and adolescents in the United States, 2001–2003. Pediatrics 121(6): e1470–e1477

McKenney JK, Heerema-McKenney A, Rouse RV (2007) Extragonadal germ cell tumors: a review with emphasis on pathologic features, clinical prognostic variables, and differential diagnostic considerations. Adv Anat Pathol 14(2):69–92

357 Late Effects of Cancer Chemotherapy in Children

Susan J. Lindemulder

Introduction

Overall 5-year survival rates for childhood cancer in developed countries is approaching 80%, and while the overall survival rates for childhood cancer in developing countries is significantly lower, improvements are being made. These improved survival rates are the result of improvements in treatment, access and delivery of care, adherence to treatment regimens, and improvements in supportive care. As the survival rates continue to grow globally there is a growing population of children, adolescents, and young adults who are at risk for late effects related to their cancer therapy.

While children generally tolerate the acute effects of cancer therapy relatively well compared to adult patients, cancer therapy received at an early age can lead to complications that may not be seen for many years. The Childhood Cancer Survivor study follows a large cohort of long-term childhood cancer survivors treated in the United States and found that 65% of patients had at least one chronic health condition, and 28% had a severe or life threatening health condition. These results are being confirmed by large cohort studies of long-term survivors, being conducted in multiple other countries around the world.

The late effects of childhood cancer therapy involve almost every organ in the body including the heart, lungs, kidneys, gastrointestinal tract, musculoskeletal system, hearing, and vision. There are also effects on growth and development, neurocognitive function, potential for future fertility, and psychosocial impact.

Treatment Summary

Given the wide variety of medications and other modalities utilized in treating childhood cancer and the multiple treatment protocols being used, the potential for late effects can vary greatly between different survivors of childhood cancer. There are many approaches to delivery of survivorship care, but all approaches require an accurate outline of what treatment the patient has received. This is commonly referred to as a Cancer Treatment Summary. ➋ *Table 357.1* details the items that should be included. The treatment summary should be created by the primary oncologist after the treatment is complete and is reviewed with the patient. This can then be used by any provider in combination with published screening guidelines such as the Children's Oncology Group Long-Term Follow-Up Guidelines to guide follow-up care and screening.

Common Late Effects

Some of the most common late effects are detailed in the rest of this chapter and are summarized in ➋ *Table 357.2.*

Infection

Children and adolescents often require at least one transfusion of a blood product during the course of their cancer treatment. Exposure to blood products increases the risk of transmission of blood born infections including Hepatitis B, Hepatitis C, Human Immunodeficiency Virus (HIV), and others. Screening of the blood supply varies by country with regard to the types of infection screened and the methods by which screening is done.

According to the World Health Organization (WHO) 2007 Blood Safety Survey, 42 countries collected less than 25% of their supply from voluntary unpaid donors (considered the safest source) and 31 countries reported still using paid donations (the least safe source). WHO recommends that at minimum, all blood be screened for HIV, Hepatitis B, Hepatitis C, and syphilis but 41 one out of 162 countries are not able to screen all donated blood for one or more of these infections.

Given these statistics, practitioners should determine whether the patient received any blood product during treatment and where that transfusion was given. Based on transfusion information, information regarding other

Abdelaziz Y. Elzouki (ed.), *Textbook of Clinical Pediatrics*, DOI 10.1007/978-3-642-02202-9_357,

Table 357.1
Components of a cancer treatment summary

Component	Description
Patient information	• Patient name
	• Date of birth
	• Treating institution
Diagnosis information	• Initial diagnosis including stage and site
	• Date of initial diagnosis
	• Date of relapse including site
	• Second cancers including diagnosis, site, and date (if applicable)
Chemotherapy	• List all chemotherapy agents and route (IV, IM, IT)[a]
	• Cumulative doses for anthracyclines, alkylators, bleomycin and others if available
	• When methotrexate or cytarabine were given, include dose or designate high dose or low dose
Radiation	• List all radiation sites
	• For each site, date and dose
Surgeries	• Procedure and date
Stem cell transplant	• Type of transplant and date
	• Graft-versus-Host disease prophylaxis and treatment
Therapy completion	• Date last therapy was received

[a]*IV* Intravenous, *IM* intramuscular, *IT* intrathecal

high risk health behaviors, living in a hyperendemic area, and available blood product screening information, patients may need to be tested for one or more infectious complications. All screening can be done on a sample of peripheral blood. Recommended screening for Hepatitis B is a Hepatitis B Surface antigen and Hepatitis B core antibody, for Hepatitis C is a Hepatitis C Antibody, and for HIV is antibodies for HIV-1 and HIV-2.

Cardiopulmonary

Pulmonary fibrosis and interstitial pneumonitis with resultant restrictive or obstructive lung disease can occur after treatment with various chemotherapy agents or after receiving radiation to the chest. The most recognized chemotherapy agent causing pulmonary effects is bleomycin, but other agents including carmustine (BCNU), lomustine (CCNU), and busulfan are also recognized as having these effects. These agents produce effects in a dose-dependent fashion with higher doses and more intensive treatment regimens resulting in higher risk. Chemotherapy combined with radiation doses greater than 15 Gy are associated with the highest risk.

Some patients will have clinical symptoms of pulmonary disease including cough, shortness of breath, dyspnea on exertion or wheezing, but many are diagnosed through screening pulmonary function testing, which shows lung volumes consistent with either restrictive or obstructive disease or decreased DLCO. Patients at risk should be interviewed yearly for symptoms such as chronic cough and shortness of breath. They should be evaluated by a physical exam and, where available, patients should have baseline pulmonary function testing with follow-up testing for abnormal results or new clinical symptoms.

Cardiac late effects are emerging as a growing concern as the survivor population ages. All cause cardiovascular events and are behind only cancer recurrence and development of second malignancies as a leading cause of mortality in this population. The mechanism and pathology vary with treatment exposure. Anthracycline chemotherapeutic agents cause cardiomyopathy with potential for congestive heart failure and radiation produces effects such as valvular disease, pericardial disease, and coronary artery disease.

Anthracycline chemotherapy agents include doxorubicin, daunorubicin, idarubicin, mitoxantrone, and epirubicin. They are thought to cause damage and death of cardiac myocytes during treatment. This leads to hypertrophic changes in the remaining myocytes, ultimately leading to inadequate left ventricular mass and decreased function. While some patients experience an acute decrease in function during treatment, this effect is often not seen for years, on average at least 15–20 years, and onset can be insidious or clinically dramatic. The risk of cardiomyopathy increases with increasing cumulative anthracycline dose, defined in doxorubicin dose equivalents.

Radiation to the heart can increase the risk of cardiomyopathy when part of a treatment regimen that includes anthracycline chemotherapy, but radiation alone causes pericardial disease, valvular disease and coronary artery disease. It is important to remember that many radiation fields include the heart. In addition to the obvious fields of chest, whole lung, mediastinal, mantle and total body, fields such as flank, spleen, whole abdomen, and paraaortic also include the heart. The risk increases with increasing dose and is highest for those who have received greater than 30 Gy (with anthracycline) or 40 Gy (without anthracycline). Other medical conditions that often result

Table 357.2

Common long-term effects, risk factors, and screening recommendations[a]

Late effect	Therapy exposure	Screening recommendations
Cataracts	Corticosteroids, busulfan, radiation (orbit) Modifiers: combined treatment, higher radiation dose	– Yearly fundoscopic and visual acuity exam – Full ophthalmologic exam for those exposed to radiation
Dental problems	Chemotherapy, radiation Modifiers: younger age (<5 years)	– Dental exam and cleaning every 6 months
Hearing loss	Cisplatin (highest risk with cumulative dose $\geq$360 mg/m^2), radiation (cranial) Modifiers: combined treatment, other ototoxic drugs (aminoglycosides, loop diuretics), younger age (<4 years)	– Baseline audiology exam – Routine follow-up audiology exam if hearing loss is detected
Pulmonary fibrosis	Bleomycin (highest risk with cumulative dose $\geq$400 U/m^2), carmustine, radiation (chest) Modifiers: combined treatment, younger age	– Yearly exam and history – Baseline pulmonary function testing (spirometry and DLCO) – Repeat pulmonary function testing as indicated
Cardiomyopathy/ congestive heart failure	Anthracyclines (highest risk with cumulative dose $\geq$300 mg/m^2), high dose cyclophosphamide, radiation (heart) Modifiers: combined treatment, younger age, female gender, obesity, pregnancy	– Yearly exam and history – Baseline echocardiogram – Interval echocardiograms determined by risk (every 1–5 years)
Blood-borne illness (Hepatitis B, C or HIV)	Transfusion of unscreened blood product Modifiers: living in hyperendemic area, other lifestyle high risk behaviors	– Hepatitis B surface antigen and hepatitis B core antibody – Hepatitis C antibody – HIV 1 and 2 antibodies – Other as indicated
Impaired sexual maturation/function	Alkylating agents, radiation (craniospinal, pelvic, gonadal) Modifiers: combined treatment	– Yearly exam for secondary sexual characteristics – Baseline evaluation (LH, FSH, estrodiol, testosterone) timing dependent on age and gender – Additional evaluations as indicated (semen analysis)
Secondary leukemia or myelodysplastic syndrome	Epipodophyllotoxins (etoposide), alkylating agents, anthracyclines Modifiers: older age, less than 5 years from exposure	– Yearly CBC until 10 years from exposure
Neurocognitive deficits	Intrathecal chemotherapy, cranial radiation Modifiers: combined treatment, female gender, younger age	– Baseline neuropsychological testing – Vigilance regarding educational and vocational progress
Renal/urinary	Cyclophosphamide, ifosfamide, cisplatin, radiation (abdomen/pelvis) Modifiers: combined treatment, higher dose	– Yearly blood pressure – Baseline BUN, creatinine, electrolytes and urinalysis – Follow-up as indicated for risk
Growth	Cranial radiation or radiation to epiphyses of long bones Modifiers: younger age, higher radiation dose, surgery to the suprasellar region	– Measurement of height and weight every 6 months until sexual maturity – Referral to endocrine for growth hormone evaluation if cross one percentile on growth curve

Table 357.2 (Continued)

Late effect	Therapy exposure	Screening recommendations
Musculoskeletal	Corticosteroids, high-dose methotrexate, radiation	- Encourage good calcium and vitamin D intake - Baseline bone density evaluation at maturity - Follow-up bone density evaluation as indicated
	Modifiers: combined treatment, older age, prolonged corticosteroids, growth hormone deficiency, hypogonadism	

[a]Screening recommendations taken from Children's Oncology Group Long-Term Follow-Up Guidelines for Survivors of Childhood, Adolescent, and Young Adult Cancers, www.survivorshipguidelines.org

from treatment can potentiate the cardiovascular risks including hypertension, obesity, dyslipidemia, and diabetes mellitus.

Screening for cardiovascular disease should include a yearly interview for symptoms of shortness of breath, dyspnea on exertion, orthopnea, chest pain, palpitations, and abdominal symptoms for younger patients. A complete physical exam should include careful evaluation of the heart for murmur, extra heart sounds (S3, S4 and increased P2), and pericardial rub and careful evaluation for signs of cardiac failure including rales, wheezes, jugular venous distention, and peripheral edema. Screening testing should include echocardiograms at intervals from every year to every five years depending on risk, a baseline EKG, and periodic fasting glucose and lipid profiles.

Genitourinary

Genitourinary late effects are generally related to specific chemotherapy agents or single kidney status after surgery. The chemotherapy agents with the most potent renal effects are cisplatin and ifosfamide. Both agents damage the ability of the kidney to filter efficiently. Cisplatin damages the distal renal tubule causing electrolyte wasting of magnesium, calcium, potassium, and sodium. Ifosfamide damages the proximal renal tubules causing wasting of potassium, phosphorus, glucose, protein, and bicarbonate (Fanconi's renal syndrome). Treatment with multiple chemotherapy agents increases risk, as does concomitant treatment with other nephrotoxic antibiotics or medications, radiation, or surgery. Children should be screened yearly with a blood pressure, creatinine, blood urea nitrogen, and chemistries, as well as urinalysis. Electrolyte replacement should be given to patients with ongoing wasting. Patients should be counseled to avoid further injury to the kidneys including avoiding nephrotoxic medications and injury to the remaining kidney (if single kidney status), and early treatment for hypertension and urinary tract infections.

Treatment with the chemotherapy agents, cyclophosphamide and ifosfamide, can cause hemorrhagic cystitis during treatment due to the accumulation of the toxic metabolite acrolein in the bladder. Bladder cancer can develop in patients who have received these agents or radiation to the pelvis. Yearly urinalysis should be done to evaluate for microscopic hematuria.

Musculoskeletal

Chemotherapy agents including corticosteroids and antimetabolite chemotherapy such as methotrexate can lead to musculoskeletal abnormalities, most notably osteoporosis or osteopenia which increase risk for future fracture. This risk is potentiated by the evidence that increasing proportions of the general population are calcium and vitamin-D deficient. In survivors of childhood cancer, these effects can also be increased due to treatment-related gonadal and growth-hormone deficiency, hyperthyroidism, chronic wasting of calcium and phosphorus due to treatment-related renal injury, and by increased body weight.

Another source of chemotherapy-related musculoskeletal damage is avascular necrosis (AVN) related to treatment with corticosteroids. AVN typically occurs during treatment but new cases can be diagnosed for many years after treatment. Clinically, children usually present with pain and limitation of activity. The large joints of the lower extremities, hip and knee, are most commonly affected, but AVN can occur in any bone.

Radiation to any bone or soft tissue can result in poor growth and tissue wasting which can contribute to the chemotherapy-related effects as well as producing effects in isolation. Children should be screened by interview yearly for symptoms of bone pain and a careful physical exam of all bones and tissues looking for asymmetry or decreased range of motion. All children should be encouraged to maximize calcium and vitamin-D intake and possibly have vitamin-D levels measured in the blood. Medicines to increase bone density are not currently approved for use in children, except in extreme circumstances. Any bony abnormality or concern for AVN should be further evaluated by plain x-ray or MRI with referral for surgical intervention as indicated.

Sensory

Platinum-based chemotherapy agents can cause long term ototoxicity. The hearing loss is sensorineural loss, but may also manifest as tinnitus or vertigo. The risk of hearing loss is increased when treatment occurs before the age of 4 years and when chemotherapy is combined with radiation or other ototoxic agents such as aminoglycoside antibiotics or loop diuretics. Children who have risk for hearing loss should undergo yearly interview for symptoms of hearing difficulty, tinnitus or vertigo as well as a complete audiological evaluation to follow loss. There should also be an emphasis on preventing further injury including avoidance of loud noises, using ear protection where indicated and avoiding further exposure to ototoxic medications.

Some treatment regimens can result in visual impairment. Children treated with chemotherapy agents such as busulfan or long-term corticosteroids are at life-long risk for the development of cataracts. This risk is increased when radiation to the total body, brain, head, or orbit was also given. Corticosteroid treatment can also increase the risk for developing glaucoma. Radiation increases the risk of chronic dry eye (Sjogren's syndrome) due to effects on the lacrimal glands. Children who have risk for these complications should be screened through a collaborative effort between ophthalmology and the primary provider and early intervention should be considered for any visual disturbance with the ultimate goal of preserving vision.

Dental

Treatment regimens including chemotherapy and radiation therapy can cause damage to or loss of teeth. Chemotherapy agents can damage the enamel of the teeth leading to an increase in the number of dental caries a patient experiences. This damage is seen in the erupted teeth, as well as the unerupted teeth. High dose chemotherapy regimens can also lead to the loss or misalignment of the adult teeth if treatment was received at a young age. Radiation therapy contributes to dental damage if the salivary glands are in the field of radiation. Damage to the salivary glands causes a decrease in saliva production leading to chronic dry mouth. The saliva plays an important role in cleaning the mouth and a decrease in saliva potentiates the damage done by other agents. It is recommended that all patients receive regular dental evaluation every six months for preventative maintenance and early intervention for dental caries.

Growth and Development

Children show a significant decreased in linear growth during and after cancer therapy. Most often, this decrease is due to radiation therapy. Chemotherapy alone can lead to decreased growth velocity while on treatment, but this is usually temporary and children experience an increased linear growth velocity after treatment and often catch up to children of a similar age.

Radiation therapy can contribute to decreased linear growth in a number of ways. First, whole brain radiation can damage the hypothalamus or pituitary gland leading to short stature. Risk factors include increasing dose, greater than 18 Gy and younger age children (age less than 5 years) showing more damage. This is thought to occur due to growth hormone deficiency or disturbance in the gonadal axis leading to early closure of the epiphyseal growth plates. Radiation also decreases linear growth through a direct effect on bones including the spine and femoral heads. This direct inhibition can lead to impaired growth locally, sometimes resulting in asymmetric growth patterns (decreased sitting height, decreased leg length, etc.). These effects are seen at doses of 20 Gy to the epiphyses.

Children at risk for decreases in linear growth should be followed carefully. If possible, height should be measured at least twice yearly until sexual maturation is complete. An accurate height should be obtained and recorded on a standardized growth curve and followed for trends. If a patient has a risk factor and crosses percentiles or is less than the third percentile, early referral for an endocrine evaluation is recommended.

Neurocognitive Function

The effects of cranial radiation on neurocognitive functioning are well documented. There is evidence that some chemotherapeutic agents also have an impact on neurocognitive functioning. These agents include intrathecal chemotherapy such as intrathecal methotrexate, high-dose cytarabine, and high-dose methotrexate. A wide array of neurocognitive effects have been described and can vary as the patient ages. Vigilance is recommended with regard to academic performance and vocation. When possible and available, neuropsychological evaluation early in treatment with repeat testing over time can inform intervention to help with deficits.

Fertility

Exposure to various chemotherapy agents and radiation in males produces gonadal dysfunction by damage to both the germ cells and leydig cells in the testicle, resulting in variable effects on spermatogenesis, testosterone production, and sexual function. As with males, exposure to chemotherapy and radiation produces impairment of gonadal function of the ovary in females. All chemotherapy agents are thought to pose some degree of risk but the largest risk is seen after treatment with the alkylating agents (cyclophosphamide, ifosfamide, procarbazine, etc.). These agents are commonly used for all cancers but notably for treatment of Hodgkin's lymphoma and solid tumors. Cumulative doses of cyclophosphamide greater than 7.5 g/m^2 are thought to greatly increase the risk for future infertility. Both the testicle and ovary are radiosensitive such that even low doses can impact function and radiation to the brain can interfere with the normal hypothalamic-pituitary-gonadal axis function, also resulting in impaired gonadal function.

There has been a focus on developing treatment regimens which limit the dosing of agents thought to have the highest impact on fertility outcomes, but this is not always possible. This has most notably been attempted in the treatment for Hodgkin's lymphoma. Other approaches are pretreatment fertility preservation techniques such as sperm cryopreservation for post-pubertal males and embryo cryopreservation for females with an identified partner and time to complete the in vitro fertilization process. Currently there are not good options for pre-pubertal males and females and females without identified partners.

Second Cancers

Longitudinal cohort studies of childhood cancer survivors from multiple countries have consistently demonstrated an increased risk of second cancers. This risk shows a steady increase with increasing time since completion of treatment. Treatment with chemotherapy agents can increase the risk for development of acute myelogenous leukemia or myelodysplatic syndromes. The chemotherapy agent, etoposide, appears to pose the greatest risk but this is seen with multiple categories of chemotherapy including the anthracyclines, alkylating agents, and the heavy metals. This risk appears to be greatest in the first 5 years from diagnosis and is thought to be virtually gone after 10 years. Screening recommendations include a yearly Complete Blood Count (CBC) for 10 years after treatment and follow-up for clinical symptoms.

The risk for other second cancers is mainly due to radiation exposure. There is increased risk for any skin cancer, soft tissue, or bone tumor in a previously irradiated field and this requires close monitoring for suspicious skin lesions and masses. In particular, radiation to the breast tissue increases the risk for development of breast cancer and this has been most notable in survivors of Hodgkin's lymphoma who underwent chest radiation. Women with a history of radiation to breast tissue should begin annual screening mammogram and/or breast MRI usually at the age of 25 years. Similarly, there is an increased risk of colorectal cancer in those patients who previously received radiation to the abdomen or pelvis and screening colonoscopy should begin usually at the age of 35 years. There should be a low threshold for investigation of any unusual mass or lesion in a previous radiation field.

Conclusion

As therapy improves for childhood cancer, there is a growing population of childhood cancer survivors at risk for late effects related to their treatment. Providers caring for these patients must be aware of these late effects and the screening recommendations to provide optimal care and prevent future morbidity and mortality.

References

Adams MJ, Lipschultz SE (2005) Pathophysiology of anthracycline- and radiation-associated cardiomyopathies: implications for screening and prevention. Pediatr Blood Cancer 44:600–606

Bath LE, Sallace WH, Critchley HO (2002) Late effects of the treatment of childhood cancer on the female reproductive system and the potential for fertility preservation. BJOG 109(2):107–114

Bertolini P, Lassalle M, Mercier G et al (2004) Platinum compound-related ototoxicity in children: long-term follow-up reveals continuous worsening of hearing loss. J Pediatr Hematol Oncol 26(10): 649–655

Bhatia S, Blatt J, Meadows AT (2006) Late effects of childhood cancer and its treatment. In: Pizzo PA, Poplack DG (eds) Principles and practice of pediatric oncology, 5th edn. Lippincott Williams & Wilkins, Philadelphia

Busch MP, Kleinman SH, Nemo GJ (2003) Current and emerging infectious risks of blood transfusions. JAMA 289(9):959–962

Chow EJ, Friedman DL, Stovall M et al (2009) Risk of thyroid dysfunction and subsequent thyroid cancer among survivors of acute lymphoblastic leukemia: a report from the Childhood Cancer Survivor Study. Pediatr Bood Cancer 53:432–437

Gerl A, Muhlbayer D, Hansmann G et al (2001) The impact of chemotherapy on Leydig cell function in long term survivors of germ cell tumors. Cancer 91(7):1297–1303

Green DM, Grigoriev YA, Bin N et al (2001) Congestive heart failure after treatment for Wilms' tumor: a report from the National Wilm's Tumor Study Group. J Clin Oncol 19(7):1926–1934

Greer FR, Krebs NF (2007) Optimizing bone health and calcium intakes of infants, children and adolescents. Pediatrics 117(2):578–585

Howell SJ, Shalet SM (2005) Spermatogenesis after cancer treatment: damage and recovery. J Natl Cancer Inst Monogr 34:12–17

Kadan-Lottick NS, Zeltzer LK, Liu Q et al (2010) Neurocognitive functioning in adult survivors of childhood non-central nervous system cancers. J Natl Cancer Inst 102(12):881–893

Kaste SC (2004) Bone-mineral density deficits from childhood cancer and its therapy. A review of at-risk patient cohorts and available imaging methods. Pediatr Radiol 34(5):373–378

Kaste SC, Goodman P, Leisenring W et al (2009) Impact of radiation and chemotherapy on risk of dental abnormalities. Cancer 115(24): 5817–5827

Kenney LB, Laufer MR, Grand FD et al (2001) High risk of infertility and long term gonadal damage in males treated with high dose cyclophosphamide for sarcoma during childhood. Cancer 91(3): 613–621

Kersun LS, Wimmer RS, Hoot AC et al (2004) Secondary malignant neoplasms of the bladder after cyclophosphamide treatment for childhood acute lymphoblastic leukemia. Pediatr Blood Cancer 42(3):289–291

Knight KR, Kraemer DF, Neuwelt EA (2005) Ototoxicity in children receiving platinum chemotherapy: underestimating a commonly occuring toxicity that may influence academic and social development. J Clin Oncol 23(34):8588–8596

Leung W, Hudson MM, Strickland DK et al (2000) Late effects of treatment in survivors of childhood acute myeloid leukemia. J Clin Oncol 18(18):3273–3279

Lipschultz SE, Lipsitz SR, Dalton VM et al (2005) Chronic progressive cardiac dysfunction years after doxorubicin therapy for childhood acute lymphoblastic leukemia. J Clin Oncol 23(12):2629–2636

Lipschultz SE, Alvarez JA, Scully RE (2008) Anthracycline associated cardiotoxicity in survivors of childhood cancer. Heart 94(4):525–533

Oeffinger KC, Mertens AC, Sklar CA et al (2006) Chronic health conditions in adult survivors of childhood cancer. N Engl J Med 355(15):1572–1582

Oeffinger KC, Nathan PC, Kremer LC (2010) Challenges after curative treatment for childhood cancer and long-term follow-up of survivors. Hematol Oncol Clin North Am 24(1):129–149

Robison LL (2009) Treatment-associated subsequent neoplasms among long-term survivors of childhood cancer: the Childhood Cancer Survivor Study experience. Pediatr Radiol 39(Suppl 1):S32–S37

Sala A, Barr RD (2007) Osteopenia and cancer in children and adolescents: the fragility of success. Cancer 109(7):1420–1431

Schwartz CL, Hobbie WL, Constine LS et al (eds) (2005) Survivors of childhood and adolescent cancer. Springer, Heidelberg

Sklar CA, Mertens AC, Mitby P et al (2006) Premature menopause in survivors of childhood cancer: a report from the Childhood Cancer Survivor Study. J Natl Cancer Inst 98(13):890–896

Smith MA, Rubinstein L, Anderson JR et al (1999) Secondary leukemia or myelodysplastic syndrome after treatment with epipodophyllotoxins. J Clin Oncol 17(2):569–577

Stohr W, Paulides M, Bielack S et al (2007) Ifosfamide-induced nephrotoxicity in 593 sarcoma patients: a report from the late effects surveillance system. Pediatr Blood Cancer 48(4):447–452

Van Leeuwen BL, Kamps WA, Jensen HW et al (2000) The effect of chemotherapy on the growing skeleton. Cancer Treat Rev 26(5):363–376

Whelan KF, Stratton K, Kawashima T et al (2010) Ocular late effects in childhood and adolescent cancer survivors: a report from the Childhood Cancer Survivor Study. Pediatr Blood Cancer 54(1):103–109

Willers E, Webber L, Delport R et al (2001) Hepatitis B-A major threat to childhood survivors of leukaemia/lymphoma. J Trop Pediatr 47(4): 220–225

www.beyondthecure.org. Beyond the Cure: Information for Survivors of Childhood Cancer

www.candlelighters.org. American Childhood Cancer Organization

www.ltfu.stjude.org. Long-Term Follow-Up Study

www.survivorshipguidelines.org. Long Term Follow-Up Guidelines for Survivors of Childhood, Adolescent and Young Adult Cancers, Version 3.0, 2008

www.who.int/mediacentre/factsheets/fs279/en/. Global Blood Safety and Availability: Facts and Figures from the 2007 Blood Safety Survey

Section 22

Neurology

Generoso G. Gascon

358 Clinical Approach to Infants, Children, and Adolescents with Neurologic Problems

Generoso G. Gascon

Neurological symptoms comprise approximately 10% of presenting complaints to primary care practitioners, family medicine physicians, and general pediatricians. Generalists can manage these efficiently by developing a systematic approach. This chapter takes a developmental, age-related, symptom-oriented approach to evaluating and managing a child presenting with neurologic complaints. Detailed treatment and management of specific disease entities mentioned in this introductory chapter is covered in the subsequent chapters.

The clinical approach needs to be flexible, depending on the age of the patient, and the informants giving the history. The setting, whether it is the normal newborn nursery, neonatal or pediatric intensive care unit, the emergency room, the hospital clinic or private office determines the pace and sequence of different parts of history taking and the neurological examination. A complete history and neurological examination need not be done in the first encounter. A focused neurological exam, sufficient enough to make an acute management decision, whether diagnostic or therapeutic, is appropriate for an acute triage situation, such as the emergency room. The presenting problem, whether acute or chronic, and the setting also influence the amount of time spent explaining the working diagnosis and management plan, as well as that spent on educating and counseling patients and families.

In this chapter the developmental ages introduced are arbitrarily divided into:

The neonate
The infant and toddler
The preschool child
Elementary school child
The middle school child
The high school child and adolescent

Clinical Approach to the Newborn with Neurological Problems

The most common acute neonatal neurological symptoms in the neonatal intensive care unit (NICU) are seizures, with or without impaired sensorium, qualifying as encephalopathy. The most common etiologies are hypoxia and/or ischemia, infection, stroke, metabolic abnormalities (hypoglycemia, hypocalcemia). Less common are metabolic diseases like aminoacidurias (maple syrup urine disease), organic acidurias (methylmalonic and propionic aciduras), and urea cycle and fatty acid oxidation disorders. Rarely, genetic epilepsies (benign familial neonatal convulsions) present in the newborn period.

In the normal newborn nursery, the common problems for which neurological consultation is sought are brachial plexus palsy (Erb's), and various involuntary movements that mimic seizures, such as benign familial neonatal myoclonus, benign nocturnal myoclonus, jitteriness, abstinence syndromes, or phasic movements normally seen in active (rapid eye movement [REM]) sleep.

History and examination of the newborn are covered in detail in the ➲ Chaps. 360, "Neonatal Neurological Disorders" and ➲ 361, "Neonatal Seizures".

History in the NICU is most commonly obtained from the bedside nurses, though the neonatologist poses the question. Parents need to be queried for the prenatal and perinatal history, and family history. One symptom, seizures, is highlighted here.

Seizures. The first important decision is to decide whether the events observed are, in fact, seizures. If so, the next decision is to classify the seizures, whether only of one kind, such as focal motor, or of many different kinds, such as focal clonic, myoclonic, focal onset but migrating, or subtle seizures. This can be done by retrospective history from the observing nurses or parents, or prospective

Abdelaziz Y. Elzouki (ed.), *Textbook of Clinical Pediatrics*, DOI 10.1007/978-3-642-02202-9_358,

observation using seizure charts. In tertiary care centers that have the technology and neurological expertise, the gold standard is continuous video-EEG monitoring.

Classifying seizures has a practical aspect. Focal clonic seizures bode, generally, for a good prognosis, because focal clonic seizures are often secondary to a transient metabolic abnormality, such as hypocalcemia. Myoclonic and subtle seizures bode for a guarded prognosis since they are usually due to hypoxia-ischemia, neurometabolic disease or brain dysgenesis.

For those working in secondary or tertiary care centers, having a once yearly teaching session with nurses on the classification of neonatal seizures, using videotapes of such seizures, if available, would be a good practice for obtaining consistent and accurate observations. Bedside nurses and nurse practitioners should be sensitized to the onset, progression of movements, whether there is more than one kind of seizure, duration, and postictal findings.

Neurological Examination

In the *general physical examination*, most important for neurology are size and shape of the head and dysmorphic features. The tape measure surrounds the head from the occipital protuberance to the forehead. Head circumference is plotted on a standard growth chart. Recognizing dysmorphic facial features may, by itself, make a diagnosis; for example, Down syndrome, Zellweger syndrome (see Genetics section and chapters).

The *mental status* exam in the newborn is essentially a determination of the level of consciousness or sleep state and general responsiveness. In a two to three-day full term infant, parts of the Brazelton neonatal assessment exam can be applied, in a clinical fashion.

Cranial nerve examination. The most important functions to determine immediately are vision (C.N. II) and hearing (C.N. VIII); then, the muscles necessary for sucking and swallowing (motor V, VII, IX, X, XII).

Motor examination. The most reliable motor exam is performed while the neonate is in Brazelton State 4. States 1 and 2 are sleep states (active and quiet sleep). State 3 is drowsiness-arousal. State 4 is awake, relaxed, and alert. State 5 is awake and active. State 6 is awake, active, and crying.

Developmental reflexes. The most important newborn developmental reflex is the Moro. It is best elicited by cradling the newborn in the horizontal supine position, with one hand under head, then suddenly letting the head drop in neck extension. There are two parts to the Moro: initial abduction and extension, then adduction and flexion, of the arms. One looks for its presence or absence. If present, any asymmetry is noted, then that suggests a hemi-syndrome.

The asymmetric tonic neck reflex (ATNR) is not normally present in the newborn, but is usually seen between 2 and 6 months of age. If present, it is abnormal because it is too obligatory. Other developmental reflexes that should be present, and best elicited about the third day of life after the neonate has "recovered" from the trauma of birth, are the grasp and traction responses, elicited by the pull-to-sit maneuver, watching also for excessive head lag. Plantar grasps are elicited by pushing the thumb into the balls of the feet and watching the toes flex. Placing and stepping reactions are elicited by holding the infant in the vertical suspension position and brushing the dorsum of the feet up against the examining bed. Automatic walking is elicited by holding the newborn upright, then pulling forward with the infant leaning forward, letting the toes brush the examining bed.

One sign, hypotonia, is highlighted here.

Hypotonia may occur with or without weakness, may be variable according to state, and may even coexist with increased tone (for example, axial hypotonia with appendicular spasticity). Central hypotonia must be distinguished from peripheral/neuromuscular causes. Weakness may be lateralized (as in a hemiplegia), or localized (as in a brachial plexus palsy, or congenital absence of the depressor anguli oris). Weakness may be bilateral and localized, as in Moebius syndrome (bilateral peripheral facial palsies).

Generalized profound hypotonia is seen in some metabolic diseases (peroxisomal disorders like Zellweger's, aminoacidurias like non-ketotic hyperglycinemia (NKH)). Neuromuscular diseases like congenital myotonic dystrophy, congenital myasthenia, and congenital myopathies, present in the newborn period with hypotonia, and definite weakness. CAVEAT: Some diseases have both brain and muscular involvement, such as mitochondrial disorders, and rare congenital muscular dystrophies (Fukuyama, muscle-eye-brain disease).

Ancillary Investigations

In many hospitals in the USA and around the world, newborn screening for treatable congenital metabolic diseases by sending blood spots for tandem mass spectroscopy, usually in regional laboratories, and other blood tests (thyroid) is now being done. This is an enormous advance in the prevention and early treatment of otherwise crippling and disabling diseases (see ➋ Chap. 38, "Disorders of Organic Acid and Amino Acid Metabolism").

Continuous video-EEG monitoring is the gold standard not only for diagnosis, but also to follow results of treatment, in neonatal seizures, since clinical-EEG dissociation is not uncommon in neonatal seizures.

Doppler ultrasound is noninvasive and portable, and is particularly useful for intracranial hemorrhages and conditions which change ventricular size. CT brain adds gray-white matter differentiation, with higher resolution than ultrasound, and fast acquisition speed. CT angiography has increasing utility in stroke. MRI, with its various sequences–FLAIR, DWI, along with its permutations–MRS, MRV, and MRA, gives the highest resolution, visualizes the brainstem, and has the advantage of being repeatable without exposing the infant to radiation. Neuroimaging in hypoxic ischemic encephalopathy is discussed in detail in the ➲ Chap. 360, "Neonatal Neurological Disorders".

Infant and Toddler (Up to 3 Years of Age)

The general approach to history taking in the infant and toddler with a neurological problem is to elicit a prenatal and perinatal history that might point to possible brain damaging events, an interval history since birth for acquired brain damaging events, and a family history that might point to genetic or familial conditions. The examination is both a neurodevelopmental assessment as well as a neurological examination (see ➲ Chap. 42, "Normal Child Development").

Milestones: The two most important milestones that physicians can determine just from history and examination are motor and speech/language. Infants should be rolling over by 4 months, sitting alone by 6 months, reaching out at 6 months, and walking alone by 14 months. A shovel grasp is followed by a pincer grasp by the early second year.

Regarding speech, babies should be cooing at 3 months, interactive babbling till 7–8 months, consonant-vowel combinations, like "da-da" by 8–9 months, single words by 16 months, short sentences by 24 months. Conditioning games such as waving bye-bye, "peek-a-boo," clapping hands occur around 12 months. Putting blocks into a 3-hole form board is usually achieved by 18 months. However, these milestones may be achieved at different times in cultures with infant-raising practices different from that of North America (see ➲ Chap. 49, "Global Perspectives on Child Development and Behavior").

Examination

In this age group, the exam needs to seem like play in order to establish rapport. The least invasive items, such as testing the teloreceptors (hearing and vision) should be done first. Examination items that require actual handling of the baby—muscle tone (pull-to-sit maneuver), deep tendon reflexes, and the developmental reflexes should be done last.

Measuring head circumference and looking at the shape of the head is mandatory. Nowadays, with the standard of practice being to advise mothers to lay infants supine to lessen the risk of sudden infant death syndrome (SIDS), the incidence of positional plagiocephaly, flattening of the skull posteriorly, is increasing. This needs to be recognized early, since molding helmets are not effective after the sutures have fused, after about 8 months of age. Microcephaly and macrocephaly usually requires that the head circumference be two standard deviations above or below the mean expected for that age. Another clinical guideline would be whether there is a 50 percentile difference between head circumference and length or weight. In babies with enlarged heads, and in geographic areas where CT head scans are not easily available, percussing the skull and listening for a "cracked pot" sign due to split sutures can still be useful. Auscultating for bruits, using the bell portion of a stethoscope, over the orbits and the skull may detect vein of Galen malformations or large arteriovenous malformations.

Of the four items of classical physical diagnosis, observation, palpation, percussion, and auscultation, observation is the most important at this age. Observations include the interrelatedness between the baby and parents and the baby and the examiner, degree of eye contact, presence of spontaneous speech, and nonverbal communication (pointing, gestures) in toddlers who have delayed speech.

General: Specific parts in the general physical examination that may suggest neurological disease are the skin, looking for neurocutaneous stigmata, and the abdominal exam, looking for hepatosplenomegaly.

Occasional café-au-lait spots are fairly common, but six or more should raise suspicion for neurofibromatosis Type I, in which case parents' skin should be examined. Ultraviolet light by a Wood's lamp can bring out the vitiliginous or hypopigmented spots of tuberous sclerosis, particularly in light-skinned patients. Hepatosplenomegaly would raise the possibility of a storage disease (see ➲ Chap. 39, "Lysosomal Storage Diseases").

When a toy is held before the child, one can watch to see if only one hand reaches out, suggesting hemiparesis, and whether tremor is present. In observing crawling, a hemiparesis is suggested if the infant pulls forward using only one side of the body. Walking on tiptoes suggests a spastic diparesis, muscular dystrophy involving calf muscles, or autism.

Cranial nerves: Infants are more likely to follow visually interesting objects, such as the distorted human face, finger puppets, or rotating concentric circles, such as pinwheels. Similarly, hearing behavior can be elicited with a bell, a clacker, or toys that reproduce animal sounds. Infants turn their head toward sound at 6 months. Prior to that they may merely become still and have an alert, listening facial expression.

Developmental reflexes: The ATNR, elicited by turning the head of the supine infant to one side, appears about 2 months and should disappear completely by 6 months. The ATNR begins to recede at 4 months, when the body-righting reflex replaces it. At 6 months, the infant is transitioning from the reflexes of a quadripedal animal, to that of a bipedal animal who stands on two legs in the upright position.

The first bipedal reflexes appear at 6 months. If the infant in the sitting position is suddenly pushed backward, the legs should kick out; if the infant is pushed sideways to either side, the arms should thrust out sideward. The parachute response appears at 8 months. It is elicited by holding the infant at the chest, face down, and propelling toward the examining table. Both arms should suddenly thrust forward (as if to break a fall) at the same time. This is a good reflex to observe any asymmetries that suggest hemiparesis. Proximal weakness at the shoulder girdle can be determined by leaving the child momentarily in the resulting wheelbarrow position, and see if the baby can bear its weight, temporarily.

Common Problems

Common problems in the infant and toddler are:

1. Delayed development.
2. Seizures. The most severe epilepsy syndromes are infantile spasms; Lennox-Gastaut; and infantile myoclonic epilepsies. The most common seizure disorder, however, is febrile seizures (see ➲ Chaps. 361, "Neonatal Seizures" and ➲ 362, "Epilepsy in Infancy and Childhood").
3. Breath-holding spells (see ➲ Chaps. 361, "Neonatal Seizures" and ➲ 362, "Epilepsy in Infancy and Childhood").
4. Movement disorders. Most common are transient tics, dystonic-like postures secondary to gastroesophageal reflux, similar to Sandifer syndrome (see ➲ Chap. 363, "Movement Disorders").
5. Sleep-related rhythmic movement disturbances (head-banging, tremors upon awakening, shuddering attacks), parasomnias (night terrors at age 3) (see ➲ Chap. 364, "Sleep and Its Disorders in Childhood").

Delayed development. (For the perspective of developmental pediatricians, see ➲ Chap. 42, "Normal Child Development", and Nancy Lamphear, Disorders of Learning and Attention.) The physician must distinguish between global developmental delay and specific developmental delay. Global usually means in two or more domains, usually specified as motor, language, social, and adaptive. When the etiology is neurological, delayed motor development, most commonly, has a cerebral cause, the most important of which is cerebral palsy–atonic in infancy, which may evolve into diplegic, hemiplegic, or choreoathetotic. Motor developmental arrest and/or deterioration, with relative preservation of mental functions, point to neuromuscular conditions such as spinal muscular atrophy, muscular dystrophy, or congenital myopathies.

Delayed language development, with preservation of motor function, intact hearing, and normal intelligence, may signify a developmental language disorder (developmental dysphasia). Delayed language may also suggest an autistic spectrum disorder, particularly if there is language regression in the second year of life. Language regression may also occur in rare conditions like the Landau-Kleffner syndrome and Continuous Spike Waves in Slow Wave Sleep (CSWSS).

At some point, usually in the preschool years, if an infant who is globally delayed shows no evidence of catching up to a normal developmental curve, mental retardation, mild, moderate, or severe needs to be considered. Although the Bayley Infant Scales are used by psychologists, formal IQ testing does not begin to be reliable until the preschool age, when the Wechsler Pre-Primary Scale for Children (WPPSI) is available. However, the primary care physician can approximate IQ, using the concept of DQ (developmental quotient). The formula is:

$$DQ = \text{developmental age}/\text{chronological age} \times 100.$$

For example, if an infant is 12 months old, and has the first bipedal reflexes and is just beginning to sit unsupported (6 month developmental milestones), the motor DQ is $6/12 \times 100$, or 50 (on borderline between moderate to mildly delayed, if parallel to IQ). This should lead to a recommendation for infant stimulation programs.

Because of the reported worldwide increase in prevalence of the autistic spectrum disorders, autism needs to be distinguished from mental retardation. The American Academy of Pediatrics, in its July, 2006 policy statement, recognizes the benefits of early detection. It recommends developmental screening at 9, 18, 24, and 30 months.

Table 358.1
Absolute indications for diagnostic referral for autism

No babbling by 12 months
No gesturing (pointing, wave bye-bye) by 12 months
No single words by 16 months
No 2 word spontaneous phrases (not echolalia) by 24 months
Loss of ANY language or social skills

There is some controversy about what constitutes quality screens, although the Denver Developmental Screening Tests are commonly used in practice. In the state of Massachusetts, screening for autism is mandated at 18 months, with a choice of various standardized screens, although the M-CHAT is probably the most widely used (Table 358.1).

The "Parents' Evaluations of Developmental Status (PEDS)" is a screening questionnaire that can be easily completed by parents in a few minutes in the waiting room. Printed in English, Spanish, and Vietnamese, additional translations like Hmong, Somali, Russian, Chinese, Thai, etc, can be licensed by e-mailing the publisher. The online application also offers the Modified Checklist of Autism in Toddlers (M-CHAT), automated scoring and ICD-9 codes.

Developmental screens requiring direct elicitation of children's skills are the Bayley Infant Neurodevelopmental Screener (BINS), the Brigance Screens II, and the Battelle Developmental Inventory Screening Test (BDIST), 2nd edition. Busy pediatricians rarely have the time to administer these, so in practice, they are most often administered by psychologists, although office personnel such as nurses, nurse practitioners, and probably even medical assistants could probably be trained to do these. Internationally, for validity and reliability, screens like these, and, I.Q. tests for later ages, should be standardized for language and culture.

In the USA, pediatricians can refer infants with developmental delays for publicly funded Early Intervention services, where developmental specialists, physical and occupational therapists, speech and language therapists provide services in the home, up to the age of 3 years. After the age of 3, if delays have not resolved, children are eligible for early education services in the public schools, where individual education plans (IEPs) are made and carried out. These services are a resource for pediatricians, as well as sources for obtaining up to date ongoing observations of developmental progress.

Developmental regression should always bring up the possibility of a progressive encephalopathy, discussed in detail in the chapter by G. Gascon.

The Preschool Child (3–6 Year Olds)

The approach to history taking is to listen carefully to the concerns of parents, other caretakers in the home, and elicit histories, when appropriate, from day care workers or preschool teachers. If complaints are unfocused, the physician's task is to help the historians clarify their concerns and priorities. The initial explicit chief complaint may mask underlying implicit concerns that are not verbalized, for fear that the child may have something viewed as devastating, such as mental retardation or autism.

The common problems at this age are global and specific developmental delays, febrile seizures and breath holding spells, and behavioral problems, from high functioning autistic spectrum disorders, to disruptive behavioral disorders, which may present first with hyperactivity and impulsivity (Attention Deficit Hyperactivity Disorder [ADHD] plus). The term "sensory integration problems" is not a diagnosis by itself, but is seen in different disorders such as autism or in children with obsessive-compulsive traits or disorder.

With video capabilities practically universal in cell phones and digital cameras, parents can help, in questions of seizures or abnormal involuntary movements, by recording the events. Having them keep sleep logs can establish a baseline, as well as help in diagnosis (see Chap. 364, "Sleep and Its Disorders in Childhood").

Asking children what television shows they watch, and asking them to name favorite characters, asking parents whether the child pays attention and follows the story lines, laughs at the appropriate situations, and a sense of humor can reveal intelligence.

Asking about how well the child plays with playground equipment, such as swings, slides, and jungle gyms, as well as when the child was able to ride a tricycle and a bicycle can give a good idea about motor coordination. How complicated a puzzle the child can manage tells something about visual perceptual motor skills. Asking about favorite toys and how the child plays with them and with other children can give an idea of rigidity, imagination, symbolic play, and development of parallel versus interactive play.

Accident proneness and sleep difficulties in this age group, particularly difficulty falling asleep after going to bed (increased sleep latency), are not uncommon antecedents of ADHD.

Finally detailed family histories and drawing a three generation family pedigree, looking not only for single gene disorders, but also paroxysmal and neuropsychiatric disorders, should be routine.

Neurological Examination

At this age one still approaches the examination in the office as if it is play. Having toys in the examining room appropriate for this developmental age helps, for example, puzzles, form boards for visual perceptual motor and fine motor coordination; cars, trains, dolls, a doll house if space warrants for imaginative play; large balls for general motor coordination. These reinforce the ambience of a child-friendly environment, put the child at ease, and enhance cooperation in the more formal parts of the neurological examination performed later.

Much can be learned from observing the child with these toys, while obtaining the history from the parents. Special attention to speech and language is important, to distinguish developmental articulation problems from developmental language disorders and the characteristic disorders of pragmatics in the language of high functioning autistic children. Whether they can remember words while singing and keep in tune should be noted. Universal songs, like the "Happy Birthday" song, are part of the repertoire.

The simplest pre-academic readiness skills to predict early literacy skills is the ability to name colors and letters of the alphabet., which nowadays is usually achieved before kindergarten. By then most middle class children have book awareness, having been exposed to books being read to them by parents, and some early phonics.

In pre-academic math skills, one to one correspondence, that is, the ability to match numbers to objects (one sock to one shoe), counting from one to ten, and understanding of measurement, length and weight, big and small, and some elementary understanding of money predict acquisition of elementary mathematics.

Visual perceptual motor skills can be tested by having the child copy shapes–circle (age 3), distinguishing + and x (cross from x) (age 4), triangle (age 5), square (age 6), diamond (age 7), British flag (age 8). Another way is putting together and taking apart constructional toys, like Legos and building blocks. Spatial relations. Up/down, in front of/behind, over/under.

In gross motor testing, children should be able to stand on one foot for a few seconds, and then hop in place for a few hops, at 4 years. They should be able to kick a soccer ball. Throwing a small ball like a baseball may still not be accurate. Preferred handedness and footedness should be noted.

Common Problems

Global Developmental Delay

Global developmental delay is taken to mean delay in at least two of the four usual domains–motor, language, social, and adaptive. In the preschool child, persisting global developmental delays since infancy would warrant etiological investigation for mental retardation or autism, if not previously done.

The American Academy of Neurology has published a practice parameter with an algorithm on how to proceed stepwise. Nonsyndromic mental retardation, characterized by the absence of associated morphologic, radiologic, or metabolic features, comprises the majority of cases. The genetic factors underlying nonsyndromic MR are not presently understood. The present standard of care, therefore, is to order the highest resolution chromosome studies available, chromosomal microarrays. Since Fragile-X Syndrome accounts for a significant fraction of MR and the characteristic morphological features are not obvious at this age, fragile-x gene studies are recommended.

As of early 2009, linkage and cytogenetic analyses have identified 29 X-linked and five autosomal recessive genes associated with nonsyndromic mental retardation, which account, however, for less than 10% of cases. Autosomal dominant genes have yet to be identified. However, *de novo* chromosomal rearrangements, usually involving a change in copy number of genomic regions, are the most commonly recognized cause of mental retardation. This suggests that monoallelic lesions are sufficient to cause MR, and therefore raises the possibility that *de novo* genetic lesions, such as point mutations, may explain a number of cases of MR. Nonsyndromic MR is not amenable to linkage or association approaches, and therefore relies on the sequencing of candidate genes. The hypothesis that *de novo* mutations of autosomal genes, involved in synaptic plasticity, recently found support in the discovery of mutations in SYNGAP1.

Specific Developmental Delay

Specific developmental delays are delays in one domain only. When two, or more, domains are involved, however, the question arises on whether these are independent, comorbid specific delays, rather than global developmental delay, which often implies cognitive subnormality.

For example, specific delays in language, that is, developmental language disorders, may be comorbid with

ADHD, or visual-perceptual motor difficulties, or excessive incoordination (developmental coordination disorder), in a cognitively normal child. Language delay must be distinguished from language regression, the loss of previously acquired speech and language. The differential diagnosis then includes progressive encephalopathy, autistic regression, Landau-Kleffer syndrome or Continuous Spike Waves in Slow Wave Sleep (CSWSS).

In the motor sphere, arrest and regression, as in the dystrophinopathies (Duchenne-Becker muscular dystrophy), need to be distinguished from just delay, as in spastic diparesis due to nonprogressive encephalopathies (cerebral palsy).

Behavioral Problems

Behavioral issues, like persisting temper tantrums, sleep issues like parasomnias, and hyperactivity always bring up the question as to whether these are still within the wide variation of normal behavior at this age, or whether they are at risk behaviors for other disorders. The child with disruptive behavior may just be having prolonged "terrible two's," but then again, may be exhibiting the beginnings of an oppositional-defiant disorder.

Incessant hyperactivity and impulsivity, excessive tantrums, more than the terrible two's, irritability, easy to anger yet repentant and overly loving afterward, cruelty to pets, hitting out to peers in day care, rapid mood swings, sometimes multiple in a day, suggest a severe disorder of mood regulation in the bipolar spectrum. However, one should make this diagnosis with caution, in the absence of a family history of bipolar disorder.

Higher functioning autistic disorders, like pervasive developmental disorder not otherwise specified (PDD. NOS), may have escaped detection before the age of three, but should not be missed in the preschool child. These two disorders – autism and childhood bipolar disorder, parallel the two poles of mental illness in adolescents and adults, schizophrenia and affective disorders (depression, bipolar disorder).

Paroxysmal Disorders (See Gaitanis Chapter)

The most common paroxysmal disorders in the preschool age group are febrile seizures and breath holding spells (BHS). Assuming that seizures with fever are not symptomatic of a CNS infection like meningitis or encephalitis, and they are not focal in onset, they would be classified as simple febrile seizures. However, they may be an expression of a familial genetic syndrome, generalized epilepsy febrile seizures plus, if there are other members of the family with febrile seizures and generalized epilepsies. Fortunately, response to antiepileptic medications for generalized seizures is very good.

The course needs to be watched, however, because, rarely, myoclonic and non-febrile generalized convulsions may follow febrile seizures, simple or complex, with developmental arrest, and evolution into the syndrome of severe myoclonic epilepsy (SME, Dravet syndrome).

This is also the age where the two most common benign epilepsies of childhood may begin, benign Rolandic epilepsy and benign occipital epilepsy (the Gastaut type).

BHS are either cyanotic (blue type), where the child cries so hard, often stimulated by denial of something she/he wants, that they turn blue, hold their breath, and then go limp. Pallid syncope (the pale type) usually occurs after sudden, unexpected painful stimuli, such as hitting the head, or stubbing a toe, where the child turns white, then falls limp. Sometimes tonic stiffening occurs, but this is usually an anoxic seizure, caused by temporary ischemia of the brain stem, mimicking "brain stem fits." Rarely does a convulsive seizure occur after a breath-holding episode, and the coexistence of both must be considered.

Screens

The same screening tests mentioned in the previous section (0–3 years old), except for the Bayley Infant Neurodevelopmental Screen, are still applicable as developmental screening tests for the preschool child (age 3–6 years).

Elementary School Child (KG Through 3rd Grade)

At this age many children are able to describe their symptoms. So, to establish rapport with the child, start with the child. Greet the child first, start with some easy banter (Whose idea was it that you come to see me? How's school?) This emphasizes that they are the center of attention, even though much of the rest of the visit may be eliciting history from the parents, and later giving information and counseling. Determine whether the child's chief concerns are the same as the parents. This gives some idea of their awareness of the presenting complaint.

In the examination, starting off with gross motor activities often loosens up the patient. Ordinary walking,

walking on tiptoes, heels, side of the feet, hopping on one foot, walking tandem, also doubles as an initial screening exam, looking for hemisyndromes and general coordination. Starting right off with mental status questions may intimidate the child and should be left till later when the child is at ease.

Common Problems

Problems often presenting for the first time at this age are absence seizures versus nonepileptic staring, tics, headaches, and learning and behavioral disorders.

Attention Deficit Hyperactivity Disorder (ADHD)

History-taking in ADHD focuses first on eliciting a history of the four major symptoms–short attention span, distractibility, impulsivity and hyperactivity, and determining whether they occur in two different environments, usually home and school and whether such behavior occurs in social settings (family gatherings, playground, play dates, and organized sports activities). Whether these are occurring in the physician's office requires observation of the child while taking a history from the parents, and watching how the child responds to commands during the physical/neurological exam. Do you have to repeat commands (inattention)? Does the child start to respond before you finish giving a command (impulsivity)? Does the child interrupt the doctor-parent conversation inappropriately (verbal impulsivity)? Does the child wander around the room touching things inappropriately (hyperactivity)?

There are questionnaires which can be filled out by parents before a physicians' visit, but some, like the Vanderbilt parent and teacher assessment scales, are proprietary and take time for the primary care physician to score. A common one used by schools in the USA is the Conners rating scales, which may come already scored to the physician, if the school is the instigator for the referral.

Special examinations looking for minor neurological dysfunction ("soft sign exams") again usually take more time than a busy pediatrician has, if he/she has not been trained in such exams, and interpretation depends on experience, and is best left to subspecialists (like developmental pediatricians, pediatric neurologists, or developmental neuropsychiatrists).

Headaches (See Ken Mack chapter)

The PedMIDAS (Pediatric Migraine Disability Scale) questionnaire, filled out by parents or patients prior to a visit, will cut down history-taking time, since it asks about frequency and severity of headaches, and degree of disability, as manifested by days missed going to school or other social or sports events.

In history taking the temporal profile of a headache distinguishes between two major patterns; that of a typical migraine attack (rapid rise, slower resolution, over hours), and that of tension-type headaches (low grade waxing and waning). At this age, however, recurrent headaches are almost always migraine-vascular.

If a verbal description of a visual aura is unclear, the child can be asked to draw it, using colored pencils or crayons, on a plain sheet of white paper. Children find it difficult to describe the quality of the headache pain. Nonverbal clues – milking hands or pounding fists that connote a throbbing or pulsating quality help. Another tactic is to give the child multiple choices – squeezing, bursting, sharp and stabbing, throbbing or pounding.

Learning Disorders

By third grade, learning disabilities should be evident – in reading (dyslexia) or arithmetic (dyscalculia). A specific learning disability is a marked delay in the acquisition of basic academic skills (reading, writing, arithmetic) despite normal intelligence, adequate hearing and vision, and adequate teaching. Operationally, schools usually use the criteria of, for example, reading level 2 years below grade level (see Nancy Lamphear, Disorders of Learning and Attention).

Neurobehavioral Disorders

The primary care physician can be aided in suspecting these conditions by using rating scales, such as:

Vanderbilt Parent and Teacher Assessment Questionnaires (ADHD, Oppositional Defiant Disorder, Conduct Disorder, Anxiety, Depression)
PARS (Pediatric Anxiety Rating Scale)
YMRS (Young Mania Rating Scale), for bipolar spectrum disorders
YBOCS (Yale-Brown Obsessive Compulsive Scale), children's version
Weinberg Affective Scale, for depression
Australian Asperger Scale, for Asperger's Disorder

Epilepsy

Common epilepsy syndromes apt to occur at this age are primary generalized absence seizures (Petit Mal Epilepsy) and benign Rolandic epilepsy. Non-epileptic staring, usually in children with attention deficit disorders are often mistaken by school personnel for absence seizures. Absence seizures can often be elicited in the office by having the child hyperventilate for at least 1 min One can determine that there is loss of consciousness by reciting a nursery rhyme ("one, two buckle my shoe, three, four, shut the door," etc.) and asking the child what she recalls hearing, if anything. Both of these epilepsy syndromes have characteristic epileptiform EEG patterns – synchronous and symmetrical three cycles per second spike waves in absence seizures, and sharp waves or spikes in the central-temporal areas that are sleep-activated.

For any kind of seizure syndrome, the use of seizure calendars which log seizure type and frequency, are a useful management tool.

The Middle School Child (4th Through 7th Grades)

At this age, children can give histories and usually cooperate with a formal neurological exam.

Common Office Problems

1. ADHD, inattentive subtype (attention deficit disorder without hyperactivity)
2. Migraine, and its variants
3. Syncope
4. Neuropsychiatric disorders – anxiety, OCD, Asperger's disorder

ADHD, Inattentive Subtype

This syndrome usually does not come to the attention of teachers until the middle school years. It affects girls more than boys and often presents as "underachieving for their potential" or "reading comprehension" difficulties, when there has been no earlier dyslexic difficulties. Executive function deficits become more evident. Executive skills are mediated through the frontal lobe, the last part of the brain to fully develop, and their deficits appear in middle school because of the requirement for more planning and organizational skills. It shows up in deficient homework management, low grades because of not handing in book reports, theme papers, or science projects on time. Medications alone do not correct executive dysfunction. Some schools recognize this by offering organizational skills training classes, but many children need daily monitoring at school and at home. Behavior management techniques, that is, the use of reward and punishment, are not effective. Executive function skills have to be taught.

Migraine and Variants

Idiopathic stabbing headaches, also called "ice pick headaches" or "indomethacin responsive headaches" can be missed, because they present as head pains more than headaches. Acute confusional migraine tends to occur around puberty and early adolescence. Headache calendars, which log frequency, severity, presence of triggers, and results of medication can clarify history taking.

Neuropsychiatric Disorders

Asperger's disorder may not be diagnosed until this period when the magnitude of social skills deficits becomes recognized. Delay in diagnosis is often due to the high I.Q.'s these children have. Parents commonly say "he has no friends," is considered weird, has "off the wall" conversational talk, and highly focused interests. Guidance counselors and school psychologists may offer social skills training classes.

Anxiety disorders, obsessive-compulsive disorder (OCD) may also become evident, if disruptive behavior is a symptom. Children with suspected neuropsychiatric disorders usually take too much time to be handled well by primary care physicians, and should, therefore, be referred to developmental pediatricians, pediatric neurologists with interest in behavioral neurology, or child and adolescent psychiatrists.

Tics which may have been minor may now become more prominent and evoke secondary emotional reactions. More likely, the highly associated disorders are apt to emerge as obstacles in school performance; particularly ADHD, but also OCD.

High School and Adolescents

As much as possible, histories should be obtained by talking directly with adolescents alone, separate from the parents. This immediately establishes that they are the focus of attention, not their parents, but also conveys to them their responsibility for managing their condition. One has to judge the capacity to introspect, and therefore, the reliability of their views. Parents can be called in later, prior to performing the neurological exam, to hear "their side of the story."

A characteristic adolescent issue is sleep. A detailed review of systems checklist filled out before the office visit can insure that the primary care physician does not miss an issue like sleep, which may not be the initial chief complaint. A complaint of fatigue or ADHD-like symptoms affecting school performance might be traced to sleep deprivation.

Another characteristic issue with adolescents is compliance – in keeping headache, seizure, or sleep logs, or even doctor's appointments, as well as in taking medication. The motivation to keep a driver's license can be used to insure compliance with taking antiepileptic medication.

Substance abuse, particularly alcohol, can be the reason for a variety of neurological symptoms, and should be inquired about in the history.

In the neurological examination, at this age a good adult type mental status examination can be done, testing orientation; immediate, short-term, and long-term memory, digit span forward and backward, serial-7 subtractions from 100, a three word retention test, interpretation of proverbs, and general information. Adolescents are also able to fully cooperate in detailed muscle testing.

Common Problems

Head Trauma – Concussions (See Chapter by Tsze and Chun)

With children and adolescents participating more and more in recreational and competitive contact sports such as football (both American and soccer), basketball, ice hockey, and lacrosse, the long-term consequences of repeated concussions has emerged as a major concern. Return to play guidelines have been changing over the years, starting with the Cantu concussion grading schemes and two subsequent international modifications, to the relatively recent use of guidelines for trainers to use on the field at the time of the accident, then on the sidelines, and then the use of ImPACT (immediate post-concussion assessment and cognitive testing). ImPACT is a computer administered neuropsychological test battery, originated at the University of Pittsburgh that measures aspects of attention, memory, reaction time, and processing speed. Athletes are not returned to play until testing has returned to their baseline, obtained at the start of the season. Even then, return to play involves a gradual return, from light aerobic, full aerobic, light contact, to full contact participation.

Chronic Daily Headache syndrome (See Chapter by Ken Mack)

A majority, about 60%, are due to transformed migraine. The rest is due to tension-type headaches, or a mixture of migraine and tension-type. Emotional factors may be present – anxiety, depression. Medication overuse may have contributed to the formation of this pattern. It is defined as headaches occurring at least 15 days out of 30, for at least 3 months. The primary care physician needs to recognize this syndrome early because it is very difficult to break and warrants referral to a neurologist or specialty headache clinic.

The most common complicated migraine syndrome at this age is the basilar migraine syndrome, commonly affecting mid-teenage females. The other occurring in puberty or early adolescence is acute confusional migraine.

Special headache examination

1. Tap over frontal, maxillary, ethmoid sinuses, for acute sinusitis.
2. Examine for possible cranio-cervical junction problems. Hold a palm on the head, then pound slightly on the palm with the other fist. Ask for any pain when testing face-turning (sternocleidomastoid) and trapezius against resistance. Check for a Lhermitte Sign.
3. Palpate occipitalis and frontalis muscles for isometric contraction, as in muscle contraction (tension-type) headaches.
4. Have patient keep jaw open, while trying to close, or push from either side for temporal-mandibular joint problems.
5. Check the fundus, looking primarily for papilledema, as in pseudotumor cerebri.

Syncope

Vasovagal syncope is the most common cause. There is often a history of breath holding spells in early childhood, a family history of syncope, and of migraine. What they have in common is they are all disorders of neurovascular instability. Cardiac syncope, due, for example, to the Long Q-T syndrome, will require an EKG and pediatric cardiology consultation. Orthostatic syncope can be documented by tilt table tests.

A special form of vasovagal syncope, reflex syncope, may occur at this age. This is fainting triggered by physically or emotionally painful stimuli, such as drawing blood or hearing bad news. A preceding history of pallid syncope, the pale type of breath holding spells, in early childhood can often be elicited.

Epilepsy

The generalized epilepsy syndromes that can begin at this age are generalized convulsions upon awakening, juvenile absences, and juvenile myoclonic epilepsy (JME) Complex partial seizures due to temporal lobe epilepsy (TLE) often begin at this age. A surgically treatable epilepsy, if refractory to antiepileptic drugs, is TLE due to mesial temporal sclerosis occurring in patients with early childhood history of febrile seizures.

Conversion Reactions

Pseudoseizures are not an uncommon symptom at this age. They may be psychogenic, but the challenge here is that patients who present with pseudoseizures often also have true epilepsy. Other common conversion symptoms are inability to stand and walk, called astasia-abasia, which looks like a pseudo-ataxia; sensory symptoms because the sensory examination, relying on subjective responses, may be a subtle presentation of demyelinating disease; and intermittent weakness, even with a normal neurological examination, may be an early presentation of myasthenia gravis. DOPA-responsive dystonia may be missed if the patient is examined in the morning, and the diurnal pattern is not appreciated.

Demyelinating Disease (See Tanuja Chitnis Chapter)

Although relatively rare, multiple sclerosis can present for the first time in adolescence. More common are post-infectious demyelinating diseases, such as Guillain-Barre syndrome, transverse myelitis, or acute demyelinating encephalomyelopathy (ADEM).

ADHD Complications

By this time the behaviors which comprise conduct disorder, which are essentially pre-delinquent behaviors (fire setting, cruelty to animals), should have been recognized and treated, because conduct disorder complicating earlier ADHD is the most important risk factor for the subsequent development of substance abuse, delinquent and criminal behavior. By the same token neuropsychiatric disorders which may have presented in early childhood with an ADHD symptom complex and disruptive behavior, which may evolve into the bipolar disorder spectrum, are a risk for impulse control problems ("anger issues") and even explode into homicide, witness the Columbine school mass shootings.

Disorders Occurring at any Age

Some neurological disorders can occur at any age, but may have different etiologies at different ages:

Stroke
Demyelinating disorders, post-infectious like ADEM, transverse myelitis, Guillain-Barre syndrome
Head trauma
Progressive encephalopathies
CNS infections
Acute toxic-metabolic encephalopathies

Seizure incidence is greatest in early childhood and late life, but partial or focal seizures, or focal-onset secondarily generalized seizures can occur at any age due to any congenital or acquired focal brain structural lesion, such as brain tumors, vascular malformations, gliosis, secondary to cerebral contusions, CNS infections, progressive cerebral degenerative disease, or stroke.

Modifications of Clinical Approach According to Clinical Setting

In the Emergency Room

The priorities are – *Treatment first (save life and limb) then diagnosis.* Cone down on the chief presenting complaint, perform a focused exam, treat immediately if necessary (for example, status epilepticus), and then go back to get more complete history of the present illness, family history (draw a family pedigree), prenatal/perinatal/developmental history, allergies (Table ➲ *358.2*).

In the P ICU

The priorities are *stabilization, recovery, and then acute rehabilitation* (See ➲ Chap. 379, "Pediatric

Table 358.2
Pediatric neurologic emergencies

Status epilepticus
Status migrainosus
Metabolic-toxic coma
Acute stroke
Acute weakness
Acute ataxia
Head and spinal cord trauma

Neurorehabilitation"). Intensivists put much reliance on monitoring devices for vital signs, cardiac and respiratory functions. Patients cannot have a "complete neurological exam" because they often have impaired consciousness or are in coma, and because of the monitoring equipment, intubation, and IV lines they cannot be moved. The mental status exam is essentially a classification of the level of consciousness, and standardized scales, such as the pediatric version of the Glasgow Coma Scale. Of the cranial nerve examination, reaction to visual threat, which can come centrally or peripherally, is a gross way to ascertain vision and field defects. The ophthalmoscopic exam needs to be repeated frequently to look for papilledema, which supplements intracranial pressure monitoring. The motor examination is limited to observation of spontaneous movement and passive range of movement for muscle tone. Sensory examination is limited to applying noxious stimuli, often to gauge level of consciousness, rather than test for distribution of sensory loss. Criteria for brain death can be found in the ➔ Chap. 365, "Coma".

In the Office

The priorities are *screening, diagnosis, and prevention.* For the busy pediatrician, developmental screening is easiest with parent-answered questionnaires, filled out prior to the visit or in the waiting room. Equipping the examining room with developmental toys, or having a playroom, enhances the "child friendliness" of the doctor's office.

Primary care physicians need to become familiar with school and community resources for early intervention, preschool early education, rehabilitation facilities with multidisciplinary services like physical therapy, occupational therapy, and speech and language therapy, parent education and support groups, and consumer organizations in the USA like the Epilepsy Foundation, the Muscular Dystrophy Association, Children and Adults with Attention Deficit Disorder, the Tourette Syndrome Association, or their equivalents in the rest of the world.

Perspectives

Common diseases are common, and physicians should think of these first, before looking for exotic or rare causes.

However, what is common and what is rare depends on which part of the world one practices. Subacute sclerosing panencephalitis is endemic in Turkey, India, and the Philippines, while so rare to the point of near extinction in North America. Glutaric aciduria Type 1 is a relatively common organic aciduria in Saudi Arabia, while relatively rare in North America (except among the Amish) and Europe. Tuberculomas are common in South and Southeast Asia, while a rarity in North America. Genetic neurometabolic diseases are common in the Middle East, while rare in North America. The neurologic complications of AIDS may be seen more frequently in Africa, where HIV is still an epidemic and where the latest combination of drugs is not highly available. Neurocysticercosis is much more common in Central and South America, than in North America. Seizures and epilepsy, headaches, and cerebral palsy are common neurological problems in children all over the world. A relatively rare disease, spinal muscular atrophy, is still the most common neuromuscular disease of infancy and early childhood throughout the world.

In developed countries, where the premium on education as a means of upward mobility in society is high, ADHD, learning and neurobehavioral problems take up a large portion of the office practice of pediatricians. In developing countries where the health care mind-set, in providers as well as patients, is often crisis-oriented, and centers around life and death issues, developmental neuropsychiatric disorders may receive short shrift.

The art of medicine begins with attentive listening to the patient and family. The primary care physician needs to inquire about the psychosocial and environmental circumstances in which they live, their dietary habits, and, in genetic diseases, elicit a detailed family history and draw a three-generation family pedigree. A 10+ systems review completes the history taking. This brings into conscious differential diagnosis the possibility that symptoms attributable to the nervous system are manifestations of a systemic disease. Symptoms in other systems, together with neurologic signs and symptoms can bring to mind a syndrome or disease involving multiple systems.

An important trend that will make it easier for primary care practitioners in office practice to care efficiently for their patients is the use of hospitalists devoted entirely to inpatient care, freeing more time for the office-based physician to practice preventive measures and counseling. Another growing trend is the use of electronic medical records, which will reduce medication errors, avoid duplication in laboratory studies and investigations, and ease communication between specialists and primary care physicians.

Developmental Screening Tests

Pediatrics, 2006 (July), 118(1):413 Table of developmental screening tests.

Medical Diagnostic Thinking

Jerome Groopman, How Doctors Think, Houghton Mifflin, Boston, 2007.

Websites

www.icnapedia.org ("wikipedia" for pediatric neurology)
http://www-personal.umich.edu/~leber/c-n/ (This site aims to coordinate the available internet resources in Child Neurology, both for professionals and patients.)
www.genetests.org (tells you which clinical and research labs in the world are doing genetic tests)
www.clinicaltrials.gov (for ongoing studies)
www.cochrane.org/reviews (for evidence-based medicine)
www.mdconsult.com (requires subscription)
www.epocrates.com (resource for drug dosages, adverse reactions, drug interactions; for Epocrates Online, requires registration)
www.medicalive.net Pediatric Neurological Examination—Introduction (09:34) and Pediatric Neurological Examination—3 months (09:16), Google Videos

References

Barkovich AJ (2005) Pediatric Neuroimaging, 4th edn. Lippincott, Williams & Wilkins, Philadelphia, PA

Brazelton TB (1973) Neonatal behavioral assessment scale. Clinics in Developmental Medicine, no 50. Spastics International Medical Publications, London

Coffey CE, Brumback RA (2006) Pediatric neuropsychiatry. Lippincott, Williams and Wilkins, Philadelphia, PA

Filipek PA, Accardo PJ, Ashwal S et al (2000) Practice parameter: screening and diagnosis of autism. Neurology 35:468–479

Friedman MJ, Sharieff GQ (2006) Seizures in Children. Pediatr Clin N Am 53(2):257–277

Gascon G, Ozand PT, Cohen B (2007) Aminoacidopathies, organicacidopathies, mitochondrial enzyme defects and other metabolic errors. In: Goetz C, (ed) Textbook of clinical neurology, 3rd edn. W.B. Saunders, Philadelphia, PA

Greene RW (1998) The explosive child. Harper Collins, New York

Hamdan F, Gauthier J, Spiegelman D et al (2009) Mutations in SYNGAP1 in autosomal nonsyndromic mental retardation. NEJM 360 (6):600–605

Jan MMS (2007) Neurological examination of difficult and poorly cooperative children. J Child Neurol 22:1209–1213

O'Tuama L, Dickstein D, Neeper R, Gascon G (1999) Functional neuroimaging in pediatric neuropsychiatry. J Child Neurol 14 (4):207–221

Pellock JM, Meyer EC (1993) Neurologic emergencies in infancy and childhood. Butterworth-Heinemann, Boston

Remmel K, Bunyan R, Olson W, Gascon G, Brumback R (2003) Handbook of symptom oriented neurology, 3rd edn. Mosby-Yearbook, St. Louis

Shevell M, Ashwal S, Donley D et al (2003) Practice parameter: evaluation of the child with global developmental delay. Neurology 60:367–380

Wilens TE (2009) Straight talk about psychiatric medications for kids. Guilford, New York for their patients is the use of hospitalists devoted entirely to inpatient care, [illegible] time for the office [illegible] to proceed [illegible] measures and [illegible] records, which will [illegible] [illegible]

[illegible] Screening Tests

[illegible]

[illegible]

[illegible]

[illegible]

[illegible] history [illegible] doing [illegible] requires [illegible]

[illegible] Pediatric Neurological Examination [illegible] and Pediatric Neurological [illegible] months (09:10) Google [illegible]

References

[illegible] (2005) [illegible] Williams & Wilkins [illegible]

[illegible] (1983) [illegible] developmental [illegible]

[illegible] Lippincott, [illegible]

[illegible] examination of difficult and poor [illegible] 22:1209–1215

[illegible] (1998) The [illegible]

[illegible] (2003) Prevalence [illegible] with [illegible]

359 Congenital Brain Malformations and Hydrocephalus

John N. Gaitanis

Classification

This chapter arranges cortical malformations according to the earliest embryological stage in which the abnormality has its origin. Yet, this is an artificial distinction since the stages of cortical development overlap in time and lack discrete boundaries. Moreover, some gene defects exert influence in more than one developmental stage. Thus, the classification system presented here will undoubtedly be modified as understanding of these conditions evolves.

Overview of Embryology

The brain and spinal cord form from the dorsal aspect of the embryo in the third and fourth weeks of gestation through neurulation, the process of neural tube formation. In the fifth and sixth weeks, prosencephalic development, the process by which the brain takes shape, begins. Cortical formation in humans spans weeks 8–24 of gestation and can be divided into stages of cell proliferation (both neural and glial precursor cells are formed), neuronal migration (cells travel to their designated destination), and cortical organization (cell networks are determined). Myelination is the final step of brain development and continues well beyond birth. As noted above, assigning strict temporal divisions is misleading, since different stages take place concurrently.

Disorders of Neurulation

Fusion of the neural tube begins at the level of the hindbrain (medulla and pons) and proceeds rostrally and caudally. Failure of rostral fusion results in dysraphic states of the brain (anencephaly and encephalocele), and incomplete caudal fusion causes spinal dysraphism (myelomeningocele). The anterior end of the neural tube closes by 24 days and posterior closure happens by day 26. Disorders of neurulation differ in severity depending on the timing of the disruption. The most severe disorder, craniorachischisis totalis, in which the brain and spinal cord fail to develop because of a complete absence of neurulation, occurs no later than 20–22 days of gestation. Anencephaly, a complete failure of anterior neural tube closure resulting in an absence of brain formation, occurs no later than 24 days. Encephalocele, a restricted failure of anterior neural tube closure, happens around day 26. Likewise, myelomeningocele, a restricted failure of posterior neural tube closure, also occurs by day 26.

Myelomeningocele is the most clinically important disorder of neurulation since patients with it usually survive. Its incidence in the United States is approximately 0.2–0.4 per 1,000 live births. The neurological features of myelomeningocele relate to the level of involvement, presence of hydrocephalus, and other associated malformations.

Impairment of motor, sensory, and sphincter function relates directly to the level of involvement. Ambulation is one of the most important clinical concerns, and retained strength of the iliopsoas and quadriceps muscles are required for walking. Lesions at or below S1 rarely affect ambulation, whereas higher defects, above L2, almost always do. Among patients with intermediate lesions (L3, L4, L5), approximately half will walk, but braces or other assistive devices may be required.

Hydrocephalus is seen in approximately 90% of patients with lumbar lesions. The usual signs of increased intracranial pressure (lethargy, irritability, limited upward gaze, rapidly expanding head circumference) are not essential for diagnosis and are present in only 15% of newborns with myelomeningocele. If clinical signs are present, they usually develop 2–3 weeks after birth and are almost certain to be present by 6 weeks. Their frequent absence necessitates serial neuroimaging for the prompt diagnosis of hydrocephalus. Infants demonstrating hydrocephalus at birth require shunt placement immediately following myelomeningocele closure. The closure stops CSF leakage, and can therefore worsen hydrocephalus if a shunt is not placed.

When myelomeningocele and hydrocephalus are combined with inferior displacement of the medulla and lower

Abdelaziz Y. Elzouki (ed.), *Textbook of Clinical Pediatrics*, DOI 10.1007/978-3-642-02202-9_359,

cerebellum through the foramen magnum, it is termed the Arnold–Chiari malformation (Chiari type II). Other features of this disorder include elongation and thinning of the upper medulla and pons and bony defects of the foramen magnum, occiput, and upper cervical vertebrae. Brain stem and cortical malformations are common. Resulting brainstem dysfunction is a significant cause of morbidity and mortality. It may result in apnea, stridor, cyanotic spells, and dysphagia. The overall mortality rate in patients with brainstem dysfunction is 21%, but when all four symptoms are present, the mortality rate is as high as 60%. Cortical malformations are an important cause of morbidity such as intellectual disability and epilepsy. They are also very common in patients with Arnold–Chiari malformations, being present in as many as 92%.

Disorders of Prosencephalic Development

Prosencephalic development is the process by which the forebrain takes shape. It begins during the fifth week and continues through the second and third months of gestation. Prosencephalic development influences formation of the face, so severe disruptions at this stage result in facial anomalies. Development of the forebrain can be divided into three stages: formation, cleavage, and midline development. The resulting disorders depend on the stage affected.

Holoprosencephaly

In holoprosencephaly (HPE), disruption of the roof plate and absence of hemispheric separation result in a single, large, forebrain ventricle. In its most severe form, alobar HPE, the brain is a single spherical structure with a common ventricle and a malformed cortical mantle. The optic nerves are dysplastic and the olfactory bulbs and tracts may be absent. The hypothalamus does not separate normally into two halves. Facial anomalies, ranging from cyclopia to a single central incisor, are observed. Less-severe forms, semilobar and lobar HPE, have milder degrees of the same anomalies. For instance, in semilobar HPE, the frontal and parietal lobes remain fused and the interhemispheric fissure is only present posteriorly. In contrast, with lobar HPE most of the left and right hemispheres and lateral ventricles are separated and fusion is seen only at the most ventral aspect of the frontal lobes.

Clinical severity relates to the degree of structural change. Neurological dysfunction inversely correlates with the degree of hemispheric separation, with less separation resulting in greater impairment. Endocrinopathies correlate with the severity of hypothalamic separation. Associated cortical malformations frequently cause epilepsy, which is often refractory. Careful attention to neuroimaging is necessary for providing an accurate prognosis.

HPE is a heterogeneous condition, with both genetic and environmental causes. The most common environmental cause is maternal diabetes, which carries a 1% risk of HPE. Cytogenetic abnormalities account for approximately 25–50% of cases, with trisomy 13 and 18 being the most common. Single-gene mutations are found in roughly 25% of patients. Several genes are known to be causative. The first gene discovered, the sonic hedgehog gene at 7q36, is the most common. The evaluation typically begins with a karyotype followed by molecular genetic testing if the karyotype is unremarkable.

Abnormalities of midline prosencephalic development are less severe than HPE. They include agenesis of the corpus callosum and septo-optic dysplasia (SOD). Agenesis of the corpus callosum can be either partial or complete. With partial agenesis, the posterior portion is more affected. It is commonly associated with other brain anomalies including Arnold–Chiari II malformations and neuronal migration disorders. SOD, on the other hand, is characterized by optic nerve hypoplasia in combination with the absence of the septum pellucidum and pituitary dysfunction. Clinically, it presents with visual impairment, endocrinopathies, or both. The causes are heterogeneous, including both environmental and genetic etiologies (➋ *Fig. 359.1*).

Disorders of Neuronal Proliferation

Neuronal proliferation takes place between the second and fourth months of gestation. Neurons and glia have their origin in the ventricular and subventricular zones. In the earliest phases of neuronal proliferation, neuronal-glial stem cells divide to form further stem cells. Later, stem cell division becomes asymmetric so that one daughter cell is postmitotic, while the other remains a stem cell. Eventually, fewer and fewer stem cells are produced and all of the neurons within the proliferative unit are postmitotic. Abnormal neuronal proliferation results in conditions characterized by too many or too few neurons.

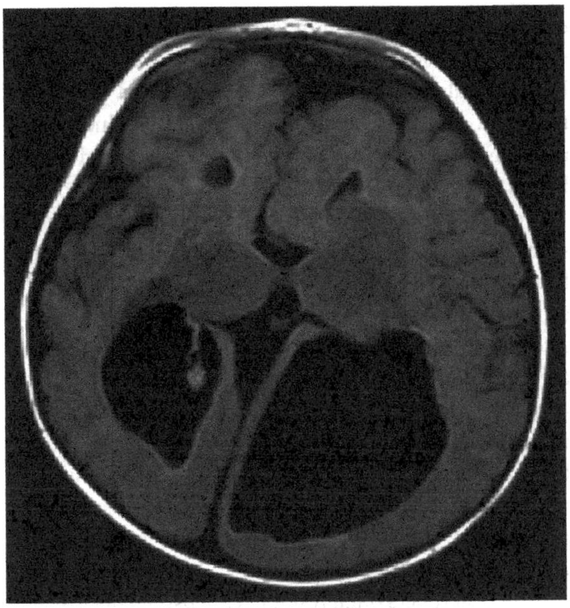

Figure 359.1
Agenesis of the corpus callosum with colpocephaly

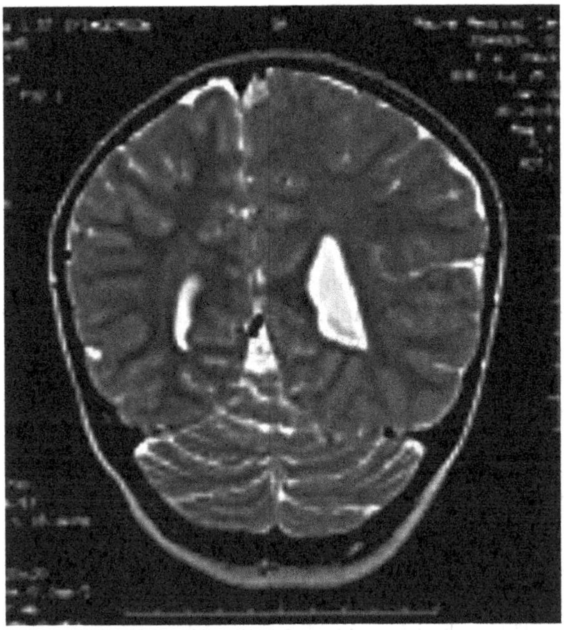

Figure 359.2
Hemimegalencephaly

Decreased Proliferation

Microcephaly/microlissencephaly primary microcephaly (microcephaly vera) is diagnosed when the head circumference at birth is three or more standard deviations below normal. Primary microcephaly is a heterogeneous condition and can be caused by in utero brain injury or from a genetically determined reduction in neuronal proliferation. Most genetic forms are recessively inherited. Microcephaly is sometimes associated with a more simplified gyral pattern or, in severe cases, with a smooth cortex, termed microlissencephaly. Seizures and global developmental delays are uniformly present.

Disordered Proliferation

Hemimegalencephaly

When there is enlargement of just one cerebral hemisphere, it is termed hemimegalencephaly. It probably results when a disturbance of cellular differentiation and proliferation interacts with the genetic expression of body symmetry. In addition to increased size of the affected hemisphere, neuroimaging may reveal abnormal gyration, ventriculomegaly, and increased T2 signal of the white matter. Histology reveals disorganized cortical lamination, subcortical heterotopia, and large, dysmorphic neurons, termed balloon neurons. The opposite hemisphere may be normal or have mild dysplasia and heterotopia. All patients have epilepsy, and hemispherectomy is often required for intractable cases (*Fig. 359.2*).

Abnormal neuronal differentiation/maturation in abnormalities of maturation or differentiation, neurons exhibit immature or glial features. Balloon neurons contain abnormally large amounts of cytoplasm and stain for both neuronal and glial markers, indicating a failure to commit to a specific cell lineage. Balloon and dysplastic neurons are seen in cortical dysplasia and in the cortical hamartomas of tuberous sclerosis complex. Evidence of disrupted neuronal migration, including disorganized or absent lamination, malpositioned neurons, and heterotopic neurons within the white matter, are also present in these disorders. Such conditions must, therefore, involve abnormalities of both maturation and migration, indicating that dysplastic and balloon neurons lack the cellular machinery to migrate properly through the cortical plate.

Tuberous Sclerosis Complex

Tuberous sclerosis complex (TSC) is a multisystem, dominantly inherited condition. It has a high rate of spontaneous mutations and approximately half of all patients do not have an affected parent. Two genes have been cloned for TSC. Both result in similar clinical features. The TSC1 gene, located on chromosome 9q34, codes for a novel protein called hamartin, which indirectly links the cell membrane to the cytoskeleton. TSC2, located at chromosome 16p13.3 encodes for the protein tuberin, which may function in cellular signaling pathways. Hamartin and tuberin interact together as part of a larger protein complex which functions to negatively regulate mTOR. When tuberin or hamartin is nonfunctional, mTOR is active, resulting in increased cell growth and proliferation. Rapamycin acts as an mTOR inhibitor and has shown efficacy in the treatment of subependymal giant cell astrocytomas in patients with TSC (➔ *Fig. 359.3*).

The clinical diagnosis of TSC is divided into three subheadings: definite, probable, and suspect based on the type and number of abnormalities. The clinical expression of TSC is based on the location and severity of organ involvement. The primary targets are the skin, kidneys, heart, and central nervous system. Hypopigmented macules are the most common skin lesions and are present in as many as 90% of affected patients. Adenoma sebaceum, an angiofibromatous lesion occurring in a butterfly

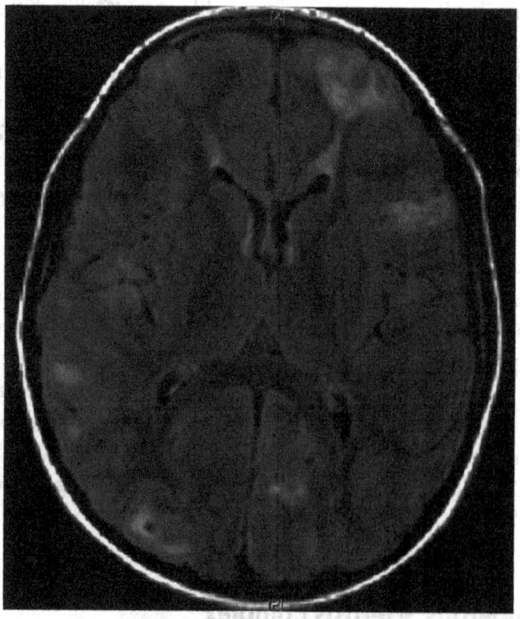

Figure 359.3
Tuberous sclerosis in a 4-year-old girl with multiple, bilateral cortical tubers

distribution about the nose and cheeks, is seen in 50%. Other skin lesions include the shagreen patch over the lumbosacral region, café au lait spots, and subungual fibromas. Tumors are common and include renal angiomyolipomas, cardiac rhabdomyomas, and retinal hamartomas.

In the brain, the characteristic features include cortical hamartomas (cortical tubers), subependymal hamartomas (subependymal nodules), and giant cell astrocytomas. Cortical tubers are firm and nodular, with a consistency resembling the potato tubers for which they are named. On MRI, cortical tubers appear as enlarged, atypically shaped gyri with abnormal signal intensity in the subcortical white matter. Microscopically, they resemble focal cortical dysplasia with disorganized lamination and balloon neurons. Beneath the cortex, subependymal nodules are at risk of transforming into subependymal giant cell astrocytomas.

Cortical tubers often result in epilepsy. Under 1 year of age, infantile spasms predominate. Vigabatrin is a particularly effective treatment for infantile spasms in TSC patients, and is widely considered to be first-line therapy in this setting. Later in life, generalized tonic–clonic seizures predominate, but simple and complex partial seizures are also common. Refractory epilepsy is a common problem in TSC; surgical resection of an epileptogenic cortical tuber is possible, and is most successful when a single epileptogenic area is identified.

The presence of epilepsy is a predictor of cognitive impairment – this is particularly true when seizures develop under 2 years of age or when infantile spasms occur. Cognitive impairment can also be predicted by the burden of cortical tubers, with more tubers correlating with greater impairment.

Autism is common in patients with TSC. It is more likely to develop in those with temporal tubers, seizure onset before age 3, or a history of infantile spasms. Attention, language, and behavioral problems are also observed. In general, TSC patients who are cognitively normal are seizure free and vice versa.

Subependymal nodules are common in TSC and consist of periventricular collections of small cells resembling candle drippings. In some instances, they transform into subependymal giant cell astrocytomas (SEGAs). SEGAs typically develop in the region of the foramen of Monro and can obstruct cerebral spinal fluid flow, resulting in hydrocephalus. Presenting symptoms include headache, vomiting, obtundation, or focal neurological deficits. Early recognition is important. Incompletely calcified periventricular nodules greater than 5 mm and nodules demonstrating gadolinium enhancement are at greater

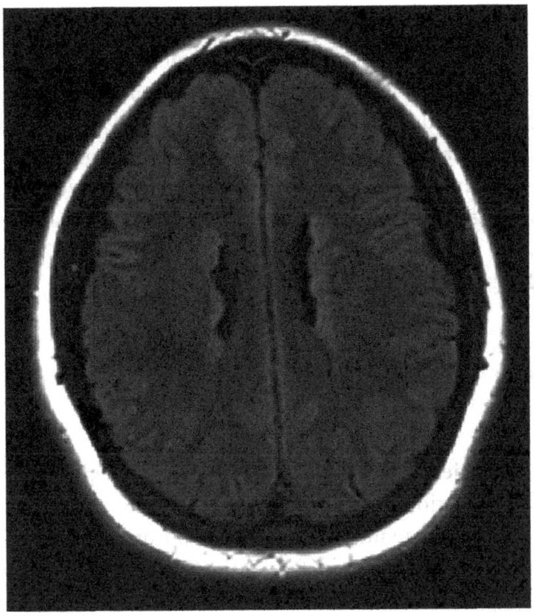

Figure 359.4
Periventricular nodular heterotopia in a 20-year-old woman

risk of transformation. Yet, the most important criterion for recognizing SEGAs is a progressive enlargement of the lesion. Neuroimaging is recommended prior to 2 years to screen for such lesions, and yearly follow-up may be necessary if suspicious periventricular nodules are observed (*Fig. 359.4*).

Focal Cortical Dysplasia

Focal cortical dysplasia (FCD) is essentially indistinguishable from the cortical tubers of TSC. Macroscopically, the lesions display wide gyri and blurring of the gray–white junction. Microscopic findings include disordered cortical lamination with dysplastic neurons and balloon cells. The underlying white matter is hypomyelinated and contains radially oriented balloon cells. The histology of FCD resembles tuberous sclerosis to such an extent that they have been postulated to be the same entity, with FCD representing a forme fruste of TSC. On MRI, FCD are slightly hyperintense on T2-weighted sequences. The hyperintense regions have a funnel-shaped appearance, with the base of the funnel oriented toward the pial surface and the tip extending to the white matter. Seizures resulting from FCD are commonly refractory to pharmacotherapy and surgical resection may be required to control the seizures.

Hypomelanosis of Ito

The brain malformations of hypomelanosis of Ito (HI) include abnormalities of neuronal differentiation (cortical dysplasia and hemimegalencephaly) and migration (heterotopia and polymicrogyria). The skin lesions of HI consist of whorls and streaks of decreased pigmentation, which follow the lines of Blaschko. There are no preceding inflammatory or vesicular eruptions as in incontinentia pigmenti, and the palms, soles, and mucous membranes are spared. The skin lesions are more prominent over the ventral surface of the torso and on the flexor surface of the extremities. They may be unilateral and exibit a midline cutoff. In patients with HI and hemimegalencephaly, the skin lesions are contralateral to the brain abnormality. Systemic manifestations include ophthalmologic, cardiac, musculoskeletal, and genital anomalies.

The neurological manifestations include epilepsy and mental retardation. Generalized tonic–clonic seizures are the most common, but infantile spasms, focal, and myoclonic seizures are also observed. Autistic behaviors are sometimes seen and are usually present in children with epilepsy. Pathology may reveal polymicrogyria, heterotopia, cortical dysplasia, or hemimegalencephaly. The etiology of HI is likely to be heterogeneous since several different choromosomal abnormalities have been associated with it.

Schizencephaly

The term "schizencephaly" refers to a cleft extending between the pial and lateral ventricular surfaces. Lining the cleft on both sides are polymicrogyria (abnormally small gyri). The presence of polymicrogyria helps distinguish this malformative lesion from the destructive disorder porencephaly, which has a similar appearance. Schizencephaly is heterogeneous in appearance. Lesions vary in size from small close-lip to large open-lip malformations. They may occur in one or both hemispheres. Possible etiologies are similarly heterogeneous. Environmental causes include fetal hypotension, exposure to organic solvents, and viral infections. Vascular anomalies have also been reported in association with schizencephaly. Familial cases exist, indicating a genetic mechanism in some patients. Mutations in the homeobox gene EMX2 have been reported in some cases.

The clinical severity relates to the degree of structural involvement. Unilateral clefts commonly present with hemiparesis and mild cognitive delay. Bilateral clefts, on the other hand, are associated with quadriparesis and significant cognitive impairment. Likewise, the size of the lesion is an important determinant of outcome. For example, patients with large or medium open-lip schizencephaly display significantly worse motor and intellectual function than patients with close-lip or small open-lip lesions. The severity of epilepsy, however, is generally unrelated to the structural findings.

Disorders of Neuronal Migration

Neuronal migration takes place between the third and fifth months of gestation. During migration, postmitotic neurons move from the ventricular and subventricular layers to their final sites within the cerebral cortex. Migration occurs in radial (perpendicular to the pial surface) and tangential (parallel to the pial surface) fashions.

Heterotopia

Heterotopia are collections of ectopic neurons located outside of the cortex. Unlike cortical dysplasia, the neurons within heterotopia are normal. On imaging, heterotopia are isointense with normal gray matter, lacking the abnormal signal intensity seen in dysplasia. The cortex overlying heterotopia is abnormally thin with shallow sulci.

Familial periventricular heterotopia (PH) are characterized by periventricular nodules of neurons resting beneath an otherwise normal-appearing cortex. In PH, some neurons migrate fully to form a normal-appearing six-layer cortex, while others have a complete failure of migration and remain in nodular collections within the subependymal region. Most patients have normal intelligence, but epilepsy is common and generally develops in the midteenage years.

Familial PH commonly displays X-linked dominant inheritance and is lethal in hemizygous male embryos. Approximately half of patients have a de novo mutation. Because epilepsy is mild or absent in approximately one-quarter of all patients, a family history is not always confirmed until neuroimaging of a patient's mother is performed. PH results from a mutation of the filamin A (FLNA) gene, which encodes a large actin-binding protein involved in structuring actin networks at the leading edge of motile cells.

Lissencephaly

Lissencephaly refers to a paucity of normal gyri and sulci resulting in a "smooth brain." It is a heterogeneous condition, which is traditionally divided into two pathologic subtypes: classical (type I) and cobblestone (type II). Radiographically, the cortex appears smooth in both types, but beyond that, few similarities exist. Classical lissencephaly results from an arrest of neuronal migration, whereas cobblestone lissencephaly results from overmigration. In both cases, lissencephaly is associated with epilepsy and severe developmental delay (➲ *Fig. 359.5*).

Classical Lissencephaly (Agyria–Pachygyria Complex)

Most patients with classical (type I) lissencephaly have a combination of agyria (a total absence of gyri) and pachygyria (a reduced number of abnormally large gyri). Radiographically, the surface of the brain appears smooth in agyria, with diminished white matter and shallow sylvian fissures. In pachygyria, gyri are reduced in number and are abnormally broad and flat. Microscopically, agyria has a disorganized outer cortical layer and a thick layer of ectopic neurons in the periventricular region, whereas pachygyria displays better cortical organization. Clinical severity is largely related to the degree of structural abnormality, with greater gyral simplification resulting

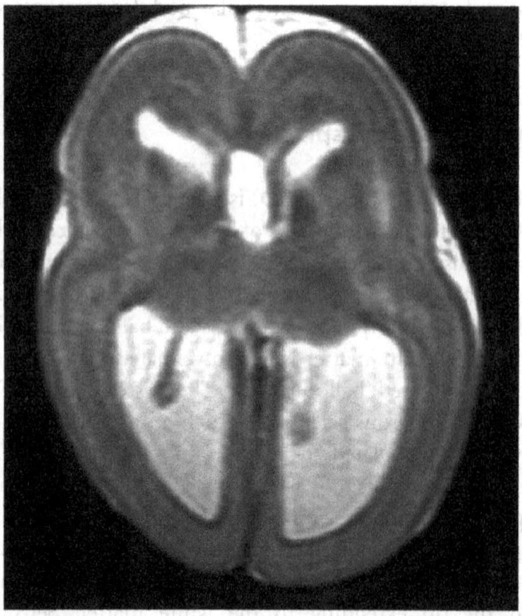

Figure 359.5
Classical lissencephaly in a patient with Miller–Dieker syndrome

in greater neurological impairment. In agyria, neurodevelopmental disabilities are severe. Patients exhibit mental retardation, spastic quadriparesis, and microcephaly. Epilepsy is universal and infantile spasms are a particularly common seizure type. In patients with pachygyria, epilepsy and developmental delays are common but are less severe. Electroencephalography reveals characteristic, high-voltage beta activity.

Classical lissencephaly is most commonly caused by a disruption of the platelet-activating factor, acetylhydrolase gene (PAFAH1B1; also known as LIS1) located on chromosome 17p13.3. Almost all patients have spontaneous, heterozygous deletions of LIS1, which are not present in the parents. The risk of having a second affected child is therefore low. When a large deletion occurs, other congenital anomalies (craniofacial, renal, cardiac, or gastrointestinal malformations) can result and together are termed the Miller–Dieker syndrome.

Abnormalities of the doublecortin (DCX or XLIS) gene, located on the X chromosome, are also known to cause classical lissencephaly. In hemizygous males, the phenotype is nearly indistinguishable from LIS1. Yet, in heterozygous females, a disorder termed double cortex (DC), also known as subcortical band heterotopia, results (➋ *Fig. 359.6*). In DC, the outer cortex displays normal six-layered architecture, but an inappropriate accumulation of neurons exists in the subcortical white matter. Random inactivation of the X chromosome accounts for this pattern. Half of the neurons express a normal copy of the doublecortin gene and undergo normal migration, whereas the other half express the mutant copy and remain arrested in the subcortical white matter. In males, only one X chromosome exists, so the mutation affects all neurons. Hence, the more severe phenotype of classical lissencephaly occurs in males.

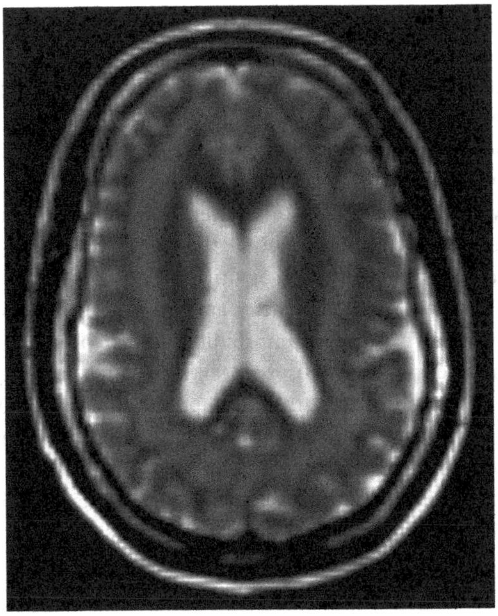

Figure 359.6
Double cortex (subcortical band heterotopia) in a 6-year-old girl with a heterozygous mutation of the doublecortin gene

Cobblestone (Type II) Lissencephaly

Cobblestone lissencephaly develops from an overmigration of neurons beyond the pial surface and onto the overlying subarachnoid tissue. Cobblestone lissencephaly is associated with congenital muscular dystrophy and eye abnormalities in Fukuyama congenital muscular dystrophy (FCMD), Walker–Warburg syndrome (WWS), and muscle–eye–brain disease (MEB). These disorders result from an impairment of glycosylation. They affect O-mannosylation, which is important to brain, nerve, and skeletal muscle, accounting for the distribution of involved tissues in these disorders.

Of all three disorders, WWS has the most severe phenotype and is often fatal in the first year of life. Genetically, WWS is recessively inherited. MEB is also an autosomal recessive condition and is most prevalent in Finland. The clinical severity is intermediate to WWS and FCMD as is the radiographic appearance. FCMD is the mildest of the three disorders. It presents with hypotonia and global developmental delays. Seizures develop in the first year of life in half of patients. FCMD is seen primarily in Japan, where 94% of the affected individuals share a common haplotype, indicating a single founder in the Japanese population. Patients who are homozygous for the founder mutation have a higher residual activity of fukutin and a milder phenotype than patients with a spontaneous point mutation on the second allele (compound heterozygotes).

Symmetric Polymicrogyria

Polymicrogyria is thought to develop at the latest stages of neuronal migration. It often results from external causes such as intrauterine cytomegalovirus infection or impairments in placental perfusion. Genetic causes also exist and tend to result in focal but symmetrical lesions in the frontoparietal, perisylvian, or parieto-occipital regions. Epilepsy and cognitive delays are common among all of the syndromes; additional symptoms depend upon the specific areas involved.

Disorders of Myelination and Cortical Organization

Cortical organization and myelination are the final steps of brain development and continue well after birth. Abnormalities at these stages may be less obvious on neuroimaging than earlier malformations, but they nonetheless have profound effects. Cognitive and motor impairments are associated with both abnormalities; spasticity is more specific to problems with myelination, whereas hypotonia is more likely in disorders of cortical organization.

Cortical organization begins in the fifth month of gestation and continues through the first several years of life. Abnormalities of cortical organization are commonly associated with mental retardation. The most consistent anatomical correlates of mental retardation are dendritic anomalies, such as deficient branching. Such abnormalities cannot be detected by neuroimaging, explaining why many patients with mental retardation have normal MRIs.

Myelination begins in the second trimester of pregnancy and continues into adulthood. Myelination is impaired when oligodrendrocytes are deficient in number or in myelin deposition around axons. Insufficient oligodendrocytes are observed in periventricular leukomalacia, in which differentiating oligodendroglia are injured and therefore unable to produce myelin. Other disorders, such as hypothyroidism, malnutrition, and organic acidopathies, cause functional impairment of myelination. Primary disturbances of myelination are distinguished from leukodystrophies in that leukodystrophies result from injury to previously myelinated axons.

Neurofibromatosis Type I

The primary disorder in neurofibromatosis relates to oncogene regulation and tumor formation. Given the white matter abnormalities in NF, it is categorized here as a disorder of myelination, but increased gray matter volume is also seen, highlighting a larger disorder of brain overgrowth in neurofibromatosis.

Neurofibromatosis type 1 (NF1), also known as peripheral neurofibromatosis, is an autosomal-dominant, single-gene defect affecting multiple organ systems. The NF1 gene localizes to chromosome 17q11.2 and encodes the protein product neurofibromin. The incidence of NF1 ranges between 1 in 3,000 and 1 in 4,000. Approximately 50% of patients with NF1 lack a family history and likely represent new mutations. The diagnosis is based on NIH consensus criteria and requires two or more of the following: six or more café au lait spots (0.5 mm or larger in prepubertal and 1.5 mm or larger in postpubertal individuals), two or more neurofibromas of any type or one plexiform neurofibroma, axillary or groin freckling, two or more Lisch nodules, optic nerve glioma, dysplasia of the sphenoid bone or long bone cortex, or a first-degree relative with NF1. Of these features, café au lait spots are the most easily recognized and are often the presenting feature of the disease. They are evenly pigmented macules, which increase in size and number with age. They may be the only sign present in infancy, making a definitive diagnosis difficult to establish until later in life.

In childhood, the most common complication of NF1 is cognitive impairment. A broad range of effects are seen including low IQ, behavioral problems, and learning disabilities. IQ scores in NF1 patients have a bimodal distribution; some children have intellectual impairment, whereas others do not. This separation may have its basis in the white matter T2 hyperintensities, also known as unidentified bright objects (UBOs), common to NF1 patients. They represent dysplastic glial proliferation and aberrant myelination in the underdeveloped brain. When compared to children without T2 hyperintensities, those with the lesions have significantly lower mean values for IQ and language scores and significantly impaired visuomotor integration and coordination. T2 hyperintensities in childhood are also a predictor of cognitive dysfunction in adulthood. A correlation is also seen between increased white matter volume and visual-perceptual deficits, suggesting that brain overgrowth is a factor in the associated cognitive deficits.

Tumors and malignancies are common in NF1, and are a major cause of morbidity. Neurofibromas, the tumors for which the disorder takes its name, are peripheral nerve sheath tumors with unpredictable growth patterns. They are benign tumors without risk of malignant transformation, and typically develop in adolescence. Although they are unlikely to cause neurological deficit, spinal neurofibromas arising from the dorsal nerve roots can lead to severe pain. Plexiform neurofibromas, on the other hand, are more likely to be present at birth. They can be found anywhere within the body and cause a variety of presenting symptoms depending on their location. Serious complications include pain, spinal cord compression, and spread to the orbit with resulting sphenoid wing dysplasia and pulsating exophthalmos. Plexiform neurofibromas can undergo transformation to malignant peripheral nerve sheath tumors.

Optic nerve gliomas are pilocytic astrocytomas involving the optic nerve, chiasm, or tract. They usually develop prior to age 7 and can be insidious in their onset. Yearly ophthalmologic assessments are important for early diagnosis and management of these tumors. Abnormalities on the ophthalmologic exam necessitate an MRI. Other malignancies observed in NF1 include CNS tumors (particularly astrocytomas), pheochromocytomas, and leukemia. Given the prevalence of tumors in NF1, it should come as no surprise that neurofibromin functions as a tumor suppressor protein, the loss of which promotes tumor formation.

The workup for NF1 is aimed at the early identification of potential complications, with tumor formation being the main concern. The American Academy of Pediatrics Committee on Genetics recommends yearly physical examinations and ophthalmologic assessments. The physical examination focuses on the organ systems involved. The skin is screened for new neurofibromas or plexiform neurofibromas. Blood pressure is followed to assess for renal or endocrine abnormalities. A skeletal examination looks for pseudoarthrosis of the tibia, bowing of the long bones, scoliosis, and orbital defects. The neurological examination may reveal macrocephaly, learning disabilities, or cognitive impairment. The ophthalmologic evaluation helps exclude optic nerve gliomas, choroidal hamartomas, and Lisch nodules.

Neurofibromatosis Type II

Like NF1, neurofibromatosis type II (NF2) is an autosomal-dominant, single-gene deficit, which, in NF2, localizes to chromosome 22. The gene product, merlin, also has tumor suppressor function. Tumors and malignancies are, therefore, common in both conditions. Beyond that, few similarities exist. Café au lait spots are rarely seen in NF2 and neurofibromas are uncommon. NF2 is much less common than NF1, with an incidence of only 1:30,000–1:40,000.

Common tumors in NF2 include schwannomas (which are usually multiple), meningiomas, ependymomas, and gliomas. Vestibulocochlear schwannomas are particularly common and sometimes bilateral. Roughly half of NF2 patients present because of hearing loss, tinnitus, and vertigo resulting from a vestibulocochlear schwannoma. The peak age of diagnosis is the third decade. In children, ocular abnormalities are the most common presenting symptoms. These are caused by hamartomas of the retina, optic nerve sheath meningiomas, or juvenile posterior subcapsular lenticular opacities. Meningiomas at a young age should also raise a suspicion of NF2. Schwannomas and ependymomas may develop in the spine, in which case back pain and paraplegia may result.

Vascular Disorders

The following disorders result from vascular abnormalities, and therefore cannot be organized within the embryological classification presented above even though each results in developmental abnormalities of the brain.

Bilateral Parasagittal Parieto-Occipital Polymicrogyria

Unlike the other symmetrical polymicrogyria syndromes, bilateral parasagittal parieto-occipital polymicrogyria is unlikely to have a genetic basis. Of the patients described, none had a familial distribution. Given that the lesion occurs in a vascular watershed region, perfusion failure is postulated to be the cause. All patients develop seizures and cognitive abilities range from normal to mild retardation.

Incontinentia Pigmenti

Incontinentia pigmenti is a rare, X-linked, dominant, neurocutaneous disorder with the onset of skin changes in the first 6 weeks of life. The cutaneous disorder follows a characteristic evolution from vesicular to verrucous to hyperpigmented and finally atrophic changes. The vesicles and bullae from the original eruption in infancy later give rise to the characteristic swirling pattern of hyperpigmentation. Hair, nail, dental, and ophthalmologic abnormalities are also observed. Neurologically, these infants may develop epilepsy, mental retardation, microcephaly, spasticity, or ataxia. The gene for incontinentia pigmenti is NEMO (NF-kappaB essential modulator)/IKKgamma (IkappaB kinase-gamma) and is located on Xq28. NEMO is 200 kilobases proximal to the factor VIII locus and is important for immune, inflammatory, and apoptotic pathways. The disorder is lethal in most males, accounting for its 20:1 female-to-male predominance. Males with IP have been described, but commonly have only a limited distribution. Somatic mosaicism is a likely mechanism in such cases.

Sturge–Weber Syndrome

Sturge–Weber syndrome is characterized by angiomata of the leptomeninges and skin. The cutaneous lesion, also known as a port-wine stain, typically involves the ophthalmic and maxillary distributions of the trigeminal nerve. The leptomeningeal angiomata may be either unilateral or bilateral, but unilateral lesions are more common. The specific neurological effects are dependent on the location of the lesion, which is most commonly parietal or occipital. Neurological impairment results from stasis and a vascular steal phenomenon. Laminar cortical necrosis with neuronal loss, gliosis, cerebral atrophy, and calcifications are seen histologically. The calcifications take on a classic train-track appearance on plain films and CT. MRI, if done, should be performed with gadolinium to allow for diagnosis of the angiomata. The clinical manifestations include hemiparesis, stroke-like episodes, mental retardation, epilepsy, and headaches. Epilepsy is present in 75–90% of patients, and the seizures are typically focal. Many patients have refractory epilepsy, in which case cortical resection or hemispherectomy are considered. An important non-neurological effect is glaucoma, which can occur at any age.

Conclusion

For children with disorders of nervous system development, there are few specific therapeutic interventions available beyond physical, occupational, and speech therapy and remedial education. Epilepsy resulting from brain malformations is often refractory to pharmacotherapy, but surgical resection of epileptogenic cortical malformations may be an option for some of these children. A crucial role for the treating physician is to provide counseling and guidance. This is particularly important in newly diagnosed children whose parents are burdened by uncertainty. A thoughtful, compassionate approach to the radiographic and genetic assessment can offer the parents insight into their child's condition, and the genetic evaluation is particularly important for purposes of family planning.

References

Barkovich AJ, Kjos BO (1992a) Nonlissencephalic cortical dysplasias: correlation of imaging findings with clinical deficits. AJNR Am J Neuroradiol 13:104–106

Barkovich AJ, Kjos BO (1992b) Schizencephaly: correlation of clinical findings with MR characteristics. AJNR Am J Neuroradiol 13: 104–106

Barkovich AJ, Kuzniecky RI, Dobyns WB, Jackson GD, Becker LE, Evrard P (1996) A classification scheme for malformations of cortical development. Neuropediatrics 27:59–63

Barkovich AJ, Kuzniecky RI, Jackson GD, Guerrini R, Dobyns WB (2001) Classification system for malformations of cortical development. Neurology 57:2168–2178

Cardoso C, Leventer RJ, Ward HL et al (2003) Refinement of a 400-kb critical region allows genotypic differentiation between isolated lissencephaly, Miller–Dieker syndrome, and other phenotypes secondary to deletions of 17p13.3. Am J Hum Genet 72:918–930

Franz DN, Leonard J, Tudor C, Chuck G, Care M, Sethuraman G, Dinopoulos A, Thomas G, Crone KR (2006) Rapamycin causes regression of astrocytomas in tuberous sclerosis complex. Ann Neurol 59:490–498

Inoki K, Corradetti MN, Guan KL (2005) Dysregulation of the TSC-mTOR pathway in human disease. Nat Genet 37:19–24

Smahi A, Courtois G, Vabres P et al (2000) Genomic rearrangement in NEMO impairs NF- kappaB activation and is a cause of incontinentia pigmenti. The international incontinentia pigmenti (ip) consortium. Nature 405:466–472

Tassi L, Colombo N, Garbelli R et al (2002) Focal cortical dysplasia: neuropathological subtypes, EEG, neuroimaging and surgical outcome. Brain 125:1719–1732

Taylor DC, Falconer MA, Bruton CJ, Corsellis JAN (1971) Focal dysplasia of the cerebral cortex in epilepsy. J Neurol Neurosurg Psychiatry 34: 369–387

Toda T, Kobayashi K, Kondo-Iida E, Sasaki J, Nakamura Y (2000) The Fukuyama congenital muscular dystrophy story. Neuromuscul Disord 10:153–159

360 Neonatal Neurological Disorders

William D. Brown · Mara G. Coyle

Introduction

At no time in life are the limitations of the neurological assessment more obvious than during the neonatal (0–28 days) period. The reflex hammer, light, and bell do no justice to the transformation taking place within the nervous system. Myelination exposes already present reflexes to the possibility of change and allows for new abilities to evolve, though the function of many unmyelinated systems is well established and acquisition of function is not always related to the occurrence of myelination. Within related functional systems, myelination generally progresses in a predictable pattern from the neuron along the axon in the direction of information flow, with the important exception of the optic system that proceeds in the reverse direction (see ➔ *Table 360.1*). In this context, the neurologist is frequently called upon to interpret the meaning of subtleties within the examination, and to divine prognosis from them. Rapid advancement in imaging techniques is allowing for more informed divination, but the use of technology to inform clinical judgment is necessarily imprecise.

This is not to say that the neurologist or pediatrician is without tools. Assessment of the neonate begins with an accounting of antecedent events that may or may not modify the clinical situation. Family history and the maternal medical history prior to pregnancy may be relevant. The quality of the gestational environment – maternal nutrition, exposure to prescription or over-the-counter medications, drugs of abuse, or physical trauma – should be assessed. Perinatal factors such as the use of forceps or vacuum extractors, the presence of a nuchal or knotted umbilical cord, placental abruption, or need for emergency caesarean section could be important to the neurological outcome. If cardiopulmonary resuscitation of the infant is required, a detailed chronological recitation of events should be reviewed.

Basic Physical Examination

The physical examination begins with simple observation, using the presence or absence of dysmorphic features or skeletal abnormalities, the facial appearance, and head shape and size to determine further actions. This examination is best performed during times of quiet wakefulness as is found between feedings although in the preterm or acutely ill neonate such an opportunity may not exist.

In order to interpret physical findings, accurate gestational age estimates are important. First trimester ultrasound examination is the most accurate way of estimating gestational age, with a range of error of 3 days. Additional methods used to estimate gestational age include the date of the mother's last menstrual period and the Dubowitz or Ballard examination, all of which have a range of error in the postnatal period of ± 2 weeks.

Healthy term infants will present a position of limb flexion while preterm or sick term infants are likely to appear more flaccid. Growth parameters should be documented at the time of delivery in order to determine if the infant is appropriate, small, or large for gestational age. This determination may direct the clinician to look for size-specific patterns of medical and neurological complications. Large for gestational age infants (LGA, birthweight >2 SD above the mean for age), for example, are at risk for hypoglycemia, polycythemia, and shoulder dystocia with or without brachial plexus injuries, while growth-restricted infants are at risk for long-term developmental and academic morbidities, including a fivefold to tenfold risk of death.

For those infants suspected of being small for gestational age (SGA, birthweight <2 SD below the mean for age), the occipital frontal circumference (OFC, measured using the middle of the forehead and the inion as reference points) will determine if they are symmetrically or asymmetrically growth restricted, an important distinction since variations in growth imply a risk for certain morbidities. Growth restriction affects up to 10% of all newborn infants, but it should be remembered that an infant designated as having intrauterine growth retardation can still be size-appropriate for gestational age.

When *symmetric* growth restriction is present (weight, length, and head circumference all <10th percentile for age) the cause is often related to chromosomal anomalies,

Abdelaziz Y. Elzouki (ed.), *Textbook of Clinical Pediatrics*, DOI 10.1007/978-3-642-02202-9_360,

Table 360.1
Correlation of brain and organ development with neurological function and gestational age in neonates

Gestational age (weeks)	Organ development	Brain development			Neurological function		
		Sulci and Fissures	Gyri	Myelination	Arousal	Examination	Reflexes
20–21		Rolandic, collateral superior temporal; Germinal matrix still increasing in size	Parahippocampal, superior temporal	Medullary and pontine MLF			
22				Mesencephalic MLF			
23				Medullary MLF, trapezoid body	Eyes tend to remain closed, opening briefly only in response to sustained noxious stimulation		
24	Surfactant formation begins	Pre- and postrolandic, middle temporal, interparietal, superior frontal, lateral occipital; Germinal matrix begins rapid phase of volume loss at 26 weeks, losing half of volume between 26 and 28 weeks of gestational age	Pre- and postrolandic, middle temporal, superior and inferior parietal lobules, superior and middle frontal, superior and inferior occipital, cuneus and lingual, fusiform	Inferior cerebellar peduncle, spinal trigeminal tract, pontine and mesencephalic lateral lemniscus, pontine medial lemniscus			
25				Pontine medial lemniscus		Extraocular movements present to Dolls' eyes maneuver	Extraocular movements present to Doll's Eye maneuver
26				Pontine and mesencephalic superior cerebellar peduncle		Blinks to light	
27	Pulmonary primitive alveoli appear			Parasagittal cerebellum		Response to noxious stimulus present	Pectoralis major reflex present
28		Inferior temporal, inferior frontal	Inferior temporal, triangular, medial and lateral orbital, callosomarginal, transverse temporal, angular and supramarginal, external occipitotemporal	Ansa lenticularis, amiculum	Eyes tend to remain closed, opening for prolonged periods of time with gentle stimuli; eyes open spontaneously	Sucking and swallowing but not breathing coordinated; resistance to passive limb manipulation minimal	Blinks or startles to sudden noise, rooting reflex present; palmar grasp present

29	Glomerular filtration rate 0.3–0.5 cm^3/min			Optic tract, capsule red nucleus			
30	Active alveolation begins; glomerular filtration rate 0.5–1.0 cm^3/min					Pupils may constrict to light	Cold calorics cause ipsilateral eye deviation
31							
32	Bowel motility allows passage of contrast through small bowel to colon;	Marginal, secondary superior, middle, inferior frontal, temporal, parietal, occipital, insular; germinal matrix involution nearly complete	Paracentral	Posterior limb internal capsule, optic chiasm	Eyes open spontaneously, with roving eye movements present; sleeping and waking periods are observable	Eyes closed as long as light shone in them; visual fixation present, pupils consistently constrict to light, spontaneous movements present; some lower extremity flexor tone present	Incomplete response to Moro
33							Achilles, patellar, biceps, thigh adductor, brachioradialis reflexes present
34				Corona radiata, mesencephalic corticospinal tract		Visual tracking present; sucking, swallowing, and breathing coordinated for limited oral feeding	
35				Transpontine middle cerebellar peduncle, pontine corticospinal tract, pyramid		Some visual pattern preference present	Tonic neck response present

Table 360.1 (Continued)

Gestational age (weeks)	Organ development	Brain development			Neurological function		
		Sulci and Fissures	Gyri	Myelination	Arousal	Examination	Reflexes
36	Bilirubin no longer found in amniotic fluid	Secondary transverse and inferior temporal and cingulate, tertiary superior, middle inferior frontal and superior parietal sulci; germinal matrix absent	Anterior and posterior orbital		Crying may accompany waking periods	Flexor tone present in upper and lower extremities; head remains briefly upright when held in sitting position	Head turning to noxious stimulation of face
37						Visual orientation to light, opticokinetic nystagmus present	Classic Moro reflex present; placing and stepping reflexes present. Palmar grasp strong enough to lift trunk off the bed
38				Cingulum, anterior limb internal capsule, rostral optic radiation and lateral mesencephalic peduncle, cerebellar hemisphere			
39							
40	Glomerular filtration rate (<24°) 2–3.5 cm^3/h; (>72°) 4–8 cm^3/h	Secondary orbital, callosomarginal, and insular, tertiary inferior temporal and superior and inferior occipital			Orients to both visual and auditory stimuli	Visual fixation and following present; acuity 20/150; flexion tone obvious; fists remain closed; little head lag when pulled to sit;	Symmetric unsustained ankle clonus and Babinski reflex present

Adapted from (1) Kuban KC, Skouteli HN, Urion DK, Lawhon GA (1986) Deep tendon reflexes in premature infants. Pediatr Neurol 2(5):226–271
(2) Gilles FH, Leviton A, Dooling EC (1983) The developing human brain. John Wright PSG, Littleton
(3) Saint-Anne Dargassies S (1977) Neurological development in the full-term and premature infant. Excerpta Medica, New York
(4) Volpe JJ (2008) Neurology of the newborn, 5th edn. Saunders/Elsevier, Philadelphia
(5) Brazleton TB (1973) Neonatal behavioral assessment scale. J.B. Lippincott, Philadelphia
(6) Amiel-Tison C, Davis SW (1991) Newborn neurologic examination. In: Rudolph AM, Hoffman JIE (eds) Pediatrics, 19th edn. Appleton & Lange, Norwalk

environmental toxic exposures especially alcohol, and intrauterine infections. These infants are at risk for neurodevelopmental delay, neurosensory deficits, and academic impairment.

Asymmetric growth restriction results in weight and length measures below the 10th percentile for age, but preserves head growth. This occurs in the last trimester and is usually associated with placental insufficiency. These infants are at a significant disadvantage with respect to growth potential and cognitive performance. More than 80% of these infants will "catch up" in their growth during the first year, but those who do not by age 2 years have an even chance of being short adults. For both symmetric and asymmetric growth-restricted infants, the ratio of head circumference to birth weight × 100 (cephalization index) has the most significant correlation with both neurodevelopmental status and cognitive performance by 10 years of age.

In addition to the OFC, the shape of the head should be assessed. Excess scalp edema, swelling, or subgaleal hemorrhage can contribute to the circumference so the OFC should be remeasured after their resolution. Head shape may also affect the circumference, as is seen in the various craniosynostoses: premature closure of the sagittal suture will result in dolichocephaly while early closure of the coronal sutures results in brachycephaly. The majority of children with these lesions do not have associated genetic syndromes. The presence of visible cutaneous tracts, dimples, or palpable subcutaneous masses should raise the suspicion of an encephalocele or tumor, especially when they are in the midline near the nasion or inion. The spine should be inspected to look for dimples, pimples, pits, and tufts of hair, with the level of suspicion for associated spinal dysraphism (lipomas, spina bifida, dermal sinuses, and tethered spinal cord) increasing with more rostral lesions.

Palpation of the skull is important when traumatic lesions such as a cephalohematoma, caput succedaneum, or skull fracture are suspected. The diamond-shaped anterior fontanel should be flat and its center gives way to gentle manual compression, while the borders of the triangular posterior fontanel may not always be appreciated particularly if the sutures are overriding. The presence of a large or bulging fontanel can suggest a skeletal dysplasia or increased intracranial pressure. The final assessment of the head should include the hair pattern. The location of the hairline (widow's peak, low hairline), absence or sparsity (alopecia), quality (wiry, curly, twisted), or color of the hair (gray, blonde, white forelock) is important to note, as these may be associated with genetic or metabolic disorders.

Evidence of minor malformations such as abnormally positioned or rotated ears or eyes, syndactyly, or polydactyly should suggest the possibility of a major systemic malformation since there is a 90% chance of a major malformation when three or more "minor" malformations are identified. When examining the mouth, particular attention should be given to the palate and tongue. A large tongue can be seen in multiple disorders with neurological implications including hypothyroidism, *Beckwith–Wiedemann Syndrome*, and lysosomal storage disorders, while fasciculations of the tongue can be seen in lower motor neuron disease such as Werdnig–Hoffmann (*spinal muscular atrophy, type I*). A high arched palate in a newborn implies hypotonia preceding delivery.

Dermatoglyphics are the dermal ridges on the palmar aspect of the digits, palms, and soles; when abnormal, a variety of syndromes are implicated. The two general categories of dermatoglyphic alterations are an aberrant pattern or unusual frequency or disruption of a typical pattern on the fingertips.

Organomegaly can be seen in infectious diseases as well as storage disorders. The skin exam is important when considering infectious illnesses (petechiae, purpura) or neurocutaneous disorders. Loose or redundant skin can be seen in the SGA infant with a paucity of subcutaneous fat, or in connective tissue disorders such as *Ehlers–Danlos Syndrome*. Disorders of skin color (hyperpigmented, hypopigmented, café-au-lait, nevi) may, depending upon their number or distribution, represent a multitude of diagnoses or be of no clinical significance. Vascular malformations such as the strawberry hemangioma may not always be evident right at birth, or be quite obvious. A port wine stain or capillary hemangioma on the face should always suggest diagnosis of leptomeningeal capillary venous angiomatosis, which can be associated with seizures or glaucoma.

The shape of the thorax may suggest the presence of neurological disease. A narrow superior thorax with a flared, wider base suggests the possibility of pulmonary hypoplasia and respiratory weakness associated with spinal muscular atrophy.

Evaluation of the extremities should include the presence or absence of contractures or arthrogryposis. Limitation of movement in utero can be due to a primary neurological abnormality (meningomyelocele, anencephaly, holoprosencephaly), a muscle disorder (fetal myopathies, myotonic dystrophy, muscle agenesis), a joint or tissue disorder (synostosis, lack of joint development, laxity of joint), or external constraint as is seen in twin or triplet pregnancies.

Neurological Examination

Level of Arousal

The neurological assessment is best performed without overhead lighting directly in the neonate's eyes, as this will in many cases preclude the examiner's ability to visualize the retina and optic disk, or to obtain papillary reflexes. If the infant will not open the eyes, then it will not be possible to make any statements about visual tracking or fixation or to record the presence or absence of even basic observations such as nystagmus or papillary responses. The notion of a level of arousal in a newborn infant does not have the same meaning as in an older infant, but Brazleton's descriptions of six states of arousal: (1) deep sleep (eyes closed, no spontaneous movements except for respirations, limbs flaccid), (2) quiet sleep (eyes closed, eye movements present rare spontaneous limb or head movements, limbs demonstrate some tone), (3) active sleep (frequent spontaneous movements, eyes closed), (4) quiet awake (eyes open, rare spontaneous movements), (5) active awake (eyes open, spontaneous limb movements), and (6) crying – are useful in consideration of an infant's arousal state. Most normal term infants tend to fluctuate between the active sleep and quiet awake states, with other states achieved only briefly or with stimulation. The infant with an encephalopathy, drug toxicity, or neonatal abstinence will tend to assume one of the other states, and be more difficult to coax to the quiet awake or active sleep states. Coaxing may require a soothing voice, dimming of the lights, a gentle touch, pacifier, swaddling, or pharmacological intervention; the difficulty or ease with which calming may be induced may also shed light on the infant's "state."

Habituation

Habituation is the extinction of an observed behavioral response to repetitive external stimulation and may be considered in the assessment of the neonate. A blinking response to light or glabellar tapping, withdrawal of the foot to stroking, or the sudden upper extremity extension and abduction response to noise (Moro reflex) are examples of reflex behaviors that are normally present. Repetition of the stimulus in a normal newborn will reliably produce a response over a limited number of trials (usually 4–8), but then the response disappears. Obligatory occurrence of the response beyond this is abnormal and suggests an impairment of neurological functioning, but should be considered in the context of the rest of the examination.

Eye Examination

Any attempts to examine the eyes should be done in a quiet, darkened room, with the intensity of the ophthalmoscope at the minimum to allow for adequate visualization; high intensity halogen light sources will simply produce lid closure, a resistant baby, and a frustrated examiner. The infant should be swaddled, recently fed if possible, and held in front of the examiner at a 45° vertical angle to facilitate spontaneous eye opening and looking. Retinal hemorrhages may occasionally be seen after a vaginal delivery; their presence is important to note along with the presence of a normal optic disk. Optic atrophy may be the first indication that a more significant neurological disorder such as septo-optic dysplasia may be present. Ipsilateral dilation of the pupil in response to noxious stimulation of the skin is the ciliospinal reflex and may be very useful to the examiner when the integrity of the spinal cord is in doubt as the pupillary dilation response will be absent at spinal segments below the level of the lesion.

Convincing demonstration of visual tracking may require a bright red or highly contrasting white and black object such as a ring target since visual acuity of the newborn is poor. A dimmed pinpoint or penlight light source moved across the visual field in a darkened room may also elicit a visual "grasping" reflex. The twisted end of a sterile cotton swab may be used when necessary to elicit a corneal reflex. Using the vertical axis of the examiner as a reference, clockwise or counterclockwise rotation of the baby will produce leftward or rightward deviation of the infant's eyes, respectively, for the duration of the rotation.

The Face

Useful landmarks are the nasolabial folds, angles of the mouth, and eye lids. Observation of facial symmetry should be performed during differing arousal states, with the quiet awake and crying states most useful. A common source of concern is drooping of the lower portion of the mouth, noted best when the infant cries. When this is the only abnormality on examination, the most likely explanation is hypoplasia or aplasia of the depressor anguli oris muscle of the *opposite* side rather than a central parenchymal or peripheral nerve injury. The presence of a triangular or persistently open mouth should suggest the possibility of a myopathy or muscular dystrophy. The palpebral fissure is the vertical distance between the upper and lower eyelids, and may be difficult to assess in the recently delivered infant due to edema of the eyelids; attempts to pry the eyelids open will generally result in their eversion. When the eyes are open, the presence or absence of unilateral or bilateral ptosis should be combined with the eye examination to determine whether the ptosis is likely to be related to a focal brain stem or nerve injury rather than generalized weakness as is seen in maternally acquired or congenital myasthenia gravis. Pinching the toes may produce crying: this is a good opportunity to compare the symmetry of movement of both sides of the face as well as the nasolabial folds and forehead creases to the spontaneous facial movements of the awake infant at rest.

The Oropharynx

In utero movements of the tongue will tend to mold the hard palate into a gentle arch during gestation; when oropharyngeal or lingual muscle strength is deficient, the palate develops into a shape like a furrow with a high arch and narrowed distance between the maxillary alveolar ridges. Insertion of a finger into the mouth of a term baby will induce a sucking reflex wherein the finger is forced into the hard palate by the tongue and an undulating anterior to posterior movement of the tongue is combined with a suctioning action. The undersurface of the tongue is a good place to look for muscle fasiculations suggestive of anterior horn cell disease in the weak patient. Mechanical or sensory stimulation of the soft palate, posterior tongue, or superior oropharynx will produce coughing or gagging in the awake infant. The presence of a cleft in the soft or hard palate should alert the observer to the possibility of other midline malformations affecting the hypothalamus or pituitary when clinically suspected. The presence of a single midline incisor or the absence of the upper lip frenulum should raise suspicions that a disorder of prosencephalic development such as holoprosencephaly is present.

The Ear

The shape, size, and orientation of the auricles should be noted; the superior attachment of the ear should be tangential to a line extended from one lateral eye canthus to the other. Malformations of the ear should suggest the possibility of branchial arch anomalies and raise suspicions of accompanying malformations of the middle and inner ear. These may be easily confirmed by computed tomography of the temporal bones. The external auditory meatus receives sensory input from four nerves: the second and third cervical, trigeminal, and vagus nerves. The presence of aberrant sensory input from the vagus nerve may rarely account for unexplained coughing or gagging when the external auditory meatus is stimulated. Bedside tests of audition with a bell, shouting, or a striking of the bed with an open palm are unreliable predictors of intact hearing; any suspicions that a hearing deficit is present should be confirmed by auditory evoked potentials.

Motor Examination

No voluntary motor movements are possible in the newborn of any gestational age, so the traditional methods of assessing muscle strength may not be applied. All movements are involuntary, reflex, or spontaneous; it is the spontaneous movements that are most relevant to the condition of the nervous system. Small for gestational age and premature infants will normally have decreased muscle bulk which in turn affects the ability to hold up the head or resist traction maneuvers, and this may falsely suggest muscle weakness. When hypotonia is present, care must be taken not to assume that muscles must therefore have diminished strength, for both hypotonia and normal strength may be simultaneously present.

Traction maneuvers are the traditional method to assess motor tone in the newborn as well as to make a subjective estimate of relative muscle strength. In the lower extremity the malleoli are grasped between the thumb and first fingers with the baby supine, and the heel is gently lifted upward until the buttocks begins to leave the bed. The popliteal angle so generated is noted, and compared with normal values enumerated by Amiel-Tison for each gestational age. An angle less than specified suggests increased tone; greater suggests relative hypotonia. A similar procedure is possible for the upper extremities: the wrist is gently pulled upward until the shoulder comes off the bed, and the angle at the elbow estimated.

There is by necessity some subjectivity involved in these assessments of tone, leading some authors to question their usefulness. However, observation of posture alone does not always inform the examiner of the degree of muscle tone present since an assessment of tone (intrinsic resistance to passive movement offered by the ligaments, tendons, and muscles) requires actually moving the limbs. Spasticity (an increase in the degree resistance to passive movement when the velocity of induced movement is increased) is rarely present in the newborn, as its appearance implies a passage of time in weeks or months since the causative injury occurred; when marked hypertonia, rigidity, or spasticity is present, other causes such as severe diffuse cerebral injury, meningitis, posterior fossa lesion, increased intracranial pressure, or the pharmacological abstinence syndrome should be suspected. Finally, hypertonia may be present because of excessive intrinsic muscle contractions seen with myotonic and paramyotonic disorders as well as hyperkalemic periodic paralyses.

Reflexes

Three general categories of reflexes are present in the infant: tendon reflexes, postural reflexes, and brain stem reflexes. Tendon reflexes are generally easy to obtain at the pectoralis, biceps, knee, and ankle jerks. In the term newborn, reflex spread (occurrence of a muscle contraction more than one joint away from the tested reflex) in the form of crossed adductors at the knees is normally present as is ankle clonus, though clonus is always abnormal when sustained or asymmetric. Postural reflexes are the intrinsic changes in tone or posture induced by movement, tactile stimuli, or the position of a body part. These include the rooting, glabellar, palmomental, palmar and plantar grasping, Moro, tonic neck, righting, placing and stepping, Landau, Galant, Santmyer swallow, vertical and horizontal suspension reflexes. Postural reflexes generally disappear with time and may reappear late in life either as a part of normal aging or in the context of various progressive or degenerative disorders as "release" phenomena. Brain stem reflexes have been described elsewhere in this chapter. The presence or absence and symmetry of the reflex responses should be noted.

Sensation

The sensory examination is of limited value in the newborn, as there are few ways to determine whether stimulation is perceived. Gradations of sensory stimulation (tickling, touching, firm pressure, or forceful pinching) may be used to generate responses varying from toe flexion, head turning, limb withdrawal, or crying, and are of most use in two situations: determining level of responsiveness and in assessing whether sensation is present in a paretic limb.

Clinical Problems

The seven categories are:

1. Excessive spontaneous motor movements
2. Diminished spontaneous motor movements
3. Alteration of mental status
4. Changes in head size and pressure
5. Hypoxic-ischemic encephalopathy
6. Imaging abnormalities
7. Brain death determination

Excessive Movements (Non-epileptic)

Jitteriness

Neonates often display abnormal movements that may suggest the possibility of seizures such as jitteriness, excessive startling, pedaling or stepping movements of the limbs, oral-lingual-buccal movements, or transient dystonic posturing. The traditional definition of seizures requires that neuronal paroxysmal discharges as documented by the electroencephalogram accompany the behavior in question. When such discharges are present, the diagnosis of seizures is not in doubt. When discharges cannot be documented in the neonate, however, the diagnosis of seizures is called into question but not necessarily excluded. This particular situation is discussed in the chapter on neonatal seizures. This section concerns movements that are *not* epileptic in origin.

Jitteriness is a low frequency, large amplitude tremulousness of the limbs and jaw that may be both spontaneous and provoked by innocuous visual, sensory, or auditory stimulation. Eye movements and gaze are normal, and help to distinguish jitteriness from seizures. While jitteriness may be regarded as a sign of central nervous system irritability, it may also be seen in up to 40% of normal term newborn infants. Tendon reflexes, a spontaneous Moro, and clonus are concomitantly exaggerated and easy to elicit. Gentle suppression of the limb movements with the examiner's hand will generally inhibit jitteriness; when it does not, seizures should be suspected. The more common causes of jitteriness include perinatal asphyxia, hypocalcemia, hypoglycemia, hypoxic-ischemic encephalopathy, and drug withdrawal. Correction of hypocalcemia or hypoglycemia will usually abolish jitteriness.

Neonatal Abstinence

Infants withdrawing from maternal drug exposure may develop seizures if their abstinence is severe, but more often they have tremors, jitteriness, and irritability, and are very difficult to console due to a heightened level of arousal with persistent crying. The common maternally used drugs known to cause neonatal abstinence include opiates, cocaine, benzodiazepines, nicotine, and the selective serotonin reuptake inhibitors. Many infants may require only environmental comfort measures to reduce the symptoms, while others require pharmacotherapy. Opiates alone or in conjunction with phenobarbital are used to treat opiate withdrawal, while phenobarbital is the drug of choice for non-opiate withdrawal. Withdrawal behaviors typically appear within the first 3 days of life, although withdrawal signs and symptoms sufficient to require medication have been reported to occur as late as 1 week of age and may persist for months. While only small amounts of maternal opiates are known to cross into breast milk, if an opiate-using mother nurses her infant then abruptly stops, the infant can develop withdrawal symptoms.

Myoclonus and Clonus

Myoclonus is a sudden, brief contraction of a muscle or muscle groups. It can be generalized and can occur in the neonate as a non-epileptic paroxysmal phenomenon. Benign neonatal sleep myoclonus occurs only with (non-rapid eye movement) sleep and begins in the first week of life, with episodes lasting several minutes. They may be provoked during sleep by jarring or rocking the bed or by exposure to benzodiazepines, and disappear upon awakening. EEG is normal with no electrographic correlate, and spells generally end before the third month of life. No other neurological or developmental impairment is present.

In otherwise healthy full-term infants, persistent multifocal clonic movements appearing toward the end of the first week of life and lasting a day or so (rarely up to 2 weeks) may suggest benign idiopathic neonatal seizures or "fifth day fits." This poorly understood condition has a generally good prognosis and a normal outcome, though the paroxysms may progress to status epilepticus and require anticonvulsants.

Hyperekplexia is an exaggerated provoked startling followed by rigidity and stiffness. Innocuous sensory stimulation brings the resting infant into an appearance of repeated startling, then increasing truncal and extremity tone, jitteriness, and dystonic posturing. Apnea may result when stiffness is excessive, and in this way hyperekplexia may be life threatening. "Breaking" the tone by forcibly overcoming the stiffness may abort the attack, and benzodiazepines may prove to be useful in reducing all symptoms. EEG during the attacks shows no electrographic correlate. Hyperekplexia has been linked to abnormal functioning of the alpha-1 subunit of glycine receptors, with inhibition of the inhibitory interneurons within the brain stem reticular formation resulting in excessive startling.

When cerebral anoxia is both prolonged and severe and the resulting encephalopathy profound, persistent spontaneous and stimulus-evoked myoclonus (Lance–Adams syndrome) may be present. The myoclonic jerks in this circumstance are generalized, frequent, and give the appearance of status epilepticus, though the electroencephalogram shows no accompanying paroxysmal discharges; anticonvulsants generally have no effect and do not modify the neurological outcome, which is uniformly poor.

Torticollis

There are two components to true torticollis: there is a tilting of the head on the neck as well as a cervical rotational component so that the chin is turned toward the shoulder. Head tilting alone should not be considered as torticollis; other causes for head tilting such as nuchal or posterior fossa masses, anatomical anomalies of the craniovertebral junction, or cervical vertebral malformations should be investigated. Shortening or limitation of movement of the ipsilateral sternocleidomastoid muscle is the final common pathway to torticollis, with the precipitating causes ranging from intrauterine malpositioning or constraint and breech presentation to intramuscular fibrosis with or without hemorrhage. When fibrosis is present, palpation of the affected muscle or ultrasound may identify the lesion. Physical therapy in most cases will result in improvement, as long as both rotational components of the torticollis are addressed independently. Untreated or unrecognized torticollis may lead to ipsilateral usually posterior plagiocephaly and may rarely result in anterior displacement of the ear, ipsilateral forehead, temporomandibular joint, and orbit.

Opisthotonos

The opisthion is the anatomic posterior-most point of the foramen magnum. In opisthotonic posturing, the head is persistently and abnormally retroflexed about this point (retrocollis), and the trunk is arched posteriorly due to abnormal contraction of the midline truncal extensor muscles. Opisthotonos may be seen in meningismus, in the presence of large posterior fossa mass lesions, in aminoacidopathies, urea cycle defects, organic acidurias, disorders of trace elements, the porphyrias, and when intracranial pressure is elevated. Opisthotonic posturing should not be confused with the similar but more transient posturing of the term infant delivered with a face presentation. Opisthotonos has been associated with acute bilirubin encephalopathy and kernicterus, but in this circumstance is more of a dystonic posturing of extrapyramidal origin than a phenomenon related to obstruction of cerebrospinal flow or meningeal inflammation.

In the newborn period and during infancy, gastroesophageal reflux is commonly associated with more transient episodes of opisthotonic and frankly dystonic truncal posturing. This association is frequently mislabeled as the Sandifer syndrome and has entered common usage this way although Sandifer's original description was in older children with both episodic dystonia and hiatus hernia; when the hernia was surgically corrected, the movement disorder disappeared. Episodic opisthotonus or dystonia in a newborn may be easily confused with seizures and may have no direct relationship with feeding, though prone positioning frequently exacerbates the reflux and subsequent motor behaviors. Treatment with histamine-2 receptor blocking agents does not generally reduce reflux, but may reduce the acidity of the refluxed fluid. Pharmacologic agents that modify gastrointestinal motility are more effective treatments for reflux, especially when combined with reverse Trendelenburg positioning of the infants. Some commonly used agents such as metoclopramide must be used with care, since drug-induced extrapyramidal side effects may be difficult to differentiate from the GER-induced dystonic or opisthotonic posturing.

Myotonia

Myotonia is a transient but sustained (seconds long) contraction of a muscle or muscle group in response to percussion. This is most easily done with a triangular (Taylor) or ball type (Tromner) reflex hammer. The thenar eminence of the hand is the most accessible group of muscles, with percussion producing a visible tonic opposition of the thumb. Percussion of other large muscles such as the biceps or quadriceps may not result in visible movements, though palpation of the just-percussed muscle will easily detect the local contraction. Myotonia is most closely associated with myotonic dystrophy; when myotonic dystrophy is present in the newborn period, the most likely genetic donor is the mother as discussed later in the chapter.

Muscle Fasciculations

Fasciculation is a spontaneous irregular contraction of the muscles subserved by a motor unit, and does not generally result in visible movement of a joint, the contractions limited instead to the muscle itself. Fasciculations are best observed in the newborn on the undersurface of the tongue of the newborn. Irregular contractions of the superior surface of the tongue of the otherwise normal newborn should not be confused with the "bag-of-worms" appearance of the inferior tongue surface in the infant with anterior horn cell or lower motor neuron disease. In type I *spinal muscular atrophy*, the presence of significant weakness, reduced or absent tendon reflexes, and abnormal shape of the thorax are regularly present and should suggest the diagnosis.

Deficiency of Movement

Brachial Plexus Injuries

In the newborn, deficiency of movement implies muscle weakness. Weakness can be of myogenic or neurogenic origin, and be limited to a single limb or portion of the body or be generalized. When weakness is isolated to a single limb, the weakness is unlikely to be myogenic. Paresis of a single arm at delivery is a fairly common cause for neurological consultation, especially in large infants or when excessive traction has been applied to the arm during delivery. There are five spinal segments and nerve roots from which the brachial plexus originates: cervical segments 5–8 and the first thoracic. These nerve roots combine to form upper, middle, and lower nerve trunks which, with the insertion of the roots into the spinal cord, are the most common sites of injury when traction is excessive.

Two general patterns of injury are seen in the term infant. When upper cervical roots (C5, C6) are injured, the pattern of weakness is as originally described by Erb: weakness or paresis of shoulder abduction and external rotation, biceps, brachioradialis, and supination. Wrist and finger extensors may sometimes be weak as well. Ipsilateral diaphragmatic weakness may be present when the C4 and C3 roots are simultaneously affected. The biceps reflex is absent in the affected arm, and the Moro is typically asymmetric. The best way to demonstrate the Moro is as he originally described it: to strike the bed next to the infant with the palm of the hand. Finger and palmar grasp reflexes are unaffected in Erb palsy.

When the lowermost roots and trunks of the brachial plexus are injured, the distal upper extremity is paretic with no finger or wrist movements elicitable, as described by Klumpke. This is an uncommon injury in the newborn, for whom a lack of finger movements usually implies a lesion involving the entire origin of the plexus at the spinal roots. In this circumstance an ipsilateral Horner syndrome is typically present.

While outcome is generally good unless nerve roots are avulsed, treatment options are limited and intended to minimize the possibility of joint contractures developing during the weeks or months required for recovery at a time when the infant is simultaneously growing. Range of motion exercises for all of the upper extremity joints including the shoulder, and splinting, where necessary, are generally sufficient. Most infants have recovery of function to the point where a routine neurological examination shows no deficits by 6 months of age, with the majority of improvement within the first few weeks to months. When weakness is present still at 6 months of age, a permanent degree of weakness becomes increasingly likely. Surgical intervention should be considered earlier rather than later, although the most appropriate time of surgery is still uncertain. The first consideration of neurosurgical referral for lysis of fibrotic tissue, neuromas, and grafting of viable roots should be considered at 2 months of age so that surgical intervention by 4 months of age can be performed in the event that weakness still has not improved.

Lumbosacral Plexus Injuries

Paralysis of a leg is seldom seen in the newborn, and occurs when traction of the leg during frank breech deliveries results in injury to the lumbar (L2-4) or sacral (L4-S3) plexuses. The rarity of this injury should lead to consideration of other causes such as occult dysraphism, though spinal dysraphism is very unlikely to involve a single limb alone. Prognosis for complete recovery is much less optimistic for the paretic leg than for the acutely paretic arm in the newborn.

Unilateral Facial Weakness

Congenital aplasia or hypoplasia of the depressor anguli oris results in an abnormal appearance of the crying or, in an older infant, smiling face. The corner of the mouth does not move inferolaterally, giving the illusion of a contralateral facial weakness. This is usually an isolated phenomenon, but may rarely be associated with other congenital defects or as a sign of the *Cayler cardiofacial syndrome* in which various cardiac defects may be present.

The facial nerve is vulnerable to traumatic injury; its emergence from the stylomastoid foramen just inferior and medial to the inferior attachment of the ear and subsequent branching to supply the muscles of facial expression makes it especially susceptible to compressive injury by external forces. Unilateral facial weakness is most frequently noticed shortly after delivery and involves both the upper and lower halves of the face. A flattening of the nasolabial fold and forehead creases may be noted, especially during crying, and feeding may be complicated by the leakage of milk from the ipsilateral corner of the mouth. In the context of the use of forceps during delivery, mechanical pressure on the nerve at its emergence may result in weakness, but facial weakness can also be seen when no forceps or vacuum-assisted extraction has occurred. Prolonged intrauterine impaction of the angle of the jaw onto the ipsilateral shoulder, a bony projection of a twin, or the maternal sacrum may result in a facial paresis; in such cases the normally excellent prognosis for a complete recovery is not as optimistic. Treatment with artificial tears or forced closure of the ipsilateral eyelids with gauze and tape is directed at preventing corneal ulcerations because of the inability to blink.

Bilateral Facial Weakness

Paresis of both sides of the face is evident when the child has an expressionless face even when provoked to the point of crying by noxious stimulation. Acquired transient weakness in the form of maternal myasthenia gravis should be differentiated from other forms of generalized motor weakness such as myotonic and other muscle dystrophies, and from the *Möbius sequence*, classically described as the presence of bilateral facial and abducens paresis in a newborn. The source of the paresis is aplasia or hypoplasia of two or more pairs of cranial motor nuclei within the dorsum of the brain stem, so the classic signs of the Möbius sequence should provoke a clinical search for weakness mediated by involvement of the other cranial nerves including the hypoglossal nerve which will affect feeding. Causation is unknown, and may be developmental or acquired. Treatment is directed at finding a method of feeding that allows for sufficient intake, since inability to seal the lips around a nipple poses a major hazard to the infant. Associated incomplete eyelid closure is managed in the same way as in unilateral facial paresis.

Ophthalmoplegia

Ophthalmoplegia and ptosis may occur independently, and can be acquired or "congenital." In contrast to older children with myasthenia gravis, infants with maternally acquired transient myasthenia gravis do not typically have either ophthalmoplegia or ptosis, presenting instead with hypotonia, generalized weakness, and feeding difficulties in the first hours of life. Administration of cholinesterase inhibitors may be necessary for this condition, one that generally abates by 3 weeks of age. Cholinesterase inhibitors may or may not be useful in the treatment of *congenital* myasthenic syndromes, which are *not* transient and *do* present with prominent ptosis and ophthalmoplegia.

The congenital myasthenic syndrome comprises a heterogeneous group of rare disorders that reflect genetically determined defects of the neuromuscular junction, with only a few generating clinical suspicion in the newborn period and are discussed later in the chapter in the section on Weakness.

Waxing and waning paresis of extraocular muscles in the newborn, especially in the presence of other signs such as internuclear ophthalmoplegia, facial weakness, or glossopharyngeal dysfunction should suggest the possibility of a metabolic encephalopathies such as *maple syrup urine disease.*

The clinical signs of Möbius sequence have already been discussed, and should be differentiated from congenital third nerve palsy, familial congenital ptosis, and the Duane syndrome, in which the pareses are generally restricted to the oculomotor system. In the *Duane retraction syndrome*, there is partial abduction of the eye and upon attempted abduction, retraction of the globe of the eye into the orbit causing the palpebral fissure to narrow. This is caused by a usually unilateral absence of the abducens nerve along with its nucleus in the pons. There is often an accompanying fibrosis of the lateral rectus muscle, linking this syndrome with other conditions leading to fibrosis of the extraocular muscles such as Congenital Fibrosis of the Extraocular Muscles (*CFEOM*) in which the eyes are fixed in a position of strabismus, and ptosis is prominent. Coaxing the newborn infant to voluntarily move the eyes in order to make any of these clinical diagnoses is difficult; the examiner may have to resort to the use of oculovestibular maneuvers, caloric stimulation of the tympanic membranes, or retreat to a dark room as described in the section on the neurological examination.

Laryngeal, Vocal Cord, and Pharyngeal Weakness

Abnormalities of sucking, swallowing, crying, and breathing are not uncommon in the newborn. Apart from the normal developmental evolution of the coordination of sucking, swallowing, and breathing in the preterm infants, the presence of such dyscoordination in the term infant may be life threatening. The laryngeal nerve has two branches of interest, the recurrent laryngeal and superior branches. The recurrent branch may be injured when the thyroid cartilage is forced against the cricoid cartilage during prolonged lateral neck flexion in utero or during delivery causing unilateral vocal cord paresis and an abnormal stridorous cry. The superior branch may be similarly compressed by the thyroid cartilage against the hyoid bone, causing trouble with swallowing and a substantial risk of aspiration with feeding. Isolated pharyngeal weakness is probably more common than the literature would suggest, and is not always evident until the first feeding when cyanosis, choking, and aspiration simultaneously appear (*Table 360.2*). The most useful diagnostic testing is with direct laryngoscopy and videofluoroscopy; magnetic resonance imaging is necessary when other malformations are present, there are focal neurological findings on examination, or when cerebral malformations are suspected.

Hemiparesis and Stroke

Hemiparesis resulting from large middle cerebral arterial infarctions may be clinically unapparent in the neonate, with no obvious limb use asymmetry until the infant begins to crawl or walk. The cause of large cerebral arterial

Table 360.2
Pattern of clinical signs and symptoms of laryngeal and pharyngeal dysfunction

	Laryngeal	Vocal cord	Pharynx
Aspiration	+	+	+
Choking with feeding	+	+	+
Cyanosis with feeding	–	–	+
Diaphragmatic paresis	+/–	–	–
Dysphonia	+	+	–
Respiratory distress with feeding	+	–/+	+
Stridor	+	+	–

infarctions, which occur in more than 5% of infants, remains unknown in the majority of cases. Ischemic stroke is more common in the newborn than in older children, and has been estimated to occur in 1 of every 4,000 live births. Although the timing of stroke discovered in the newborn period has been considered as *fetal* (focal ischemic, thrombotic, and/or hemorrhagic event occurring between 14 weeks gestation and the onset of labor resulting in delivery) or *neonatal* (occurring between labor resulting in delivery and 28 days of life), this distinction may be somewhat arbitrary since clear etiologic or prognostic differences for strokes in these two epochs are not present. Most infarctions are ischemic and unilateral, with the majority of these involving the middle cerebral artery. The remainder is related to hemorrhage and cerebral venous sinus thrombosis. Unexplained is why the left middle cerebral arterial distribution is affected more commonly than the right side. Infarction from arterial occlusion is more common in the term than the preterm infant with the incidence increasing from 5% of infants between 28 and 32 weeks gestational age to 15% in infants between 37 and 40 weeks.

Two patterns of arterial occlusion are present on neuroimaging when hemiparesis is present, and they do offer some guidance in an investigation of cause. Most identifiable causes are related to adverse maternal conditions (i.e., diabetes, hypercoagulable states, anticonvulsant or warfarin use, gastroenteritis with fever, idiopathic thrombocytopenic purpura), pregnancy disorders (i.e., preeclampsia, abruption, in utero growth retardation, twins, oligohydramnios, chorioamnionitis), or fetal disorders (i.e., TORCH-type infections, Rh isoimmunization, alloimmune thrombocytopenia, protein C deficiency).

The presence of multiple arterial infarctions should suggest the possibility of congenital heart disease, polycythemia (venous hematocrit of >65% or hemoglobin >22 g/100 mL in a symptomatic term infant), disseminated intravascular coagulation, or perinatal distress.

Single artery distribution infarctions should raise the possibility of a focal arterial vascular anomaly or thrombotic occlusion, ischemic proliferative vasculopathy when twins are present, or vasospasm related to maternal substance abuse, especially cocaine.

When the infarctions are remote, there is an increasing recognition that genetic factors may be present, such as the *hypoprothombinemia, 5, 20-methylenetetrahydrofolate reductase*, and *COL4A1* genetic deficiencies. The latter has been associated with familial cases of *porencephaly.*

Mechanical occlusion of cerebral arteries may occur during or after delivery, resulting in ischemic parenchymal injury and focal neurological symptoms. When the neck is hyperextended and rotated, the lumen of the internal carotid artery may be narrowed or occluded as it passes over the lateral portion of the upper cervical vertebrae. A similar injury may occur in the *posterior* circulation during hyperextension and rotation of the neck. At birth, the foramen magnum is almost its adult size, but both the lateral mass of the atlas and the atlantooccipital condyle are hypoplastic. These conditions result in a narrowing of the spinal canal within the atlas. In addition, the ligaments between atlas, occiput, and axis are lax, so that the vertebral arteries are vulnerable to compression between the bony lamina of the atlas and the exoccipital bone when even mild hyperextension of the neck occurs. The compressed vertebral arteries will reduce blood flow to the brain stem, cerebellum, and upper cervical cord, and may result in stroke.

Acute strokes of either venous or arterial origin most often present as focal motor seizures involving a single extremity rather than hemiparesis, and have been estimated to account for up to 10% of all seizures in neonates.

Weakness associated with remote (weeks to months old) arterial occlusions may not be immediately apparent. The abrupt appearance of weakness in an arm and leg (face is usually not affected) when normal movement had been documented previously should suggest an acute arterial occlusion and should provoke a more energetic investigation as to cause than remote occlusions, for which an etiology can only rarely be discovered. A suggested diagnostic panel is given in ➲ *Table 360.3.* One purpose of a diagnostic workup, even when the chances of discovery of an etiology is unlikely, is to estimate the risk of stroke recurrence. Recurrent thromboembolism, acute ischemic stroke, and cerebral venous sinus thrombosis do occur, and are more likely when factors promoting thrombosis such as complex congenital heart disease, sepsis, or hypovolemia are present.

Treatment of neonatal stroke is supportive. The safety of medical thrombolysis is unproven in the neonate, and the deployment of agents to promote thrombolysis such as unfractionated or low molecular weight heparin is not common. The exception to this is when cardiac or multiple systemic thrombi or a clear tendency to prothrombosis is present. Low platelet counts and coagulation factor deficiencies should be corrected. Vitamin K should always be administered to the newborn, especially when exogenous pharmacological agents such as warfarin, barbiturates, or phenytoin have been administered to the mother during the pregnancy or when biliary atresia is present.

Outcome and prognosis in neonatal stroke is variable, with estimates of disability differing widely. A "normal" outcome is possible, but so too is mild to dense

Table 360.3
Prothrombotic laboratory evaluation of the newborn

Humoral factors (Blood, Serum)
Complete blood count[a]
Prothrombin and partial Thromboplastin time (PT, PTT)[a]
International normalized ratio (INR)[a]
Electrolytes[a]
Proteins C and S activity[a]
Activated protein C resistance screen[a]
Homocysteine[a]
Factor VIIIc
Lipoprotein a
Antibodies
Antiphospholipid antibody screen
Antithrombin III activity[a]
Genetic Deficiencies
Factor V Leiden mutation[a]
Prothrombin 20210 gene defect
Methylene tetrahydrofolate reductase (MTHFR), C677T[a], A1298C gene defects
Plasminogen activator inhibitor-1 gene 4G/5G polymorphism
Imaging
Computed tomography brain (CT)[a]
CT angiography or venography
Magnetic resonance (MR) imaging brain; include diffusion weighted imaging[a]
MR angiography, venography
Echocardiogram[a]

[a]Minimum recommended testing; remaining tests where available and suggested by history. The removed volume of blood necessary for testing may be excessive in small or very premature neonates and force prioritization of tests or preclude obtaining all studies on a timely basis

hemiplegia. Most children with a history of neonatal stroke will learn to walk independently before the end of the second year of life. Epilepsy after the neonatal period, even when seizures are the presenting sign of stroke, is uncommon. Cognitive impairment may range from severe to none at all. The possibility of clinically and academically significant disabilities should be anticipated including cognitive and learning deficits, non-progressive impairment of motor functioning (cerebral palsy), sensory and visual deficits, and epilepsy. When hypoxic-ischemic injury is complicated by or superimposed upon stroke, outcome is generally worse.

Paraparesis

Simultaneous weakness of both legs is rarely seen in the neonate. Congenital malformations of the caudal spinal cord, conus medullaris, and cauda equina may produce variable degrees of asymmetric weakness, tendon reflexes, and sensory impairment, making it difficult to differentiate central from peripheral causes of paraparesis on clinical grounds alone. Cerebral lesions may produce weakness of the legs. Parasagittal primary motor cortex corresponding with the lower extremities may be injured after prolonged hypotension and hypoperfusion, causing a borderzone infarction between the middle and anterior cerebral arterial supplies. Arm weakness may be similarly produced with more lateral anatomical displacement of the borderzone area. Cystic or hydrocephalic disruption of periventricular white matter tracts in the preterm infant will produce bilateral leg weakness although this is not generally clinically apparent in the newborn period. Disruption of the spinal cord may occur when excessive spinal traction has taken place during delivery, and cause a flaccid weakness and areflexia below the torn spinal segment.

Quadriparesis, Generalized Weakness, and Hypotonia

Quadriparesis is rare in the neonate. Posterior fossa lesions and upper cervical spinal cord injuries should be suspected and excluded by appropriate neuroimaging. Quadriparesis should be differentiated from generalized weakness and hypotonia wherein the presence of muscle tone can generally be documented. When it is present in the newborn period, quadriparesis due to compressive or disruptive spinal cord injuries results in a relative *absence* rather than an *increase* of tone. Spasticity and hypertonia following quadriparesis will frequently appear in the weeks to months after injury but are not seen during the first month of life unless the cerebral injury has preceded delivery by the same time interval.

Inability to move the limbs may occur when their joints are limited in their excursion as is seen in the clinical entities described by the term *arthrogryposis multiplex congenita*. This is not a single disease but a final common clinical observation for a number of disorders that may affect any part of the nervous system. Many additional congenital anomalies are often present along with the joint limitations and reflect underlying muscle hypotrophy or atrophy, weakness, and hypo- or areflexia. More than 150 distinct clinical syndromes are known to result in the physical finding of arthrogryposis. Talipes equinovarus, micrognathia and retrognathia, clinodactyly, and camptodactyly occur when there is insufficient in utero movement of the joints; polyhydramnios and a high arched palate with narrowed alveolar ridges reflect weakness and lack of movement of the muscles of deglutition. Arthrogryposis has been associated with central nervous system malformations at every level, from migrational disorders in the brain and cerebellum to dysplasia of anterior horn cells and meningomyelocele in the spinal cord, to myasthenic syndromes, merosin-related dystrophies, glycogen storage disorders, and mitochondrial cytopathies affecting muscle, to hypomyelination syndromes affecting the peripheral nerves.

Transient maternally acquired myasthenia gravis occurs in as many as one in five infants born to myasthenic mothers. The weakness is usually apparent within the first hours of birth, but may become evident after an initial brief period during which no weakness can be observed, and may rarely become evident as late as the second postnatal day. The predominant clinical feature is feeding difficulty, with sucking and swallowing problems quickly leading to respiratory distress. Mechanical ventilatory support and gavage or nasogastric tube feedings are required in about one in three infants. The remainder of treatment is generally supportive since duration of symptoms does not generally last for more than 3 weeks. Circulating maternal acetylcholine receptor protein antibodies may be transmitted across the placenta to the infant and exert their pathogenic effect on acetylcholine receptors at the postsynaptic muscle membrane causing receptors to be degraded, displacing acetylcholine from the receptors, and inducing local degradation of the receptor expressing muscle membrane via complement. Diagnosis is made clinically, and may be confirmed by demonstrating an electrodecremental response to repetitive stimulation on electromyography. Expertise in neonatal electromyography is not widely available, and is not therefore practical for the vast majority of hospitalized infants throughout the world. An alternative confirmatory procedure is the test administration of an anticholinesterase agent such as the short acting edrophonium (0.15 mg/kg administered intravenously in fractions over a several minute period after an initial dose of 0.03 mg/kg) or the longer acting neostigmine methylsulfate (0.04 mg/kg administered intramuscularly or subcutaneously). Each medication yields a positive result when clinical improvement in the form of sucking or swallowing, crying, breathing, or facial movement is seen. The duration of improvement is short lived, with edrophonium-induced improvement appearing within 5 min and persisting for up to 15 min. Neostigmine-induced improvements may not appear for up to a half hour after administration. For administration of either anticholinesterase there is risk of excessive muscarinic side effects, and so atropine should be simultaneously available at the moment of injection.

Neonatal maternally acquired myasthenia gravis is a transient phenomenon; while the infant may become quite ill and require complete ventilatory and feeding support, improvement will occur and prognosis for normal outcome is excellent. It is common practice to use exogenous anticholinesterase medications such as neostigmine (intravenous dose of 0.04 mg/kg or nasogastric dose of 0.4 mg/kg) a half hour before feedings for the first weeks of life.

A complete discussion of the congenital, non-acquired myasthenic syndromes is beyond the scope of this chapter. More than a dozen such syndromes are known, variously affecting individual steps within the pathway associated with the assembly of acetylcholine, its vesicles within the presynaptic terminal, or its receptor on the postsynaptic membrane. A clinical response to the administration of acetylcholinesterase may not be seen in the congenital myasthenic syndromes, and should not be used to exclude the diagnosis that requires electrophysiologic investigation.

Other genetic causes of generalized hypotonia include myotonic dystrophy and Prader–Willi syndrome; these are common enough that genetic testing should be considered in all infants presenting in the neonatal period with symmetric muscle weakness and hypotonia. In *Prader–Willi syndrome*, hypotonia is severe, reflexes diminished or absent, feeding and crying weak, and subtle dysmorphic features such as a narrow bifrontal diameter, almond shaped eyes, small mouth, or hypogonadism present. There is frequently a history of diminished movement preceding delivery.

Although *congenital myotonic dystrophy* is an autosomal dominant disorder, when it is present in the newborn the parent contributing the trait is almost always the mother. It is one of a number of disorders known to be associated with an increased number of CTG trinucleotide repeats, in this case in an unstable DNA sequence on the 3′ untranslated end of the myotonic dystrophy gene on chromosome 19. While paternal transmission of the gene does rarely occur in the newborn period, maternal transmission is the rule, and the severity of disease is highly correlated with the total number of repeats. With each female transmission, the number of repeats increases, further worsening severity and causing symptoms earlier in life, a phenomenon referred to as anticipation. Prognosis is dependent at some level on the number of CTG repeats, and further determined by the severity of weakness, respiratory compromise, gastrointestinal motility, and cognitive impairment universally present. The *mother's* appearance should therefore give the first clinical clues as to the potential presence of myotonic dystrophy in the hypotonic infant; upon shaking her hand at the first meeting, her hand may not immediately release its clasp due to myotonia.

Diaphragmatic Paresis

Persistent unexplained respiratory difficulty in the first hours of life may be caused by unilateral diaphragmatic paralysis. Cyanosis and arterial blood gas determinations may suggest the possibility of hypoventilation and congenital heart or primary pulmonary disease. Routine chest radiographs may not show the familiar hemidiaphragmatic elevation characteristic of paresis in the older child or adult. After an initial period of respiratory distress, there may be a stabilization or improvement with oxygen supplementation, but a more severely paretic infant may instead acutely deteriorate. Diagnosis is made by ultrasonic or fluoroscopic real time imaging of respirations, demonstrating the paradoxical upward movements of the affected hemidiaphragm with breathing. Any such imaging will yield a false negative result if positive pressure ventilation is in use at the time of the test. Diaphragmatic paralysis results from injury to the 3rd, 4th, and 5th cervical nerve roots, and thereby complicates about 5% of brachial plexus injuries, but it may occur without arm weakness as well. Long-term prognosis depends upon the response to ventilatory interventions such as intermittent positive pressure ventilation, but when it becomes clear that there has been no improvement, surgical plication of the hemidiaphragm may be indicated.

Alteration of Consciousness

Encephalopathy

The traditional definition of encephalopathy as the clinical condition resulting when any two of (1) seizures, (2) alteration in the state of consciousness, or (3) alteration in cognition or personality are present cannot be applied easily to infants, for whom changes in cognition are not possible to detect and personality is not present. Instead, neonatal encephalopathy may be better defined as a condition in which there is altered consciousness, difficulty in initiating and maintaining spontaneous respirations, and associated depression of reflexes and muscle tone with or without seizures. Major categories of causes for neonatal encephalopathy can be separated into *intrinsic* deficiencies (genetic, enzymatic, subcellular organelle dysfunction) and *acquired* disorders (infection, cerebral hemorrhage or thrombosis, hypoxic-ischemic).

The clinician should be aware that other conditions such as congenital heart disease, neuromuscular disorders, congenital myopathies, and cerebral malformations may give the infant the *appearance* of an encephalopathy because of accompanying profound hypotonia or weakness when an *actual* encephalopathy, best determined by electroencephalography, is absent.

Important enzymatic deficiencies producing encephalopathy in the newborn, especially the amino and organic acidopathies, are covered in the chapter on metabolic disorders. These generally evolve over the first days of life, and yield as clues altered levels of glucose, ammonia, serum ketones, and sometimes an obvious clinical deterioration after feedings. Deficient levels of glucose, sodium, calcium, and magnesium are commonly present in the newborn and need to be recognized and treated before the encephalopathy is corrected.

Incipient or evolving infection, especially in the context of diminished peripheral perfusion, tachycardia, and hypotension should always be considered as an emergent cause for encephalopathy. A well-appearing infant can be dead in a matter of hours from certain bacterial infections, with Group B *Streptococcus*, *Escherichia coli*, and *Klebsiella* being the most notorious. A complete septic workup including lumbar puncture, blood cultures, and urine culture is necessary to identify and properly isolate the offending bacterium. Congenital cytomegalovirus and herpesvirus infections are usually readily identifiable in retrospect on clinical grounds but may pose diagnostic dilemmas if they are not considered or when typical ocular or cutaneous lesions are absent.

Herpesvirus infections are usually acquired during delivery when asymptomatic maternal vaginal lesions are present, when there are active lesions in a mother not known to have had prior herpes infections (type II), or from infected hospital personnel or family members handling the infant (type I). The resulting symptoms in the newborn appear by the end of the first week of life in the form of poor feeding and lethargy. Irritability or its opposite, somnolence, is followed by focal seizures with rapid progression to stupor and coma. Lumbar puncture should be performed in all such infants with care taken to distinguish traumatic lumbar puncture (many red cells, clear, colorless supernatant) from the xanthochromia, white blood cell pleocytosis, and elevated protein in cerebrospinal fluid when herpes is present. Treatment with acyclovir should never be postponed or delayed until laboratory testing or PCR results are returned as the acyclovir is viro*static* rather than viro*cidal*, and the hemorrhagic encephalitis-induced destruction of brain parenchyma is already under way. Prognosis in such an event is grave.

Intracranial Hemorrhage and Post Hemorrhagic Hydrocephalus

Intracranial hemorrhage is an important cause of altered mental status and neurological debilitation in the newborn, and has many sources. Subdural, subarachnoid, intraparenchymal, and intraventricular hemorrhages are the most common. During vaginal delivery, especially when vacuum extractors are applied, the relative motion of the bones of the deforming cranial vault may exert traction on the major venous sinuses affixed to them. The confluence of the straight and transverse sinuses, vein of Galen, and the free tentorial edges at the junction of the double layered falcine and tentorial dura is especially vulnerable to tearing, with leakage of venous blood into the juxtatentorial or parafalcine spaces. There may be a rapid and extensive accumulation of venous blood, with a full fontanel, depressed level of consciousness, skew eye deviation, pupillary asymmetry, abnormal response to light, and nuchal rigidity. Coma, fixed dilated pupils, and respiratory rhythm disturbances follow over the next hours. A similar progression of events follows the disruption and displacement of the occipital bone (occipital osteodiastasis) with difficult breech deliveries; in this circumstance, the transverse sinuses or the vein of Galen may be disrupted and death follows.

Subdural blood may appear in the *infratentorial* space without producing any clinical symptoms and be noted incidentally upon routine neuroimaging. Blood also may slowly accumulate in the posterior fossa leading to signs of brain stem dysfunction (apnea, bradycardia, eye deviations) and compression (irritability or lethargy, full fontanel, increasing OFC) suggestive of increased intracranial pressure. No clinical signs may be present when subdural blood appears in the *supratentorial* space or there may be clinical signs (hemiparesis, eye deviation, dilated pupil) of an evolving herniation when the volume of blood is large. The volume of subdural blood present may be easily underestimated on neuroimaging, especially when the width of the observed blood on MR or CT slices is small but the number of images showing blood present is large.

Subarachnoid hemorrhages are relatively common in the newborn. They may be seen incidentally on imaging in an infant with no clinical signs, or be associated with focal seizures in an otherwise healthy looking infant. Diagnosis is made by CT or MRI, and may be suspected when the spinal fluid of an infant with seizures shows an excessive number of RBCs and an elevated protein. Lumbar puncture is usually done in such an infant for other reasons such as to exclude infection and the abnormal CSF is found incidentally; care should be taken to differentiate this clinical presentation from that described in extensive subdural supratentorial or infratentorial hemorrhage, for which lumbar puncture may provoke cerebral herniation. Prognosis in most cases of subarachnoid hemorrhage is generally good and seizures can be expected to remit spontaneously.

Intraparenchymal hemorrhage in the newborn is not uncommon and disproportionately affects premature infants, with the most premature among them bearing the greatest risk. Primary hemorrhage may be conceptually distinguished from hemorrhage that secondarily complicates venous infarction or ischemic parenchyma, but from a clinical and management standpoint there is little to distinguish them. The cerebellar hemisphere is a common location for hemorrhage in very premature infants, and produces signs and symptoms similar to infratentorial subdural hemorrhage already described. CT and MRI are preferred to ultrasound at documenting the extent and location of cerebellar hemorrhage. Surgical intervention other than ventriculoperitoneal shunting when obstructive hydrocephalus complicates cerebellar hemorrhage does not demonstrate clear advantages over medical management in term infants, and probably contributes to morbidity and mortality in preterm infants. Recent evidence suggests that prior assumptions regarding the benign nature of cerebellar hemorrhage are incomplete. Long-term follow-up of such infants suggests that there is a markedly increased risk of significant cognitive impairment including pervasive developmental disorder, and reflects an evolving recognition of the importance of the cerebellum to cognitive processes other than coordination including emotional affect, language development, and mathematical abilities.

Intraventricular hemorrhages are relatively common in the term infant, and should not be confused with the entity of the same name as applied to premature infants. The latter should be more appropriately described as germinal matrix hemorrhages, even when blood within the germinal matrix escapes into the ventricle. In term infants, the source for the intraventricular blood is usually the choroid plexus. Some authors have attributed the source of intraventricular blood in term infants to the germinal matrix, although the normal involution of the germinal matrix is mostly complete by 32 weeks, and the germinal matrix is absent by 36 weeks (see Table 360.1). Another locus of intraventricular hemorrhage in the term infant is the thalamus. Venous sinus thrombosis in the vein of Galen and straight and transverse sinuses may be complicated by thalamic infarction and secondary hemorrhage, suggesting a role for coagulation disorders in the genesis of intraventricular hemorrhage. Outcome is dependent upon the degree to which symptoms are present and medical or surgical intervention is necessary.

Changing Head Size and Increased Intracranial Pressure

Hydrocephalus

Small intraventricular hemorrhages in the term newborn may be asymptomatic; larger hemorrhages may obstruct CSF outflow and be complicated by hydrocephalus. Other neonatal causes of obstructive hydrocephalus such as aqueductal stenosis will generally be apparent upon delivery. Clinical evidence of increased intracranial pressure includes a tense or bulging fontanel, splitting of coronal, sagittal, or metopic sutures, apnea, bradycardia, extraocular dysmotility, hypertonia, lethargy or irritability, and blood oxygen desaturations. A head circumference growth velocity of more than 2 mm/day is highly suggestive, and ultrasound or CT/MRI is confirmatory.

Hydrocephalus may require medical or surgical intervention. Ventriculoperitoneal shunting is the conventional management for obstructive and communicating hydrocephalus. Surgical shunting adversely affects outcome, especially when it is performed in very small infants or complicated by infection and the subsequent need for external ventricular drainage and repeated shunt revisions. Management should therefore be directed towards minimizing the need for surgical intervention.

A common practice has been to perform serial lumbar punctures, despite a lack of evidence that such a practice reduces the need for later surgical intervention or disability. The small volume of the CSF space relative to the size of the patient should be considered, and excessive amounts of CSF should not be removed without increasing the likelihood of producing clinically significant apnea, bradycardia, or blood oxygen desaturations. Extraction of less than 20 mL/kg of CSF at a rate of less than 1 mL/kg/min is recommended to minimize the risk of iatrogenic symptoms. Pharmacological reduction of CSF production with acetazolamide and diuretics does not yield any measurable clinical benefit and may worsen outcome. Another strategy for the management of hydrocephalus is to use an Ommaya reservoir. This is an implanted device with a subcutaneous reservoir and a tubular channel that can be inserted into the ventricular space. When CSF continues to accumulate to the point where head circumference continues to grow excessively and symptoms of increased intracranial pressure recur, an Ommaya reservoir can be placed to allow easier access for repeated CSF removal. In expert neurosurgical hands, complication rates are low, even in very small infants. Daily taps of 10 mL/kg from the reservoir are recommended in the first days after implantation, with up to 20 mL/kg once or twice a day after this to control head enlargement. If this degree of CSF removal still fails to control excessive head enlargement and head circumference growth exceeds 2 mm/day, ventriculostomy may be necessary. Prognosis is heavily dependent upon the need for ventriculoperitoneal placement, duration of the hydrocephalus before recognition and treatment, and the occurrence of surgical complications.

When the degree of head enlargement due to hydrocephalus is large and ventriculoperitoneal shunting is required, the acute relative reduction in the size of the dilated ventricles can result in a collapse of the head with overriding bony sutures and redundancy of the scalp. If the degree of collapse is excessive, bridging cortical veins may be ruptured and subdural bleeding may occur as a complication. This is less likely to occur when more gradual reduction of head size occurs for other reasons such as cerebral parenchymal dissolution and absorption after severe global parenchymal injury due to infection, prolonged asphyxia, ischemia, or bilateral hemispheric infarction.

Hypoxia, Ischemia, and Encephalopathy

Acquired newborn encephalopathy is the final manifestation of a number of pathophysiologic sequences, only one of which is hypoxic-ischemic injury. Pure ischemia (insufficient blood flow) or hypoxia (insufficient quantity of dissolved blood oxygen) virtually never occur in isolation, since both are almost always accompanied by hypercarbia. This in turn influences cerebral arterial caliber via autoregulation, a response that may be lost when hypercarbia is progressive – especially in the ventilated preterm newborn.

Ischemia not only fails to deliver a sufficient supply of oxygen to the tissues but it prevents the removal of the metabolic byproducts of aerobic metabolism, allowing local accumulation of toxic metabolites including lactic acid and excitatory neurotransmitters, as well as the loss of ionic homeostasis. ATP and phosphocreatine are depleted, impaired osmoregulation follows, and calcium is released activating tissue lipases, proteases, and endonucleases. This first phase of hypoxic-ischemic injury is best viewed as a failure of energy production and supply.

A second phase of injury can occur at a later time and differs from this first failure of energy production and supply in that it occurs in the absence of cerebral acidosis. In this phase, the initiating event alters cerebral metabolic pathways linking neuronal and glial protein synthesis, growth factor production, and inflammatory byproducts to produce parenchymal injury. The most obvious form of this type of injury is when asphyxia is present. Although the complication of asphyxia is as old as childbirth, our understanding of it is incomplete in part because it is defined in so many disparate ways in the literature, making comparisons of treatment strategies and outcomes difficult. The most recent consensus definition of neonatal asphyxia is that of the American Academy of Pediatrics and the College of Obstetricians and Gynecologists: (1) fetal acidemia, (2) umbilical cord pH <7.0, (3) Apgar score of 0–3 after 5 min, (4) neurological dysfunction, and (5) multisystem organ dysfunction.

The occurrence of asphyxia as defined does *not* inevitably lead to permanent injury such as cerebral palsy, since so many other variables also influence outcome. These include the extent of encephalopathy present along with obstetric risk factors, perinatal events, and neonatal signs. Genetic factors may also play an important role in long-term outcome. Heterozygosity for endothelial protein C receptor single nucleotide polymorphism in term infants and possession of the variant A allele of interleukin 8 and heterozygosity for the β-2 adrenergic receptor in preterm newborns have been associated with the spastic diplegic form of cerebral palsy.

The interval between the first and second phases of cerebral energy depletion does provide an opportunity for therapeutic intervention. Numerous treatments have been proposed with generally disappointing results (see *Table 360.4*). Benefits of various treatments demonstrated in animal models of asphyxia do not generally translate well into the human newborn, so that none of the interventions listed can be endorsed as effective or recommended as a standard of care for the asphyxiated newborn.

This leaves supportive care as the treatment standard, with careful attention to ventilatory and blood gas management, fluid and electrolyte status, maintenance of perfusion, and careful manipulation of serum glucose levels so that they neither drop below 40 mg/dL nor rise above 200 mg/dL. Both hyperglycemia and hypoglycemia will worsen the extent of cerebral parenchymal injury due to hypoxia and ischemia.

There has been recent interest in and research into the possibility that cerebral cooling of the asphyxiated newborn may be a treatment modality that can be implemented before the second stage of energy depletion occurs. Using highly selected cohorts, both systemic cooling and systemic + head cooling have been shown to reduce adverse outcome, with a relative risk for death or moderate/severe disability of 0.69 compared with control groups. Target core temperatures in both studies were 33.5–35°C achieved by cooling over a 2 h period for a duration of 72 h. The rate of rewarming was 0.5°C/h in

Table 360.4
Proposed pharmacological therapeutic interventions for hypoxic-ischemic encephalopathy

Intervention	Proposed mechanism of effect			
	FRI/S	NMDA	CCB	Misc
Allopurinol	+			
Catalase	+			
Desferoxamine	+			
Destromethorphan		+		
Dizocilpine (MK-801)		+		
Erythropoietin				+
Flunarizine			+	
Ketamine		+		
Insulin growth factor-1				+
Magnesium		+		
Minocycline				+
Monosialoganglioside GM_1				+
Nerve growth factor				+
Nicardipine			+	
Nimodipine			+	
Oxypurinol		+		
Phencyclidine (PCP)		+		
Phenobarbital				+
Platelet activating factors				+
Superoxide dismutase	+			

HIE hypoxic-ischemic encephalopathy, *NMDA* N-methyl-D-aspartate antagonist, *FRI/S* free radical inhibitor/scavenger, *CCB* calcium channel blocker, *Misc* miscellaneous both studies. In both studies, cooling was started before 6 h of age. Further investigation and standardization of selection criteria are necessary before brain cooling can be widely deployed as an intervention for hypoxic-ischemic encephalopathy in a non-research setting.

Neuroimaging Abnormalities in the Neonate

A full recitation of possible acquired cerebral imaging abnormalities in the newborn is beyond the scope of this chapter. Congenital infections and malformations are covered in other chapters. The use of neuroimaging in the setting of three common brain injuries in the neonate, however, will be described. These are germinal matrix hemorrhage, hypoxic-ischemic encephalopathy, and periventricular leukomalacia.

Germinal Matrix Hemorrhages

Between 10 and 20 weeks gestation, the subependymal germinal matrix is interposed between the caudate nucleus, the caudothalamic groove, and the ventricle, and is the primary generator of cerebral neuronal and glial cell precursors during this time. By 23 weeks, the germinal matrix (GM) begins an involution that will not be completed until about 36 weeks, with the process mostly completed by 32 weeks gestation (see ➋ *Table 360.1*). The dissolution of the GM is an apoptotic process taking place within a gelatinous structure that is devoid of arteries, veins, or capillaries. The GM does have a disorganized sponge-like internal structure that is suffused with blood, and has major vessels such as the superior thalamostriate (terminal) vein embedded within it. The minimum age of viability of the premature neonate unfortunately coincides with the occurrence of the weeks long dissolution of the GM; the unique generative and devolving structure of this metabolically active tissue poses an especially high risk for hemorrhage (➋ *Table 360.5*).

Some GM hemorrhages may occur prenatally, but the majority of all GM hemorrhages occur within the first 72 h of life in a preterm infant who may be critically ill. For this reason the most commonly deployed neuroimaging tool is ultrasound, with an initial scan performed in a preterm newborn at 24° and again at 72°, with follow-up scans at a week and at hospital discharge. Grading the severity of germinal matrix hemorrhages is based upon the schema as first described by Papile, and best visualized by cranial ultrasound. Grade I GM hemorrhages are confined to the anatomical boundaries of the subependymal germinal matrix. The greatest volume of the GM is anatomically correlated with the greatest volume of the caudate nucleus at its head in the frontal portion of the lateral ventricle, but the GM does follow the head, body, and tail of the caudate into the temporal horn of the ventricle so that GM hemorrhages may rarely be seen in the temporal GM.

Grade II GM hemorrhages differ from Grade I in that blood escapes from the GM into the cerebrospinal fluid *without* causing ventricular dilatation. In a Grade III hemorrhage, not only does blood escape into the ventricle, but the resulting impairment of cerebrospinal drainage through the narrow aqueduct of Sylvius and of absorption through the arachnoid granulations causes ventricular enlargement.

Grade IV GM hemorrhage should not properly be considered as an "extension" of a Grade III hemorrhage since its pathological correlate, periventricular hemorrhagic infarction, has a different set of antecedent risk factors and markedly different implications for prognosis. In addition to the destruction of local white matter, the germinal matrix is itself ablated with consequences for cerebral development as production of neuronal and glial precursors is still under way. Grade IV GM hemorrhage significantly increases the risk of permanent neurological injury, with major cognitive and motor deficits likely if the infant survives the initial injury.

Hypoxic-Ischemic Encephalopathy

Imaging abnormalities suggestive of hypoxic-ischemic encephalopathy (HIE) will not occur without a suggestive clinical history, but imaging can be quite helpful. Magnetic resonance imaging (MR) is the most useful diagnostic tool in the setting of HIE. Important advantages of MR over other imaging modalities in this setting include superior anatomical resolution and localization and, based upon the pattern of abnormality seen, an ability to make inferences about the mechanism of injury.

Three general patterns of cerebral injury related to HIE may be seen in the *term* infant. These are (1) parasagittal arterial borderzone lesions, (2) structure-specific ("selective") neuronal necrosis, and (3) focal or multifocal neuronal necrosis. The first of these is associated with pre- or perinatal systemic hypotension of sufficient duration to impair distal flow of cerebral arteries and, because major cerebral arteries (middle [MCA], anterior [ACA], posterior [PCA]) in their termini supply the same parenchymal tissues, those tissues are deprived of blood flow and are susceptible to injury. Parasagittal cortex and adjacent

Table 360.5
Selected disorders with genetic correlation

Disorder	Gene	OMIM™	Gene location
Beckwith–Wiedemann syndrome	BWS	130650[a]	11p15.5, 5q35
Cardiofacial syndrome of Cayler	ACF	125520[b]	22q11
CFEOM	CFEOM1	135700[a]	12q12
COL4A1	COL4A1	120130[c]	13q34
Convulsions, benign familial infantile	BFIC3	607745[a]	2q23-q24.3
Duane retraction syndrome	DURS1	126800[b]	8q13
Ehlers–Danlos syndrome	EDS	130050[a]	2q31
Epilepsy, Benign Neonatal	KCNQ3	121200[a]	20q13.3
Hyperexplexia	GLRA1	149400[a]	14q24, 11p15.2-p15.1, 5q32, 4q31.3
Maple syrup urine disease	MSUD	248600[a]	7q31-q32, 1p31, 6q14, 19q13.1-q13.2
5,10-Methylenetetrahydrofolate reductase	MTHFR	607093[c]	1p36.3
Myasthenia syndrome, congenital	CMS1D	608931[a]	7p12-p11, 17p13-p12, 11p11.2-p11.1, 9q31.3-q32
Myotonic dystrophy	MDPK	160900[a]	19q13.2-q13.3
Möbius syndrome	MBS	157900[b]	13q12.2-q13
Prader–Willi syndrome	PWS	176270[a]	15q12, 15q11-q13
Prothrombin	F2	176930[d]	11p11-q12
Ptosis, congenital	PTOS2	300245[b]	Xq24-q27.1
Spinal muscular atrophy type I	SMA1	253300[a]	5q12.2-q13.3

OMIM Online Mendelian Inheritance in man based upon the text *Mendelian Inheritance in Man*, authored and edited by Dr. Victor A. McKusick and a team of science writers and editors at Johns Hopkins University and elsewhere. *Mendelian Inheritance in Man* is now in its 12th edition. See McKusick VA (1998) Mendelian Inheritance in Man. 12th edn. Johns Hopkins University Press, Baltimore. http://www.ncbi.nlm.nih.gov/sites/entrez?db=omim

[a]Usually a phenotype and not representing a unique locus
[b]A confirmed Mendelian phenotype or phenotypic locus for which the underlying molecular basis is not known
[c]A gene of known sequence
[d]A phenotype with a gene of known sequence

subcortical white matter are affected with a posterior to anterior severity gradient due to the additional susceptibility of the posterior cortex to injury since this is the borderzone between three (MCA, ACA, PCA) rather than two (MCA, ACA) arteries. An unrecognized nuchal umbilical cord with restriction of arterial flow represents one possible cause.

The duration and extent of the hypoxic-ischemic event will influence the type of injury seen on imaging. Very severe, very prolonged events will lead to diffuse injury of the entire neuraxis, with diffuse neuronal necrosis present. When the duration of the event is less prolonged, and the extent moderate to severe, "selective" injury to the cerebral cortex, basal ganglia (putamen in the term, globus pallidus in the preterm infant), and thalamus is prominent. Severe but less lengthy events will lead to a different pattern of "selective" necrosis involving the basal ganglia, thalamus, and brain stem with relative sparing of the cerebral and cerebellar cortex. Event etiologies include uterine rupture, placental abruption, and umbilical cord prolapse.

Focal and multifocal cortical necrosis is readily distinguished from the parasagittal and selective patterns because the associated injury occurs within an arterial vascular distribution rather than a regional injury that does not conform to a particular arterial or venous supply. Systemic circulatory insufficiency at any time prior to, during, or immediately after delivery promotes this type of hypoxic-ischemic parenchymal injury.

Periventricular Leukomalacia

Two general patterns of periventricular white matter injury may be imaged in neonates. The first is a blush of periventricular white matter echogenicity seen on cranial ultrasound. The location of the echogenicity is adjacent to the frontal horns and atria of the lateral ventricles. This early finding has an MR correlate of increased T1W, T2W, and FLAIR signal. The second pattern is that of small or sometimes large cystic cavitations (leukomalacia) in the same anatomical distribution. It is likely that these two patterns represent opposite ends of a continuum of injury that begins with focal areas of *microscopic* white matter gliosis and necrosis, and ends with *macroscopic* cystic degeneration of periventricular white matter. While white matter gliosis is commonly seen in the brains of *dead* premature infants, the incidence of cystic periventricular leukomalacia (PVL) in *live* preterm infants is by comparison rare. So too is the observation of PVL in the *neonate*, as this imaging finding has few clinical correlates in the newborn period, and is most commonly documented in infants with emerging neurological deficits or signs *after* the neonatal period.

Neonatal Brain Death Determination

Death occurs when the heart stops, the lungs no longer allow for respiration, *and* the brain ceases to function. With modern therapy, the heart and lungs can recover from injury and remain functional for extended periods of time, leaving a need to better define when brain functioning has ceased *and no recovery is possible.* The American Bar Association, the American Medical Association, the National Conference of Commissioners on Uniform State Laws, the President's Commission for the Study of Ethical Problems in Medicine and Biomedical and Behavioral Research and the Academy of Pediatrics (AAP) have all endorsed the following language in determining brain death: "An individual who has sustained either (1) irreversible cessation of circulatory and respiratory functions or (2) irreversible cessation of all functions of the entire brain including the brain stem, is dead. A determination of death must be made in accordance with accepted medical standards."

In the United States, as in most countries, the clinical neurological exam is the standard used to determine whether brain death has occurred. There are two important prerequisites that must be satisfied before determining that brain death has occurred. The first is that all possible alternative causes for the clinical presentation of brain inactivity be excluded, and the second is that the examination must be unchanged at two different points in time. Therefore, the following conditions must be excluded: toxic and metabolic disorders, use of sedative-hypnotic or paralytic drugs, hypothermia, and hypotension.

In the neonate, the maternal and perinatal history is important in helping to rule out reversible or remediable causes of coma. According to the Special Task Force convened by the AAP, the criteria used in older children to confirm brain death are useful in the *term* infant (≥38 weeks) but not until 7 days *after* the insult, as the brain death examination and understanding the proximate cause of the insult can be difficult to determine prior to this time.

Application of these criteria to the *preterm* infant is much more difficult. Hypotonia and apnea, for example, may be normal findings in the very preterm infant, so that there are no indisputable criteria for these patients. The British Pediatric Association believes that it is difficult to confirm brain death at all in the *full-term* newborn, and does not recognize an acceptable definition of brain stem death in the *preterm* infant.

The clinical examination for brain death determination in the term newborn has the following minimum elements:

1. Normothermia (≥36.5°C) and normal blood pressure (or positive fluid balance in the previous 6 h) must be present.
2. Intoxicant levels are within a range that would not normally be expected to interfere with consciousness. Sedative drugs, aminoglycosides, tricyclic antidepressants, anticholinergics, antiepileptic drugs, or neuromuscular blocking agents should all be considered.
3. Absent pupillary responses to light and ciliospinal stimulation. Pupils should be fixed and either midposition or dilated.
4. Absence of spontaneous eye movements.
5. Absence of evoked eye movements (caloric, oculovestibular stimulation). Caloric stimulation is generally performed with cold water to minimize the possibility of thermal injury. A minute after water infusion should be allowed before determining a negative response, and 5 min allowed between sides.
6. Absence of facial or tongue movements, as well as absent swallowing, cough, gag, sucking, and rooting reflexes. Stimulation of the posterior pharynx should elicit no response.
7. Absent corneal reflexes.
8. Absent spontaneous motor movements. Reflex withdrawal to noxious stimulation and reflex myoclonus are allowable.
9. Absent respiratory activity. This requires the completion of an apnea test upon conclusion of the second clinical examination. Pure oxygen is delivered into the trachea. Arterial PO_2, PCO_2, and pH are determined

after 5 min. If PCO_2 is 60 mm Hg or is $\geq$20 mm Hg greater than baseline, and no respiratory movements are present, the apnea test is positive, supporting the diagnosis of brain death. If respiratory movements occur, the test is negative, and brain death is not supported.

10. Two examinations separated by at least 48 h must show identical findings.
11. Additional testing is not necessary unless anatomical abnormalities of the face, brain, or pharynx are present, cardiac dysrhythmias during the apnea testing, or other factors preclude the completion of the examination. In that case confirmatory testing may be deployed.

Confirmatory testing may include EEG, nuclear brain scanning, somatosensory evoked potentials, transcranial Doppler ultrasonography, and angiography. These may be of limited utility in the newborn, and have the potential to be unhelpful, so their use should be carefully considered. Cerebral angiography is rarely used in newborns, and is not recommended due to the small size of the patient and the potential for severe renal injury. Somatosensory evoked potentials (SEP) may show the absence of N20-P22 responses, but few neurophysiologists have any experience with SEP in newborns and the test interpretations may be unreliable.

EEG and radionuclide scanning may be misleading as well, since in newborns both types of tests can fail to confirm clinically determined brain death in nearly half of cases. Persisting EEG activity may be present even when brain death is certain, so EEG activity does not obviate the diagnosis of brain death. Conversely, electrocerebral silence does not always imply brain death, particularly when phenobarbital levels are supratherapeutic ($\geq$25 mg/dL), hypothermia is evident, or a brain malformation is present. Term infants who meet clinical criteria for brain death for 2 days, and preterm infants who meet clinical criteria for brain death for 3 days do not survive independent of their EEG or cerebral blood flow status, so an unchanged clinical examination remains the most reliable indicator of an irreversible lack of brain function.

Despite the absence of clear and clinically reliable criteria for the determination of brain death in critically ill preterm newborn infants, neurological prognosis is grave when brain activity is persistently absent, and this needs to be clearly imparted to the family who is invested on many levels in the decision making process, the outcome, and subsequent care of the child.

References

American Academy of Pediatrics, American College of Obstetricians and Gynecologists Care of the neonate (2002) Guidelines for perinatal care, 5th edn. Elk Grove Village, American Academy of Pediatrics

American College of Obsetetricians and Gynecologists and American Academy of Pediatrics (2003) Neonatal encephalopathy and cerebral palsy: defining the pathogenesis and pathophysiology. American College of Obstetricians and Gynecologists Distribution Center, Washington, DC

Barmadi MA, Moossy J, Shuman RM (1979) Cerebral infarcts with arterial occlusion in neonates. Ann Neurol 6:495–502

Gibson CS, MacLennan AH, Dekker GA, Goldwayer PN, Sullivan TR, Munroe DJ, Tsang S, Stewart C, Nelson KB (2008) Candidate genes and cerebral palsy: a population based study. Pediatrics 122: 1079–1085

Gluckman PD, Wyatt JS, Azzopardi D et al (2005) Selective head cooling with mild systemic hypothermia after neonatal encephalopathy: mulitcentre randomized trail. Lancet 365:663–670

Limperopoulos C, Bassan H, Gavreau K, Robertson RL, Sullivan NR, Benson CB, Avery L, Stewart J, Soul JS, Ringer SA, Volpe JJ, du Plessis AJ (2007) Does cerebellar injury in premature infants contribute to the high prevalence of long-term cognitive, learning and behavioral disability in survivors? Pediatrics 120:584–593

Perlman JM (2008) Neurology: neonatology questions and controversies. Saunders/Elsevier, Philadelphia

Roach ES, Golomb MR, Adams R, Biller J, Daniels S, deVeber G, Ferriero D, Jones B, Kirkham FJ, Scott RM, Smith ER (2008) Management of stroke in infants and children a scientific statement from a special writing group of the American Heart Association Stroke Council and the Council of Cardiovascular Disease in the Young. Stroke 39(9):2644–2691

Shankran S, Laptook AR, Ehrenkranz RA et al (2005) Whole body hypothermia for neonates with hypoxic-ischemic encephalopathy. N Engl J Med 353:1574–1584

Task Force for the Determination of Brain Death in Children (1987) Guidelines for the determination of brain death in children. task force for the determination of brain death in children. Arch Neurol 44(6):587–588

361 Neonatal Seizures

Juan Piantino · John N. Gaitanis

Definitions

Seizures are self-limited clinical events resulting from an abnormal and excessive firing of cortical neurons. Neonatal seizures (NS) occur within the first 4 weeks of life in a full-term infant and up to 44 weeks from conception in premature infants. Neonatal seizures can be classified as symptomatic, cryptogenic, or idiopathic. Symptomatic seizures are associated with identifiable brain insults. Cryptogenic seizures are believed to be symptomatic, but the underlying insult has not been confirmed. Idiopathic seizures are not associated with an underlying brain lesion and are generally presumed to be genetic in origin. Most seizures in neonates are focal, arising from one region of the brain, or multifocal, arising independently from multiple different regions. Generalized seizures, which originate in deep midline structures and spread rapidly through both hemispheres, are uncommon in neonates. The clinical appearance of seizures can be described as tonic, clonic, myoclonic, or subtle. Tonic seizures involve sustained contraction of one or more muscle groups, whereas clonic seizures refer to contraction alternating with relaxation with a frequency generally ranging between 1 and 3 Hz. Myoclonic seizures involve a rapid, nonrhythmic jerking movement of one or more extremities. Subtle seizures are the most difficult to clinically diagnose. They involve alterations of behavior, motor, or autonomic function that can be difficult to distinguish from normal neonatal patterns. Examples of subtle seizures include bicycling or sucking movements, extraocular movement abnormalities, and apneic spells.

Etiology

In the neonatal period, the development of seizures most often represents a manifestation of an underlying neurological insult (➋ *Table 361.1*). However, in some cases, NS occur in the absence of any identifiable cause. Identification and treatment of the primary cause of NS is the most important determinant of outcome. Four major etiologic groups have been described in previous classifications: neonatal encephalopathy (including hypoxic-ischemic encephalopathy), metabolic disturbances, CNS or systemic infections, and structural brain lesions (see ➋ *Table 361.1*).

Neonatal Encephalopathy

Neonatal encephalopathy is a heterogeneous syndrome characterized by central nervous system dysfunction, affecting term or near-term infants ($\geq$36 weeks gestation). These infants may have an abnormal state of consciousness (i.e., hyper-alertness, irritability, lethargy, obtundation), respiratory difficulties, hypotonia, or seizures. The causative factors of neonatal encephalopathy are varied, and although its true incidence is unclear, birth asphyxia is a well-known contributor to this condition. Administration of chest compressions for >1 min, onset of regular respirations >30 min after birth, and a base deficit >16 mmol/L on any blood gas analysis within the first 4 h from birth are predictors of severe adverse outcome (death or severe disability).

Permanent neurologic sequelae vary from learning difficulties and attention deficit, to cerebral palsy, epilepsy, visual impairment, and severe cognitive and developmental disorders. The severity of neonatal encephalopathy can be categorized as follows: mild (hyper-alertness, hyper-exitability, normal muscle tone, no seizures), moderate (hypotonia, decreased movements, and seizures), and severe (stuporous, flaccid, absent primitive reflexes, and frequent seizures). There is a correlation between the degree of encephalopathy and neurologic outcome. Mild neonatal encephalopathy carries a good prognosis, with a high probability of normal neurological outcome. Moderate encephalopathy carries a 20–35% risk of later sequelae. Neonates with severe encephalopathy have a 75% mortality risk in the neonatal period, and neurologic consequences are almost universal in this group. In addition to clinical predictors,

Abdelaziz Y. Elzouki (ed.), *Textbook of Clinical Pediatrics*, DOI 10.1007/978-3-642-02202-9_361,

Table 361.1

Most common causes of neonatal seizures (From UCSF Intensive Care House Staff Manual)

Cause	Usual age at onset	Preterm	Term
Hypoxic-ischemic encephalopathy	<3 days	+++	+++
Metabolic			
Hypoglycemia	<2 days	+	+
Hypocalcemia			
Early onset	2–3 days	+	+
Late-onset	>7 days	+	
Hypomagnesemia (often with hypocalcemia)			
Hyper/hyponatremia			
Drug withdrawal	<3 days	+	+
Local anesthetic toxicity			
Pyridoxine (vitamin B6) dependency			
Disorders of small molecules (amino acid, organic acid, and urea cycle disorders)			
Disorders of subcellular organelles (mitochondrial and peroxisomal disorders)			
Intracranial infection			
Bacterial meningitis (*E. coli*, Group B Strep., *Listeria*)	<3 days	++	++
Viral encephalitis (Herpes simplex, Enterovirus)			
Intrauterine infection (CMV, Toxoplasm., HIV, Rubella, Syphilis)	>3 days	++	++
Cerebral vascular			
Intraventricular hemorrhage	<3 days	++	
Primary subarachnoid bleed	<1 day		++
Subdural/epidural hematoma			
Focal ischemic necrosis (stroke)	Variable		++
Sinus thrombosis	Variable		+
Developmental defects			
Neurocutaneous disorders (tuberous sclerosis complex, incontinentia pigmenti)	Variable	++	++
Epilepsy syndromes			
Epileptic encephalopathies (early myoclonic encephalopathy, early infantile epileptic encephalopathy)			
Benign familial neonatal convulsions			

Relative Frequency: +++ = most common; ++ = less common; + = least common. If no +, then uncommon

MRI and EEG abnormalities have been linked to poor neurologic outcome.

Metabolic Disturbances

Metabolic abnormalities are among the most common causes of seizures in the neonatal period. Electrolyte imbalances such as hypocalcemia, hypomagnesemia, and hypoglycemia have been linked to the development of seizures. In addition, rare but potentially treatable metabolic causes of seizures are biotinidase and pyridoxine deficiency. Inborn errors of metabolism such as aminoacidurias, urea cycle defects, and organic acidurias are other rare causes of neonatal seizures.

CNS Infections

Bacterial as well as viral infections are common causes of seizures in the newborn period. Infectious agents

Table 361.2
Diagnostic workup for neonatal seizures (From Tharp: Neonatal seizures)

Serum glucose, calcium, magnesium, ammonia, lactate, pH, and a complete chemistry panel
Cerebrospinal fluid
Cranial ultrasound
EEG with perfusion of pyridoxine
Toxicology screen
Urine organic acids, serum and cerebrospinal fluid amino acids
Maternal and fetal titers for congenital infection
CT scan (hemorrhage and calcium) or MRI scan (cerebral dysgenesis, stroke)

transmitted vertically during pregnancy also put neonates at risk for developing seizures (➋ *Table 361.2*).

Structural Brain Lesions

Structural brain lesions such as hemorrhages (intracerebral, subarachnoid, and intraventricular), infarctions, and anomalies of brain development are associated with seizures.

Epidemiology

The incidence of seizures in neonates is higher than in any other age group and is estimated to be 1–3.5 per 1,000 live births in full-term newborns. In the third world, the risk may be much higher. One study in rural Kenya reported an incidence of 39.5 per 1,000 live births. Preterm infants have the greatest risk, with an incidence as high as 227 per 1,000 live births. In the first world, the most common etiology is hypoxic-ischemic encephalopathy, which accounts for approximately two-thirds of cases. In third world countries, infectious causes are more common and account for up to three-fourths of cases. The risk of seizures is higher in male infants. Other risk factors for seizures in full-term newborns include nulliparity, diabetes, maternal infection, or fever, and delivery after 42 weeks gestation.

Pathogenesis

The mechanisms underlying neonatal seizures are distinct from those of other age groups. There are several major differences between neonatal and adult brains that are relevant to the development of seizures. In the balance between inhibition versus excitation, the neonatal brain tends toward excitation. This shift occurs, in part, because neurotransmitter systems are not yet fully developed.

Inhibition

Gamma-aminobutyric acid (GABA) is the primary inhibitory neurotransmitter of the central nervous system. Unlike glutamate receptors, which may have reduced expression in neonates, GABA receptors are present very early in development and are even expressed at embryonic stages. Once released into the synaptic cleft, GABA binds to its target receptors on the postsynaptic cell. Two classes of GABA receptors exist: ionotropic and metabotropic. Activation of ionotropic GABA(A) receptors results in opening of the ion channel, which, in adults, causes influx of chloride. Yet, in neonates, intracellular Cl^- concentrations are elevated when compared to adults. Hence, activation of GABA(A) receptors results in an efflux rather than an influx of Cl^-. The net result is that GABA(A) activation is excitatory in the neonate rather than inhibitory. This paradoxical effect of GABA receptor activation in newborns results from the developmental expression of the two Cl^- transporters responsible for determining intracellular Cl^- levels. In neonates, the Na+-K+-Cl^- cotransporter (NKCC1), which causes Cl^- influx, is highly expressed. Conversely, expression of the K+-Cl^- cotransporter (KCC2), resulting in Cl^- efflux, is virtually absent. The net result is an elevation of intracellular Cl^- in newborns. Hence, activation of GABA receptors in neonates results in Cl^- efflux and is thus excitatory. GABA becomes inhibitory as neuronal efflux of Cl(–) increases throughout development.

Excitation

Considering the rapid rate of learning and development in newborns, it should come as no surprise that neonatal brains are balanced toward excitation. Glutamate, the most abundant free amino acid in the brain and the predominant excitatory neurotransmitter of the central nervous system, is necessary for synaptogenesis and plasticity. It contributes to learning and memory through use-dependent changes in synaptic function, such as long-term potentiation and depression. Glutamate receptors can be divided into two types: ionotropic and metabotropic. Ionotropic receptors are cation channels with varying permeabilities for Na^+ and Ca^{2+}. By contrast, metabotropic glutamate receptor (mGluR) activation occurs through second-messenger pathways. For the most part, glutamate receptors are overexpressed in the developing brain, and the timing of that heightened expression overlaps with the ages of greatest seizure susceptibility. Thus, an overexpression of glutamate receptors may predispose the neonate to heightened excitation and seizure susceptibility.

Glutamate transporters, referred to as excitatory amino acid transporters (EAATs), are necessary for ending glutamatergic transmission and keeping glutamate levels below a toxic range. EAATs are present in both neurons and glia. Dysfunction of glutamate transporters can result in cell death and has been implicated in a number of neurological disorders, including epilepsy. Both temporal and regional differences occur throughout development in the expression of EAATs. Hypoxic-ischemic encephalopathy, the most common cause of neonatal seizures, induces a loss of glutamate transporters in specific brain regions, such as the CA1 region of the hippocampus. Such reductions in EAATs further promote excitotoxic injury and seizures. This is observed in animal models in which diminished expression of glutamate transporters results in a reduced seizure threshold.

Clinical Manifestations

In neonates, seizures are difficult to recognize since they often mimic non-epileptic behaviors (See *Table 361.3*). Thus, video EEG is often required to confirm the diagnosis. The most difficult type of seizures to diagnose are termed subtle seizures. These consist of behavioral, motor, or autonomic alterations that appear similar to normal newborn behaviors. They include chewing, bicycling, ocular movements, and apnea. The sudden or sustained onset of these behaviors combined with their frequent recurrence help distinguish them from non-epileptic events. The most reliable seizures to diagnose clinically are clonic seizures. They consist of rhythmic movements (generally ranging between 1 and 3 Hz) of one or more extremities. They are also likely to have an EEG correlate. Tonic seizures, which involve sustained muscular contraction, may involve one extremity or the whole body. Myoclonic seizures, on the other hand, consist of rapid jerking movements and may be either focal, multifocal, or generalized. Myoclonus can also result from non-epileptic causes in newborns.

Neonatal seizures are further characterized by their relationship to findings on EEG (See *Table 361.4*). An electrographic seizure is a discrete event visualized on EEG that has a definable beginning, middle, and end.

Table 361.3

Clinical characteristics, classification, and presumed pathophysiology of neonatal seizures (From Mizrahi EM, Kellaway P (1998) Diagnosis and management of neonatal seizures. Lippincott-Raven, Philadelphia, p 181. Copyright © 1998 Lippincott Williams & Wilkins)

Focal clonic
Repetitive, rhythmic contracts of muscle groups of the limbs, face, or trunk
May be unifocal or multifocal
May occur synchronously or asynchronously in muscle groups on one side of the body
May occur simultaneously, but asynchronously on both sides
Cannot be suppressed by restraint
Pathophysiology: epileptic
Focal tonic
Sustained posturing of single limbs
Sustained asymmetrical posturing of the trunk
Sustained eye deviation
Cannot be provoked by stimulation or suppressed by restraint
Pathophysiology: epileptic
Generalized tonic
Sustained symmetrical posturing of limbs, trunk and neck
May be flexor, extensor or mixed extensor/flexor
May be provoked or intensified by stimulation
May be suppressed by restraint or repositioning
Presumed pathophysiology: nonepileptic
Myoclonic
Random, single, rapid contractions of muscle groups of the limbs, face, or trunk
Typically not repetitive or may recur at a slow rate
May be generalized, focal, or fragmentary
May be provoked by stimulation
Presumed pathophysiology: may be epileptic or nonepileptic
Spasms
May be flexor, extensor, or mixed extensor/flexor
May occur in clusters
Cannot be provoked by stimulation or suppressed by restraint
Pathophysiology: Epileptic
Motor Automatisms
Oral-buccal-lingual movements
Random and roving eye movements or nystagmus (distinct from tonic eye deviation)
Progression movements (rowing, swimming, bicycling)
May be provoked or intensified by stimulation
Presumed pathophysiology: nonepileptic

Table 361.4
Classification of neonatal seizures based upon electroclinical findings (Modified from Mizrahi EM, Clancy RR (2000) Neonatal seizures: early-onset seizure syndromes and their consequences for development. Ment Retard dev Disabil Res Rev 6:229. Copyright © 2000 Wiley-Liss)

Clinical seizures with a consistent electrocortical signature (pathophysiology epileptic)
Focal clonic
Unifocal
Multifocal
Hemiconvulsive
Axial
Focal tonic
Asymmetrical truncal posturing
Limb posturing
Sustained eye deviation
Myoclonic
Generalized
Focal
Spasms
Flexor
Extensor
Mixed extensor/flexor
Clinical seizures without a consistent electrocortical signature (pathophysiology presumed nonepileptic)
Myoclonic
Generalized
Focal
Fragmentary
Generalized tonic
Flexor
Extensor
Mixed extensor/flexor
Motor automatisms
Oral-buccal-lingual movements
Ocular signs
Progression movements
Complex purposeless movements
Electrical seizures without clinical seizure activity

Electroclinical seizures are those clinical seizures that occur in correlation with electrographic seizure activity. If the seizure does not correlate with EEG seizure activity, it is denominated clinical only. A significant number of infants have electrographic seizures only. These seizures occur in infants who have severe encephalopathy, those who have received antiepileptic drugs (AEDs), or in infants with drug-induced paralysis.

Diagnosis

As mentioned above, neonatal seizures are symptomatic and most likely secondary to an underlying abnormality. More rarely, these seizures are part of a more extensive epilepsy syndrome. Four neonatal syndromes have been described: benign neonatal convulsions (BNC), benign neonatal familial convulsions (BNFC), early myoclonic encephalopathy (EME), and early infantile epileptic encephalopathy (EIEE). The first two syndromes are considered benign, and are associated with relatively good prognosis and survival. The latter two exhibit a suppression-burst pattern on EEG and are categorized as catastrophic for their poor prognosis.

Benign Neonatal Convulsions

The cause of this syndrome, which comprises 2–7% of all neonatal seizures, is unknown; however, acute zinc deficiency in the cerebrospinal fluid (CSF) of affected neonates as well as rotavirus infection have been postulated as possible etiologies. The seizures affect mostly term or near-term infants after an uneventful pregnancy and delivery, and with no family history of seizures. The incidence is higher in the first 7 days of life, with 90% occurring between days 4 and 6. The seizures are brief and self-limited, although some evolve to prolonged seizures. They are most commonly focal clonic or focal tonic, and usually recur in a period of 24–48 hours. EEG findings associated with these seizures include nonreactive rhythmic activity, discontinuity, interhemispheric asynchrony, and multifocal sharp waves. This pattern is known as "theta pointu alternant"; it is nonspecific, and is seen only in 60% of the patients. Due to the resemblance of this syndrome with other seizure types, this diagnosis remains a diagnosis of exclusion, after other most common etiologies have been ruled out. Diagnostic criteria have been proposed for this syndrome, which include an Apgar score greater than 7 at 1 min, a typical interval between birth and seizure onset (4–6 days), a normal neurologic examination before and between the seizures, normal laboratory findings (e.g., metabolic studies, neuroimaging, and cerebrospinal fluid analysis), and no family history of neonatal seizures. The treatment of these seizures is similar to other seizures in the neonatal period. If AEDs are used, they can be stopped once the infant is beyond the 24–48 hours period of recurrence risk. The prognosis of this syndrome is relatively good in terms of neurologic status, development, and postneonatal epilepsy. However, some data suggest a variable outcome, with 15% of infants manifesting transient "psychomotor delay" at 4–6 months of age, implying that the seizures may adversely affect the infant.

Benign Familial Neonatal Convulsions (BFNC)

This is an autosomal dominant disorder that affects approximately 14.4 per 100,000 live births. There are two types of BFNC: EBN1 is the result of a mutation in the voltage-gated potassium channel KCNQ2, whereas EBN2 is the result of a deletion in the chromosome 8q24, which encodes for another potassium channel known as KCNQ3. This syndrome is characterized by focal or multifocal clonic or tonic seizures, a family history of neonatal seizures, and no other neurologic abnormalities. It is characterized by brief seizures, which in some cases may recur until the age of 2–3 months, when spontaneous resolution typically occurs. The interictal EEG is usually normal. The treatment of this syndrome is similar to that of other neonatal seizures. Even if this syndrome is thought to be benign, recent data suggests an increased rate of postnatal epilepsy in these patients.

Early Myoclonic Encephalopathy (EME)

This disorder peaks in the early neonatal period. Its etiology is unknown, but it has been associated with inborn errors of metabolism, such as non-ketotic hyperglycemia, D-glycemic academia, methylmalonic academia, propionic academia, and hyperammonemia due to carbamyl phosphate synthetase deficiency. This syndrome is characterized by myoclonic seizures in the first week of life. This is followed by partial seizures, myoclonus, infantile spasms, and infrequently, tonic seizures. The EEG shows a characteristic suppression burst pattern (S-B; bursts of spikes, sharp waves, and slow activity lasting 5–6 s, alternating with 4- to 12-s periods of attenuation), that progresses to a hypsarrythmic pattern or a markedly abnormal background with multifocal spikes and sharp waves. Neonates with this syndrome present with an altered state of consciousness, with manifestly delayed milestones, hypotonia, and microcephaly from cerebral atrophy. The myoclonus present at birth tends to resolve; however, the focal motor seizures become refractory to antiepileptic therapy. Approximately 50% of the infants die, most within the first year of life. The focal motor seizures are treated with standard AEDs.

Early Infantile Epileptic Encephalopathy

This disease is characterized by intractable tonic seizures in the neonatal or infantile period. On EEG, a suppression-burst pattern is seen. The bursts are relatively prolonged (2–6 s) and shorter periods of suppression is seen when compared to EME. There is associated synchronization with the tonic spasms, with an initial high-voltage slow wave followed by generalized fast activity. The EEG abnormalities in EME and EIEE are similar, and the etiologies may overlap. The majority of anomalies associated with EIEE, however, are structural in origin, that is, porencephaly, Aicardi's syndrome, cerebral atrophy, hemimegalencephaly, dentate-olivary dysplasia, and migrational defects. Inborn errors of metabolism are rarely associated with EIEE. This is in contrast to disorders associated with EME, which are mostly metabolic in origin. This syndrome occurs during the first months of life. Affected infants have an abnormal neurological exam, with spasticity, motor asymmetries, and developmental delay. Tonic spasms are the predominant seizure type. Additional seizures include focal motor seizures and hemiconvulsive seizures. Erratic myoclonus is absent in EIEE, which is in contrast with EME where it is an early characteristic, and tonic spasms occur late in the disease. Several different approaches have been implemented in the treatment of EIEE, including AEDs, steroids, ACTH, and vitamin B6. The outcome, however, is still poor, with approximately a 50% mortality during infancy, and survivors being severely affected and sometimes progressing to develop infantile spasms.

Differential Diagnosis

Normal behaviors of the newborn sometimes raise suspicion of seizures. Nonspecific random movements, including sucking, coughing, and gagging, are among these behaviors. Neonates may also experience normal myoclonus during REM as well as non-REM sleep. Jitteriness, a tremulous movement that is suppressible when holding the limb, is normal in newborns and is generally not a manifestation of seizure activity. Apnea, bradycardia, and tonic posturing can be seen from gastroesophageal reflux (Sandifer syndrome). A barium swallow or pH probe may be required to confirm this diagnosis. Hyperekplexia, an exaggerated startle response to an unexpected stimulus, may resemble generalized myoclonus. However, hyperekplexia is non-fatigable, and can be elicited repeatedly by finger tap on the infant's glabella.

Treatment

The first step in treatment is to assess the general medical condition of the child, beginning with airway, breathing, and circulation. It is important to determine the underlying etiology of the seizures, since some conditions can result in brain injury if not treated promptly. Meningitis and hypoglycemia are two particularly important conditions to consider. After medically stabilizing the patient, antiseizure medications should be initiated to prevent recurrence. Pharmacotherapy is generally continued until the underlying cause has resolved, the seizures have subsided, and the patient is fully alert. Achieving these conditions often requires 1–3 months.

CNS Infection

Treatment of infection, if present, is of extreme importance in controlling seizures in the neonate. Broad spectrum antibiotics in high doses should be instituted after CSF has been obtained to evaluate for the presence of meningitis. In neonates, the first choice of antibiotics is ampicillin (100 mg/Kg/dose) and gentamycin (dose in accordance with gestational age).

Metabolic Abnormalities

Hypoglycemia, hypocalcemia, and hypomagnesemia are common electrolyte imbalances that should be corrected promptly. Pyridoxine dependency must also be considered in refractory seizures and can be diagnosed by administering intravenous pyridoxine (100 mg; the dose may be repeated four times to a total of 500 mg if needed) under EEG monitoring. If pyridoxine dependency is present, the seizures and epileptic changes on EEG will resolve within seconds of administration. Folinic acid–responsive seizures should also be considered in refractory cases, and may be combined with pyridoxine.

Institution of Antiseizure Medications

The acute treatment of neonatal seizures is not different from the management of any other emergency (see

Table 361.5
Long-term outcome of neonatal seizures (From Tharp: neonatal seizures)

High mortality (30%) and morbidity (50% of survivors)
Approximately 30% of survivors develop epilepsy
Worst outcome in infants with hypoxic – ischemic encephalopathy, meningitis, and cerebral dysplasia
Better outcome with transient neonatal hypocalcemia, idiopathic and familial seizures, and stroke
Neonatal EEG, neurologic examination, and imaging results are best predictors of outcome

Table 361.6). After airway, breathing, and circulation have been addressed, and the above-mentioned causes of seizures have been investigated and treated, the physician is left with the decision of whether to institute antiseizure medications. In so doing, there are a few issues that need to be considered. Not all the clinical events in the neonate are seizures in origin, and may therefore not require treatment. Further, some benign causes of neonatal seizures are transient and resolve without associated morbidity. In these cases, instituting therapy will expose the neonate to medication side effects with limited benefit. More aggressive seizures, on the other hand, can be associated with severe neurological impairment and future morbidity. Such seizures therefore require treatment.

Phenobarbital

As stated above, this is the first drug of choice in the treatment of neonatal seizures. Phenobarbital is metabolized in the liver, and eliminated by the kidney. In infants with impaired function of these two organs, such as HIE patients, phenobarbital levels can be elevated and cause toxicity. Additionally, as the neonate matures, the metabolism of this drug augments, and the levels drop. This has the potential to cause breakthrough seizures. Phenobarbital levels should be monitored in neonates to avoid this phenomenon.

Phenytoin

This drug has variable pharmacokinetics in the developing neonate, with potential for subtherapeutic levels. Therefore, phenytoin levels should be monitored and its dose should be adjusted to each particular patient. In a randomized trial comparing phenobarbital and phenytoin, both drugs controlled seizures in less than 50% of patients.

Table 361.6

Doses of AEDs (Reproduced with permission from Mizrahi EM, Kellaway P (1998) Diagnosis and management of neonatal seizures. Lippincott-Raven, Philadelphia, p 181. Copyright © 1998 Lippincott Williams & Wilkins)

Drug	Loading	Maintenance	Average therapeutic range	Apparent half-life
Diazepam	0.25 mg/IV (bolus)	May be repeated 1–2 times		31–54 h
	0.5 mg/kg (rectal)			
Lorazepam	0.05 mg/kg (IV) (over 2–5 min)	May be repeated		31–54 h
Phenobarbital	20 mg/kg IV (up to 40 mg)	3–4 mg/kg in two doses	20–40 mcg/L	100 h after day 5–7
Phenytoin	20 mg/kg IV (over 30–45 min)	3–4 mg/kg in 2–4 doses	15–25 mcg/L	100 h (40–200)

Other Antiseizure Medications

Third-line antiseizure medications that have been tested include clonazepam, lidocaine, midazolam, and paraldehyde. Oral AEDs have also been employed including carbamazepine, primidone, valproate, vigabatrin, and lamotrigine. There is little known regarding the efficacy of these therapies, but some have shown promise in limited trials. In one study, 13 out of 13 newborns who failed to achieve seizure control on phenobarbital or phenytoin were seizure-free following the addition of midazolam. No adverse effects of the medication were reported and the patients demonstrated improved neurodevelopmental outcome. In a pilot study of levetiracetam monotherapy, six out of six neonates were seizure-free within 6 days of starting it. In a smaller case series, three infants, aged 2 days to 3 months, exhibited seizure freedom and had no side effects on levetiracetam. In a recent survey of child neurologists, 73% recommended treatment of neonatal seizures with either levetiracetam or topiramate, although adverse reactions were felt to occur more frequently from topiramate.

Prognosis

Neonatal seizures are mostly self-limited and disappear when the provoking insult resolves. Many infants, however, will experience seizure relapses after a seizure-free period. Other patients will continue to have seizures without a seizure-free interval. Epileptogenesis (the development of epilepsy) has been observed in several animal models of neonatal seizures. Rodent models of seizures and status epilepticus in the first 2–3 postnatal weeks generally cause very little cell death, and the synaptic sprouting associated with cell death in adult models of epilepsy are not observed in most neonatal models. Furthermore, neuronal death may not be observed even when epileptogenesis occurs. Initially, it was assumed that the lack of neuronal death indicated a relative absence of sequelae. More recently, however, the changes following neonatal seizures have come to be recognized as functional rather than structural. For example, limbic cognitive deficits are seen following neonatal seizures despite the absence of pathological abnormalities. Thus, a dissociation exists between pathological and functional deficits following neonatal seizures, and cell death may not be required for functional injury or subsequent epilepsy to occur within the hippocampal/limbic network. The long-term outcome of NS is illustrated in *Table 361.5.*

Prevention

Prevention of neonatal seizures centers on reducing known causes of brain injury. These include, but are not limited to, hypoxic-ischemic encephalopathy, intracranial hemorrhage, CNS infection, hypoglycemia, and stroke. Prompt recognition of hypoglycemia and infection are particularly important since these conditions worsen if not treated early. For causes of brain injury that are more difficult to avoid, neuroprotection may play a role in the future. A major development in the treatment of perinatal hypoxic-ischemic encephalopathy, the most common cause of neonatal seizures, is the administration of therapeutic hypothermia to prevent neuronal injury. In a recent meta-analysis that examined the 18-month outcome of newborns with HIE, therapeutic hypothermia significantly reduced the risk of death and neurodevelopmental disabilities, such as cerebral palsy and psychomotor retardation. In the largest study reviewed in that meta-analysis, there was a nonsignificant trend toward reduced rates of continued seizures in survivors (12/116 vs. 16/116, *P* value 0.42). A longer period of follow-up may be required to determine if epilepsy rates are truly improved in patients receiving hypothermia.

References

Auvin S, Pandit F, De Bellecize J, Badinand N, Isnard H, Motte J, Villeneuve N, Lamblin MD, Vallee L (2006) Benign myoclonic epilepsy in infants: electroclinical features and long-term follow-up of 34 patients. Epilepsia 47(2):387–393

Barnett A, Mercuri E, Rutherford M, Haataja L, Frisone MF, Henderson S, Cowan F, Dubowitz L (2002) Neurological and perceptual-motor outcome at 5–6 years of age in children with neonatal encephalopathy: relationship with neonatal brain MRI. Neuropediatrics 33(5):242–248

Biagioni E, Mercuri E, Rutherford M, Cowan F, Azzopardi D, Frisone MF, Cioni G, Dubowitz L (2001) Combined use of electroencephalogram and magnetic resonance imaging in full-term neonates with acute encephalopathy. Pediatrics 107(3):461–468

Clancy RR (1996) The contribution of EEG to the understanding of neonatal seizures. Epilepsia 37(Suppl 1):S52–S59

Co JPT, Elia M, Engel J, Guerrini R, Mizrahi EM, Moshe SL, Plouin P (2007) Proposal of an algorithm for diagnosis and treatment of neonatal seizures in developing countries. Epilepsia 48(6):1158–1164

Dehan M, Quillerou D, Navelet Y, D'Allest AM, Vial M, Retbi JM, Lelong-Tissier MC, Gabilan JC (1997) Convulsions in the fifth day of life: a new syndrome? Arch Fr Pédiatr 34(8):730–742

Di Capua M, Fusco L, Ricci S, Vigevano F (1993) Benign neonatal sleep myoclonus: clinical features and video-polygraphic recordings. Mov Disord 8(2):191–194

Finer NN, Robertson CM, Richards RT, Pinnell LE, Peters KL (1981) Hypoxic-ischemic encephalopathy in term neonates: perinatal factors and outcome. J Pediatr 98(1):112–117

Goldberg HJ, Sheehy EM (1982) Fifth day fits: an acute zinc deficiency syndrome? Arch Dis Child 57(8):633–635

Herrmann B, Lawrenz-Wolf B, Seewald C, Selb B, Wehinger H (1993) Fifth day convulsions of the newborn infant in rotavirus infections. Monatsschr Kinderheilkd 141(2):120–123

Hill A (1991) Current concepts of hypoxic-ischemic cerebral injury in the term newborn. Pediatr Neurol 7(5):317–325

Holmes GL (1997) Epilepsy in the developing brain: lessons from the laboratory and clinic. Epilepsia 38(1):12–30

Lacey JL, Henderson-Smart DJ (1998) Assessment of preterm infants in the intensive-care unit to predict cerebral palsy and motor outcome at 6 years. Dev Med Child Neurol 40(5):310–318

Lombroso CT (1974) The treatment of status epilepticus. Pediatrics 53(4):536–540

Mizrahi EM, Clancy RR (2000) Neonatal seizures: early-onset seizure syndromes and their consequences for development. Ment Retard Dev Disabil Res Rev 6:229

Mizrahi EM, Kellaway P (1987) Characterization and classification of neonatal seizures. Neurology 37(12):1837–1844

Mizrahi EM, Kellaway P (1998) Diagnosis and management of neonatal seizures. Lippincott-Raven, Philadelphia, p 181

Mizrahi EM, Watanabe K (2002) Symptomatic neonatal seizures. In: Roger J, Bureau M, Dravet Ch (eds) Epileptic syndromes in infancy, childhood and adolescence. John Libbey, London, pp 16–17

Okumura A, Watanabe K, Negoro T, Hayakawa F, Kato T, Maruyama K, Kubota T, Suzuki M, Kurahashi H, Azuma Y (2006) Long-term follow-up of patients with benign partial epilepsy in infancy. Epilepsia 47(1):181–185

Robertson CM, Finer NN, Grace MG (1989) School performance of survivors of neonatal encephalopathy associated with birth asphyxia at term. J Pediatr 114(5):753–760

Ronen GM, Penney S, Andrews W (1999) The epidemiology of clinical neonatal seizures in Newfoundland: a population-based study. J Pediatr 134(1):71–75

Rose AL, Lombroso CT (1970) A study of clinical, pathological, and electroencephalographic features in 137 full-term babies with a long-term follow-up. Pediatrics 45(3):404–425

Shah PS, Beyene J, To T, Ohlsson A, Perlman M (2006) Postasphyxial hypoxic-ischemic encephalopathy in neonates: outcome prediction rule within 4 hours of birth. Arch Pediatr Adolesc Med 160(7): 729–736

Shankaran S, Woldt E, Koepke T, Bedard MP, Nandyal R (1991) Acute neonatal morbidity and long-term central nervous system sequelae of perinatal asphyxia in term infants. Early Hum Dev 25(2):135–148

Takeuchi T, Watanabe K (1989) The EEG evolution and neurological prognosis of neonates with perinatal hypoxia [corrected]. Brain Dev 11(2):115–120

Volpe JJ (1989) Neonatal seizures: current concepts and revised classification. Pediatrics 84(3):422–428

Watanabe K, Hara K, Miyazaki S, Kuroyanagi M, Asano S, Kondo K, Kuno K, Jose H, Iwase K (1977) Electroclinical studies of seizures in the newborn. Folia Psychiatr Neurol Jpn 31(3):383–392

362 Epilepsy in Infancy and Childhood

John N. Gaitanis

Definitions

Seizures are self-limited clinical events resulting from an abnormal and excessive firing of cortical neurons (➋ *Table 362.1*). They manifest as transient motor, sensory, autonomic, or psychic symptoms with or without an alteration of consciousness (➋ *Table 362.2*). *Epilepsy*, on the other hand, is a condition characterized by recurrent, unprovoked seizures. Epilepsy does not constitute a single entity and is instead a heterogeneous group of disorders, with multiple etiologies and clinical manifestations. Subdivisions of epilepsy are based upon the etiology or the clinical features. The International League Against Epilepsy published a classification system for seizures in 1981, and for epilepsies in 1989. In it, epilepsy is categorized as either *localization-related* (focal onset beginning over one region of brain) or *generalized* (having a simultaneous onset over both hemispheres). Epilepsy is further subdivided as *idiopathic* (no underlying cause other than a possible hereditary predisposition), *symptomatic* (a consequence of a known or suspected disorder), or *cryptogenic* (presumed to be symptomatic, but the cause is unknown). This classification scheme is based largely on clinical and electroencephalographic data. Significant advances in molecular biology, neuroimaging, and genetics have since taken place and will likely play a role in the development of future classification schemes.

When seizures are so frequently repeated or so prolonged as to create a "fixed and enduring epileptic condition," they are termed status epilepticus (SE). The most commonly chosen duration for seizures to qualify as SE has been 30 min, based on the belief that seizures persisting longer than that result in brain injury. More recently, however, an "operational" definition of SE has been proposed as 5 min or more of continuous seizures or "two or more discrete seizures between which there is incomplete recovery of consciousness." This definition, which applies primarily to GCSE, may be used clinically to direct treatment and help avoid refractory SE.

Etiology

Epilepsy is a heterogeneous condition with a multitude of etiologies (➋ *Table 362.3*). Idiopathic and cryptogenic etiologies account for 60–70% of cases while symptomatic causes account for 30–40%. These rates are similar in industrialized and developing countries. Idiopathic epilepsies have an underlying genetic basis. Many idiopathic cases result from channelopathies, which impair neurotransmission. Others involve genes that are important for broader aspects of development, which may also result in mental retardation, autism, or brain malformations. Symptomatic etiologies of epilepsy, on the other hand, develop following brain injury. In children, perinatal insults are important causes and include hypoxic-ischemic encephalopathy, stroke, intracranial hemorrhage, periventricular leukomalacia, and hypoglycemia. Later in childhood, head trauma, infections, and brain tumors are more common. In developing nations, neurocystercircosis is a particularly important cause and may account for as many as 60% of first-time seizures and one-third of symptomatic epilepsies.

Epidemiology

Epilepsy is estimated to affect 50 million people worldwide, and it accounts for 1% of the global burden of disease. In industrialized countries, its prevalence ranges between 4 and 10 active cases per 1,000 persons. Prevalence estimates are only slightly higher in the developing world, ranging between 3.8 and 15.4 per 1,000. The incidence of epilepsy, however, is noticeably higher in developing nations. It ranges between 114 and 190 per 100,000 in developing countries, but is only 24–53 per 100,000 in industrialized nations. Developing countries have higher mortality rates for epilepsy, accounting in part for the disparity in incidence and prevalence data.

The age of onset also differs between regions. In industrialized countries, the onset of epilepsy occurs at the extremes of life, whereas in developing nations, the onset

Abdelaziz Y. Elzouki (ed.), *Textbook of Clinical Pediatrics*, DOI 10.1007/978-3-642-02202-9_362,

Table 362.1
Seizure terminology

Seizure: A clinical event, displaying signs or symptoms, resulting from an abnormal and excessive discharge of cortical neurons
Epilepsy: Recurrent, unprovoked seizures
Generalized: The initial seizure discharge involves a large number of neurons throughout both hemispheres and the clinical manifestations indicate bilateral onset
Partial: The initial seizure discharge involves a limited number of neurons in just one hemisphere
Simple: A seizure that does not cause alteration in consciousness
Complex: A seizure involving alteration in consciousness
Idiopathic: Epilepsy with a genetic cause
Cryptogenic: Non-idiopathic epilepsy without a known cause
Symptomatic: Non-idiopathic epilepsy with a known cause (usually a brain insult or other lesion)
Tonic: Sustained posturing of a body part
Clonic: Rhythmic jerking of a body part
Myoclonic: Brief, irregular contractions of a body part
Atonic: An abrupt loss of muscle tone
Tonic-clonic: Tonic activity alternating with clonic movements
Absence: A transient discontinuation of activity with loss of awareness

Table 362.2
Seizure classification

I. Partial (Focal)
A. Simple
1. Motor
2. Sensory
3. Autonomic
4. Psychic
B. Complex
II. Generalized
A. Absence
1. Typical
2. Atypical
B. Myoclonic
C. Clonic
D. Tonic
E. Tonic-clonic
F. Atonic

is highest in young and middle-aged adults. Parasitic diseases, more endemic in the developing world, likely account for this difference.

The incidence of status epilepticus ranges between 18.1 and 41 per 100,000 patients per year. In the United States, this amounts to 102,000–152,000 cases and 22,000–42,000 deaths annually.

Pathogenesis

The pathogenesis of epilepsy is as varied as the etiologies. Idiopathic and symptomatic causes of epilepsy have entirely different mechanisms of disease. Symptomatic epilepsy results from brain injury, whereas idiopathic forms result from genetic alterations involving proteins necessary for normal neurotransmission. Idiopathic epilepsy is therefore less likely to reveal neuroimaging abnormalities and more likely to be associated with a family history of epilepsy. There is considerable genotype-phenotype heterogeneity within genetic causes of epilepsy, even within the same family.

For example, mutations of the sodium channel gene, SCN1A, result in six different phenotypes, ranging from generalized epilepsy with febrile seizures plus syndrome (GEFS+) on the milder end of the spectrum to severe myoclonic epilepsy of infancy at the severe end. SCN1A codes for the alpha subunit of the neuronal voltage-gated sodium channel. The alpha subunit forms the membrane pore of sodium channels. There is some correlation between genotype and phenotype. Mutations resulting in premature protein truncation are more likely to lead to a severe phenotype whereas missense mutations are associated with milder phenotypes.

Multiple ion channels are now known to play a role in epilepsy. They include the sodium channel genes SCN1A and SCN1B, potassium channel mutations of KCNQ2 and KCNQ3, chloride channel mutations in CLCN2, and calcium channel impairments of CACNB4. Genetic alterations of neurotransmitter receptors, such as the GABA receptor genes GABRD and GABRG2, also result in epilepsy. Just as mutations of a single gene result in varied phenotypes, mutations of two completely unrelated genes can lead to identical phenotypes. GEFS+, for example, can result from mutations of SCN1A, SCN1B, SCN2A, SCN9A, GABRG2, or GABRD. Confirmation of the specific genetic cause may be clinically useful when determining the correct treatment plan. Sodium channelopathies,

Table 362.3
Etiologies of epilepsy

Symptomatic
Perinatal brain injury
HIE
PVL
ICH
Hypoglycemia
Stroke
Infection
Neurocystercircosis
Meningitis
Encephalitis
Trauma
Stroke
Hemorrhagic
Ischemic
Metabolic (i.e., MELAS)
Inborn errors of metabolism
Mitochondrial disorders
Lysosomal disorders
Peroxysomal disorders
Amino and organic acidopathies
Urea cycle disorders
Congenital brain malformations
Lissencephaly
Polymicrogyria
Focal cortical dysplasia/tuberous sclerosis
Heterotopia
Idiopathic
Channelopathies
Generalized epilepsy with febrile seizures plus
Childhood absence epilepsy
Juvenile myoclonic epilepsy
Chromosomal disorders
Trisomy 21
Wolf–Hirschhorn syndrome (4p-)
Ring Chromosome 20
Single gene disorders
Rett syndrome (MECP2, CDKL5, FOXG1)
Angelman's syndrome
Unverricht–Lundborg disease
Autosomal-dominant nocturnal frontal lobe epilepsy
Benign familial neonatal seizures
Cryptogenic
Undiagnosed cases associated with other neurological disorders such as autism, mental retardation, apraxia, or other developmental delays

for example, may worsen with sodium channel–blocking agents such as carbamazepine and phenytoin. Genetic confirmation is also helpful when counseling families.

Symptomatic epilepsy, on the other hand, results from environmental rather than genetic causes. Traumatic, ischemic, and infectious insults all result in epilepsy. Epilepsy develops from different types of injury through common mechanisms. Breakdown of the blood-brain barrier (BBB) is observed in brain injury. When the BBB is disrupted, intravascular albumin leaks into the extracellular space, resulting in glial dysfunction. Without proper glial function, glutamate cannot be cleared from the extracellular space. Elevation of glutamate results in hyperexcitability and an influx of intracellular neuronal calcium, which in turn causes neuronal injury and seizures. The initial injury, caused in part by excessive glutamatergic activity, is followed by a latent period, during which time no seizure activity takes place. During that period, pathophysiological and structural alterations are occurring which will later culminate in epilepsy. Further understanding of how injury leads to epileptogenesis may provide targeted treatments, which can prevent the onset of epilepsy.

Excessive glutamatergic activity also plays a role in the development of status epilepticus. As an illustration of this, an outbreak of toxic encephalopathy caused by ingestion of mussels contaminated with domoic acid, a glutamate analogue, caused prolonged seizures in many of the affected patients. Excitatory amino acids, especially glutamate, also contribute to the neuronal injury caused by SE. As seizures persist, there is also downregulation of inhibitory mechanisms, further contributing to SE. GABA-A receptors become less susceptible to the GABA agonist effects of benzodiazepines. This causes refractoriness to treatment with the GABA-acting medications, benzodiazepines and barbiturates.

Pathology

Temporal lobe structures, particularly the hippocampus and amygdala, are the most susceptible regions to epileptogenesis following brain injury. The resulting neuronal loss and fibrillary gliosis of the mesial temporal structures is termed mesial temporal sclerosis (MTS). MTS is the most common pathological finding in patients with temporal lobe epilepsy and is seen in 65% of temporal lobectomy specimens. In approximately one-third of patients with MTS, dual pathology is observed. Additional findings may include dysplastic neuroepithelial tumors, cavernous angiomas, caudate atrophy, inflammatory changes, and focal cortical dysplasia. The significance of dual pathology is not known, but it calls into question whether MTS is the cause or effect of active epilepsy. Neuronal migration disorders, for instance, may predispose the patient to febrile seizures, which later result in MTS. Alternatively, the pathological changes seen in MTS can mimic dysplastic tissue, erroneously pointing toward a dual diagnosis. A final possibility is that both dysplastic tissue and MTS share a common embryological origin, and that both act together in the development of epilepsy.

Clinical Manifestations

Epilepsy should be suspected whenever a patient reports transient, repetitive, and stereotyped symptoms. Seizure semiology, the signs and symptoms of how a seizure is expressed, differs depending on the seizure type. Partial seizures involve a localized region of the cerebral cortex, and their symptoms reflect the area of involvement. For example, occipital seizures result in visual hallucinations whereas frontal seizures are more likely to cause motor symptoms. There are two main subdivisions of partial-onset seizures: simple and complex. Simple partial seizures do not involve impairment of consciousness. The symptoms can include sensory, motor, autonomic, or psychic (emotional sensation, dream-like state, or déjà vu) changes. Complex partial seizures, on the other hand, involve impairment of consciousness. They typically manifest as behavioral arrest and may involve staring or automatisms (repetitive movements such as chewing, lip smacking, or fumbling with hands). The patient often has no memory for these behaviors. Simple and complex partial seizures can secondarily generalize into generalized tonic-clonic seizures. Distinguishing between a primary versus secondary generalized seizure can be difficult. Secondary generalized seizures are recognized by a preceding aura, which represents a simple partial seizure preceding generalization. Primary generalized seizures, on the other hand, are not associated with a preceding aura.

There are six major categories of generalized seizures: absence, tonic, clonic, myoclonic, tonic-clonic, and atonic (see ➋ *Table 362.2*). Absence seizures are often difficult to distinguish from complex partial seizures since both manifest as staring spells. When compared to complex partial seizures, absence seizures are shorter (under 20 s), occur more frequently (often multiple times daily), and are less likely to be associated with automatisms or a prolonged postictal state. Many patients with primary generalized epilepsy experience more than one generalized seizure type. In juvenile myoclonic epilepsy, for example, patients exhibit generalized tonic-clonic, myoclonic, and absence seizures.

Just as seizures can take multiple forms, status epilepticus also presents in varied ways. *Generalized Convulsive Status Epilepticus* is the most dramatic and life-threatening form of SE. Fortunately, it is readily recognizable. It may begin with a partial seizure (simple or complex) that generalizes secondarily, or it can start as a generalized convulsion. There may be tonic and clonic movements, typically bilateral and symmetric, although the onset may occur on just one side. Consciousness is always impaired from the time the seizure generalizes. Afterward, the patient is stuporous. If the patient does not recover from the postictal stupor within a reasonable time, the possibility of continuing epileptic brain activity must be considered. This sort of decoupling of the electrical and motor systems constitutes "subtle" nonconvulsive SE, sometimes with just twitching or blinking or even no movement at all. Electroencephalography (EEG) is often helpful in confirming this.

Diagnosis

The diagnosis of seizures begins with a careful history. A detailed description of the episode, focusing on its onset, progression, time course, and recovery, helps establish if seizures are a likely etiology. If parents have a video camera, recordings of the event are particularly helpful in determining its clinical characteristics. The physical examination looks for neurological dysfunction, as might be present in a symptomatic etiology. Laboratory evaluations search for items missed on the history and examination. Two studies are particularly valuable: electroencephalography (EEG) and magnetic resonance imaging (MRI). EEG measures the brain's electrical activity. Transient electrical disruptions (spike waves or slowing) can indicate a predisposition for seizures and help determine if the seizures are focal or generalized. In addition, the appearance of abnormalities can be specific for particular seizure types or epilepsy syndromes. EEG is far from a perfect test, and can be normal in as many as 50% of patients with known epilepsy. Similarly, patients without a history of seizures can display EEG abnormalities. Thus, the study has to be interpreted within its clinical context. Prolonged inpatient or ambulatory EEG, both of which can be combined with video, is an effective way to capture an event and confidently diagnose epilepsy. MRI provides a structural assessment of the brain, helping to determine if an epileptic focus is present. It is particularly useful in patients with a focal seizure onset, localized exam, or lateralized EEG abnormalities.

Once a diagnosis of seizures has been established, it is incumbent upon the treating physician to establish whether the patient's seizure type and EEG characteristics fall within a well-described epilepsy syndrome. These are important to recognize since each syndrome exhibits a characteristic treatment response and prognosis.

Febrile Seizures are the most common form of childhood seizures, affecting between 2% and 4% of all children. They occur between 6 months and 5 years of age, but the peak incidence is 18 months. Febrile seizures can be divided into simple and complex types. Simple febrile seizures are generalized, last less than 15 min, and do not recur within a 24-h period. All others are considered complex. Overall, one-third of children with a first febrile seizure will experience a recurrence. Risk factors for recurrence include a family history of febrile seizures and an age of onset less than 18 months. In children with febrile seizures, the overall risk of later epilepsy is approximately 2%. This risk is higher in the presence of neurological or developmental abnormalities, complex febrile seizures, or a family history of epilepsy.

Severe myoclonic epilepsy of infancy (SMEI or Dravet Syndrome) can mimic febrile seizures early in its course. Seizures begin in the first year of life. They are often associated with a fever and can be prolonged. By age 2, multiple seizure types develop, including atypical absence, complex partial, and myoclonic. The child is initially developmentally appropriate, but a decline occurs between 1 and 4 years of age. By age 4, most children exhibit intractable seizures and developmental delays. In approximately 80% of patients, the condition occurs from mutations of SCN1A (see section on ➋ Pathogenesis). Mutations of SCN1A are also found in patients with febrile seizures and Generalized Epilepsy with Febrile Seizures Plus (GEFS+) syndrome.

Infantile spasms are one of the most worrisome epilepsy syndromes, since the seizures are subtle and the prognosis is often poor (➋ *Fig. 362.1*). They typically develop during the first year, with a peak age of onset between 4 and 6 months. Brief (1–5 s), symmetric contractions of the trunk with extension and elevation of the arms and tonic extension of the legs characterize the typical spasm. They occur in clusters shortly after waking. During a cluster, the infant may appear irritable. The triad of infantile spasms, hypsarrhythmia (a chaotic EEG pattern), and developmental regression is termed West's syndrome. The *Lennox–Gastaut syndrome* will develop in as many as 50% of children with infantile spasms. This syndrome, which occurs between 1 and 7 years of age, is comprised of mixed seizure types, cognitive decline, and a slow spike and wave pattern on EEG (<3 Hz) (➋ *Figs. 362.2* and ➋ *362.3*).

Absence seizures are common to three epilepsy syndromes: childhood absence epilepsy, juvenile absence epilepsy, and juvenile myoclonic epilepsy. *Childhood absence epilepsy* develops between 4 and 10 years of age and manifests with brief (5–15 s) periods of behavioral cessation or staring spells (➋ *Fig. 362.4*). They can be exacerbated by hyperventilation. This can be a useful feature when diagnosing absence seizures in the office or EEG laboratory. The EEG reveals generalized 3 Hz spike and slow wave discharges in association with the clinical event. *Juvenile absence epilepsy* is similar, but has a later age of onset (6–10 years) and a greater frequency of generalized tonic-clonic seizures than childhood absence epilepsy. *Juvenile myoclonic epilepsy* has an onset between 12 and 18 years, and patients exhibit absence, generalized tonic-clonic, and myoclonic seizures. The myoclonic jerks typically occur in the early morning hours. The EEG displays fast (3.5–6 Hz), generalized spike and wave or polyspike and wave activity.

Benign childhood focal seizures account for 22% of children with epilepsy. These syndromes develop in school age and are outgrown in adolescence. They are characterized by their semiology, EEG features, and absence of neuroimaging abnormalities. The most common of these conditions is *benign epilepsy with centrotemporal spikes* (BECTS), which represents approximately 15% of all childhood epilepsies (➋ *Fig. 362.5*). The most common seizure type is simple partial, involving motor or sensory symptoms of the hands or face. Generalized tonic-clonic seizures may also develop. Both seizure types commonly occur during sleep. The characteristic EEG pattern includes broad centrotemporal spikes that show an anterior-to-posterior dipole. In *Panayiotopoulos syndrome* (PS), children develop autonomic symptoms, with vomiting being the most common. Patients may appear restless or agitated during a seizure, and usually become confused or unresponsive over its course. Two-thirds of the seizures begin in sleep, and they are often prolonged (lasting greater than 30 min). EEG in PS reveals multifocal, high-amplitude, sharp slow wave complexes that shift between regions and hemispheres, but predominate in the occipital leads. *Idiopathic childhood occipital*

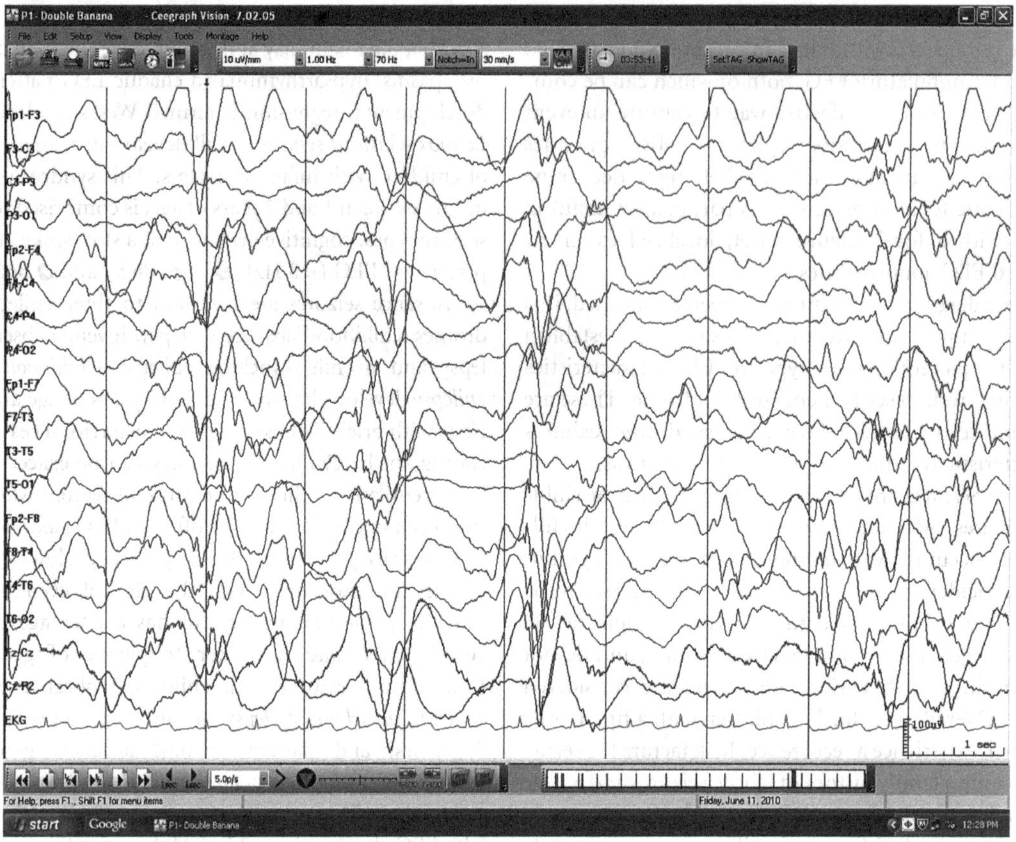

Figure 362.1
Twelve-month boy with infantile spasms. The interictal EEG shows a discontinuous background with high voltage delta slowing and spike waves interrupted by periods of voltage attenuation

epilepsy of Gastaut (ICOE-G) is also characterized by occipital spike waves on EEG. They are sometimes observed only in sleep and may be intermixed with centrotemporal discharges. The semiology differs from PS and is characterized by visual hallucinations, blindness, or both. The seizures are short, lasting 1–3 min, and occur frequently (sometimes daily). They may be followed by a postictal headache which is indistinguishable from migraine. ICOE-G is outgrown later than the other benign focal epilepsies of childhood, and may sometimes evolve into atypical absence epilepsy (➋ *Fig. 362.6*).

Differential Diagnosis

The first challenge in evaluating a patient with suspected seizures is to determine if the clinical events are epileptic or nonepileptic in etiology. There are several nonepileptic events (NEE) that resemble seizures, and the considerations change based on the patient's age.

The diagnosis of seizures is hardest to make in neonates, in whom subtle nonspecific clinical findings, such as eye deviation, apneas, bicycling, or buccolingual movements, may be the only manifestations. Many of these subtle signs are easily misdiagnosed. Suspected seizures are actually NEE in as many as 90% of neonates. The clinical event with the greatest specificity for epileptic seizures is focal clonic activity, which is epileptic in approximately 44% of newborns. Jitteriness, on the other hand, is nearly always a nonepileptic phenomenon. Because of the difficulty in confidently diagnosing seizures in the neonate, video EEG is often required.

In infancy, tonic posturing is a common event, and is often misdiagnosed. Without other associated signs or symptoms, tonic posturing is epileptic only 30% of the time. One common nonepileptic cause in infants is Sandifer syndrome. This refers to abnormal tonic posturing of the neck, trunk, or limbs, resulting from gastroesophageal reflux. There is often a temporal association with feeds, or there is a past history of spitting up or feeding intolerance. A gastrointestinal evaluation is needed to confirm this diagnosis.

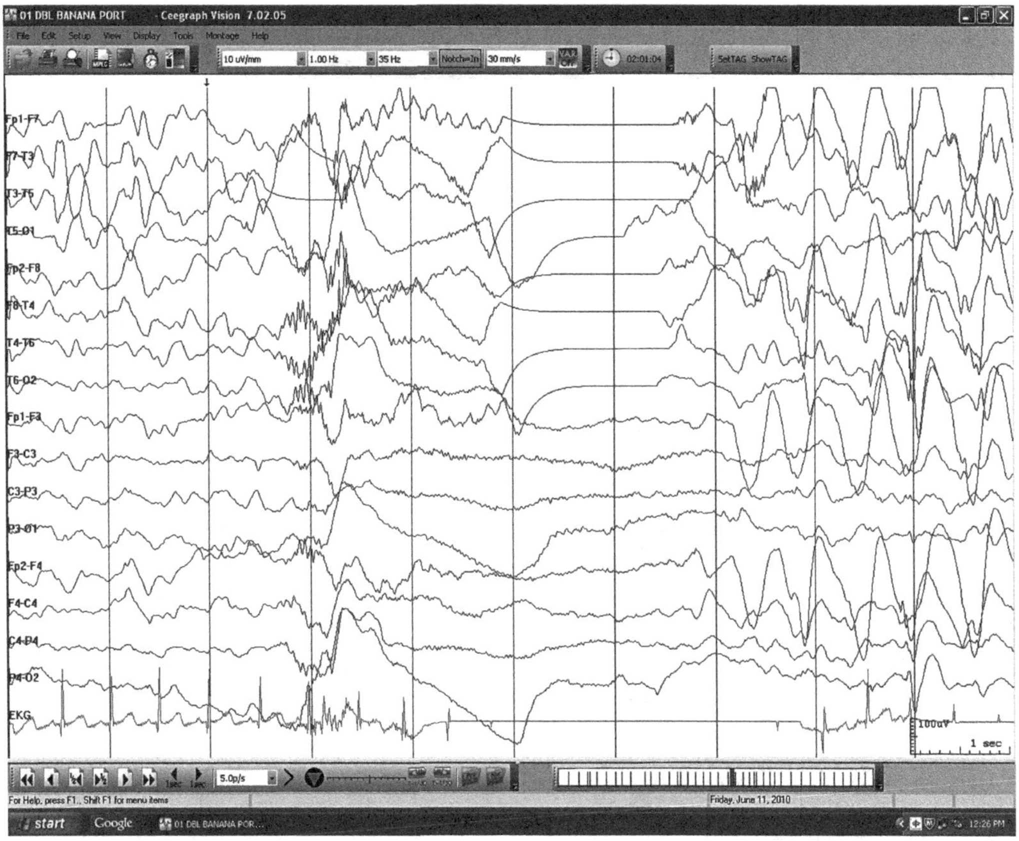

Figure 362.2
Twelve-month boy with infantile spasms. During his clinical spasms, there is a generalized decrement of the background activity with superimposed fast frequencies

Myoclonus is another event that is frequently misdiagnosed. Although myoclonic epilepsies can develop in infancy, there are two nonepileptic myoclonic syndromes that must be considered. These are benign neonatal sleep myoclonus and benign myoclonus of infancy. In benign neonatal sleep myoclonus, focal, multifocal, or generalized myclonic movements occur only during sleep. Each movement is brief, lasting a second or less, but the events may cluster. They end abruptly upon awakening. The movements usually begin in the first month and subside by 6 months of age, rarely persisting into childhood. The infant is otherwise neurologically normal. Benign myoclonus of infancy, on the other hand, begins at a later age (between 3 and 15 months) and involves tonic or myoclonic movements during wakefulness. The course is self-limited, and the events usually regress by age 2.

In early childhood, breath-holding spells are a common event. They may develop as early as infancy and will resolve prior to school age. Although most occur in response to an upsetting incident, the preceding cause is sometimes not observed by the parent. The child will display a color change, either pallor or cyanosis. Some children will have convulsive movements mimicking seizures and many are followed by a period of lethargy.

Later in childhood, most NEE can be distinguished from seizures based on a careful history or direct observation of the spells. Some include movement disorders such as motor tics, paroxysmal choreoathetosis, or focal dystonias. Narcolepsy, staring spells, complicated migraines, and syncope can also be difficult to distinguish from seizures. If all other causes have been excluded, psychogenic seizures must be considered. Many children with psychogenic seizure have epileptic seizures as well, so video EEG is often required for diagnosis.

Treatment

Once a correct diagnosis of epilepsy has been made, there are several reasons to consider treatment: (1) Reduce the risk of

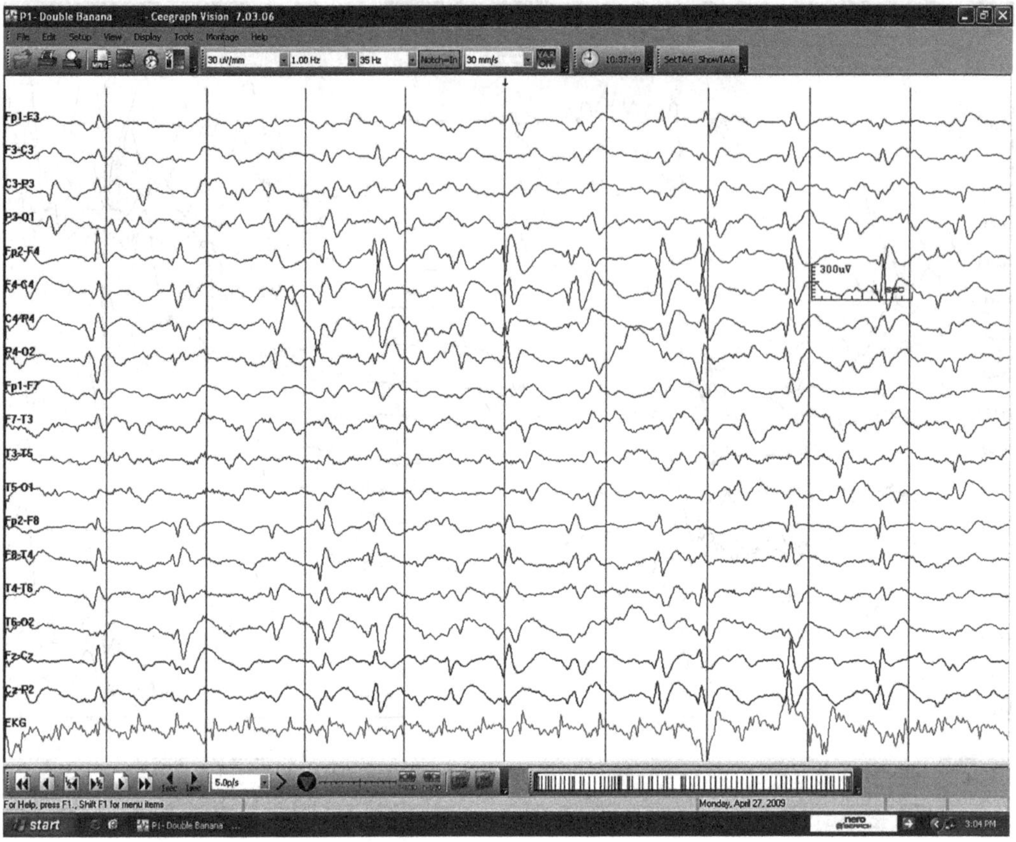

Figure 362.3

Seven-year-old boy with a history of infantile spasms and profound global developmental delays. He has multiple seizure types including generalized tonic-clonic, atypical absence, and drop spells. His EEG shows prolonged runs of slow spike and slow waves (approximately 1–2 Hz) and frequent delta slowing

epilepsy-induced injury. (2) Lessen the risk of prolonged seizures (status epilepticus). (3) Prevent sudden unexplained death in epilepsy (which is fortunately a rare occurrence in children). (4) Lessen cognitive effects from frequent seizures. (5) Improve the patient's overall quality of life. As with any medical intervention, the benefits that the patient derives from treatment will need to outweigh potential risks. The decision to treat is individualized and based on both seizure (type, frequency, duration) and patient (age, compliance, level of activity) specific factors.

Because epilepsy treatment is aimed at prevention, a decision to treat cannot be made without first estimating the recurrence risk (see section on ➋ Prognosis). Once a decision has been made to treat, choosing the right antiepileptic drug (AED) becomes the next major consideration (➋ *Table 362.4*). The optimal choice for a given patient depends on many factors, the two most important of which are efficacy and side effects. Efficacy differs based on the seizure type. For each seizure phenotype, there are first-, second-, and third-line treatments (➋ *Table 362.5*). There is often more than one accepted first-line therapy. Deciding which therapy has the most favorable side-effect profile helps narrow this choice down to a single agent. Other important considerations include the frequency of dosing, ease of administration, and cost. In children, taste and the availability of a liquid or chewable preparation can be among the most important considerations since they impact greatly on compliance.

The seizure type is very important when choosing the correct AED. Generalized seizures respond best to broad-spectrum medications, and can be exacerbated by medications geared toward partial seizures, such as carbamazepine. Matching the correct treatment to the individual epilepsy syndrome is also important.

In febrile seizures, epidemiologic data indicate that the seizures are benign, so aggressive treatment measures are

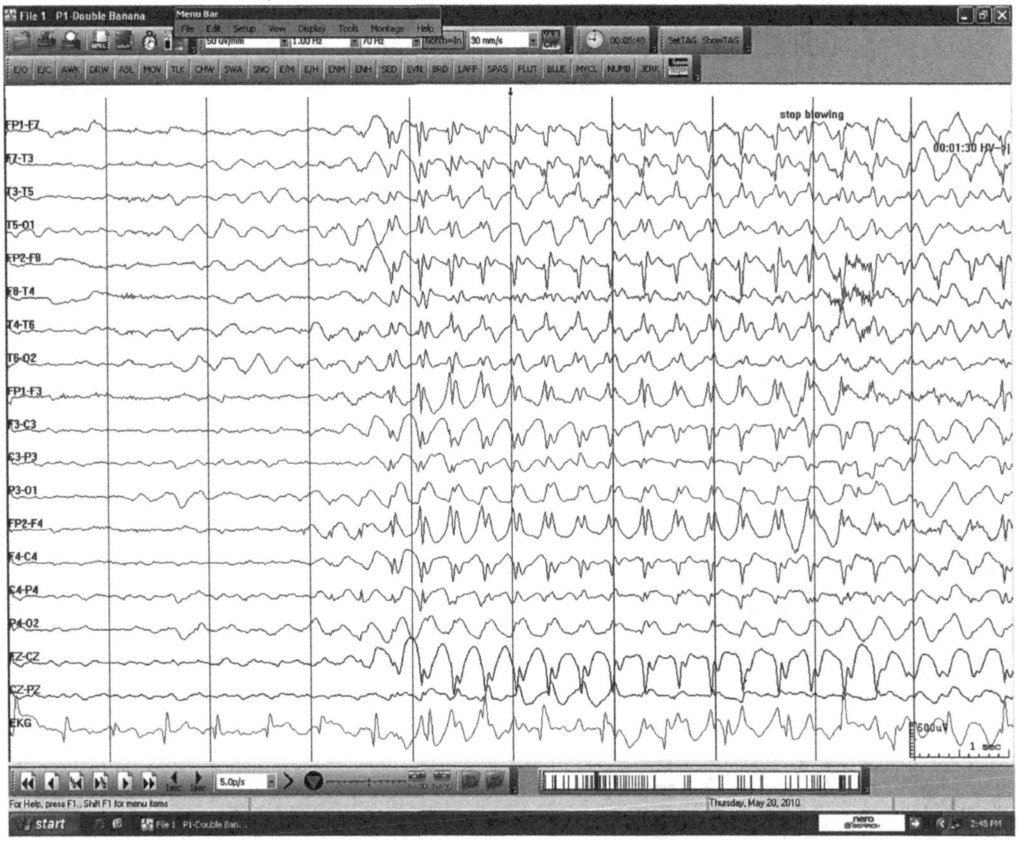

Figure 362.4
Eight-year-old girl with absence epilepsy. During her staring spells, bursts of generalized, 3 Hz spike and slow waves are seen on EEG

not required. The simplest preventative strategy is to use analgesics during febrile illnesses, although this approach has not demonstrated efficacy in clinical trials. Diazepam can also be given during febrile illnesses, but this results in only a modest reduction in recurrence. Additionally, rectal diazepam can be used acutely to abort a prolonged febrile seizure. Daily prophylaxis is rarely used in febrile seizures. Phenobarbital and valproic acid are effective for this purpose, but both have potential side effects. Treatment with a daily antiepileptic agent is therefore reserved for only the most severe cases.

Some patients initially diagnosed with febrile seizures go on to develop SMEI. Since this syndrome results from a mutation of voltage-gated sodium channel, sodium channel–blocking medications, such as carbamazepine and lamotrigine, can exacerbate seizures and should be avoided. Levetiracetam, topiramate, and stiripentol all offer better treatment success. The ketogenic diet can also be an effective option.

In infantile spasms, two treatment options are most effective: ACTH and vigabatrin. A course of pyridoxine may also be considered to exclude pyridoxine-dependent seizures. The Lennox–Gastaut syndrome may evolve from infantile spasms, and can be very refractory to treatment. Valproate and felbamate are two of the more effective options in this condition. The ketogenic diet can be effective in some patients, and vagus nerve stimulation may help prevent drop spells.

In absence seizures, ethosuximide is typically the first-line agent, but valproate and lamotrigine are also effective. In juvenile absence epilepsy and juvenile myoclonic epilepsy, valproate, levetiracetam, and lamotrigine are all effective options to consider.

For benign childhood focal seizures (PS, BECTS, and ICOE-G), treatment is optional since there is no evidence that the long-term prognosis is worse in untreated children. Daily prophylaxis depends largely on the presence of generalized convulsive seizures, since the simple partial seizures are typically not harmful. In ICOE-G, seizures can be

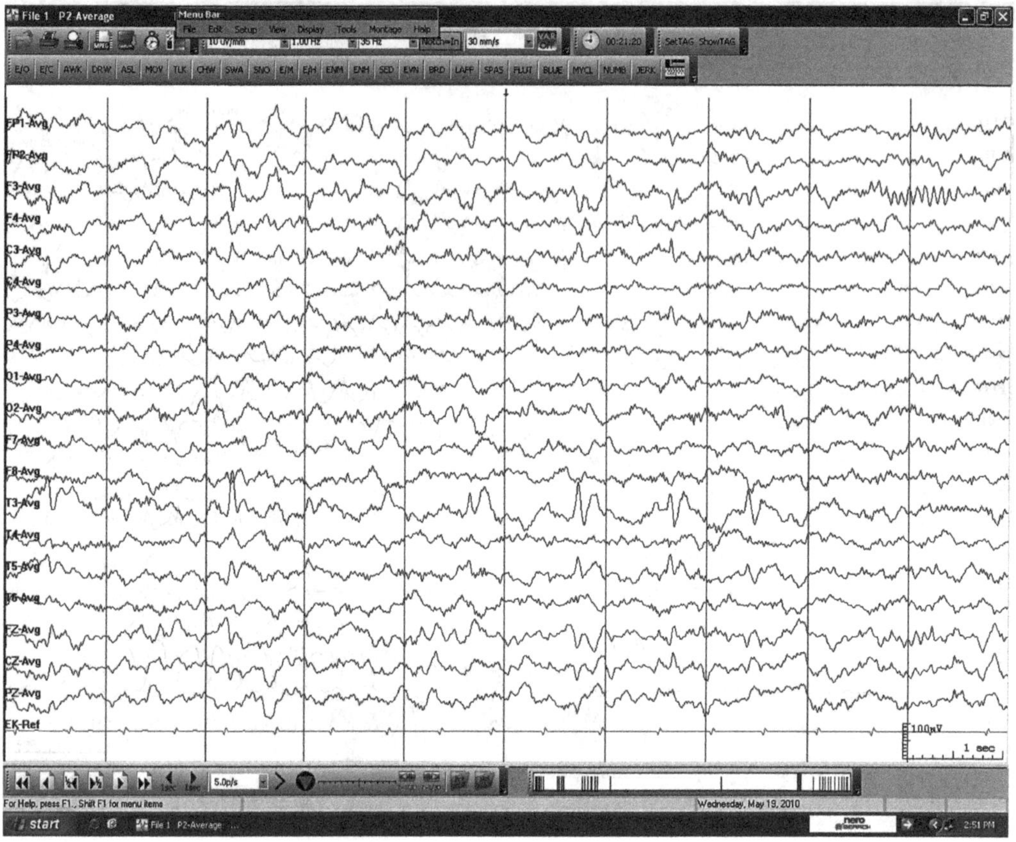

Figure 362.5
Seven-year-old boy with BECTS. His seizures are nocturnal and begin with a clicking sound of the throat followed by clonic activity of the face and hand. The involved side alternates between seizures. His EEG shows sleep-activated spike and slow waves over the left central and temporal regions (T3, T5, C3) which are accompanied by positive deflections over the frontal leads (F3) indicating a tangential dipole

frequent and may generalize, so continuous treatment is most needed more often in this syndrome than it is in PS and BECTS. If instituted, therapy consists of medications proven to be effective in partial seizures, and may include carbamazepine or valproic acid. In general, carbamazepine is preferred in the USA, and valproic acid has greater use in Europe. Newer medications, including gabapentin, lamotrigine, and levetiracetam, may also be effective. For BECTS, sulthiame is particularly effective and can normalize the EEG, but may result in cognitive impairment.

Regardless of which medication is chosen, the goal is the same – for the patient to be free of both seizures and side effects. With careful administration of the right medication, this goal can usually be achieved. In general, most AEDs are started at a low dose and increased gradually. This allows for early detection of side effects. If side effects occur, the dose is lowered. If seizures return, the dose is raised. If neither is present, no dose change is required. Unfortunately, some patients will have continued seizures and side effects, in which case, a medication change is generally needed.

Of patients who have never received an AED, approximately 47% will become seizure free with the first medication given. If a second drug is needed, only 13% will respond. If a third drug is used, the response rate is only 4%. A high initial seizure frequency before treatment, slowing on the EEG, and a symptomatic etiology are risk factors for developing medically intractable epilepsy.

After a patient has failed multiple AEDs, non-medication therapies must be considered. There are three non-medication options that are commonly used: the ketogenic diet, vagal nerve stimulator, and epilepsy surgery. All involve a multidisciplinary approach and require a comprehensive epilepsy center for their implementation and management.

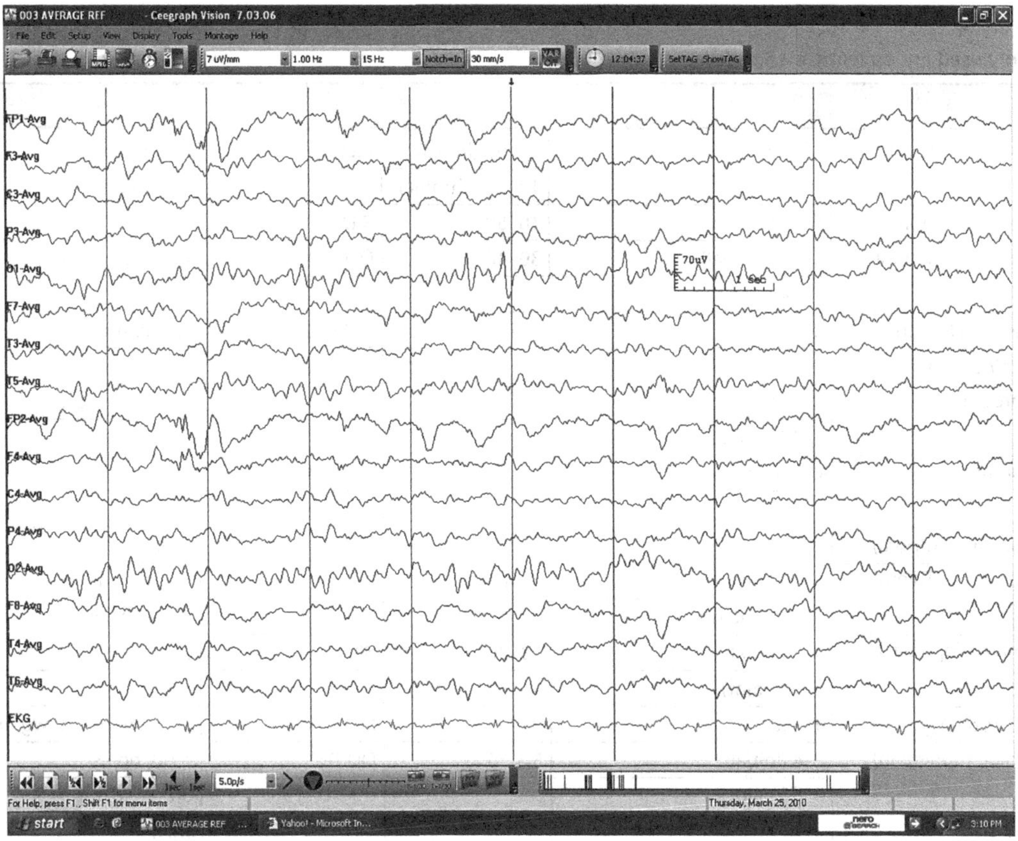

Figure 362.6

Nine-year-old boy with ICOE-G. His seizures cause him to wake from sleep with transient blindness followed by a headache. The EEG shows spike waves over the left occipital region (O1)

For status epilepticus, the ideal treatment acts rapidly, has long-lasting effects, produces little sedation, is easy to administer, safe, inexpensive, and can be pharmacologically reversed if needed. No single medication possesses all of these criteria, but the key requirements can usually be met.

In the largest prospective study on early treatment of SE, the Veterans Affairs Status Epilepticus Cooperative Study Group performed a randomized, double-blinded, multicenter trial using four i.v. treatments for status epilepticus: diazepam (0.15 mg/kg) followed by phenytoin (18 mg/kg), lorazepam (0.1 mg/kg), phenobarbital (15 mg/kg), and phenytoin (18 mg/kg). In patients with generalized convulsive status epilepticus, lorazepam had the best success rate, but this was statistically significant only when compared to phenytoin alone. No significant differences were observed among any of the four treatments with subtle SE. All of these trials lend support to intravenous lorazepam as initial therapy for SE.

An appropriate approach is to initiate therapy with lorazepam 0.1 mg/kg. If seizures persist, then phenytoin (20 mg/kg) or fosphenytoin (20 mg/kg phenytoin equivalents) should follow, with an additional 5–10 mg/kg of phenytoin/fosphenytoin if needed. In many cases, phenobarbital (20 mg/kg initially followed by an additional 5–10 mg/kg if needed) follows, with induction of anesthesia if the seizure persists beyond that. With the low success rate for subsequent drugs in the VA study, it is reasonable to consider moving on to definitive treatment with high-dose barbiturates, benzodiazepines, or propofol if SE remains refractory.

Prognosis

There are many ways to assess prognosis in patients with epilepsy. The most direct outcome measure is quantification of the seizures themselves. This includes an examination of seizure frequency, relapse rates following drug withdrawal, and the probability of outgrowing the condition. Assessment of comorbidities is also important, including developmental delays, intellectual impairment, and psychiatric disorders.

Table 362.4
Commonly used antiepileptic medications

Agent	Pediatric dose (mg/kg/day)	Half-life (h)[a]	Dosing schedule	Side effects
Carbamazepine (Tegretol)	10–35	25–65 (initial)	BID-QID	r, hep, bd, s,n
		12–17 (chronic)		dip, hypn, ost
Clonazepam(Klonopin)	0.01–0.2	18–50	BID-TID	s, a, h, b
Ethosuximide (Zarontin)	10–15 (initial)	30–40	QD-TID	gi, n, an, s, d, b
	15–40 (maint)			r, bd
Gabapentin (Neurontin)	30–60	5–7	TID-QID	s, d, a, ny, wg
Lamotrigine (Lamictal)				
Off valproate:	0.6 (initial)	7	BID	r, hep, d, a, s, n
	5–15 (maint)			
On valproate:	0.15 (initial)	45	QD-BID	
	1–5 (maint)			
Levetiracetam (Keppra)	20–60	6–8	BID	s, d, ha, b
Oxcarbazepine (Trileptal)	8–10 (initial)	8–10	BID	r, hep, s, diz, n
	20–50 (maint)			dip, a, ha, hyp
Topiramate (Topamax)	1–3 (initial)	18–30	BID	s, an, ks, ps, wl
	5–9 (maint)			
Valproic acid (Depakote)	15–60	9–20	BID-QID	hep, bd, n, s, d, wg, hl, r, gi
Zonisamide (Zonegran)	2–4 (initial)	50–70	QD-BID	r, bd, hep,s
	4–8 (maint)			diz, an, n, ha
				wl, ks

r rash, *hep* hepatotoxicity, *bd* blood dyscrasia, *n* nausea, *ny* nystagmus *dip* diplopia, *hypn* hyponatremia, *ost* osteomalacia, *s* sedation, *a* ataxia, *h* hyperactivity, *d* dizziness, *b* behavioral difficulties, *gi* gastrointestinal distress, *an* anorexia, *ha* headache, *ks* kidney stones, *ps* psychomotor slowing, *wg* weight gain, *hl* hair loss, *wl* weight loss, *maint* maintenance
[a]Half-life is based on monotherapy and assumes normal renal function.

Other measures of clinical significance are quality of life and mortality risk in epilepsy patients. Some childhood epilepsy syndromes are labeled as "benign." The use of this term refers to the prognosis of the seizures themselves, and not to the severity of associated conditions. For example, BECTS is often associated with motor or language delay. These features can have profound effects on patients, yet the condition is still labeled as "benign" since the seizures are characteristically outgrown.

Overall, the recurrence risk following a first unprovoked seizure in childhood ranges between 44% and 64%. The recurrence risk is highest in patients with an abnormal neurological examination, an abnormal electroencephalogram, or a remote-symptomatic etiology. In patients with only a single non-symptomatic seizure who have a normal examination and EEG, the risk of recurrent seizures is low (approximately 25%), and observation off of antiepileptic medications is generally favored. Should a second seizure occur, the recurrence risk jumps to approximately 79%. Thus, treatment is often started following a second seizure.

When seizures remain in remission on antiepileptic medications, the question of when to end treatment arises. Of patients who have been seizure free for over 2 years, 60–75% will remain seizure free when medication is withdrawn. A remote-symptomatic etiology and an abnormal EEG portend a higher relapse risk. Moreover, some epilepsy syndromes, such as juvenile myoclonic epilepsy, have a high relapse rate requiring a prolonged treatment course whereas others, such as BECTS, have no chance of relapse once outgrown. The ultimate decision of withdrawing antiepileptic medications is therefore dependent on individual patient factors. Overall, following 2 years of seizure remission on medication, roughly two-thirds of children will remain seizure free following discontinuation of their antiseizure treatment. If seizures are to recur, they will do so within 1 year in 60–80% of patients. Late recurrences (greater than 2 years after stopping AEDs) can develop, but are rare.

Table 362.5
Which medications for which seizure types?

Seizure type	First-line therapy	Second-line	Third-line
Partial (all types)	CBZ, OXC	LTG, VPA, GBP	TGB, ZNS, PB, LAC
		TPM, PHT, LEV	
Generalized			
Tonic-clonic	VPA, LEV	LTG, TPM, PHT	PB, ZNS
Myoclonic	VPA, LEV	LTG, CZP	PB, ZNS
Tonic	VPA, LEV	LTG	CZP, TPM, ZNS
Absence (Before age 10)	ESM[a]	VPA, LTG	ZNS, TPM
(After age 10)	VPA	LTG, LEV	ESM, TPM, ZNS
Epilepsy syndromes			
CAE	ESM	VPA, LTG, LEV	ZNS, TPM
JAE	VPA	LTG, LEV	ESM, TPM, ZNS
JME	VPA, LTG, LEV	TPM, ZNS	CZP, PHT
Lennox–Gastaut	VPA	LTG, TPM, LEV	CZP, ZNS, FBM, RUF
Infantile Spasms	ACTH, VGB	VPA, TPM, TGB, CZP	FBM, ZNS, LEV
BECTS	CBZ, GBP	VPA, PHT, CBZ, LEV	LTG, TPM

ACTH Adrenocorticotropic hormone, *CZP* clonazepam(Klonopin), *CBZ* carbamazepine(Tegretol), *GBP* gabapentin(Neurontin), *ESM* ethosuximide (Zarontin), *FBM* felbamate(Felbatol), *LEV* levetiracetam(Keppra), *LTG* lamotrigine(Lamictal), *OXC* oxcarbazepine(Trileptal), PB phenobarbital, *PHT* phenytoin(Dilantin), *TGB* tiagabine (Gabitril), *VGB* vigabatrin(Sabril), *ZNS* zonisamide(Zonegran), *RUF* rufinamide, *LAC* lacosamide, *CAE* childhood absence epilepsy, *JAE* Juvenile absence epilepsy, *JME* Juvenile Myoclonic Epilepsy, *BECTS* Benign Epilepsy of Childhood with Centrotemporal Spikes

[a]Assuming no convulsive seizures.

Overall, the prognosis for most epilepsy patients is favorable. Approximately two-thirds will achieve long-term remission of greater than 5 years, and nearly half of those will do so off of medications. Positive predictors for remission include a rapid response to therapy (greater than a 75% seizure reduction within 3 months), and idiopathic epilepsy. Remission is less likely in patients with an underlying structural cause or abnormal EEG. When followed into adulthood, children with epilepsy are at greater risk of school dropout and unemployment, and are less likely to be married or have children.

Prevention

Strategies for epilepsy prevention differ depending on the etiology. In genetic epilepsies, the only form of prevention currently available is family counseling. The recurrence risk can be as high as 50% for autosomal-dominant inheritance or less than 1% for spontaneous mutations involving only a single child within the family. Diagnostic confirmation through genetic testing now makes it possible to provide an accurate risk assessment prior to family planning. As genetic causes are better understood, treatment strategies directed at the mechanisms of disease may offer potential for averting epilepsy onset.

Symptomatic causes of epilepsy offer the greatest prospects for prevention. Since symptomatic causes generally develop following known brain injury, the possibility exists of either averting the injury or disrupting epileptogenesis following the insult. In children, neonatal causes of brain injury, such as hypoxic-ischemic encephalopathy and complications from prematurity, are major preventable etiologies. In adults, stroke is the most common identifiable etiology, and can be avoided through lifestyle modifications and management of hypertension and hypercholesterolemia.

In the third world, cysticercosis remains a major cause of epilepsy and is potentially eradicable. Since the only animal reservoirs are humans and pigs, breaking the life cycle of *Taenia solium* is possible. Strategies include concomitant treatment of both human and porcine populations. In pigs, treatment with oxfendazole is effective and confers protection for at least 3 months. Other strategies include immunization of pigs and improved meat inspection.

If the injury itself cannot be prevented, perhaps the mechanisms of epileptogenesis, which follow the injury, can be. Presently, no such interventions are known to exist, but many are theorized. One possibility is to initiate antiseizure medications immediately following injury, and prior to the development of seizures. Current data for head trauma suggests that, although prophylactic treatment may reduce early seizures, it does not prevent late seizures or reduce neurological disability. Similar conclusions are observed following brain tumors and strokes. Given those results, antiseizure medications are not routinely started prior to the development of seizures, but more research is needed in this area. A different approach is to use neuroprotective agents immediately following injury in an effort to prevent epilepsy and improve neurological outcome. To date, no such agents have demonstrated proven clinical efficacy in reducing injury or preventing epilepsy. Stem cell therapy also offers potential. In a rat model of pilocarpine-induced epilepsy, intravenous transplantation of bone marrow mononuclear cells prevented the development of chronic seizures and reduced neuronal loss. One challenge to bringing such therapies to clinical use is the increased time and cost of studying epileptogenesis as the primary outcome. Since it can take years for epilepsy to develop, the use of biomarkers for epileptogenesis may be the best solution to making such trials feasible.

References

Carpio A, Hauser A (2009) Epilepsy in the developing world. Curr Neurol Neurosci Rep 9:319–326

Chacon LM, Estupinan B, Pedre LL et al (2009) Microscopic mild focal cortical dysplasia in temporal lobe dual pathology: an electrocorticography study. Seizure 18:593–600

Commission on Classification and Terminology of the International League Against Epilepsy (1981) Proposal for revised clinical and electroencephalographic classification of epileptic seizures. Epilepsia 22:489–501

Commission on Classification and Terminology of the International League Against Epilepsy (1989) Proposal for revised classification of epilepsies and epileptic syndromes. Epilepsia 30:389–399

Hauser WA, Anderson VE, Lowenson RB et al (1982) Seizure recurrence after a first unprovoked seizure. N Engl J Med 307:522–528

Lowenstein DH, Bleck T, Macdonald RL (1999) It's time to revise the definition of status epilepticus. Epilepsia 40:120–124

Millichap JJ, Koh S, Laux LC, Nordli DR (2009) Dravet syndrome: when to suspect the diagnosis. Neurology 73:e59–e62

Mitchell LA, Jackson GD, Kalnins RM et al (1999) Anterior temporal abnormality in temporal lobe epilepsy: A quantitative MRI and histopathologic study. Neurology 52:327–336

National Institutes of Health Consensus Conference (1990) Surgery for epilepsy. JAMA 264:729–733

Panayiotopoulos CP, Michael M, Sanders S et al (2008) Benign childhood focal epilepsies: assessment of established and newly recognized syndromes. Brain 131:2264–2286

Seiffert E, Dreier JP, Ivens S et al (2004) Lasting blood–brain barrier disruption induces epileptic focus in the rat somatosensory cortex. J Neurosci 24:7829–7836

Shinnar S, Berg AT, Moshe SL et al (2004) Discontinuing antiepileptic drugs in children with epilepsy: a prospective study. Ann Neurol 35:534–545

Sillanpaa M, Jalava M, Kaleva O et al (1998) Long-term prognosis of seizures with onset in childhood. N Engl J Med 338:1715–1722

Treiman DM, Meyers PD, Walton NY et al (1998) A comparison of four treatments for generalized convulsive status epilepticus. Veterans Affairs Status Epilepticus Cooperative Study Group. N Engl J Med 339:792–798

363 Movement Disorders

Yasser Awaad

Movement disorders in childhood have received little attention, especially when compared with such conditions as epilepsy or neuromuscular disorders. The information on movement disorders in childhood is scattered in multiple neurological and pediatric journals. This chapter attempts to put together information from these various sources in a form accessible to clinically oriented pediatricians.

Only disorders of children and adolescents under 18 years of age are dealt with. The differences in movement disorders between children and adults are striking. The clinical manifestations of extrapyramidal disease are profoundly influenced by the age of onset. A good example is the difference between Huntington disease in adults and children. Moreover, a number of disease processes occur almost exclusively in the pediatric age, for example, transient disorders. So the prevalence of the various movement disorders in children, their clinical presentation, course, prognosis, and management differ considerably from those in adults.

Movement disorders are syndromes characterized by impaired voluntarily movement, presence of involuntary movements, or both. There may be targeting and velocity of intended movements, abnormal involuntary movements, abnormal postures, or excessive normal-appearing movements at inappropriate or unintended times. Movement disorders in children include athetosis, chorea, dystonia, myoclonus, Parkinsonism, stereotypies, tics, and tremor. Movement disorders may be accompanied by weakness, spasticity, hypotonia, ataxia, apraxia, and other motor deficits, although many authors do not include these accompanying deficits among the movement disorders.

Movement disorders have been divided into hyperkinetic disorders in which there is excessive movement, and hypokinetic disorders in which there is a paucity of movement. Hyperkinetic disorders consist of abnormal, repetitive involuntary movements and include most of childhood movement disorders such as chorea, dystonia, myoclonus, stereotypies, tics, and tremor. Hypokinetic disorders are primarily akinetic or rigid. The primary syndrome in this category is Parkinsonism, occurring mostly in adulthood as Parkinson disease or one of the many forms of secondary Parkinsonism. In children, hypokinetic disorders are much less common than hyperkinetic disorders.

Abnormalities of movement that are presumed to be due to central nervous system disorders are typically divided into two primary categories: pyramidal and extrapyramidal. Many authors consider only the extrapyramidal symptoms to be movement disorders. "Extrapyramidal diseases" is the oldest but has fallen into disuse because of its lack of precision. The term includes other systems of control of movement that are not usually termed extrapyramidal, for example, the cerebellum. Pyramidal symptoms typically involve weakness, specific patterns of weakness, or spasticity. Pyramidal symptoms are thought to be due to injury to the pyramidal tract, including the corticospinal tract, and therefore to represent, to some extent, the effect of a denervated spinal cord. Extrapyramidal disorders are often described as everything that is not a pyramidal disorder. In particular, the term usually includes disorders of movement that are not due to weakness.

"Disorders of the basal ganglia" is also inadequate as not all abnormal movements are the result of involvement of these structures, and, conversely, lesions of the basal ganglia can manifest with cognitive deficit rather than with movement disorders. For these reasons, the term "movement disorders" seemed least inadequate, as it is merely descriptive and does not imply any hypothesis regarding the anatomical location of defects.

Movement disorder terminology has been well defined for adults but less so for children. Therefore, it is likely that movement disorders are underreported in children and that there is inconsistent terminology. Recently there have been attempts to provide specific definitions of childhood hypertonic disorders, including dystonia and rigidity. The prevalence in children of different types of hypertonic disorders, as well as other movement disorders, is not well known, although there have been studies investigating this in certain populations. Consistent definitions of non-hypertonic disorders in childhood are not yet available.

In adult movement disorders, it is frequently helpful to divide disorders into primary and secondary disorders, although there is no consistent definition of these terms. Many authors refer to disorders as primary if there is only a single dominant symptom and the underlying cause is presumably genetic or is due to an identified gene; however, the existence of a single symptom in childhood movement disorders is probably the exception rather than the rule.

Abdelaziz Y. Elzouki (ed.), *Textbook of Clinical Pediatrics*, DOI 10.1007/978-3-642-02202-9_363,

Since Sydenham in 1686 identified the first disease characterized by a movement disorder, a long time has elapsed and, especially in the past 35 years, knowledge of the pathophysiology of abnormal movements has increased extraordinarily as a result of better understanding of neurotransmitter function, of modern neuroimaging techniques (especially MRI but also functional neuroimaging with MR spectroscopy, PET, and functional MR), and of the advent of molecular genetics. This last not only provides new bases for neurological classification, previously based exclusively on clinical/pathological data, but also raises the hope of prevention and possible cure of genetically determined movement disorders.

Although new disorders are being identified with such methods, progress in patient care has remained rather patchy, and much has to be done to improve the management of many movement disorders. Therapeutic difficulties are even greater where children are concerned. The consequences on learning and on the neurological and psychological development of children with chronic movement disorders are largely unknown. Even drug doses are often poorly established and extrapolated from adult practice, even though there are well-known differences in the handling of pharmacological agents between children and adults.

Movement disorders in children differ from those in adults in several important aspects. Perhaps the most important is that movement disorders in childhood are primarily symptoms of other diseases, rather than diseases by themselves. In adults, dystonia and Parkinsonism are usually due to primary dystonia or idiopathic Parkinson's disease, respectively. However, dystonia or Parkinsonism in children is more likely to be a feature of underlying static or progressive neurologic disorder. Diagnosis in children is complicated by the fact that many symptoms have more than one cause, and any particular underlying pathophysiology may lead to complex combinations of symptoms. The diagnostic evaluation in children is guided by symptoms, but the existence of a large class of diseases that can lead to the same set of symptoms often necessitates a broad etiologic evaluation. There may be specific etiologic treatments and symptomatic treatments, both of which may be beneficial in an individual child. In particular, many of the causes of childhood movement disorders do not yet have any specific treatment, yet symptomatic treatment for the resulting movement disorder can be extremely helpful and lead to improvement in quality of life.

Another distinction between movement disorders in adults and children is that many adult neurologic disorders can be attributed to anatomically localized injury, but childhood disorder frequently results from a global or multifocal injury that may affect particular cell types, receptor types, or metabolic pathways. Therefore in children, the injury is open sparse but global, with manifestations across multiple areas of function, including sensorimotor and cognitive functions.

The clinical manifestations of movement disorders will depend on the child's developmental stage. The same illness may present differently depending on the age at onset of symptoms. Detection of a progressive disorder may be complicated by superimposition of a progressive disorder on the natural improvement of function that is expected throughout childhood. Therefore, a child with a progressive movement disorder may continue to develop new skills despite falling further and further behind in age-appropriate behavior. The presence of a movement disorder may affect the current and continuing development of the child's normal motor and cognitive abilities. Therefore, an acute illness may have developmental consequences that outlast the duration of the injury itself.

Classification of the movement disorder based on temporal pattern is essential for diagnosis. It is also important to define the context in which the movements occur. Although it is often helpful to list the characteristics of the movements, the diagnosis relies on pattern recognition, and the clinician must see the movements. If the movements are not apparent during the neurologic examination, repeating the examination at another time or obtaining video recordings of the movements is essential. The widespread availability of video cameras has substantially improved diagnosis of movement disorders.

When approaching a patient with a movement disorder, it is helpful to determine the answers to some key questions:

1. Is the number of movements excessive (hyperkinetic) or diminished (hypokinetic)?
2. If hyperkinetic, do the individual movements appear normal or abnormal?
3. Is the movement paroxysmal (sudden onset and offset), continual (repeated again and again), or continuous (without stop)?
4. What is the developmental stage of the child, and has the development been normal?
5. How does voluntary movement affect the movement disorder? Are the symptoms and signs present at rest (body part supported against gravity), with maintained posture, with action, with approach to a target (intention), or a combination?
6. Has the movement disorder changed over time?
7. Do environmental stimuli or emotional states precipitate, exacerbate, or alleviate the movement disorder?
8. Is the patient aware of the movements?

9. Can the movements be suppressed voluntarily?
10. Are the movements heralded by a premonitory sensation or urge? (It may be helpful to ask the patient, "Why do you do that?")
11. Does the movement disorder abate with sleep?
12. Are there other findings on the examination suggestive of focal neurologic deficit or systemic disease?
13. Is there a family history of a similar or related condition?

Laboratory tests, imaging, and other diagnostic testing should be based on the specific movement disorder. There is no universal "movement disorder workup" because the causes are varied and some movement disorders (e.g., tics) are rarely symptomatic of an underlying disease (➲ *Table 363.1*).

Movement disorders may be difficult to characterize unless other symptoms and behavioral context are taken into account. Chorea can resemble myoclonus. Dystonia can resemble spasticity. Paroxysmal movement disorders such as dystonia and tics may resemble seizure. Movements in some contexts may be normal and in others may indicate underlying pathology. For example, frequent eye blinking can be perfectly normal and appropriate in one setting, but excessive in another (tics). Movements that raise concern about a degenerative disorder in older children (progressive myoclonus) may be completely normal in an infant (benign neonatal myoclonus). Thus, it is important to view the movement disorder in the context of a complete history and neurologic examination.

Table 363.1
Phenomenologic classification of movement disorders

Movement disorder	Brief description
Athetosis	Slow, continuous writing movements of distal body parts, especially the fingers and hands
Chorea, ballism	Chaotic, random, repetitive, brief, purposeless movements. Rapid but not as rapid as myoclonus. When very large amplitude affecting proximal joints, choreic limb movements are often called *ballism*
Dystonia	Repetitive, sustained, abnormal postures typically have a twisting quality
Myoclonus	Sudden, brief, shock-like movements that may be repetitive or rhythmic
Parkinsonism	Hypokinetic syndrome characterized by a combination of reset tremor, slow movement (bradykinesia), rigidity, and postural instability
Stereotypy	Patterned, episodic, repetitive, purposeless, rhythmic movements
Tics	Stereotyped intermittent, sudden, discrete, repetitive, nonrhythmic movements, most frequently involving head and upper body
Tremor	Rhythmic oscillation around a central point or position involving any one body part or more than one

The etiology of movement disorders in children is extensive and is discussed further below. The most common cause of secondary disorders is likely to be cerebral palsy, with a prevalence of 2 per 1,000. However, cerebral palsy itself represents a constellation of both injuries and symptoms (Surveillance of Cerebral Palsy in Europe, 2002). Cerebral palsy can be associated with almost all forms of childhood movement disorders, and despite the lack of an ongoing destructive process, the clinical picture may change during the development. The diagnosis and management of cerebral palsy is complex.

Specific types of movement disorders may represent injury to particular localized regions of the central nervous system. Ataxia most likely results from injury to the cerebellum or its inflow and outflow. Bradykinesia most likely occurs with injury to the substantia nigra or striatum of the basal ganglia leading to either presynaptic or postsynaptic failure of dopaminergic transmission. Chorea occurs in severe cortical injury or basal ganglia injury, particularly if the subthalamic nucleus is involved. Dystonia most likely involves injury to basal ganglia, but the possibility of cortical or cerebellar abnormalities cannot be excluded as contributors. Myoclonus most likely involves cortical, brainstem, or spinal injury to gray matter. The localization of tremor depends on the type, but some forms of tremor involve cerebellum or brainstem circuits. Tic disorders probably involve an abnormality of the basal ganglia, but cortical mechanisms may also contribute.

Treatment of childhood movement disorders is based primarily on symptomatology independent of the underlying cause. When a specific treatment for the underlying cause is available, certainly this should be applied, but in many cases such treatment is only partly effective. The goal of symptomatic treatment is to break the connection between the pathophysiology and the expression of clinical impairment.

It is essential to ask both the child and the parents for the most significant cause of disability. In some children, the impairment that is most evident to the clinician is not the primary cause of disability. Sometimes treatment of a disability is more effective, less time-consuming, and less risky than attempts to treat the underlying pathophysiology, and therefore it is essential to be certain that any treatment addresses the needs and goals of the child and family. In particular, it is usually neither necessary nor possible to treat all symptoms. It is most helpful to pick specific goals and to monitor progress toward those goals. In many cases, a team approach has been found to be helpful, particularly when there are multiple impairments leading to disability, and the team approach allows appropriate focusing and selection of interventions. In some individuals, a supportive environment and adaptive equipment are more effective than any medical intervention.

TIC Disorders and Tourette Syndrome

Tic disorders and related conditions are among the most common clinical conditions encountered by pediatric neurologists. The evaluation and management of these conditions is usually fairly straightforward and may follow predictable, relatively simple paradigms. On the other hand, more complex cases require considerable effort, numerous treatment strategies, and intensive management of patients and families. Gilles de la Tourette syndrome (TS) is a chronic neuropsychiatric disorder characterized by the presence of involuntary motor and phonic tics that wax and wane. Once considered a rare disorder, the prevalence of TS is estimated to be up to 1% of children and adolescents. In his late nineteenth-century description, Georges Gilles de la Tourette suggested a familial pattern and a psychogenic origin. Since then, there is further evidence for a genetic inheritance pattern, but accumulating data support a neurobiological disorder than emotional basis. In addition, those children with TS often suffer from a variety of concomitant psychopathologies, including obsessive–compulsive disorder, attention-deficit hyperactivity disorder, mood disorders, episodic outbursts, learning difficulties, sleep abnormalities, and other behavioral problems. Although the presence of neurobehavioral problems is not required for the diagnosis of TS, they are very common, and their clinical impact on the affected patient is often more significant than the impact of the tics themselves. The physician caring for a child with tics and complex psychopathologies must be able to recognize the various problems, understand their individual complexities, and develop an appropriate treatment plan.

Dystonia

Description

Dystonia is defined as a movement disorder in which involuntary sustained or intermittent muscle contractions cause twisting and repetitive movements, abnormal postures, or both.

Dystonia usually occurs only during voluntary movement or with voluntary maintenance of a posture of the limbs or body. For example, flexion of the fingers to hold a pen may lead to flexion of additional fingers, extension of the wrist, or movements of the opposite hand or the neck.

There is often no abnormal muscle tone in children with dystonia. A dystonic limb may or may not have increased resistance to movement, it may be either stiff or floppy, or change with time.

Focal dystonia is described if only one body part is involved, such as a hand, foot, or the neck. On the other hand, if two contiguous parts are involved, such as the face and neck, then it is termed a "segmental dystonia." If two noncontiguous parts of the body are involved, such as the face and one leg, it is termed a "multifocal dystonia." Hemidystonia involves one half of the body. If both legs, as well as one additional body part are involved, then it is termed "generalized dystonia." A focal dystonia that progresses to become generalized or generalized dystonia itself are the most common patterns observed in children.

Dystonia may occur at rest or with action and it may be triggered by the movement of other body parties. Task-specific dystonia occurs only rarely in children.

Primary dystonia includes the genetic dystonias, and some adult onset, focal dystonias, is not due to another disease. When dystonia is due to another identified disease, then it is called "secondary dystonia." Secondary dystonia is due to different causes, for example, cerebral palsy, metabolic disease, or head trauma.

The mechanism of dystonia is understood. Studies in humans and animals have not been able to find a good explanation that can relate particular injuries to the emergence of dystonic symptoms. Dystonia is frequently associated with injury to the basal ganglia, in particular the sensory-motor regions of the putamen. In children, dystonia may also occur with decreased dopamine as occurs in dopa-responsive dystonia (DRD). Low dopamine level can cause many childhood dystonias. Acute dystonic reactions in children and adults are caused by medications that selectively block the dopamine receptors in the indirect pathway. These reactions are treated with anticholinergic medications that may increase the effectiveness of dopamine in both the direct and indirect pathways (➲ *Tables 363.2* and ➲ *363.3*).

Examination

The child must be observed at rest, during the action of the parts of the body affected by dystonia, as well as actions unrelated to the dystonia. For example, a child with foot dystonia must be observed while sitting, standing, walking, and performing tasks with the hands. Mental distraction is helpful to elicit the dystonia. Distractions may help to determine the specific triggers for the dystonic movements and also assist in evaluating if other body parts are subtly affected. It is important to test the child during certain activities (reaching movements of the arms, speaking, and tongue movement).

When dystonia is present at rest, it is important to examine children when they are as relaxed as possible. Any stress or discomfort may worsen the symptoms.

Muscle tone is not usually increased in children with dystonia; it might be increased and there will be difficulty in differentiating dystonia from spasticity or rigidity. This will be difficult when dystonia and spasticity are simultaneously present (e.g., cerebral palsy). It is equally important to examine for other movement disorders, such as ataxia or myoclonus, which might lead to a specific diagnosis.

Dystonia is usually not present during sleep. Stiffness of the limbs during sleep suggests possible spasticity or fixed joint contractures. Dopa-responsive dystonia may improve

Table 363.2
Etiologic classification of dystonia

Primary: Dystonia is the only neurological sign and evaluation does not reveal an identifiable exogenous cause or other inherited or degenerative disease	*Secondary*: Variety of lesions, mostly involving the basal ganglia and/or dopamine synthesis
Childhood- and adolescent-onset	*Inherited non-degenerative (dystonia plus)*
• DYT1: Autosomal-dominant with reduced penetrance (approx. 30%), early limb-onset with predominant family phenotype	• Dopa-responsive dystonia (DRD): due to DYT5 and other genetic defects
• Other genes to be identified	• Myoclonus-dystonia: due to DYT11 and possibly other genetic defects
	• Rapid-onset dystonia-Parkinsonism due to DYT12
Adult onset	*Inherited degenerative*
• DYT7: Autosomal-dominant, cervical onset in adult life	Autosomal-dominant, autosomal-recessive, X-linked (DYT3), mitochondrial
• Other genes to be identified	
Mixed phenotype	*Degenerative disorders of unknown etiology*
• DYT6, DYT13: Autosomal-dominant, early- and late-onset, with possible cranial, cervical, and sometimes limb-onset and variable spread	• Parkinson's disease
• Other genes to be identified	• Progressive supranuclear palsy
	• Corticobasal ganglionic degeneration
	Acquired
	• Drugs (dopamine receptor blockers), other toxins
	• Head trauma
	• Stroke, hypoxia
	• Encephalitis, infectious, and post-infectious
	• Tumors
	• Peripheral injuries
	Other movement disorders with dystonic phenomenology
	• Tics, paroxysmal dyskinesias (DYT8, 9, 10)
	Psychogenic dystonia

Table 363.3
Classification of genetic loci associated with dystonia

Gene	Location	Inheritance	Phenotype	Gene Product
DYT1	9q34	AD	Early limb-onset PTD	Torsin A
DYT2	Not mapped	AR	Early onset	
DYT3	Xq13.1	XR	Lubag dystonia/Parkinsonism	Not identified
DYT4	Not mapped	AD	Whispering dysphonia	
DYT5	14q22.1	AD	DRD/Parkinsonism	GCHI
DYT6	8p21-p22	AD	"Mixed" cranial/cervical/limb-onset	Not identified
DYT7	18p	AD	Adult cervical	Not identified
DYT8	2q33-25	AD	PDC/PNKD	Not identified
DYT9	lp21	AD	Episodic choreoathetosis/ataxia with spasticity	Not identified
DYT10	16	AD	PKC/PKD (EKDI & 2)	Not identified
DYT11	7q21	AD	Myoclonus-dystonia	Epsilon-sarcoglycan
DYT12	19q	AD	Rapid-onset dystonia-Parkinsonism	Not identified
DYT13	lp36	AD	Cervical/cranial/brachial	Not identified
DYT14	14q13	AD	DRD	Not identified

Abbreviations: *AD* autosomal-dominant, *AR* autosomal-recessive, *XR* X-linked recessive, *PTD* primary torsion dystonia, *DRD* DOPA-responsive dystonia, *PDC* paroxysmal dystonic non-kinesigenic choreoathetosis, *PNKD* paroxysmal non-kinesigenic dystonia, *PKC* paroxysmal kinesigenic choreoathetosis, *PKD* paroxysmal kinesigenic dyskinesia, *GHC*1 GTP Cyclohydrolase 1

upon awakening in the morning or after a nap; but the symptoms worsen throughout the day. Other forms of dystonia may be worse upon morning awakening.

Dystonia has several genetic causes with autosomal-dominant inheritance. Therefore, a thorough family history of dystonia or other neurological diseases is very important. The onset of dystonia is important, but dystonia may start many years after the causative event. Toxin exposure and medications use (neuroleptics and psychiatric medications) must be investigated. Such medicines may cause dystonia even after they have been stopped. Autosomal-dominant inheritance is caused by too many different genes. The most common genes are DYT1 (9q34, encodes torsinA) and DYT5 (14q22.1-2, encodes GTP cyclohydrolase I, causing Dopa-responsive dystonia or Segawa's disease). DYT2 can cause an autosomal-recessive trait. DYT3 causes an X-linked dystonia-Parkinsonism syndrome of Lubag (Xq13). The familial rapid-onset dystonia-Parkinsonism is linked to chromosome 19.

Structural lesions like cerebral palsy, kernicterus, hypoxic injury, head trauma, encephalitis, tumors, basal ganglia stroke, Moyamoya disease, and congenital malformations can cause dystonia.

Different neurodegenerative diseases can cause dystonias like Fahr's disease (or basal ganglia calcification), pantothenate-kinase associated neurodegenerative disease (PKAN, formerly neurodegeneration with brain iron accumulation type I, formerly Hallervorden–Spatz disease, PANK2 gene at 20p12.3-p13), Huntington's disease (Westphal variant, IT15-4p16.3), spinocerebellar ataxias (SCAs), neuronal ceroid lipofuscinosis, Rett syndrome, Tay–Sachs disease, Sandhoff's disease, Niemann–Pick type C, metachromatic leukodystrophy, striatal necrosis, Leigh's disease, neuroacanthocytosis, vitamin E deficiency, HARP syndrome (hypoprebetalipoproteinemia, acanthocytosis, retinitis pigmentosa, and pallidal degeneration), Pelizaeus–Merzbacher disease, and ataxia telangiectasia (AT).

Other chemical and metabolic disorders like glutaric aciduria, acyl-CoA dehydrogenase deficiency dopa-responsive dystonia or DRD (biopterin metabolic defect DYT5 or tyrosine hydroxylase deficiency), dopamine agonist-responsive dystonia (or ALAD: aromatic L-amino acid decarboxylase deficiency), mitochondrial disorders, Wilson's disease, homocystinuria, GM1 gangliosidosis, metachromatic leukodystrophy, Lesch–Nyhan disease, methylmalonic aciduria, and tyrosinemia could lead to dystonia.

Different drugs and toxins can induce dystonia, for example, neuroleptic and antiemetic medications (haloperidol, Thorazine, olanzapine, risperidone, quetiapine, promethazine, prochlorperazine, etc.), calcium channel blockers, stimulants (amphetamine, cocaine, ergot alkaloids, etc.), anticonvulsants (carbamazepine, phenytoin, etc.), thallium, manganese, carbon monoxide, ethylene glycol, cyanide, methanol, and wasp sting. Drug- or toxin-induced dystonia may occur while taking the drug or months after stopping the drug. Other paroxysmal disorders could induce dystonia, paroxysmal kinesogenic choreoathetosis (PKC), paroxysmal non-kinesogenic choreoathetosis (PNKC), familial periodic paralysis, exercise-induced dystonia, complex migraine, alternating hemiplegia, and paroxysmal torticollis of infancy.

There are some disorders that misdiagnosed as dystonia, like tonic seizures (including paroxysmal nocturnal dystonia caused by nocturnal frontal lobe seizures); syringomyelia; Arnold–Chiari malformation type II; atlantoaxial subluxation; posterior fossa mass; cervical spine malformation (including Klippel–Feil anomaly); ocular skew deviation with vertical double vision causing neck twisting, juvenile rheumatoid arthritis; Sandifer's syndrome (gastrointestinal disorder associated with hiatus hernia in infants); spasmus nutans; tics; self-stimulation; spasticity; myotonia; rigidity; stiff-person syndrome; Isaac's syndrome; startle disease (hyperexplexia); neuroleptic malignant syndrome; and psychogenic disorders.

The investigation of dystonia depends on the specific type of dystonia. In hemidystonia MRI will show a localized injury to the brain, often at or before birth.

In many cases, dystonia will start before early adulthood without obvious cause, and then become progressively worse. In these cases, there may be a genetic mutation in the *DYT1* gene. The child should be tested for the presence of this gene, particularly if symptoms began in the foot and progressed to other areas of the body.

Metabolic causes for dystonia are treatable and should be excluded. Dopa-responsive dystonia (DRD) is a rare disorder of the enzyme pathway responsible for synthesizing dopamine. DRD is tested by measuring chemicals in the CSF and in the blood, following an oral dose of phenylalanine (known as the phenylalanine loading test).

Metabolic disorders, such as Wilson's disease, amino acid or organic acid disorders, and lysosomal storage diseases may be tested for in certain children. An MRI is helpful during the workup for many metabolic diseases.

Treatment

It is recommended that any child with unexplained dystonia should receive a trial of L-dopa therapy (➋ *Table 363.4*). If the child does have DRD, the response is often dramatic and further testing may be arranged. L-dopa may also be helpful in some children with dystonia due to cerebral palsy, or perhaps in other metabolic disorders or structural abnormalities.

Table 363.4
Treatment Options for Dystonia

Oral Medication
1. L-dopa therapy
2. Trihexyphenidyl (Artane®)
3. Diazepam (Valium®)
4. Clonazepam (Klonopin®)
5. Valproate (Depakote®)
6. Baclofen
7. Carbamazepine (Tegretol®)
8. Reserpine or tetrabenazine (Nitoman®, not available in the USA)
Choice of the best regimen is usually by trial and error. It is difficult to predict which medicine will be most effective for a particular child
Botulinum toxin injections
For focal dystonias
Deep brain stimulation (DBS)
Particularly in children who have a mutation in the *DYT1* gene
Intrathecal baclofen pump (ITB therapy)
A very promising treatment
Other surgical procedures
1. Tendons lengthening or cutting muscles
2. Dorsal rhizotomy

Trihexyphenidyl (Artane®) is the most commonly used medication for children with dystonia. Sometimes requires very high doses of 50 mg or 100 mg per day, or even more in some children. Slow titration will help to tolerate the medicine with relatively few side effects. Other medicines that have used include diazepam (Valium®), clonazepam (Klonopin®), valproate (Depakote®), baclofen, carbamazepine (Tegretol®), reserpine, or tetrabenazine (Nitoman®, not available in the USA). Choice of the best regimen is usually by trial and error. It is difficult to predict which medicine will be most effective for a particular child.

Focal dystonias can be treated with botulinum toxin injections into those specific muscles. The goal of the injections is to reduce the symptoms of dystonia, without causing significant muscle weakness. Toxin injections usually need to be repeated every 3–6 months.

Deep brain stimulation (DBS) has been used to improve dystonia particularly in children who have a mutation in the *DYT1* gene. Implantation of the stimulator electrode in the globus pallidus led to gradual resolution of symptoms over 2–12 months.

Intrathecal baclofen pump (ITB therapy) is a very promising treatment. Although originally developed as a treatment for spasticity, recent results suggest that there may be benefit in dystonia as well.

Other surgical procedures like tendons lengthening or cutting muscles help to reduce the effect of the dystonic muscles. Dorsal rhizotomy, cutting the sensory nerves from muscles where they enter the spine is helpful; however, this procedure is more likely to improve spasticity, rather than dystonia.

Dopa-Responsive Dystonia

Other names for dopa-responsive dystonia *(DYTS)* include *dystonia-Parkinsonism syndrome*, *dystonia with diurnal variation*, and *Segawa disease*. The cause of the syndrome is either of two different genetic abnormalities. The inheritance of one type is as an autosomal-dominant trait and the other is as an autosomal-recessive trait. The dominant type is due to mutations in the gene for guanosine triphosphate cyclohydrolase 1, the cofactor for tyrosine hydroxylase, and the recessive form is due to mutations in the tyrosine hydroxylase gene. Most reported cases of "juvenile Parkinsonism" are probably variants of dopa-responsive dystonia.

Clinical Features

Marked variation in expressivity occurs between affected members of the same kindred and even between monozygotic twins. Age at onset is usually between 4 and 8 years but ranges from infancy to 12 years. Incorrect diagnosis of early onset cases is common; cerebral palsy is the common misdiagnosis. The initial feature is nearly always a gait disturbance caused by leg dystonia. Flexion at the hip and knee and plantar flexion of the foot cause toe walking. Flexor and extensor posturing of the arms develop. Finally, Parkinsonian features, such as cogwheel rigidity, masklike faces, and bradykinesia, appear. The disease reaches a plateau in adolescence. Postural or intention tremor occurs in almost half of patients, but typical Parkinsonian tremor is unusual.

Diurnal fluctuation in symptoms occurs in more than half of patients. Symptoms improve considerably on awakening and worsen later in the day. Movement and exercise exacerbate dystonia in some patients. Other disorders with exercise-induced dystonia as the main or only clinical feature may be expressions of the same genetic error.

Diagnosis

Dopa-responsive dystonia may be difficult to differentiate from other genetic disorders with dystonia because of phenotypic variation among family members. Diagnosis by mutation analysis is available. Important clues to diagnosis are features of Parkinsonism without other neurological signs, diurnal variation in severity of symptoms, exacerbation of symptoms with exercise, and response to levodopa.

Management

A small dose of levodopa usually provides immediate and complete relief in most patients, even when initiating treatment long after symptoms begin. No other dystonia responds so well. Initiate carbidopa-levodopa therapy at the lowest possible dose, and slowly increase the dose until a response is established. Long-term therapy is beneficial and required; symptoms return after discontinuing the drug. Trihexyphenidyl, in doses lower than ordinarily needed to treat also idiopathic torsion dystonia, and bromocriptine are partially effective.

Chorea

Chorea is a hyperkinetic movement disorder characterized by frequent, brief, and purposeless movements that tend to flow from one body part to another body part in an unpredictable manner. The affected child often appears fidgety or restless and unable to sit still. The word "chorea" comes from the Greek word for dance. The jerky movements of the feet or hands are often similar to dancing or piano playing. Chorea and ballismus are a spectrum sharing the same differential diagnosis. When chorea is severe, the movements may cause flailing motions of the arms or legs that results in throwing whatever is in the hand or falling to the ground. This form of severe chorea is referred to as "ballism." Akathisia can appear as chorea, but it is the result of a sense of a need to move, whereas chorea refers to involuntary movements. Choreaic movements can be sudden and jerky or can be more continuous and flow-in. Choreiform is often used to describe the benign piano-playing movements seen in normal young children when arms are extended during the neurologic exam. When chorea is the primary manifestation, a substantial differential diagnosis can be obtained. Athetosis is a slower writhing and twisting movement. Choreoathetosis is a movement of intermediate speed, between the quick, flitting movements of chorea and the slower, writhing movements of athetosis. Choreoathetosis is the most common form in children. Choreoathetosis tends to worsen with attempts at movement and often occurs only while the child is attempting to move. Chorea may affect the hands, feet, trunk, neck, and face. In the face, they often lead to nose wrinkling, continual flitting eye movements, and mouth or tongue movements. These disorders may be distinguished from tics, as tics tend to repeat the same set of movements. In addition, the child often describes a "buildup" in the need to make the tic, with a sense of release afterward. There is no such sense of release following chorea; the movements are continually changing and flowing from one body part to another.

Etiologies

Chorea can be classified into primary (inherited) and secondary (acquired) disorders. Primary causes include essential chorea and benign familial (hereditary) chorea. Autosomal-dominant, recessive, and X-linked inheritances have been described. Huntington's disease is the most famous inherited cause of chorea; the autosomal-dominant transmission of a triplet repeat (CAG) at the Huntington site on chromosome 4. Huntington's disease rarely presents in childhood with chorea. Juvenile-onset Huntington's disease (also known as the Westphal variant) is characterized by Parkinsonism (bradykinesia and rigidity) and dystonia. The number of CAG triplet repeats predicts the onset of Huntington's disease. The normal repeat number is <35. When the number is >70, onset of symptoms occurs at less than 18 years of age. The majority of chorea in childhood is secondary or acquired. Many causes of secondary chorea have been identified, but for most patients chorea is not the only sign or symptom. The most common cause of chorea in childhood is acute rheumatic fever (ARF). Other causes include metabolic disorder (hypo- or hypernatremia, hypocalcemia, hyperthyroid, pregnancy, or hypo- or hyperglycemia), perinatal brain injury (cerebral palsy), infectious or peri- or post-infectious disease (acute disseminated encephalomyelitis, viral encephalitis, and celiac disease), other autoimmune disease (systemic lupus erythematosus [SLE] or antiphospholipid antibody [APLA] syndrome), vascular disorders (Moyamoya syndrome, or basal ganglia stroke), toxins (methanol, carbon monoxide, manganese), other heredodegenerative disorders (Wilson's disease, ataxia telangiectasia, Niemann–Pick type C disease, Friedreich's ataxia, Machado–Joseph disease, gangliosidoses, other lysosomal storage diseases), and disorders of intermediary metabolism (glutaricaciduria, Lesch–Nyhan syndrome). Chorea can be the manifestation of conversion. It is very important to note that because behavioral changes are often observed as part of rheumatic chorea, one must avoid misconstruing the chorea of Sydenham's chorea as psychogenic. Common iatrogenic causes of chorea or exacerbations of extant chorea include dopamimetics, antiepileptics (e.g., phenytoin), antidepressants (e.g., selective serotonin reuptake inhibitors), methylphenidate (and other stimulants), antihistamines, anticholinergics, calcium channel blockers, digoxin, and oral estrogens.

Diagnostic Evaluation

A diagnostic test for treatable causes includes: throat culture with rapid group A ®-hemolytic streptococcal (GABHS) testing, serum antistreptolysin O and antideooxyrobonuclease (AntiDNase) B titers, electrocardiogram, echocardiogram, thyroid function tests, complete blood count (for acanthocytes), antinuclear antibody test, erythrocyte sedimentation rate, electrolytes (i.e., sodium, potassium, chloride, bicarbonate), magnesium, calcium, serum ceruloplasmin, APLAs (including lupus anticoagulant, anticardiolipin, and anti-®2 glycoprotein 1), urine drug screen, and urine pregnancy test, uric acid, quantitative immunoglobulin (ataxia telangiectasia), α-fetoprotein, serum amino acid, urine organic acid, and arterial (or cerebrospinal fluid) lactate and pyruvate testing, Epstein–Barr virus titers, Lyme disease titers, human immunodeficiency virus, serum calcium, and genetic testing for Friedreich's ataxia, spinocerebellar ataxia type 3 (Machado–Joseph disease), and possibly dentatorubropallidoluysian atrophy (DRPLA). Brain magnetic resonance imaging (MRI) with and without contrast is recommended in order to look for structural abnormalities, such as those related to a tumor, stroke, metabolic or degenerative disorders, or a previous injury due to low oxygen.

Sydenham's (Rheumatic) Chorea

Chorea is one of the major Jones criteria for the diagnosis of ARF. The revised Jones criteria indicate the presence of chorea without any other criteria is sufficient to make the diagnosis of ARF. The development of ARF after a GABHS infection is thought to occur in only 1–2% of those infected. Only a fraction of those patients with ARF will develop Sydenham's chorea. Sydenham's chorea is most common in children aged 5–15 years old. There is enough evidence that suggests individuals who develop ARF have a genetic susceptibility. There is a roughly 2:1 female predominance after age 10. Typically, the clinical manifestations of Sydenham's chorea begin several weeks to several months after a GABHS infection

The onset is insidious, with gradually progressive clumsiness and behavior and personality change, usually with emotional labiality, aggression, impulsivity, and obsessive–compulsive behaviors. The emotional labiality and personality change presents the most salient morbidity. The typical natural history of Sydenham's chorea is weeks to months of a waxing and waning course, with ultimate resolution of the chorea. Some individuals have behavioral changes that persist for months. Relapse of chorea can occur with or without subsequent GABHS infection. Therefore, it can be very difficult to distinguish between recurrences and relapse. There is a recognized increased risk of relapse associated with pregnancy (chorea gravidarum), oral contraceptives, and probably with intercurrent infection other than GABHS. Ten to twenty percent of patients, and perhaps as many as 50%, have a relapsing course. Recurrence and relapse provoke consideration of whether prophylactic penicillin is effective and whether follow-up investigations of cardiac function are needed. An additional confounding factor is that pharyngeal carriage of GABHS is common and is not necessarily eradicated by antibiotic prophylaxis. Therefore, surveillance testing for GABHS may produce false-positives. Certainly, signs, such as new murmur or abnormal rhythm, and symptoms, such as fatigue, palpitations, and shortness of breath, demand cardiac reassessment.

The diagnosis of Sydenham's chorea is made on the basis of clinical history and can be supported by laboratory data. However, laboratory data should be viewed as ancillary, not confirmatory. Most children with Sydenham's chorea have positive serology (antistreptolysin O and AntiDNase B antibodies) for GABHS, but over 25% are serologically negative. Most children with Sydenham's chorea have negative throat cultures for GABHS. MRI scans occasionally show signal abnormalities in the basal ganglia, but a clear clinical-radiographic linkage has not been seen. Therefore, structural imaging is neither diagnostically sensitive nor specific for Sydenham's chorea. Presence of carditis or valvitis or other manifestations of ARF supports the diagnosis of Sydenham's chorea. Every child thought to have Sydenham's chorea should be evaluated for rheumatic heart disease. Cerebrospinal fluid parameters in Sydenham's chorea have not been well studied. ARF remains a quintessential example of post-infectious or peri-infectious autoimmune disease. Although anti-brain antibodies have been recognized in a proportion of Sydenham's chorea patients for 30 years, the nature of the pathogenic mechanism has only recently been elucidated. Specifically, sera from patients with active Sydenham's chorea contain antibodies directed at brain lysoganglioside and GABHS glucosamine. Thus, there appears to be a direct effect of antibody on neuronal cell signaling, perhaps leading to inappropriate release of striatal dopamine.

SLE and APLA Syndrome

Chorea is an uncommon sign of SLE. When it is the only sign of SLE, it remains so for years. Less than 10% of children will have chorea, 50% are younger than 16 years of age. Usually it will have a poor prognosis. Chorea of SLE is clinically identical to that seen in ARF. Treatment of the underlying SLE is indicated. Chorea in SLE may be iatrogenic (drug-induced). Haloperidol may be effective for SLE chorea, but the other treatments for Sydenham's chorea may also be effective. The chorea of APLA syndrome is indistinguishable from that of SLE. Autoimmune mechanisms for chorea should include investigations for (antiphospholipid antibodies lupus anticoagulant, anticardiolipin, and anti-®2 glycoprotein 1), even if recurrent venous or arterial thrombosis have not occurred.

Chorea Associated with Viral Encephalitis

Post- or peri-infectious chorea is common and is very difficult to treat. There might be an MRI signal abnormalities in deep gray matter brain structures, such as basal ganglia and thalamus, as part of an aseptic meningitis or meningoencephalitis as well as in acute disseminated encephalomyelitis.

Wilson's Disease

Wilson's disease (hepatolenticular degeneration) is rare, but it has to be ruled out because it is treatable. It is an autosomal-recessive disease on chromosome 13, resulting in deficient ceruloplasmin; it leads to an intracellular accumulation of copper in the brain (particularly the basal ganglia) and liver. When Wilson's disease presents with chorea, hepatic function is already compromised. Slit-lamp examination often reveals copper deposits in the margin of the iris (Kayser–Fleischer ring). Although abnormal copper accumulation begins at birth, the symptoms of Wilson's disease may not become apparent until late childhood or adolescence. In all patients, copper initially accumulates in the liver. This may cause acute or chronic hepatitis or liver cirrhosis. The degree of liver involvement is variable and may range from mild elevations of certain liver enzymes to complete liver failure. Associated symptoms may include fatigue, anorexia, weight loss, generalized weakness, ascites and abdominal swelling, or jaundice. Other findings may include hepatomegaly, splenomegaly, or both (hepatosplenomegaly). In general, the younger the age at symptom onset, the greater the degree of liver involvement. In patients with Wilson's disease, neurologic symptoms seem to be predominant after age 20.

Many individuals with Wilson's disease experience symptoms associated with damage to the nervous system. These symptoms usually become apparent during the second decade of life or, in some patients, during the third decade; however, such findings have been known to appear as late as age 50. Neurologic abnormalities rarely occur in patients younger than age 10. These neurologic symptoms may include tremor of the head, arms, or legs; generalized dystonia; and bradykinesia, particularly those of the tongue, lips, and jaw. Patients may also experience clumsiness, ataxia, or slowness of finger movements and loss of fine motor skills. Tremor or trembling may be present in one hand or leg and gradually progress to involve all four limbs. Speech may become increasingly slurred or slowed (dysarthria). The voice may also have a hoarse or "whispering" quality (whispering dysphonia). In some patients, swallowing may become increasingly difficult (dysphagia).

Psychiatric problems also occur in some individuals with Wilson's disease. These may include increasing agitation and irritability, mood swings, hysteria, neurotic anxiety, bizarre behaviors, or depression accompanied by thoughts of suicide. A relatively small percentage of people with Wilson's disease may experience dementia or, in severe cases, psychosis (e.g., manic-depressive disease, schizoaffective disorder, or schizophrenia).

The goal of drug therapy in individuals with Wilson's disease is to remove excess copper from the body and prevent ongoing copper accumulation and deposition. Therefore, drug therapy must be continued throughout life. Inadequate treatment or disruption of drug therapy may result in life-threatening complications or irreversible organ damage. The initial approach is the removal of excessive copper with chelating agents. The most common agent used for this purpose is D-penicillamine (Cuprimine®, Depen®). D-penicillamine depletes pyridoxine or Vitamin B6 from the body. Therefore, dietary supplementation with pyridoxine is required. The side effects of D-penicillamine range from minor disturbances to severe or life-threatening complications, such as aplastic anemia, immune complex nephritis, systemic lupus erythematosus, or myasthenia gravis. In some individuals, neurologic symptoms may worsen during penicillamine therapy. Other chelating agents used are trientine (Syprine) as well as a drug known as tetrathiomolybdate. There are indications that neurologic symptoms may not worsen during tetrathiomolybdate therapy. Ongoing maintenance therapy usually involves use of zinc acetate (Galzin®), which blocks the absorption of copper in the intestines and promotes the elimination of copper in the stool. Patients with Wilson's disease must avoid copper-rich foods such as cocoa, chocolate, liver, mushrooms, nuts, and shellfish and ensure that their copper intake is restricted to less than 1 mg/day. Liver transplantation may be considered in patients with severe, overwhelming (fulminant) liver disease. Other treatment is symptomatic and supportive.

Chorea of Hyperthyroidism

Hyperthyroidism must be ruled out in any patient with chorea or hyperkinesis. Treatment of hyperthyroidism is dictated by the etiology. The chorea secondary to hyperthyroidism is indistinguishable from that of other causes. Manifestations of hyperthyroid disease, such as weight loss, anxiety, and altered thermoregulation, may be helpful in diagnosis.

Treatment

The decision to treat the Chorea should be granted if symptoms bother the child or interfere with activities of daily living. If chorea is secondary to a treatable etiology, such as hyperthyroidism, SLE, or drug reaction, treatment of the underlying disease may alleviate the chorea. If the child is taking any medications that can cause or worsen chorea, these should be tapered and discontinued, if possible. Dopamine blockers (such as neuroleptics) and presynaptic depleters for neurotransmitters (such as reserpine and tetrabenazine) have been used to treat Chorea. These drugs selectively enhance the function of the indirect pathway by blocking the inhibitory effect of dopamine on this pathway. However, the incidence of side effects in children from neuroleptics has been reported to be as high as 20%. Therefore, it is often safer to start with an alternative medication, such as a benzodiazepine, particularly clonazepam, diazepam, or clobazam. Hypotension is a side effect of the presynaptic depleters. Neuroleptics have significant side effects (tardive dyskinesia, weight gain, prolongation of the QT interval). Tetrabenazine is a very effective medication for chorea, but it is not available in the USA. The antiepileptic drug valproate is considered to be an effective treatment for chorea, but reports vary.

Its mechanism of action is not known but may be through nonspecific – aminobutyric acid (GABA) potentiation. Other GABA-mimetic medications, such as baclofen and clonazepam, appear to have efficacy as well.

Treatment of Syndeham's chorea depends on the disability associated with the chorea. In many cases, the chorea causes only mild disability and symptomatic treatment is not required, because Syndeham's chorea is usually self-limited. When treatment is acquired, antiepileptics like valproate can be effective and are usually associated with fewer side effects than phenothiazines or butyrophenones. Benzodiazepines may be used. Symptomatic treatment for 2–4 months is usually sufficient. Corticosteroids, intravenous immunoglobulin, or plasma exchange have been used on the basis of the presumptive autoimmune mechanism. Antibiotic prophylaxis to prevent GABHS recurrence is recommended to prevent carditis or valvitis, not to prevent chorea. The cardiac manifestations of ARF cause a great deal of morbidity (and mortality) and are irreversible. Penicillin still is the first-line treatment for prevention. Penicillin intramuscular injection of 1.2 million units of benzathine G. can be administered as a monthly, oral form (e.g., Pen V®) and can be given at 250 mg twice daily. The antibiotic sulfadiazine is another option. Patients allergic to penicillin and sulfadiazine, erythromycin can be administered at 250 mg orally bid. The duration of treatment has not been determined, but the American Heart Association recommendations are available. Patients with carditis or valvitis, but no persistent cardiac or valve disease, prophylaxis should continue for 10 years from diagnosis, or "well into adulthood" (whichever is longer). For patients with cardiac disease, the duration of prophylaxis should be for at least 10 years subsequent to the prior episode and until the patient is older than 40 years of age. For patients without cardiac disease (the most common scenario), prophylaxis should continue for 5 years or until 21 years of age.

Pediatric Movement Disorders: Myoclonus

Description

Myoclonus is "sudden, brief, jerky, shock-like, involuntary movements." The movements are quite rapid and may be triggered by attempts at voluntary movement, sensory stimulation, or startle. Myoclonus may cause rhythmic jerks, in which case, it is termed a "myoclonic tremor." Myoclonus is categorized based upon the likely source of movement. Such sources include cortical or subcortical areas or the spinal cord.

Cortical myoclonus is thought to be due to a lack of inhibition in the sensory or motor cortex. Subcortical myoclonus is often due to abnormalities in the brainstem; spinal myoclonus is presumed to be due to abnormalities in spinal inhibitory circuits. Myoclonus may be severely disabling, particularly when it is triggered by movement. In some cases, it may also be very mild. The most common example of a mild myoclonus is sleep myoclonus. In this form of myoclonus, children or adults have occasional brief jerks of an arm or a leg; these "jerks" occur while the individual is falling asleep. Negative myoclonus is a sudden involuntary relaxation of a muscle, rather than a contraction; this is thought to be due to mechanisms similar to those of sleep myoclonus. Cortical reflex myoclonus is triggered by attempts to obtain a knee jerk or other tendon reflex. Epilepsia partialis continua is a type of focal epilepsy that causes myoclonic tremor. Myoclonus is often associated with epilepsy; there is a particular class of degenerative disorders called "progressive myoclonus epilepsies (PME)" in which the association of myoclonus and epilepsy is common.

Examination

As with other movement disorders, it is important to determine which parts of the body are affected by myoclonus. It may occur in a single limb, the neck, the back, or the face. In other cases, it may affect the entire body. When severe, myoclonus may cause the child to fall. It is important to determine whether symptoms improve or worsen with voluntary activity. This is often tested by observing the child attempting to drink from a cup. In some cases, a myoclonic jerk may be caused by an unexpected, loud noise or a gentle tap on the tip of the nose or on the forehead.

To test for negative myoclonus, also known as asterixis, children are asked to extend their arms with the wrists back or to perform some other movement that requires holding the limb against gravity. In this way, a sudden loss of muscle contraction causes the hand or the arm to fall in a downward direction. Since myoclonus may occur along with other movement disorders, it is important to look for evidence of dystonia, tremor, ataxia, or spasticity. It is also important to look for opsoclonus, which is a random, dance-like jerking of the eyes in all directions. This eye movement occurs in the opsoclonus-myoclonus-ataxia syndrome.

Mechanism

The mechanism of myoclonus is not well understood. Cortical myoclonus is possibly a disorder of decreased inhibition in the cortex. The frequent association with seizure disorders suggests that there may be a common cause for myoclonus and some types of epilepsy. However, the reason for the reduced inhibition is not known. The mechanism of subcortical and spinal myoclonus is even less well understood. A group of disorders called "startle syndromes" probably involves hyperexcitability of the normal brainstem startle circuits and decreased inhibition in spinal circuits. This may be due to a mutation in the receptor for the neurotransmitter glycine.

Etiology

Etiological Classification of Myoclonus

Physiological
- Anxiety-induced
- Exercise-induced
- Sleep jerks and nocturnal myoclonus

Essential

Epileptic

Symptomatic
- Postcentral nervous system injury
  - Hypoxia
  - Trauma
  - Stroke

Basal ganglia degenerations
- Idiopathic torsion dystonia
- Hallervorden–Spatz disease
- Hepatolenticular degeneration (Wilson's disease)
- Huntington disease

Drug-induced
- Carbamazepine
- Levodopa
- Tricyclic antidepressants

Lysosomal storage diseases

Metabolic encephalopathies
- Dialysis syndromes
- Disorders of osmolality
- Hepatic failure
- Renal failure

Myoclonic encephalopathy
- Idiopathic
- Neuroblastoma

Spinal cord tumor

Spinocerebellar degenerations

Toxic encephalopathies

Viral encephalitis

Physiological

Sleep myoclonus, benign myoclonus of infancy

Essential Myoclonus

Familial essential myoclonus, essential myoclonus-dystonia, stimulus-sensitive myoclonus

Epileptic

Juvenile myoclonic epilepsy, progressive myoclonic epilepsies, epilepsia partialis continua, Rasmussen's encephalitis, early infantile myoclonic encephalopathy, infantile spasms (West syndrome), Lennox–Gastaut syndrome, benign familial myoclonic epilepsy, Angelman syndrome.

Idiopathic epilepsy without any other neurological problem may have myoclonus as a major clinical expression. This includes entities such as benign myoclonus of infancy, myoclonic absences, juvenile myoclonic epilepsy of Janz, and photosensitive epileptic myoclonus. In such instances, the jerks are usually generalized and occur spontaneously, are frequently facilitated by lack of sleep, alcohol, etc., and may be triggered by visual stimuli.

Myoclonus may also be present in patients with generalized tonic-clonic epilepsy in the setting of a progressive encephalopathy (progressive myoclonic epilepsy), which will be discussed in another section.

Symptomatic

- *Fixed injury*: Carbon-monoxide poisoning, hypoxic injury or near-drowning (Lance-Adams syndrome), heatstroke, trauma, stroke, and electrocution
- *Storage/degenerative*: Sialidoses (cherry-red-spot myoclonus), lipidosis, lysosomal storage disease (Niemann–Pick type C, Tay–Sachs, Sandhoff's), other storage disorders (neuronal ceroid lipofuscinosis), pantothenate-kinase associated neurodegenerative disease (PKAN, formerly neuronal brain iron accumulation

type 1, formerly Hallervorden–Spatz disease), Wilson's disease, Lafora body disease, Rett syndrome, Baltic myoclonus, spinocerebellar ataxias (SCAs), dentatorubropallidoluysian atrophy (DRPLA), multiple sclerosis, and mitochondrial disorders (e.g., myoclonic epilepsy with ragged-red fibers [MERRF] and others)
- *Infections/para-infectious*: New-variant Creutzfeldt–Jacob disease (nvCJD), subacute sclerosing panencephalitis (SSPE), viral encephalitis, and *Streptococcus*
- *Endocrine*: Hyperthyroidism, hyponatremia, and hypoglycemia
- *Structural*: Tumors that irritate the brain in a direct manner, tumors that release chemicals into the blood (as in abdominal or thoracic neuroblastoma [which causes the opsoclonus-myoclonus-ataxia syndrome]), and palatal myoclonus (with injury to the Guillain–Mollaret triangle in the brainstem or cerebellum)
- *Drug-induced/toxins*: Antiseizure medications (valproate, carbamazepine, etc.), antidepressants (amitryptaline, nortryptaline, desipramine, fluoxetine, sertraline, lithium, etc.), stimulants (amphetamine, dexedrine, methylphenidate, some asthma inhalers, caffeine, etc.), liver toxic medications, respiratory depressants, corticosteroids, amiodarone, acyclovir, bismuth, thallium, and L-dopa
- *Associated with systemic illness*: Dialysis, renal failure, liver failure, pulmonary disease, and carbon dioxide intoxication

Workup

Myoclonus may be tested by looking at the electrical activities in brain and affected muscle(s). Electromyography (EMG) of the muscles typically shows the duration and frequency of the myoclonic bursts, and whether these bursts spread to other spinal segments (as is seen in propriospinal myoclonus). It may also be helpful in determining whether jerking movements occur simultaneously in more than one limb, or whether they flow gradually down the body. In cortical myoclonus, there may be an excessively large brain electrical response to electrical stimulation of the hands or feet. This response is tested by using somatosensory-evoked potentials (SSEPs). In some cases, it is also possible to demonstrate the myoclonic electrical signal in muscle following a tendon tap. This may be helpful in diagnosing cortical reflex myoclonus.

In any form of myoclonus, it is important to look for a cause. Any medication or toxin that could produce the symptoms should be removed if possible. Family history needs to be investigated and metabolic studies may be appropriate, particularly if there are other symptoms or if symptoms become progressively worse. Metabolic tests may include screening for treatable disorders such as Wilson's disease. Since myoclonus may be a symptom of general systemic illness, including liver failure and some types of tumors, it is important to screen for general health problems. In particular, in the opsoclonus-myoclonus syndrome, the child should have a CT or nuclear medicine scan of the chest and abdomen as well as blood and urine tests. These tests look for evidence of a neuroblastoma tumor. If there is a suspicion of an epilepsy syndrome, an electroencephalogram (EEG) is recommended. Brain MRI is important to look for tumors, stroke, malformations, or other structural lesions near the cortex, brainstem, or cerebellum. This is particularly true if the myoclonus is focal or if the child is suspected of having the syndrome of epilepsia partialis continua. Since certain viral infections can cause myoclonus, a spinal tap is sometimes needed for this diagnosis.

Many cases of essential myoclonus or essential myoclonus-dystonia will improve with small amounts of alcohol. Although this is useful for diagnosis, it is not helpful for long-term treatment.

Treatment

- If a specific cause can be found, then the myoclonus will usually resolve if treatment of the underlying disease is effective. Immune-mediated myoclonus (such as occurs in opsoclonus-myoclonus) usually requires treatment with oral steroids such as prednisone, in addition to removal of the tumor if one is found.
- Intravenous immunoglobulin and plasmapheresis has also been attempted in some cases. Juvenile myoclonus epilepsy usually responds to valproate, and may require lifelong treatment. Symptomatic treatment usually includes benzodiazepines such as clonazepam or diazepam. Cortical myoclonus may respond to valproate, piracetam, or lamotrigine. There are reports of myoclonus due to a hypoxic event responding to 5-hydroxy-tryptophan (5HT), and this may be helpful in other causes as well. Carbamazepine may worsen myoclonus and should be avoided.

Startle Disease or Hyperekplexia

Excessive startle or complex motor reactions in response to sudden unexpected stimuli occur in startle disease or hyperekplexia. When severe, there may be generalized muscle contraction resulting in postural instability and falls. After the fall, there is recovery of normal tone and control. The attacks are worsened by stress and fatigue and ameliorated by central nervous system (CNS) depressants. Hyperekplexia may be sporadic or familial with dominant inheritance (chromosome 5q). Disorders such as the Jumping Frenchmen of Maine, Latah, and Myriachit probably represent variants of startle disease. Abnormal startle and hyperekplexia have also been described in brainstem lesions. In the neonatal variety of startle disease, slight stimuli induce a nonepileptic convulsion that may be tonic or clonic or a mixture of the two. A quivering vocalization precedes the silence when a profound syncope ensues, with subsequent anoxic seizure. The clinical diagnosis is made by the nose-tap test: percussion of the tip of the nose induces an obvious startle. Ictal treatment is by repeatedly flexing the baby (face to knee); further episodes are prevented by clonazepam or clobazam.

Benign Nocturnal Myoclonus

Sudden jerking movements of the limbs during sleep occur in normal people of all ages. They appear primarily during the early stages of sleep as repeated flexion movements of the fingers, wrists, and elbows. The jerks do not localize consistently, stop with gentle restraint, and end abruptly with arousal. When prolonged, the usual misdiagnosis is focal clonic or myoclonic seizures. The distinction between nocturnal myoclonus and seizures or jitteriness is that it occurs solely during sleep, it is not activated by a stimulus, and the EEG is normal. Treatment is not required. Anticonvulsant drugs may increase the frequency of benign nocturnal myoclonus by causing sedation.

Benign Myoclonus of Infancy

Many series of patients with infantile spasms include a few with normal EEG results. These infants cannot be distinguished from others with infantile spasms by clinical features because the age at onset and the appearance of the movements are the same. The spasms occur in clusters, frequently at mealtime. Clusters increase in intensity and severity over weeks or months, and then abate spontaneously. After 3 months, the spasms usually stop altogether, and although they may recur occasionally, no spasms occur after 2 years of age. Affected infants are normal neurologically and developmentally and remain so afterward. The term "benign myoclonus" suggests that the spasms are an involuntary movement rather than a seizure. A normal EEG result distinguishes this condition from other types of myoclonus in infancy. No other tests are required. Treatment is not required.

Tremor

Tremor is a rhythmic, involuntary back-and-forth oscillation of part of the body. Tremor in children may be caused by many disorders including familial essential tremor, focal epilepsy, or a psychogenic movement disorder. Tremor is often seen with ataxia, dystonia, or myoclonus. Physiologic tremor is the normal shaking that occurs when people attempt to exert large forces or lift heavy objects. If a child has weakness, this type of tremor may be accentuated. Ataxia may lead to tremor when the inaccurate movements are corrected and then repeatedly over corrected.

Tremor may occur at rest, while maintaining a fixed arm position or posture (postural tremor) or with movement or kinetic, action, or intention tremor.

Tremor may occur in the hands, feet, back, neck, face, voice, or other parts of the body. The frequency of the tremor may be described by the number of cycles per second, or Hertz (Hz). Tremor may appear suddenly, or worsen gradually over months or years. Most types of tremor disappear during sleep, only to return the next day upon awakening. Tremor is often associated with other neurological disorders; therefore, it is important to look for the cause of tremor.

In familial essential tremor, the onset may occur at any age. Once started, this type of tremor often continues or becomes slowly worse with time. Some family members may notice that the tremor improves briefly after drinking alcohol. This type of tremor is usually postural, and may be particularly evident while the child attempts to eat or drink from an open cup.

Types of Tremor

There are still many controversial issues with regard to tremor. The Movement Disorder Society has suggested definitions as well as clinical and syndromic classifications of tremors. Because of the numerous etiologies for tremor, a practical etiologic classification or a valid physiologic classification is not available.

Tremor is a rhythmic, involuntary, oscillatory movement of a body part. The amplitude and frequency of tremor is not crucial to this definition. For practical purposes, the following categories are presented.

Resting Tremor

Resting tremor occurs in a body part that is supported in such a way that skeletal muscle activation is neither necessary nor intended. Resting tremor is mostly found in Parkinson's disease and other basal ganglia disorders. This is a rarity in childhood and will not be considered further here.

Action Tremor

Tremors not occurring at rest are categorized as action tremor. This occurs during any voluntary contraction of skeletal muscle. The most relevant forms of action tremor are postural tremor, kinetic tremor, and intention tremor.

Postural Tremor

Postural tremor occurs during an attempt to hold a body part motionless against the force of gravity.

Kinetic Tremor

These are tremors occurring during any voluntary movement.

Tremor During Target-Directed Movements (Intention Tremor)

Classic intention tremor is present when amplitude increases during visually guided movements toward a target at the determination of the movement. It can be inferred that a disturbance of the cerebellum and its afferent or efferent pathway is present. The type and distribution of the tremors in hyperthyroidism and due to sympathomimetic drugs correspond to those of physiologic tremor; most drug-induced tremors are a mixture of postural and kinetic tremors.

Essential Tremor

Essential tremor (ET) is the most frequent movement disorder. Patients exhibit a mixed postural and kinetic tremor without other neurologic abnormalities. The upper limbs are predominantly involved. Other body parts are less commonly involved. Many patients with ET inherit the disease through an autosomal-dominant gene; however, the ratio of hereditary versus sporadic ET is unknown. This diagnosis can be made on clinical grounds if this tremor type is of long duration. The "red flags" are rapid onset, unilateral tremor, rest tremor, and gait disturbance.

Examination

The child is examined to determine which body parts are affected, as well as the frequency and amplitude of the tremor. The tremor is observed while the child is at rest, while holding a posture against gravity (e.g., as with the arms outstretched), and while reaching for targets. Tremor may be accentuated by attempting to drink from a nearly full cup of water. It may be difficult to distinguish myoclonic or dystonic tremor from "true" tremor. Frequently, the distinction depends upon whether or not other symptoms are present, such as dystonic posturing or stimulus sensitivity. In dystonic tremor, there is often a "null point" or a position of the joint at which the tremor disappears, and then reverses direction as the joint is moved farther. The child's strength must be assessed, as enhanced physiologic tremor may become more apparent if there is muscle weakness. Family history of tremor is important, as several types of tremor, myoclonus, or dystonia may be inherited. It is also important to look for medications or toxins that are known to cause tremor (such as valproate, sympathomimetics, or centrally acting substances). The following information should also be obtained in the history taking and examination: past history of neurologic disorders, type of tremor, onset, asymmetry, evidence of systemic disease (e.g., hyperthyroidism), and evidence of additional neurologic symptoms (such as dystonia, gait disturbance).

Mechanisms

There are probably many mechanisms that may cause tremor. In some cases, there is alternating muscle activity in the flexors and extensors about a joint. This suggests the presence of an oscillatory signal in the nervous system. In other cases, there is rhythmic contraction or relaxation of a single muscle or group of muscles. Tremor may be generated in muscles, when they are strongly contracted, the spinal cord, the brainstem, the basal ganglia, as in Parkinson's disease, and the cortex. Occasionally, anxiety and hyperthyroidism might increase tremors in children.

Workup

The workup of tremor depends upon the specific type of tremor and its possible cause. Any medications that may worsen tremor should be avoided, if possible. If the constellation is typical for ET, no additional investigations (neuroimaging) are mandatory. If the tremor had sudden onset, an MRI of the head may be able to show a stroke, multiple sclerosis, or other lesion. Treatable conditions, in particular hyperthyroidism and Wilson's disease, should be considered. Wilson's disease may present in the first decade as hemolytic anemia or as a hepatic problem; a neurologic presentation is not encountered before the second decade and not as an isolated tremor. Electroencephalogram (EEG), which measures electrical activity in the brain, is important if there is a suspicion that the tremor is due to focal seizures. If there has been gradual onset, it is important to check electrolytes, including glucose, calcium and magnesium, thyroid function, copper in the urine (for Wilson's disease), and possibly the amount of adrenaline metabolites (for pheochromocytoma). If Parkinsonian features are present, a trial of L-DOPA may be helpful. Rarely, an EMG may help to determine if the tremor is more likely to be due to dystonia or myoclonus. Tests for myoclonus, including EEG with back-averaging and SEP (somatosensory-evoked potentials), may help to confirm the presence of dystonia or myoclonus. If there is a family history of tremor, it may be helpful to try the use of alcohol. This is often tried with an adult family member, rather than the child. If the tremor improves with alcohol, this suggests that it will also improve with other medications such as primidone.

Treatment

There is no general treatment for tremor per se. Mild tremor does not require treatment. If there is a specific illness such as Parkinson's or Wilson's disease, tremor will improve with appropriate therapy. For the underlying condition ET may be improved with propranolol (0.5–1.5 mg/kg bodyweight) and primidone. However, most children and adults with ET are not functionally impaired and manage without drug treatment. Medication can be limited to particular (stressful) events. In all cases, the child should start with a very small dose. The dose should be increased gradually in order to avoid side effects. Long-term use of primidone, which is metabolized, in part, to phenobarbital, is probably not desirable. If the tremor is felt to be psychogenic, then psychotherapy may be helpful in determining and avoiding any psychiatric triggers for the movement. Patients especially adolescents have to avoid certain dietary products like caffeine, recreational drugs, and alcohol.

Non-movement Disorders of Infancy and Childhood

Movement disorders can be classified as transient, paroxysmal, and chronic. Transient movement disorders (TMDs) are simply defined as those that stop over time. In a review by Fernandez-Alvarez (1998), 19% of 356 children under the age of 18 with movement disorders had a TMD. Most common in infancy, TMDs are readily recognized with experience. The generally benign and transient nature of these disorders has resulted in a lack of understanding (but no shortage of theories) as to the underlying cause in most cases. The following discussion approaches the TMDs on the basis of their age of presentation. The aim is to provide a practical approach to the recognition of the more common TMDs. There is insufficient space to discuss the possible theoretical basis of most of these conditions.

The differentiation between a transient and a paroxysmal movement disorder is clearly somewhat artificial as many of the latter diminish or stop with time.

Benign Neonatal Sleep Myoclonus

Benign neonatal sleep myoclonus (BNSM) was described by Coulter and Allen in 1982. Myoclonic jerks confined to sleep start in the neonatal period. They abruptly stop with arousal and are never seen in the awake state. The jerks are most frequent during NREM sleep but may appear during all stages. They may be unilateral or bilateral and often appear in short clusters and shift sides. The severity of individual jerks and duration of clusters may vary considerably. The EEG is normal both during the jerks and interictally. Detailed neurophysiological studies with back-averaging have not been performed.

Rocking the basinet or crib, touch and simple restraint do not abolish the jerks and may actually induce them. Neurological examination and metabolic investigations are normal. BNSM is more common in preterm newborns. Usually the jerks cease by 2–7 months of age. A recent report described completely normal follow-up in five siblings with BNSM seen 3–10 years after remission. The relationship between BNSM and benign myoclonus of early infancy (BMEI) is not clear, although in one series 2/21 patients with BNSM were reported to have developed BMEI on follow-up.

Benign Myoclonus of Early Infancy

Benign myoclonus of early infancy (BMEI) was described by Lombroso and Fejerman in 1977. The usual age of presentation is between 3 and 15 months. The history is suggestive of infantile spasms with episodes of limb stiffening occurring in clusters. However, unlike infantile spasms the episodes usually occur in the awake state rather than in drowsiness and are often provoked by excitement or frustration.

There are rarely more than 10 events in a cluster, whereas with established infantile spasms many more episodes can be seen. There is no developmental delay or regression and the neurological examination is normal. Interictal EEG is normal.

Typically there were tonic spasms of the limbs with associated shuddering-like movements of the trunk. EMG of the tonic limb spasms revealed durations as long as 2 s. The EEG was normal during the spasms. Therefore the term "myoclonus" is probably not appropriate for these events. There was a close similarity between BMEI and "nonepileptic reflex tonic seizures," a condition described by the same group where sustained tonic contractions occur only when the infant is held in someone's arms.

The jerking episodes become more prominent for a few weeks or months after onset but, within an average of 3 months, decrease considerably in most infants. They disappear spontaneously by 2 years of age. Antiepileptic drugs do not stop the episodes.

Most of the cases have been sporadic; however familial occurrence has been reported.

As well as infantile spasms, the differential diagnosis includes benign myoclonic epilepsy of infancy, when there are generalized ictal and interictal EEG abnormalities.

Transient Idiopathic Dystonia of Infancy

This condition was first reported by Willemse in 1986 and other reports followed. Onset is usually in the first 6 months. There is dystonic posturing of an upper limb and sometimes the trunk or a leg. The typical arm posture is forearm pronation with hyperflexion of the wrist. When prone, the affected arm often rests on the dorsum of the hand. Typically, the posture disappears with intentional movement, for example, when reaching out to grab an object. Motor and mental development is usually normal. The posturing usually stops before the age of 2 years. Some cases seem to have more prominent dystonia and a more prolonged clinical course. Genetic factors may have a role.

Symptomatic forms of dystonia are not uncommon in the first year of life and investigations are usually required, but the normal development and the lack of functional abnormality suggest idiopathic dystonia. Investigations have been reported to be normal, including imaging and tests for metabolic disorders. However, one report has documented a decreased perfusion of the basal ganglia and left temporomesial cortex using SPECT and decreased glucose metabolism in the basal ganglia and cerebellum in one patient. Worsening of the dystonic posturing apparently induced by cisapride, a 5-HT receptor antagonist, has been described in two patients.

Beltran and Coker described transient dystonia beginning in the newborn period to 3 months of age in four infants exposed to cocaine in *utero*. Torticollis was a particular feature. Angelini described nine patients with paroxysmal episodes of dystonia involving limbs and trunk. The episodes lasted minutes to hours. It is not clear if this is the same condition.

Benign Paroxysmal Torticollis

Snyder first reported this condition in 1969. Drigo et al. have recently reported a large series of 22 patients. It is characterized by recurrent episodes of torticollis without persistent or obligatory head tilt, followed by subsequent spontaneous resolution. Onset is usually in the first year often between 2 and 8 months of age but sometimes as early as in the first week of life or as late as 30 months. Attacks tend to occur frequently at the onset (1–2 months) and sometimes with a striking regularity.

Truncal posturing (retrocollis and tortipelvis) may also be seen. A few cases have been familial. The episodes last from 10 min to 14 days, may recur two or three times a month, and involve either side. Drigo et al. have suggested the attacks can be subdivided into the more common "periodic torticollis" lasting hours or days and a "paroxysmal" form lasting only minutes and accompanied by ptosis and mydriasis. Many episodes appear in the morning and may be precipitated by postural changes, for example, changing from the upright to the supine position. There may be a prodrome of irritability, pallor, ataxia, distress, or vomiting prior to the attack. Ataxia may be a dominant feature. Neurological examination between attacks is normal. In most cases the attacks stop by 2–3 years of age without treatment. EEG and neuroimaging are normal. The pathophysiology of benign paroxysmal torticollis is subject to speculation. The observation of eye rolling or deviation in some cases suggests labyrinthine involvement. Abnormal oculo-vestibular function has also been suggested. Some believe that benign paroxysmal torticollis is related to benign paroxysmal vertigo and is a migraine equivalent and may precede these conditions. In a recent report, two of four patients belonged to kindred with familial hemiplegic migraine and linked to the CACNA I A mutation giving further support that BPT may be a "migraine equivalent" or a channelopathy.

Children with apparent benign paroxysmal torticollis need to be carefully investigated. The differential diagnosis includes seizures, vertigo, gastroesophageal reflux, and Sandifer's syndrome, dystonic reaction to drugs, posterior fossa, and craniocervical junction abnormalities (basilar impression, platybasia, atlantoaxial instability, Arnold–Chiari malformation, and Klippel–Feil syndrome). Vestibular testing may be difficult to perform and interpret in young children. EEG during the paroxysms is normal. Neuroimaging studies are necessary to exclude congenital and acquired lesions involving the craniocervical region.

Treatment with dimenhydrinate. Meclizine and chlorpromazine has not been successful. The prognosis, however, is favorable and follow-up studies suggest spontaneous resolution in most cases.

Shuddering Attacks

Shuddering attacks are benign paroxysmal spells of childhood that can mimic epileptic seizures. They may superficially resemble several seizure types, including tonic, absence (typical and atypical), and myoclonic seizures. The pathophysiology is unknown, although a relationship with essential tremor has been postulated. The origin is unclear, but shuddering attacks are not epileptic in nature. Incidence is unknown, but shuddering attacks are relatively uncommon. These episodes are usually benign and non-disabling. They are not associated with increased morbidity or mortality and tend to remit spontaneously. No sex predilection is reported. The condition is seen in older infants and young children.

Parents describe the paroxysmal episodes of shuddering attacks as a sudden flexion of the neck and trunk and adduction of the arms. A shiver-like movement of the trunk ("like a chill") occurs, and the body may stiffen. Consciousness does not seem to be altered, but this can be difficult to confirm. The episode usually lasts 5–15 s. Unlike epileptic seizures, shuddering attacks do not occur during sleep. General and neurological examination findings are normal. The cause is unknown. A relationship with essential tremor has been postulated because there may be an increased frequency of essential tremor in the families of these children.

Absence seizures, benign childhood epilepsy, complex partial seizures, dizziness, vertigo and imbalance, epilepsy, juvenile myoclonic, essential tremor, febrile seizures, frontal lobe epilepsy, psychogenic nonepileptic seizures, seizures, and epilepsy: overview and classification, simple partial seizures, syncope and related paroxysmal spells and tonic-clonic seizures. No laboratory studies are helpful for the diagnosis of shuddering attacks. EEG, brain CT scan, or MRI may be performed because epileptic seizures are in the differential diagnosis. However, the results of these studies are normal.

Reviewing the appearance of a typical episode as captured on video camera by the parents is helpful in suggesting the diagnosis; however, prolonged electroencephalography (EEG) video monitoring to record a typical episode definitively differentiates shuddering attacks from epileptic seizures. Recordings of the spells confirm that typical characteristics of an episode are 5–10 s of shiver-like movements of the trunk and limbs with no impairment of consciousness and no EEG discharge during the episode. A normal EEG result helps to rule out an epileptic origin. Ambulatory EEG without video recording is useful for diagnosis because it records the EEG, but not the clinical event, although eyewitnesses marking the event with a pushbutton can vouch that the event was the kind in question. Routine EEG results are typically normal. In most cases, no treatment is necessary for shuddering attacks. Occasionally, if the episodes are unusually frequent or disabling, treatment may be attempted. However, there is no consistently effective treatment. Antiepileptic drugs are ineffective. Propranolol can be helpful in isolated cases, although pediatric dosages are not established. Infants and children with shuddering attacks are typically referred to a neurologist to check for possible seizures. Shuddering attack episodes tend to remit. A relationship to essential tremor occurring later in life has not been definitively established. The primary care physician should educate the family concerning the benign nature of this condition and the excellent long-term prognosis.

Sandifer Syndrome

Sandifer syndrome involves spasmodic torsional dystonia with arching of the back and rigid opisthotonic, posturing, mainly involving the neck, back, and upper extremities, associated with symptomatic gastro esophageal reflux, esophagitis, or the presence of hiatal hernia. Pediatric neurologists may be the first to see patients with Sandifer syndrome because the primary care provider and the parents may believe that the spasms represent seizures. Pediatric emergency department physicians, pediatric neurologists, and gastroenterologists see patients with this complex with some frequency. The syndrome is most certainly under recognized, and delays in diagnosis are due to atypical presentations or cases in which the diagnosis is not part of the differential. The true pathophysiological mechanisms of this condition remain unclear. The incidence is unknown, although there is some suggestion that in clinical practice, it occurs in less than 1% of children with gastroesophageal reflux. Mortality is not typically associated with Sandifer syndrome. Morbidity consists of the discomfort associated with this syndrome. Infants may lose weight if persistent or severe gastroesophageal reflux disease (GERD) is present. Associated morbidities may also include the presence of a hiatal hernia and esophagitis. Race does not seem to influence incidence. No sex predilection is recognized. Typically, Sandifer syndrome is observed from infancy to early childhood. Peak prevalence is in individuals younger than 24 months. Children with mental impairment or spasticity may experience Sandifer syndrome into adolescence. Sandifer syndrome is most commonly mistaken for seizures. The child typically appears to have an alteration in mental status associated with the tonic posturing. A relationship with feeding may suggest a diagnosis of Sandifer syndrome, which commonly occurs after feeding. The child may have a sudden rotation of the head and neck to one side and the legs to the opposite side with a stretched out appearance. Typically, the back is arched posteriorly with hyperextension of the spine and elbows may be flexed and held posteriorly with hyperextended hips. Torticollis may be present. Although the intermittent stiff tonic posture and periods of crying and apparent discomfort may suggest seizures, in many cases the rhythmic clonic component, which may be present in seizures, is not described. Various stiff, bizarre postures can be observed.

- Typically, the duration of the posture is 1–3 min.
- This brief, paroxysmal pattern of posturing accounts for the fact that the movement observed in Sandifer syndrome may be mistaken for seizures.
- During the posture, the infant may become very quiet or, less commonly, become very fussy. Fussiness and evident discomfort is most commonly observed as the posture abates.
- If a significant volume of gastroesophageal reflux is observed, even without actual vomitus, some infants and children may manifest evidence of respiratory tract irritation as well, including cough, wheezing, and stridor, depending on the degree and volume of reflux.

In children with Sandifer syndrome without mental impairment, the examination findings are normal. Children with Sandifer syndrome with mental impairment often have evidence of spasticity and may be diagnosed with cerebral palsy. Sandifer syndrome in infants is most commonly associated with normal examination findings. Sandifer syndrome in older children may be associated with mental impairment. Dysfunction of the lower esophagus is thought to be the most common precipitating factor. In some children, a cause cannot be found. Gastroesophageal reflux disease (GERD) with varying degrees of esophageal inflammation is common. Esophageal dysmotility, characterized by low-amplitude waves, lack of normal propagation, and low lower esophageal sphincter (LES) pressure, is not the cause but most likely the consequence of esophagitis: gastroesophageal reflux, seizure, infantile spasms, tonic seizures, torticollis, and dystonia. In patients with Sandifer syndrome, pH monitoring is useful in demonstrating gastroesophageal reflux and in clarifying any temporal association of reflux and posturing. Barium swallow studies are used less frequently, although they may be useful in documenting anatomy and the possible association with hiatal hernia. Cranial MRI is helpful in defining the nature of the neurologic deficits in children with mental impairment. Video-EEG monitoring helps differentiate seizures from posturing related to reflux and can be combined with a pH probe study to demonstrate the nature of the spells. Endoscopy may confirm anatomy via visualization and allows biopsy samples to be obtained to confirm mucosal changes due to esophagitis.

Sandifer syndrome does not require treatment unless the spasms are the result of gastroesophageal disease significant enough to interfere with growth and feeding. In the latter case, therapy should be directed toward the specific cause (see ➔ Chap. 178, "Gastroesophageal Reflux"). The American Gastroenterological Association has issued recent guidelines for the management of gastroesophageal reflux disease (GERD). The primary aim of medical care is to identify Sandifer syndrome. This can be accomplished most often by soliciting a careful history of the times of day the spasms occur and the precipitating causes. If recognizing the complex is difficult, then video-EEG monitoring may be of value. Often, parent education and explanation regarding the nature of the spasms are all that is required in treatment of this condition. If the patient does have pathologic gastroesophageal reflux or complications from gastroesophageal reflux such as esophagitis, then therapy for gastroesophageal reflux, or specifically for esophageal peptic disease, is indicated. Muscle relaxants could be used in patients with Sandifer syndrome in whom a GI cause has been excluded and seizure-like postures are causing distress and discomfort for the patient or their family. However, muscle relaxants have not been demonstrated to relieve the seizure-like manifestations of Sandifer syndrome.

In cases with severe, confirmed gastroesophageal disease that is interfering with growth and development, some evidence suggests that fundoplication may alleviate symptoms (➋ *Fig. 363. 1*).

Primary consultations should be with a gastroenterologist. If any doubt surrounds the nature of the seizure-like activity or if the child has underlying neurological impairment, a consultation with a pediatric neurologist could be beneficial. When gastroesophageal reflux is discovered, treatment must be directed at the reflux.

Therapeutic response for the treatment of gastroesophageal reflux disease may take as long as 2 weeks. If treatment is successful, weight increases and vomiting episodes decrease. Prokinetic agents are used to augment cholinergic activity. Prokinetic pharmacotherapy is often used before acid suppression therapy in children without evidence of esophagitis because of the predominance of motility-related problems over increased acid (and regurgitation over pain) in the pathogenesis and presentation. Different medications have been used to treat this disorder. Dopaminergic antagonist (Metoclopramide (*Reglan*)) that works by increasing LES tone gastric emptying stimulates muscular activity, leading to decrease in reflux. *Antacids* are agents used as diagnostic tools in providing symptomatic relief in infants. Associated benefits include symptomatic alleviation of constipation (aluminum antacids) or loose stools (magnesium antacids). *H2 receptor antagonists* like antacids are agents that do not reduce the frequency of reflux, but they decrease the amount of acid in the refluxate by inhibiting acid production. All are equipotent when used in equivalent doses. They work best in patients with nonerosive esophagitis. Because of proton pump inhibitor (PPI) superiority, H2 blockers are reserved for use in patients unable to tolerate PPIs. *Ranitidine* (*Zantac*) inhibits histamine stimulation of the H2 receptor in gastric parietal cells, which reduces gastric acid secretion, gastric volume, and hydrogen ion concentrations. *Famotidine* (*Pepcid*) competitively inhibits histamine at H2 receptor of gastric parietal cells, resulting in reduced gastric acid secretion, gastric volume, and hydrogen ion concentrations. *Proton pump inhibitors* are agents indicated in patients who need complete acid suppression (e.g., infants with chronic respiratory disease or neurological disabilities). Administer with the first meal of the day (children with nasogastric or gastrostomy tubes may have granules mixed with an acidic juice, then flush tubes to prevent blockage). *Omeprazole* (*Prilosec*) decreases gastric acid secretion by inhibiting the parietal cell H^+/K^+ -ATP pump. It is used for the short-term treatment (4–8 weeks) of GERD. Lansoprazole (*Previcid*) *suppresses* gastric acid secretion by specific inhibition of the (H+, K+)-ATPase enzyme system (i.e., proton pump) at the secretory surface of the gastric parietal cell. It blocks the final step of acid production. The effect is dose-related and inhibits both basal and stimulated gastric acid secretion, thus increasing gastric pH. *Esomeprazole magnesium* (*Nexium*), S-isomer of omeprazole, inhibits gastric acid secretion by inhibiting H^+/K^+-ATPase enzyme system at secretory surface of gastric parietal cells. Used in severe cases of and patients not responding to H2 antagonist therapy. Sandifer syndrome is not life threatening. Many patients with the condition eventually outgrow the spasms in later childhood. The diagnosis of Sandifer syndrome should not be made without

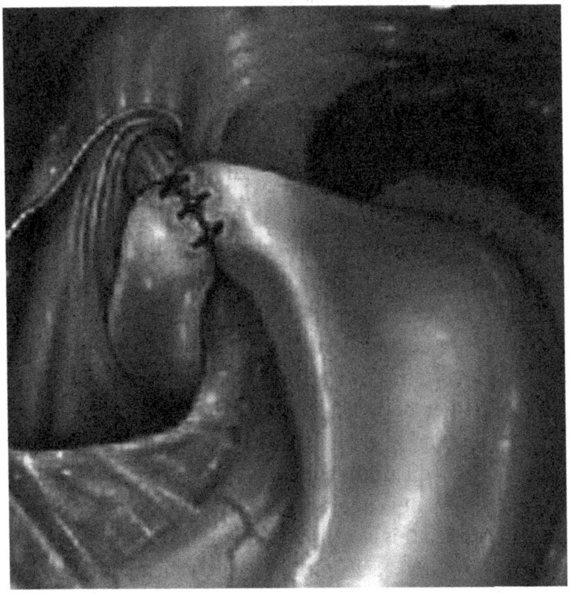

Figure 363. 1

adequate study. It is important to exclude infantile spasms, require relatively rapid treatment and management. In infantile spasms, a hypsarrhythmia pattern is observed on EEG.

Stereotypies in Normal Children

A wide variety of repetitive movements is readily recognized by parents as part of normal development and these are not considered as TMDs. Body rocking occurs in 6–19% of normal young children, thumb-sucking in 21%, nail-biting in around 12% of preschool children, and hair twisting in approximately16% of normal children.

Stereotypic movements are well recognized among neurologically impaired children, for example, in autism and Rett syndrome. However, they are also commonly seen in children without major neurological impairment. They are the most common movement disorder of childhood after tics. Tan et al. defined stereotypies as "involuntary coordinated, patterned, repetitive, rhythmic, non-reflex non-goal directed motor activity that is carried out in exactly the same way during each repetition." They described ten normal children with stereotypies.

Seven were boys. Only two of the ten children seemed to be completely normal, the others had mild learning difficulties, speech problems, and attention-deficit disorder.

The onset of the stereotypies was at 12 months or younger in five of the children. The oldest age of onset was 6 years. A large variety of movements were seen. The commonest were arm flapping and leg shaking. The movements appeared when the child was excited, stressed, bored, or unoccupied. Follow-up was available to a maximum age of 11 years in nine children and the stereotypies had completely stopped in only two.

Stereotypies usually appear earlier than tics. Typically, the same basic movement persists over time although often with elaboration. This is in contrast to tics, where there is usually a constant changing, with one tic dominating for a while and then another taking over. The phenomenology of a stereotypic movement may be identical to that of a complex tic or a compulsion. The child's description of the event may help in the differentiation. There may be a sense of pleasure obtained from performing the stereotypy. This is in contrast to the feeling of physical discomfort and need to perform a tic to relieve the discomfort. Older children may report the association of obsessive thoughts with a compulsion.

Stereotypies may superficially resemble seizures but calling the child or interacting with them, for example, by tickling, can immediately stop the movements. There is generally no need to attempt treatment. Even if the movements persist for a number of years, over time, the child tends to restrict the movements to times when they are not observed by others, for example, when they are alone in their bedroom.

Self-stimulation (Infant Masturbation)

Infant masturbation is usually only a diagnostic problem in young girls as it is readily recognized in boys. Infant masturbation can be mistaken for epileptic seizures, abdominal pain, and paroxysmal dystonia. Typically, the legs are tightly opposed and the feet crossed at the ankles.

There may also be mechanical pressure over the suprapubic or pubic area. Pelvic thrusting may be prominent. Irregular breathing, facial flushing sweating, irritable cries, and grunting give an impression that the child is in pain. The episodes can last minutes to several hours. A fixed and glazed look may give the impression of altered consciousness but the episode can usually be stopped immediately by picking up the child. This may produce annoyance and resumption of the activity as soon as the child is put down again. Multiple observers have suggested that the infant experiences orgasm and this is often followed by exhaustion, or sleep giving the impression of a postictal state.

Still and many others, since, postulated that the behavior begins after an episode of local vulval irritation, which sensitizes the child to pleasurable sensations arising from genital stimulation. Some young girls persist in the activity for many hours a day (so-called malignant masturbators). Sexual abuse, family stress, deprivation of affectionate parental physical contact, parental feelings of guilt, anger, shame, or perception of the child as vulnerable have all been suggested as underlying causes with very limited proof.

There are few follow-up studies. Bakwin described three girls. One continued to perform the movements at 4 years of age. Another stopped at 6–7 months and there had been no recurrence up to age 8 years. The third child, at 12 months carried a large rag doll with her constantly and repeatedly threw it to the floor and would rhythmically press her body against it "as in the sexual act." By 4 years, she rarely exhibited the behavior and when last seen was a medical student.

No treatment is necessary. It is important to explain to the parents that this is a normal behavior, more pronounced in some children. Self-stimulation is a better term than masturbation, which carries with it thousands of years of both moral and medical prejudice. Considerable explanation may be required to prevent the use of unsuccessful coercive measures to try to stop this benign activity.

Midazolam Withdrawal Syndrome

Midazolam infusions have been increasingly used in intensive care units to provide sedation and analgesia for critically ill children. Sudden cessation of the midazolam can result in a withdrawal syndrome characterized by altered state of consciousness, restlessness, irritability, vomiting, tremors, and choreoathetoid and dystonic movements. This may occur more frequently when the midazolam is combined with fentanyl. In this setting, investigations are required to exclude metabolic disorders and nonconvulsive status epilepticus, but the possibility of a withdrawal syndrome should be kept in mind as it may be more common than is generally recognized.

Conclusion

The transient movement disorders of childhood are a distinctive group of disorders that are not rare. Over a number of years of practice, most general pediatric neurologists become familiar with them. They are usually seen in infants. Most require some investigation but recognition allows a limitation of what otherwise could be a very expensive diagnostic workup. They are a satisfying group of disorders to deal with, as most need no specific treatment and settle with time. The long-term neurological outcome is generally good, although some children subsequently are found to have learning and attention problems.

References

Anca MH, Giladi N, Korczyn AD (2004) Ropinirole in Gilles de la Tourette syndrome. Neurology 62:1626

Awaad Y (1999) Tics in Tourette syndrome: new treatment options. J Child Neurol 14:316

Awaad Y, Michon A, Minarik S (2005) The use of levetiracetam to treat tics in children and adolescents with Tourette syndrome. Mov Disord 20(6):714–718

Awaad Y, Minarik MA, Minarik S (2007) Long term follow-up use of levetiractam to treat tics in children and adolescents with Tourette syndrome. Pediatr Neurol 5:209–214

Awaad Y, Michon AM, Minarik S, Rizk T (2009) Levetiracetam in Tourette syndrome: a controlled double-blind, placebo study. Accepted J Pediatr Neurol

Brazis PW, Masdeu JC, Biller J (2007) Localization in clinical neurology, 5th edn. Lippincott Williams & Willkins a Wolter Kluwer business, Philadelphia

Burne JA, Carleton VL, O'Dwyer NJ (2005) The spasticity paradox: movement disorder or disorder of resting limbs? J Neurol Neurosurg Psychiatry 76:47

Carod-Artal FJ, Vargas AP, Marinho PB et al (2004) Tourettism, hemiballism and juvenile Parkinsonism: expanding the clinical spectrum of the neurodegeneration associated to pantothenate kinase deficiency (Hallervorden-Spatz syndrome). Rev Neurol 38:327

Caviness JN, Brown P (2004) Myoclonus: current concepts and recent advances. Lancet Neurol 3:598

Chmelik E, Awadallah N, Hadi FS et al (2004) Varied presentation of PANDAS: a case series. Clin Pediatr (Phila) 43:379

Cif L, Valente EM, Hemm S et al (2004) Deep brain stimulation in myoclonus-dystonia syndrome. Mov Disord 19:724

Conry JA (2004) Pharmacologic treatment of the catastrophic epilepsies. Epilepsia 45(Suppl 5):12

Coubes P, Cif L, El Fertit H et al (2004) Electrical stimulation of the globus pallidus internus in patients with primary generalized dystonia: long-term results. J Neurosurg 101:189

Dale RC, Church AJ, Surtees RA et al (2004) Encephalitis lethargica syndrome: 20 new cases and evidence of basal ganglia autoimmunity. Brain 127:21

Dias-Anzaldua A, Joober R, Riviere JB et al (2004) Tourette syndrome and dopaminergic genes: a family-based association study in the French Canadian founder population. Mol Psychiatry 9:272

Doodley JM, Hayden JD (2004) Benign febrile myoclonus in childhood. Can J Neurol Sci 31:504

Eapen V, Fox-Hiley P, Banerjee S et al (2004) Clinical features and associated psychopathology in a Tourette syndromecohort. Acta Neurol Scand 109:255

Eltahawy HA, Saint-Cyr J, Giladi N et al (2004) Primary dystonia is more responsive than secondary dystonia to pallidal interventions: outcome after pallidotomy or pallidal deep brain stimulation. Neurosurgery 54:613, discussion, 619

Fenichel G (2005) Clinical pediatric neurology; a signs and symptoms approach, 5th edn. Elsevier Saunders, Philadelphia

Fernandez-Alvarez E, Aicardi J (2001) Movement disorders in children, International Review of Child Neurology Series edition. Mac Keith Press, London

Germano IM, Gracies JM, Weisz DJ et al (2004) Unilateral stimulation of the subthalamic nucleus in Parkinson disease: a double-blind 12-month evaluation study. J Neurosurg 101:36

Gilbert DL, Batterson JR, Sethuraman G et al (2004) Tic reduction with risperidone versus pimozide in a randomized, double-blind, crossover trial. J Am Acad Child Adolesc Psychiatry 43:206

Hayflick TM, SJ JJ (2004) Clinical heterogeneity of neurodegeneration with brain iron accumulation (Hallervorden-Spatz syndrome) and pantothenate kinase-associated. Mov Disord 19(1):36–42

Hoekstra P, Steenhuis M, Kallenberg C et al (2004) Association of small life events with self reports of tic severity in pediatric and adult tic disorder pastirents: a prospective longitudinal study. J Clin Psychiatry 65:426

Hong JJ, Rippel CA, Yoon DY et al (2004) Comparison of anti-basal ganglia antibodies in PANDAS and Tourette syndrome. Ann Neurol 56(Suppl 8):S129

Jankovic J, Madisetty J, Vuong KD (2004) Essential tremor among children. Pediatrics 114:1203

Jin R, Zheng RY, Huang WW et al (2004) Study on the prevalence of Tourette syndrome in children and juveniles aged 7–16 years in Wenzhou area. Zhonghua Liu Xing Bing Xue Za Zhi 25:131

Kirsh DB, Mink JW (2004) Psychogenic movement disorders in children. Pediatr Neurol 30:1

Kurlan R, Kaplan EL (2004) The pediatric autoimmune neuropsychiatric: disorders associated with streptococcal infection (PANDAS) etiology for tics and obsessive-compulsive symptoms: hypothesisi or entity? Practical considerations for the clinician. Pediatrics 113:883

Kyriagis M, Grattan-Smith P, Scheinberg A et al (2004) Status dystonicus and Hallevorden-Spatz disease. Treatment with intrathecal baclofen and pallidotomy. J Pediatr Child Health 40:322

Langbehn DR, Brinkman RR, Falush D et al (2004) A new model for prediction of the age of onset and penetrance of hantingston disease based on CAG length. Clin Genet 65:267

Lanzi G, ZAMBRINO c, Termine C et al (2004) Prevalence of tic disorders among primary school students in the city of Pavia, Italy. Arch Dis Child 89:45

Lesperance P, Djerroud N, Diaz Anzaldua A et al (2004) Restless legs in Tourette syndrome. Mov Disord 19:1084

Loiselle CR, Lee O, Moran TH et al (2004) Striatal microinfusion of Tourette syndrome and PANDAS sera: failure to induce behavioral changes. Mov Disord 19:390

Lotze TE, Wilfong AA (2004) Zonisamide treatment for symptomatic infantile spasms. Neurology 62:296

Mackay MT, Weiss SK, Webber AT et al (2004) American academy of neurology; child neurology society. Practice parameter: medical treatment of infantile spasms. Report of the American Academy of Neurology and the Child Neurology Society. Neurology 62:1668

Mahone EM, Bridges D, Prahme C et al (2004) Repetitive arm and hand movements (complex motor stereotypies in children). J Pediatr 145:391

Mankes JH, Sarnat HB (2001) Child neurology, 6th edn. Lippincott Williams & Willkins, Philadelphia

March JS (2004) Pediatric autoimmune neuropsychiatric disorders associated with streptococcal infection (PANDAS): implications for clinical practice. Arch Pediatr Adolesc Med 158:927

Maria B (2002) Current management in child neuroplogy, 4th edn. BC Decker, Hamilton

MedLink Neurology [editor@medlink.com]

Miller J, Singers HS, Waranch HR (2004) Behaviour therapy for the treatment of stereotypic movements in non-autistic children. Ann Neurol 56(Suppl 8):S109

Montagna P (2004) Sleep-related non-epileptic motor disorders. J Neurol 251:781

Nikkhah G, Prokop T, Hellwig B et al (2004) Deep brain stimulation of the nucleus ventralis netermedius for Holmes (rubral) tremor and associated dystonia caused by upper brainstem lesions Report of two cases. J Neurosurg 100:1079

O'Riordan S, Raymund D, Lynch T et al (2004) Age at onset as a factor in determining the phenotype of primary torsion dystonia. Neurology 63:1423

Oliveira JR, Spiteri E, Sobrido MJ et al (2004) Genetic heterogeneity in familial idiopathic basal ganglia calcification (Fahr disease). Neurology 63:2165

Patten J (2000) Neurological differential diagnosis, 2nd edn. Springer, London

Peppe A, Pierantozzi M, Bassi A et al (2004) Stimulation of the subthalamic nucleus compared with the globus pallidus internus in patients with Parkinson disease. J Neurosurg 101:195

Pranzatelli MR, Travelstead AL, Tate ED et al (2004) B-and T-cell markers in opsoclonus-myoclonus syndrome: immunophenotyping of CSF lymphocytes. Neurology 62:1526

Rho JM (2004) Basic science behind the catastrophic epilepsies. Epilepsia 45(Suppl 5):5

Richardson MA, Small AM, Read LL et al (2004) Branched chain amino acid treatment of tardive dyskinesia in children and adolescents. J Clin Psychiatry 65:92

Robinson D, Smith M, Reddy R (2004) Neuroacanthocytosis. Am J Psychiatry 161:1716

Rosser T (2007) Pediatric neurology a case-based review. Lippincott Williams & Willkins a Wolter Kluwer business, Philadelphia

Schule B, Kock N, Svetel M et al (2004) Genetic heterogeneity in ten families with myoclonus-dystonia. J Neurol Neurosurg Psychiatry 75:1181

Shibasaki H, Hallett M (2004) Electrophysiological studies of myoclonus. Muscle Nerve 31:157

Singer H (2005) Tourette syndrome: behavior to biology. Lancet Neurol 4:149

Singer HS, Loiselle CR, Lee O et al (2004a) Anti-basal ganglia antibodies in PANDAS. Mov Disord 19:406

Singer HS, Lioselle CR, Lee O et al (2004b) Anti-basal ganglia antibodies in PANDAS. Mov Disord 19:406

Snider T, Grand L (2002) Air pollution by nitrogen oxides. Elsevier, Amsterdam

Snider La, Swedo SE (2004) PANDAS: current status and directions for research. Mol Psychiatry 9:900

Stephens RJ, Bassel C, Sandor P (2004) Olanzapine in the treatment of aggression and tics in children with Tourette's syndrome – a pilot study. J Child Adolesc Psychopharmacol 14:255

Swaiman KF, Ashwal S, Ferriero DM (eds) (2010) Pediatric neurology: principles and practice, 4th edn. C.V. Mosby Co., Philadelphia

Tate Ed, Allison TJ, Pranzatelli MR et al (2005) Neuroepidemiologic trends in 105 US cases of pediatric opsoclonus-myoclonus syndrome. J Pediatr Oncol Nurs 22:8

Temel Y, Visser-Vandewalle V (2004) Surgery in Tourette syndrome. Mov Disord 19:3

Thomas M, Jankovic J (2004) Psychogenic movement disorders: diagnosis and management. CNS Drugs 18:437

Turny F, Jedynak P, Agid Y (2004) Athentosis or dystonia? Rev Neurol 160:759

Uncini A, De Angelis MV, Di Fulvio P et al (2004) Wide expressivity variation and high but no gender-related penetrance in two dopa-responsive dystonia families with a novel GCH-1 mutation. Mov Disord 19:1139

Van Toorn R, Weyers HH, Schoeman JF (2004) Distinguishing PANDAS from Sydenham's chorea: case report and review of the literature. Eur J Paediatr Neurol 8:211, 12:2587

Watts R, Koller WC (2004) Movement disorders; neurologic principles and practice, 2nd edn. McGraw Hill, New York

Zippel J, Harding FW, Lagrange M (1992) The stress of playing God. In: Mildor E (ed) Explorations in geopolitics, 4th edn. Wiley, New York, pp 103–104

364 Sleep and Its Disorders in Childhood

Jonathan Lipton · Sanjeev Kothare

Introduction

Sleep disorders are common in pediatrics and a major cause of both child and parental morbidity. It is estimated that approximately 25% of children experience a sleep problem during childhood. Epidemiologic data increasingly suggest that children in the United States do not get the adequate sleep for optimum academic, physiological, psychological, and social functioning. Insufficient sleep can have profound, potentially detrimental physiological and metabolic effects, and associate with an increase in symptoms of anxiety or depression, impairment of attention mechanisms, and behavioral problems. Even modest sleep loss in school-age children results in an increased risk of obesity consistent with sleep deprivation experiments in healthy young adults that result in the metabolic syndrome. It has been estimated that there is a 226% increase in health care utilization in children with obstructive sleep apnea. This represents a significant financial burden further underscoring the importance of childhood sleep disorders as a public health problem.

Sleep Structure and Physiology

Sleep can operationally be defined as a *reversible* behavioral state of quiescence characterized by a relative lack of motor activity, decreased level of consciousness, and an increased arousal threshold as an adoption of species-specific, state-dependent postures. Sleep is not a single "offline" physiological condition but rather a dynamic series of connected, yet distinct, behavioral and physiological states (➊ *Table 364.1*). Sleep is divided between rapid eye movement (REM) sleep and non-REM (NREM) sleep. NREM is further subdivided into N1, N2, and N3 manifest as progressive slowing and synchronization of the electroencephalogram. REM sleep, in contrast, is characterized by a relative activation of the cortex with reemergence of certain waking EEG frequencies, eponymic, rapid, phasic, eye movements, fluctuations in heart rate and respirations, and a decrease muscle tone on EMG. A night's sleep has a remarkably stable, developmentally specific architecture.

Sleep Architecture from Birth to Adolescence

Sleep is the primary activity of the brain during early development, and also to a large extent during childhood and adolescence, accounting for about 40% of an average day's behavior. Significant changes in sleep architecture occur throughout early childhood. While changes occur across the entire lifespan, the most significant changes occur within the first few years (➊ *Figs. 364.1* and *364.2*).

Newborn (0–3 months). The normal newborn sleeps 16–20 h per day. Sleep generally occurs in 1–4 h periods, followed by 1–2 h wake periods. Classic EEG patterns are not present in the first months of life, and sleep staging is divided equally into active sleep and quiet sleep.

Infants (3–12 months). NREM stages 1 through 3/4 can be identified, and sleep is entered through one of these stages. The proportion of REM sleep begins to decline around 3 months of age (➊ *Figs. 364.1* and *364.2*). Throughout the first 12 months of life, total sleep time (TST) decreases to about 14 h per day. Sleep consolidation into a 6–8 h nighttime period occurs in about 75% by age 9 months and in nearly all children by 12 months. Naps persist about twice a day in 2–4 h blocks.

Toddlers (1–3 years). TST decreases to about 12 h per day with one nap per day, but the duration of the nap decreases to 1–3 h. Up to 25% of toddlers have sleep problems with bedtime resistance and frequent night awakenings. Behavioral insomnia of childhood is the primary sleep disorder in this age group.

Preschool (3–6 years). TST may decrease slightly and generally is 11–12 h per day. Most children stop taking naps by age 5. Bedtime resistance, nightmares, and nighttime fears are common in this age group. Obstructive sleep apnea syndrome (OSAS) and arousal parasomnias peak during this stage.

School-aged children (6–12 years). Children still require 10–11 h of sleep, with rare naps. Sleep problems in this group include insufficient sleep, bedtime resistance, OSAS, and poor sleep hygiene. Sleep restriction in this age group has been related to behavioral problems.

Adolescence (13–18 years). Sleep requirements are 8–9 h (➊ *Fig. 364.3*), however most adolescents are sleep deprived due to social and school activities. Delayed

Abdelaziz Y. Elzouki (ed.), *Textbook of Clinical Pediatrics*, DOI 10.1007/978-3-642-02202-9_364,

Table 364.1
Sleep stages

Stage	Polysomnographic characteristics	Behavioral characteristics
Wake	Alpha rhythm (8–13 Hz) over occipital region with eye closure attenuating with eye opening, rapid eye blinks, EMG variable	Variable
NREM 1 (N1)	Low amplitude theta (4–7 Hz), vertex waves, slow conjugate eye movements	Light sleep
NREM 2 (N2)	K complexes, sleep spindles	Limb movements commonly seen
NREM 3/4 (N3)	Slow high amplitude delta frequency (0.5–2 Hz) adopts at least 20% of 30 s epoch	Highest arousal threshold
REM	Variable low amplitude mixed frequency, runs of central theta (e.g., sawtooth waves), alpha, rapid phasic eye movements, decreased muscle tone, variability heart rate and respirations	Dreaming, paralysis of extremities

NREM non-rapid eye movement, *REM* rapid eye movement

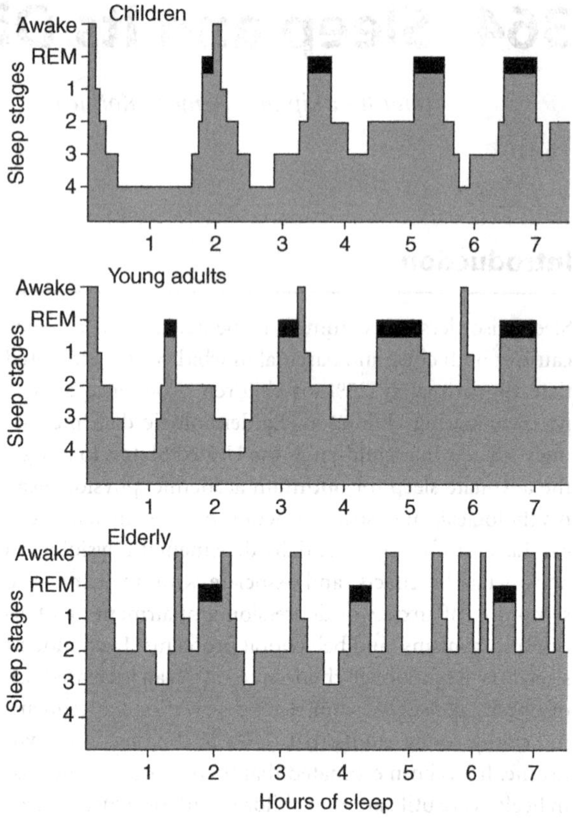

Figure 364.1
Sleep architecture changes with age **(Modified from Mindell JA, Owens JA (2003) A clinical guide to pediatric sleep: diagnosis and management of sleep problems in children and adolescents. Lippincott Williams and Wilkins, Philadelphia)**

sleep phase syndrome, OSAS, insufficient sleep, insomnia, restless legs syndrome (RLS), periodic limb movements of sleep (PLMS), and narcolepsy are seen in this age group (see below).

Mechanisms of Sleep

The biological mechanisms that govern sleep are still largely mysterious. A "two-process" model has been widely adopted that predicts the interaction between homeostatic sleep drive ("Process S") and the circadian timing system ("Process C") (➋ *Fig. 364.3*). Process S is manifest as sleep drive (or sleep "pressure") that accrues proportionally to the duration of wakefulness and dissipates rapidly during sleep. Thus, sleep drive is predicted to be greatest just before sleep and least just after sleep. Process C refers to the 24-h (circadian) periodic oscillations of sleep propensity regulated by the endogenous and autonomous circadian timing mechanism. The core circadian clock comprises an evolutionarily conserved transcriptional, translational, and posttranslational feedback loop that is chiefly orchestrated by the master circadian regulator in the suprachiasmatic nucleus (SCN) of the hypothalamus (➋ *Fig. 364.4*). The SCN is both necessary and sufficient to synchronize the biological clock. The endogenous clock is precisely entrained to the geophysical world by various *zeitgebers* ("time-givers"), including the light-dark cycle, feeding cues, and social interactions. Importantly, the circadian clock appears to be ubiquitous, present in most if not all tissues. The mechanisms by which the central timekeeper in the SCN conveys synchronizing information to peripheral tissues remain obscure.

Neuroanatomy and Neurochemistry of Sleep

The neuroanatomical substrates of arousal comprise monoaminergic nuclei in the brainstem including

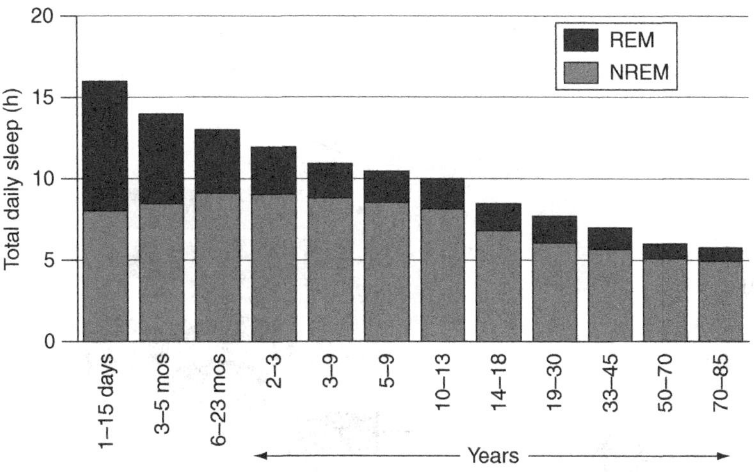

Figure 364.2
Ontogeny of REM/NREM sleep **(Modified from Roffwarg HP, Muzzio JN, Dement WC (1966) Ontogenic development of the human sleep–dream cycle. Science 152:604–619)**

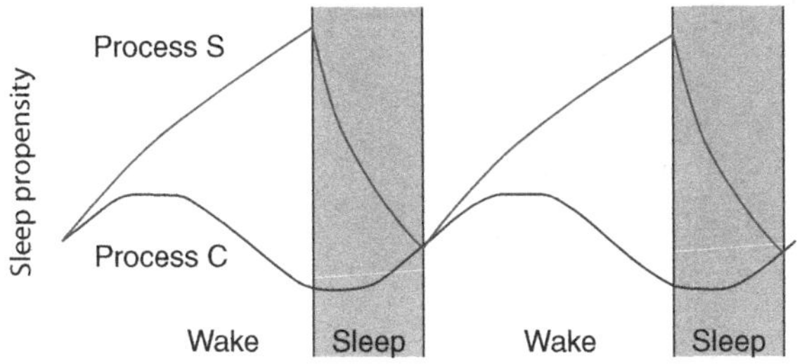

Figure 364.3
The two process model of regulation in sleep propensity. **Shown is the relationship of the circadian timing mechanism (Process C) to homeostatic sleep drive (Process S). Note that homeostatic drive is always greatest just before sleep and least just after sleep. Importantly, in the hours before sleep note opposite effects of Process C and Process S on sleep propensity; this can result in significant insomnia in the hours prior to the appropriate bedtime**

the locus coeruleus (noradrenergic), dorsal raphe (serotonergic), tuberomamillary nucleus (histaminergic), ventral periaqueductal gray (dopaminergic), and pedunculopontine nucleus (cholinergic) that project toward the basal forebrain and thalamus (➲ *Fig. 364.5*). The ventro-lateral preoptic nucleus (VLPO), containing GABA-ergic and galanin-ergic nuclei appears to be a final common pathway in the stimulation of sleep as lesions in this region result in profound insomnia. The stability of state transitions between sleep and wake is modulated by the orexin/hypocretin system that originates in the lateral hypothalamic nucleus. Dysfunction of this system results in narcolepsy. Several sleep-promoting factors have been identified including adenosine, tumor necrosis factor-α, and interleukin-1. The precise mechanism by which the experience of clinical sleepiness arises, however, remains poorly understood.

Physiological Correlates of Sleep States

Sleep influences most major physiologic systems including breathing, cardiovascular function, the endocrine system, and muscle tone. Heart rate, blood pressure, and respiratory rate decrease dramatically during NREM sleep but extraordinary variability in both pulse and respirations are seen in phasic REM sleep. There is an increase in hypoxic ventilatory response during REM sleep as well as a modification of the hypocapnic control of respiration. These phenomena may contribute to the physiological instability associated with REM–NREM transitions as well as sleep–wake transitions.

Core body temperature (Tb) shows a circadian variation independent of sleep. The amplitude of temperature variation is about one degree. Secondly, there is a reduction in the body's thermal set point (the result of increased heat dissipation and decreased heat generation). In REM sleep, there is an absence

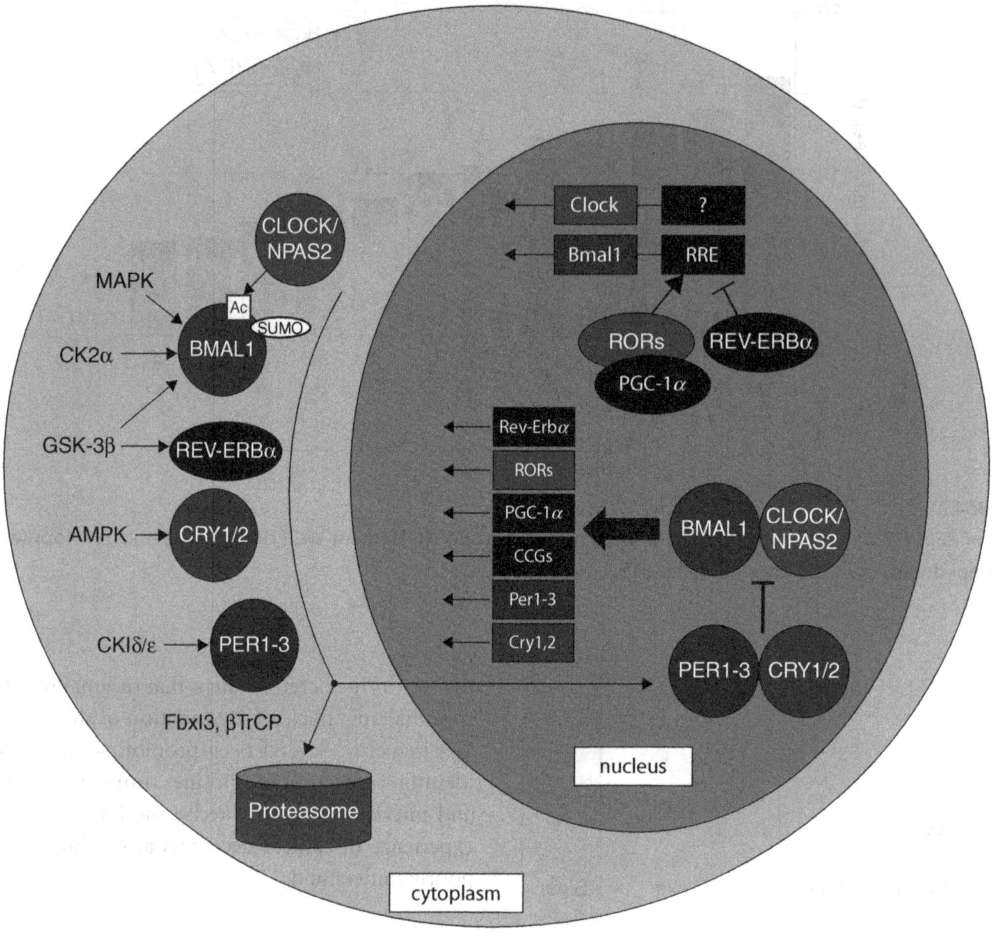

Figure 364.4

Schematic of the molecular clock transcriptional-transalational feedback loop. The "positive limb" is initiated by binding of BMAL1:CLOCK/NPAS2 heterodimers in the nucleus that activate the transcription of clock-controlled genes (CCGs). Upon translation in the cytoplasm, several of these CCGs, including the PERs and CRYs re-enter the nucleus, and inhibit the activity of the BMAL1:CLOCK complex, closing the feedback loop. Note that clock proteins undergo extensive post-translational modification that contribute importantly to their dynamics

of thermoregulatory response, resulting in effective poikilothermy and a drifting of Tb toward environmental temperature.

Slow-wave sleep is associated with secretion of growth hormone independent of circadian time. Sleep onset (and possibly slow-wave sleep) is associated with inhibition of thyroid-stimulating hormone and of the adrenocorticotropic hormone–cortisol axis, an effect that is superimposed on the prominent circadian rhythms in the two systems.

The pineal hormone melatonin is under direct modulation by the circadian pacemaker via a complex neuroanatomical pathway starting with the retinohypothalamic tract and traversing the SCN and cervical sympathetic chain. Melatonin is predominantly secreted at night independently of sleep and thus may represent a biological signature of circadian time. Exogenous melatonin increases sleepiness and sleep duration when administered in adults attempting to sleep during daylight hours (when endogenous melatonin is low). Melatonin has been used for sleep-onset and sleep maintenance insomnia in children, however neither effectiveness nor safety of long-term use have been established.

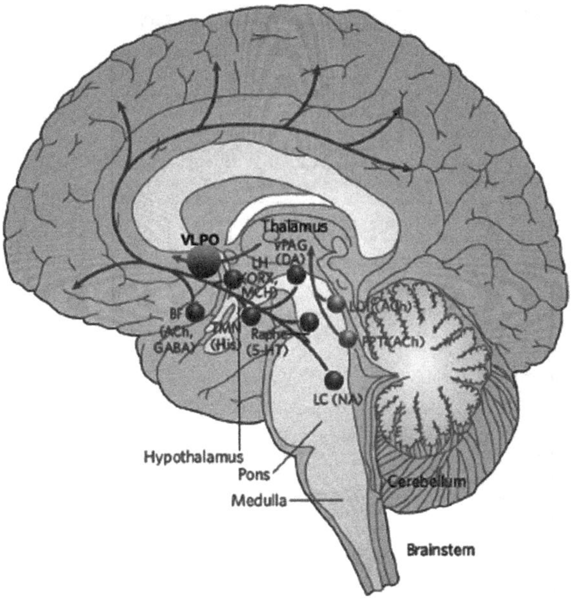

Figure 364.5
Neuroanatomy of sleep and wakefulness. TMN **tuberomamillary nucleus,** ***LC*** **locus coeruleus,** ***PPT*** **parapontine tegmentum,** ***LDT*** **lateral dorsal tegmentum,** ***vPAG*** **ventral periaqueductal gray,** ***BF*** **basal forebrain,** ***VLPO*** **ventral lateral preoptic area,** ***Ach*** **acetylcholine,** ***DA*** **dopamine (Modified after Saper, C et al** ***Nature*** **2005)**

Evaluation of Sleep Disorders in Children

Studies have shown that despite recognizing the importance of sleep, most pediatricians do not feel comfortable identifying and treating sleep disorders.

Assessment of sleep disorders should include:

Sleep history – difficulty going to bed, initiating or maintaining sleep, excessive daytime sleepiness and nocturnal awakenings, unusual behaviors at night, snoring and difficulty breathing, schedules on weekdays and weekends, and napping. Validated questionnaires such as the "BEARS" algorithm, Pediatric Daytime Sleepiness Score (PDSS), and the Pediatric Sleep Questionnaire (PSQ) can be useful for assessment of age-specific subjective sleep parameters.

Medical and psychiatric history – asthma, allergies, gastroesophageal reflux disease (GERD), chronic lung disease, sickle cell disease, epilepsy, headaches, cerebral palsy, developmental delay, ADHD, autism, depression, bipolar disorder, and anxiety.

Family history – sleep-disordered breathing, narcolepsy, sleep-related movement disorders.

Developmental screen and assessment of school functioning and behavioral assessment.

Physical examination, especially:

Growth parameters: height, weight, BMI

ENT exam: looking for deviated septum, adenotonsillar hypertrophy, adenoid facies, or oropharyngeal crowding.

Neurologic exam: especially in children with excessive sleepiness and seizures.

Polysomnography (PSG)

A PSG is a continuous recording of EEG, EKG, EOG (electro-oculogram), respiratory effort using chest and abdominal belts, airflow, gas exchange and end tidal CO_2, electromyogram, snore microphone, and pH probe (*Fig. 364.6*).

A PSG is warranted to investigate causes of excessive daytime sleepiness such as sleep-disordered breathing, sleep fragmentation due to frequent nocturnal arousals from PLMS, bruxism, GERD, the etiology of episodic nocturnal phenomena (e.g., parasomnias versus nocturnal seizures), or as a screening tool prior to a test for excessive daytime sleepiness such as the multiple sleep latency test (MSLT).

Sleep logs. Sleep logs give an estimate of the number, duration, and timing of daily episodes of nocturnal sleep, daytime naps, and wake periods.

Actigraphy. Actigraphy has been widely recognized as a low-cost, home-based tool for screening of sleep disorders, especially circadian rhythm disorders or behavioral insomnias. Actigraphy data is limited by the confounding of influences of immobility during wakefulness or, conversely, sleep-related movements.

Multiple Sleep Latency Test (MSLT)

The MSLT is a validated objective measure of the ability or tendency to fall asleep. It is indicated as part of the evaluation of patients with suspected narcolepsy and idiopathic hypersomnia. This test involves five 20-min opportunities to nap during the day with each nap being separated by 2 h. The sleep onset for each nap is determined as sleep latency. A sleep latency between 5 and 10 min indicates mild/moderate daytime sleepiness, whereas <5 min indicates severe daytime sleepiness). Onset of REM sleep within 15 min of sleep onset is determined as SOREMP (sleep onset REM period) (*Fig. 364.7*).

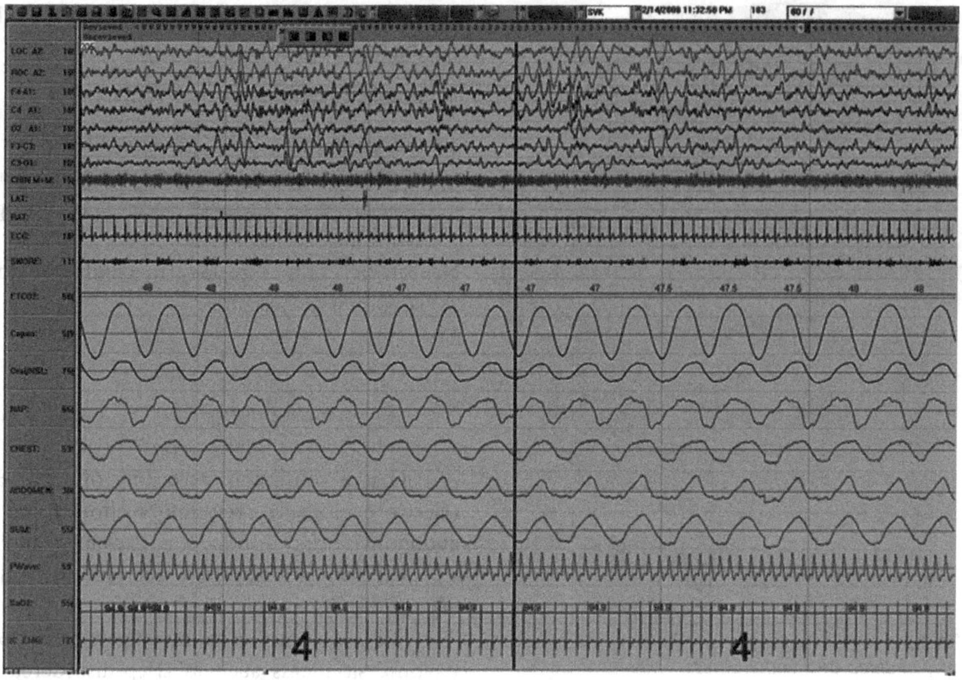

Figure 364.6
Normal polysomnography. From *top* to *bottom*: *LOC/ROC* left and right oculography; EEG (next 5 lines). Green = chin EMG. *LAT* and *RAT* left and right anterior tibialis EMG, respectively. ECG, snore microphone, $EtCO_2$, capnography; *NAP* nasal air pressure; chest and abdomen movement and sum of two; oxygen saturation, *IC EMG* intercostals EMG

Disorders of Sleep Onset and Maintenance in Children

Insomnia

Insomnia is defined by repeated difficulty with sleep initiation, duration, consolidation, or quality despite adequate time and opportunity for sleep that results in some form of daytime impairment (defined as at least one of the following: fatigue, attention or concentration impairment, poor school performance, vocational dysfunction, mood disturbance or irritability, daytime sleepiness, decreased motivation or initiative, proneness for errors, tension, headaches, or gastrointestinal symptoms in response to sleep loss, or concerns or worry about sleep). Insomnia can be difficult to assess in young children because signs and symptoms are expressed by caregivers with limited accuracy and reliability. Population-wide studies suggest that there is a high prevalence of children getting inadequate sleep. Parental or child self-reported problems with sleep initiation or maintenance in school-age children varies from 30% to 41%. Finally, insomnia can have a profound effect on family dynamics and, conversely, familial distress can be a risk factor for development of insomnia, even into adulthood.

The Primary Insomnias

Infants and toddlers. The most common cause of sleeplessness in the youngest children – with estimated prevalence of 10–30% – is behavioral insomnia of childhood (BIC). BIC can been subdivided into two: (1) sleep-onset association type characterized by a child's dependency on stimulation or objects for return to sleep (e.g., parental touch, coddling, co-sleeping, or pacifier) and (2) learned-onset type typically characterized by stalling at bedtime secondary to inadequate limit setting.

Preschool-aged children (3–5 years). Bedtime resistance and sleep onset insomnia are common in preschool children as an expanding communicative palette results in further limit-testing behavior. Differential diagnosis for insomnia includes anxiety disorder, post-traumatic stress disorder (PTSD), child abuse, and use or acute disuse of medications that interfere with REM sleep such as clonidine or selective serotonin reuptake inhibitors (SSRIs).

Problems with sleep hygiene are a common cause of insomnia in this age group frequently secondary to duration of time in bed that exceeds the child's sleep requirement. This frequent phenomenon results in varying constellations of sleep fragmentation with nocturnal

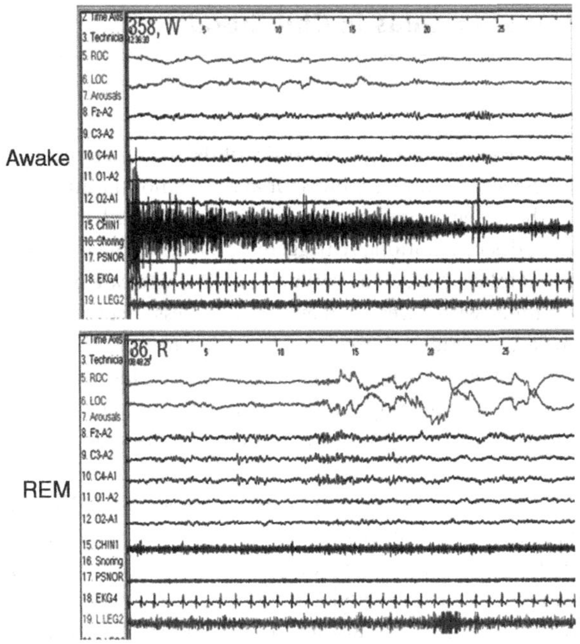

Figure 364.7
MSLT montage comparing appearance of wake to REM sleep

arousals, sleep onset insomnia, and an exacerbation of behavioral difficulties associated with sleep.

School-age children (6–11 years). Inadequate sleep and poor sleep hygiene are common in school-age children as the increased social, educational, and parental demands are made of them. Bedtime resistance, shortened sleep duration, and sleep-onset delay are common in this age group.

Adolescents (12–18 years). Hormonal changes that accompany adolescence have been hypothesized to result in the prominent changes in adolescent sleep patterns that include reduced daytime alertness, delayed sleep phase syndrome (DSPS) with delayed bedtimes, and reduced sleep timing (see below). A combination of increased autonomy and the psychosocial, familial, and educational demands of adolescent life also promote poor sleep hygiene.

Psychophysiological insomnia. Characterized by a heightened level of arousal in bed, psychophysiological insomnia often manifests as excessive anxiety about sleep, heightened inability to relax in bed, or an ability to sleep better away from home can also present in adolescents.

Idiopathic insomnia. The term idiopathic insomnia refers to a relatively rare uncommon condition characterized by lifelong insomnia without identifiable cause, with usual onset in childhood or adolescence, and strong family history. In children, it must be distinguished from behavioral insomnia and should always remain a diagnosis of exclusion. Patients with idiopathic insomnia can be distinguished from normal short sleepers because the latter are not distressed by relatively reduced total sleep time.

Secondary or Comorbid Insomnia

Medical and Psychiatric Conditions. Several medical conditions may impair sleep onset or maintenance including pain, colic, otitis media, asthma, allergies, gastroesophageal reflux, sickle cell disease, fibromyalgia, and cancer. It can be particularly difficult to distinguish sleep dysfunction as a contributing cause as opposed to a symptom of an underlying psychiatric disorder. Anxiety disorders, major depression, and post-traumatic stress disorder should always be considered in the differential diagnosis of insomnia. In older children and adolescents, use of alcohol and other recreational drugs should be explored as possible causes for insomnia.

Neurological Conditions. Children with neurological conditions are at particular risk of insomnia. Attention-deficit disorder (ADD) with or without hyperactivity has been repeatedly identified as either the cause or a symptom of sleep onset and/or sleep maintenance insomnia. Low ferritin levels (less than 50 ng/mL) have been associated with both ADD and sleep-related movement disorders (see below). Sleep and epilepsy have a mutual relationship with sleep quality strongly affecting seizure control. Many anti-convulsants alter sleep macroarchitecture and can also contribute to both sleep initiation and maintenance difficulties. For unknown reasons, insomnia is common in children with autistic spectrum disorders (ASD). Insomnia is common in children with cerebral palsy (CP) and those with severe visual impairment are especially affected. Sleep maintenance is extremely disrupted in Angelman syndrome and Rett syndrome; however, little is known about the underlying pathophysiology. Finally, children with the rare Smith–Magenis syndrome demonstrate circadian cycle inversion and may suffer from significant insomnia.

Circadian Rhythm Sleep Disorders (CSRD)

Circadian oscillations are the manifestation of an endogenously working clock that has, in each individual, a genetically specified period. Yet, the circadian system is extraordinarily plastic and responds to environmental cues – so-called zeitgebers (or “time-givers”) including light, food, and social interactions – that serve to synchronize the clock with geophysical and sociobiological time.

CSRDs result from a misalignment of the endogenous clock with the socially mandated schedule and can result from: (1) environmentally imposed behavior or cues such as shift work, jet lag, or a dearth of normal light/dark cues; (2) decreased sensitivity to synchronizing cues such as light (e.g., with blindness); and (3) genetic variability in the biological clock itself that renders a relatively short or long period or inappropriate responsiveness to *zeitgebers.*

Delayed Sleep Phase Syndrome (DSPS). DSPS is the most common CSRD in the pediatric population, especially adolescents (prevalence ~7%), and is characterized by a delay in the phase of circadian clock mechanism relative to local time. DSPS presents with sleep-onset insomnia, daytime sleepiness, and sleep deprivation until the restrictions on the mandated schedule are relieved (e.g., during the weekend) and the circadian phase is "expressed." When patients with DSPS are permitted to sleep without restriction, sleep is normal, differentiating it from psychophysiological insomnia. Delays in melatonin secretion, changes in core body temperature, and sleep/wake cycle have been demonstrated in DSPS patients. Treatment has focused on resetting the circadian clock (chronotherapy) by advancing sleep times and/or light therapy in which subjects are exposed to bright light at the same time every morning after the normal physiological temperature nadir. Pharmacologically, exogenous melatonin administered prior to desired sleep time has been shown to have efficacious hypnotic and phase-shifting effects.

Advanced Sleep Phase Syndrome (ASPS). ASPS refers to a condition in which an individual falls asleep and wakes early relative to local time. A tendency toward relative phase advancement occurs with normal aging. True ASPS is uncommon however, and may have a strong genetic basis. Mutations in two regulators of the "negative limb" of the circadian feedback loop – *Per2* and *CK-1ε* – have been identified in familial cohorts (➋ *Fig. 364.2*).

Blindness. Because blind individuals do not benefit from the entraining influences of light on the endogenous circadian clock, they may exhibit a "free-running" rhythm in which the circadian phase cycles independently of local time often resulting in severe insomnia. Melatonin has proven valuable as an exogenous entraining signal in these patients. A free-running circadian rhythm is extremely rare in sighted individuals.

Jet Lag Disorder and Shift Work Disorder. Children are not frequently exposed to jet lag or regular shift work. Both can result in chronic sleep disruption secondary to misalignment of internal clock with local time.

Hypersomnias in Childhood

Narcolepsy

Narcolepsy is a disabling disorder of sleep characterized by excessive daytime sleepiness for at least 3 months duration in the absence of another primary sleep disorder and/or episodes of emotionally triggered cataplexy. The presence of cataplexy (i.e., a paroxysmal, bilateral decrease of muscle tone) with excessive daytime sleepiness is sufficient to make a diagnosis. Narcolepsy has other features that vary in prevalence including hypnagogic (occurring with falling sleep) or hypnopompic (occurring with waking) hallucinations, sleep paralysis, and an urge to sleep that is often uncontrollable.

Narcolepsy has an estimated prevalence in the United States of 0.8 per 100,000; however, the prevalence is higher in Japan and lower in Europe. It is more common in women and has a bimodal age of diagnosis: the first peak occurs at about 15 years and the second, smaller peak, at about 36 years. Narcolepsy with cataplexy can be familial. Interestingly, about 85–95% of patients with narcolepsy with cataplexy carry the HLA DQ1B*0602 haplotype, suggesting a genetic predisposition to the disease (importantly however, 99% of individuals with this haplotype do not have narcolepsy).

Elegant genetic studies in narcoleptic dogs in conjunction with molecular studies in mouse models have identified the orexin/hypocretin system as the culprit signaling defect in narcolepsy. The orexins are a family of neuropeptides produced exclusively in the lateral nucleus of the hypothalamus. These orexinergic neurons make extensive projections both caudally into the brainstem arousal system and rostrally into the basal forebrain (➋ *Fig. 364.5*). In *postmortem* brains from patients with narcolepsy with cataplexy, an absence of orexin-expressing neurons has been noted. It has been hypothesized that orexins stabilize the transitions between REM and NREM sleep. Thus, loss of orexinergic signaling results in sleep-state instability with frequent and abrupt wake/REM transitions, sleep fragmentation, and the other associated symptoms of the disease. The underlying mechanisms of cataplexy remain controversial. Orexin levels in the cerebrospinal fluid (CSF) of patients with narcolepsy with cataplexy are severely reduced or undetectable. Importantly, individuals with narcolepsy *without* cataplexy have normal CSF orexin levels.

The diagnosis of narcolepsy is made on clinical grounds. Supporting tests of sleepiness such as the MSLT are recommended. A mean sleep latency of less than 8 min and presence of two or more sleep-onset REM periods on an MSLT is supportive of a diagnosis of narcolepsy. These values are not validated for children. Diagnosis can be difficult in the pediatric population, especially in young children. Misdiagnoses include laziness, attention-deficit, epilepsy, opposition-defiant disorder, depression, tics, and even psychosis.

Consolidation of nocturnal sleep and control of cataplexy are the treatment goals of narcolepsy therapy. Optimization of sleep hygiene is a required first step. Scheduled daytime naps can be remarkably helpful. Sleep-stabilizing medication such as sodium oxybate is increasingly used. Stimulants such as modafinil or amphetamine derivatives (e.g., methylphenidate or dextroamphetamine) can effectively offset daytime sleepiness and limit unwanted diurnal sleep bouts. Sodium oxybate (or g-hydroxybutyrate), a GABA-B receptor agonist, is approved for treatment of cataplexy and is also beneficial in sleep consolidation, daytime fatigue, and possibly hypnagogic hallucinations. Sodium oxybate is not approved for children; however, it has been used off-label. Cataplexy can be controlled with selective serotonin/noradrenaline reuptake transporters and their derivatives (e.g., venlafaxine) or with second-generation tricyclic antidepressants (e.g., clomipramine or desipramine).

Other causes of cataplexy. Niemann–Pick disease C, Prader–Willi Syndrome, and myotonic dystrophy can present with cataplexy and should be differentiated from idiopathic narcolepsy with cataplexy.

Other Hypersomnias

Idiopathic hypersomnia. Idiopathic hypersomnia is an incompletely defined disorder reserved for daytime sleepiness in the absence of cataplexy or identifiable cause; it is always a diagnosis of exclusion.

Kleine–Levin syndrome. This rare disorder is characterized by relapsing–remitting episodes of hypersomnia, cognitive disturbances, and behavioral disturbances usually of primal functions including hyperphagia and hypersexuality. Between episodes, sleep and wake behavior are normal. Hypersomnia episodes may last for a few days to several weeks. The cause of this syndrome remains obscure. Symptomatic cases of Kleine–Levin syndrome associated with structural brain lesions have been reported, but most cases are idiopathic. The syndrome is often linked to an antecedent respiratory illness of presumed viral origin.

Pediatric Parasomnias

Definitions

Parasomnias are defined as undesirable physical events or experiences that occur during entry into sleep, during sleep, or during arousals from sleep. They are classified as (1) disorders of arousals from non-rapid eye movement (NREM) sleep, (2) parasomnias associated with rapid eye movement (REM) sleep, and (3) other parasomnias.

Disorders of Arousal from NREM Sleep

Most disorders of arousals occur during slow wave sleep (SWS) during incomplete transitions into wakefulness, and are characterized by automatic behavior, altered perception of the environment, and variable degree of amnesia for the event. They tend to occur in the first third of the night when SWS is more prominent. The EEG during the episodes demonstrates an admixture of theta, delta, and alpha frequencies. They are felt to be due to a faulty switch that prevents normal sleep cycle progression. They are brought out by sleep deprivation, medications, noisy or stimulating environments, stress, fever, and sleep fragmentation due to obstructive sleep apnea (OSA) or periodic limb movements of sleep (PLMS). Several studies suggest a genetic predisposition to some of the arousal parasomnias.

Evaluation should include a complete description of the event, time of night when they happen, frequency of episodes, recollection of the event by the child, and presence during daytime naps. Information regarding whether the movements are rhythmic and stereotypical, associated with eye deviation, and focal tonic clonic activity may support an epileptic origin to the events. Examination should focus on looking for evidence of upper airway obstruction such as adeno-tonsillar hypertrophy, mid-facial hypoplasia, and retrognathia. In appropriate cases, a video-EEG may be indicated to rule out seizures. Overnight polysomnography is indicated when there is concern for an intrinsic sleep disorder like OSA or PLMS, rather than to document the parasomnia per se.

Management usually includes reassurance, securing the environment, voidance of known precipitants such as sleep deprivation, caffeinated drinks, and avoiding any attempts of restraining or awakening the child during the episode which may actually be counterproductive. Medications should be reserved for protracted cases with no associated sleep disorders, frequent events or those associated with a threat for injury. Low-dose clonazepam or tricyclic antidepressants for a short duration have been used with good success in such cases.

Sleep walking (somnambulism): Occurs in up to 17% of children, highest at 12–13 years of age, and with equal frequencies amongst males and females. It is further classified as calm or agitated subtype, with the former more common in children. The major concern during these benign behaviors is risk for injury.

Confusional arousals: Occur mainly in infants and toddlers, in up to 17.3% of the population. A typical event begins with moaning, evolving to confusion, and agitated behavior lasting 5–15 min. Attempts to wake up the child fully are unsuccessful.

Sleep Terrors: Occurs in 1–6% of children with peak frequency between 4 and 8 years of age. The child may sit up suddenly and scream with a blood-curdling battle cry. There is an expression of intense fear on the face and is accompanied with autonomic activation including mydriasis, tachycardia, and diaphoresis. Some children may report indistinct recollections of threat such as monsters, spiders, and snakes from which they have to defend themselves. In most cases, however, there is no recollection of the event. The event may last from a few minutes up to 20 min. Most cases go into a natural remission by adolescence.

Nocturnal seizures: Parasomnias must be differentiated from nocturnal seizures. Frontal lobe seizures are especially important since they occur predominantly in sleep, sometimes many times per night, and are characterized by stereotypical movements, thrashing of entire body, vocalizations, and dystonic posturing lasting 20 s to a few minutes with minimal postictal drowsiness or confusion. Paroxysmal nocturnal dystonia, which is now considered to be a frontal lobe seizure, is characterized by an arousal from NREM sleep, accompanied with dystonic posturing, bizarre movements of the extremities, and vocalization, with minimal EEG correlation due to a deep-seated focus of seizure onset in the mesial frontal region.

REM Parasomnias

Nightmares. These are characterized by vivid dreams in the second half of the night with intense feelings of terror or dread that typically awaken the child from sleep. The child can be easily aroused, with good recollection of the event. They are frequently seen between the ages of 3 and 6 years. Prevalence ranges from 30% to 90% for occasional and 5–30% for frequent episodes. In children, psychiatric disorders are seen more often in those experiencing nightmares than those without nightmares. They may also be a marker for a history of sexual abuse in children and adolescents.

REM sleep behavior disorder (RBD). This disorder is characterized by enacting of unpleasant and combative dreams with complex movements that can be vigorous and violent due to lack of REM sleep atonia. The disorder occurs more often in the sixth or seventh decade in males, and may precede onset of Parkinson's disease, or progressive supra-nuclear palsy. The disorder is uncommon in children, but may be seen in association with use of selective serotonin reuptake inhibitors like fluoxetine, or accompanying narcolepsy, and Tourette's syndrome. RBD responds very well to clonazepam given at bedtime.

Recurrent isolated sleep paralysis. This is characterized by a generalized inability to speak, or to move the trunk, head, and limbs that occur during the transitional period between sleep and wakefulness. The episodes are brief and transient, but may be accompanied with vivid hallucinations which make them very distressing. Usually seen with narcolepsy, they may be seen as an isolated form in otherwise healthy individuals, with a strong family history in some cases.

Sleep-related hallucinations. These are characterized as vivid dreams, or perceptions not based in reality, that occur at sleep onset (hypnagogic hallucinations) or on awakening (hypnopompic hallucinations) that occur in otherwise healthy individuals, but are frequent seen as part of the symptoms of narcolepsy. They may be visual, tactile, auditory, or kinetic in nature. They probably represent brief intrusion of REM sleep into NREM sleep or wakefulness.

Sleep-related enuresis. Nocturnal enuresis (bedwetting) refers to involuntary passage of urine while asleep. It occurs in almost 15–25% of children at 5 years of age, more often in boys, and in almost 1–3% of adolescents. It may be classified as primary (when present from birth) or secondary (with periods of at least 6 months of dryness prior to recurrence of enuresis) and nocturnal or diurnal. Three major pathological factors have been considered as possible etiologies: Group 1, volume dependent with polyuria; Group 2, detrussor dependent, with involuntary detrussor contractions, and small urinary bladder; Group 3, with decreased arousability. There are strong associations of enuresis with genetic and familial factors, and high prevalence of secondary enuresis in children with OSA. Treatment involves removal of inciting factors, reassurance, behavioral programs, and use of nasal desmopressin, or oral tricyclics like imipramine.

Exploding head syndrome. It is a harmless but potentially terrifying situation usually occurring while a patient is falling asleep, and is characterized by a terrifying loud noise, accompanied by myoclonic jerks, or the perception of a flash of light. Events are very brief. There is no headache or pain accompanying these episodes; and they can begin in childhood. No treatment is needed.

Sleep-related eating disorder. Usually seen accompanying sleep walking and daytime eating disorder, it is characterized by out-of-control eating binges, predominantly of carbohydrate-containing diets, 2–3 h after sleep onset, with no recall of the event subsequently. They can be seen to begin in childhood, but are more often seen in teenage years and adulthood. These behaviors have recently been described in association with use of hypnotics like zolpidem.

Catathrenia. Also called nocturnal groaning, this can occur in REM or NREM sleep during expiration in clusters of 2 min to an hour, ending with a snort, and accompanied with changes in heart rate. The onset may begin during childhood or adolescence. The exact etiology is unknown, and no specific therapy has been found to be effective.

Sleep starts. Also called hypnic jerks, these are sudden whole body jerks experienced by individuals during sleep–wake transition. Variations include sensory; auditory, including exploding tinnitus; and visual sensations, which may occur without the motor jerks. No treatment other than reassurance is necessary for them.

Sleep-sex disorders. Inappropriate sexual behavior occurring during sleep without conscious awareness has been reported in adults, with onset around adolescence in some cases.

Sleep-talking. Is very common in the general population, and can occur in REM or NREM sleep with a strong familial and genetic propensity.

Hypnic headaches. This is characterized by diffuse headache occurring 4–6 h after sleep onset at a consistent time, lasting 30–60 min, seen in older adults accompanied by nausea but no other autonomic features.

Rhythmic Movement Disorders of Sleep

Restless Legs Syndrome (RLS) and Periodic Limb Movements of Sleep (PLMS)

RLS is a common sensorimotor disorder of unclear cause characterized by (1) an urge to move the limbs often in association with an unpleasant sensation, (2) the urge to move is worse at night or occurs only at night, (3) the urge to move is present while at rest, and (4) the urge to move or unpleasant sensation is relieved by movement. Diagnosis can be extremely challenging in children. Periodic limb movements of sleep (PLMS), a related disorder, is diagnosed almost exclusively by 0.5–5 Hz limb movements seen during polysomnography and thus, most patients with PLMS are unaware of the presence of the movements (➲ *Fig. 364.8*). When PLMS is associated with sleep disturbance and daytime sleepiness, it is referred to as periodic limb movement disorder (PLMD). RLS and PLMS, like other disorders that potentially alter sleep quality and duration can have demonstrable impact on cognitive function, mood, neurological status, and quality of life. Primary RLS is idiopathic whereas secondary RLS has been associated with iron deficiency, pregnancy, end-stage renal disease, neuropathy, and certain medications.

Epidemiology. The prevalence in the pediatric population has been estimated at about 2% in 8–17 year olds in the United States and United Kingdom. Thus, RLS affects an estimated 984,000 of the school-age pediatric population in the United States. The prevalence of PLMS in children is unknown. While RLS and PLMS can exist independently of one another in the same individual, many patients with RLS also have PLMS.

Diagnosis. For children over the age of 12, adult definitions of RLS apply. Because of the difficulty of expressing sensory symptoms in younger children, modifications to the adult diagnostic criteria have been adopted (➲ *Table 364.2*).

Etiology and Associations. In children with confirmed RLS, a history of RLS in a biological parent can be found in more than 70%, suggesting that genetic factors may play a prominent causative role. Polymorphisms in at least four independent loci have been identified that confer increased risk of PLMS and/or RLS. Whether these polymorphisms will provide insight into the etiology and neuropathology of RLS is unclear. Both RLS and PLMS are associated with attention-deficit hyperactivity disorder (ADHD) and interestingly, all three disorders have been associated with iron deficiency, suggesting that iron metabolism may represent a common pathophysiological pathway. The prevalence of ADHD or ADHD symptoms in patients with RLS symptoms is 18–26% whereas the converse prevalence of RLS (or RLS symptoms) in patients with ADHD is 10.5–44%, again supportive of mechanistic overlap between these disorders.

Treatment. The primary treatment of RLS and PLMS are the dopaminergic agonists ropinirole and pramipexole; however, neither has been approved for use in children. Serum ferritin below 50 ng/mL has been associated with increased severity of RLS; furthermore, supplemental iron administration has demonstrated benefit in RLS.

Head banging. Also called *jactatio capitis nocturna*, it is now classified as a rhythmic movement disorder of sleep

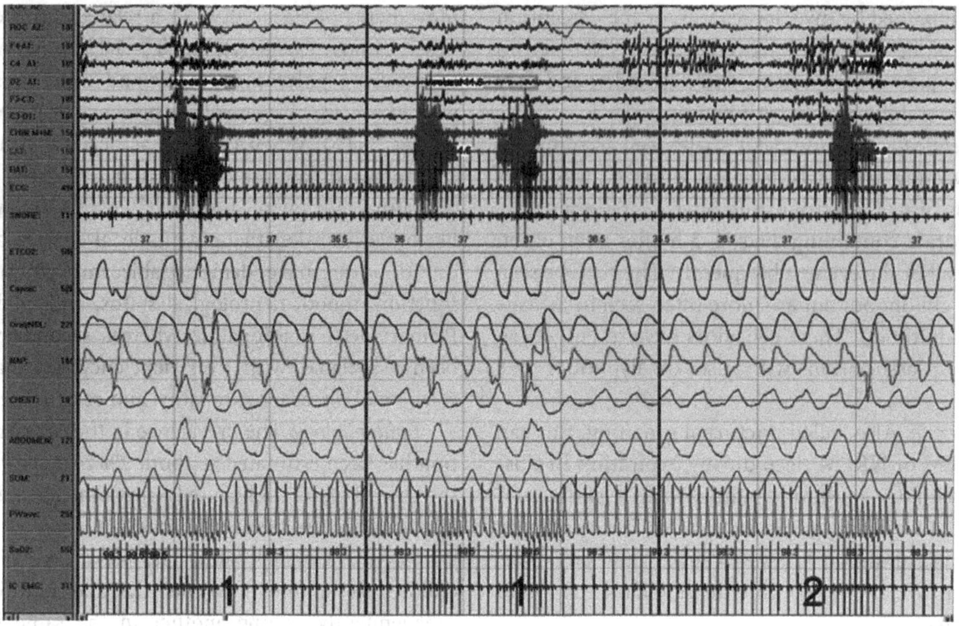

Figure 364.8
***Polysomnographic characteristics of periodic limb movements of sleep*. Note high amplitude paroxysmal activity of both legs lasting 1–2 s per movement**

Table 364.2
Criteria for making the diagnosis of definite RLS in children

1. The child meets all four essential adult criteria for RLS (the urge to move the legs, is worse during rest, relived by movement and worse during the evening and at night)
2. The child relates a description in his or her own words that is consistent with leg discomfort (the child may use terms such as "oowies," "tickle," "spiders," "boo-boos," "want to run," and "a lot of energy in my legs" to describe the symptoms. Age-appropriate descriptors are encouraged)
Or
1. The child meets all four essential adult criteria for RLS
2. Two of the three following supportive criteria are present
(a) Sleep disturbance for age
(b) A biologic parent or sibling has definite RLS
(c) The child has a polysomnographically documented periodic limb movement index of 5 or more per hour of sleep

and is characterized by rhythmic movements of head and body at sleep onset in infants and toddlers. It is seen more often in children with developmental disability and autism, but may be seen in normal children. No specific treatment other than reassurance is indicated.

Bruxism. The prevalence of bruxism (teeth grinding) is 14–17% in childhood, decreasing over the lifespan. Sleep-related bruxism without clear cause is termed primary, whereas secondary sleep-related bruxism may be associated with the use of psychoactive medications, recreational drugs or a variety of medical disorders. It can lead to abnormal wear of teeth, jaw muscle pain, or temporal headache. Dental examination and oral appliance may be indicated. The cause of bruxism is unknown; however, it may represent a motor manifestation of sleep-disordered breathing.

Sleep-Disordered Breathing: Obstructive Sleep Apnea

Obstructive sleep apnea syndrome (OSAS) was first reported in children over 30 years ago; however, it remains underdiagnosed despite strong evidence of increasing incidence. OSAS is a form of sleep-disordered breathing (SDB) that comprises one end of a spectrum of sleep-associated changes in upper airway resistance that in its most severe form constitutes recurrent hypoxia and subsequent arousals from sleep. OSAS is diagnosed on polysomnography by the presence of obstructive apneas (absence of airflow for at least two breaths) or hypopneas

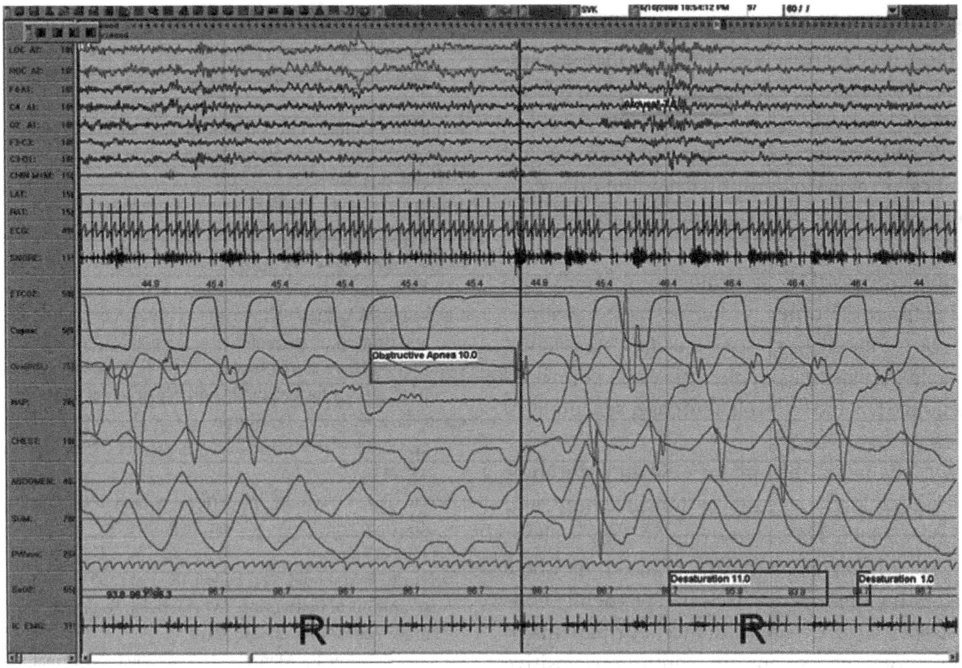

Figure 364.9

Polysomnographic characteristics of obstructive sleep apnea. Note diminution and then absence of oral thermistor (oral) and nasal air pressure (NAP) followed by an EEG arousal, brisk recovery breath, and delay of desaturation

(a greater than 30% reduction in baseline nasal airflow with an associated decrease in oxyhemoglobin saturation of at least 3%) and in children, an apnea-hypopnea index (AHI = (number of apneas + number of hypopneas)/total sleep time) of greater than one per hour (➋ *Fig. 364.9*). Recurrent respiratory effort–related arousals (RERAs; defined as a decrease in airflow without associated desaturation) occurring in the absence of frank hypopnea, apnea, or gas exchange abnormalities is referred to as upper airway resistance syndrome (UARS). UARS has been hypothesized to result from a decreased arousal threshold in relation to respiratory fluctuations during sleep.

Epidemiology. OSAS affects 2–3% of middle school children and as many as 13% of children aged 3–6 years. Importantly, the prevalence may be two- to fourfold higher in vulnerable populations: children with adenotonsillar hypertrophy, craniofacial anomalies, African-American race, preterm birth, and relatively low household income may have increased odds of having OSAS. In children, OSAS has been associated with adverse cardiovascular and metabolic outcomes: higher blood pressure, left ventricular hypertrophy, higher C-reactive protein, and increased insulin resistance. Whether these associations translate into increased risk of disease in adulthood remains unknown.

Symptoms. Symptoms of OSAS include snoring, mouth breathing, daytime sleepiness, frequent nocturnal arousals, and cognitive-behavior problems, especially attention-deficit, mood impairment, and poor school performance.

Pathophysiology. The pathophysiology of pediatric OSA includes neurophysiological, anatomical, and mechanical factors that conspire to increase upper airway resistance during sleep. Studies have demonstrated a correlation between the degree of airway narrowing and apnea-hypopnea index (AHI). Anatomic causes of upper airway narrowing such as adenotonsillar hypertrophy are the most common cause of pediatric OSA. Increased airway collapsibility during inspiration has been described in children with OSA suggesting either increased airway compliance or abnormal neuromuscular compensatory changes in pressure oscillation during sleep-associated breathing.

Obesity. Body mass index is among the strongest predictors of both presence and severity of OSAS in adults. Several studies have demonstrated that incremental increases in AHI correlate with increases in body mass index (BMI). Childhood overweight (>95% of BMI for age) and obesity are rising at an alarming rate with prevalence tripling over the past two decades. The Cleveland Family Study demonstrated a 4.6-fold increase in OSA in overweight children compared to normal weight children. This odds ratio may increase even further when adolescents age 13–16 years are considered as a separate cohort. The mechanisms by which obesity increases OSAS risk are likely multiple and may include impairment of airway and lung mechanics or velopalatal insufficiency and do not, in contrast to adults, appear to be related to parapharyngeal fat deposition.

Association with metabolic syndrome. Adolescents with obesity and SDB are 6.5 times as likely to have metabolic syndrome (a constellation of insulin resistance, dyslipidemia, hypertension, and obesity) when compared to those without SDB and controlled for age, sex, preterm status, and race.

Treatment. The initial therapy for OSA in both obese and non-obese children is surgical tonsillectomy and adenoidectomy (T&A). The success rate of T&A is about 85%; however, efficacy is markedly reduced in obese children suggesting that obesity itself independently contributes to sleep-related airway resistance. For patients in whom T&A do not resolve symptoms, continuous positive airway pressure (CPAP) delivered via a mask interface is extremely effective in stenting the airway. CPAP initiation can be difficult in certain children, especially those with neurodevelopmental disorders. Other therapies include oral appliances that advance the mandible, rapid maxillary expansion, and reconstructive surgeries such as maxillary mandibular advancement and uvulo-palato-pharyngioplasty.

Central sleep apnea. Central sleep apnea (CSA) is defined as the absence of airflow accompanied by a lack of effort to breath. CSA likely results from abnormal neurological control of breathing. CSA after the postnatal period should prompt investigation of central nervous system (CNS) causes including congenital causes (i.e., central alveolar hypoventilation syndrome), infection, structural lesions (e.g., Arnold–Chiari malformation, midline tumors, holoprosencephaly), or peripheral disorders such as myasthenia gravis or motor neuron disease (e.g., spinal muscular atrophy).

References

Allen RP, Picchietti D, Hening WA et al (2003) Restless legs syndrome: diagnostic criteria, special considerations, and epidemiology. A report from the restless legs syndrome diagnosis and epidemiology workshop at the National Institutes of Health. Sleep Med 4:101–119

American Academy of Sleep Medicine (2005) International classification of sleep disorders: diagnostic & coding manual, 2nd edn. American Academy of Sleep Medicine, Westchester

American Thoracic Society (1999) Cardiorespiratory sleep studies in children. Establishment of normative data and polysomnographic predictors of morbidity. Am J Respir Crit Care Med 160:1381–1387

Amin RS, Kimball TR, Kalra M et al (2005) Left ventricular function in children with sleep-disordered breathing. Am J Cardiol 95: 801–804

Arnulf I, Lin L, Gadoth N et al (2008) Kleine-Levin syndrome: a systematic study of 108 patients. Ann Neurol 63:482–493

Borbely AA (1982) A two process model of sleep regulation. Hum Neurobiol 1:195–204

Carskadon MA, Vieira C, Acebo C (1993) Association between puberty and delayed phase preference. Sleep 16:258–262

Carskadon MA, Acebo C, Jenni OG (2004) Regulation of adolescent sleep: implications for behavior. Ann NY Acad Sci 1021:276–291

Chemelli RM, Willie JT, Sinton CM et al (1999) Narcolepsy in orexin knockout mice: molecular genetics of sleep regulation. Cell 98: 437–451

Chervin RD, Dillon JE, Bassetti C et al (1997) Symptoms of sleep disorders, inattention, and hyperactivity in children. Sleep 20: 1185–1192

Chervin RD, Archbold KH, Dillon JE et al (2002) Associations between symptoms of inattention, hyperactivity, restless legs, and periodic leg movements. Sleep 25:213–218

Connor JR, Boyer PJ, Menzies SL et al (2003) Neuropathological examination suggests impaired brain iron acquisition in restless legs syndrome. Neurology 61:304–309

Czeisler CA, Richardson GS, Coleman RM et al (1981) Chronotherapy: resetting the circadian clocks of patients with delayed sleep phase insomnia. Sleep 4:1–21

Dahlitz M, Alvarez B, Vignau J et al (1991) Delayed sleep phase syndrome response to melatonin. Lancet 337:1121–1124

Dauvilliers Y, Arnulf I, Mignot E (2007) Narcolepsy with cataplexy. Lancet 369:499–511

Farber JM (2002) Clinical practice guideline: diagnosis and management of childhood obstructive sleep apnea syndrome. Pediatrics 110: 1255–1257, author reply 1255–1257

Fregosi RF, Quan SF, Kaemingk KL et al (2003) Sleep-disordered breathing, pharyngeal size and soft tissue anatomy in children. J Appl Physiol 95:2030–2038

Fricke-Oerkermann L, Pluck J, Schredl M et al (2007) Prevalence and course of sleep problems in childhood. Sleep 30:1371–1377

Fuller PM, Gooley JJ, Saper CB (2006) Neurobiology of the sleep-wake cycle: sleep architecture, circadian regulation, and regulatory feedback. J Biol Rhythms 21:482–493

Gozal D, Kheirandish-Gozal L (2007) Neurocognitive and behavioral morbidity in children with sleep disorders. Curr Opin Pulm Med 13:505–509

Gregory AM, Caspi A, Moffitt TE et al (2006) Family conflict in childhood: a predictor of later insomnia. Sleep 29:1063–1067

Guilleminault C, Eldridge FL, Simmons FB et al (1976) Sleep apnea in eight children. Pediatrics 58:23–30

Hibbs AM, Johnson NL, Rosen CL et al (2008) Prenatal and neonatal risk factors for sleep disordered breathing in school-aged children born preterm. J Pediatr 153:176–182

Ievers-Landis CE, Redline S (2007) Pediatric sleep apnea: implications of the epidemic of childhood overweight. Am J Respir Crit Care Med 175:436–441

Johnson EO, Roth T, Schultz L et al (2006) Epidemiology of DSM-IV insomnia in adolescence: lifetime prevalence, chronicity, and an emergent gender difference. Pediatrics 117:e247–e256

Kotagal S (2009) Parasomnias in childhood. Sleep Med Rev 13:157–168

Kotagal S, Silber MH (2004) Childhood-onset restless legs syndrome. Ann Neurol 56:803–807

Kryger MH, Roth T, Dement WC (eds) (2005) Principles and practice of sleep medicine. WB Saunders, Philadelphia

Kushida CA, Littner MR, Morgenthaler T et al (2005) Practice parameters for the indications for polysomnography and related procedures: an update for 2005. Sleep 28:499–521

Lin L, Faraco J, Li R et al (1999) The sleep disorder canine narcolepsy is caused by a mutation in the hypocretin (orexin) receptor 2 gene. Cell 98:365–376

Liu X, Liu L, Owens JA et al (2005) Sleep patterns and sleep problems among schoolchildren in the United States and China. Pediatrics 115:241–249

Lumeng JC, Somashekar D, Appugliese D et al (2007) Shorter sleep duration is associated with increased risk for being overweight at ages 9 to 12 years. Pediatrics 120:1020–1029

Marcus CL, Omlin KJ, Basinki DJ et al (1992) Normal polysomnographic values for children and adolescents. Am Rev Respir Dis 146: 1235–1239

Montgomery-Downs HE, O'Brien LM, Gulliver TE et al (2006) Polysomnographic characteristics in normal preschool and early school-aged children. Pediatrics 117:741–753

Moore M, Allison D, Rosen CL (2006) A review of pediatric nonrespiratory sleep disorders. Chest 130:1252–1262

Morgenthaler T, Alessi C, Friedman L et al (2007) Practice parameters for the use of actigraphy in the assessment of sleep and sleep disorders: an update for 2007. Sleep 30:519–529

Neuberger HR, Bohm M, Mewis C (2006) Sleep apnea and heart disease. N Engl J Med 354:1086–1089, author reply 1086–1089

Nixon GM, Thompson JM, Han DY et al (2008) Short sleep duration in middle childhood: risk factors and consequences. Sleep 31:71–78

O'Brien LM, Gozal D (2004) Neurocognitive dysfunction and sleep in children: from human to rodent. Pediatr Clin N Am 51:187–202

O'Brien LM, Holbrook CR, Mervis CB et al (2003) Sleep and neurobehavioral characteristics of 5- to 7-year-old children with parentally reported symptoms of attention-deficit/hyperactivity disorder. Pediatrics 111:554–563

O'Brien LM, Mervis CB, Holbrook CR et al (2004a) Neurobehavioral implications of habitual snoring in children. Pediatrics 114:44–49

O'Brien LM, Mervis CB, Holbrook CR et al (2004b) Neurobehavioral correlates of sleep-disordered breathing in children. J Sleep Res 13: 165–172

Owens JA (2001) The practice of pediatric sleep medicine: results of a community survey. Pediatrics 108:E51

Owens JA, Spirito A, McGuinn M et al (2000) Sleep habits and sleep disturbance in elementary school-aged children. J Dev Behav Pediatr 21:27–36

Owens JA, Rosen CL, Mindell JA (2003) Medication use in the treatment of pediatric insomnia: results of a survey of community-based pediatricians. Pediatrics 111:e628–e635

Picchietti DL, Stevens HE (2008) Early manifestations of restless legs syndrome in childhood and adolescence. Sleep Med 9:770–781

Picchietti D, Allen RP, Walters AS et al (2007) Restless legs syndrome: prevalence and impact in children and adolescents–the Peds REST study. Pediatrics 120:253–266

Redline S, Tishler PV, Schluchter M et al (1999) Risk factors for sleep-disordered breathing in children. Associations with obesity, race, and respiratory problems. Am J Respir Crit Care Med 159:1527–1532

Redline S, Storfer-Isser A, Rosen CL et al (2007) Association between metabolic syndrome and sleep-disordered breathing in adolescents. Am J Respir Crit Care Med 176:401–408

Rosen CL, Larkin EK, Kirchner HL et al (2003) Prevalence and risk factors for sleep-disordered breathing in 8- to 11-year-old children: association with race and prematurity. J Pediatr 142:383–389

Rosenthal NE, Joseph-Vanderpool JR, Levendosky AA et al (1990) Phase-shifting effects of bright morning light as treatment for delayed sleep phase syndrome. Sleep 13:354–361

Sack RL, Brandes RW, Kendall AR et al (2000) Entrainment of free-running circadian rhythms by melatonin in blind people. N Engl J Med 343:1070–1077

Saper CB, Chou TC, Scammell TE (2001) The sleep switch: hypothalamic control of sleep and wakefulness. Trends Neurosci 24:726–731

Saper CB, Scammell TE, Lu J (2005) Hypothalamic regulation of sleep and circadian rhythms. Nature 437:1257–1263

Schormair B, Kemlink D, Roeske D et al (2008) PTPRD (protein tyrosine phosphatase receptor type delta) is associated with restless legs syndrome. Nat Genet 40:946–948

Sheldon SH, Ferber R, Kryger MH (eds) (2005) Principles and practice of pediatric sleep medicine. Saunders, Philadelphia

Simakajornboon N, Gozal D, Vlasic V et al (2003) Periodic limb movements in sleep and iron status in children. Sleep 26:735–738

Smaldone A, Honig JC, Byrne MW (2007) Sleepless in America: inadequate sleep and relationships to health and well-being of our nation's children. Pediatrics 119(Suppl 1):S29–S37

Stefansson H, Rye DB, Hicks A et al (2007) A genetic risk factor for periodic limb movements in sleep. N Engl J Med 357:639–647

Stein MA, Mendelsohn J, Obermeyer WH et al (2001) Sleep and behavior problems in school-aged children. Pediatrics 107:E60

Stradling JR, Thomas G, Warley AR et al (1990) Effect of adenotonsillectomy on nocturnal hypoxaemia, sleep disturbance, and symptoms in snoring children. Lancet 335:249–253

Tasali E, Ip MS (2008) Obstructive sleep apnea and metabolic syndrome: alterations in glucose metabolism and inflammation. Proc Am Thorac Soc 5:207–217

Tauman R, O'Brien LM, Ivanenko A et al (2005) Obesity rather than severity of sleep-disordered breathing as the major determinant of insulin resistance and altered lipidemia in snoring children. Pediatrics 116:e66–e73

Tauman R, Gulliver TE, Krishna J et al (2006) Persistence of obstructive sleep apnea syndrome in children after adenotonsillectomy. J Pediatr 149:803–808

The international classification of sleep disorders, 2. (eds) (2006) American Academy of Sleep Medicine, Westchester

Toh KL, Jones CR, He Y et al (2001) An hPer2 phosphorylation site mutation in familial advanced sleep phase syndrome. Science 291:1040–1043

Watanabe T, Kajimura N, Kato M et al (2003) Sleep and circadian rhythm disturbances in patients with delayed sleep phase syndrome. Sleep 26:657–661

Winkelmann J, Schormair B, Lichtner P et al (2007) Genome-wide association study of restless legs syndrome identifies common variants in three genomic regions. Nat Genet 39:1000–1006

Xu Y, Padiath QS, Shapiro RE et al (2005) Functional consequences of a CKIdelta mutation causing familial advanced sleep phase syndrome. Nature 434:640–644

Zintzaras E, Kaditis AG (2007) Sleep-disordered breathing and blood pressure in children: a meta-analysis. Arch Pediatr Adolesc Med 161:172–178

Kotagal S (2009) Parasomnias in childhood. Sleep Med Rev 13:1[illegible]
Kotagal S, Silber MH (2004) Childhood-onset restless legs syndrome. Ann Neurol 56:803–807
[illegible] Dement [illegible] (2005) [illegible] and [illegible] Saunders [illegible]
[illegible] (2005) Practice parameters [illegible] for [illegible] polysomnography and related procedures [illegible] Sleep [illegible]
[illegible] The sleep disorder [illegible]
[illegible] [illegible]–376
[illegible] Owens [illegible] School [illegible] 1132(4)–249
[illegible] Rosen [illegible] review [illegible]
[illegible]

Redline S, [illegible] A, Rosen CL et al (20[illegible]) [illegible] between [illegible] sleep-disordered breathing in adolescents. Am J Respir Crit Care Med 1[illegible]:401–[illegible]
Rosen [illegible] (2003) Prevalence and risk factors for [illegible] sleep-disordered breathing in 8- to 11-year-old children [illegible] Pediatr 142:[illegible]
Rosenthal [illegible] Am J [illegible] Sleep [illegible] for delayed sleep phase syndrome. Sl[illegible]
Sack RL, Brandes RW, Kendall AR et al (2000) Entrainment of free-running circadian rhythms by melatonin in blind people. N Engl J Med 343:1070–1077
Saper CB, Chou TC, Scammell TE (2001) The sleep switch: hypothalamic control of sleep and wakefulness. Trends Neurosci 24:726–731
Saper CB, Scammell TE, Lu J (2005) Hypothalamic regulation of sleep and circadian rhythms. Nature 437:1257–1263
[illegible]
Stores [illegible] N Engl J Med [illegible]
[illegible]

365 Coma

David J. Michelson · Stephen Ashwal

Case History

A woman left her house at 1:45 pm to go shopping, leaving her 11-month-old son in the care of her two teenaged children. An hour later her 16-year-old son called her in a panic, crying that his "little brother is dead." Paramedics were called and arrived within 4 min to find the little boy pulseless and apneic. The boy's 15-year-old sister explained that she had found him with his head in a bucket she had been using to mop the floors. The paramedics started chest compressions and mask ventilation with 100% oxygen. They transported the boy to a nearby emergency room, where he was intubated and given three successive intravenous doses of epinephrine. A spontaneous pulse was first recovered after 35 min of resuscitation. His temperature was 90°F (32°C), his pupils were fixed and dilated, and he had no corneal or gag reflex or facial grimace to pain. His first arterial blood gas showed a pH of 6.72 and a base deficit of 31 mEq/L, and he was given multiple boluses of normal saline and bicarbonate. He had episodes of body stiffening that were concerning for seizures and was given an intravenous loading dose of phenobarbital and transferred to a tertiary care center for further management. His initial head CT showed mild cerebral edema (➋ *Fig. 365.1*). He was weaned off of mechanical ventilation and from all sedating medications, but he continued to lie in bed with his eyes closed, unresponsive to voice, with only flexion of the right arm with noxious compression of the sternum. His pupils were minimally reactive to light, and he had brisk oculocephalic reflexes, but his eyes were disconjugate at rest, and he demonstrated no visual tracking. Magnetic resonance imaging of the brain done on the fifth day of hospitalization showed brightness on diffusion and T-2 weighted images bilaterally in the thalami, basal ganglia, and subcortical white matter (➋ *Figs. 365.2–365.4*). Magnetic resonance spectroscopy showed N-acetyl aspartate to creatine ratios more than four standard deviations below the mean for age in cortical and subcortical gray matter and a small amount of lactate in the occipital gray matter (➋ *Figs. 365.5* and ➋ *365.6*). At the parents' request, the boy had a gastrostomy tube placed, and he was discharged 2 months later to their care in a condition best described as a coma due to a severe global hypoxic-ischemic brain injury.

Definition/Classification

Coma is a disease state of persistent unconsciousness that derives from the ancient Greek word for deep sleep. Patients may *awaken* from coma into normal consciousness or into other pathological states of altered or depressed consciousness, but this awakening does not occur in response to external stimuli of any kind. In coma, dysfunction of the brain prevents the generation of arousal and awareness, the two necessary components of full consciousness. The severe metabolic and structural injuries capable of causing coma carry a high risk of death and severe long-term neurological disability.

A patient who is fully conscious demonstrates both arousal or wakefulness and awareness of both their internal states, such as hunger, thirst, and pain, and their external world, such as it comes to them through visual, auditory, tactile, olfactory, or gustatory stimulation. Patients who are said to be *falling into* a coma show gradually decreasing levels of awareness, attention, and arousal, such that increasingly intense stimulation is required for them to show any response as they become lethargic, stuporous, and obtunded, and finally, comatose.

Most patients are only comatose for a short time, typically a period of several days to weeks, before either dying from their medical problems or beginning to show signs of improvement. When improvement occurs in arousal alone, with patients regaining spontaneous eye-opening and sleep–wake cycles but lacking clear signs of awareness of their internal or external state, purposeful action, or communicative ability, the condition is described as a *vegetative state.* If awareness partially recovers but is insufficient for consistent communication, a patient may be described as being in a *minimally conscious state.* Some patients recover from coma dramatically, passing quickly from lower to higher levels of function. Other patients remain in a prolonged or *permanent* vegetative or minimally conscious state.

Abdelaziz Y. Elzouki (ed.), *Textbook of Clinical Pediatrics*, DOI 10.1007/978-3-642-02202-9_365,

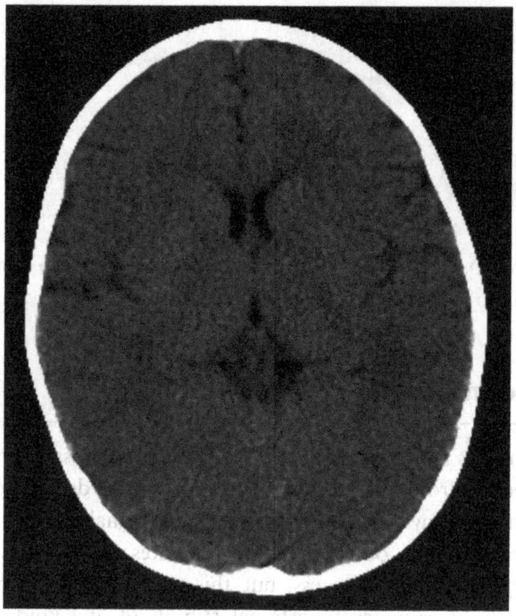

Figure 365.1
Eight hours after an 11-month-old boy suffered cardiopulmonary arrest, computed tomography showed loss of the distinction between the cortical gray and subcortical white matter with relative hypodensity of the supratentorial structures, suggesting bihemispheric cerebral edema

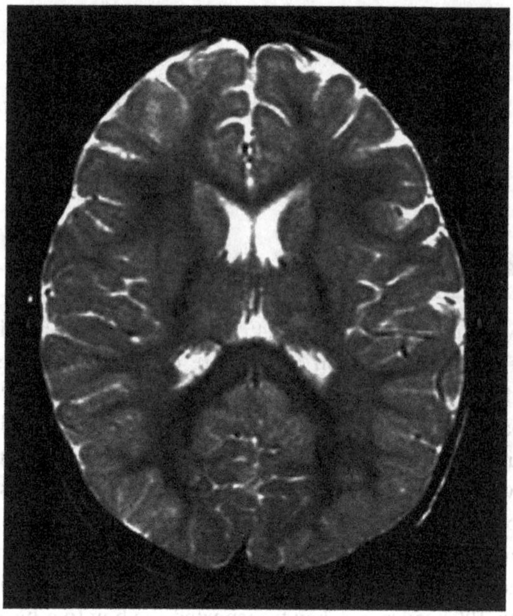

Figure 365.2
Five days after an 11-month-old boy suffered cardiopulmonary arrest, magnetic resonance imaging showed brightness on T2 weighted (***Fig. 365.2*****) and diffusion weighted (** ***Fig. 365.2*****) axial sequences and darkness on the apparent diffusion coefficient map (** ***Fig. 365.3*****) within the bilateral subcortical white matter, corpus callosum, basal ganglia, and thalami, consistent with diffuse hypoxic-ischemic injury**

Other disorders of consciousness include *delirium*, in which arousal may be heightened or depressed but in which attention and awareness fluctuate rapidly, and *akinetic-mutism*, in which arousal may be normal, but patients demonstrate minimal signs of attention and awareness only intermittently. The *locked-in syndrome* is often discussed with disorders of consciousness because it can mimic coma in many ways. Patients in a locked-in state are fully awake and aware but have motor impairments that make it difficult or impossible for them to demonstrate this on examination. Patients with psychiatric illnesses such as depression and schizophrenia may present with *catatonia* or *pseudocoma*, demonstrating dramatically reduced voluntary behavior and responsiveness, although they maintain normal consciousness and lack any structural or metabolic disturbance of brain function.

Brain death is also frequently discussed in association with coma. It was initially described by French physicians as a *state beyond coma* in which all signs of consciousness and all brainstem reflexes, including the respiratory drive, are irrevocably destroyed by injury. In most countries, this has come to be accepted as an alternative to cardiorespiratory arrest for defining the end of life. The major distinctions between the disorders of consciousness are outlined in *Table 365.1* and the differences between the vegetative and minimally conscious states are outlined in *Table 365.2.*

Etiology

Arousal is initiated and sustained by a complex neuronal network that widely distributes multiple sensory and circadian inputs to the cerebral cortex. Awareness and full consciousness likely arise from the integrated processing of this input in the polymodal association areas of the cortex. Coma can occur with relatively small structural injuries to the brainstem, more widespread cortical or subcortical injuries to both cerebral hemispheres, or diffuse metabolic disturbances that cause generalized impairment of neuronal function.

There are four main anatomical structures involved in the generation of arousal: the brainstem, thalamus, basal forebrain, and hypothalamus. Within the brainstem, the

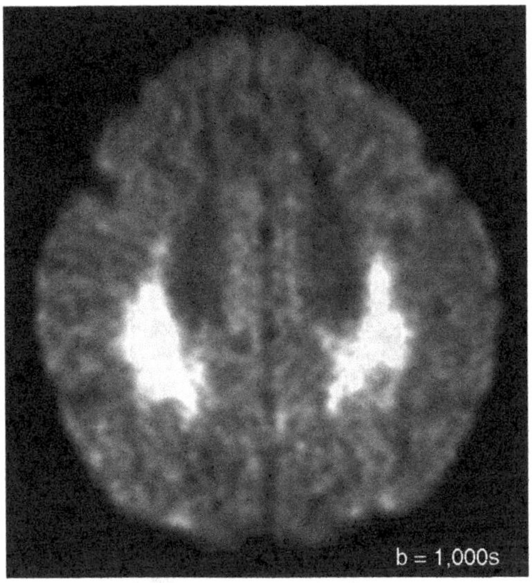

Figure 365.3
Five days after an 11-month-old boy suffered cardiopulmonary arrest, magnetic resonance imaging showed brightness on T2 weighted (*Fig. 365.2*) and diffusion weighted (*Fig. 365.2*) axial sequences and darkness on the apparent diffusion coefficient map (*Fig. 365.3*) within the bilateral subcortical white matter, corpus callosum, basal ganglia, and thalami, consistent with diffuse hypoxic-ischemic injury

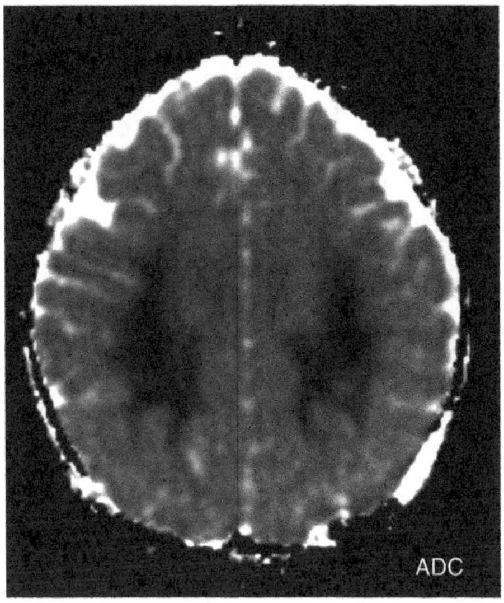

Figure 365.4
Five days after an 11-month-old boy suffered cardiopulmonary arrest, magnetic resonance imaging showed brightness on T2 weighted (*Fig. 365.2*) and diffusion weighted (*Fig. 365.2*) axial sequences and darkness on the apparent diffusion coefficient map (*Fig. 365.3*) within the bilateral subcortical white matter, corpus callosum, basal ganglia, and thalami, consistent with diffuse hypoxic-ischemic injury

ascending activating system (AAS) composed of excitatory glutamatergic neurons within the upper pontine and lower midbrain tectum relays a variety of stimuli along two pathways, the first to the thalamus and the second to the basal forebrain. Other structures and neurotransmitters from the brainstem, the pedunculopontine tegmental and laterodorsal nuclei (acetylcholine), locus ceruleus (noradrenaline), midline raphe nuclei (serotonin), and substantia nigra pars compacta (dopamine) modify arousal through both cortical and subcortical (thalamus, basal forebrain, and striatum) connections.

The thalamus participates in the generation of arousal through circuits which relay specific sensory inputs to the cortex and through nonspecific output from midline, medial, and intralaminar nuclei. The basal forebrain arousal system consists of the nucleus basalis of Maynert, the substantia innominata, the diagonal band of Broca, the magnocellular preoptic nucleus, the medium septum, and the globus pallidus. These structures receive input from the brainstem and hypothalamus and assist in the maintenance of the waking state via cholinergic excitation of the thalamus and cortex.

The hypothalamus contains histaminergic nuclei, predominantly in the tuberomammilary and posterior regions, which influence the activity of basal forebrain and thalamocortical neurons. The periforniceal and lateral areas of the hypothalamus contain neurons that secrete orexins (hypocretins), which not only influence nearby histaminergic, noradrenergic, and serotonergic neurons but also have widespread arousal-promoting connections throughout the cerebral cortex.

The functional correlates of altered consciousness have been examined through advanced imaging studies of cerebral metabolism in conditions of physiologic (sleep), pharmacologic (anesthesia), and pathologic unconsciousness. The most consistent change across etiologies is the deactivation of the polymodal association cortices, including the bilateral lateral frontal, medial frontal, parietotemporal, posterior parietal, precuneal, and posterior cingulate areas. The posterior cingulate in particular shows early and dramatically decreased metabolism in unconsciousness, even beyond that seen in the thalamus, and it has the highest basal metabolism in normal conscious wakefulness.

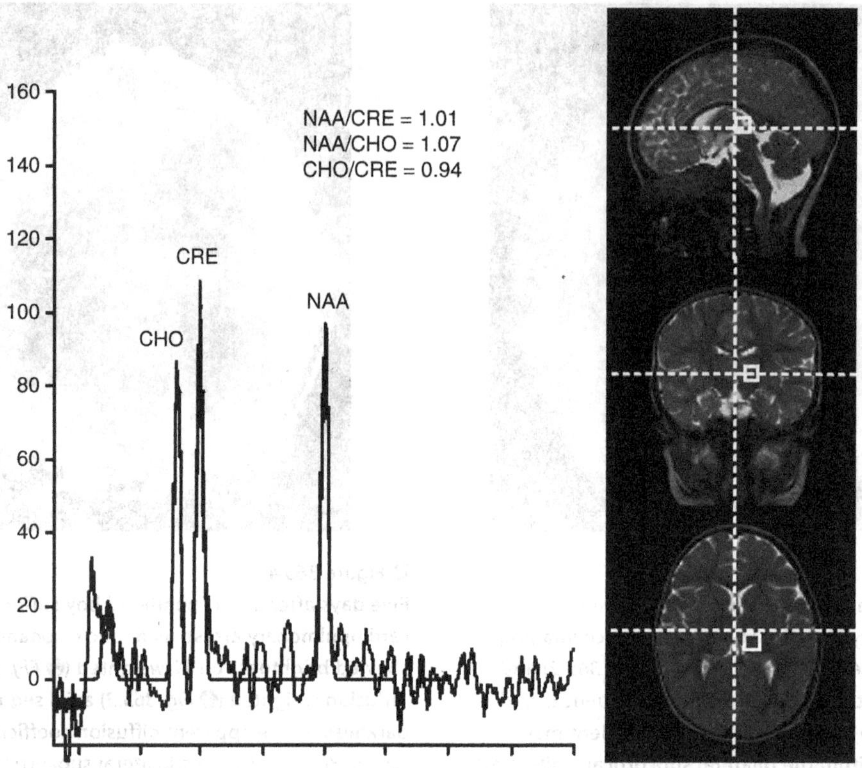

Figure 365.5
Five days after an 11-month-old boy suffered cardiopulmonary arrest, magnetic resonance spectroscopy showed NAA/Cr ratios more than four standard deviations below the mean in the occipital gray matter (*Fig. 365.5*) and left thalamus (*Fig. 365.6*). A small lactate peak was also discernible in the occipital cortex, consistent with the injury being due to ischemia

In most cases of coma, such as those resulting from severe traumatic brain injury, global hypoxic ischemic injury, or the progression of a previously known disease state, the etiology is clear from the initial history and physical examination. An unexplained coma is a true medical emergency and such patients require immediate testing for treatable causes. A listing of broad categories for the etiology of coma, along with subcategories and specific examples, is given in *Table 365.3.*

Epidemiology

In the United States, coma has a yearly incidence of approximately 60 per 100,000 children, and cases are fairly evenly divided between traumatic and non-traumatic causes of brain injury. A prospective, population-based study of non-traumatic coma in the United States from 2001 found that infection was responsible for 38% of pediatric cases, with *Neiserria meningitidis* being the most commonly identified organism. Toxic ingestions, both accidental and non-accidental, were responsible for 10% of all cases and for 35% of cases among adolescents. Seizures, congenital heart disease, brain malformations, accidental drowning, diabetes, and inborn errors of metabolism were among the other common etiologies of non-traumatic coma in children. A smaller but more recent study from India also found infection to be the most common cause of pediatric non-traumatic coma. Sixty percent of cases were attributed to infections and *Mycobacterium tuberculosis* was the most commonly identified organism.

In their now landmark study from 1984 of 500 adults with coma of initially unknown cause, Plum and Posner found that 65% had diffuse metabolic causes, usually from poisonings and intoxications. They also found that 20% had supratentorial mass lesions, including 77 hemorrhages and 9 infarctions, and that 13% had infratentorial lesions, which were mainly brainstem infarctions. Eight of their patients had psychiatric pseudocoma.

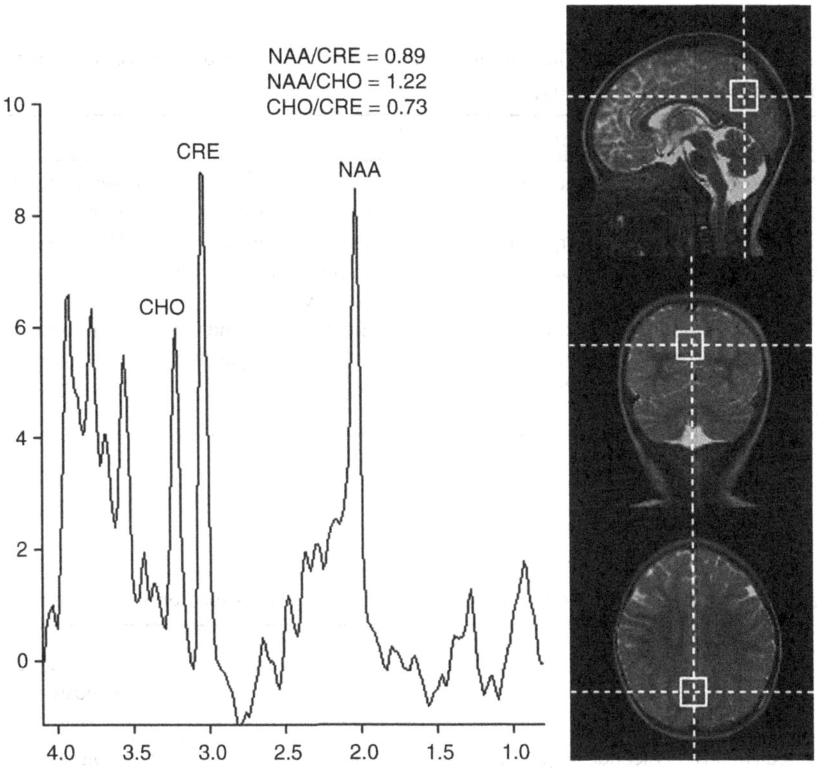

Figure 365.6
Five days after an 11-month-old boy suffered cardiopulmonary arrest, magnetic resonance spectroscopy showed NAA/Cr ratios more than four standard deviations below the mean in the occipital gray matter (***Fig. 365.5*** **) and left thalamus (** ***Fig. 365.6*** **). A small lactate peak was also discernible in the occipital cortex, consistent with the injury being due to ischemia**

Table 365.1
Disorders of consciousness. The disorders of consciousness discussed in the text are differentiated from normal by the degree to which arousal, awareness, and motor function are impaired

Condition	Arousal	Awareness	Motor function
Normal consciousness	Normal	Normal	Normal
Locked-in syndrome	Normal	Normal	Low to absent
Akinetic-mutism	Normal	Low	Intermittent
Delirium	High or low	Low	High or low
Lethargy	Mildly low	Mildly low	Mildly low
Stupor	Moderately low	Moderately low	Moderately low
Obtundation	Severely low	Severely low	Severely low
Coma	Absent	Absent	Low
Vegetative state	Variable	Absent	Low
Minimal consciousness	Variable	Low	Low
Brain death	Absent	Absent	Absent

Table 365.2
Vegetative and minimally conscious states. The diagnostic criteria for these disorders of consciousness have been put forward by the American Academy of Neurology

Vegetative state	Minimally conscious state
No evidence of self- or environmental awareness, with demonstration of all of the following: • No evidence of sustained, reproducible, purposeful, or voluntary behavioral responses to visual, auditory, tactile, or noxious stimuli • No evidence of language comprehension or expression • Intermittent wakefulness occurring with sleep–wake cycles • Sufficiently preserved autonomic function to survive with supportive care	Limited but reproducible evidence of self- or environmental awareness, demonstrated by one of the following: • Purposeful movements or affect expressions in response to relevant environmental stimuli that are not purely reflexive • Simple command following, gestural or verbal yes/no responses (regardless of accuracy), or intelligible verbalization

Table 365.3
Etiologies for coma. Broadly defined etiologic categories for coma, along with subcategories and specific examples

Category	Subcategory	Examples
Non-structural	External toxins	Carbon monoxide, cyanide, ethylene glycol, lead, methanol, mushrooms, thallium
	Medications	Alcohol, amphetamines, anticholinergics, antipsychotics, barbituates, bromides, lithium, monoamine oxidase inhibitors, opioids, paraldehyde, phencyclidine, salicylates, sedative hypnotics
	Organ failure	Hyper- or hypocalcemia, cortisolism, glycemia, natremia, tension, thermia, or thyroidism; hyperammonemia, hypercapnea, hypoxia, ketoacidosis, porphyria, uremia, Wernicke encephalopathy
	Infections	Cerebral malaria, encephalitis, meningitis, post-infectious encephalitis, sepsis, syphilis, typhoid fever
	Other	Postictal state
Structural – symmetrical	Supratentorial	Bilateral anterior cerebral or carotid artery occlusion, hydrocephalus, thalamic hemorrhages, traumatic brain injury
	Infratentorial	Basilar artery occlusion, midline brainstem tumor, pontine hemorrhage
Structural – asymmetrical	Supratentorial	Acute disseminated encephalomyelitis, adrenoleukodystrophy, cerebral abscess, cerebral vasculitis, chemotherapy-related leukoencephalopathy, Creutzfeldt–Jakob disease, disseminated intravascular coagulation, fat embolization, hemispheric mass (tumor, bleed, and abscess) with herniation, intracerebral bleeds, massive or bilateral infarctions, progressive multifocal leukoencephalopathy, multiple sclerosis, nonbacterial thrombotic (marantic) endocarditis, pituitary apoplexy, subacute bacterial endocarditis, thrombophlebitis, thrombotic thrombocytopenic purpura
	Infratentorial	Brainstem hemorrhage, brainstem infarction

Clinical Evaluation

The initial assessment and management of a comatose patient should address the adequacy of basic life support functions, ensuring that the patient has a patent airway and adequate respiration, oxygenation, and circulation.

Patients with an altered level of consciousness can aspirate oral secretions and thus may require prophylactic intubation and ventilation even when the underlying cause of their coma has not otherwise compromised their respiratory function. Patients with a traumatic or unknown cause of coma should be assumed to have a spinal cord injury until proven otherwise and treated with appropriate spinal precautions. Initial measurement of blood sugar as well as repeated measurements of the vital signs, including temperature, arterial blood gas determination (hypoxia, hypercarbia), blood pressure, heart rate, and respiratory rate, aid in the diagnosis and avoidance of correctable causes of further injury. Some patients will require urgent medical or surgical interventions before they are stable enough for a detailed neurodiagnostic evaluation.

All patients should be given high concentrations of supplemental oxygen until continuous oxygen saturation monitoring is possible. In patients with known diabetes, coma of unknown etiology, or measured hypoglycemia (less than 60 mg/dL), treatment with supplemental glucose is warranted. A 0.5 g/kg intravenous bolus of dextrose should be given using a 10% solution in neonates, a 25% solution in children under 30 kg, and a 50% solution in larger children. Unlike adult patients, who may have unrecognized chronic malnutrition, children do not require intravenous thiamine prior to receiving intravenous dextrose to prevent Wernicke encephalopathy. The benefits of treating coma due to hypoglycemia outweigh any theoretical drawback of giving supplemental glucose to patients with anoxic or ischemic brain injury. Diabetics with hypoglycemia should also be given a 0.1 mg/kg (maximum 1 mg) intravenous dose of glucagon.

Intravenous naloxone hydrochloride should be given to patients with coma of unknown etiology at a dose of 0.1 mg/kg (maximum 2 mg) to reverse possible accidental or intentional opioid toxicity. Most children are at little risk for the severe withdrawal effects, which can be precipitated by naloxone use in patients with established opioid dependence.

A detailed and systematic general physical examination, done once the patient has been stabilized, can help determine the underlying cause of coma. The sections that follow review some of the more important considerations.

Vital Signs

Hypotension will cause loss of consciousness when the mean arterial blood pressure drops below levels for which cerebral autoregulation can maintain adequate cerebral blood flow. Hypotension may result from shock, poisoning, or damage to the medullary pressor center. Hypotension due to hypovolemia, whether from dehydration or hemorrhage, is associated with peripheral vasoconstriction and cool extremities. Hypotension due to septic shock and Addisonian crisis is associated with peripheral vasodilation and warm extremities.

Severe hypertension will overwhelm the autoregulatory capacity of cerebral blood vessels and lead to vasogenic edema and hemorrhagic infarction. Hypertension may be seen with renal disease, poisoning, or as an adaptive response to any cause of increased intracranial pressure (ICP). The Kocher–Cushing reflex response to increased ICP, frequently referred to as *Cushing's triad*, consists of hypertension, bradycardia, and irregular respirations and is caused by compression or ischemia of the medullary pressor center.

Bradycardia can also be seen with myocardial injury and with poisonings, such as with beta-blockers or cholinergic agonists. Tachycardia may result from hypotension, hyperthyroid storm, fever, anemia, hypoxia, and poisoning with stimulants and anticholinergics.

Respiratory depression can be seen with poisonings and with carbon dioxide retention from impaired pulmonary gas exchange. Tachypnea can be seen with hypoxia, fever, and various causes of metabolic acidosis, including sepsis, diabetic ketoacidosis, renal failure, hepatic failure, and poisonings with such substances as methanol, ethylene glycol, paraldehyde, and salicylates. Damage to the basal forebrain, thalami, or hypothalamus may result in *Cheyne-Stokes respirations*, with slowly alternating hypoventilation and hyperventilation. The emergence of such a respiratory pattern in a comatose patient may be an early sign of central herniation.

Other abnormal respiratory patterns can be seen with brainstem injuries and can be seen sequentially during central herniation. Damage to the low midbrain ventral to the aqueduct of Sylvius or of the upper pons ventral to the fourth ventricle can cause *central neurogenic hyperventilation*. Hyperventilation in comatose patients is far more commonly caused by compensation for metabolic acidosis or hypoxia. Metabolic acidosis, such as with diabetic ketoacidosis, can cause *Kussmaul breathing*, with deep, regular respirations. Lesions of the dorsolateral tegmentum of the middle and caudal pons medulla may cause *apneustic breathing*, in which the patient breathes inward quickly, pausing at full inspiration. *Cluster breathing* shows great variability in the pauses between breaths and can be seen with lower pontine tegmental lesions. Progressively irregular respiratory rate and rhythm may be referred to as *ataxic or agonal breathing*, seen with damage to the reticular formation of the dorsomedial medulla, at times immediately prior to the onset of complete apnea.

Fever may occur as a result of subarachnoid hemorrhage, intraparenchymal hemorrhage, or hypothalamic injury. Fever can also result from heatstroke, thyroid storm, and from poisonings such as with anticholinergic toxicity, neuroleptic malignant syndrome, or serotonin syndrome. Shivering without sweating is suggestive of fever of neurologic or toxic etiology. However, fever is usually a sign of infection and, in a comatose patient, it should prompt consideration of a diagnosis of meningitis or encephalitis, whether or not meningismus is present. Fever may be absent when infection occurs in young infants or in the setting of renal failure, hypothyroidism, or immunocompromise. Empirical use of broad spectrum intravenous antibiotics at meningitic doses is preferable to waiting for the results of cerebrospinal fluid (CSF) testing by lumbar puncture. In patients with altered consciousness or any focal neurological disturbance, use of computed tomography (CT) of the brain is favored, if available, to look a supratentorial mass lesion that might lead to the lumbar puncture precipitating downward transtentorial herniation and brainstem compression.

Hypothermia is usually due to cold exposure but can also be caused by sepsis, hypothyroid coma, hypopituitarism, Wernicke encephalopathy, lesions of the posterior hypothalamus, and poisonings such as with barbiturate overdose. Hypothermia is more likely to be due to a neurological cause in patients who are sweating but not shivering. Several well-described toxidromes are summarized in ➋ *Table 365.4*.

Head, Eyes, Ears, Nose, Throat, and Neck

The head and neck examination may reveal occult signs of trauma, such as scalp laceration, scalp edema or hematoma, or depressed skull fracture. Anterior basal skull fracture may cause bruising around the orbits (*raccoon eyes*) and temporal bone fracture may cause bruising over the mastoid portion of the bone (*Battle's sign*) but these findings may first appear several days after injury. Signs of meningismus, including nuchal rigidity, may be masked by coma but generally indicate meningeal irritation, which can occur with meningitis, inflammation of surrounding structures (e.g., retropharyngeal abscess), carcinomatosis, subarachnoid hemorrhage, or transtentorial herniation. Patients with hypothyroidism or hyperthyroidism may have a generally enlarged, asymmetrical, or nodular thyroid gland.

Edema of the conjunctiva or eyelids suggests fluid overload, as occurs in congestive heart failure, or reduced osmotic pressure, as occurs with hypoalbuminemia or nephrotic syndrome. Sunken orbits would suggest severe (>10%) dehydration. Conjunctival petechiae can be seen with thrombophilia as well as with fat embolism, as may occur after long bone fracture from trauma or surgery. The sclerae may become icteric with hyperbilirubinemia and liver disease. The lenses may show band keratopathy with hypercalcemia or cataracts with hypocalcemia. Brown Kayser–Fleischer rings at the margin of the iris are seen with copper deposition in patients with Wilson's disease.

The funduscopic examination may show the chronic effects of long-standing medical conditions, such as hypertension or diabetes, or reveal acute changes such as papilledema due to increased ICP, retinal hemorrhages from trauma, retinal edema from methyl alcohol poisoning, or grayish retinal deposits from lead poisoning.

The otoscopic exam may reveal a middle ear infection or evidence of a fracture through the temporal bone with evidence of hemotympanum or CSF otorrhea. Clear or serosanguinous drainage from the ear canal or nose can be tested for glucose or, more specifically, beta trace protein (prostaglandin B synthase) or beta-2-transferrin, to identify CSF leakage.

The patient's breath may suggest alcohol intoxication, diabetic ketoacidosis, or acetone, phenol, or salicylate ingestion (fruity acetone odor); uremia (ammonia odor); hepatic encephalopathy (musty odor or *fetor hepaticus*); arsenic, phosphorus, organophosphate, or thallium poisoning (garlic odor); cyanide poisoning (bitter almond odor); or oral, pharyngeal, or sinus infection (foul odor). Examination of the oral cavity may find lacerations of the tongue to suggest convulsions or blue-black gingival staining to suggest bismuth, mercury, or lead poisoning.

Skin

A comprehensive head-to-toe and back-to-front inspection of the skin, hair, and nails may show signs of dehydration, drug exposure, trauma, or infection. The skin may be hot and dry in the setting of heatstroke or anticholinergic poisoning or hot and sweaty as part of the sympathetic response to hypotension or hypoglycemia. The relevance of various skin findings to the etiology of coma is reviewed in ➋ *Table 365.5*.

Other General Examination

Cardiac auscultation can reveal arrhythmias and murmurs associated with structural heart disease, cardiomyopathy,

Table 365.4

Toxidromes with coma. The characteristic changes associated with various categories of poisonings

Toxidrome	Pupils	Cardiovascular - - - - - Respiratory	Temperature - - - - - Skin	Other	Examples
Anticholinergics	Dilated	Tachycardia, hypertension - - - - - Tachypnea	Hyperthermia - - - - - Dry and flushed	Dry mucous membranes, quiet bowel sounds, urinary retention, myoclonus and seizures	Antihistamines, tricyclic antidepressants, cyclobenzaprine, orphenadrine, antiparkinson agents, antispasmodics, phenothiazines, atropine, scopolamine, belladonna alkaloids (Jimson Weed)
Sympatho-mimetics	Dilated	Tachycardia, hypertension, widened pulse pressure - - - - - Tachypnea, Hyperpnea	Normal - - - - - Diaphoresis	Tremors, hyperreflexia, seizures	Cocaine, amphetamines, ephedrine, pseudoephedrine, phenylpropanolamine, theophylline, caffeine
Hallucinogens	Dilated	Tachycardia, hypertension - - - - - Tachypnea	Hyperthermia - - - - - Normal		PCP, LSD, mescaline, psilocybin, MDMA, MDEA
Opioids	Small	Bradycardia, hypotension - - - - - Bradypnea, pulmonary edema	Hypothermia - - - - - Needle marks		Opioids (heroin, morphine, methadone, oxycodone, hydromorphone), diphenoxylate
Sedative-hypnotics	Small	Bradycardia, hypotension - - - - - Bradypnea, hypopnea	Hypothermia - - - - - Normal	Hyporeflexia	Benzodiazepines, barbiturates, carisoprodol, meprobamate, glutethimide, alcohols, zolpidem
Cholinergics	Small	Bradycardia, hypertension or hypotension - - - - - Tachypnea or bradypnea	Normal - - - - - Diaphoresis	Salivation, urinary and fecal incontinence, diarrhea, emesis, lacrimation, GI cramps, bronchoconstriction, fasciculations, seizures	Organophosphate and carbamate insecticides, nerve agents, nicotine, pilocarpine, physostigmine, bethanecol, urecholine
Serotonin syndrome	Dilated	Tachycardia, hypertension - - - - - Tachypnea	Hyperthermia - - - - - Diaphoresis and flushing	Tremor, myoclonus, hyperreflexia, trismus, rigidity, diarrhea	MAOIs, SSRIs, meperidine, dextro-methorphan, TCAs, L-tryptophan
Tricyclics	Dilated	Tachycardia, hypertension then hypotension, arrhythmias and cardiac conduction disturbances - - - - - Hypopnea	Hyperthermia - - - - - Normal	Seizures, myoclonus, choreoathetosis	Amitriptyline, nortriptyline, imipramine, clomipramine, desipramine, doxepin

Table 365.5
Skin changes in coma. Various skin findings which may be seen in association with unexplained coma and examples of the underlying causes

Skin change	Underlying cause
Antecubital needle marks	Opioid abuse
Pale skin	Anemia or hemorrhage
Sallow, puffy appearance	Hypopituitarism
Hypermelanosis	Porphyria, Addison's disease, chronic nutritional deficiency, disseminated malignant melanoma, chemotherapy
Generalized cyanosis	Hypoxemia, carbon dioxide poisoning
Grayish-blue cyanosis	Methemoglobin (aniline or nitrobenzene) intoxication
Localized cyanosis	Arterial emboli, vasculitis
Cherry-red skin	Carbon monoxide poisoning
Icterus	Hepatic dysfunction, hemolytic anemia
Petechiae	Disseminated intravascular coagulation, thrombotic thrombocytopenic purpura, drugs
Ecchymosis	Trauma, corticosteroid use, abnormal coagulation from liver disease or anticoagulants
Telangiectasia	Chronic alcoholism, vascular malformations of the brain
Vesicular rash	Herpes simplex, varicella, Behcet's disease, drugs
Petechial-purpuric rash	Meningococcemia, gonococcemia, staphylococcemia, *pseudomonas* infection, subacute bacterial endocarditis, allergic vasculitis, purpura fulminans, Rocky Mountain spotted fever, typhus, fat emboli
Macular-papular rash	Typhus, *Candida* infection, *Cryptococcus* infection, toxoplasmosis, subacute bacterial endocarditis, staphylococcal toxic shock, typhoid, leptospirosis, *Pseudomonas* sepsis, immunological disorders, systemic lupus erythematosus, dermatomyositis, serum sickness
Ecthyma gangrenosum	*Pseudomonas* sepsis
Splinter hemorrhages, Osler's nodes, gangrene of digits	Subacute bacterial endocarditis, anemia, leukemia, sepsis

and valvular disease associated with endocarditis. Peritoneal lavage may be required to exclude hemorrhagic abdominal injury in a comatose patient with known or suspected trauma. Bowel sounds are hypoactive in many acute abdominal conditions and with anticholinergic poisoning. Hyperactive bowel sounds are seen with acetylcholinesterase inhibitor toxicity.

Hepatomegaly is seen with right heart failure, lysosomal and glycogen storage disorders, and hepatic tumors. A nodular or hard liver edge can be seen with hepatic tumors and with cirrhosis. Splenomegaly can be seen with portal hypertension, hematological malignancies, infections, and collagen vascular diseases. Ascites can be seen in association with liver disease, right heart failure, and ovarian cancer.

Breast, testicular, and rectal examination may reveal primary tumors. Stool testing for occult gastrointestinal bleeding may indicate a bowel carcinoma. Gastrointestinal bleeding can precipitate hyperammonemic encephalopathy in patients with cirrhotic liver failure. Generalized lymphadenopathy can be seen with hematologic malignancy, infections, immunodeficiency states, collagen vascular diseases, hyperthyroidism, Addison disease, and drug reactions. Localized adenopathy suggests a nearby malignancy or infection.

Level of Consciousness

The state of consciousness should be described in detail to avoid ambiguity. The patient should be tested with cues of increasing intensity, with stimulation progressing from verbal to visual to noxious, and the maximal response should be recorded. Voluntary eyelid and vertical eye movements are sometimes preserved in locked-in syndromes due to anterior brainstem injuries and should be tested for in all patients with apparent coma.

The Glasgow Coma Scale (GCS) records the best eye opening, motor, and verbal response of the patient and is in widespread use in emergency rooms and intensive care units around the world. The verbal response scale has been modified for preverbal children in the Pediatric Coma Scale (PCS) (➋ *Table 365.6*). The GCS and PCS correlate with long-term morbidity and mortality but have low predictive value as single measures of the severity of injury. One significant drawback of these scales is that patients who are intubated or who have suffered severe facial trauma will necessarily score lower in the eye opening and verbal subscales. Another is that neither of the scales directly records brainstem reflexes, such as the pupillary light reflex, that are strongly predictive of the outcome.

Pupillary Reflexes

Normal pupillary dilation in dim light depends on intact sympathetic efferents which arise in the hypothalamus, synapse in the thoracic level of the spinal cord, synapse again in the superior cervical sympathetic ganglion, and then travel along with the internal carotid arteries to the ciliary ganglia and the pupillodilator muscles of the iris. Constriction of the pupils in response to light depends on the afferents from the optic nerves reaching their projections to the parasympathetic Edinger–Westphal nuclei of the midbrain tectum and on the efferent nerves arising there and traveling along the surface of the oculomotor nerves to the ciliary ganglia and the pupillosphincter muscles of the iris.

Thalamic lesions, pontine lesions, and toxic-metabolic causes of coma that impair sympathetic inputs to the pupils leave them small, even pinpoint, but reactive. The reaction to light may be so slight as to require magnification, such as through an otoscope, to observe. Lesions along the sympathetic pathway can also cause *Horner syndrome*, a triad of ipsilateral miosis, mild ptosis due to denervation of the superior and inferior tarsal muscles of the eyelids, and anhydrosis of the face, neck, and arm. Midbrain lesions that interrupt both sympathetic and parasympathetic pathways result in fixed and irregular midposition pupils which may be unequal. An injury to the midbrain or to the third nerve that only affects parasympathetic function causes the ipsilateral pupil to be large and unresponsive to light. A sluggishly reactive pupil may be due to partial compression of the oculomotor nerve and occurs early during uncal herniation, prior to pupillary dilation and oculomotor palsy. Pupillary abnormalities can be of a fixed nature due to prior ocular or neurological injury or may be transient due to seizures

Table 365.6
Coma scales. The components and scores for the Glasgow Coma Scale and Pediatric Coma Scale are outlined

Sign	GCS	PCS	Score
Eye opening	Spontaneous	Spontaneous	4
	To command	To sound	3
	To pain	To pain	2
	None	None	1
Verbal response	Oriented	Age-appropriate vocalization, smile, or orientation to sound	5
	Confused, disoriented	Irritable, consolable, uncooperative, aware of the environment	4
	Inappropriate words	Irritable, inconsistently consolable	3
	Incomprehensible sounds	Inconsolable, unaware of the environment, restless, agitated	2
	None	None	1
Motor response	Obeys commands	Obeys commands, spontaneous movements	6
	Localizes pain	Localizes pain	5
	Withdraws	Withdraws	4
	Abnormal flexion to pain	Abnormal flexion to pain	3
	Abnormal extension to pain	Abnormal extension to pain	2
	None	None	1
Best total score			15

or ophthalmic or systemic medications with effects on the autonomic nervous system.

Ocular Movements

Normal conjugate ocular motility, whether spontaneous or reflexive, requires intact function of the brainstem from the vestibular nuclei at the pontomedullary junction to the oculomotor nuclei in the midbrain. Its presence helps to reduce suspicion for a brainstem injury as a primary cause of coma. The resting position of the eyes when the patient is maximally stimulated may show a discrepancy in eye position, representing weakness of one of the extraocular muscles. Oculomotor or third nerve palsy from a midbrain lesion or from compression of the nerve results in severe ptosis and downward and lateral deviation of the eye. Abducens or sixth nerve palsy results in inward deviation of the eye and can result from an injury to the nucleus in the pons or to compression of the nerve anywhere along its extensive course, which can be due to increased ICP. Trochlear or fourth nerve palsies are inapparent in comatose patients. Conjugate eye deviations at rest are usually due to lesions that disrupt the input to the lateral gaze centers adjacent to the abducens nuclei (parapontine reticular formations) from the contralateral frontal eye fields in the premotor cortex. Downward deviation of the eyes is seen not only in midbrain injury, particularly compression of the midbrain tectum but also in hepatic failure and some other metabolic causes of coma. Downward and inward deviation of the eyes, such that patients appear to be looking at their nose, can occur with thalamic or subthalamic lesions. Conjugate upward deviation of the eyes is not a particularly helpful sign for the localization of lesions causing coma.

Nystagmus can be a sign of an irritative or epileptogenic cause of coma, which can occur in isolation or with other subtle motor signs of seizure activity such as twitching movements of the eye, eyelid, face, jaw, or tongue. Vertical *ocular bobbing*, whether upward or downward, generally indicates diffuse and severe brain injury. When the bobbing involves rapid downward jerking and a slow return to midposition, in association with lateral gaze paralysis, it is typically due to an acute pontine injury. *Ocular flutter*, with conjugate horizontal saccades, is reflective of dysfunction of the cerebellum.

Reflexive ocular movements can be elicited by sudden, rapid head turning (oculocephalic reflex), or by cold water irrigation of the ear canals (vestibuloocular reflex). The oculocephalic reflex clearly cannot be tested in patients with a known or possible cervical spine injury. When the oculocephalic reflex is preserved, the eyes move conjugately in a direction opposite to the direction the head turns, as would be required to maintain gaze fixation. This is sometimes referred to as the *doll's eye* reflex or phenomenon being positive, but due to ambiguity regarding these terms the ocular response should simply be described. Caloric testing is done with the patient supine, with the head raised 30° from horizontal to maximally stimulate convection currents in the endolymph of the lateral semicircular canal. The ear canal is visualized to ensure that it is unobstructed, and that the tympanic membrane is intact, and 10 mL of ice-cold water is slowly instilled. When the vestibuloocular reflex is intact, the eyes will show conjugate deviation toward the cold ear canal. Corrective nystagmus away from the slow deviation and back to a point of visual fixation is seen only in conscious subjects. Irrigation of the ear canals with warm water causes slow conjugate eye deviation away from the warmed canal in the comatose patient and additional nystagmus back toward the point of visual fixation in the conscious patient. The mnemonic COWS (cold opposite, warm same) refers to the fast phase of the nystagmus seen in conscious patients. Simultaneous bilateral cold water irrigation would result in slow downward eye deviation and simultaneous bilateral warm water irrigation would cause slow upward eye deviation. Oculocephalic and caloric testing can be abnormal due to diffuse brainstem lesions, individual cranial nerve palsies, restrictive eye disease, including severe globe and eyelid edema, or vestibular dysfunction due to ototoxic, sedative, paralytic, or anticholinergic medications.

Motor Exam

The purposeful and reflexive movements of the limbs are helpful localizing signs in the examination of the comatose patient. Flaccid hemiparesis with conjugate gaze toward the paralysis indicates a pontine lesion affecting the contralateral pyramidal tract and the ispilateral abducens nucleus. Flaccid hemiparesis with conjugate gaze away from the paralysis can occur with a supratentorial lesion disrupting the contralateral pyramidal tract and corticobulbar tract to the parapontine reticular formation. Generalized flaccidity can be seen early with any cause of coma, including diffuse supratentorial injuries, brainstem injuries, or metabolic encephalopathies. Hypertonicity of the limb muscles due to injury to the motor system, whether unilateral or generalized, usually takes time to develop.

Decorticate posturing is flexion at the elbow and wrist, adduction of the shoulder, and extension of knee and ankle. Its presence indicates disruption of corticospinal tracts above the rubrospinal pathway from the midbrain (upper limb flexion) and the vestibulospinal pathway from the pontomedullary junction (upper and lower limb extension). *Decerebrate posturing* is extension at the elbow and wrist, adduction and internal rotation of the shoulder, and extension of the knee and ankle. Bilateral decerebrate posturing is usually due to bilateral midbrain or pontine lesions that disrupt the corticospinal and rubrospinal tracts, leaving the vestibulospinal pathways unopposed. Bilateral decerebrate posturing is a far more ominous sign than decorticate posturing or unilateral posturing of either kind, which can be seen with transient injuries anywhere along the motor system.

Posturing may sometimes be mistaken for tonic or clonic seizure activity but it needs to be recognized because it may indicate progressive brainstem compression due to an expanding posterior fossa mass lesion or to transtentorial herniation. Convulsive movements due to seizures may be overt but also can be quite subtle, particularly in established refractory status epilepticus. Myoclonus that is non-rhythmic and not generalized can occur with many metabolic causes of coma, including global hypoxic-ischemic encephalopathy or hepatic encephalopathy. Myoclonus that is rhythmic and generalized can occur with anoxic injury and is predictive of a dismal outcome when caused by myoclonic status epilepticus. Rhythmic myoclonus due to a brainstem injury and tonic posturing due to hypocalcemia can also mimic epileptic convulsions.

Limb movements in response to local pain should be tested and recorded, although many such responses are mediated by spinal reflexes that can easily be mistaken for purposeful withdrawal and are generally unhelpful for defining the cause or severity of coma. Withdrawal of an arm from a painful stimulus that includes abduction at the shoulder is reliably non-reflexive and indicates some preservation of the spinothalamic and corticospinal tracts. Purely reflexive withdrawal of the arm can be as complex as to include adduction of the shoulder, flexion of the elbow, and pronation of the arm. The complex but purely reflexive withdrawal of the leg known as the *triple flexion response* includes flexion of the hip, flexion of the knee, and dorsiflexion of the ankle. The extensor plantar reflex of the foot or *Babinski sign* is nonlocalizing and can be seen in coma from any cause.

Brain Herniation

The Monroe–Kellie hypothesis states that because the volume of the skull is fixed, when there is an increase in the volume of any one of the intracranial contents (brain, blood, CSF), there must be a compensatory decrease in the volume of the others. This will hold true for an infant with unfused sutures if the changes in volume and pressure are too great or rapid for suture widening to accommodate. In the setting of an expanding intracranial mass lesion such as a subdural hematoma, for example, there will initially be a compensatory decrease in CSF volume due to the compression of lateral ventricles and arachnoid cisterns, and a decrease in cerebral blood volume due to the compression of cerebral veins and sinuses. When the hematoma is small, these compressible spaces allow increases in volume to have little effect on the ICP and the system is described as compliant. When these spaces are maximally compressed, however, the system loses its compliance. Further and relatively small increases in hematoma volume will cause more dramatic increases in ICP and dangerous displacements of arterial blood and brain tissue.

Caudal displacements of brain tissue include *uncal herniation* of the medial temporal lobe beneath the tentorium and *central herniation* of the diencephalon through the tentorium and of the brainstem through the foramen magnum. Comatose patients with known or suspected increased ICP must be watched carefully for signs of these forms of life-threatening herniation. In most, in the setting of an expanding lateral mass lesion, there is a lateral shift of the diencephalon away from the mass and compression of the third nerves against the tentorium. Typically, this involves the third nerve ipsilateral to the mass lesion, but the contralateral third nerve can be affected first, or both nerves can be affected simultaneously. Early compression leads to dysfunction of the more superficially located parasympathetic fibers to the eye and to a dilated and nonreactive pupil. Further compression of the third nerve leads to ptosis and a fixed lateral and downward gaze. With further lateral displacement of the diencephalon and midbrain, there is a compression of the cerebral peduncles of the midbrain against the tentorium, causing signs of pyramidal tract dysfunction such as hemiplegia or decorticate posturing. This may occur on either side but usually occurs first in the contralateral cerebral peduncle, causing the *Kernohan's notch phenomenon*, with pyramidal dysfunction in the limbs ipsilateral to the mass lesion. Loss of the sympathetic input to the eye from the diencephalon will cause a previously dilated pupil to become midposition but remain nonreactive. Severe lateral displacement will finally lead to actual herniation of the most medial portion of the temporal lobe (uncus) through the tentorium and to caudal displacement of the brainstem through the foramen magnum or central herniation.

Central herniation can also occur directly with the downward displacement of the diencephalon, such as might be caused by bilateral mass lesions, including obstructive hydrocephalus. The signs of central herniation may evolve in a rostrocaudal fashion, with loss of midbrain function being followed by loss of pontine and then medullary function. Early signs of midbrain dysfunction include deepening coma, loss of sympathetic inputs to the eyes that leave them small but reactive to light, loss of reflexive vertical gaze, and bilateral corticospinal tract dysfunction with weakness or posturing. Lower midbrain injury can cause further loss of parasympathetic inputs to the eyes that leave them midpositioned and nonreactive to light, more complete loss of eye movements mediated by the third nerve nuclei, and loss of the rubrospinal tract that causes posturing to become decerebrate. Central neurogenic hyperventilation is sometimes, but infrequently, seen with midbrain compression. Diencephalic and midbrain injuries in an unventilated patient are more likely to present with a Cheyne-Stokes pattern of respiration.

Involvement of the pons and midbrain will lead to a loss of virtually all cranial nerve reflexes, flaccid paralysis with loss of all posturing, and increasingly dysfunctional respiratory patterns described as apneustic, ataxic, and, finally, agonal. Central herniation does not always progress in a slow or stepwise fashion, and medullary signs of severe autonomic dysfunction may be present early. Herniation may progress precipitously soon after the first signs of increased ICP are noted and the structural injuries associated with the brainstem signs outlined above may be irreversible. Close monitoring and early intervention are needed to manage increases in ICP. The measures available for decreasing ICP are outlined in *Table 365.7.*

Table 365.7
Interventions to decrease ICP

Decrease cerebral blood volume
30° head elevation in neutral position
Hyperventilation to a pCO_2 of 25–30 mmHg
Anesthetic agents (barbiturates, propofol) to reduce $CMRO_2$
Paralytic agents to reduce resistance to ventilation
Analgesic agents to reduce agitation
Prevention of hyperthermia with aggressive cooling measures
Decrease extracellular fluid and CSF volume
Osmotic diuretics (mannitol, 3% saline)
Loop diuretics (furosemide)
Corticosteroids (dexamethasone)
Carbonic anhydrase inhibitors (acetazolamide)
Intraventricular drainage of CSF
Decrease/ameliorate intracranial brain tissue volume
Decompressive lesionectomy
Decompressive resection of adjacent brain tissue
Decompressive craniectomy and dural expansion

History

Ideally, a clinical history will be obtained concurrently by the physician or other team members while the patient is being transported, stabilized, and put through initial examinations and laboratory tests. Attempts should be made to contact those who may know about the patient's past medical history or who may have witnessed the events leading up to the patient's loss of consciousness. A family member or bystander may have witnessed trauma or seizures. Others caring for the child may be aware of a past history of disease predisposing to loss of consciousness or be aware of the presence and time course of any prodromal symptoms. Complaints from the child suggestive of increased ICP or meningeal irritation, such as headache, nausea, vomiting, photophobia, or nuchal rigidity, would suggest subarachnoid hemorrhage, meningitis, or hydrocephalus. Symptoms such as dyspnea or chest pain would suggest a respiratory, cardiac, or neuromuscular disorder. Symptoms of cranial nerve dysfunction such as diplopia, dysphagia, dysarthria, and dizziness would suggest direct brainstem injury or compression from a posterior fossa mass.

If the loss of consciousness remains unexplained, the child's environment should be evaluated for the presence of illicit drugs or prescription medications that may have been accidentally or intentionally ingested. Children failing to emerge from anesthesia after surgery should be investigated for such surgical complications as fat embolism, adrenal insufficiency, hypothyroid coma, and opioid overdose.

Pseudocoma

There are several findings on examination of the eyes inconsistent with unconsciousness that are helpful in identifying patients who are either purposefully feigning coma or appear unarousable as a manifestation of psychiatric illness. A history of prior psychiatric illness or of precipitation of the apparent coma by a stressful event should be taken into account but do not exclude medical causes of coma. In true coma, passive eyelid opening will not induce movement of the eyes and the eyelids will close slowly and gradually when released. In pseudocoma, patients will often actively resist eye opening, either forcefully, attempting to keep their eyes tightly shut, or subtly, inducing a Bell's phenomenon of upward eye rolling during eyelid opening. When released, the eyelids will close quickly or hesitantly. Nystagmus with the vestibuloocular reflex test is not seen in true coma. The severe vertigo and nausea induced by cold caloric testing may *awaken* a patient with pseudocoma.

Diagnostic Testing

Laboratory Testing

The testing that should be done for all patients with unexplained coma should begin with a bedside test of blood glucose, followed by formal laboratory testing of serum glucose as well as a complete blood cell count (CBC), a chemistry panel that measures serum electrolytes (Na, K, Cl, HCO3, Ca, Mg, Phos) and renal function (BUN, Cr) and liver function tests (ALT, AST, Alk Phos, Tbili, Albumin, Ammonia, PT, PTT). Tests for accidental and intentional toxic ingestions should include a screening urine test for common drugs of abuse and serum tests for alcohol, salicylates, acetaminophen, and tricyclic antidepressants. These tests will identify around 80% of all toxic overdoses. Additional testing can be ordered through urine thin layer chromatography or specific serum tests when there is a suspicion that a patient had access to other potentially toxic compounds.

An arterial blood gas will help in the identification and differentiation of metabolic and respiratory disturbances associated with altered consciousness (*Table 365.8*).

Inborn errors of metabolism may be hinted at by abnormalities in the screening laboratory tests such as hypoglycemia, metabolic acidosis, or hyperammonemia but will require more detailed testing for identification. Small amounts of plasma, serum, and urine should be collected, frozen, and saved for later analysis when a child presents with a possible inborn error of metabolism, as testing after the child has been stabilized may be less diagnostic. Secondary analysis can include measures of urine ketones, amino acids, and organic acids, plasma lactate and pyruvate, plasma amino acids, and serum acylcarnitine profiles.

Other tests can be ordered depending on clinical suspicion or when the cause of coma remains obscure after other assessments are done. These tests include blood cultures, urine cultures, and lumbar puncture for CSF culture regarding possible infection and thyroid function and cortisol studies regarding possible endocrine disorders. Neuroimaging should be performed prior to lumbar puncture to look for any evidence that the procedure could precipitate herniation, such as midline shift, a posterior fossa mass, or loss of any of the cisternal spaces (suprachiasmatic, basilar, superior cerebellar, quadrigeminal plate). Lumbar puncture should also be deferred in the presence of an uncorrected coagulopathy. The serum cortisol level should be elevated in the stressful setting of coma and a low to normal value should prompt further laboratory testing for adrenal insufficiency. Patients who have suffered generalized trauma or who

Table 365.8

Arterial blood gas and respiratory rate evaluation. Interpretation of the respiratory rate and arterial blood gas results

Respiratory rate	Metabolic pattern	ABG results	Causes
Increased	Metabolic acidosis	pH < 7.35 $PaCO_2 < 30$ mmHg $HCO_3 < 17$ mmol/L	Uremia, diabetic ketoacidosis,lactic acidosis, poisoning with salicylates, methanol, and ethylene glycol
Increased	Respiratory alkalosis	pH > 7.45 $PaCO_2 < 30$ mmHg $HCO_3 > 17$ mmol/L	Hepatic failure, acute sepsis, acute salicylate poisoning, cardiopulmonary disease with hypoxemia, psychogenic hyperventilation
Decreased	Respiratory acidosis	pH < 7.35 (acutely) $PaCO_2 > 90$ mmHg $HCO_3 > 17$ mmol/L	Respiratory failure due to CNS disease, neuromuscular disease, or cardiopulmonary disease
Decreased	Metabolic alkalosis	pH > 7.45 $PaCO_2 > 45$ mmHg $HCO_3 > 30$ mmol/L	Vomiting, alkali ingestion

remain immobile for a prolonged period of time should be monitored for elevated serum creatine kinase levels indicating rhabdomyolysis.

Electrocardiography

In addition to continuous monitoring of the heart rate, comatose patients should undergo electrocardiography to identify myocardial infarction, arrhythmia, or conduction disturbance that may indicate an electrolyte abnormality or toxidrome prior to confirmation by blood tests.

Computed Tomography and Magnetic Resonance Imaging

Following stabilization, the patient with unexplained coma should undergo neuroimaging. A CT scan of the brain without contrast can be obtained rapidly in most medical centers and visualizes most abnormalities that would require immediate intervention, including intracranial hemorrhage, hydrocephalus, cerebral edema, and impending herniation. MRI is superior to CT in identifying acute stroke, diffuse axonal injury, and lesions of the posterior fossa but its use is limited by the longer image acquisition times, need for patient immobility, and patient inaccessibility within the scanner. MRI done with special sequences, including diffusion weighted imaging, diffusion tensor imaging, and proton spectroscopy can identify abnormalities in patients with unexplained coma and can contribute to the assessment of a child's prognosis for recovery, as discussed below.

Electroencephalography

An electroencephalogram (EEG) can identify seizure activity in patients suspected to be unconscious due to status epilepticus, including those who have prolonged depressed consciousness following a witnessed seizure. The presence of focal epileptiform discharges, slowing, or suppression on EEG suggests an underlying focal lesion as may occur with hemorrhage, infection, or stroke. Temporal lobe periodic lateralized epileptiform discharges (PLEDs) are frequently seen with herpes simplex encephalitis but are nonspecific. Metabolic encephalopathies associated with hepatic or renal failure are often associated with frontally predominant triphasic, high-amplitude slow waves. EEG activity that is generally slow or suppressed is a nonspecific indicator of brain dysfunction but does exclude pseudocoma; such patients will typically have EEG findings consistent with normal wakefulness.

Prognosis

The diagnostic evaluation of a patient in coma will often result in sufficient information to provide an estimate of the degree of brain injury that has occurred and of the level of recovery that can be expected. Other than patients who meet the clinical criteria for brain death, however, there are rarely situations in which the neurologist can have certainty regarding either survival or neurological prognosis. Nevertheless, giving families early estimates of the likelihood of a good recovery will help to prepare them to understand later, more definitive declarations regarding prognosis and to make decisions about the appropriateness of future resuscitative efforts.

Many academic reports of outcomes in children use qualitative terms such as good or poor without tying them to quantitative measures that would be comparable between studies. The majority of studies of brain injury in adults report overall long-term outcomes using the simple five-category Glasgow Outcome Scale (GOS), describing patients as either dead, vegetative and unresponsive, severely disabled and dependent on others, moderately disabled but able to live independently, or doing well enough to return to work or school. When the GOS is used, the upper two categories are often considered good outcomes. An eight-category version, the GOS Extended, subdivides each of the three higher categories into halves to further distinguish levels of disability. Other measures that are frequently reported in adults include the 8-item Disability Rating Scale, the 12-item Functional Independence Measure (FIM), and the 8-category Rancho Los Amigos Scale of cognitive function. Scales of global outcome developed for children include the six-category Pediatric Cerebral Performance Category Scale Score, the WeeFIM, and the KOSCHI (King's Outcome Scale for Childhood Head Injury) score.

There is a considerable difference in the general prognosis for coma that is drug induced, otherwise non-traumatic, or traumatic in origin. For drug-induced coma, a good recovery can usually be expected for patients identified early and provided with good supportive care. Brain injury is usually secondary to at least potentially avoidable metabolic or systemic derangements such as hypotension, hypoxia, or hypoglycemia. For non-traumatic coma due to hypoxic-ischemic injury and for traumatic coma, the clinical features present during the initial resuscitation may not be highly predictive of outcome, but a number of clinical, laboratory, and radiological findings in subsequent days have been found to help predict a favorable or unfavorable outcome.

Non-traumatic Coma

The prognosis for patients in coma secondary to non-traumatic and non-drug-induced reasons is generally poor, with only 15% of patients recovering independent function. The outcome for children with coma due to hypoxic-ischemic encephalopathy, as might occur following cardiopulmonary arrest, is significantly worse than for those with potentially reversible metabolic encephalopathies, as might be seen with hepatic or renal failure. Naturally, more extensive structural brain injury is correlated with poorer outcome, as is the length of time of coma before some degree of recovery is seen. A child's age does not predict the degree of recovery in most analyses.

A practice parameter published by the AAN regarding the prognosis of comatose adults following resuscitation for cardiac arrest identified a number of clinical and laboratory findings that show evidence of being very highly predictive of a poor outcome, including (1) absent pupillary or corneal reflexes or absent or extensor motor responses to stimulation after 3 days, (2) myoclonic status epilepticus within the first day, (3) bilaterally absent cortical somatosensory evoked potentials (SSEP) in the first 3 days, and (4) a serum neuron-specific enolase level greater than 33 ng/L. There was evidence to suggest that the presence of burst-suppression, generalized suppression, or generalized epileptiform discharges on EEG was associated with a poor prognosis but was not specific enough to be used for outcome prediction.

Studies of the outcomes of resuscitation for cardiopulmonary arrest in children have shown that a number of clinical factors are associated with a poorer prognosis. Mortality and morbidity is generally higher in patients with cardiac arrest rather than respiratory arrest. In one study, 57% of 21 children with pure respiratory arrest died before leaving the hospital and 10% were severely impaired or dead a year later, while 92% of 80 children suffering cardiac arrest died prior to leaving the hospital and another 4% were in a vegetative state or had died a year later. Another study of 599 children with out-of-hospital combined cardiopulmonary arrest showed that only 8.6% survived to hospital discharge and that few of them had good neurological outcomes.

Cardiac and cardiopulmonary arrests that occur in hospital have a better rate of survival and of good neurologic outcome. One study of 880 children found that 27% survived to discharge and that the majority of survivors had good neurologic function at the time of discharge. Cardiopulmonary resuscitation that continues for more than 10–15 min or requires more than one bolus of epinephrine suggests a poor prognosis, but there have been cases with good outcomes despite 60 min of resuscitation for children with in-hospital arrest or ice-water submersion.

Few findings on the initial physical examination have been found to be as predictive of outcome from hypoxic-ischemic coma as those seen after 24 h. Poor outcomes were seen in all children with absent pupillary responses after 24 h in one study and in all children without purposeful movement or normal brainstem reflexes in another, but there have also been reports of children with better outcomes despite these findings. Along these lines, while lower GCS scores are associated with poorer outcomes, with one study finding that none of the children who had a GCS of 3 or 4 after the first 24 h had a good recovery, there are reported exceptions and predicting outcomes using a child's GCS score at the scene, or on admission is even less accurate. The effect of paralytic or sedative medications must be taken into account when assessing these physical findings.

Several studies have suggested that somatosensory evoked potential (SSEP) testing in children with severe hypoxic-ischemic brain injury is as useful as in adults with cardiac arrest for accurately predicting poor outcome when there is no cortical response. However, other studies have shown this finding to have a specificity of 92–95% and sensitivity of 61–75% for poor outcomes, making its clinical use far more problematic in children than in adults. Other electrophysiologic studies, including EEG, brainstem auditory evoked potentials, and visual evoked potentials, are all even more prone to error in predicting outcome, although severe abnormalities show a correlation with poorer outcomes. Conversely, initial or follow-up EEGs showing little to no slowing or suppression, normal reactivity to stimuli, or normal sleep rhythms in comatose survivors of hypoxic-ischemic injury have been correlated with favorable outcomes, suggesting a potential prognostic value to repeated or continuous monitoring.

Studies of the use of MRI for predicting outcomes for children in coma from hypoxic-ischemic injury have found that there is a greater sensitivity and specificity to abnormal findings 3–4 days after the injury, with one showing universally poor outcomes (vegetative state or death) for children with T2 hyperintensity within the brainstem or within both the cortex and basal ganglia. Studies of magnetic resonance spectroscopy have found that severely depressed N-acetylaspartate levels and elevated lactate levels are also associated with poorer neurological outcomes.

Traumatic Coma

Children with traumatic coma can have a good outcome despite prolonged coma and generally do better than children with non-traumatic coma, but this makes predicting long-term prognosis even more difficult.

The most accurate predictors in early research studies were age, the GCS score on presentation and within the first week, and the presence or absence of pupillary reactivity. A recent study of 309 children compared the predictive value of the GCS score, other clinical variables including injuries to other organs, and the results of head CT scans and found that the GCS score was the best predictor of survival, with few children with an initial GCS score of 3 or 4 showing better than moderate disability. CT findings of cerebral edema and intracranial hemorrhage were also associated with poorer outcomes.

One study of children with severe traumatic brain injury showed continued clinical improvement after hospital discharge with the number of children who were independent in all areas of function increasing over an average of 2 years from 37% to 65%. Another study found that cognitive impairments in children who had survived for more than 1 year after suffering severe TBI were better predicted by the duration of coma measured as the time to follow commands, than by the initial GCS score. Other studies have shown that the duration of posttraumatic amnesia is also a better predictor than the GCS score for long-term cognitive impairment.

Additional predictors of poorer recovery include open head injuries, multiple skull fractures, deeper, more diffuse and more severe brain injury on neuroimaging, increased ICP, fever, seizures, and unstable blood pressure. For infants, a non-accidental etiology of the head trauma is often associated with signs of secondary ischemic brain injury and is predictive of greater morbidity and mortality.

Persistent Vegetative State

Children who awaken from coma into a vegetative state have some chance to regain consciousness; most who do will do so early in their recovery and will continue to have severe disability. When the vegetative state persists for more than 1 month following non-traumatic coma, or for more than 3 months after traumatic coma, improvements are very unlikely. Survival in the vegetative state is precarious and requires meticulous medical and nursing care, but recovery to a state of independence is almost unheard of for patients in such a state for more than a year and has never been reported for patients in a persistent vegetative state for 3 years. There are a significant number of patients who are initially misdiagnosed as being vegetative but later reclassified as being in a minimally conscious state following repeated and more detailed evaluations that consider the possibility of fluctuating levels of consciousness and limitations on interactions due to sensory deficits. Most of the older reports of patients making surprisingly good recoveries from the vegetative state were likely minimally conscious patients who had been misdiagnosed as vegetative. However, there have been more recent reports of the use of functional brain imaging to identify vegetative patients with preserved receptive language function who did make exceptional late recoveries.

Brain Death

The clinical requirements on physicians for declaring a child as having died from brain death are fairly consistent across most regions of the world, although, when surveyed, knowledge of these requirements and documentation of the examinations performed is often incomplete. The difficulties that physicians face in presenting a diagnosis of brain death to a child's family are universal. Although brain death has been used in clinical practice since the 1970s, families are likely to have little familiarity with the concept and to see ambiguity in the ongoing use of cardiopulmonary support systems, especially when physicians persist in referring to them as providing *life support*.

The diagnosis of brain death requires that there be an irreversible cause of injury to the brain that precludes any chance for recovery of consciousness. In a few countries, including the United Kingdom, it is sufficient for the injury to involve only the brainstem, although in most countries, including the United States, there is a requirement for *whole brain* death that involves both the brainstem and the cerebral hemispheres.

With the loss of all brainstem function, there should be no spontaneous movements, postures, or convulsions, no movements in response to stimulation other than those mediated by spinal reflexes, no brainstem reflexes including pupillary, corneal, oculocephalic, vestibuloocular, or gag reflexes, and no spontaneous respiration despite elevation of the partial pressure of CO_2 from at or below 40 mmHg to above 60 mmHg on arterial blood gas testing, or a 20 mmHg elevation from an initial level above 40 mmHg. For a purely clinical diagnosis to be accurate, the examination cannot be confounded by factors that interfere with the examination, such as facial trauma, or that might induce unresponsiveness, such as significant hypothermia, hypotension, metabolic disturbance, or significantly elevated serum levels of sedating or paralyzing medications. When the clinical examination is limited in any way, confirmation can be obtained using a radionucleotide scan that shows absent cerebral blood flow. Confirmatory testing with EEG to show electrocerebral silence has been recommended for children under 1 year of age but this test is prone to being influenced by metabolic derangements and is less helpful in the setting of confounding circumstances.

Following brain death, patients frequently develop cardiac and cardiovascular instability despite intensive supportive care. Continuous intravenous infusion of vasopressin has been found helpful in preventing the severe diuresis and hypotension resulting from the loss of pituitary function. Patients whose organs are not being maintained for donation can be withdrawn from artificial support, with intravenous drips, ventilators, and all monitors turned off to allow families a period of time with their child before the absence of a heartbeat is confirmed by a physician through auscultation and palpation and the absence of cardiac activity is documented by an electrocardiogram. In rare instances when there have been reasons to continue supportive care indefinitely, organ failure usually occurs in less than a week, although there are bodies that have been maintained following brain death for months or years.

References

Abend NS, Licht DJ (2008) Predicting outcome in children with hypoxic ischemic encephalopathy. Pediatr Crit Care Med 9:32–39

ANA Committee on Ethical Affairs (1993) Persistent vegetative state: report of the American Neurological Association Committee on Ethical Affairs. Ann Neurol 33:386–390

Bansal A, Singhi SC, Singhi PD et al (2005) Non traumatic coma. Indian J Pediatr 72:467–473

Beca J, Cox PN, Taylor MR et al (1995) Somatosensory evoked potentials for prediction of outcome in acute severe brain injury. J Pediatr 126:44–49

Biarent D, Bingham R, Richmond S et al (2005) European resuscitation council guidelines for resuscitation 2005. Section 6. Paediatric life support. Resuscitation 67(S1):S97–S133

Booth CM, Boone RH, Tomlinson G, Detsky AS (2004) Is this patient dead, vegetative or severely neurologically impaired? Assessing outcome for comatose survivors of cardiac arrest. JAMA 291:870–879

Boveroux P, Bonhomme V, Boly M et al (2008) Brain function in physiologically, pharmacologically, and pathologically altered states of consciousness. Int Anesthesiol Clin 46:131–146

Bowker R, Green A, Bonham JR (2007) Guidelines for the investigation and management of a reduced level of consciousness in children: implications for clinical biochemistry laboratories. Ann Clin Biochem 44:506–511

Bratton SL, Jardine DS, Morray JP (1994) Serial neurologic examinations after near drowning and outcome. Arch Pediatr Adolesc Med 148:167–170

Brenner T, Freier MC, Holshouser BA et al (2003) Predicting neuropsychologic outcome after traumatic brain injury in children. Pediatr Neurol 28:104–114

Brenner RP (2005) The interpretation of the EEG in stupor and coma. Neurologist 11:271–284

Carpentier A, Galanaud D, Puybasset L et al (2006) Early morphologic and spectroscopic magnetic resonance in severe traumatic brain injuries can detect "invisible brain stem damage" and predict "vegetative states". J Neurotrauma 23:674–685

Carter G, Butt W (2005) A prospective study of outcome predictors after severe brain injury in children. Intensive Care Med 31:840–845

Chadwick O, Rutter M, Brown G et al (1981) A prospective study of children with head injuries. II. Cognitive sequelae. Psychol Med 11:49–61

Cheliout-Heraut F, Sale-Franque F, Hubert P et al (1991) Cerebral anoxia in near-drowning of children. The prognostic value of EEG. Neurophysiol Clin 21:121–132

Chiaretti A, Antonelli A, Genovese O et al (2008) Nerve growth factor and doublecortin expression correlates with improved outcome in children with severe traumatic brain injury. J Trauma 65:80–85

Christophe C, Fonteyne C, Ziereisen F et al (2002) Value of MR imaging of the brain in children with hypoxic coma. AJNR Am J Neuroradiol 23:716–723

Chung CY, Chen CL, Cheng PT et al (2006) Critical score of Glasgow Coma Scale for pediatric traumatic brain injury. Pediatr Neurol 34:379–387

Claret-Teruel G, Palomeque-Rico A, Cambra-Lasaosa JR et al (2007) Severe head injury among children: computed tomography evaluation as a prognostic factor. J Pediatr Surg 42:1903–1906

Di H, Boly M, Weng X et al (2008) Neuroimaging activation studies in the vegetative state: predictors of recovery? Clin Med 8:502–507

Dubowitz DJ, Bluml S, Arcinue E et al (1998) MR of hypoxic encephalopathy in children after near drowning: Correlation with quantitative proton MR spectroscopy and clinical outcome. AJMNR Am J Neuroradiol 19:1617–1627

Ducrocq SC, Meyer PG, Orliaguet GA et al (2006) Epidemiology and early predictive factors of mortality and outcome in children with traumatic severe brain injury: experience of a French pediatric trauma center. Pediatr Crit Care Med 7:461–467

Evans BM, Bartlett JR (1995) Prediction of outcome in severe head injury based on recognition of sleep related activity in the polygraphic electroencephalogram. J Neurol Neurosurg Psychiatry 59:17–25

Ewing-Cobbs L, Levin HS, Fletcher JR et al (1990) The Children's Orientation and Amnesia Test: relationship to severity of acute head injury and of recovery of memory. Neurosurgery 27:683–691

Fischer C, Luauté J, Adeleine P, Morlet D (2004) Predictive value of sensory and cognitive evoked potentials for awakening from coma. Neurology 63:669–673

Fisher CM (1969) The neurological evaluation of the comatose patient. Acta Neurol Scand 45(S36):1–56

Galloway NR, Tong KA, Ashwal S et al (2008) Diffusion-weighted imaging improves outcome prediction in pediatric traumatic brain injury. J Neurotrauma 25:1153–1162

Geocadin RG, Eleff SM (2008) Cardiac arrest resuscitation: neurologic prognostication and brain death. Curr Opin Crit Care 14:261–268

Giacino JR, Smart CM (2007) Recent advances in behavioral assessment of individuals with disorders of consciousness. Curr Opin Neurol 20:614–619

Giacino JT, Ashwal S, Childs N et al (2002) The minimally conscious state: definition and diagnostic criteria. Neurology 58:349–353

Hakimi R, McDonagh DL (2008) Unconsciousness in the intensive care unit: a practical approach. Int Anesth Clin 46:171–173

Hoesch RE, Koenig MA, Geocadin RG et al (2008) Coma after global ischemic brain injury: Pathophysiology and emerging therapies. Crit Care Clin 24:25–44

Jagannathan J, Okonkwo DO, Yeoh HK et al (2008) Long-term outcomes and prognostic factors in pediatric patients with severe traumatic brain injury and elevated intracranial pressure. J Neurosurg Pediatr 2:240–249

Johnson AR, DeMatt E, Salorio CF (2009) Predictors of outcome following acquired brain injury in children. Dev Disabil Res Rev 15:124–132

Kirkham FJ, Newton CRJC, Whitehouse W (2008) Pediatric coma scales. Dev Med Child Neurol 50:267–274

Lescot T, Galanaud D, Puybasset L (2009) Exploring altered consciousness states by magnetic resonance imaging in brain injury. Ann N Y Acad Sci 1157:71–80

Levin HS, Eisenberg HM, Wigg NR et al (1982) Memory and intellectual ability after head injury in children and adolescents. Neurosurgery 1:668–673

Lin M, Sciubba DM, Carson BS et al (2009) Increased Intracranial Pressure. In: Maria BL (ed) Current management in child neurology, 4th edn. BC Decker, New York, pp 681–687

Lucas da Silva PS, Reis ME, Aguiar VE (2008) Value of repeat cranial computed tomography in pediatric patients sustaining moderate to severe traumatic brain injury. J Trauma 65:1293–1297

MacDonald ME, Liben S, Franco A et al (2008) Signs of life and signs of death: brain death and other mixed messages at the end of life. J Child Health Care 12:92–105

Mandel R, Martinot A, Delepoulle F et al (2002) Prediction of outcome after hypoxic-ischemic encephalopathy: a prospective clinical and electrophysiologic study. J Pediatr 141:45–50

Martin C, Falcone RA (2008) Pediatric traumatic brain injury: an update of research to understand and improve outcomes. Curr Opin Pediatr 20:294–299

Mathur M, Petersen L, Stadtler M et al (2008) Variability in pediatric brain death determination and documentation in Southern California. Pediatrics 121:988–993

McKenny-Fick NM, Ferrie CD, Livingston JH et al (2009) Prolonged recovery of consciousness in children following symptomatic epileptic seizures. Seizure 18:180–183

Nadkarni VM, Larkin GL, Peberdy MA et al (2006) First documented rhythm and clinical outcome from in-hospital cardiac arrest among children and adults. JAMA 295:50–57

Pampiglione G, Chaloner J, Harden A et al (1978) Transitory ischemia/anoxia in young children and the prediction of quality of survival. Ann N Y Acad Sci 315:281–292

Paterakis K, Karantanas AH, Komnos A et al (2000) Outcome of patients with diffuse axonal injury: the significance and prognostic value of MRI in the acute phase. J Trauma 49:1071–1075

Posner JB, Saper CB, Schiff ND et al (2007) Plum and Posner's diagnosis of stupor and coma, 4th edn. Oxford University Press, New York

Ramachandrannair R, Sharma R, Weiss SK et al (2005) Reactive EEG patterns in pediatric coma. Pediatr Neurol 33:345–349

Rescuscitation ILCo (2005) Part 6: paediatric basic and advanced life support. Resuscitation 67:271–291

Salorio CF, Slomine BS, Guerguerian AM et al (2008) Intensive care unit variables and outcome after pediatric traumatic brain injury: a retrospective study of survivors. Pediatr Crit Care Med 9:47–53

Schindler MB, Bohn D, Cox PN et al (1996) Outcome of out-of-hospital cardiac or respiratory arrest in children. N Engl J Med 335:1473–1479

Shewmon DA (1998) Chronic "brain death": meta-analysis and conceptual consequences. Neurology 51:1538–1545

Soddu A, Boly M, Nir Y et al (2009) Reaching across the abyss: recent advances in functions magnetic resonance imaging and their potential relevance to disorders of consciousness. Prog Brain Res 177:261–274

Tasker RC, Boyd S, Harden A et al (1988) Monitoring in non-traumatic coma. Part II: Electroencephalography. Arch Dis Child 63:895–899

Thakker JC, Splaingard M, Jzu J et al (1997) Survival and functional outcome of children requiring endotracheal intubation during therapy for severe traumatic brain injury. Crit Care Med 25:1396–1401

The Multi-Society Task Force on PVS (1994) Medical aspects of the persistent vegetative state. N Engl J Med 330:1499–1508

Vavilala MA, Muangman S, Tontisirin N et al (2006) Impaired cerebral autoregulation and 6-month outcome in children with severe traumatic brain injury: preliminary findings. Dev Neurosci 28:348–353

Weiss N, Galanaud D, Carpentier A et al (2007) Clinical review: prognostic value of magnetic resonance imaging in acute brain injury and coma. Crit Care 11:230–242

Weschler B, Kim H, Gallagher PR et al (2005) Functional status after childhood traumatic brain injury. J Trauma 58:940–949

Wijdicks EFM, Hijdra A, Young GB et al (2006) Practice Parameter: Prediction of outcome in comatose survivors after cardiopulmonary resuscitation (an evidence-based review): Report of the Quality Standards Subcommittee of the American Academy of Neurology. Neurology 67:203–210

Wijdicks EFM (2007) 10 questions about the clinical determination of brain death. Neurologist 13:380–381

Wijdicks EFM, Cranford RE (2005) Clinical diagnosis of prolonged states of impaired consciousness in adults. Mayo Clin Proc 80:1037–1046

Wong CP, Forsyth RJ, Kelly TP et al (2001) Incidence, aetiology, and outcome of non-traumatic coma: a population based study. Arch Dis Child 84:193–199

Young GB (2009) Coma. Ann N Y Acad Sci 1157:32–47

Young GB, Pigott SE (1999) Neurobiological basis of consciousness. Arch Neurol 56:153–157

366 Acute, Subacute, and Chronic Progressive Encephalopathies

Generoso Gutierrez-Gascón

Introduction

Definitions and Exclusions

For purposes of this chapter, "encephalopathy" will mean *a disorder in which there is an altered mental state, which, depending on the type and severity, can include loss of cognitive function, personality changes, inability to concentrate, confusion, delirium, stupor, or coma.* It does not refer to a single disease, but to a syndrome of global brain dysfunction, which can be caused by many different illnesses, both systemic, secondarily affecting the brain, and primary in the brain itself. The onset may be acute, subacute, chronically progressive, or static. This chapter will not discuss the static or nonprogressive encephalopathies such as the mental retardation or cerebral palsy syndromes, nor will it discuss neuropsychiatric disorders such as the autistic spectrum disorders (See Dr. Pamela High's section on ➋ Developmental and Behavioral Disorders). Furthermore, it will exclude traditional acute infectious etiologies such as viral encephalitis (e.g., Herpes Simplex encephalitis), bacterial and fungal meningitis, toxic encephalopathies from ingested heavy metals like lead, accidental poisoning, drug ingestion in suicide attempts, or inhaled toxins, such as carbon monoxide.

Encephalopathies discussed in this chapter are likely to be seen by pediatricians and primary care practitioners throughout the world, although some are seen in some parts of the world more than others. For example, HIV encephalopathy (AIDS) is not uncommon in Africa and south Asia, and subacute sclerosing panencephalitis (SSPE) in Turkey and India, but early cases of the encephalopathy associated with the H1N1 influenza pandemic, though first described in Mexico and southern California, have been seen throughout the world.

Classification

This chapter will arbitrarily discuss encephalopathies by age group (infancy and early childhood, mid-childhood, and late childhood/adolescence), with stratification by clinical course (acute, subacute, chronic progressive) (See ➋ *Tables 366.1* and ➋ *366.3*).

Etiology and Clinical Presentation

Etiologies discussed in this chapter include inborn errors of metabolism, lysosomal storage disorders, epileptic encephalopathies, infection-related such as acute toxic encephalopathy and Reye syndrome, immune-mediated, slow virus infections, and progressive encephalopathic degenerative diseases. Because there are many different etiologies, the disturbance in mental status may be accompanied by other neurological symptoms or signs, such as seizures, ataxia, weakness, movement disorders or visual loss, depending on the part of the brain affected. The mental status change, especially in the progressive encephalopathies, may also be expressed as specific higher cortical dysfunction, such as aphasia, apraxia, or agnosia, before progression to a dementia. Dementia is defined as a loss of previously acquired cognitive and/or behavioral function and is central to the neurodegenerative diseases.

Management

Adopting a mind set of searching for treatable and reversible etiologies can focus the diagnostic and treatment approach. The neuropathologic substrate, particularly in the acute toxic-metabolic encephalopathies, is usually cerebral edema. This can be indicated by CT brain findings of decreased attenuation periventricularly and in subcortical white matter or increased T2 signal intensity on brain MRI. Functional techniques such as magnetic resonance spectroscopy (MRS) and positron emission tomography (PET), single photon emission computerized tomography (SPECT) show the pathophysiology better, but are not widely available in non-tertiary care centers and in the developing world. CSF findings may show increased

Abdelaziz Y. Elzouki (ed.), *Textbook of Clinical Pediatrics*, DOI 10.1007/978-3-642-02202-9_366,

Table 366.1
Acute, subacute, and progressive encephalopathies in infancy and early childhood

Age	Acute	Subacute	Progressive
Infancy/early childhood	Hypoxic-ischemic	Biotinidase deficiency	Tay–Sachs
	Aminoacidurias Organic acidurias Urea cycle	Early myoclonic encephalopathy	Sandhoff
			GM1 gangliosidoses
		Ohtahara syndrome	NCL[a]
	Vitamin-dependent	FIRES[b]	Infantile
	Fatty acid oxidation	Leigh's disease	Late infantile
	Neurotransmitter	MELAS[c]	Juvenile
		MERRF[d]	Mucolipidoses
			MPS[e]
			Hurler
			Hunter
			San Filippo
			Leukodystrophies
			Krabbe
			Metachromatic
			Austin
			Pelizaeus-Merzbacher
			Canavan
			Alexander
			POLG-related
			Alpers-Huttenlocher
			MCHS[f]
			Aicardi–Goutieres

[a]Neuronal ceroid lipofuscinosis
[b]Febrile infection-related epilepsy syndrome
[c]Mitochondrial encephalomyelopathy, lactic acidosis, stroke-like episodes
[d]Myoclonic epilepsy with ragged red fibers
[e]Mucopolysaccharidoses
[f]Myocerebrohepatopathy

opening pressure, no pleocytosis, and normal protein. Electroencephalography (EEG) reveals diffuse slow background activity of low or high voltage, indicating depressed brain functioning. If an inborn error of metabolism is suspected, blood for amino acid determination by gas-liquid chromatography (GLC), urine for organic acid determination by gas chromatography-mass spectroscopy (GCMS), or better yet, a blood spot on filter paper to be sent to a regional or national laboratory for tandem mass spectroscopy (tandem MS) should be obtained. Also, samples for blood pH, electrolytes, lactate, pyruvate, ammonia, glucose, carnitine, liver function tests, and CSF for lactate and pyruvate should be obtained. For possible future studies, samples of the following should be stored frozen: 3 ml of CSF for future possible studies such as neurotransmitter metabolites, polymerase chain reaction (PCR) amplification for viral DNA fragments, immunoglobulins, oligoclonal bands, myelin basic protein, and measles-specific antibody titers; 5 ml of urine; and 5 ml of blood (−20°C), 1 ml in a fluoride tube and the rest in a heparinized tube. Until a specific diagnosis is made, if the initial tests suggest an organic aciduria, broad spectrum cofactor supplementation for possible treatable and reversible acute encephalopathies can be given without risk of adverse reactions. A starting combination is thiamine (300 mg plus per day), biotin (50 mg twice a day), riboflavin (100 mg/kg/day), and L-carnitine (100 mg/kg/day in three divided doses). If a mitochondrial disease of

Table 366.2
Progressive genetic encephalopathies

Age	Gray matter	White matter
Infancy/early childhood	Gangliosidoses, GM1, GM2	Leukodystrophies
	NCL,[a] infantile, late infantile	Krabbe
	Nieman-Pick	Metachromatic
	Gaucher, infantile	Canavan
	Mucolipidoses	Alexander
	Hurler, Hunter	Austin
	San Filippo	Pelizaeus–Merzbacher
	POLG[b] disorders	Leukoencephalopathies
	Alpers–Huttenlocher	Vanishing white matter
	Myocerebrohepatopathy	Megancephalic with subcortical cysts
	Aicardi–Goutieres	Neuroaxonal dystrophy, Type 1
	Pompe (glycogen storage disease Type 1)	
Late childhood/ adolescence	NCL, juvenile (Kufs)	Adrenoleukodystrophy
	Nieman Pick Type C	
	Sialidosis Type 1 (cherry-red spot-myoclonus)	
	Huntington's	
	Wilson's	
	PANK2[c], Neurodegeneration with brain iron accumulation	

[a]NCL neuronal ceroid lipofuscinosis
[b]POLG polymerase gamma gene
[c]PANK2 pantothenate kinase gene

oxidative phosphorylation is suspected, one can add vitamin K, vitamin C, and coenzyme Q. Specific therapy can then await specific diagnosis (See Chap. 38, "Disorders of Organic Acid and Amino Acid Metabolism" by Ozand and Al-Essa).

The specific etiology, pathogenesis, genetics, neuropathology, clinical manifestations, diagnostic investigations, differential diagnosis, and treatment will be discussed, when appropriate, for the individual diseases that are not otherwise discussed elsewhere in this book, such as in the section on Inborn Errors of Metabolism (Pinar Ozand), Chap. 360, "Neonatal Neurology" (William Brown and Mara Coyle), or Chap. 362, "Epilepsy" (John Gaitanis). For single gene disorders, prenatal diagnosis is possible through amniocentesis or chorionic villus sampling. If the single gene mutation in a progressive debilitating or fatal disease is already known in a family, having been identified in a previously affected child, and abortion is not an option, preimplantation genetic diagnosis (PIGD), using in vitro fertilization (IVF) techniques, can be utilized as preventive treatment, in IVF centers with technically qualified obstetricians and geneticists.

Web-Based Resources for Physicians

For readers who desire in-depth information beyond this chapter, web-based resources are the quickest way to access information at the point of service, since computers and internet access are now available almost everywhere, except in the most remote locations. For diagnostically puzzling patients whose presentations suggest some kind of chromosomal, genetic or unrecognized syndrome, www.simulconsult.com can be helpful in narrowing down differential diagnostic possibilities. For more detailed descriptions of genetic diseases with Mendelian inheritance, consult OMIM (Online Mendelian Inheritance in Man) at www.ncbi.nlm.nih.gov/omim. For succinct information on clinical presentation and management of any genetic disease, click on "Gene Reviews" in www.genetests.org. For information on availability of molecular genetic testing, on a clinical or research basis, for any of the genetic diseases discussed in this chapter, click on "Laboratory Directory" in www.genetests.org. For information on ongoing clinical trials, consult www.clinicaltrials.gov. For evidence-based

Table 366.3
Acute, subacute, progressive encephalopathies, mid-childhood and adolescence

Mid-childhood	Infection-related Acute toxic, Reye–Johnson, Influenza-associated Acute necrotiz Encephalopathy, ADEM[a], AHLE[b], Hepatic encephalop, Uremic encephalop, Hypertensive, Hypoglycemic	Cerebral malaria Trypanosomiasis, Epileptic encephal, ESESS[c], Landau-Kleffner, CSWS[d]	Adrenoleukodystrophy, Nieman-Pick Type C, Juvenile Huntington's
Adolescence	Acute Confusional Migraine, Immune-mediated: Hashimoto's, Rassmussen's, AERRPS[e], DESC[f], NORSE[g]	Nonconvulsive status epilepticus	SSPE[h]
			HIV[i]
			PMFL[j]
			Wilson's disease
			Hallervorden–Spatz
			Progressive myoclonic epileptic encephalop: Sialidosis Type 1, Unverricht-Lafora, MERRF[k]

[a]Acute demyelinating encephalomyelitis
[b]Acute hemorrhagic leukoencephalitis
[c]Electrical status epilepticus in slow-wave sleep
[d]Continuous spike waves in sleep
[e]Acute encephalitis with refractory, repetitive partial seizures
[f]Devastating epileptic encephalopathy in school-aged children
[g]New onset refractory status epilepticus
[h]Subacute sclerosing panencephalitis
[i]Human immunodeficiency virus
[j]Progressive multifocal leukoencephalopathy
[k]Myoclonic encephalopathy, ragged red fibers

information on efficacy of treatments, consult www.cochranereviews.com.

Infancy and Early Childhood

Acute Encephalopathies

Hypoxic-ischemic encephalopathy (HIE)
Inborn errors of metabolism
- Aminoacidurias
- Organic acidurias
- Urea cycle disorders
- Vitamin-dependent disorders
- Fatty acid oxidation (FAO) disorders
- Neurotransmitter-related disorders

Neonatal encephalopathy describes an obtunded newborn with abnormal pediatric Glasgow Coma Scale, often experiencing seizures and exhibiting hypotonia. In developed countries, 2–3 per 1,000 live term birth infants develop acute, moderate to severe encephalopathy. Rates are 10 times that in less developed nations (See *Table 366.1*).

Most commonly *hypoxic-ischemic encephalopathy (HIE)* is the cause. Neonatal encephalopathy and HIE are covered in the Chap. 360, "Neonatal Neurology" by William Brown and Mara Coyle Brown, and in the Neonatology section.

It is in this age group that *the inborn errors of metabolism (IEM)* are most likely to present. The devastating metabolic diseases of the newborn are discussed in the chapter by P. Ozand and M Al-Essa, on Disorders of Amino and Organic Acidurias. The aminoacidurias, such as non-ketotic hyperglycinemia, organic aciduras such as methylmalonic and propionic acidemia, fatty acid oxidation disorders and vitamin-dependent disorders, such as pyridoxine dependency present as neonatal encephalopathies in developed countries, but are much more common in populations where there are large families and a high rate of consanguineous marriages.

Moammar et al. report that in the Eastern Province of Saudi Arabia, over 25 years, IEM had a cumulative incidence of 150/100,00 live births. Small-molecule disorders were diagnosed in 134/248 patients (54%). Organic acidurias were the most common (48/248 patients; 19%), methylmalonic aciduria being the most frequently observed (13/48 patients; 27%). Lysosomal storage diseases were diagnosed in 74/248 patients (30%), of which mucopolysaccharidosis was the most frequently observed (28/74; 38%).

Fatty Acid Oxidation Disorders (FAO)

Medium-chain acyl Co-A dehydrogenase deficiency (MCAD)
Very long chain acyl Co-A dehydrogenase deficiency (VLCFA)
Multiple acyl Co-A dehydrogenase deficiency (Glutaric aciduria Type 2)

Medium-, long-, and short-chain acyl-CoA dehydrogenase deficiencies (MCAD, LCAD, SCAD) are due to defects of the β-oxidation spiral. The encephalopathic presentations are acute toxic encephalopathy with nonketotic hypoglycemia in infancy and toddlerhood provoked by fasting (primarily MCAD), the syndrome of nonketotic hypoglycemia plus very low plasma carnitine and absent dicarboxylicaciduria (carnitine transport defects), and sudden infant death (SIDS). MCAD is the most common mitochondrial β-oxidation disorder, occurring in 1/10,000 to 1/20,000. Children usually present between ages 3 and 15 months. A common presentation is vomiting, lethargy, followed by fasting and associated with a preceding viral gastrointestinal or respiratory infection. In the emergency room, it presents as an acute toxic encephalopathy or coma, with hypoketotic hypoglycemia, hyperammonemia, and abnormal liver function tests. Serum carnitine is low, urine acycarnitines are increased. The differential diagnosis includes other fatty acid oxidation disorders, exogenous toxin ingestion, and true Reye syndrome. Management utilizes10% dextrose intravenously, L-carnitine 100 mg/kg/day orally in divided doses, frequent short feeds. Prognosis: the risk of death with first episode is about 20%. If treatment is delayed, developmental retardation, behavioral problems, seizures, and failure to thrive may result. Preventive treatment: living siblings should be screened with acylcarnitine profiles and subsequent siblings should be screened in the neonatal period.

For further discussion of MCAD, as well as other FAOs – very long chain acyl-CoA dehydrogenase deficiency, multiple acyl-CoA dehydrogenase deficiency (glutaric aciduria Type 2), see chapter by Ozand and Al-Essa, ➲ Chap. 38, "Disorders of Organic Acid and Amino Acid Metabolism".

Neurotransmitter-Related Disorders

These disorders are due to a relative deficiency or excess of a neurotransmitter. Two of these disorders present as encephalopathy in the neonatal period – biopterin-dependent PKU and non-ketotic hyperglycinemia. In biopterin-dependent PKU, the etiology causing encephalopathy *is 6-PTS deficiency (6-pyruvoyltetrahydropterin synthase). In non-ketotic hyperglycinemia,* it is the excessive glycine (a CNS neurotransmitter), due to defects in various components of the mitochondrial glycine cleavage enzyme system, that causes the seizures and encephalopathy in the acute neonatal presentation. Clinical presentation and treatment are discussed in the chapter by Ozand and Al-Essa, ➲ Chap. 38, "Disorders of Organic Acid and Amino Acid Metabolism".

Other

Other rare miscellaneous acute encephalopathies to be mentioned but not discussed here are acute chemotherapy-related leukoencephalopathy, usually in leukemia patients treated with methotrexate, and bronchiolitis-associated encephalopathy in critically ill infants, seen in pediatric intensive care units.

Subacute Encephalopathies

Biotinidase deficiency
Epileptic encephalopathies
- Early myoclonic encephalopathy
- Early infantile epileptic encephalopathy (Ohtahara syndrome)
- Febrile infection-related epilepsy syndromes (FIRES)

Mitochondrial disorders (of oxidative phosphorylation)
- Subacute necrotizing encephalomyelopathy (Leigh's disease)
- Mitochondrial encephalomyopathy, lactic acidosis, stroke-like episodes (MELAS)
- Myoclonic epilepsy with ragged red fibers (MERRF)

Biotinidase Deficiency

This subacute to progressive encephalopathy is mentioned because it is eminently treatable, by giving biotin, L-carnitine, and Polycitra. In areas of the world where neonatal metabolic screening is done, the encephalopathy can be prevented because of early diagnosis and treatment. The disorder is described in the chapter by Ozand and Al-Essa, ➲ Chap. 38, "Disorders of Organic Acid and Amino Acid Metabolism".

Epileptic Encephalopathies

The epileptic encephalopathies are disorders that present as seizures of various kinds that are refractory to medication treatment and are accompanied by developmental behavioral arrest or regression. In infancy, these are the infantile spasms or West syndrome, in early childhood, the Lennox Gastaut syndrome and Severe Myoclonic Epilepsy (Dravet syndrome). These are discussed in the ➋ Chap. 362, "Epilepsy" (John Gaitanis). Two epileptic encephalopathies appear in the neonatal period – early myoclonic encephalopathy and early infantile epileptic encephalopathy with burst-suppression, or Ohtahara syndrome.

Other Selected Epileptic Encephalopathies

Early Myoclonic Encephalopathy (Neonatal Myoclonic Encephalopathy). This clinical-EEG syndrome presents in the neonatal period with partial or fragmentary erratic myoclonus, massive myoclonias, and frequent partial motor seizures. The EEG displays complex spike bursts, sharp waves, and slow waves, separated by flattening of the background and localized discharges, so-called suppression bursts. These become more apparent in sleep and may persist into late childhood, after a transient hypsarrhythmia in late infancy. The etiology is usually nonstructural/ metabolic, for example, non-ketotic hyperglycinemia. Treatment is directed at the etiology. Symptomatic suppression of seizures with antiepileptic drugs is rarely successful in this refractory epileptic encephalopathy. Prognosis is severe, with early death, or severe and profound psychomotor retardation.

Early Infantile Epileptic Encephalopathy with Burst-Suppression (Ohtahara Syndrome). Tonic spasms are the main seizures, often appearing in clusters. Suppression bursts appear in both wake and sleep. They evolve into hypsarrhythmia at 3–4 months of age and West syndrome, then eventually to diffuse slow spike waves and the Lennox–Gastaut syndrome. The etiology most commonly is structural brain lesions such as prenatal cerebral dysgenesis. Prognosis is dire, with early death or marked psychomotor retardation and seizure intractability, despite treatment with ACTH, corticosteroids, vigabatrin, or ketogenic diet.

Febrile Infection-Related Epilepsy Syndrome (FIRES), A Nonencephalitic Epileptic Encephalopathy. Previously healthy children develop prolonged or recurring seizures lasting days after fever onset, usually with respiratory or nonspecific infections. CSF shows no pleocytosis and no pathogens. EEG usually reveals diffuse slowing or multifocal discharges. Neuroimaging is normal and no inflammation is seen on brain biopsies, when done. The course is dire. A.van Baalen reported only two recovered in a series of 22 children in Germany. Two died, two had behavioral disturbances, eight continued with impaired consciousness, and eight developed medically refractory epilepsy. The pathogenesis is likely neuronal hyperexcitation rather than inflammatory cerebral damage.

Mitochondrial Disorders: Disorders of Oxidative Phosphorylation

Leigh's disease
MELAS (mitochondrial encephalomyopathy, lactic acidosis, and stroke-like episodes)
MERRF (myoclonic epilepsy associated with ragged red fibers)

Leigh's Disease (Subacute Necrotizing Encephalomyelopathy)

Leigh syndrome is a relatively common disease. About one-half are diagnosed before the age of 6 months. A previously healthy infant begins with brain stem signs such as poor feeding, sucking, and swallowing, and supranuclear ophthalmoplegia. A central hypoventilation syndrome is prominent early. Seizures may occur early, movement disorders late. Developmental arrest and then deterioration follows. Diagnosis is made by noting the typical course, elevated CSF lactate and pyruvate, and a typical distribution on brain MRI of paramedian T2 increased intensity lesions in brainstem, cerebellum, and basal ganglia. Magnetic resonance spectroscopy (MRS) reveals elevated lactate peaks in these lesions. The differential diagnosis includes the organic acidurias presenting as progressive encephalopathy like glutaric aciduria type 1, biotinidase deficiency, and biopterin-dependent PKU, the primary lactic acidoses, atypical peroxisomal disorder, and infantile neuraxonal dystrophy. Leigh's disease is caused by mitochondrial DNA as well as autosomal recessive, nuclear coded DNA mutations. Although several enzyme complexes of the respiratory chain, primarily in Complex IV, are involved, the most commonly reported defect is in the ATPase6 gene at mtDNA position 8993, causing defective ATP production. The pathology consists of spongy degeneration, demyelination, gliosis, necrosis, with relative sparing of neurons, and capillary proliferation. Treatment is primarily supportive and symptomatic. Metabolic treatment using mitochondrial "cocktails" have been used, with inconclusive results. These usually include biotin 50 mg/day or more, thiamine 300 mg/day or more, coenzyme Q10, vitamin K, and vitamin C. Dichloroacetate has been used to lower serum lactate levels. Patients with pyruvate dehydrogenase complex deficiency may respond to the ketogenic diet. The prognosis is grave, this being a fatal disease, although there may be periods of arrest of progression.

MELAS – Mitochondrial Encephalomyopathy, Lactic Acidosis, and Stroke

MELAS (mitochondrial encephalomyopathy, lactic acidosis, and stroke-like episodes) is a multisystem disorder typically beginning usually between 2 and 10 years of age. Development is usually normal, though stature may be short. The most common initial symptoms are generalized tonic-clonic seizures, recurrent headaches, anorexia, and recurrent vomiting. Exercise intolerance or proximal limb weakness can present early. Sensorineural hearing loss is common. Stroke-like episodes of recurrent transient hemiparesis or cortical blindness may be associated with altered consciousness. Motor abilities, vision, and mentation are impaired by adolescence.

The diagnosis rests on a combination of clinical findings and molecular genetic testing. Mutations in the mitochondrial DNA (mtDNA) gene *MT-TL1* encoding $tRNA^{Leu(UUR)}$ are causative. The most common mutation, present in over 80%, is an A-to-G transition at nucleotide 3243. Mutations can usually be detected in mtDNA from leukocytes. However, because of heteroplasmy in mitochondrial disorders, the pathogenic mutation may be undetectable in leukocytes but can be detected in other tissues, such as cultured skin fibroblasts grown from skin biopsies or, most reliably, skeletal muscle obtained from muscle biopsy.

No specific treatment for MELAS exists. Sensorineural hearing loss has been treated with cochlear implantation. Seizures respond to antiepileptics. Coenzyme Q10 and L-carnitine have been beneficial in some individuals.

MELAS is transmitted by usually asymptomatic mothers. A male with a mtDNA mutation cannot transmit it to any of his offspring. A female (affected or unaffected) transmits the mutation to all of her offspring. Prenatal diagnosis for MELAS is available if a mtDNA mutation has previously been detected in the mother.

MERRF – Myoclonic Epilepsy, Ragged Red Fiber Syndrome

MERRF is a multisystem disorder characterized by myoclonus, which is often the first symptom, followed by generalized epilepsy, ataxia, weakness, and dementia. Onset is usually in childhood, occurring after normal early development. Common findings are hearing loss, short stature, optic atrophy, and cardiomyopathy with Wolff–Parkinson–White (WPW) syndrome. Less common are pigmentary retinopathy and lipomatosis.

The clinical diagnosis of MERRF is based on the clinical history and exam of myoclonus, generalized epilepsy, ataxia, and ragged red fibers (RRF) in the muscle biopsy. The mitochondrial DNA (mtDNA) gene *MT-TK* encoding $tRNA^{Lys}$ is the gene most commonly associated with MERRF. The most common mutation, present in over 80% of affected individuals with typical findings, is an A-to-G transition at nucleotide 8344 (m.8344A>G). Mutations are usually present in all tissues and can be detected in mtDNA from blood leukocytes. However, because of "heteroplasmy" in mitochondrial disorders, the pathogenic mutation may be undetectable in mtDNA from leukocytes and may only be detected in other tissues, such as cultured skin fibroblasts from skin biopsy or, most reliably, skeletal muscle obtained by muscle biopsy.

Levetiracetam, clonazepam, zonisamide, and valproic acid (VPA) have been used to treat the myoclonic epilepsy. However, VPA may cause secondary carnitine deficiency and should be avoided or if used, L-carnitine must be added. Coenzyme Q_{10} (100 mg 3 × /day) and L-carnitine (1,000 mg 3 × /day) are often used in hope of improving mitochondrial function.

Mitochondrial genetics dictates that the mother of an affected child usually has the mtDNA mutation and may or may not have symptoms. The father is not at risk for having the disease-causing mtDNA mutation. If a male has an mtDNA mutation, he cannot transmit it to his children. A female with the mutation (whether affected or unaffected) transmits the mutation to all of her offspring. Prenatal diagnosis for MERRF is possible if an mtDNA mutation from the mother has been identified.

Progressive Encephalopathies

Incidence

Progressive encephalopathy (PE) in children is a heterogeneous group of diseases mainly composed of metabolic diseases, but consists also of neurodegenerative disorders where neither metabolic nor other causes are found. In an epidemiologic study from Norway by Stromme P et al. from 1985 to 2003, 84 PE cases were registered in Oslo, with 28 different diagnoses. The age-specific incidence rates per 100,000 were 79.89 (<1 year), 8.64 (1–2 years), 1.90 (2–5 years), and 0.65 (>5 years). Furthermore, 66% (55/84) of the cases were metabolic, 32% (27/54) were neurodegenerative, and 2% (2/84) had HIV encephalopathy. In regard to presentations by age group, 71% (60/84) of the cases presented at <1 year, 24% (20/84) were late infantile presentations, and 5% (4/84) were juvenile presentations. Neonatal onset was more common in the metabolic (46%) (25/55) compared to the neurodegenerative group (7%) (2/27). Unspecified neurodegenerative disease occurred in 20% (17/84) of all cases. Overall two-thirds of the cases were metabolic, of which almost half presented in the neonatal period.

One way to conceptualize the progressive genetic encephalopathies in infancy and early childhood is to consider whether progressive degeneration at the onset occurs primarily in the gray matter or in the white matter (See *Table 366.2*, Progressive Genetic Encephalopathies).

Although the disturbance in mental status, usually heralded by developmental arrest and then deterioration, may seem similar, early accompanying neurological symptoms/signs differ. Most of the lysosomal storage diseases are primarily gray matter diseases, because symptoms are due to abnormal storage of metabolic products in neurons. Seizures present early in the course. These are best exemplified by the GM2 gangliosidoses (Tay–Sachs, Sandhoff) and the neuronal ceroid lipofuscinoses. In the white matter diseases (leukodystrophies or leukoencephalopathies), there is progressive degeneration, or hypomyelination, of myelin, and present with long tract (pyramidal) signs early in the course.

Lysosomal Storage Diseases

GM2 gangliosidoses (Tay–Sachs, Sandhoff)
GM1 ganlgiosidoses
Neuronal ceroid lipofuscinosis, Infantile Form (Santavuori), Late Infantile (Jansky–Bielslchowsky), juvenile (Batten–Spielmeyer–Vogt)
Mucolipidoses
Mucopolysaccharidoses (Hurler, Hunter, San Filippo)
Leukodystrophies
- Globoid Cell leukodystrophy (Krabbe disease)
- Metachromatic Leukodystrophy
- Multiple Sulfatase Deficiency (Austin's disease)

These disorders, all presenting in the neonatal and early childhood period, are discussed in the Chap. 39, "Lysosomal Storage Diseases", by Ozand and Al-Essa.

Other Leukodystrophies, Leukoencephalopathies

The term leukoencephalopathies is a broad one which includes any disorder which primarily affects brain white matter or myelin, and so includes disorders of hypomyelination or dysmyelination. The leukodystrophies are inherited disorders characterized by progressive degeneration of the white matter of the brain.

Ozand and Al-Essa (Chap. 39, "Lysosomal Storage Diseases" chapter) discuss the traditional leukodystrophies:
- Globoid cell leukodystophy (Krabbe's disease)
- Metachromatic leukodystrophy (MLD)
- Multiple sulfatase deficiency (Austin's disease)

Other leukodystrophies discussed here are:
- Pelizaeus–Merzbacher disease
- Canavan's disease
- Alexander's disease

Two relatively recently described leukoencephalopathies are:
- Vanishing white matter disease
- Megalencephalic leukoencephalopathy with subcortical cysts

Pelizaeus–Merzbacher Disease (PMD)

PMD is an x-linked leukodystrophy secondary to mutations in the proteolipid protein (PLP) gene, which presents in infancy or early childhood, with "wheeling" nystagmus, hypotonia, and impaired cognition. Hypotonia evolves into spasticity, the nystagmus disappears but cerebellar ataxia, choreoathetosis may appear, as well as optic atrophy. Death occurs in the second to third decade. A connatal form presenting in the first 3 months of life has a much more severe course, with laryngeal stridor, and early death. The clinical diagnosis is based on clinical signs and symptoms, diffuse T2 hyperintensity of the brain MRI, an x-linked inheritance pattern, and finding mutations of the PLP1 gene. Abnormalities of the PLP gene also cause a phenotypically different entity, spastic paraplegia type 2 (SPG 2), which presents at a later age. Treatment is symptomatic and supportive, aimed at preventing secondary complications with multidisciplinary surveillance. Although *PLP*1-related disorders are inherited in an x-linked manner, *de novo* mutations have been reported. Males with the PMD phenotype do not reproduce; males with the SPG2 phenotype may have children. All daughters of a male proband will be carriers; no sons will inherit the mutation. All sons of a female carrier are at a 50% risk of inheriting the mutation and having the disease; all daughters are at a 50% risk of being carriers. Carrier testing for at-risk relatives and prenatal testing for pregnancies at increased risk are possible in families in which the disease-causing *PLP*1 mutation has been identified.

Canavan Disease (CD)

In CD, macrocephaly begins in the first year of life, with failure to sit and marked hypotonia, which eventually evolves into spasticity. In CD, there is diffuse T2 hyperintensity of the white matter which on magnetic resonance spectroscopy shows markedly elevated NAA (n-acetylaspartic acid). Urine shows acetylaspartic aciduria. ASPA is the only gene associated with CD. Three common mutations account for approximately 99% of the disease-causing alleles in Ashkenazi Jewish patients and approximately 50–55% of disease-causing alleles in non-Jewish patients. There is a later presenting rare juvenile form of CD. CD is inherited as an autosomal recessive. This disease is the next targeted disease for prevention by genetic screening of the population at risk, Ashkenazi Jews, following the decreasing incidence of Tay–Sachs disease because of genetic screening.

Alexander Disease (AD)

The classical presentation, the infantile form, affects 51% of patients with AD. It presents in the first 2 years of life with megalencephaly, frontal bossing, psychomotor deterioration, seizures, pyramidal signs, and hydrocephalus due to aqueductal stenosis. There is also a neonatal form, a juvenile form, onset 4–10 years, affects about 23%, and an adult form (about 24%) with wide variability of symptoms. Children with the infantile form survive from weeks to years; with the juvenile form, to the 20s and 30s. In AD, increased T2 hyperintensity predominates in the frontal lobes. Brain biopsy shows inclusion bodies (Rosenthal fibers) in astrocytes. *GFAP*, which encodes glial fibrillary acidic protein, is the only gene currently known to be associated with AD. Molecular genetic testing has eliminated the need for diagnostic brain biopsy. Treatment is symptomatic and supportive.

Vanishing White Matter Disease (Childhood Ataxia with Central Hypomyelination)

Vanishing white matter (VWM) is one of the most prevalent inherited childhood leukoencephalopathies, but this may affect people of all ages, including neonates and adults. It is a progressive disorder clinically dominated by cerebellar ataxia and in which minor stress conditions, such as fever or mild trauma, provoke major episodes of neurologic deterioration. Typical pathological findings include increasing white matter rarefaction and cystic degeneration, oligodendrocytosis with highly characteristic foamy oligodendrocytes, meager astrogliosis with dysmorphic astrocytes, and loss of oligodendrocytes by apoptosis. Vanishing white matter is caused by mutations in any of the genes encoding the five subunits of the eukaryotic translation initiation factor 2B (eIF2B), EIF2B1 through EIF2B5. eIF2B is an ubiquitously expressed protein complex that plays a crucial role in regulating the rate of protein synthesis. Vanishing white matter mutations reduce the activity of eIF2B and impair its function to couple protein synthesis to the cellular demands in basal conditions and during stress. Reduced eIF2B activity leads to sustained improper activation of the unfolded protein response, resulting in concomitant expression of proliferation, prosurvival, and proapoptotic downstream effectors. Consequently, VWM cells are constitutively predisposed and hyperreactive to stress. VWM genes are housekeeping genes, so it is surprising that the disease is primarily a leukoencephalopathy. The pathophysiology of selective glial vulnerability in VWM remains poorly understood.

Megalencephalic Leukoencephalopathy with Subcortical Cysts (MLC)

MLC is an autosomal recessive disease characterized by infantile-onset macrocephaly, often in combination with mild gross motor developmental delay and seizures, gradual onset of ataxia, spasticity, and sometimes extrapyramidal findings. Mental deterioration is late and mild. Some die in the second and third decades of life, others are alive in their forties.

Magnetic resonance imaging (MRI) shows diffusely abnormal and swollen cerebral white matter and subcortical cysts in the anterior temporal or frontoparietal areas. On follow-up, atrophy ensues. Approximately 80% of MLC patients have mutations in MLC1, the only gene associated with MLC. Sequence analysis detects mutations in approximately 60–70% of affected individuals. Two phenotypes can be distinguished among the non-MLC1 mutated MLC patients: a classical and a benign phenotype. Management utilizes antiepileptic drugs for seizures, physical therapy for motor dysfunction, and special education.

The differential diagnosis is essentially that of white matter diseases that present with a large head, namely, Canavan's disease (CD), due to aspartoacylase deficiency, and Alexander's disease. Both present in the first year of life and are inherited in an autosomal recessive fashion. Neuroimaging differentiates these from each other and from MLC.

POLG (DNA Polymerase Gamma) – Related Disorders

POLG-related disorders comprise a continuum of overlapping phenotypes that were clinically defined long before their molecular basis was known. Mitochondrial DNA is replicated by DNA polymerase gamma. Onset of the *POLG*-related disorders ranges from early childhood to late adulthood. Diagnostic criteria do not exist. Two POLG-related diseases that occur in early childhood with encephalopathy are Alpers–Huttenlocher syndrome (AHS) and childhood myocerebrohepatopathy spectrum (MCHS). Establishing the diagnosis requires identification of two disease-causing *POLG* mutations, for each of these syndromes.

Alpers–Huttenlocher Syndrome (AHS)

AHS affects approximately one of every 51,000 and is characterized by childhood-onset progressive severe encephalopathy with intractable epilepsy and hepatic failure. As the illness progresses, neuroimaging shows gliosis initially in occipital areas and generalized brain atrophy. Molecular genetic testing consists of targeted mutation analysis and sequence analysis. The p.Ala467Thr mutation is the most common *POLG* mutation associated with AHS and is found in almost half of all affected individuals. Two other specific mutations tested are p.Trp748Ser and p.Gly848Ser. These are found in 70% of AHS patients. The rest require full-sequence analysis of both POLG alleles.

Depletion of mitochondrial DNA (mtDNA) develops in clinically affected tissues causing a mitochondrial oxidative-phosphorylation defect. The central nervous system regions affected in AHS are the same as those affected by Leigh syndrome but typically evolve in the reverse order. In AHS, the gliosis is most severe and occurs earliest in the cerebral cortex, followed by the cerebellum, basal ganglia, and brain stem.

Treatment is symptomatic and supportive. Valproic acid (Depakene®) and sodium divalproex (Depakote®) should be avoided. Because other anticonvulsants have also been implicated in accelerating liver deterioration, liver enzymes should be monitored every 2 to 4 weeks after introducing any new antiepileptic medications.

Childhood Myocerebrohepatopathy Spectrum (MCHS)

MCHS presents between the first few months of life up to about age 3 years with developmental delay or dementia, lactic acidosis, and a myopathy with failure to thrive. Other features of a mitochondrial disorder that may be present include liver failure, renal tubular acidosis, pancreatitis, cyclic vomiting, and hearing loss. Seizures are not present, at least early in the disease course.

Aicardi–Goutieres Syndrome (AGS)

AGS is an early-onset encephalopathy that results in severe mental and physical handicap. A subgroup of infants with AGS presents at birth with abnormal neurologic findings, hepatosplenomegaly, elevated liver enzymes, and thrombocytopenia, a picture similar to congenital infection. Otherwise, affected infants present at variable times after the first few days of life, frequently after a period of apparently normal development. Typically, they demonstrate the subacute onset of a severe encephalopathy characterized by extreme irritability, intermittent fevers, loss of skills, and slowing of head growth. Between 20% and 50% of affected individuals have generalized tonic-clonic or focal tonic seizures. As many as 40% have chilblain skin lesions on the fingers, toes, and ears.

The most important clinical laboratory tests are CSF examination for number of white cells and concentrations of interferon alpha and neopterin. These are most likely to be informative early in the disease and are frequently normal after the first few years of life. CSF IFN-α concentration is greater than 2 IU/mL (normal: <2 IU/mL). Lymphocytosis is defined as more than 5 lymphocytes/mm^3 CSF. Typical values range from 5 to 100 lymphocytes/mm^3. CSF concentrations of neopterin (and less so biopterin) are frequently raised in molecularly proven AGS. Levels of the neurotransmitter metabolites 5HIAA, HVA, and 5MTHF are normal.

The diagnosis can be confirmed in children with typical clinical findings, calcification of the basal ganglia and white matter on CT brain scan and leukodystrophic changes in brain MRI, and identifiable mutations in one of the four known causal mutations. Mutations in *TREX1*, *RNASEH2A*, *RNASEH2B*, and *RNASEH2C* are identified in approximately 80% of individuals.

Management includes chest physiotherapy and treatment of respiratory complications; attention to diet and feeding methods to assure adequate caloric intake and avoid aspiration; and seizure control. Infants should be monitored with repeat ophthalmologic examinations in the first few months for glaucoma. Older children should be followed for evidence of scoliosis, insulin-dependent diabetes mellitus, and hypothyroidism.

Most AGS is inherited in an autosomal recessive manner. Most individuals with AGS do not reproduce. Prenatal testing is possible for pregnancies at increased risk if the disease-causing mutation(s) in the family have been identified. Rarely, AGS can be caused by *de novo* autosomal dominant mutations in *TREX1*.

Neuronal Ceroid Lipofuscinoses (NCLs)

The neuronal ceroid-lipofuscinoses (NCLs) are the most common hereditary progressive neurodegenerative diseases. The prevalence is about 1.5–9 per million population. The incidence ranges from 1.3 to 7 per 100,000 live births, depending on the country.

The NCLs are inherited lysosomal storage disorders presenting early with seizures, then intellectual and motor deterioration, progressive blindness, and death. They are to be differentiated from other disorders called in old terminology "the familial amaurotic idiocies," of which Tay–Sachs, Sandhoff's diseases (the GM2 gangliosidoses) are the prototype. NCLs and GM2 gangliosidoses commonly present in infancy or late infancy, with seizures and visual loss. However, the blindness in GM2 gangliosidoses is due to macular degeneration with a cherry red spot (cerebromacular degeneration) on opthalmoscopic examination, while in the NCL's, progressive blindness is due to retinitis pigmentosa (cerebroretinal degeneration).

Phenotypes have been characterized clinically by age of onset and order of appearance of the clinical features: infantile neuronal ceroid-lipofuscinosis (INCL, Santavuori), late-infantile (LINCL, Jansky–Bielschowsky), juvenile (JNCL, Batten–Spielmeyer–Vogt), adult (ANCL, Kuf's disease), and Northern epilepsy (NE, progressive epilepsy with intellectual disability). The clinical presentations of INCL, LINCL, and JNCL are discussed in the ➲ Chap. 39, "Lysosomal Storage Disorders" chapter by Ozand and Al-Essa. The differential diagnosis, genetics, diagnostic tests, and management are discussed here.

Differential Diagnosis

For INCL, Santavuori type (infantile onset):

Tay–Sachs and Sandhoff diseases, Leigh syndrome, Rett syndrome, the infantile peroxisomal disorders (infantile Rhefsum's, neonatal adrenoleukodystrophy), subacute presentations of non-ketotic hypoglycinemia, pyridoxine dependency, CSF glucose transporter deficiency (Devivo syndrome), Niemann–Pick disease types A and B. The distinguishing feature usually is lack of retinal degeneration in these disorders. The differential diagnoses are as follows:

For LINCL, Jansky–Bielschowsky type (late infantile onset):

The epileptic encephalopathies, particularly Severe Myoclonic Epilepsy of Infancy (Dravet syndrome) and Lennox-Gastaut syndrome, and other lysosomal storage disorders.

For JNCL, Batten–Spielmeyer–Vogt type (juvenile onset):

MELAS, MERRF, juvenile onset GM2 gangliosidoses.

The retinal degeneration of JNCL differs from classic retinitis pigmentosa in that in JCNL there is loss of central vision first, not peripheral, and rapidly progresses, with total blindness in 1–2 years.

Genetics

All are inherited as autosomal recessive.

For INCL, Santavuori type: Age of onset 6–24 months. Major gene involved is PPT1.

For LINCL: Classic Jansky–Bielshcowsky type: Onset 2–4 years, major gene is TPP1.

But, there are less common variants:

- Finnish variant: Onset 4–7 years. Gene is CLN5.
- Early juvenile variant: Onset 18 months to 8 years. Gene is CLN6.
- Other variants: Onset 3–7.5 years. Genes are MFSD8, CLN8, CTSD, PPT1.

For JNCL: Batten–Spielmeyer–Vogt: Classic presentation, gene is CLN3.

Rarer variants: Genes are PPOT1, TPP1, CLN9.

Diagnosis

With a good pediatric hematopathologist, diagnosis can be made clinically by electron microscope analysis of lymphocytes in the buffy coat, achieved by centrifuging a sample of blood, which reveal curvilinear or fingerprint bodies or granular osmophilic deposits typical of NCL. Such storage material can also be seen by obtaining ganglion cells through rectal biopsy or conjunctival biopsy, although analyzable samples are technically difficult to obtain. Skin biopsies can also be sampled. White blood cells and cultured skin fibroblasts can be examined for three enzymes: PPT1 (palmitoyl-protein thioesterase 1), TPP-1 (tripeptidyl peptidase 1), and CTSD (cathepsin D). Molecular genetic testing utilizes targeted mutation analysis or sequence analysis.

Management

Treatment is symptomatic and supportive. Drugs used may be antiepileptics, anti-dystonia drugs such as trihexyphenidyl, benzodiazepines for spasticity, antidepressants, and antipsychotics. Phenytoin and carbamazepine need to be avoided because they may activate seizures and and increase rate of deterioration. Lamotrigine can exacerbate myoclonus and seizures, particularly in the late infantile form.

Mid-Childhood

Acute Encephalopathies

Infection-related encephalopathies
- Acute toxic encephalopathy
- Reye–Johnson syndrome
- Influenza-associated encephalopathy
  - Acute necrotizing encephalopathy
- ADEM
- AHLE
- Metabolic encephalopathies
  - Hepatic encephalopathy
  - Uremic encephalopathy
  - Hypertensive encephalopathy (PRES, posterior reversible encephalopathy syndrome)
  - Hypoglycemic encephalopathy

Infection-Related Encephalopathies

Acute Toxic Encephalopathy

Acute toxic encephalopathy results from bacterial toxins from a number of agents: *Bordetella pertussis, Shigella, Campylobacter jejunum, Salmonella, Bartonella henseke.* It presents with acute change in mental status, but is not due to infectious encephalitis or meningitis. The treatment is antibiotics directed at the infectious agents.

Reye–Johnson Syndrome

Reye–Johnson syndrome (See ➋ Chap. 217, "Hepatopathies and Reye Syndrome") presents 3–5 days after a viral infection, often influenza, as an acute change in mental status associated with hypoglycemia, hyperammonemia, fatty infiltration of the liver, and cerebral edema. Four clinical and EEG stages have been postulated in the past, with patients recovering if in Stage 1 or 2, equivocal in Stage 3, almost always progressing to death in Stage 4. The association of aspirin and Reye syndrome is now considered spurious, and the rise and fall in the incidence of Reye syndrome remains unexplained.

The biochemical explanation for Reye-like symptoms is a generalized disturbance in mitochondrial metabolism, eventually resulting in metabolic failure in the liver and other tissues. The etiology of "classical" Reye syndrome is unknown. Hypothetically, the syndrome may result from an unusual response to the preceding viral infection, which is determined by host genetic factors but can be modified by a variety of exogenous agents.

For the past decade or so, reported cases of Reye or Reye-like syndromes have usually had a biochemical explanation, usually the fatty acid oxidation disorders. The treatment of Reye syndrome was always supportive, with the therapeutic aim of reducing cerebral edema.

Influenza-Associated Encephalopathy

Influenza-associated encephalitis/encephalopathy is an uncommon but potentially more serious complication widely reported in Japanese populations, although cases from other East Asian countries, North America, and Europe have been described. Clinical manifestations are diverse, and typically involve febrile seizures and abnormal behaviors in mild cases, with rapid evolution through decreased consciousness to coma in severe forms. Influenza is also a known trigger for a number of rarely encountered, yet often serious, CNS diseases, including Reye–Johnson syndrome. In cases of serious disease, the prognosis is often poor, with outcomes including death or severe neurological sequelae.

Acute necrotizing Encephalopathy (ANE). First described by Mizuguchi et al., ANE occurs early after influenza A and H1N1 infection and presents with encephalopathy and seizures, no CSF pleocytosis, no elevated blood ammonia, and symmetrical multifocal brain lesions and hypoxia, intoxication, hemolytic uremic syndrome, metabolic and neurodegenerative disorders have been ruled out. Most cases occurred in children younger than 5 years of age of Asian origin. Sporadic cases have been reported in Europe and North America. Brain MRI using T2 weighted images, diffusion-weighted imaging (DWI), and apparent diffusion coefficient (ADC) maps show symmetrical lesions in the pons, thalami and geniculate bodies, with swelling. Pathology shows necrosis with petechiae in thalamus and tegmentum of the pons and myelin pallor in cerebellar and cerebral subcortical white matter.

Pathogenesis of IAE is not fully understood but may involve viral invasion of the CNS, proinflammatory cytokines, metabolic disorders, or genetic susceptibility. An autosomal dominant viral acute necrotizing encephalopathy (ANE) was recently found to have missense mutations in the gene Ran-binding 2 (RANBP2).

Acute Disseminated Encephalomyelomyelitis (ADEM)

Acute disseminated encephalomyelitis (ADEM) is a diffuse, monophasic demyelinating disease that follows either a viral infection or, rarely, a viral immunization. Symptoms typically develop a week or two after the antecedent infection and include headache, lethargy, and coma. The clinical course is rapid, and as many as 20% of those affected die; the remaining patients recover completely. ADEM is discussed in detail, and AHLE briefly, by Tanuja Chitnis, ➲ Chap. 375, "Parainfectious and Autoimmune Disorders".

Acute Hemorrhagic Leukoencephalomyelitis (AHLE)

Acute hemorrhagic leukoencephalomyelitis of Weston Hurst is a rare fulminant disorder typically affecting young adults and children and is thought to be a hyperacute form of ADEM. AHLE often presents with abrupt onset of fever, neck stiffness, seizure, and/or focal neurologic signs several days following a viral illness or vaccination. The illness is preceded by a recent episode of upper respiratory infection, most often of unknown cause. The differential diagnosis considers a direct central nervous system infection or a toxic ingestion. Pathology shows lesions much more severe than those of ADEM and includes destruction of small blood vessels, disseminated necrosis of white and gray matter with acute hemorrhage, fibrin deposition, and abundant neutrophils. Scattered lymphocytes are seen in foci of demyelination. An autoimmune pathophysiology is likely, with immune cross-reactivity between myelin basic protein moieties and various infectious agent antigens. Although treatment is not well-established; some authors report that a combination of immunosuppressant medications and/or therapeutic plasma exchange may be of benefit. Prognosis is severe, with death in days to a week after symptom onset. Significant residuals remain in the few who survive.

Hepatic Encephalopathy (See chapter on ➲ Liver Failure). Specific neurologic features in *hepatic encephalopathy* are asterixis, and an EEG pattern of triphasic waves upon a slow background, although the latter is nonspecific and may be seen in other encephalopathies. The toxin most implicated is ammonia. The most important component of managing a child with hepatic encephalopathy is basic intensive care with regulation of fluid status, glucose, and electrolyte homeostasis. Specific management includes measures to reduce serum ammonia concentrations, and the prevention and prompt treatment of complications. Methods to reduce ammonia target various steps in its metabolism. This includes reducing its production in and absorption from the intestine and promoting its metabolism in the liver. Specific pediatric care issues, approaches to treatment of fulminant hepatic failure, the role of artificial liver support devices, and decision for liver transplantation are beyond the scope of this chapter.

Uremic Encephalopathy. In *uremic encephalopathy* (See chapter on ➲ Chronic Renal Failure), hypertension is often associated (see chapter on ➲ Hypertension in Children), and the syndrome of posterior reversible encephalopathy (PRES) is seen. Pavlakis, et al. assert that PRES is just a new name for hypertensive encephalopathy. Clinical presentation is usually with seizures, headache, visual disturbances including cortical blindness, and encephalopathy. PRES is a clinical-neuroradiological syndrome, with bilateral posterior parietal-occipital increased T2 and FLAIR signal intensities, which resolve over time. PRES has been reported with a number of different conditions in normotensive children – cancer chemotherapy, usually leukemia, systemic lupus erythematosus, measles vaccination, glomerulonephritis, vasculitis, immunosuppressive treatment, renal failure and eclampsia, but it is likely that a comorbid acute hypertensive episode has occurred. The rise in blood pressure is probably rapid, and may be brief, so that it may not have been clinically observed before the clinical/radiological picture emerges. Jones BV et al. postulate that children develop hypertensive encephalopathy at lower absolute pressures than adults owing to the relative "left shift" of their range of cerebral blood flow autoregulation. Neuroradiological perfusion techniques that were applied in their patients support vasodilatation, rather than vasoconstriction and edema, as the primary pathogenic event, with breakdown of blood-brain barrier, and extravasation of protein and fluid. Arterioles situated a short distance from the cortical surface are most affected, and sympathetic nervous activity affords protection from these effects. The posterior circulation has significantly less sympathetic innervation than the carotid circulation, which may explain why the majority of lesions in hypertensive encephalopathy are found in the vascular territory of the posterior circulation. The syndrome is reversible, if secondary complications, such as hemorrhage into the leukoencephalopathic areas, do not occur.

Hypoglycemic Encephalopathy. The multiple different causes of hypoglycemia in infants, children, and adolescents are discussed in the chapter on ➲ Hypoglycemia. Encephalopathic presentations of hypoglycemia vary in different ages. Neonates may be asymptomatic. Older children may show palpitations, perspiration, and pallor, with a feeling of weakness and hunger if hypoglycemia is rapid, which usually precede encephalopathic manifestations like disorientation, confusion, headache, inability to concentrate, somnolence, and seizures. If blood glucose levels dip to 10 mg/dL or less, coma ensues, with pupillary dilatation, bradycardia, hypotonia, and shallow breathing. The pathogenesis may involve energy depletion, accumulation of metabolites from nonglucose metabolism, and changes in levels of neurotransmitters. Pathologically, laminar necrosis of the cerebral cortex has long been described, the hippocampus being particularly sensitive.

Recent studies have also reported extensive lesions in cerebral white matter and reversible lesions in the splenium of the corpus callosum (Gallucci M), thought to be due to cytotoxic edema. The management requires prompt glucose replacement, whatever the etiology, with thiamine supplementation. In malnourished patients, niacin, to prevent pellagra, should also be given.

Subacute Encephalopathies

Two parasitic diseases are worth discussing here, since their presentations are essentially with encephalopathy.

Cerebral malaria
Trypanosomiasis (African sleeping sickness)
Epileptic encephalopathies
- Electrical status epilepticus in slow-wave sleep (ESESS)
- Landau–Kleffner syndrome
- Continuous spike waves in slow-wave sleep (CSWS)

Cerebral Malaria (See chapter on Malaria)

Cerebral malaria is a rapidly progressive encephalopathy with a 20% mortality in the pediatric population. This means 80% of children survive, but often with neurological residuals. Although rare relative to the total number of infections, cerebral malaria significantly contributes to approximately 1,000,000 deaths per year and disproportionately affects children less than 6 years of age in sub-Saharan Africa.

A cardinal feature of the pathology is the massing of red cells containing *Plasmodium falciparum* toward the end of its life cycle within the cerebral capillaries. Adhesion of these parasitised red cells to endothelium, an event which may initiate cerebral malaria, is being studied at the molecular level. Basic pathogenesis in mouse models and human studies focus on cytokines, inflammation, cytoadherence, and endothelial activation. Coagulation is variably important, but it is most likely the end point of a series of processes.

One model of pathogenesis is cytokine storm and TNF activation. Lessons from the mouse model and in vitro tissue culture have definitely demonstrated that the endothelium must be stimulated via inflammatory/activation agents before the ligands on the surface are sufficient for sequestration to occur. The correlation of retinal and cerebral pathology suggests that those pediatric patients with features of malarial retinopathy who survive must have had similar changes in the brain including ring hemorrhages. However, anti-TNF agents applied when patients are in coma have not proven effective. They probably have to be given before the TNF cascade begins.

Low levels of nitric oxide, and its precursor arginine, have been found, in cerebral malaria, suggesting that less localized nitric oxide is available to provide for vascular dilatation, which subsequently leads to endothelial activation, upregulation of proadherent molecules, and damage of alternative pathways, including activation of superoxide dismutase. This suggests the possibility of L-arginine as a treatment.

Clinical presentation is a diffuse, febrile encephalopathy, with nonfocal signs, in a *P. falciparum* endemic area (or in travelers who have recently been in such an area). The incubation period is usually 10–18 days. The fever may be intermittent, irregular, or continuous. Generalized seizures occur in 50%, nuchal rigidity rarely occurs, and bilateral pyramidal tract signs when severe, which may proceed to decorticate and decerebrate posturing. Most important is examination of the fundus. Ophthalmoscopic examination to evaluate the retinas in comatose children greatly increases the accuracy of diagnosis of cerebral malaria. It is also a measure of prognosis in patients with evidence of retinopathy with or without papilledema and is a tool for stratifying or triaging patients into treatment or further diagnostic workup. The pediatric retinal findings are peripheral whitening, orange and white vessels, hemorrhages, and papilledema.

Regarding treatment, chloroquin is used for non-*falciparum* malaria. But there is now widespread resistance in endemic areas. All cases *of falciparum* malaria must be admitted for therapy owing to the high mortality of the disease. Falciparum malaria is treated with atovaquone-proguanil (Malarone) or quinine sulfate plus doxycycline, tetracycline, or clindamycin. Cerebral malaria is treated with intravenous quinidine. Since 1991, quinidine gluconate has been the only parenterally administered antimalarial drug available in the United States. A loading dose of 6.25 mg base/kg (10 mg salt/kg) of quinidine gluconate is infused intravenously over 1–2 h, followed by a continuous infusion of 0.0125 mg base/kg/min (0.02 mg salt/kg/min). At least 24 h of quinidine infusion is recommended. Once the patient can take oral medication, and the parasite density is less than 10%, the treatment course is completed with oral quinine at a dosage of 10 mg salt/kg every 8 h. The combined treatment course of quinidine/quinine is 7 days, if the disease was acquired in Southeast Asia, and for 3 days if from South America and Africa. The availability of artemisinin combination therapy in adults across most of Africa produces more rapid cures with no definitive drug failures at present. However, the resistance and delayed clearance patterns seen in Southeast Asia and Africa are worrying for emerging resistance. Clinical trials with artemisinin compounds have shown decreased mortality in adults with severe disease after 48 h of treatment, compared to quinine. No such studies in pediatric patients have been published and almost all mortality in children with cerebral malaria occurs within the first 48 h. Regarding prevention, the RTS,S vaccine trials ongoing in multiple African nations are showing positive results with decreases in both disease incidence and severe disease.

African Trypanosomiasis (Sleeping Sickness)

Sleeping sickness is caused by two organisms: in East Africa, *Trypanosoma brucei rhodesiense,* which causes the more severe form, and in West Africa, *Trypanosomoa brucei gambiense.* They are transmitted by tsetse flies, who feed primarily on wild animals, causing a painful, red swelling at the site of the bite. The infection then spreads through the blood circulation, causing episodes of fever, headache, sweating, and swelling of the lymph nodes. When it reaches the brain, behavioral changes such as fear and mood swings occur, followed by headache, fever, delirium, and asthenia. Patients experience drowsiness during the day, but nighttime insomnia. Symptoms may include anxiety, headache, mood changes, and an uncontrollable urge to sleep. West African trypanosomiasis is primarily a problem in rural populations, and tourists rarely become infected with *T. b. gambiense.* East African trypanosomiasis is an occupational hazard for persons such as game wardens who work in areas where infected wild animals and vectors are present, and in occasional tourists who visit game parks.

Patients without CNS involvement are treated with suramin. The protocol is available through the Centers for Disease Control (CDC). Patients who have positive lumbar punctures should be treated with melarsoprol, a trivalent arsenic compound which, however, has significant toxicity. It can cause hepatotoxicity, cardiac arrhythmias, albuminuria, vomiting, abdominal pain, peripheral neuropathy, and paraplegia. Arsenic encephalopathy occurs in as many as 10% of treated patients and is frequently fatal. The 5–10% risk of mortality from the therapy is outweighed by the risk of the disease. The mortality of CNS African trypanosomiasis is 100%. As is true for suramin, melarsoprol is only available in the United States through the CDC.

Other regimens being explored include a combination chemotherapy, eflornithine alongside nifurtimox, to decrease the time frame and overall dosing of eflornithine, in order to reduce the risk of emerging drug resistance. A nitroheterocycle, fexinidazole, whose trypanocidal activity was first shown nearly 30 years ago, has entered clinical trials. The World Health Organization has declared a campaign to eradicate human African trypanosomiasis.

Epileptic Encephalopathies

Electrical status epilepticus in slow-wave sleep (ESESS)
Landau–Kleffner syndrome (LKS)
Continuous Spike Wave in Sleep (CSWS)

ESESS is an EEG finding and is defined as epileptiform discharges occurring in 80–85% of nocturnal slow-wave sleep. The terms continuous spike wave in slow-wave sleep (CSWS) and Landau–Kleffner syndrome (LKS) describe the clinical epileptic syndromes, among others, that can be seen with ESESS.

LKS is a disorder of uncertain etiology, presenting usually in early childhood, with subacute loss of both comprehension and production of language over weeks to months, where seizures occur concurrently or after language loss begins, and a behavioral change occurs with hyperactive, impulsive, and inattentive behavior. Seizures are usually mild and easy to control, but suppression of seizures does not necessarily herald recovery of language function. The initial language loss often appears as an auditory verbal agnosia, but other childhood aphasia syndromes may occur. Although anecdotal papers have reported remarkable reversal of seizures and language loss with IV or oral steroids, IV IgG, high-dose diazepam, ketogenic diet, or multiple subpial transaction, no controlled studies have been done, and many children with LKS have long-standing language and learning disabilities lasting into adulthood. The reacquisition of oral language is aided by use of visual systems, such as signing.

Although there is an overlap between LKS and CSWS, children with CSWS present with a more global regression, have more problematic epilepsy, and have EEG foci located predominantly in frontotemporal or frontocentral regions. In contrast, children with LKS present with language, not cognitive, loss, have fewer seizures, and the EEG foci are said to be predominantly in the posterotemporal regions. Reports from Japan tout high-dose valproic acid or a combination of valproic acid and ethosuximide as causing remission of CSWS in 2/3 of their patients. Other reports from Europe report levetiracetam as being the most effective AED, causing remission in 40% of patients. Most reports agree that early age of onset and longer duration of ESESS in CSWS bode for poor prognosis.

Chronic Encephalopathies

Adrenoleukodystrophy
Niemann–Pick Type C (see Ozand and Al-Essa chapter on ➋ Lysosomal Storage Diseases)
Juvenile Huntington's disease

Adrenoleukodsystrophy (ALD)

ALD is a disorder where a defective enzyme, lignoceroyl-coenzyme A interrupts the normal β-oxidation of very long chain fatty acids (VLCFAs) in the peroxisomes, resulting in the accumulation of the C-26 and above VLCFAs, a main component of myelin. Excess VLCFAs stimulate adjacent astrocytes and macrophages, which initiate a tumor necrosis factor cytokine cascade which results in demyelination. ALD is an x-linked disorder, the gene *ABCD1* being mapped to Xq28. In neuroimaging studies, increased T2 and FLAIR intensity is primarily in bilateral occipito-parietal areas.

Although there is a neonatal form and an adult form, adrenomyeloneuropathy, which presents as a progressive spastic diplegia, the most common childhood presentation is between the ages of 4 and 8 years. Initial presentations are a decline in school work and ADHD-like symptoms, then early visual agnosia, cortical blindness, progressive dementia, upper motor neuron dysfunction, with adrenal insufficiency, which often predates neurological symptoms and may manifest over time as progressive darkening of the skin and requires ACTH stimulation tests for confirmation.

There is another phenotype, Addison's disease only, presenting with adrenal insufficiency usually by age 7–8 years, with no neurologic signs, but who, in about 10%, later in life usually develop adrenomyeloneuropathy. About 20% of female carriers develop mild neurological signs later in life, usually after age 35.

Diagnosis is made by the typical history, clinical neurological signs, the brain MRI, and elevated serum levels of VLCFAs. Molecular genetic testing of *ABCD1*, the only gene known to be associated with X-ALD, is clinically available.

Differential diagnosis includes other leukodystrophies like metachromatic and globoid cell leukodystrophies, other childhood dementing disorders such as NCL, the juvenile or Batten–Spielmeyer–Vogt presentation, and subacute sclerosing panencephalitis (SSPE).

Management includes replacement steroid therapy for the adrenal insufficiency, psychological, supportive, and educational support. Bone marrow transplantation is an option available for boys with the typical childhood form, who have brain MRI abnormalities, but with still preserved cognitive function (performance I.Q.>80) and a normal neurological examination. An investigational therapy is Lorenzo's oil, a 4:1 mixture of the triglycerides of oleic and erucic acid, prepared from olive oil and rapeseed oil, given to presymptomatic boys treated with Lorenzo's oil who had reduction of C26, and resulted in reduced risk of later brain MRI abnormalities. However, some still developed ALD. Lorenzo's oil remains an investigational therapy.

Juvenile Huntington's Disease

The prevalence of Huntington's disease is 3–7/100,000 in people of western European ancestry. It is much less in African blacks, Chinese, and Japanese. The highest prevalence in the world is probably in the Lake Maracaibo region of Venezuela. It is an autosomal dominant progressive degenerative disease that usually presents in midlife with chorea and slowly progressive dementia. It is due to an expansion of 36 or more CAG trinucleotide triple repeats in the Huntington gene HTT (See ➋ Movement Disorders chapter, by Yasser Awaad). In any triple repeat disease, there is the phenomenon of anticipation; that is, the disease expresses itself at younger and younger ages in subsequent generations. *Juvenile Huntington's Disease* is defined as presenting before the age of 20 years and occurs primarily through paternal transmission of HTT. In adolescents, it presents with rigidity rather than chorea, and with mental status changes such as attention and concentration problems, cognitive slowness, and impaired executive functioning, so it should be in the differential diagnosis of decrease in school performance. There may be depression, personality changes, intermittent explosiveness, and even psychosis. Seizures occur in up to 50% of children presenting before the age of 10 years. The pathology shows selective degeneration of neurons in the corpus striatum – the caudate and putamen. Brain MRI can show striatal atrophy 10 years before clinical symptoms appear. Treatment is supportive and symptomatic. Antiparkinsonian agents containing L-DOPA aimed at decreasing rigidity risk increasing chorea. Haloperidol, tetrabenazine, or benzodiazepines may suppress chorea. Psychiatric disorders can be treated with appropriate psychotropic medications. Genetic counseling is mandatory for at-risk, presymptomatic children under age 18 years. The consensus at present is not to gene-test these children because of the psychosocial, legal, and ethical implications of genetic testing of children and adolescents for a disease that has no definitive treatment.

Late Childhood – Adolescence

Acute Encephalopathies

Acute confusional migraine
Immune-mediated encephalopathies
  Hashimoto's encephalopathy
  Rassmussen's encephalitis
Other immune mediated epileptic encephalopathies
  Acute encephalitis with refractory, repetitive partial seizures (AERRPS)
  Devastating epileptic encephalopathy in school-aged children (DESC)
  New onset refractory status epilepticus (NORSE)

Acute Confusional Migraine (ACM)

Gascon and Barlow first described pubertal and early adolescent children who presented to emergency rooms with the acute onset of confusion, disorientation, and short-term memory loss lasting hours. If an EEG was done during this period, it showed high-voltage diffuse delta slowing, most prominent posteriorly. After an overnight sleep, they recovered and returned to normal. In retrospect, the presence of mild headache was elicited. Some neurologists consider these episodes similar to, if not identical with, the syndrome of transient global amnesia in adults. The differential diagnosis includes nonconvulsive status epilepticus, drug ingestion, concussion, encephalitis, or acute posychosis. Brain MRIs and CSF studies are normal. A history of migraine headaches preceding the confusional episode can be obtained, or subsequently, conventional migraine with or without aura develops (See chapter on ❯ Headache by Mack and Matarese). No treatment is necessary, since the episodes resolve spontaneously after sleep (See ❯ *Table 366.3*).

Immune-Mediated Encephalopathies

Hashimoto's encephalopathy
Rassmussen's encephalitis

Hashimoto's Encephalopathy

Hashimoto's encephalopathy is of presumed autoimmune origin and is characterized by high titers of antithyroid peroxidase antibodies. It is more common in women than in men and has been reported in pediatric, adult, and elderly populations throughout the world.

The clinical presentation may be relapsing and remitting and include seizures, stroke-like episodes, cognitive decline, neuropsychiatric symptoms, and myoclonus. Thyroid function tests are normal. Diagnosis is made first, by excluding other toxic, metabolic, and infectious causes of encephalopathy, and secondly, finding elevated titers of antithryoid antibodies. Pathological findings can suggest an inflammatory process, but features of a severe vasculitis are absent. It may be that Hashimoto's encephalopathy will be subsumed into a group of nonvasculitic autoimmune inflammatory meningoencephalopathies, such as paraneoplastic limbic encephalitis, which usually occurs in women with ovarian teratomas, who have elevated NMDA receptor antibodies. Treatment with corticosteroids is almost always successful, although relapse may occur if treatment is abruptly terminated. Intravenous immune-globulin and plasma exchange may also be effective.

Rassmussen's Encephalitis

This is a rare, disabling disease of childhood, presenting first as epilepsia partialis continua, may progress to refractory focal seizures and focal status epilepticus, hemiplegia, and dementia. Neuroimaging studies show progressive hemiatrophy of the brain. Anti Glu-R3 antibodies (against the glutamate receptor subunit 3) have been reported in some, but not all, patients. The pathology shows inflammation, with cytotoxic T cell reactions against neurons. Immunotherapy using corticosteroids, IV IgG, tacrolimus, and intraventricular alpha interferon, and plasmapheresis have temporarily arrested the course of the disease, all of which supports an autoimmune pathogenesis. Eventually, however, the patients are candidates for hemispherectomy for refractory seizures.

Other Immune-Mediated Epileptic Encephalopathies

Acute encephalitis with refractory, repetitive partial seizures (AERRPS)
Devastating epileptic encephalopathy in school-aged children (DESC)
New onset refractory status epilepticus (NORSE)

What these epileptic encephalopathies with different acronyms all have in common is an acute or subacute onset of status epilepticus after a febrile illness, with no evidence of encephalitic infection, followed by drug-resistant partial epilepsy, reported from Japan, France, the United Kingdom, and Singapore. They appear like a more acute, rapidly evolving Rassmussen's encephalitis, but not limited to a hemisyndrome. AERRPS was defined as a prolonged acute phase of more than 2 weeks, partial seizures frequently evolving into convulsive status, drug resistance, with viral encephalitis and metabolic disorders excluded. DESC was described as status epilepticus and fever at onset, later occurrence of drug-resistant epilepsy and neuropsychological deficits. Response to steroid treatment in DESC patients was unsuccessful. Specchio et al. described eight cases which overlapped with AERRPS and DESC. In two AERRPS cases, antibodies against Glu ε2 were found. In Specchio's eight cases, two had anti-GAD (glutamic acid decarboxylase), one had a CL (anti-cardiolipin) and anti-B2-GPI (anti-beta 2 glycoproteinI autoantibody), and one had ASMA (anti smooth muscle) auto-antibodies. Only one patient recovered; the rest had chronic epilepsy. Response to steroid treatment in DESC patients was unsuccessful.

Subacute Encephalopathies

Non-convulsive status epilepticus (NCSE)
- Absence status
- Psychomotor status (complex partial status epilepticus)
- Comatose patients

Nonconvulsive status epilepticus (NCSE) is defined as a state of altered mental status that can vary from confusion to obtundation to coma for at least 30 min, where an EEG records continuous or frequent electrographic seizures. It constitutes about 25% of all cases of status epilepticus, 8% in subarachnoid hemorrhage, and 8–10% in coma. In *absence status epilepticus*, the child may constantly blink the eyes or may stare blankly, and the EEG shows continuous three cycles per second spike-wave complexes. *In psychomotor status, also called complex partial status epilepticus,* in addition to an altered mental status, there may be automatisms. The EEG shows repetitive high-voltage theta waves in temporal areas. The diagnosis is verified by return to a normal state of consciousness concomitant with suppression of the EEG discharges by intravenous AEDs, usually diazepam or lorazepam. Both of these forms of NCSE present in a patient who is ambulatory, and where the differential diagnosis includes acute confusional migraine, drug ingestion, or psychosis. For primary generalized absences, if benzodiazepines do not stop the status, intravenous valproate (Depacon) is most appropriate. For psychomotor status, if benzodiazepines do not stop it, intravenous phenobarbital or phenytoin (or IM fosphenytoin) would be appropriate. General anesthesia with agents like short-acting barbiturates, propofol, or ketamine, which are options in refractory convulsive status epilepticus (CSE), are not usually necessary in NCSE.

Then there is the critically ill patient, where it occurs in 8–10% of patients in coma. There is a bimodal distribution of NCSE in critically ill patients, affecting children (age <1 year) and the elderly. It is commonly detected in an intensive care unit, after a patient has been hospitalized for overt CSE. After successful suppression of clinically observed seizures, the patient fails to wake up and this is not accounted for by medication-induced drowsiness. The estimated incidence is 15–40% after CSE. It may also occur in any patient who fails to awaken after any acute brain illness, whether an acute stroke, subarachnoid hemorrhage (incidence 8%), head injury, acute encephalitis, hypoxic-ischemic encephalopathy, or postoperatively, for example, after surgery for correction of congenital cardiac anomalies. In this setting, NCSE is diagnosed by a high index of suspicion and by continuous EEG monitoring.

The presence of NCSE is a risk for clinical deterioration and poor prognosis, independent of the original acute brain insult. Not enough studies have been done yet to determine whether early recognition and prompt suppression of electrographic seizures significantly improves outcome.

Chronic Encephalopathies

Slow virus diseases
- Subacute sclerosing panencephalitis (SSPE)
- HIV encephalopathy (See chapter on ➋ Human Immunodeficiency Virus)
- Progressive multifocal leukoencephalopathy (PMFL)

Progressive genetic encephalopathies
- Wilson's disease (see ➋ Movement Disorder chapter, Yasser Awaad)
- Juvenile Huntington's disease (See previous section in this chapter)
- Neurodegeneration with brain iron deposition (PANK2)
  - Formerly called Hallervorden–Spatz disease
- Progressive myoclonic encephalopathies
  - Unverricht
  - Lafora
  - MERRF (See previous section in this chapter)

Slow Virus Diseases

Subacute Sclerosing Panencepalitis (SSPE)
Human immunodeficiency virus (AIDS encephalopathy)
See chapter on ➋ Human Immunodeficiency Virus
Progressive multifocal leukoencephalopathy

What these all have in common is the persistence over years of a virus, in mutated form, after an initial infection, either from long known common viruses like measles, or viruses that were previously unknown but emerged in the late twentieth century, human immunodeficiency virus and papova virus. Recovery from the initial systemic infection occurs, but after a prolonged latent period, symptoms of brain dysfunction appear, and slowly progress.

Subacute Sclerosing Panencephalitis (SSPE)

SSPE is a progressive degenerative encephalopathy due to persistence in the CNS of a mutated form of the measles virus (MV). (See chapter on ➋ Measles) It is now extremely rare in the developed world, where countries have reached or exceeded 80% of the population being immunized with the measles vaccine, but still endemic in the developing world where that standard of immunization has not been reached. The viral genome consists of biased hypermutations affecting principally the matrix (M) gene. There are high CSF titers of antibodies to measles virus, with infiltrations of B and T cells into the CNS. The pathogenesis starts with measles infection at a critical stage of maturation of the CNS and immune system, usually before the age of 2 years. The infection is not contained, despite what seems like initial recovery from childhood systemic measles. There is no major histocompatibility complex in neurons. The mutations of the MV genome affect viral epitopes that are critical for recognition of infected cells. Therefore, there is a defective cytotoxic lymphocyte response and lack of viral clearance. The mutated virus lies dormant in the CNS for years until it becomes activated. What triggers the activation is not known. The pathology reveals nuclear inclusions in neurons that contain the viral antigens. Neurofibrillary tangles can be seen in neurons and oligodendrocytes. Perivascular cells are predominantly CD4+ T cells, with B cells seen more in parenchymal inflammatory infiltrates.

The typical clinical presentation usually starts with cognitive and behavioral deterioration, often mimicking the symptoms of attention deficit hyperactivity disorder, with decline in school performance, over weeks to months. Periodic myoclonus then reveals itself as sudden falls or uncontrolled periodic movements, which in the beginning may be as subtle as eye blinks or slight postural changes, but then proceed to falls. If not treated at this stage, motor and mental deterioration inexorably proceed, until a neurovegetative state or death. The stages of deterioration were first proposed by Jabbour and modified by Gascon et al. (See ➋ *Table 366.4.*)

The typical presentation discussed above can occur anywhere from mid-childhood through adolescence, and presents subacutely, followed by a chronic, progressive course.

Atypical presentations have been reported in infancy as an encephalopathy without the typical myoclonus, in childhood as an acute fulminant encephalopathy, as an ADEM presentation, and in adulthood.

The following drugs have been used in anecdotal reports: amantadine, cimetidine, corticosteroids, intravenous immunoglobulin, interferon beta, inosiplex, alpha interferon, and ribavarin. In the only published randomized, controlled treatment study, which compared oral inosiplex to combination inosiplex and intraventricular alpha interferon, carried out by the International Consortium on SSPE in Ankara, Mumbai, and Manila, there was no statistically significant difference between the two treatments. However, there was a satisfactory treatment outcome, meaning improvement or stabilization, in 34% of those treated with inosiplex alone, and 35% in those who had combined treatment. These are higher than the spontaneous remission rates of 5–10% reported in the literature. The conclusion is that neither treatment is

Table 366.4
SSPE stages

IA	Behavioral, cognitive, personality changes
IB	Myoclonic spasms – aperiodic, focal, subtle, infrequent
IIA	Myoclonic spasms – periodic, generalized, synchronous, frequent. EEG relatively normal background activity, but with PSWCs
IIB	Apraxias, agnosias, speech/language, spasticity, ataxia. Ambulatory with assistance
IIIA	Sits independently, may stand, no walking, no ADLs. Speaks less, visual difficulties. Spasms frequent, multifocal
IIIB	Bedridden, no spontaneous speech, poor comprehension, may be blind, dysphagia, chorea-ballismus-athetosis. EEG delta background; PSWCs obscured
IV	No myoclonic spasms, neurovegetative state. EEG background attenuation, no PSWCs

PSWC's periodic slow-wave complexes, ADLs activities of daily living
(Modified from Gascon et al. 1993)

Table 366.5
CSF IgG synthesis index

Total intrathecal IgG synthesis (mg/day) = [(IgGCSF − IgGserum/615)−(AlbCSF-Albserum/291) × (IgGserum/ Albserum)(0.43)] × 5

Concentrations in mg/dL, 615 and 291 are the average normal serum/CSF ratios for IgG and albumin, 0.43 the molecular mass ratio of albumin to IgG, and 5 the average daily production of CSF in deciliters (From Conrad AJ et al. 1994)

statistically superior to the other, but treatment is superior to no treatment. The critical laboratory value to follow for treatment response is the CSF IgG Synthesis Index, the best indication of immune response activation. (See *Table 366.5.*)

At this writing, although inosiplex has been available throughout the world, it has recently been approved by the FDA for restricted use in the USA. Clinical trials using ribavarin are being carried out in Japan and the Philippines.

Progressive Multifocal Leukoencephalopathy (PMFL)

PMFL is a rare slow virus infection of the brain caused by the JC virus, a common papova virus often acquired during childhood. The virus remains dormant unless certain circumstances, such as an immunosuppressive state, foster viral reactivation. Once reactivated, the virus may infect the brain and cause PML. It is a demyelinating disease caused by direct infection of oligodendrocytes by the JC virus.

It was first recognized through post-mortem examination in patients with severe illnesses, usually lymphomas or Hodgkins disease, who were immuno-compromised. Later, it was recognized as one of the superinfections in acquired immunodeficiency syndrome (AIDS) due to human immunodeficiency virus (HIV). With the advent of antiretroviral therapy, all the superinfections in AIDS have been decreasing in incidence. With the advent of neuroimaging, PML can be recognized in life through brain MRI. Recently, it has been recognized to occur in association with a drug used to treat multiple sclerosis, natalizumab, if there are multiple treatments.

The symptoms of PML may begin gradually, usually worsen rapidly, and vary depending on which part of the brain is infected. These may include difficulty with walking and other movements, decline in mental function, speech and visual difficulties. Rarely, headaches and seizures occur. Symptoms of PML are similar to the presenting symptoms of multiple sclerosis. A diagnosis of PML is made on the basis of results from magnetic resonance imaging of the brain, which shows T2-hyperintense, small to large, sometimes confluent lesions in the white matter, sparing the subcortical U-fibers. The diagnosis is confirmed by polymerase chain reaction (PCR) for JC virus in cerebrospinal fluid. The treatment is either cessation of immunosuppressive therapy in cancer patients or successful restoration of the immune system in HIV infection.

Pantothenate Kinase-Associated Neurodegeneration (PKAN)

Also called neurodegeneration with brain iron deposition (NBIA)
Formerly called Hallervorden–Spatz disease
(See also, Movement Disorders chapter by Yasser Awaad)

PKAN usually presents with dystonia, rigidity, and retinitis pigmentosa before age 10 years, and is due to progressive deposition of iron in astrocytes, microglia, and neurons of the globus pallidus. About one-fourth of patients present in adolescence, with slower progression, psychiatric symptoms, and intellectual decline.

The diagnosis is made by noting a progressive dystonia coupled with the "eye of the tiger" sign on brain MRI, a small region of hyperintensity surrounded by a rim of hypointensity in the globus pallidus, which, on coronal or transverse T2-weighted images, appears like a tiger's eye. Sequence analysis detects the mutations in PANK2, the only gene abnormality found in this disease.

Iron chelation therapy has not proven effective. The parkinsonian signs may respond to levodopa and bromocriptine, but not to anticholinergics. Botulinus toxin injections may help muscle rigidity or spasticity, as well as oral or intrathecal baclofen with a baclofen pump. Surgical approaches are ablative pallidotomy or deep brain stimulation.

Genetic counseling for the family is the same as for any autosomal recessive disease. Carrier testing for relatives at risk and prenatal testing for pregnancies at risk are possible if the disease-causing mutations have already been identified in an affected family member. The prognosis is dire, with death by age 20 years in about half of patients.

Progressive Myoclonic Epileptic Encephalopathies

Unverricht–Lundborg disease
Lafora disease

Unverricht–Lundborg Disease

Unverricht–Lundborg disease (EPM1) is an autosomal recessive neurodegenerative disease with onset from age

6–15 years, stimulus-sensitive myoclonus, action myoclonus, myoclonic seizures, and generalized convulsions. Some years after the onset, ataxia, incoordination, intentional tremor, and dysarthria develop. Individuals with EPM1 are initially mentally alert but show emotional lability, then mild cognitive decline over time. EPM1 results from defective function of cystatin B, a cysteine protease inhibitor, due to mutations in the *CSTB* gene. Brain MRI is normal. EEG shows generalized spike and polyspike/slow-wave discharges upon a slow background, and photic activation. The diagnosis can be confirmed by identifying disease-causing mutations in *CSTB* through targeted mutation analysis or sequence analysis. The differential diagnosis includes myoclonic epilepsy with ragged red fibers (MERRF) (See previous section on ➋ MERRF in this chapter), neuronal ceroid-lipofuscinosis (Kufs type), and Lafora disease. The drug of choice is valproic acid, to which clonazepam can be added. High-dose piracetam suppresses the myoclonus. Levetiracetam can suppress myoclonus and myoclonic seizures. Sodium channel blockers (carbamazepine, oxcarbazepine), GABAergic drugs (tiagabine, vigabatrin), and gabapentin and pregabalin may aggravate myoclonus and myoclonic seizures. Phenytoin aggravates neurologic symptoms and can accelerate cerebellar degeneration.

Lafora Disease

Lafora disease (LD) is a progressive degenerative disease which begins in adolescents between 12 and 17 years with symmetrical, multifocal, or generalized myoclonus and/or generalized tonic-clonic seizures. Emotional disturbance and confusion are common soon after seizures begin and are followed by dementia. Dysarthria and ataxia appear early; spasticity late. Death results a decade later from status epilepticus or complications of nervous system degeneration.

Diagnosis is usually based on the history, clinical course, and detection of mutations in the genes known to be associated with LD: *EPM2A* or *NHLRC1(EPM2B)*. Skin biopsy to detect pathognomonic Lafora bodies is sometimes necessary to confirm the diagnosis.

Of the antiepileptic drugs, phenytoin, and possibly lamotrigine, carbamazepine, and oxcarbazepine exacerbate seizures. Piracetam has been reported to be particularly effective, but is not available in the USA. Levetiracetam is the closest related drug. Treatment is otherwise supportive and aimed at preventing complications.

LD is inherited through autosomal recessive transmission. Carriers (heterozygotes) are asymptomatic. DNA testing for at-risk relatives and prenatal diagnosis for at-risk pregnancies are possible if the disease-causing mutations in the family are known.

References

Akman C (2010) Nonconvulsive status epilepticus and continuous spike and slow wave of sleep in children. Semin Pediatr Neurol 17(3):155–162

Arya R, Gulati S, Deopujari S (2010) Management of hepatic encephalopathy in children. Postgrad Med J 86:34–41

Barrett MP (2010) Potential new drugs for human African trypanosomiasis: some progress at last. Curr Opin Infect Dis 23(6):603–608

Berger JR, Houff SA (2010) Neurological infections: the year of PML and influenza. Lancet Neurol 9(1):14–17

Brouns R, De Deyn PP (2004) Neurological complications in renal failure: a review. Clin Neurol Neurosurg 107(1):1–16

Bugiani M, Boor I, Powers JM, Scheper GC, van der Knaap MS (2010) Leukoencephalopathy with vanishing white matter: a review. J Neuropathol Exp Neurol 69(10):987–996

Caplan L, Chedru F, L'Hermitte F, Mayman C (1981) Transient global amnesia and migraine. Neurology 31:1167–1170

Conrad AJ, Chiang EY, Andeen LE, Tourtellotte WW (1994) Quantitation of intrathecal measles virus IgG antibody synthesis rate: SSPE and multiple sclerosis. J Neuroimmun 54:99–108

Dabbagh O, Gascon G, Crowell J, Bamoggadam F (1997) Intraventricular interferon-alpha stops seizures in Rasmussen's encephalitis: a case report. Epilepsia 38(9):1047–1049

Dulac OJ, Chiron C (1996) Malignant epileptic encephalopathies in children. Baillières Clin Neurol 5(4):765–781

Epstein LG, Sharer LR, Joshi VV et al (1985) Progressive encephalopathy in children with acquired immune deficiency syndrome. Ann Neurol 17(5):488–496

Fedi M, Reutens D, Dubeau F, Andermann E et al (2001) Long-term efficacy and safety of piracetam in the treatment of progressive myoclonus epilepsy. Arch Neurol 58(5):781–786

Freeman J (2005) Rassmusen's syndrome: progressive auto-immune multi-focal encephalopathy. Pediatr Neurol 32(5):295–299

Gallucci M, Limbucci N, Paonessa A, Caranci F (2007) Reversible focal splenial lesions. Neuroradiology 49(7):541–544

Gascon G, Barlow C (1970) Juvenile migraine, presenting as an acute confusional state. Pediatrics 45:628–635

Gascon GG, Yamani S, Crowell J et al (1993) Combined oral isoprinosine-intraventricular alpha interferon therapy for SSPE. Brain Develop 15:346–355

Gascon G, Frosch MP (1998) Thirty-four year old female with confusion and visual loss. Case records of the Massachusetts general hospital. Weekly clinicopathological exercises. Case 15-1998. New Engl J Med 338(20):1448–1456

Gascon G, International Consortium on SSPE (2003) Randomized treatment study of inosiplex versus combined inosiplex and intraventricular interferon alpha in subacute sclerosing panencephalitis (SSPE). J Child Neurol 18:819–827

Gascon GG, Coskun CJ, Brown WD (2005) Acute confusional migraine; case series and brief review. Int J Child Neuropsych 2(2):189–194

Gascon GG, Ozand PT, Cohen B (2007) Aminoacidopathies and organic acidoopathies, mitochondrial enzyme defects, and other metabolic errors. In: Goetz CG (ed) Textbook of clinical neurology, 3rd edn. Saunders Elsevier, Philadelphia, pp 641–681

Gene Reviews, in www.genetests.org, for all leukodystrophies discussed in this chapter. Accessed 2010

Gupta S, Shah DM, Shah I (2009) Neurological disorders in HIV-infected children in India. Ann Trop Paediatr 29(3):177–181

Hindawy A, Gouda A, El-Ayyadi A et al (2007) Metabolic encephalopathy in Egyptian children. Batisl Lek Listy 108(2):75–82

Hissa Moammar, George Cheriyan, Revi Mathew, Nouriya Al-Sannaa (2010) Incidence and patterns of inborn errors of metabolism in the Eastern Province of Saudi Arabia, 1983–2008. Ann Saudi Med 30(4):271–277

House HR, Ehlers JP (2008) Travel-related infections. Emerg Med Clin N Am 26:499–516

Idro R, Newton C, Kiguli S et al (2010) Child neurology practice and neurological disorders in East Africa. J Child Neurol 25(4):518–524

Johnson GM, Scurletis TD, Carroll NB (1963) A study of 16 fatal cases of encephalitis-like disease in North Carolina children. N C Med J 14:646

Jones BV, Egelhoff JC, Patterson RJ (1997) Hypertensive encephalopathy in children. Am J Neuroradiol 18:101–106

Kohlschütter A, Bley A, Brockmann K et al (2010) Leukodystrophies and other genetic metabolic leukoencephalopathies in children and adults. Brain Dev 32(2):82–89

Kramer U, Sagi L, Goldberg-Stern H et al (2009) Clinical spectrum and medical treatment of children with electrical status epilepticus in sleep (ESES). Epilepsia 50(6):1517–1524

Lann MA, Lovell MA, Kleinschmidt-DeMasters BK (2010) Acute hemorrhagic leukoencephalitis: a critical entity for forensic pathologists to recognize. Am J Forensic Med Pathol 31(1):7–11

Lanzi G, D'Arrigo S, Drumbi G et al (2003) Aicardi-Goutières syndrome; differential diagnosis and aetiopathogenesis. Funct Neurol 18(2):71–75

Lebas A, Husson B, Didelot A et al (2010) Expanding spectrum of encephalitis with NMDA receptor antibodies in young children. J Child Neurol 25(6):742–745

Mariotti P, Lorio R, Frisullo G et al (2010) Acute necrotizing encephalopathy during novel influenza A (H1N1) virus infection. Ann Neurol 68:111–114

Milner DA Jr (2010) Rethinking cerebral malaria pathology. Curr Opin Infect Dis 23:456–463

Mizuguchi M, Abe J, Mikkaichi K et al (1995) Acute necrotizing encephalopathy of childhood: a new syndrome presenting with multifocal, symmetric brain lesions. J Neurol Neurosurg Psychiatry 58:555–561

Mocellin R, Walterfang M, Velakoulis D (2007) Hashimoto's encephalopathy: epidemiology, pathogenesis and management. CNS Drugs 21(10):799–811

Moritz ML, Ayus JC (2010) New aspects in the pathogenesis, prevention, and treatment of hyponatremic encephalopathy in children. Pediatr Nephrol 25(7):1225–1238

Ni J, Zhou LX, Hao HL et al The clinical and radiological spectrum of posterior reversible encephalopathy syndrome. J Neuroimaging 2010, June 21. [Epub ahead of print]

Ohtahara S, Yamatogi Y (2006) Ohtahara syndrome: with special reference to its developmental aspects for differentiating from early myoclonic encephalopathy. Epilepsy Res 70(Suppl 1):S58–S67

Pavlakis SG, Frank Y, Chusid R (1999) Topical review: hypertensive encephalopathy, reversible occipitoparietal encephalopathy, or reversible posterior leukoencephalopathy: three names for an old syndrome. J Child Neurol 14:277–281

Phillips RE, Solomon T (1990) Cerebral malaria in children. Lancet 336(8727):1355–1360

Pollard LM, Williams NR, Espinoza L et al (2010) Diagnosis, treatment and long-term outcomes of late-onset (Type III) multiple acyl-CoA dehydrogenase deficiency. J Child Neurol 25(8):954–960

Pugliese A, Beltramo T, Torre D (2008) Reye's and Reye's-like syndromes. Cell Biochem Funct 26(7):741–746

Hopkins SE, Somoza A, Gilbert DL (2010) Rare autosomal dominant POLG1 mutation in a family with metabolic strokes, posterior column spinal degeneration, and multi-endocrine disease. J Child Neurol 25(6):752–756

Schiffmann R, van der Knaap MS (2004) The latest on leukodystrophies. Curr Opin Neurol 17(2):187–192

Schrör K (2007) Aspirin and Reye syndrome: a review of the evidence. Paediatr Drugs 9(3):195–204

Shah R (2010) Imaging manifestations of progressive multifocal leukoencephalopathy. Clin Radiol 65(6):431–439

Sharma M, Kupferman JC, Brosgol Y (2010) The effects of hypertension on the paediatric brain: a justifiable concern. Lancet Neurol 9(9):933–940

Specchio N, Fusco L, Claps D, Vigevano F (2010) Epileptic encephalopathy in children possibly related to immune-mediated pathogenesis. Brain Dev 32:51–56

Stromme P, Kanavin OJ, Abdelnoor M et al (2007) Incidence rates of progressive childhood encephalopathy in Oslo, Norway: a population based study. BMC Pediatr 7:25. doi:10.1186/1471-2431-7-25

Sugaya N (2002) Influenza-associated encephalopathy in Japan. Semin Pediatr Infect Dis 13(2):79–84

Swoboda KJ, Hyland K (2002) Diagnosis and treatment of neurotransmitter-related disorders. Neurol Clin 20:1143–1161

Tein I (2002) Role of carnitine and fatty acid oxidation and its defects in infantile epilepsy. J Child Neurol 17(Suppl 3):3S57–3S82, discussion 3S82-3

Toovey S (2008) Influenza-associated central nervous system dysfunction: a literature review. Travel Med Infect Dis 6(3):114–124

Tucker EJ (2010) Recent advances in the genetics of mitochondrial encephalopathies. Curr Neurol Neurosci Rep 10(4):277–285

Tyler K (2010) Progressive Multifocal Leukoencephalopathy: can we reduce risk in patients receiving biological immunomodulatory therapies. Ann Neurol 68(3):271–274

van Baalen A, Häusler M, Boor R et al (2010) Febrile infection-related epilepsy syndrome (FIRES): a nonencephalitic encephalopathy in childhood. Epilepsia 51(7):1323–1328

Van der Knaap MS (2010) Megalencephalic leukoencephalopathy with cysts without MLC1 defect. Ann Neurol 67(6):834–837

Vasconcellos E, Piña-Garza JE, Fakhoury T (1999) Pediatric manifestations of Hashimoto's encephalopathy. Pediatr Neurol 20(5):394–398

Wang GF, Li W, Li K (2010) Acute encephalopathy and encephalitis caused by influenza virus infection. Curr Opin Neurol 23(3):305–311

Weber T (2008) Progressive multifocal leukoencephalopathy. Neurol Clin 26:833–854

Wong V (1997) Neurodegenerative diseases in children. Hong Kong Med J 3:89–95

367 Ataxias

S. H. Subramony

Ataxia: Definition

Ataxia refers to a syndrome of neurological dysfunction characterized by problems with balance and poor coordination of movements. Typically, it results from pathology in the cerebellum and its connecting pathways. It leads to difficulties with gait and stance, poor dexterity of limb movements, often a dysarthric speech and changes in eye movements that can produce visual symptoms such as blurry vision or a sense of oscillation of the environment called oscillopsia. Occasionally, a similar poor coordination of limb movements and imbalance can result from lesions that affect sensory input to the central nervous system, especially proprioceptive input. This is called sensory ataxia. Patients with cerebellar ataxia present with gait and balance in the absence of any demonstrable muscle weakness. Tasks requiring fine coordination such as writing, handling tools and utensils become difficult, and in the case of lower limbs, activities like biking and skating can suffer before regular walking becomes abnormal. Speech becomes slurred and appears to have abrupt changes in pitch and volume.

Neurological examination of patients with cerebellar ataxia reveals many abnormalities. Gaze-evoked nystagmus is usually seen and primary position nystagmus can also occur. For example, downbeat nystagmus in primary position is considered to be a pathognomonic sign of a lesion at the cranio-vertebral junction. Visual pursuit is abnormal and becomes jerky because pursuit of visual objects is achieved using small saccades (saccadic pursuit). Sacccades (quick, targeted eye movements) usually have normal speed with cerebellar lesions but are not accurate; they can over- or undershoot the target with subsequent corrective saccades to cancel the error (hypermetric and hypometric saccades). The dysarthria of cerebellar disease is characterized by unnecessary changes in pitch and volume and wrong emphasis on various syllables ("scanning dysarthria"). Limb motility and posture can be disturbed in several ways. There can be an action tremor that appears when a limb is maintained in sustained posture such as when the fingers are pointed at each other with elbows up. This type of tremor becomes even more overt when the limbs are moved in a purposeful, target-oriented fashion such as touching the examiner's finger and patient's nose repeatedly (finger to nose test) or the heel is slid along the shin from the knee to the ankle (heel to shin test). The oscillation of limbs in these situations is a form of kinetic tremor. A tremor of the head and trunk can occur (titubation). Also, fast movements that require accuracy result in either over- or under-reaching the target (hypermetric or hypometric movements). This can be shown by the finger chase test in which the patient is asked to touch the examiner's finger tip again and again as the latter is moved to a new location in a rapid manner. Multi-jointed movements become decomposed; the rapid pronation and supination of the forearm over the thigh is an example (dysdiadochokinesis). With increasing cerebellar dysfunction, patients have increasing sway of the body when placed in the feet together position of stance (such maneuvers as tandem stance and one foot stance become abnormal even earlier, but may not be specific). Eventually, patients tend to have a broad-based stance in their natural position. Tandem gait (heel to toe walking) becomes abnormal early with cerebellar ataxia. Later, regular gait becomes broad based, lurching and veering in quality.

With sensory ataxia, patients can have stance and gait problems and limb incoordination, but do not have speech or eye movement difficulties. The ataxia results from sensory loss (especially position and kinesthetic sense). Patients may admit to numbness, but this is not always the case. The deep tendon reflexes are lost or diminished because of the sensory fiber dysfunction. In many of the inherited types of ataxias, both sensory and cerebellar components are present. This chapter will give an outline of the various ataxic disorders with an emphasis on the genetic forms of the disease. An approach to a patient presenting with ataxia will be presented.

Etiological Classification of Ataxias

Ataxias are broadly grouped into acquired and inherited forms. Any overt structural lesions in the cerebellum and connecting pathways can lead to ataxia. These can usually be diagnosed readily when imaging studies are obtained,

Abdelaziz Y. Elzouki (ed.), *Textbook of Clinical Pediatrics*, DOI 10.1007/978-3-642-02202-9_367,

especially MRI scans of the brain. In these cases, signs of cerebellar disease are often accompanied by signs related to damage to contiguous structures being affected by the structural lesion. Signs and symptoms may be asymmetric depending on the location of the lesion. However, there are many acquired lesions of the cerebellum in which an evident lesion of the cerebellum may be lacking. ➋ *Table 367.1* lists acquired causes of cerebellar ataxia that are common in pediatric age groups.

A more difficult diagnostic situation occurs when progressive ataxia is related to an atrophic or degenerative process in the cerebellum, brainstem, and other connecting pathways. In childhood, almost all of these are related to genetic disorders. Information on the mutations and genes involved is available in many but not all of these diseases. The majority of inherited ataxias in childhood have autosomal recessive (AR) inheritance; thus the parents (who are carriers) are asymptomatic, but siblings may be affected. With small family sizes, most of these cases present as singletons. Consanguinity may be a clue to AR inheritance. Other inherited ataxias of childhood have mitochondrial or X-linked inheritance. The analysis of the pedigree may point to the mode of such inheritance, though many of these patients are also singletons. Lastly, autosomal dominant (AD) ataxias may occasionally present in childhood, though commonly they are of adult onset. The diagnostic process in childhood is particularly difficult because many inherited diseases, not usually grouped as primarily ataxic in character, can present with ataxia (in addition to other signs) in this age group. ➋ *Table 367.2* lists the inherited diseases which are conventionally classified as an ataxia. ➋ *Table 367.3* is a list of disorders usually with childhood onset in which ataxia can be a major feature, but these are not typically classified as ataxias. Lastly, a special group of ataxic diseases have onset in the neonatal period. These are classified as congenital ataxias.

Table 367.1
Acquired ataxias seen in pediatric age groups

Entities with overt structural lesions on imaging	Entities in which an overt structural abnormality is not universally seen
Tumors in the posterior fossa	Infections
	Acute cerebellar ataxia of childhood
	Post-infectious
Cranio-vertebral junction anomalies	Toxic disorders
	Chemotherapy (5FU, Ara C)
	Anticonvulsants (DPH)
Vascular disease	Sequel to hypoxic encephalopathy
Demyelinating disease	Hypothyrodism
Infections (cerebellar abscess, Bickerstaff encephalitis)	Autoimmune
	Paraneoplastic (e.g. opsoclonus-myoclonus syndrome)

Epidemiology

Ataxias are rare disorders. Epidemiological studies generally have tried to estimate prevalence of degenerative ataxias and the usual figures range up to 9.3 per 100,000. There are interesting variations in the occurrence of genetic ataxias among various geographic and ethnic groups. Thus, Friedreich's ataxia, the most common recessive ataxia is confined to Indo-European populations. There are pockets of high prevalence of certain SCAs, likely the result of isolated population kinetics: examples include high prevalence of SCA 1 among the Iakut in Siberia, SCA 2 in the Eastern provinces of Cuba, and SCA 3 in the Portuguese Azores.

In the following sections, different types of acquired and inherited ataxias are described, including their pathogenesis, clinical features, therapy, and prognosis.

Acquired Ataxias in Childhood

A number of disorders in which imaging studies can be diagnostic can have an ataxic presentation in childhood. These include posterior fossa tumors such as cerebellar astrocytomas and pontine gliomas, congenital malformations at the cranio-vertebral junction, and bacterial infections such as a cerebellar abscess. The term brainstem or Bickerstaff encephalitis is used for an acute clinical picture that includes ataxia and oculomotor palsy with added clinical signs such as obtundation and Babinski sign that distinguish the disease from Miller-Fisher variant of Guillain–Barre Syndrome (GBS). MRI often shows signal density changes in the brainstem. Vascular lesions, including ischemic strokes and malformation, can occur in the pediatric age group, but again can be diagnosed readily be imaging. Demyelinating diseases like multiple sclerosis can present with lesions in the cerebellum and connecting pathways. Ataxia in these situations usually develops fairly rapidly, and correct diagnosis leads to appropriate intervention. Other ataxias of nongenetic origin such as those related to hypothyroidism and previous hypoxic

Table 367.2
Inherited ataxias

Autosomal recessive ataxias	Autosomal dominant ataxias	X-linked ataxias	Mitochondrial ataxias
1. Friedreich ataxia (FA)	1. Spinocerebellar ataxias types 1 through 31 (There is no SCA 9 or 24)	1. Fragile X tremor ataxia syndrome (FXTAS)	1. Neurogenic weakness, ataxia, retinitis pigmentosa (NARP)
2. Ataxia with oculomotor apraxia (AOA) type 1 and 2	2. Machado–Joseph disease (MJD also known as SCA 3)	2. Other X-linked ataxias	2. Other mtDNA diseases such as MERRF, MELAS, and KSS can have ataxia as a feature
3. Ataxia telangiectasia (AT)	3. Dentatorubral-pallidoluysian atrophy (DRPLA)		
4. Ataxia with vitamin E deficiency (AVED)	4. Episodic ataxias types 1 through 6		
5. Autosomal recessive ataxia of Charlevoix-Saguenay (ARSACS)			
6. Polymerase gamma related ataxias: mitochondrial recessive ataxia syndrome (MIRAS), sensory ataxic neuropathy, dysarthria and ophthalmoplegia (SANDO), myoclonic epilepsy myopathy sensory ataxia (MEMSA)			
7. Autosomal recessive cerebellar ataxia 1 (ARCA 1)			
8. Ataxia Telangiectasia-like disorder (ATLD)			
9. Spinocerebellar ataxia with axonal neuropathy (SCAN 1)			
10. Marinesco–Sjogren syndrome			

Table 367.3
Autosomal recessive or X-linked syndromes with ataxia and other features

1. Amino acid disorders: Hartnup disease, urea cycle diseases, triple H syndrome
2. Carbohydrate disorders: pyruvate dehydrogenase complex (PDHC) deficiency
3. Storage disorders: late-onset Tay–Sachs (LOTS); Ceroid lipofuscinosis; Neimann–Pick disease, type C
4. Aceruloplasminemia
5. Eukaryotic initiation factor 2 gene related diseases (vanishing white matter disease)
6. Congenital disorders of glycosylation (CDG's)
7. Others: proteolipid protein (PLP) mutations; cerebrotendinous xanthomatosis; Regsum diseases; Giant axonal neuropathy

encephalopathy are rare, but may have cerebellar atrophy on imaging studies. The following section deals with some special types of acquired ataxias seen in children.

Acute Cerebellar Ataxia of Childhood and Post-Infectious Ataxia

Acute cerebellar ataxia (ACA) of childhood refers to a problem of involving only the cerebellum that occurs in children, usually in the setting of a preceding viral infection. Post-infectious encephalomyelitis can have ataxia as a major feature, but usually evidence for a more diffuse affliction of the nervous system including the hemispheres and spinal cord can be found. Some authors use the term acute cerebellitis (AC) to refer to a more severe disorder with associated cerebellar edema and features of increased intracranial pressure.

Pathogenesis: The speculation has been made that ACA may be a post-infectious immune phenomenon whereas AC may be the result of a direct infection.

Clinical features and diagnosis: The antecedents can be a nonspecific viral syndrome, but varicella is a trigger in many, with a peak incidence at the age of 5–6 years. A similar syndrome following Epstein–Barr virus or vaccinations has been reported in teenage years. Children with ACA develop an acute ataxic disorder that is not associated with a more diffuse process reflected by seizures, meningismus, or obtundation. CSF may show some elevation of protein, and a modest mononuclear pleocytosis and PCR may allow identification of a specific etiology such as EBV. Edema, hydrocephalus, and herniation have been described in some and may require decompressive surgery. Some authors refer to this as acute cerebellitis (AC) in which additional features of headache, menigismus, fever, and obtundation can occur. Patients with AC usually have prominent MRI abnormalities in the form of cerebellar edema and diffuse T2 hyperintensity in the cerebellar cortex, and secondary features of compression are often seen with hydrocephalus and tonsillar herniation. In contrast, MR imaging in acute cerebellar ataxia may be normal or show spotty changes in the cerebellum and its peduncles (*Fig. 367.1*).

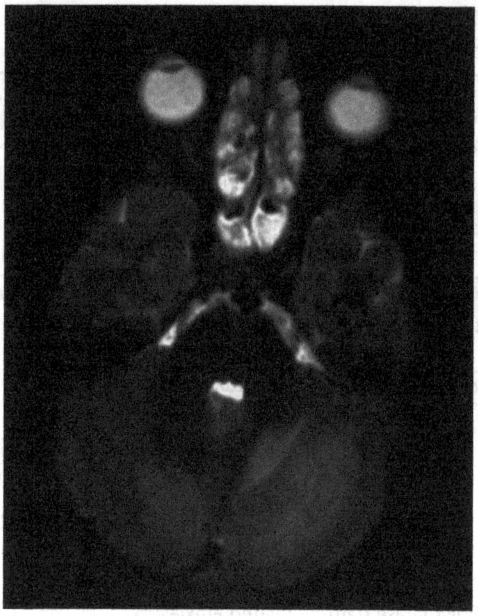

Figure 367.1
Signal density changes in cerebellar cortex in acute cerebellar ataxia of childhood (From Bruecker Y, Claus F, Demaerel P et al (2004) MRI findings in acute cerebellitis. Eur J Radiol 14:1478–1483. With permission)

Differential diagnosis: Other types of acute cerebellar or balance disorders such as tumors, demyelinating disease, toxic diseases, and inborn metabolic errors need to be considered in the acute situation. Acute labyrinthitis and migraine can present with associated balance problems.

Treatment: Patients with evolving features of intracranial hypertension obviously need careful monitoring and decompressive procedures such as posterior fossa decompression and ventriculostomy. These authors in their review also note that occasionally a direct infective agent can be identified by PCR and this may need an appropriate antibiotic. Steroids have been suggested to reduce swelling.

Prognosis: In the majority of children, the prognosis is excellent with full recovery over a few weeks to months. A minority may have residual neurological problems.

Toxic Causes of Ataxia

Alcohol which is a common cause of ataxia among adults (both acute intoxication and chronic alcoholic cerebellar degeneration) is not of particular concern in young children. However, iatrogenic ataxia related to pharmacological agents is not uncommon. Antiepileptics are particularly prone to cause ataxia when their levels are supratheraputic, though there is considerable individual variation as to the level that is cerebello-toxic. History of chronic antiepileptic use, together with inappropriate dosing or introduction of another drug that may result in an interaction, is often obtained. It is well recognized that older antiepileptics such as diphenylhydantoin and carbamazepine can produce gait ataxia and other cerebellar disturbances at toxic levels. In a meta-analysis of second generation antiepileptics (gabapentin, lamotrigine, levetiracetam, oxcarbazepine, pregabalin, tiagabine, topiramate, or zonisamide) used as adjunct therapy, all of them were found to increase the risk of imbalance with the exception of gabapentin and levetiracetam. A dose-response relation was seen with almost all of the drugs. Zacarra et al. reported that gabapentin, lamotrigine, pregabalin, topiramate, oxcarbazepine, and zonisamide were all found to produce ataxia or dizziness. Measuring drug levels may be useful to diagnose antiepileptic induced ataxia.

Some cancer chemotherapeutic agents such as 5 fluorouracil and cytosine arabinoside produce ataxia as a side effect. An acute cerebellar dysarthria has been reported with infusions of the agent irinotecan.

Opsoclonus-Myoclonus Syndrome(OMS)

This syndrome is characterized by the acute or subacute onset of imbalance and ataxia, soon followed by opsoclonus, a chaotic, irregular, and involuntary movement of the eyes ("dancing eyes").

Pathogenesis: It is likely a result of an autoimmune phenomenon triggered by an underlying neoplasm, but can be idiopathic. It has been postulated that in OMS associated with neuroblastomas, there is an immune reaction against the tumor that has cross reactivity with neuronal tissue. Antibodies against cerebellar Purkinje cell antigens have been noted in the sera of OMS patients, and some have antibodies to neurofilament and the Hu antigen.

Clinical features and diagnosis: Opsoclonic eye movements are conjugate, fast, and multidirectional and can be often precipitated by changes in fixation. This is associated with myoclonic movements and behavioral changes including usually extreme irritability, sleep disturbance, developmental regression, and sometimes loss of speech. In young children, about 50% of cases have an associated neuroblastoma, but this figure may be higher if high-resolution imaging of abdomen is obtained. In older children and adults, OMS can be associated with a direct infection such as with West Nile virus or parainfectious process or other types of malignancies such as lymphomas, lung cancer, and breast cancer. All young patients with OMS require a thorough search for neuroblastoma with high-resolution scans through the adrenals, measurement of catecholamine metabolites in urine, and metaiodobenzylguanidine (MIBG) scan.

Treatment: Apart from treatment of any neoplasm found, a number of immunomodulatory therapies such as corticosteroids and ACTH have shown benefit in many of the motor aspects of this disorder. IVIG, other immunosuppressants such as azathioprine, and plasma exchange have also been used in an anecdotal fashion. Any neuroblastoma needs to be removed. Neuroblastomas associated with OMS tend to be small and localized.

Prognosis: Opsoclonus tends to resolve even with no treatment, and the ataxic disturbance also improves, though not completely. Recovery in speech and language, as well as behavioral abnormalities, tends to be incomplete, and children often require long-term therapy for relapses. As adolescents, these children can exhibit poor school performance and behavioral difficulties such as impulse control and mood disorders. Adults with OMS tend to recover after a monophasic illness.

Cerebral Folate Deficiency

This disorder is characterized by insomnia, agitation, declining head growth, and cognitive decline. There is associated gait ataxia, speech changes, and epilepsy. Serum and RBC folate levels are normal, but CSF 5-methyl tetrahydrofolate levels are decreased. The disorder has been linked to folate receptor antibodies and defective folate transport.

Congenital Ataxias

The concept of congenital ataxia may not have an exact definition. However, these rare syndromes are characterized by onset very early in life, usually in the neonatal period, the presence of cerebellar hypoplasia rather than atrophy and often, but not always, a nonprogressive course. Cerebellar hypoplasia may be differentiated from atrophy by a small cerebellum that does not show the open pattern of folia seen with atrophy and is nonprogressive when examined serially. In a series of nonprogressive ataxia in 78 children from Sweden, no imaging abnormalities occurred in 61%. Among the rest, MRI showed varying patterns of abnormalities including focal or generalized maldevelopment, or extensive malformations consistent with Dandy–Walker syndrome, Joubert syndrome, and cerebellar hypoplasia, as well as lesions that were more consistent with acquired pathology. Some form of genetic etiology was established in close to 20%, including chromosomal abnormality, Angelman syndrome, and Joubert syndrome. Some cases had an autosomal dominant inheritance pattern (see also SCA 29). Others had what appeared to be acquired lesions, including hypoxic-ischemic pathology by imaging. Clinical picture included ataxia with delayed milestones, mental retardation in 60%, refractory and other types of visual problems in 58%, and hearing loss.

Joubert syndrome (JS) is recognized by an autosomal recessive (AR) inheritance, hypotonia, developmental delay, neonatal tachypnea or apnea, and altered eye movements. Infants have mental retardation, episodic hyperpnea or apnea, oculomotor apraxia, and later ataxia. Imaging shows a deep posterior interpeduncular fossa, prominent superior cerebellar peduncles and hypoplasia, and clefting of the superior vermis producing a molar tooth sign (➋ *Fig. 367.2*). Chance et al. in their review describe a number of related clinical phenotypes including the following: Arima syndrome (vermal hypoplasia, retinopathy, polycystic kidneys, AR inheritance); Senior–Loken syndrome (vermal hypoplasia,

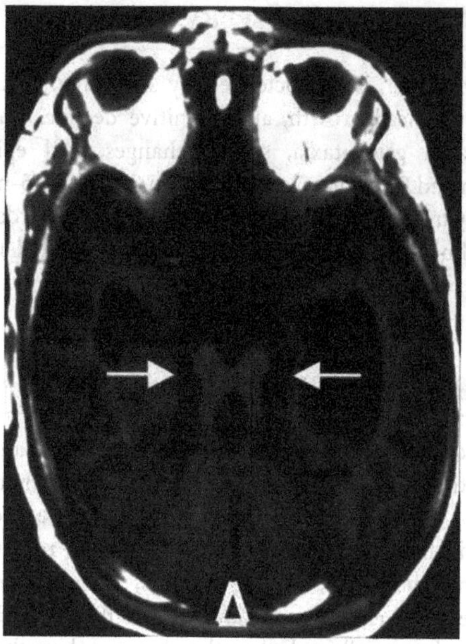

Figure 367.2
Typical molar tooth sign in patient with Joubert syndrome (From Louie CM, Gleeson JG (2005) Genetic basis of Joubert syndrome and related disorders of cerebellar development. Hum Mol Genet 14:R235–R242. With permission)

retinopathy, juvenile onset nephronophthisis, AR inheritance); vermal hypoplasia and retinopathy alone; COACH syndrome (vermal hypoplasia, coloboma, nephronophthsis, hepatic fibrosis); and vermal hypoplasia and nepheonophthisis alone. In Joubert's syndrome, there are no renal, hepatic, or other systemic features, including retinopathy.

The essential feature of many of these conditions include a characteristic set of imaging abnormalities that include a deep posterior interpeduncular fossa, prominent superior cerebellar peduncle and hypoplasia of the superior vermis that lead to a "molar tooth sign" appearance of the upper brainstem on axial images. The clinical picture in Joubert syndrome includes onset in infancy, developmental delay and hypotonia, episodic apnea and hyperpnoea, oculomotor apraxia and hypotonia. Recently, some advances have occurred in identifying genes responsible for such diseases. One variety of JS, associated with cerebral cortical abnormalities has been related to mutations in the AHI 1 gene (Abelson helper integration 1) which encodes the protein Jouberin. Another syndrome associated with nephronophthisis is related to mutations in the NPHP 1 gene, which appears to have a functional role in ciliary function.

Inherited Ataxias

Ataxias can be inherited in autosomal recessive, autosomal dominant, X-linked, and mitochondrial fashion (➋ *Table 367.2*). Childhood ataxias are predominantly autosomal recessive; this group can be further divided in to those diseases which are traditionally classified as ataxias and a second group in which ataxia forms a variable part of a more complex phenotype ("genetic-metabolic" diseases).

Autosomal Recessive Ataxias

Friedreich's Ataxia (FA)

Epidemiology: This is the most common recessive ataxia and perhaps the most common inherited ataxia among Indo-European populations.

Genetics and pathogenesis: FA results from an unstable expansion of a repeated trinucleotide (GAA) sequence within the first intron of the *FRDA* gene on chromosome 9q13-21.1. Most of the normal alleles have fewer than 10 repeats. Long normal alleles (12–40 repeats) appear to be confined to Caucasian populations and serve as the reservoir for expansion into pathogenic mutations. Expanded alleles have 66 to over 1,000 repeats. Over 95% of the affected FA patients have the GAA expansion in both alleles (homozygous expansion). Rarely, patients with clinical findings compatible with FA have only one expanded allele; such patients harbor point mutations in the unexpanded allele. Sequencing of the unexpanded allele to document a point mutation will have to be done in this situation. Point mutations located in the carboxy terminal half of the mature frataxin appear to be associated with a typical FA phenotype. However, missense mutations in the amino terminal half of the protein such as the G130V mutation appear to result in a milder phenotype with less ataxia and greater spasticity and no dysarthria. All the patients with point mutation to date have been compound heterozygotes with one expanded allele. Homozygous point mutations will cause complete lack of frataxin, and this may be incompatible with life. This has been further supported by the fact that complete knockout of the gene in animal models is embryonically lethal.

There is an inverse correlation between the size of the GAA repeat and the age at onset. This correlation is better with the smaller of the two expanded alleles. Cardiomyopathy and diabetes also tend to occur in patients with larger expansions (>700 GAA repeats). All of the variation in age at onset and severity of disease cannot be

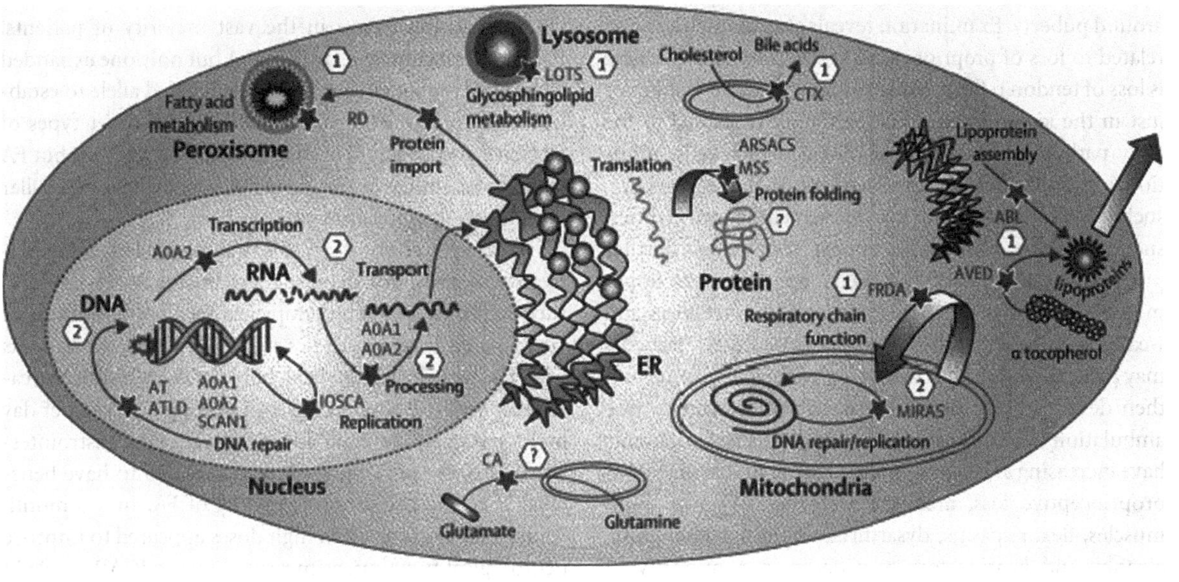

Figure 367.3

Cellular mechanisms in autosomal recessive ataxias. The pathways or sites affected by the various underlying mutations causing the different autosomal recessive ataxias are indicated by a red star. Oxidative stress and DNA repair abnormalities appear major targets in AR ataxias (Numbered 1 and 2). In FA and MIRAS, there are intrinsic mitochondrial abnormalities. In AT and AOAs, DNA repair mechanisms may be affected. ARSACS and MSS may be related to protein folding defects. Other defects depicted include peroxisomal and lysosomal defects and abnormal handling of vitamin E. *ER* endoplasmic reticulum, *FRDA* Friedreich's ataxia, *AVED* ataxia with vitamin E deficiency, *ABL* abetalipoproteinaemia, *RD* Refsum's disease, *LOTS* late-onset Tay–Sachs disease, *CTX* cerebrotendinous xanthomatosis, *MIRAS* mitochondrial recessive ataxia syndrome, *SCAN*1 spinocerebellar ataxia with axonal neuropathy, *AT* ataxia telangiectasia, *AOA*1 ataxia with oculomotor apraxia, type 1 *AOA*2 ataxia with oculomotor apraxia, type 2 *ARSACS* autosomal recessive ataxia of Charlevoix-Saguenay, *IOSCA* infantile-onset spinocerebellar ataxia, *CA* Cayman ataxia, *MSS* Marinesco–Sjögren syndrome (From Fogel BL, Perlman S (2007) Clinical features and molecular genetics of autosomal recessive cerebellar ataxias. Lancet Neurol 6:245–257. With permission)

correlated with the GAA size alone. Other genetic and possibly environmental factors may contribute to this variation. In addition, variation in clinical picture can result from somatic mosaicism of the repeat size with different tissues having significant differences in the size of the expansions.

The mutation in the FA gene leads to a partial deficiency of the protein frataxin. The reduced transcriptional efficiency of the mutated gene has been attributed to an unusual "sticky DNA" configuration of the expanded repeat. In addition, there is evidence for chromatin condensation and remodeling which can further suppress frataxin transcription. The exact role of frataxin in normal biology is still not clear, but many studies suggest that it is a mitochondrial protein (➋ *Fig. 367.3*).

Knockout of the frataxin homologue in yeast leads to accumulation of iron in the mitochondria, a finding of interest in view of the presence of iron in the cardiac muscle in human disease; more recent data suggest that such overt iron accumulation may be a late event. Activity of enzymes, such as aconitase and complex I, II, and III of the respiratory chain, that contain iron-sulfur clusters is reduced in cardiac muscle biopsies of patients with FA. The ISC synthesis defect results from the role of frataxin in the process and probably is the cause of iron accumulation. It has been hypothesized that the presence of excess iron as well as excess oxidative stress related to impaired respiratory chain function can induce oxidative stress via the Fenton reaction and cause progressive nuclear and mitochondrial damage. Frataxin may function both as an iron storage protein and as an iron chaperone with a role in ISC and heme synthesis.

Pathology: There is loss of dorsal root ganglion cells, resultant degeneration of the dorsal columns, degeneration of spinocerebellar and corticospinal tracts, and loss of cells in the cerebellar dentate nucleus.

Clinical features: Typical FA has onset before age 25 years with gait difficulties and clumsiness, usually around puberty. Examination reveals ataxia which appears related to loss of proprioceptive sense in the limbs. There is loss of tendon reflexes usually in a generalized fashion or just in the lower limbs. These findings are related to the early pathology in the dorsal root ganglion cells. Additional signs indicating involvement of the cerebellum, such as dysarthria, and eye movement abnormalities, such as square wave jerks, appear soon after. Further progression causes disabling ataxia, appearance of upper motor neuron signs such as extensor plantar reflexes and weakness in lower limbs and dysphagia. Rarely, patients may present with cardiac disease or a spinal deformity and then develop neurological disease. Patients tend to lose ambulation within 15 years of onset. At this stage, patients have increasing ataxia of upper and lower limbs, profound proprioceptive loss, areflexia, weakness of lower limb muscles, flexor spasms, dysarthria, and dysphagia. Optic atrophy and hearing loss may occur in a minority of patients. Since the FA mutation was identified, it has been noted that about 15% of patients with the mutation have onset after 25 years of age (late-onset FA or LOFA), occasionally even after 50 years of age. Others continue to retain tendon reflexes (about 10%), a finding not seen in classic cases (FA with retained reflexes or FARR). Some of these patients can be spastic in their lower limbs and have pathologically brisk reflexes.

Heart disease is common with abnormal EKG's in most patients. ECHO-cardiography shows hypertrophic cardiomyopathy in many. Cardiac symptoms, such as atrial fibrillation and occasionally a dilated cardiomyopathy with heart failure, may arise. Cardiac disease is the cause of death in a significant proportion. Skeletal abnormalities such as spinal deformities and foot deformities are common and add to ambulatory and respiratory problems. The mean age of death among patients with FA has been reported to be late in the fourth decade; this however does not take into account the more recent information on late-onset cases. Diabetes occurs in about 10% and appears to be related to both beta cell dysfunction and peripheral insulin resistance.

Diagnosis: Nerve conduction studies show absence or reduction of sensory nerve potentials in a diffuse fashion. Central motor conduction studies show abnormalities that evolve over the course of the disease and may reflect the progression of the disease. MRI scans of the brain reveal no abnormalities in the cerebellum; rather the upper cervical cord shows atrophy. Signal density changes may be seen in the posterior columns by MRI, and the cerebellar dentate has been reported to show increased iron content and volume loss. Diagnosis is confirmed by targeted mutation analysis to detect the homozygous GAA expansion found in the vast majority of patients. Patients with clinical features of FA but only one expanded allele need sequencing of their unexpanded allele to establish the presence of a point mutation. All other types of recessive ataxias figure in the differential diagnosis, but FA is the most common and does not usually have cerebellar atrophy on imaging studies.

Treatment of FA: Based on evidence for excess oxidative stress and poor defense mechanisms of FA tissue to such stress, antioxidant therapy has been tried over the last 10 years. At least 11 studies using idebenone in patients with FA have been reported until 2008. It has been reasonably well tolerated in doses of 900 mg or more per day by FA patients, the main adverse effect being gastrointestinal. At doses of 5 mg/kg/day, it appeared to have beneficial effect on the cardiomyopathy of FA. In a 6 month study, idebenone given in high doses appeared to improve neurological function, as measured by the ICARS scale in ambulatory FA patients. Newer approaches, now in experimental phase, include gene replacement and the use of molecules that may enhance frataxin production even in the presence of the GAA expansion. Recent open label experience suggests some beneficial effect from erythropoietin.

In addition, there have been many attempts at symptomatic therapy of FA patients with possible neurotransmitter replacements such as cholinergic, serotoninergic, and dopaminergic drugs which have shown variable and usually less than optimal results.

The supportive care of FA patients includes adequate rehabilitation efforts aimed at mobility, using appropriate devices. Monitoring and caring for the systemic complications are also important. Such systemic problems include skeletal deformities, cardiomyopathy, and diabetes.

Ataxia with Oculomotor Apraxia Types 1 and 2 (AOA 1, AOA 2)

Oculomotor apraxia refers to a peculiar inability to initiate saccades; eye movement recordings suggest that while saccades can be produced, they have increased latency. Children typically use head thrusts to move eyes from one target to another.

Epidemiology: Ataxia with oculomotor apraxia type 1 is likely the most common AR ataxia in Japan and second only to FA in Portugal. AOA 2 is the most frequent AR ataxia next to FA in European series.

Genetics and pathogenesis: AOA 1 results from mutations in the aprataxin (*APTX)* gene. Nonsense, missense, and splice site mutations as well as deletions have been described. Aprataxin is a nuclear protein that has an N terminal fork-head associated (FHA) domain resembling PNKP, a histidine triad (HIT) domain and a C terminal zinc finger domain. Most of the mutations affect the HIT domain. The protein may function in base excision repair, a form of single strand DNA repair mechanism. The C terminal is also known to interact with XRCC1 which plays a role in single strand break repair. It is unclear how this functional role is related to neurodegeneration in the cerebellum.

AOA 2 has been linked to mutations in the senataxin gene (*SETX*) which codes for senataxin. Many different mutations have been identified including nonsense, missense and frameshift mutations as well as deletions and duplications. The normal function of senataxin is unclear. Its C-terminal region has homology to the superfamily of helicases, so the DNA/RNA helicase function may contribute to the pathogenesis of neurological dysfunction.

Clinical features and diagnosis: AOA 1 has onset about 10 years of age, with a range from early childhood to the 20s in some cases. It causes progressive ataxia associated with MRI evidence for cerebellar atrophy. Chorea and dystonia occur in about 80% of cases. Oculomotor apraxia appears a mean of 9 years after onset and is seen in over 80% of cases. Children use head movement to fixate on eccentric targets with a head eye lag; this may result from very hypometric saccades and the need for multiple small amplitude saccades to make the movement. Mental retardation can occur in about 40% of cases. Later, patients develop a sensory motor polyneuropathy. Low albumin and high cholesterol levels occur in the majority of patients after some years. Muscle CoQ 10 levels may be decreased in some patients with AOA 1, and symptomatic improvement may occur with high-dose CoQ 10 therapy. There are no other systemic features such as telangiectasia and elevated alpha fetoprotein.

Ataxia with oculomotor apraxia type 2 is a progressive AR ataxia associated with cerebellar atrophy and an axonal polyneuropathy, which are the most prevalent features together with elevation of serum alpha fetopotein. The age at onset is around 15 years, and the disease progresses to a stage requiring significant ambulation devices in about 15 years. Oculomotor apraxia does not occur universally, being seen in about 50% cases. Ocular recordings show increased horizontal saccade latencies and hypometria. Other clinical signs noted are upper motor neuron signs in about 20%, dystonia, chorea, head tremor, and strabismus. Anheim et al. note that with a non-FA patient, the elevation of serum alpha fetoprotein to over 7 μg/l may be predictive of AOA 2. Other features that have been noted infrequently include elevation of serum CK and hypogonadotrophic hypogonadism. No other systemic features such as high risk for malignancy, telangiectasia, or radiation sensitivity are seen.

Treatment: Treatment remains purely supportive.

Ataxia with Vitamin E Deficiency (AVED)

Epidemiology: It is most common in North Africa where its prevalence approaches that of FA.

Genetics and pathogenesis: AVED results from mutations in the α tocopherol transfer protein (αTTP) gene; αTTP is involved in the hepatic handling of vitamin E facilitating the incorporation of vitamin E into very low-density lipoproteins. The mutations in the αTTP gene are variable and include missense, nonsense, frameshift, and splice site mutations; some mutations allow for residual function and thus a milder phenotype.

Clinical features and diagnosis: AVED is a childhood onset ataxia with clinical features similar to FA. The onset is usually in childhood but can be later. There is progressive ataxia and evidence for a polyneuropathy with loss of proprioception and tendon reflexes. Retinitis pigmentosa and visual loss can accompany this syndrome. Patients often have head titubation. Cardiomyopathy can occur but is less common than in FA. Vitamin E levels are very low (less than half the lower limit of normal) but are not the result of impaired absorption.

Treatment: Vitamin E supplementation allows the stabilization of the neurological features, especially when started early in the disease, but some features may show worsening despite therapy.

Abetalipoproteinemia

This disorder results from mutations in the gene *MTTP* which codes for a subunit of the microsomal triglyceride transfer protein; this results in impaired lipid absorption in the intestine including lipid soluble vitamins like vitamin E. The ataxia resembles that in AVED but is associated with evidence for malabsorption. Vitamin E and cholesterol levels are low, and apolipoprotein B is absent on lipoprotein electrophoresis. Acanthocytes are found in peripheral blood smear. Transaminases may be high and INR elevated due to vitamin K deficiency.

Cayman Ataxia

This is an autosomal recessive ataxia described from the Cayman Islands, characterized by early onset of minimally progressive ataxia and mental retardation. The gene involved is on chromosome 19p and codes for a neuron-restricted protein (Caytaxin) that contains a CRAL-TRIO motif common to proteins, including α tocopherol transfer protein, which bind small lipophilic molecules. This suggests a pathogenic similarity to AVED.

Polymerase Gamma Mutations and Ataxia

Recessive mutations in the gene encoding the alpha subunit of polymerase gamma (POLG 1), an enzyme involved in the replication of mtDNA, result in ataxia. Mitochondrial inherited recessive ataxia syndrome (MIRAS) is common in Finland and has onset from childhood to early adult life. Progressive ataxia can be associated with tremor and myoclonus. Schulte et al. recently analyzed the phenotype associated with POLG 1 mutations. Patients who had sensory ataxic neuropathy associated with dysarthria and ophthalmoplegia (SANDO) had a high (80%) prevalence of POLG 1 mutations, whereas only a quarter of patients with ataxia and neuropathy with no eye movement defects had POLG mutations. The syndrome of myoclonic epilepsy, myopathy, sensory ataxia (MEMSA) can also be associated with POLG mutations.

Infantile-Onset Spinocerebellar Ataxia (IOSCA)

This syndrome, also common in Finland, causes an infantile onset of ataxia, mental retardation, seizures, ophthalmoplegia, and neuropathy. Recessive mutations of the gene *C10orf2* which codes for Twinkle, a protein that interacts with POLG 1 in the synthesis of mtDNA have been reported in IOSCA.

Ataxia Telangiectasia

Epidemiology: The occurrence of AT has been estimated to be 1 in 20,000–100,000 live births.

Genetics and pathogenesis: The disease is caused by mutations in the ATM gene on chromosome 11. ATM codes for the ATM protein which appears to be a transducer protein involved in DNA double-strand break repair; this can explain the radiosensitivity seen in AT. ATM is a serine-threonine kinase which autophosphorylates in response to DNA double-strand break and in turn activates many substrates. AT is one of several diseases in which genes involved in DNA repair mechanisms have been implicated in cerebellar ataxia.

Clinical features and diagnosis: This disorder has its onset early in the first decade with truncal instability and impaired gait. This is followed by progressive ataxia associated with evidence for a polyneuropathy such as hypotonia and loss of reflexes. Choreiform movements are frequent. Characteristic eye movement abnormalities are seen with the need for a rapid head thrust for fixating on targets to one side with the eyes following later (eye-head lag). This is referred to as oculomotor apraxia. Telangiectasia tend to appear about 5 years of age and are most frequent on the conjunctivae (➋ *Fig. 367.4*), but can also occur over the ear lobes and popiteal fossa and other locations.

There is evidence for an immune deficiency with frequent bronchopulmonary infections. The children are at risk for malignancies, especially hematologic tumors like lymphomas and leukemias; other types of cancers occur if the patient reaches adult ages. Because of better care for infections and malignancies, the life span of AT children has increased to over 25 years. Clinical diagnosis is usually apparent, but laboratory features can further support the diagnosis. The serum α fetoprotein is usually elevated (above 10 ng/ml) and immunoglobulin levels are low. Karyotyping often shows chromosomal abnormalities, especially a 7:14 translocation. Increased sensitivity of

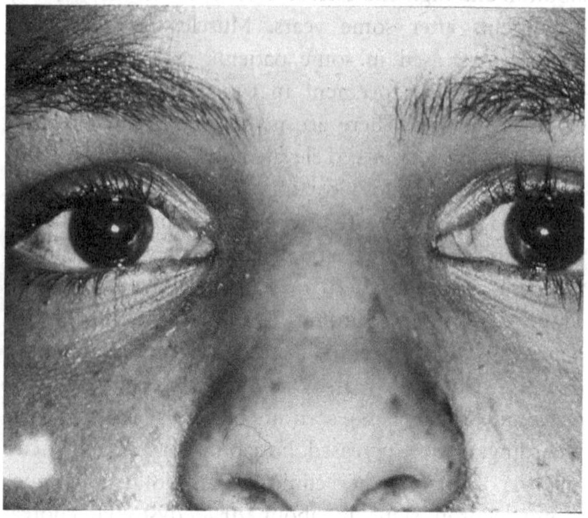

Figure 367.4
Telangiectasia of conjunctiva in ataxia telangiectasia

cultured fibroblasts to radiation can be documented by the "colony survival assay." The definitive way of establishing diagnosis is immunoblotting for the ATM protein; 90% of patients have no protein, 10% have trace amounts, and rare patients have normal ATM levels but no kinase activity ("kinase-dead") (www.geneclinics.org). Further molecular confirmation can be achieved by detecting the mutation; however, this can be difficult because of the size of the ATM gene and the lack of mutation "hot-spots." Sequence analysis of the coding regions of the ATM gene will detect 90% of the mutations but miss intronic alterations and heterozygous deletions. Also benign polymorphisms and pathogenic alterations may be difficult to distinguish. Other types of DNA-based tests include protein truncation tests (examining for premature stop codons) which can detect about 70% of the mutations and mutation scanning using DHPLC which has a sensitivity of 85%.

Treatment: Treatment remains supportive and includes appropriate rehabilitation measures. Children need to be monitored for infections and malignancies. Chronic intermittent immunoglobulin therapy is used to prevent infections, usually in those noted to have very frequent infections. Radiation therapy and investigations with high-dose X-ray exposure have to be managed with great caution and expertise as also chemotherapy because of the radiation sensitivity. Endocrinopathies such as diabetes and gonadal failure need to be looked for and treated appropriately.

Ataxia Telangiectasia-Like Disorder (ATLD)

ATLD is related to mutations in the gene coding for MRE 11, another protein involved in double-stranded DNA break repair. It has a clinical picture resembling AT, but has a milder course, no telangiectasia, and no elevation of serum α fetoprotein.

Spinocerebellar Ataxia with Neuropathy 1 (SCAN 1)

SCAN 1 is a rare disorder, reported in patients from Saudi Arabia, with onset in the second decade; ataxia is associated with sensory motor polyneuropathy, but there are no systemic features. Mutations affecting the tyrosyl-DNA-phosphodiesterase (TDP 1) gene have been identified. TDP 1 gene is involved in single strand DNA break repair.

Other DNA Repair Defects

Both xeroderma pigmentosum and Cockayne syndrome are characterized by photosensitivity. A proportion of these individuals develop neurological problems including ataxia, spasticity, cognitive decline, and seizures.

Autosomal Recessive Ataxia of Charlevoix-Saguenay (ARSACS)

ARSACS was initially identified in children with spastic ataxia among French Canadians in the Charlevoix-Saguenay province of Quebec, Canada, an inbred population with a high carrier frequency for the gene. ARSACS has since then been documented in other geographic areas such as Turkey, Japan, Spain, and Italy. Clinically, it is characterized by very early onset, prominent spasticity followed by ataxia and amyotrophy of distal muscles. Myelinated optic nerve fibers are seen in the French Canadian patients but not in others, and patients from non-Canadian regions have had a more variable phenotype. Mutations in the SACS gene, encoding a protein-labeled SACSIN, are related to ARSACS. The C terminal region of this protein has a DnaJ motif that can interact with Hsp70, and the N terminus has homology to HSp90. Thus, SACSIN may have a chaperone function involved in protein folding.

Marinesco-Sjogren Syndrome

This rare early-onset syndrome is characterized by ataxia, mental retardation, cataracts, and evidence for a myopathy. Peripheral neuropathy, epilepsy, and hypogonadism may be all seen in this disease. Mutations in the gene *SIL 1* have been described; the *SIL 1* product appears to have interactions with one of the Hsp70 chaperone proteins.

Autosomal Recessive Cerebellar Ataxia Type 1 (ARCA 1)

This term has been used to describe an autosomal recessive ataxia in a population isolate of French Canadians from Quebec. The disorder begins in young adult life (17–46 years) and causes progressive ataxia, dysarthria, and mild eye movement problems. Reflexes were normal or slightly brisk, and there was cerebellar atrophy on imaging studies. Molecular studies have revealed that this is related to mutations in the *SYNE 1* gene. It is thought that *SYNE 1* is a member of the spectrin family of cytoskeletal proteins that may be involved in anchoring actin to the plasma membrane and appears enriched in Purkinje cells.

Autosomal Recessive Cerebellar Ataxia Type 2 (ARCA 2)

This term has been used to denote cerebellar ataxia associated with CoQ 10 deficiency. CoQ 10 is a lipid soluble component of cell membranes and is involved in transport of electrons between complex I and II of the electron transport chain to complex III. Ataxia associated with deficiency of muscle CoQ 10 is heterogeneous. This combination can be seen in some patients with AOA 1 as well as in some with defined abnormalities in CoQ 10 metabolism. Ataxia is associated with pyramidal signs and mild cognitive decline. Some patients may have hypogonadism. CoQ 10 deficiency can be associated with other phenotypes such as an infantile multisystem disease, encephalomyopathy with ragged red fibers, and Leigh's syndrome. Some gene mutations have been identified in the infantile cases. The syndrome may respond to CoQ 10 replacement therapy.

Other Poorly Defined Recessive Ataxias

Among 102 patients with recessive ataxias reported by Anheim et al., extensive molecular studies led to a genetic diagnosis in only 57. The cases that could not be molecularly classified had a slightly later onset (>20 years), and milder course. Cerebellar atrophy is seen in 68% of these individuals and polyneuropathy in about 50%. A small proportion of these individuals had oculomotor apraxia and elevated alpha fetoprotein and serum CK. A number of clinically defined syndromes may be seen in this group, including ataxia with hypogonadism, deafness, and myoclonus.

Autosomal Recessive or X-Linked "Genetic-Metabolic" Diseases with Ataxia as a Feature

A number of disorders of childhood or young adult onset are not classified as an ataxia, yet often have ataxia as a feature. In many, other CNS and systemic features occur, cognitive decline or mental retardation is common, and imaging studies may be distinctive. These tend to separate them from the classical ataxias (➲ *Table 367.3*).

Cerebrotendinous Xanthomatosis

This disease is caused by mutations in the CYP 27 gene encoding 27-hydroxylase that cleaves a side chain off cholesterol and this leads to reduced bile acid synthesis and increased formation of intermediates such as cholestanol and 27-C bile alcohols. There is increased serum and tissue levels of cholestanol and tissue deposits of sterols. The clinical picture includes chronic diarrhea beginning in the first decade and a neurological syndrome that combines spastic ataxia and cognitive decline. Xanthomas can be seen by 15 years of age, usually over Achilles tendon, tibial tuberosities, or fingers (➲ *Fig. 367.5*). Juvenile cataracts are also a feature. Later in the course, osteoporosis, easy fractures, and coronary disease occur. Diagnosis can be established by clinical features and elevated serum cholestanol levels as well as by mutation analysis of CYP 27. Therapy with chenodeoxycholic acid and statins may arrest disease progression.

Urea Cycle Defects

The late-onset varieties of these can present in childhood with episodes of encephalopathy, nausea, and vomiting

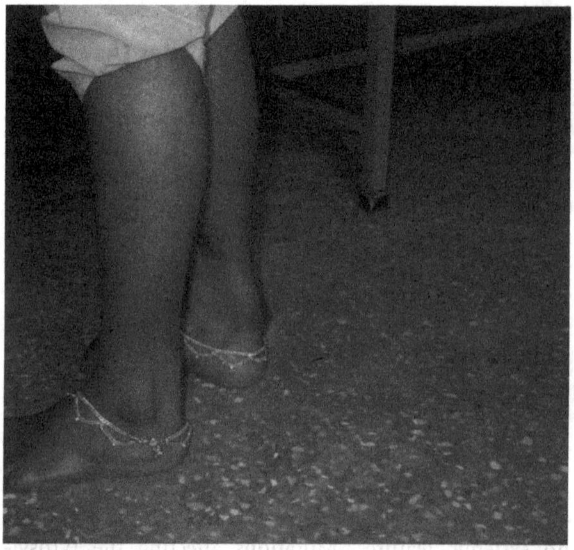

Figure 367.5
Achilles tendon xanthoma in cerebrotendinous xanthomatosis

associated with ataxia. One variety (arginase deficiency) can present with spatic paraplegia. Brain MRI may be normal or show edema during episodes. Serum ammonia is elevated to over 80 µmol.

Hartnup Disease

This disease is caused by mutations in the neutral amino acid transporter gene (SLCGA 19) and results in neutral aminoaciduria. Clinical picture includes growth delay, skin rash, diarrhea, ataxia, and psychosis. Tryptophan metabolism abnormality leading to a deficiency of serotonin has been proposed as a mechanism for the clinical picture. Diagnosis is established using plasma and urine amino acid levels.

Pyruvate Dehydrogenase Complex Deficiency

This can be X-linked or autosomal recessive depending on the component of the PDHC complex that is abnormal. The disease presents with episodic dysfunction including ataxia and encephalopathy; later, there are persistent deficits associated with cognitive decline and neuropathy. Optic atrophy is common and MRI may show putaminal necrosis in the brain. Serum and CSF lactate and pyruvate are increased with decreased lactate to pyruvate ration. Diagnosis is established by estimating PDHC activity in cultured skin fibroblasts. Therapy with high-dose vitamin B1 and ketogenic diet may help.

Late-Onset Tay–Sachs Disease (GM1 Gangliosidosis)

Though Tay–Sachs disease is typically infantile in onset, a late-onset form (age at onset 8–36 years) has been described. The clinical picture is characterized by ataxia, neurogenic weakness with atrophy and fasciculations due to anterior horn cell loss, psychosis and cognitive decline. Mutations in the hexosaminidase gene can be established and leuokocyte hexosamonidase A and total hexosaminidase levels are reduced.

Aceruloplasminemia

This disease results from mutations in the ceruloplasmin gene. Ceruloplasmin transports copper and also has ferroxidase activity that allows it to mobilize tissue iron. Both homozygous and heterozygous mutations can cause disease. The former causes ataxia, cognitive decline, chorea, Parkinosinian features, and retinal degeneration. MRI of the brain shows T2 hypointensity in the cerebral and cerebellar cortex, basal ganglia, and the dentate nucleus. Heterozygous mutations cause ataxia, tremor, and chorea with no T2 hypointensity on MRI. Serum and urine copper is low, ferrtitin high, and ceruloplasmin absent. Therapy with chelation may improve the clinical picture.

Vanishing White Matter Disease

This disorder has been linked to mutations in five eukaryotic initiating factor 2B genes (EIF 2B 1–5). Patients present with ataxia and upper motor neuron signs between 2 and 5 years of age. Episodes of rapid progression after stress have been reported. MRI is characterized by cavitating bilateral leukoencephalopathy. An adult variant of this disease has also been seen with a mean age at onset of 31 years and spasticity, ataxia, cognitive decline, and seizures. Imaging studies show cerebral atrophy, cystic breakdown of white matter, and increased T2 signal in cerebellum and corpus callosum.

Refsum Disease

A deficiency of phytanyl CoA hydroxylase results in increased phytanic acid in tissue peroxisomes. The clinical picture is characterized by a polyneuropathy associated with ataxia, hearing loss, and ichthyotic skin changes. Plasma phytanic acid is high, and a low phytanic acid diet may slow disease progression.

Giant Axonal Neuropathy

This autosomal recessive disease is characterized by onset between 2 and 7 years of age. Neurologically, there is severe ataxia, mental retardation, and sensory motor polyneuropathy with weakness and atrophy of muscles. Hair appears kinky and red. Variant phenotypes include a spastic syndrome with mild ataxia and no kinky red hair. MRI shows diffuse white matter changes in the hemispheres and cerebellum. Nerve biopsy shows distended axons with microfilament accumulation by electron microscopy. Mutations in the gene gigaxonin that is involved in microtubular stability are responsible for this condition.

Congenital Disorders of Glycosylation Syndromes (CDG Syndromes)

These are disorders characterized by defective synthesis of N-linked oligosaccharides. There are 21 enzymes in this pathway that are known to be defective in the CDG syndromes. The disorders have a wide phenotypic spectrum with developmental delay, cerebellar hypoplasia, liver disease, and abnormal fat tissue as possible manifestations. During early childhood, patients have hypotonia, ataxia, and delayed language. Peculiar slow rolling eye movements have been described. Other features that can occur include seizures, stroke-like episodes, elevated liver enzymes, coagulopathy, and joint contractures. Systemic features include hepatomegaly, proteinuria, orange peel appearance of skin, hypogonadism, and large ears. Diagnosis can be suspected by an abnormal serum transferring glycoforms detected by isoelectric focusing.

Neuronal Ceroid Lipofuscinoses

These are autosomal recessive lysosomal storage diseases of infancy and childhood which have been classified into many types. Some varieties of this such as the late infantile type, the adult onset type, and the Gypsy-Indian type are associated with ataxia, but other features such as cognitive decline, seizures, and visual loss usually dominate the clinical picture. Measuring palmitoyl priten thiesterase 1 (PPT 1) and tripeptidyl peptidae 1 (TPP1) may be useful indicators of NCL. Electron microscopy of conjunctival or skin biopsies and of the buffy coat may reveal characteristic lysosomal storage material in the form of curvilinear, fingerprint, or granular osmiophilic bodies. Genetic mutations in the genes CLN 1 through CLN 8 have been identified but diagnosis can be difficult.

Niemann–Pick Disease Type C

This is a rare autosomal recessive disease with a wide range of age at onset (perinatal period to over 15 years) and phenotypic variability related to mutations in the genes NPC 1 and 2. A wide variety of motor phenomena are seen with ataxia, dystonia, and dysarthia being very common. Cognitive decline, hearing loss, myoclonus, and seizures are seen commonly at different age groups, and vertical supranuclear gaze palsy appears to be a frequent phenomenon. Cataplexy and hearing loss also have been described. Hepatosplenomegaly is common but may need ultrasound to detect in older patients. Elevation of plasma chitotriosidase may be a diagnostic clue but not specific. Examination of tissue (bone marrow, skin, liver biopsy, lymph nodes) can reveal characteristic foam cells or sea blue histiocytes. Cultured fibroblasts can be subjected to the filipin test to detect typical perinuclear cholesterol filled vesicles. Mutation analysis of the two responsible genes (NPC 1 and 2 associated with 96 and 4% cases respectively) may establish the diagnosis, but novel polymorphisms can be difficult to distinguish from pathogenic mutations.

PLP-1 Related Disease

Classic Pelizaeus–Merzbacher disease is characterized by onset <5 years, nystagmus, hypotonia, spastic ataxia, dystonia, and decreased cognition. A milder variant causes spastic ataxia, mild cognitive decline, and neuropathy. MRI shows diffuse leukoencephalopathy. Diagnosis is established by PLP1 mutation analysis, FISH for duplication or chromosomal microarray.

Adrenomyeloneuropathy

Though this X-linked disorder typically presents as adrenoleukodystrophy in young boys with progressive cerebral and motor problems, milder phenotypes have been described in both males and females. Occasional patients may present with a spinocerebellar ataxia presentation, and imaging abnormalities in the brain may be scant. Screening for this disease by measuring very long chain fatty acids should be done in patients with ataxia in whom other causes have been excluded.

Miscellaneous Disorders

The following disorders can all be associated with ataxia in addition to other more diffuse CNS symptomatology: late-onset maple syrup urine disease, methylmalonic academia, propionic academia, isovaleric academia, arginase deficiency, and Lafora disease.

Mitochondrial Diseases with Ataxia

The term mitochondrial disease refers to a clinical disorder that is thought to have its origin in a primary defect of a respiratory chain component, whether the component is coded by a nuclear or mitochondrial gene. The phenotype of mitochondrial diseases may include both neurological and systemic features and be quite variable. Many classic phenotypic syndromes related to mtDNA mutations such as Kearns–Sayre syndrome (KSS), myoclonic epilepsy with ragged red fibers (MERRF), mitochondrial encephalomyopathy with lactic acidosis and stroke-like episodes (MELAS), neurogenic weakness with ataxia and retinitis pigmentosa (NARP) can all have ataxia as one of the features. While many of the more-recently-recognized nuclear mutations causing respiratory chain defects lead to complex neurological diseases, ataxia may be a feature of nuclear mutations resulting in multiple mtDNA deletions.

Autosomal Dominant Ataxias

Autosomal dominant (AD) ataxias with a progressive course are labeled spinocerebellar ataxia (SCA) followed by a number indicating the particular chromosomal locus or gene mutation that is responsible. At this time, SCA 1 through SCA 31 have been recognized, with the following caveats: SCA 9 was reserved for a family which appears not to have been followed up, and at the moment its status is unclear; SCA 15 and 16 have been recently found to be related to the same gene mutation; SCA 19 and 22 may be allelic diseases, but this has not been settled; SCA 24 was identified in a family which likely has a recessive mode of inheritance, and this is now called Spinocerebellar ataxia with saccadic intrusions (SCASI). The preferred name for SCA 3 is Machado–Joseph disease (MJD). Dentato-rubral pallido-luysian atrophy (DRPLA) is grouped with the ataxias, but has no SCA designation.

In addition, there are autosomal dominant ataxias in which symptoms are episodic; these are labeled as episodic ataxia syndromes (EA) with the numbers (EA 1 through 6) denoting distinct chromosomal loci. There is more experience worldwide with SCA 1, 2, 3 (MJD), 6, 7 and EA 2 than the other AD ataxias, and thus their clinical picture is better defined for the most part. With the other SCAs, clinical experience is restricted to single families or small number of families, and the phenotypic spectrum may change as more experience is accumulated.

Genetics and pathogenesis: Many of the initial gene mutations identified in the SCAs were unstable expansion of CAG triplets within coding sequences of different genes (➋ *Table 367.4*).

The CAG repeat codes for a string of glutamines and, therefore, these ataxias are also called polyglutamine ataxias. Other repeat expansions discovered to cause ataxia occurred in noncoding regions and include a CAG expansion in the promoter sequence for SCA 12, a CTG expansion in the 3'UTR for SCA 8, and an intronic ATTCT repeat expansion for SCA 10 and finally a TGGAA pentanucleotide insertion for SCA 31. More recently, identified gene mutations in the SCAs have been other types of gene alterations, including

Table 367.4
Autosomal dominant ataxias related to expanded nucleotide repeat motifs

Disease	Gene, repeat, and locus	Normal repeat numbers	Mutable normal alleles	Reduced penetrance alleles	Pathogenic alleles
SCA 1	ATXN 1, CAG, 6p23	6–44	36–38		39-91[a]
SCA 2	ATXN2,CAG,12q	<31	None		32–>200
SCA 3 (MJD)	ATXN 3, CAG, 14q	<44		45–51	52–86
SCA 6	CACNA1A, CAG,19p	<18		19[b]	20–33
SCA 7	ATXN 7, CAG, 3p	<19	28–33	34–36	37–400
SCA 8	ATXN8OS, CTG-CAG, 13q	15–50 combined $(CTA{\cdot}TAG)_n(CTG{\cdot}CAG)_n$			71–1,300[c]
SCA 10	ATXN 10, ATTCT, 22q	10–29		280–850	800–4,500
SCA 12	PP2R2B, CAG, 5q	4–32		40–62	51–78
SCA 17	TBP, CAG, 6q	25–42		43–48	49–66
DRPLA	ATN, CAG, 12p	6–35	May exist		48–93

[a]Note the overlap between upper end of normal and lower end of pathogenic range. Normal and pathogenic alleles of the same size can be distinguished by the presence of CAT interruptions in the former. The interruptions can be detected using Sfa NI restriction site testing
[b]19 repeat allele has been seen in asymptomatic elderly persons, in a person with atypical symptoms, in a homozygous individual with typical symptoms and has been shown to expand into a pathogenic range in the offspring of an individual with no symptoms
[c]Alleles of the same size can be seen in asymptomatic individuals

missense and nonsense mutations, insertions, deletions, and chromosomal duplications (➋ *Table 367.5*).

Lastly, in many SCAs chromosomal loci are known, but the mutations are yet to be identified. The EA mutations identified so far have involved missense and nonsense mutations in ion channel or transporter proteins (➋ *Table 367.6*).

The pathogenesis of the polyglutamine ataxias has been related mainly to a toxic gain of function by the product of the mutant allele. The protein product of the mutant allele has a longer glutamine tract and undergoes misfolding and aggregate formation, and this is believed to trigger many pathogenic cascades (➋ *Fig. 367.6*). Examples of such altered cellular pathways include transcriptional dysregulationn of other genes because of the presence of misfolded protein in the nucleus, colocalization of chaperone proteins with the aggregates, disruption of preoteasome pathways and mitochondrial dysfunction and apoptosis. The role of posttranslational modification of the mutant protein such as phosphorylation and the need for nuclear transport and cleavage of the protein for pathogenicity are also being investigated as possible therapeutic targets. Shutting off the mutated gene using siRNA has succeeded in reducing pathology in many model systems. Other types of therapeutic options may include targeting some of the secondary cascades triggered by the mutations.

In the case of the more-recently-discovered non-polyglutamine ataxias, a diverse series of pathogenic mechanisms may play a role. In SCA 8 and SCA 10, repeat expansions in noncoding regions of the gene may be pathogenic due to an RNA-based mechanism with the long transcript being toxic to a number of cellular mechanisms. In other diseases such as SCA 5, SCA 13, SCA 14, and SCA 27, such processes as cytoskeletal integrity, channel function, and signaling pathways may be altered.

In the episodic ataxia syndromes, mutations involve proteins that function as channels or transporters, and they appear to be examples of neuronal channelopathies. Mutant channels may express a variety of aberrant properties and produce haploinsufficiency or a dominant negative effect, leading to abnormal channel physiology.

Clinical features: In general, the SCAs have onset in young to middle adult life and are not high on the diagnostic list in pediatric age groups, though reported range of age at onset is very wide for many of the SCAs. In many of the better known SCAs which result from unstable nucleotide repeat expansions, anticipation in age at onset is prominent and onset in childhood and even neonatal period has been described. Typically, in these diseases, age at onset is inversely correlated with expansion size so that, with larger expansions, onset can be in teen or early childhood years. There are also more-recently-described SCAs unrelated to nucleotide repeat expansions with onset in early years, but with a very slow progression.

The clinical picture of the SCAs is usually dominated by cerebellar ataxia. In some, ataxia is the loan clinical finding. In others, ataxia is associated with evidence for pathology in many other neural systems including the upper motor neurons, basal ganglia, brain stem neurons, anterior horn cells, cortical neurons,and peripheral nerves. Thus, patients with these SCAs have an array of clinical signs in addition to ataxia such as brisk tendon reflexes, spasticity, Babinski signs, akinesia, rigidity, tremor of different types, oculomotor deficits of many

Table 367.5

Autosomal dominant ataxias with defined mutations unrelated to nucleotide expansions

Disease	Gene	Locus	Mutation
SCA 5	SPTBN 2	11p	Deletions, point mutation
SCA 11	TTBK 2	15q	Insertion/deletion
SCA 13	KCNC 3	19q	Point mutations
SCA 14	PRKCG	19q	Deletions, point mutations
SCA 15/16	ITPR 1	3p	Deletions, point mutations
SCA 20	Unknown	11q	Duplication
SCA 27	FGF 14	13q	Point mutations
SCA 28	AFG3L2	18p	Point mutations

AFG3L2 ATPase family gene 3-like 2 gene, *FGF* 14 fibroblast growth factor 14 gene, *ITPR 1* inosine triphosphate receptor 1 gene, *PRKCG* protein kinase C gamma gene, *KCNC 3* voltage gated potassium channel/member 3 gene, *STBPN 2* beta-III spectrin gene, *TTBK 2* tubulin tau kinase 2 gene. In SCA 20, the region duplicated has multiple genes

Table 367.6

Episodic ataxia syndromes (Modified from Manto M, Marmolino D (2009) Cerebellar ataxias. Curr Opin Neurol 22:419–429)

Disease	Phenotype	Onset	Mutation
EA 1	Very brief episodes of ataxia; interictal skeletal myokymia	Early childhood	*KCNA1*
EA 2	Ataxic episodes lasting hours; interictal nystagmus	Childhood to young adult	*CACNA1A*
EA 3	Episodic vertigo and tinnitus		Linked to 1q
EA 4	Episodic vertigo; interictal nystagmus	Late onset	
EA 6	Associated with hemiplegic migraine		
EA 7	Attacks of vertigo, weakness, slurred speech	<20 years	Linked to 19q

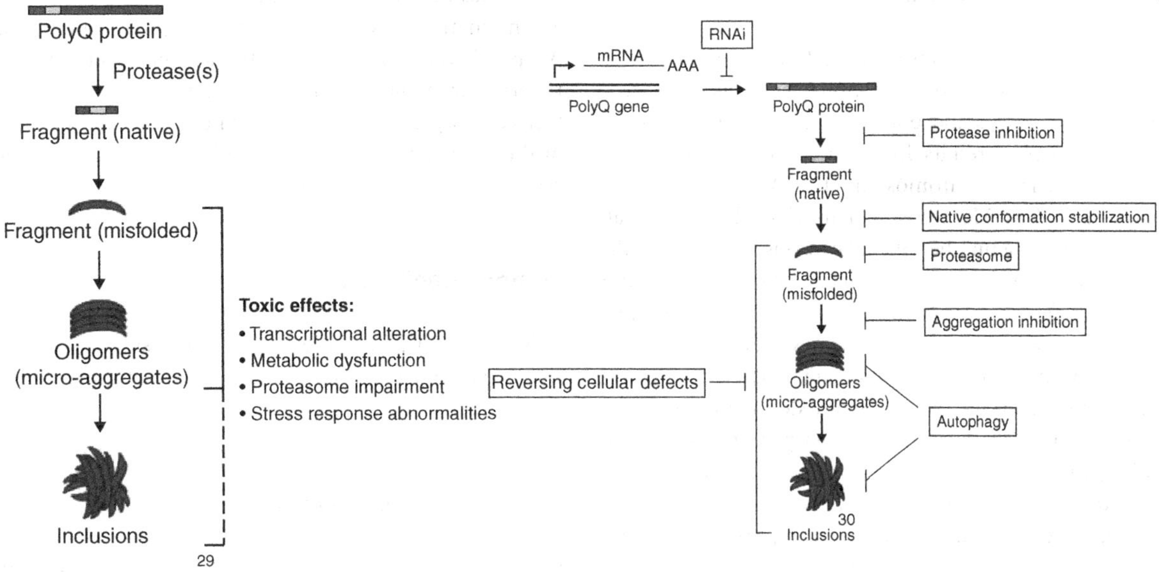

Figure 367.6

Pathogenesis of spinocerebellar ataxias related to CAG repeat expansions. The polyglutamine protein product of the mutated allele tends to misfold and form oligomers and aggregates, sometime after cleavage by proteases. Such misfolded protein can be pathogenic due to a variety of reasons, including interference with transcriptional machinery in general, and with the proteasome, chaperone, and autophagy systems. Numerous secondary events may cascade from these effects including changes in mitochondrial function, apoptosis, and abnormal calcium homeostasis. On the right, some of the potential interventions that may be useful are illustrated, including the use of siRNA to inhibit the mutant gene and therapies that may influence aggregation, autophagy, and proteasome (From Shao and Diamond 2007. With permission)

types, dysarthria, dysphagia, tongue and facial atrophy with fasciculations, muscle atrophy, cramps, muscle fasciculations, sensory loss and areflexia in varying combinations. Seizures, cognitive decline, and retinopathy with visual loss occur in some SCAs.

While the genotypic diagnosis of a particular type of SCA from clinical signs alone is very difficult, certain clinical features may be seen more typically in some SCAs. The course of the SCAs is progressive, with loss of ambulation 15–20 years after onset and death resulting from severe motor disability and resultant complications. Both the array of clinical findings and the course of the disease can be influenced by the repeat expansion size. The diagnosis of an SCA can be made by the documentation of a progressive degenerative ataxic disease with an autosomal dominant inheritance pattern. Further confirmation can be achieved by obtaining mutation analysis for the various SCA genes. In the subsequent section, the SCAs are described in brief with emphasis on those that may have a pediatric presentation.

Spinocerebellar Ataxia 1

The mean age at onset is in the fourth decade, but there is a wide range of age at onset, and childhood onset is possible. In typical cases, clinical picture is characterized by progressive ataxia, dysarthria, upper motor neuron signs, and a mild sensory polyneuropathy. Cognitive decline may occur, especially with younger age at onset. The disease is related to a CAG repeat expansion in the ataxin 1 gene on chromosome 6p.

Spinocerebellar Ataxia 2

Typically, SCA 2 has onset in the fourth decade and is characterized by progressive cerebellar signs associated with slow saccades and polyneuropathy often leading to areflexia. SCA 2 results from a CAG expansion in the ataxin 2 gene on chromosome 12q. Yis et al., Abdel-Aleem and Zaki, Moretti et al., Babovic-Vukasnovic et al. have described a number of pediatric onset cases. In addition to the typical features of ataxia, slow saccades, and loss of reflexes, the childhood cases exhibit cognitive decline and extrapyramidal features. Cases with neonatal onset have hypotonia, developmental delay, ocular problems, and dysphagia. Diagnosis of a dominant condition may be missed because the affected parent (usually the father) may be asymptomatic at the time the children get symptoms. Careful family history and drawing at least a three-generation family pedigree is important. Neonatal cases may have "hyperexpansions" of the CAG tract in the ataxin 2 gene, and these may not be detected by the usual PCR method of mutation detection. When suspicion exists, a "normal" result from such a PCR test should be followed by a Southern blot to detect hyperexpansions.

Spinocerebellar Ataxia 3 or Machado–Joseph Disease

Age at onset can vary from 5 to 75 years, but onset in childhood is rare. There is an inverse correlation between the number of repeats and age at onset, so that pediatric onset typically occurs with repeat sizes over 75 in the mutant allele. This type of early-onset disease is characterized more by extrapyramidal features, including bradykinesia, rigidity, and dystonia, together with spasticity. Ataxia may not be prominent. This has been called the type I MJD phenotype as opposed to type II, which has onset in young adult life and is characterized by ataxia and upper motor neuron findings. Type III disease is characterized by ataxia and neuropathy leading to loss of tendon reflexes. Rare patients with homozygous expansion in the ataxin 3 gene can have a severe phenotype and onset below 10 years of age, but heterozygous expansion also has led to a very early onset. Carvalho et al. reported one homozygous patient who had motor regression and dysphagia starting at age 4, followed by dystonia and spasticity with only minor ataxia.

Spinocerebellar Ataxia 4

SCA 4 has been localized to chromosome 16q and causes a combination of sensory motor neuropathy and ataxia. A "pure" cerebellar ataxia with dominant inheritance, reported from Japan, has an overlapping chromosomal locus and segregates with a single nucleotide substitution in the puratrophin gene within this region; but it is not certain whether this is allelic to SCA 4.

Spinocerebellar Ataxia 5

This dominant adult onset ataxia causes slowly progressive ataxia and has been linked to a mutation in the β spectrin gene (*SPTBN 2)*.

Spinocerebellar Ataxia 6

SCA 6 is characterized by a progressive, pure cerebellar syndrome with onset in the fifth decade and a slow course. It is related to a CAG expansion in the α subunit of the neuronal calcium channel gene (*CACNA1)*.

Spinocerebellar Ataxia 7

SCA 7 is caused by a CAG expansion in the ataxin 7 gene on chromosome 3p. It has wide range of age of onset and the considerable instability of the CAG expansion, especially on paternal transmission, often causes major anticipation in age of onset, with childhood and infantile onset. Adult onset cases are characterized by ataxia and other cerebellar signs, spasticity, and other upper motor neuron signs and a variable occurrence of visual loss related to a cone-rod dystrophy in the retina. Childhood onset has been described both in molecularly confirmed families and in the pre-molecular era. Onset below age was seen with repeat expansion sizes of over 67, and early-onset cases often have visual loss preceding the ataxia, a situation different from adult onset cases. Early-onset patients also have an accelerated course often leading to death within 5 years of onset and a clinical picture with many features other than ataxia, such as cognitive decline, muscle weakness and atrophy, myoclonus and epilepsy. Infantile onset can be associated with developmental delay, dysphagia, hypotonia, poor visual tracking, and evidence for cardiomyopathy. Similar to that in SCA 2, the "hyperexpansions" associated with such infantile onset can be missed by routine PCR testing and need Southern blotting.

Spinocerebellar Ataxia 8

The CTG expansion in ataxin 8 gene associated with SCA 8 has been seen in both sporadic cases and in some families with dominant ataxia. SCA 8 patients have ataxia, some upper motor neuron signs, and mild sensory loss. The direct role of the expansion in the causation of ataxia is still debated since the same expansion occurs with some frequency in non-ataxic individuals; both an RNA-based mechanism and a "polyglutamine" mechanism based in bidirectional transcription of the gene have been proposed.

Spinocerebellar Ataxia 10

This disease which causes a combination of ataxia and epilepsy is related to a pentanucleotide (ATTCT) expansion in the 5'untranslated region of the ataxin 10 gene and appears confined to people of central and South American ancestry.

Spinocerebellar Ataxia 11

SCA 11 has been described in a limited number of families and causes ataxia, upper motor neuron signs and abnormal eye movements. Mutations have been described in the tubulin tau kinase gene (TTBK2).

Spinocerebellar Ataxia 12

SCA 12 causes a variable combination of ataxia, tremor, basal ganglia signs, and dementia. The causative mutation is a CAG expansion in the promoter sequence of the gene PPP2R2B gene.

Spinocerebellar Ataxia 13

The limited experience with SCA 13 indicated both childhood and adult onset of very slowly progressive ataxia, sometime associated with mild mental retardation. Mutations in a potassium channel gene (KCNC3) are responsible.

Spinocerebellar Ataxia 14

This disorder results from mutations in the protein kinase C γ gene and causes a variable phenotype including childhood onset, though most patients have onset in adult life. The clinical picture has varied from one of pure cerebellar ataxia to one that has additional features including axial myoclonus, choreic movements, diplopia and gaze palsy, and facial myokymia. Rigidity, dystonia, proprioceptive loss, and slow saccades also have been noted from time to time.

Spinocerebellar Ataxia 15 and 16

SCA 15 and 16 were originally reported from Australia and Japan, respectively, but more recent findings suggest that the same gene mutation underlies these entities. The disease causes pure cerebellar ataxia, but the Japanese cases had postural tremor as well. Deletions involving two contiguous genes (SUMF1 and ITPR1) were found in the Australian kindred, but in the Japanese patients, only the ITPR1 gene was deleted, suggesting that this is the critical gene.

Spinocerebellar Ataxia 17

SCA 17 is caused by a CAG expansion in the TATA-binding protein (TBP) gene. It is a polyglutamine disorder. It has a wide range of age at onset, including childhood, and has a very variable phenotype including ataxia, extrapyramidal signs, psychiatric features, epilepsy, and dementia.

Spinocerebellar Ataxia 18

Brkanac et al. described a chromosome 7q22–q32-linked autosomal dominant condition characterized by both ataxia and a sensory motor neuropathy in a five generation American family of Irish ancestry.

Spinocerebellar Ataxia 19

Schelhaas et al. reported a family of Dutch origin with a mild ataxia, myoclonus, irregular postural tremor, and cognitive impairment. Among 11 family members with clinical data, many also had decreased proprioception and tendon reflexes. The disorder in this family was mapped to chromosome 1p21–q21 by Verbeek et al.

Spinocerebellar Ataxia 20

SCA 20 was described in an Australian family with a wide range of age at onset, prominent dysarthria and dysphonia, and the presence of calcification in the cerebellar dentate. The disease is localized to chromosome 11 and appears related to the duplication of a 260 Kb segment on chromosome 11q. Its pathogenesis remains unclear.

Spinocerebellar Ataxia 21

In a family with autosomal dominant ataxia with onset in childhood and young adult life, a new gene locus was established at chromosome 7p. In addition to ataxia, the patients had tremor, rigidity, and cognitive impairment.

Spinocerebellar Ataxia 22

Chung et al. (2003) reported a Chinese family with dominant ataxia, hyporeflexia, onset between 10 and 46 years of age and MRI showing isolated cerebellar atrophy and established a locus at chromosome 1p, overlapping that reported in SCA 19.

Spinocerebellar Ataxia 23

In a single family with adult onset dominant ataxia, the locus was mapped to chromosome 20p.

Spinocerebellar Ataxia 25

In a single family from France, Stevanin et al. noted childhood onset of a dominant ataxia with variable progression and an associated peripheral neuropathy. Linkage studies localized the disorder to chromosome 2p.

Spinocerebellar Ataxia 26

Yu et al. have a described a single family of Norwegian descent with relatively pure cerebellar ataxia with little in the way of extracerebllar signs. Age at onset was from 33 to 60 years. MRI showed cerebellar atrophy, but brainstem was spared. Genetic mapping has localized this disease to chromosome 19p13.3 adjacent to the SCA 6 locus.

Spinocerebellar Ataxia 27

This disease, related to mutations in the fibroblast growth factor 14 gene, has onset in childhood with tremulousness and then progressive ataxia which is slowly progressive. Orofacial dyskinesias, cognitive decline, and aggressive outbursts were noted in some patients.

Spinocerebellar Ataxia 28

There is limited experience with this disease in two families of Italian origin. The phenotype is characterized by juvenile onset (range 12–36), slow progression of ataxia, nystagmus, and later in the disease course, ophthalmoparesis with ptosis and slow saccades. Point mutations have been discovered in the SCA 28 gene in these two families, located on chromosome 18p.

Spinocerebellar Ataxia 29

In an Australian family with congenital, nonprogressive ataxia and "cerebellar hypoplasia" on imaging studies, Dudding et al. identified a locus on chromosome 3p.

Spinocerebellar Ataxia 30

An Australian family with dominantly inherited ataxia of late onset was mapped to chromosome 4q.

Dentato-Rubral-Pallido-Luysian Atrophy (DRPLA)

This disease with a very complex phenotype is usually classified among the ataxias. It is most prevalent in Japan, but molecularly proven DRPLA has been reported from Europe and the USA. The original African-American family in which the typical neuropathology was described many years ago is now known to carry the same mutation as the Japanese cases. DRPLA has a variable age of onset from infancy to old age and anticipation is common. With onset below 20 years of age, the clinical picture is one of seizures, myoclonus, ataxia, and intellectual decline. With older onset, the disease is characterized by ataxia, chorea, dementia, and psychiatric features. Thus, the differential diagnosis varies with age and includes the progressive myoclonic epilepsy syndromes in children and adolescents, and Huntington's disease in older persons. Diagnosis can be established by documenting an expanded CAG repeat in the atrophin 1 gene.

Episodic Ataxias

The episodic ataxias are characterized by brief, reversible attacks of ataxia of variable duration often associated with other neurological features. However, in some of them, a more persistent neurological deficit may develop or may be present from the very onset, blurring the distinction from the SCAs. Conversely, some of the SCAs (such as SCA 6) may have features reminiscent of episodic attacks. Many of the EA syndromes have pediatric onset.

Onset of EA 1 is in early childhood with very brief episodes of ataxia lasting seconds to minutes associated with a coarse tremor and dysarthria. Between attacks of ataxia, patients have skeletal muscle myokymia that may be detected clinically or only by electrophysiological studies. Children with EA 1 may have other features such as partial epilepsy, transient postural abnormalities, and tight heel cords. Some patients may have only peripheral myokymia with no ataxia, and some may have persistent cerebellar findings and cerebellar atrophy on scans. Mutations in the potassium channel gene, *KCNA 1,* have been identified in EA 1.

EA 2 also has a childhood onset in the majority of patients. Episodes of ataxia last many hours and are associated with other symptoms such as headache, nausea, vomiting, diplopia, and dysarthria. Interictally, many EA 2 patients have mild cerebellar deficits including nystagmus (often downbeating) and difficulty with tandem gait. EA 2 patients may have a progressive ataxia later in life. Unusual features have been described, including children with features of benign paroxysmal vertigo and cognitive decline associated with attention deficit disorder. In addition, the EA 2 mutations may be associated with seizures, coma, and cerebral edema after mild head trauma. EA 2 is allelic to two other diseases, familial hemiplegic migraine (FHM) and SCA 6. All of them are related to mutations in the α subunit of the neuronal calcium channel gene, *CACNA1A*; EA 2 and FHM are related to point mutations in the gene and SCA 6 to a CAG expansion.

Other EAs have been defined by the presence of familial episodic ataxia or vertigo and exclusion of the EA 1 and EA 2 mutations. EA 3 is characterized by brief episodes of ataxia and vertigo, associated with tinnitus. It has been localized to chromosome 1q42. EA 4 has been reported to produce late-onset episodic vertigo and ataxia (vestibulocerebellar ataxia) lasting many hours; linkage to EA 1 and EA 2 loci has been excluded, but no other genetic information is available. EA 5 has clinical features similar to EA 2; mutation in the $\beta 4$ subunit of the calcium channel gene, *CACNB4,* has been reported in one family. Finally, EA 6 was reported in a single child with episodes of ataxia, hemiplegia, and seizures with a mutation in an astrocytic glutamate transporter gene (*SLC1A3).* The mutation was shown to have lead to loss of function of the protein with a dominant negative effect on the wild type product by functional studies.

Treatment: EA syndromes respond to many drugs with reduction in the number of episodes. Whether these drugs prevent long-term, progressive deficits is not clear. EA 1 responds to carbamazepine, valproate, and sometimes to acetazolamide. Acetazolamide often leads to dramatic improvement in EA 2; other drugs that may ameliorate attacks include flunarazine and 4-aminopyridine.

For the SCAs, there is no proven therapy at this time. Supportive and rehabilitative care need to be organized as for many other disabling neurological illnesses. As in all genetic diseases, appropriate referral for genetic counseling is indicated.

References

Abdel-Aleem A, Zaki MS (2008) Spinocerebellar ataxia type 2 (SCA 2) in an Egyptian family presenting with polyphagia and marked CAG expansion in infancy. J Neurol 255:413–419

Amino T, Ishikawa K, Toru S et al (2007) Redefining the disease locus of 16q22.1-linked autosomal dominant cerebellar ataxia. J Hum Genet 52:643–649

Anheim M, Fleury M, Monga B et al (2009a) Epidemiological, clinical, paraclinical and molecular study of a cohort of 102 patients affected with autosomal recessive progressive cerebellar ataxia from Alsace, Eastern France: implications for clinical management. Neurogenetics 11(1):1–12

Anheim M, Monga B, Fleury M et al (2009b) Ataxia with oculomotor apraxia type 2: clinical, biological and genotype/phenotype correlation study of a cohort of 90 patients. Brain 132(Pt 10):2688–2698

Babcock M, De Silva D, Oaks R et al (1997) Regulation of mitochondrial iron accumulation by Yfh 1 p, a putative homolog of frataxin. Science 276:1709–1712

Babovic-Vuksanovic D, Snow K, Patterson MC et al (1998) Spinocerebellar ataxia type 2 (SCA 2) in an infant with extreme CAG expansion. Am J Med Genet 12:383–387

Bauer PO, Nukina N (2009) The pathogenic mechanisms of polyglutamine diseases and current therapeutic strategies. J Neurochem 110:1737–1765

Benton CS, de Silva R, Rutledge SL et al (1998) Molecular and clinical studies in SCA-7 define a broad clinical spectrum and the infantile phenotype. Neurology 51:1081–1086

Ber L, Bouslam N, Rivaud-Péchoux S et al (2004) Frequency and phenotypic spectrum of ataxia with oculomotor apraxia 2: a clinical and genetic study in 18 patients. Brain 127:759–767

Bertholon P, Chabrier S, Riant F et al (2008) Episodic ataxia type 2: unusual aspects in clinical and genetic presentation. Special emphasis in childhood. J Neurol Neurosurg Psychiatry 80:1289–1292

Boesch S, Strum B, Hering S et al (2008) Neurological effects of recombinant human erythropoietin in Friedreich's ataxia: a clinical pilot trial. Mov Disord 23:1940–1944

Bomar JM, Benke PJ, Slattery EL et al (2003) Mutations in a novel gene encoding a CRAL-TRIO domain cause human Cayman ataxia and ataxia/dystonia in the jittery mouse. Nat Genet 35:264–269

Brknac Z, Fernandez M, Matsushita M et al (2002) Autosomal dominant sensory motor neuropathy with ataxia (SMNA): linkage to chromosome...???? Am J Med Genet 114:450–457

Burke JR, Wingfield MS, Lewis KE et al (1994) The Haw River syndrome: dentatorubropallisoluysian atrophy in an African American family. Nat Genet 7:521–524

Carvalho DR, Rocque-Ferreira AL, Rizzo IM et al (2008) Homozygosity enhances severity in Spinocerebellar ataxia type 3. Pediatr Neurol 38:296–299

Catsman-Berrevoets CE, Aarsen FK, van Hemsbergen MLC et al (2009) Improvement of neurological status and quality of life in children with opsoclonus myoclonus syndrome at long term follow-up. Pediatr Blood Cancer 53:1048–1053

Chance PF, Cavalier L, Satran D et al (1999) Clinical, nosologic and genetic aspects of Joubert and related syndromes. J Child Neurol 14:660–666

Chen YZ, Benett CL, Huynh HM et al (2004) DNA/RNA helicase gene mutations in a form of juvenile amyotrophic lateral sclerosis (ALS4). Am J Hum Genet 74:1128–1135

Chung MY, Lu YC, Cheng NC, Soong BW (2003) A novel autosomal dominant spinocerebellar ataxia (SCA 22) linked to chromosome 1p21-q23. Brain 126:1293–1299

Connolly AM, Dodson WE, Prensky AL, Rust RS (1994) Course and outcome of acute ataxia. Ann Neurol 35:673–679

Cossee M, Durr A, Schmitt M et al (1999) Frataxin point mutations and clinical presentation of compound heterozygous Friedreich ataxia patients. Ann Neurol 45:200–206

Date H, Onodera O, Tanaka H et al (2001) Early-onset ataxia with oculomotor apraxi and hypoalbuminemia is caused by mutations in a new HIT superfamily gene. Nat Genet 29:184–188

De Bruecker Y, Claus F, Demaerel P et al (2004) MRI findings in acute cerebellitis. Eur J Radiol 14:1478–1483

Della Nave R, Ginestroni A, Gianelli M et al (2008) Brains structural damage in Friedreich's ataxia. J Neurol Neurosurg Psychiatry 79:82–85

Demos MK, Macri V, Farrell K et al (2009) A novel KCNA1 mutation associated with global delay and persistent cerebellar dysfunction. Mov Disord 24:778–782

DiMauro S, Schon EA (2008) Mitochondrial disorders in the nervous system. Annu Rev Neurosci 31:91–123

Dudding TE, Friend K, Schofield PW et al (2004) Autosomal dominant congenital non-progressive ataxia overlaps with the SCA 15 locus. Neurology 63:2288–2292

Esscher E, Flodmark O, Hagberg G, Hagberg B (1996) Non-progressive ataxia: origins, brain pathology and impeirments in 78 Swedish children. Dev Med Child Neurol 38:285–296

Flanigan K, Gardner K, Alderson K et al (1996) Autosomal dominant spinocerebellar ataxia with sensory axonal neuropathy (SCA 4): clinical features? And genetic localization to chromosome 16q22.1. Am J Hum Genet 59:392–399

Fogel BL, Perlman S (2007) Clinical features and molecular genetics of autosomal recessive cerebellar ataxias. Lancet Neurol 6:245–257

Fogli A, Boespflug-Tunguy O (2006) The large spectrum of eIF2B-related diseases. Biochem Soc Trans 34:22–29

Garcia-Cazorla A, Wolf NI, Serrano M et al (2009) Inborn errors of metabolism and motor disturbances in children. J Inherit Metab Dis 32:618–629

Gordon N (2009) Cerebral folate deficiency. Dev Med Child Neurol 51:180–182

Hamberg P, De Jong FA, Brandsma D et al (2008) Irinotecan-induced central nervous system toxicity. Report on two cases and review of the literature. Acta Oncol 47:974–978

Harding AE (1981) Friedreich Ataxia: a clinical and genetic strudy of 90 families with an analysis of early diagnostic criteria and intrafamilial clustering of clinical features. Brain 104:589–620

Hebert M (2008) Targeting the gene in Friedreich ataxia. Biochimie 90:1131–1139

Houlden H, Johnson J, Garner-Thorpe C et al (2007) Mutations in TTBK2, encoding a kinase implicated in tau phosphorylation, segregates with Spinocerebellar ataxia type 11. Nat Genet 39:1434–1436

Ikeda Y, Dick KA, Weatherspoon MR et al (2006) Spectrin mutations cause Spinocerebellar ataxia type 5. Nat Genet 38:184–190

Iwaki A, Kawano Y, Miura S et al (2008) Heterozygous deletion of ITPR1 but not SUMF 1 in Spinocerebellar ataxia type 16. J Med Genet 45:32–35

Jalanko A, Braulke T (2009) Neuronal ceroid lipofuscinoses. Biochim Biophys Acta 1793:697–709

Jen JC, Graves TD, Hess EJ et al (2007) Primary episodic ataxias: diagnosis, pathogenesis and treatment. Brain 130:2484–2493

Johansson J, Forsgren L, Sandgren O et al (1998) Expanded CAG repeats in Swedish Spinocerebellar ataxia type 7 (SCA 7) patients: effect of CAG repeat length on the clinical manifestations. Hum Mol Genet 7:171–176

Karen Z, Falik-Zaccai TC (2009) Cerebrotendinous xanthomatosis (CTX): a treatable lipid storage disease. Pediatr Endocrinol Rev 7:6–11

Karthikeyan G, Lewis LK, Resnick MA (2002) The mitochondrial protein frataxin prevents nuclear damage. Hum Mol Genet 11: 1351–1362

Karthikeyan G, Santos JH, Graziewicz MA et al (2003) Reduction in frataxin causes progressive accumulation of mitochondrial damage. Hum Mol Genet 12:3331–3342

Knight MA, Garner RJM, Bahlo M et al (2004) Dominantly inherited ataxia and dysphonia with dentate calcification: Spinocerebellar ataxia type 20. Brain 127:1172–1181

Krasnewich D, O'Brien K, Sparks S (2007) Clinical features in adults with congenital disorders of glycosylation type I a (CDG-I a). Am J Med Genet 145C:302–306

Labauge P, Horzinski L, Ayrignac X et al (2009) Natural history of adult-onset eIF2B-related disorders: a multicenteric survey of 16 cases. Brain 132:2161–2169

Le Ber I, Moreira MC, Rivaud-Picoux S et al (2003) Cerebellar ataxia with oculomotor apraxia type 1: clinical and genetic studies. Brain 126:2761–2672

Lodi R, Taylor DJ, Shapira AH (2001) Mitochondrial dysfunction in Friedreich's ataxia. Biol Signals Recept 10:263–270

Louie CM, Gleeson JG (2005) Genetic basis of Joubert syndrome and related disorders of cerebellar development. Hum Mol Genet 14: R235–R242

Manto M, Marmolino D (2009) Cerebellar ataxias. Curr Opin Neurol 22:419–429

Mariotti C, Gellera C, Rimoldi R et al (2004) Ataxia with isolated vitamin E deficiency: neurological phenotype, clinical follow-up and novel mutations in TTPA gene in Italian families. Neurol Sci 25:130–137

Mariotti C, Brusco A, Di Bella D et al (2008) Spinocerebellar ataxia type 28: a novel autosomal dominant cerebellar ataxia characterized by slow progression and ophthalmoparesis. Cerebellum 7:184–188

Mascalchi M, Salvi F, Piacentini S, Bartolozzi C (1994) Friedreich 's ataxia: MR findings involving the cervical portion of the spinal cord. Am J Roentgenol 163:187–191

Matthay KK, Blaes F, Hero B et al (2005) Opsoclonus myoclonus syndrome in neuroblastoma: a report from a workshop on the dancing eyes syndrome at the advances in neuroblastoma meeting in Genoa, Italy, 2004. Cancer Lett 228:275–282

McNeill A, Pandolfo M, Kuhn J et al (2008) The neurological presentation of ceruloplasmin gene mutations. Eur Neurol 60:200–205

Meir T, Buise G (2009) Idebenone: an emerging therapy for Friedreich ataxia. J Neurol 256(S1):25–30

Moreira MC, Barbot C, Tachi N et al (2001) The gene mutated in ataxia-oculomotor apraxia 1 encodes the new HIT/Zn-finger protein aprataxin. Nat Genet 29:189–193

Moreira MC, Klur S, Watanabe M et al (2004) Senataxin, the ortholog of a yeast RNA helicase, is mutant in ataxia-ocular apraxia 2. Nat Genet 36:225–227

Moretti P, Blazo M, Garcia L et al (2004) Spinocerebellar ataxia type 2 (SCA 2) presenting with ophthalmoplegia and developmental delay in infancy. Am J Med Genet A 124:392–396

Nakamura K, Jeong S-Y, Uchihara T et al (2001) SCA17, a novel autosomal dominant cerebellar ataxia caused by an expanded polyglutamine in TATA-binding protein. Hum Mol Genet 10:1441–1448

Odaka M, Yuki N, Yamada M et al (2003) Bickerstaff's encephalitis: clinical features of 62 cases and a subgroup associated with Guillain-Barre syndrome. Brain 126:2279–2290

Pandolfo M (1999) Friedreich's ataxia: clinical aspects and pathogenesis. Semin Neurol 19:311

Pandolfo M (2009) Friedreich Ataxia: the clinical picture. J Neurol 256(S 1):3–8

Pandolfo M, Pastore A (2009) The pathogenesis of Friedreich Ataxia and the structure and function of frataxin. J Neurol 256(S1):9–17

Puccio H, Koenig M (2000) Recent advances in the molecular pathogenesis of Friedreich's ataxia. Hum Mol Genet 9:887–892

Riess O, Rüb U, Pastore A et al (2008) SCA3: neurological features, pathogenesis and animal models. Cerebellum 7:125–137

Rolfs A, Koeppen AH, Bauer I et al (2003) Clinical features and neuropathology of autosomal dominant spinocerebellar ataxia (SCA17). Ann Neurol 54:367–375

Sato N, Amino T, Kobayashi K et al (2009) Spinocerebellar ataxia type 31 is associated with "inserted" penta-nucleotide repeats containing (TGGAA)n. American J Human Genet 85:544–557

Sawaishi Y, Takada G (2002) Acute cerebellitis. Cerebellum 1:223–228

Schelhaas HJ, Ippel PF, Hageman G, Sinke RJ, van der Laan EN, Beemer FA (2001) Clinical and genetic analysis of a four-generation family with a distinct autosomal dominant cerebellar ataxia. J Neurol 248:113–120

Schols L, Bauer P, Schmidt T et al (2004) Autosomal dominant cerebellar ataxias: clinical features, genetics, and pathogenesis. Lancet Neurol 3:291–304

Schulte C, Synofzik M, Gasser T, Schols L (2009) Ataxia with ophthalmoplegia or sensory neuropathy is frequently caused by POLG mutations. Neurology 73:898–900

Schulz JB, DiProspero NA, Fischbeck K (2009) Clinical experience with idebenone in Friedreich ataxia. J Neurol 256(Suppl 1):42–45

Sevin M, Lesca G, Baumann N et al (2007) The adult form of Niemann-Pick disease type C. Brain 130:120–133

Silva MC, Coutinho P, Pinheiro CD, Neves JM (1997) Serrano P Hereditary ataxias and spastic paraplegias: methodological aspects of a prevalence study in Portugal. J Clin Epidemiol 50:1377–1384

Sirven JI, Fife TD, Wingerchuck DM, Drazkowski JF (2007) Second-generation antiepileptic drugs' impact on balance: a meta-analysis. Mayo Clin Proc 82:40–47

Soong BW, Paulson HL (2007) Spinocerebellar ataxias: an update. Curr Opin Neurol 20:438–446

Stevanin G, Hahn V, Lohmann E et al (2004a) Mutation in the catalytic domain of protein kinase C γ and extension of the phenotype associated with Spinocerebellar ataxia type 14. Arch Neurol 61:1242–1248

Stevanin G, Bouslam N, Thobois S et al (2004b) Spinocerebellar ataxia with sensory neuropathy (SCA25) maps to chromosome 2p. Ann Neurol 55:97–104

Storey E, Bahlo M, Fahey M et al (2009) A new dominantly inherited pure cerebellar ataxia, SCA 30. J Neurol Neurosurg Psychiatry 80:408–411

Swift M, Heim RA, Lench NJ (1993) Genetic aspects of Ataxia Telangiectasia. In: Harding AE, Deufel T (eds) Advances in neurology, vol 61. Raven, New York, pp 115–125

Takiyama Y (2007) Sacsinopathies: sacsin-related ataxia. Cerebellum 28:1–7

Tazir M, Nouioua S, Magy L et al (2009) Phenotypic variability in giant axonal neuropathy. Neuromuscul Disord 19:270–274

Van de Leemput J, Chandran J, Knight MA et al (2007) Deletions at ITPT 1 underlies ataxia in mice and Spinocerebellar ataxia 15 in humans. PLoS Genet 3:1076–1082

Van Lierde A, Righini A, Tremolati E (2004) Acute cerebellitis with tonsillar herniation and hydrocephalus in Epstein-Barr virus infection. Eur J Pediatr 163:689–691

Van Swieten MC, Brusse E, de Graaf BM et al (2003) A mutation in the fibroblast growth factor 14 gene is associated with autosomal dominant cerebellar ataxia. Am J Hum Genet 72:191–199

Verbeek DS (2009) Spinocerebellar ataxia type 23: a genetic update. Cerebellum 8:104–107

Verbeek DS, Schelhaas JH, Ippel EF, Beemer FA, Pearson PL, Sinke RJ (2002) Identification of a novel SCA locus (SCA19) in a Dutch autosomal dominant cerebellar ataxia family on chromosome region 1p21-q21. Hum Genet 111:388–393

Vuillame I, Devos D, Schraen-Maschke S et al (2002) A new locus for Spinocerebellar ataxia (SCA 21) maps to chromosome 7p 21.3-p15.1. Ann Neurol 52:666–670

Waldvogel D, van Gelderen P, Hallet M (1999) Increased iron in the dentate nucleus of patients with Friedreich's ataxia. Ann Neurol 46:123–125

Waters MF, Pulst S (2008) SCA 13. Cerebellum 7(2):165–169

Wong A (2007) An update on opsoclonus. Curr Opin Neurol 20:25–31

Yu GY, Howell MJ, Roller MJ, Xie TD, Gomez CM (2005) Spinocerebellar ataxia type 26 maps to chromosome 19p13.3 adjacent to SCA6. Ann Neurol 57:349–354

Zacarra G, Gangemi PF, Cincotta M (2008) Central nervous system adverse effects of new antiepileptic drugs. A meta-analysis of placebo-controlled studies. Seizure 17:405–421

Zortea M, Armani M, Pastorello E, Lombardi S, Tonello S, Rigoni MT, Zuliani L, Mostacciuolo ML, Gellera C, Di Donato S, Trevisan CP (2004) Prevalence of inherited ataxias in the Province of Padua, Italy. Neuroepidemiology 23:275–280

368 Approach to Diagnosis and Treatment of a Child with Motor Unit Diseases

Mustafa A. M. Salih

Definition/Classification

The anatomical route of the lower motor neuron, which composes the motor unit, has four subunits. These subunits consist of a motor neuron in the brainstem or ventral horn of the spinal cord and its axon, which together with other axons form the peripheral nerve; the neuromuscular junction; and the group of muscle fibers innervated by a single motor neuron. Disorders affecting these motor subunits can be further subdivided into hereditary syndromes and acquired diseases, and into acute and chronic disorders.

Epidemiology

Diseases of the motor unit affect all races and are common in children. A world survey of the commoner neuromuscular diseases estimated an overall prevalence of 286 per million populations. Nevertheless, the prevalence of some disorders in particular countries, such as congenital muscular dystrophy in Finland and Japan, spinal muscular atrophy and severe childhood autosomal recessive muscular dystrophy (SCARMD, limb-girdle muscular dystrophy [LGMD]) in Middle East and North African populations, reflects inbreeding in these communities, which increases the relative incidence of recessive disorders.

Diagnostic Approach

The recent advances in molecular biology has dramatically changed the diagnostic approach to neuromuscular disorders (NMDs), paved the way for accurate genetic counseling and for potential treatment by gene or cell therapy. Yet, a careful history and physical examination remain the cornerstones that guide the molecular and other investigative tools available to the clinician.

Symptoms

In childhood, common presenting symptoms of NMDs include floppiness or hypotonia, delayed motor milestones, abnormal gait, tendency to fall, as well as muscle weakness, cramps, or stiffness. It is also important to ascertain in the history whether certain activities that the child had difficulty with remained static or deteriorated. These activities include running, climbing stairs, and getting up from the floor. Questions pertaining to increase in muscle weakness as the day progresses, fatigue on effort and improvement on rest (suggesting myasthenia), and increased disability with inactivity and improvement with activity (suggesting myotonia) are also important. History of recurrent episodes of muscle weakness points toward periodic paralysis (in channel disorders), myasthenia gravis, dermatomyositis or polymyositis, and rhabdomyolysis or relapsing polyneuropathy. The occurrence of muscle cramps with exertion and their relief by rest may be the manifestation of some of the slowly progressive forms of muscular dystrophy (MD) such as Becker MD. They also occur in metabolic disorders of muscle (glycogenosis types V and VII and lipid metabolic disorders due to carnitine palmitoyl transferase deficiency, as well as other syndromes associated with myoglobinuria). Any observed muscle enlargement (hypertrophy) or wasting should also be ascertained. Difficulty with chewing or swallowing and associated respiratory deficit or disturbed sleep (indicating sleep apnea) are also vital components of enquiry.

Detailed family history of a similar condition is essential in each case and a pedigree chart will point toward an X-linked disease when the male relatives on the maternal

Abdelaziz Y. Elzouki (ed.), *Textbook of Clinical Pediatrics*, DOI 10.1007/978-3-642-02202-9_368,

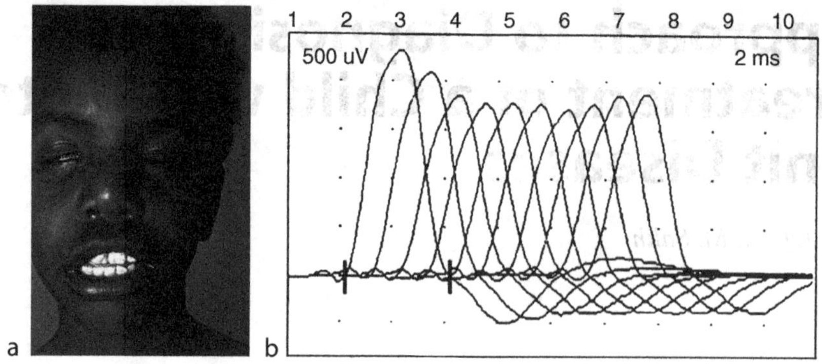

Figure 368.1
(a) Bilateral lower motor neuron facial weakness in a 12-year-old boy with fascioscapulohumeral muscular dystrophy. The patient cannot bury the eyelashes when asked to close his eyes tightly. The mouth is open with trickling saliva.
(b) Repetitive electrical stimulation of a motor nerve showing myasthenic decremental response. There is a fall-off in the size of muscle action potential of greater than 10% between the first and fifth response

side are affected. Consanguineous parents having earlier normal generations and affected siblings of both sex may be carriers of autosomal recessive conditions.

Signs

A considerable proportion of the physical examination can be done while the child is still clothed sitting in one of parent's lap. Using an examination couch and undressing a child for formal assessment invites uncooperativeness and irritability. Uncomfortable procedures, like inspecting the tongue (for fibrillations) and palatal movement of a young child should be deferred to the end. An infant can be given an object of interest to handle, like small cubes or one of the parent's keys. This activity will assess the baby's ocular motility and the pincer grasp. It will also assess coordination and ability to raise the arms against gravity. Facial expression should be noted, especially the presence of an open, drooping, or triangular mouth. Ability to raise the eyebrows on looking up speaks against lower motor neuron facial weakness. The older child can be asked to shut the eyes tightly. In the presence of facial weakness, he or she will not be able to bury the eyelashes completely (see *Fig. 368.1a*). The lower face can be assessed by asking the child to pout, blow (or whistle), smile, show the teeth, and puff out the cheeks.

Examination of the upper and lower limbs should take note of muscle bulk, tone and power, whether weakness is proximal or distal, symmetric (involving both sides of the body) or asymmetric. The Medical Research Council (MRC) scale for evaluation of muscle (*Table 368.1*) is a useful and practical guide for comparing muscle groups (proximal vs. distal) initially and during follow-up examinations.

Table 368.1
Medical research council grading scale for evaluation of muscle power

Grade	Muscle response
0	No contraction
1	Flicker of contraction
2	Active movement, with gravity eliminated
3	Active movement against gravity
4	Active movement against gravity and resistance
5	Normal power

Deep tendon reflexes are generally lost in neuropathies and in motor neuron diseases (including spinal muscular atrophy) and are diminished, but preserved, in myopathies and dystrophies. In Duchenne MD, the ankle jerks are often retained and may even be brisk until late in the disease.

Joint abnormalities should also be assessed. These can manifest as laxity of ligaments or limitation of joint movement as a result of permanent shortening (contractures). They usually take the form of flexion contractures of the hips, knees, and other joints in the non-ambulant child. In inherited peripheral neuropathies, pes cavus is the usual joint abnormality to be seen when the child is still walking. With loss of ambulation, scoliosis usually develops in various neuromuscular disorders, but can be prevented by adequate seating and other supportive measures.

Assessment of gait can start from the time an ambulant child comes into the consulting room. Toe-walking can be a transitory phenomenon in normal children but is a common feature in various neuromuscular disorders, spastic diplegic type of cerebral palsy, and hereditary spastic paraplegias. Walking on heels and heel-to-toe walking along a straight line are also useful in assessment. Ability to sit up from the supine position, get up from the floor, or from a chair are important details to elicit for examining the degree of hip girdle muscle weakness.

Following assessment of a child, it should be easy to determine whether the history and physical signs are indicative of a specific neuromuscular disorder or one outside the neuromuscular system.

Investigations

Three modalities of investigations are still used for diagnosing neuromuscular disorders. These are serum enzymes, electrophysiological procedures, and muscle and sural nerve biopsies. With the advent of molecular genetic markers, DNA analysis has become a routine definitive diagnostic test in several neuromuscular disorders, surpassing electromyography (EMG) and muscle biopsy.

Serum Enzymes

Creatine kinase (CK), which is released by damaged or degenerating muscle fibers is separated into three isoenzymes: MM for skeletal muscle, MB for cardiac muscle, and BB for brain. Serum CK determination is a very useful screening test for a suspected neuromuscular disease. (See ➋ Chap. 374, "Hereditary and Acquired Myopathies")

Electrophysiological Investigations

Nerve Conduction Studies

Motor and sensory nerve conduction can be measured by a relatively simple technique using surface electrodes. The conduction velocity is dependent on the diameter and the degree of myelination of the axon. At birth, conduction is about half of the adult value and reaches the mature value by 3–5 years of age. In peripheral neuropathies, the pathology may be primarily in the axon (axonal neuropathy) or, if in the supporting Schwan cell, it leads to segmental demyelination (demyelinating neuropathy). The nerve conduction velocity (NCV) is markedly decreased in demyelinating neuropathies. In axonal neuropathy, the NCV may be normal or slightly decreased, whereas the compound muscle action potential (CMAP) will be significantly low. Determining whether the neuropathy is demyelinating or axonal is of great help in guiding the DNA tests for the various forms of Charcot–Marie–Tooth disease (CMT, hereditary motor and sensory neuropathy [HMSN]).

In dominantly inherited demyelinating CMT, it is also important to assess the NCV in both parents and siblings, to detect subclinical cases. Post-infectious polyneuritis (Guillaine–Barre syndrome and diphtheritic polyneuropathy) may manifest as a demyelinating neuropathy. Measurement of the sensory conduction velocity and sensory action potential are useful diagnostic tools in mixed and complex neuropathies, such as CMT and Friedreich's ataxia, and in hereditary sensory and autonomic neuropathies.

Repetitive electrical stimulation of a motor nerve supplying a muscle aids diagnosis of congenital myasthenic syndromes and myasthenia gravis. Fatiguability of the muscle can be demonstrated by the falloff in the size of the muscle action potential (myasthenic decremental response) (➋ *Fig. 368.1b*).

Electromyography (EMG)

This technique is capable of showing whether a particular muscle is normal or abnormal and whether the abnormality is myopathic or neuropathic. However, it is less useful in children than in adults because it requires insertion of a needle into the belly of a muscle, and because the amount of received information is directly proportional to the degree of cooperation. It has been largely replaced by more specific diagnostic tools, namely DNA analysis (such as in Duchenne MD and spinal muscular atrophy [SMA]) and muscle biopsy. Nevertheless, EMG is the diagnostic modality of choice in muscle diseases manifesting with myotonia, including myotonia congenita, myotonic dystrophy, and Schwartz–Jampell syndrome. It shows the pathognomonic spontaneous myotonic bursts of activity with gradual decrement. A typical sound of the "dive bomber" or "departing motor cycle" sound will be heard on acoustic amplification. It is usually present in dominantly inherited congenital myotonic dystrophy, but appears later after the age of 2–3 years. The minimally affected mother of a suspected baby will usually show these pathognomonic bursts.

Muscle Biopsy

If a specific diagnosis of hereditary disease is not provided by molecular genetic testing in blood, which is currently available in many centers, a muscle biopsy is essential for establishing a definitive diagnosis in any patient with a suspected neuromuscular disorder. When interpreted by an experienced pathologist, it distinguishes between neurogenic, myopathic, and dystrophic processes. It can also indicate the type of myopathy and specify the deficient protein or enzyme.

An open biopsy, done under local anesthesia is preferable to needle biopsy, since it allows obtaining adequate tissue for additional biochemical studies, such as respiratory chain enzymes for investigating mitochondrial diseases. The vastus lateralis (quadriceps femoris) is the muscle usually sampled. Conventional paraffin sections of the biopsied specimen are not adequate, since that technique does not allow the diagnosis of many congenital and metabolic myopthies. Histochemical studies of frozen sections are, hence, obligatory. Immunohistochemistry is now essential, because it demonstrates the expression of dystrophin protein in Duchenne MD and Becker MD, as well as a number of other dystrophin-associated proteins. Deficiency of the latter causes a variety of autosomal recessive dystrophies. A portion of the biopsy specimen should be fixed in gluteraldehyde for potential electron microscopy, for diagnosis of several congenital myopathies and mitochondrial myopathy.

Sural Nerve Biopsy

The sural nerve is the most commonly biopsied nerve in neuropathies. Electron microscopy of a sural nerve sample can accurately differentiate between axonal and demyelinating neuropathies, as well as assess the types of fibers in hereditary sensory and autonomic neuropathies. Teased fiber preparations are useful in showing segmental demyelination, but are not done routinely since they are labor intensive.

Imaging of the Motor Unit

Differential involvement of muscle occurs in several neuromuscular disorders and this can be assessed by either ultrasound, computed tomography (CT), or magnetic resonance imaging (MRI). Ultrasound, performed by an experienced operator, is a rapid and practical method to apply before sampling a muscle for biopsy. However, in advanced dystrophies a muscle biopsy might need MRI guidance. The latter technique is also useful in inflammatory myopathies of infectious (bacterial and parasitic), as well as immune (dermatomyositis) origin. Imaging of the spinal cord, nerve root, and plexus is best achieved using MRI.

Respiratory and Cardiac Investigations

Respiratory function tests should be done for children with diseases of the motor unit initially and on regular follow-up. In certain conditions with fluctuating weakness, like congenital myasthenic syndromes and myasthenia gravis, sleep studies need also to be arranged to explore the possibility of the occurrence of sleep apnea and hypoventilation. Electrocardiography (ECG) is also important in the clinical evaluation of muscular dystrophies and in inflammatory and metabolic myopathies to explore an associated subclinical conduction defect or cardiomyopathy. Regular follow-up with a pediatric cardiologist (on yearly or biennial basis) and serial assessment by electrocardiography are required in muscular dystrophies and certain congenital and metabolic myopathies.

Floppy Infant Syndrome

The complex of floppiness/hypotonia is a common neurologic symptom in infancy; and the floppy infant syndrome refers to an infant with generalized hypotonia presenting at birth or in early life. The diagnostic work up is often challenging, if a systematic evaluation of infants with hypotonia is not followed. Hypotonia usually manifests as unusual postures, such as lying in frog-leg position when supine (➔ *Fig. 368.2a*). Hypotonia becomes more apparent by positioning the infant in certain ways. On ventral suspension, a floppy infant will lose the ability to maintain the head in line with body. The limbs will be dangling (➔ *Fig. 368.2b*). On pulling to the sitting position by traction on hands, prominent head lag occurs (➔ *Fig. 368.2c*). After the neonatal period, floppy infants usually present with delay in motor milestones.

A Practical Approach to Diagnosis

It has been a standard practice to decide first, whether the hypotonia is a manifestation of a motor unit disease or if it

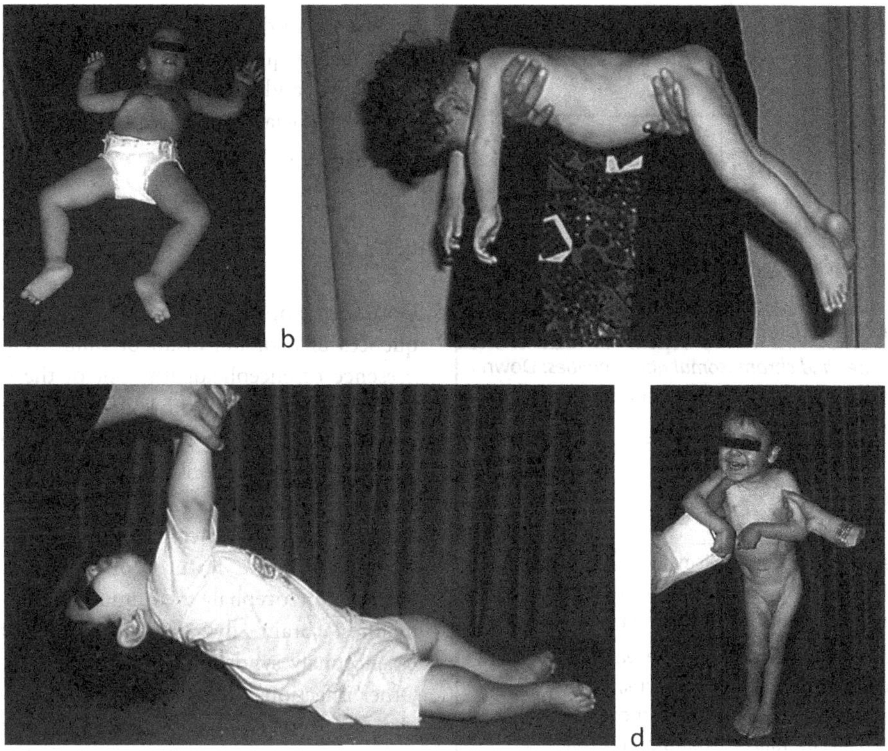

Figure 368.2
(a) A floppy infant with frog-like position when supine. (b) On ventral suspension, the limbs are dangling. (c) Prominent head lag on pulling to the sitting position. (d) Central nervous system (CNS) disorder causing floppy infant syndrome. When assessing the ability to support weight, there is scissoring of legs, flexion of elbows and clenching of the hands

is due to a disorder of the central nervous system (CNS), or another system in the body. Significant degree of weakness is usually associated with motor unit diseases. On the other hand, hypotonia without weakness includes disorders of CNS, and metabolic, nutritional, and endocrine disorders. Assessing weakness can be achieved even in very young infants by observing the spontaneous movements of the face and limbs, response to stroking the soles, and the ability to sustain passively elevated arms or legs. Other features that point to hypotonia being caused by disorders of CNS include the easily elicited (or brisk) deep tendon jerks, whereas in a disease of the lower motor unit, reflexes are typically diminished or absent. With increasing age, hypotonia is gradually replaced by hypertonia in disorders of CNS and there is persistence of neonatal reflexes such as the grasp, Moro, and tonic-neck reflex. When assessing the ability to support weight of such older infants, the legs will be kept crossed (scissoring) and there is plantar flexion of the feet. The elbows are usually flexed, hands are clenched, and the thumb is kept across the palm (fisting position) (➋ *Fig. 368.2d*).

Disorders of the CNS (Cortical, Subcortical, and Cerebellar)

Congenital or acquired disorders of the CNS account for the majority of the causes of floppy infant syndrome (➋ *Table 368.2*).

Clinical Manifestations

History: Pregnancy, Birth, and Perinatal

Important features to ascertain when considering hypotonia due to disorders of CNS include age of the mother at time of birth. Advanced age increases the chance of chromosomal disorders. Other features include history of fever, infections or teratogens especially during early pregnancy, polyhydramnios or oligohydramnios, recurrent abortions or stillbirth, and if any abnormalities were detected on screening ultrasound.

Table 368.2
Disorders of the central nervous system (CNS) manifesting as floppy infant syndrome

Static encephalopathy
Cerebral dysgenesis/dysplasia: Lissencephaly, holoprosencephaly, Joubert syndrome, pontocerebellar hypoplasia
Perinatal hypoxic/ischemic insult, kernicterus and intracranial hemorrhage
Congenital infections: TORCH
Genetic syndromes and chromosomal abnormalities: Down syndrome (Trisomy 18, Prader-Willi syndrome, Cri-du-chat [5p-] syndrome).
Metabolic disorders:
Disorders of carbohydrate metabolism: galactosemia, hereditary fructose intolerance
Disorders of amino acid metabolism: Phenylketonuria, tyrosinosis type 1, sulphite oxidase deficiency, nonketotic hyperglycinemia, argininosuccinic aciduria
Organic acidemias: Maple syrup urine disease (MSUD), methylmalonic academia, glutaric aciduria, propionic academia, malonic aciduria, multiple carboxylase deficiencies (defects in utilization of biotin).
Mitochondrial disorders: Respiratory chain and Kreb cycle disorders, Leigh's syndrome, pyruavete carboxylase deficiency, pyruvate dehydrogenase complex deficiency.
Lysosomal storage disease: Mucopolysaccharidosis, lipidosis (Gauher type 2, Nieman-pick type A, Tay-Sachs disease), mucolipidosis (sialidosis type II, I-cell disease).
Perioxosomal disorders: Zellweger syndrome, rhizomelic chondrodysplasia punctata.

The duration of pregnancy and the birthweight are also vital. Preterm delivery increases the risk of perinatal hypoxic-ischemic insult and intraventricular hemorrhage. The mode of delivery, whether assisted by ventose or through a cesarean section following difficult birth and the Apgar score 5 min after birth is important. If this is not available, asking whether the baby breathed spontaneously and cried immediately after birth gives a reasonable idea, provided the mother has not been under the effect of anesthesia for cesarean section. Difficulties in sucking and swallowing during the first 24 h after birth may reflect the severity of the hypoxic-ischemic insult. Whether the baby needed to be shifted to the neonatal intensive care unit (NICU), required mechanical ventilation or had seizures, and the duration of stay in the NICU are also salient points.

History of delayed motor, speech, or cognitive development following the neonatal period points toward genetic disorders or cerebral dysgenesis. Loss of previously acquired milestones usually heralds neurodegenerative and metabolic disorders. Seizure disorders may be associated with cerebral dysgenesis or chromosomal disorders.

Signs

Obtunded appearance of the baby may reflect consequences of neonatal insult or brain dysgenesis, and the presence of encephalopathy out of the context of birth history points toward an underlying metabolic disorder. Dysmorphic features give important clues to identifying genetic disorders. Skin examination may reveal neurocutaneous signs. Anthropometry (weight, height, and head circumference) should be routine. Obesity and short stature are features of Prader–Willi syndrome, whereas microcephaly is common in chromosome abnormalities, brain dysgenesis (e.g., microcephaly and lissencephaly syndromes), and TORCH (Toxoplasmosis, Other infections, Rubella, Cytomegalovirus, Herpes simplex virus) infections (except for congenital toxoplasmosis, which can present with hydrocephalus).

Ophthalmologic examination may reveal important diagnostic signs. Oculomotor apraxia is a feature of Joubert syndrome, ataxia telangiectasia, and ataxia-oculomotor apraxia syndromes. A cherry red spot indicates an underlying lipidosis. Retinitis pigmentosa may indicate other storage diseases, such as neuronal ceroid lipofuscinosis. Ptosis and ophthalmoplegia (or ophthalmoparesis) are found in congenital myasthenia, congenital myasthenic syndromes, and some mitochondrial disorders.

Examination of the chest, cardiovascular system, and abdomen may reveal an underlying multisystem involvement. In particular, the presence of hepatosplenomegaly may be associated with TORCH infections, glycogen storage disease, and lipidosis (e.g., Nieman–Pick disease types A and C) (Fig. 368.3a).

Spinal Cord Lesions

These lesions can follow damage to the spinal cord during delivery, the presence of a congenital tumor, or dysraphic states (tethered cord and myelomeningocele). Traumatic lesions involve either the lower cervical and upper thoracic cord with breach delivery, or the upper cervical region with cephalic presentation. Mid-forceps

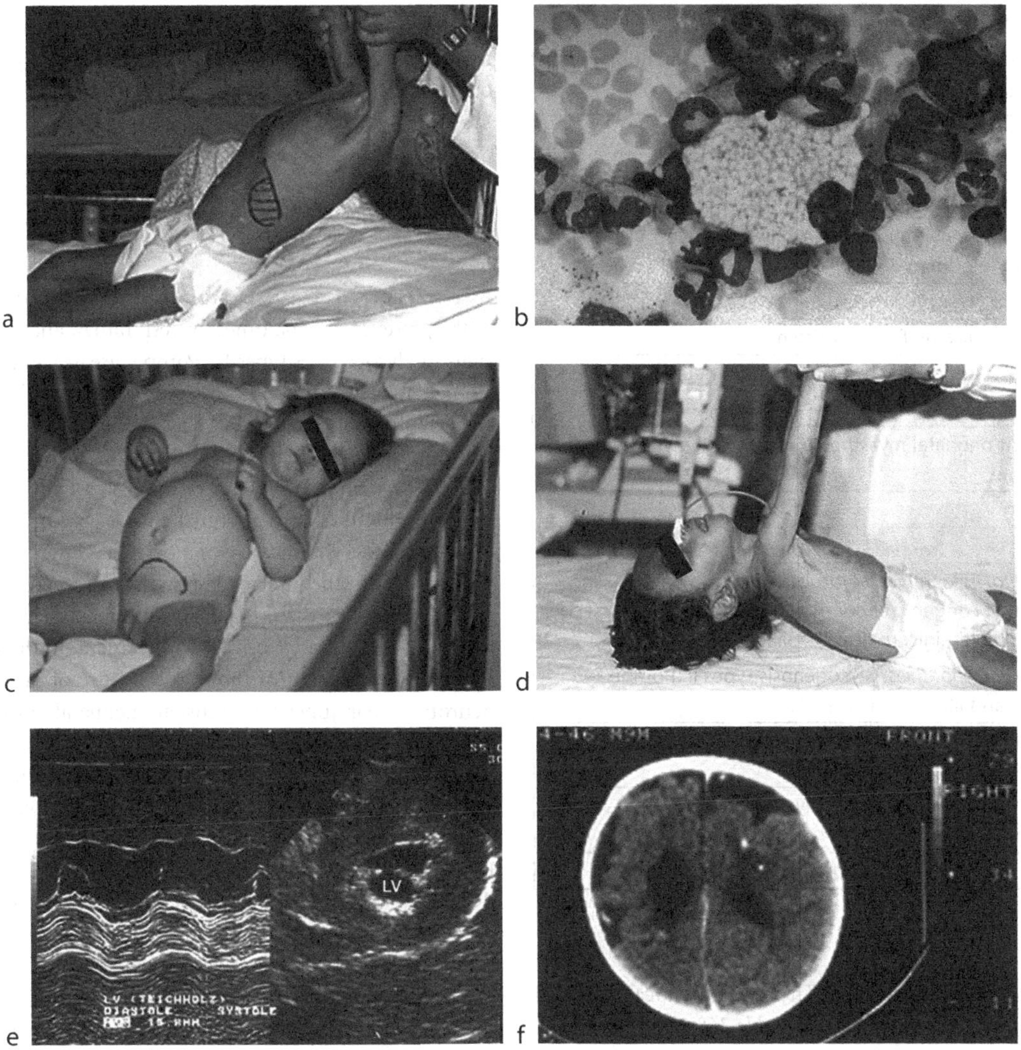

Figure 368.3
(a) Floppy infant syndrome due to Niemann-Pick disease. The enlarged liver and spleen are marked. (b) Bone marrow showed the characteristic foam cell (arrow). (c) Bladder distension associated with hypotonia due to spinal cord injury. (d) An infant with Pompe disease (glycogenosis type II). (e) Echocardiography showed hypertrophic cardiomyopathy and small left ventricle (LV). (f) Cranial computed tomography (CT) scan showing periventricular calcification and brain malformation in congenital cytomegalovirus infection (Figs. 3d and e are courtesy of Dr. Elsayed Ali)

extractions with excessive longitudinal traction or rotation are known risk factors.

The clinical picture is characterized by hypotonia, which may persist or evolve into spasticity, associated with paraplegia or tetraplegia, respiratory insufficiency or paradoxical breathing in some cases, bladder distension, impaired bowel control, pyramidal tract signs, and sensory level (➋ *Fig. 368.3c*). The lower roots of the brachial plexus may be affected and manifest with paralysis of the intrinsic hand muscles. Congenital spinal cord tumors present with similar localizing signs.

Diseases of the Motor Unit

Disorders of the motor unit account for 18–47% of the causes of the floppy infant syndrome. In these conditions, the infant has a significant degree of weakness in

Table 368.3
Diseases of the motor unit associated with the floppy infant syndrome

Anterior horn cell
Acquired: Poliomyelitis, other viral syndromes (e.g., Coxsackie A)
Hereditary: Spinal muscular atrophy (SMA) type 1 (Werdnig–Hoffman disease and SMA type 2).
Peripheral nerve
Acquired: Guillaine-Barre syndrome
Hereditary: Congenital hypomyelination neuropathy
Neuromuscular junction
Transient neonatal myasthenia, congenital myasthenic syndrome
Botulism
Muscle
Congenital myopathies: Myotubular myopathy, nemaline myopathy, congenital fiber type disproportion, central core disease, multiminicore disease, Salih myopathy
Metabolic myopathies: Glycogenosis types II (Pompe disease) and III.
Mitochondrial myopathies, lipid storage myopathies, periodic paralysis
Congenital myotonic dystrophy, neonatal Schwartz-Jampel syndrome
Congenital muscular dystrophies

association with hypotonia. The anatomic localization of these disorders is detailed in *Table 368.3*.

Clinical Manifestations

History: Pregnancy, Birth, and Perinatal

It is always pertinent to ask whether the mother has been diagnosed to have a neuromuscular disease such as myotonic dystrophy or myasthenia gravis. History of polyhydramnios is a common feature in congenital myotonic dystrophy. Diminished fetal movements may be noticed by the mother in congenital myotonic dystrophy and spinal muscular atrophy (SMA) type 1 (Werdnig–Hoffman disease). On ultrasound screening, brain abnormalities are detectable in Walker–Warburg phenotype of congenital muscular dystrophy (CMD). Arthrogryposis multiplex can also be noted. Breech presentation is common in neuromuscular births. Poor respiratory effort and difficulties in sucking and swallowing may also be a feature, as in congenital myotonic dystrophy, myotubular myopathy, nemaline myopathy, neonatal myasthenia, congenital myasthenic syndrome, and the Walker–Warburg type of CMD.

Signs

Assessment for associated features should also be done, such as the presence of hepatomegaly, respiratory, and/or cardiac signs in glycogenoses types II (Pompe disease) and III, lipid storage myopathies, and mitochondrial myopathies.

The distribution and degree of weakness may help to distinguish between the various causes of hypotonia of neuromuscular origin. Loss of antigravity movement of the limbs points toward proximal muscle weakness, whereas distal weakness is indicative of a peripheral nerve disorder. In SMA type 1, the intercostal muscles are severely affected and breathing is diaphragmatic. Tongue fasciculation is a helpful sign. Occular muscle involvement, in the form of ophthalmoplegia and/or ptosis is a feature of disorders of neuromuscular junction (transient neonatal myasthenia, congenital myasthenic syndrome, and botulism), mitochondrial myopathy, some congenital myopathies (e.g., myotubular myopathy), and myotonic dystrophy. Asymmetric ptosis is found in some cases of Salih myopathy. Facial muscle involvement is common in CMD, myotonic dystrophy, and congenital myopathies, but it is not present in SMA. Pursed-mouth appearance during crying is a feature of neonatal Schwartz–Jampel syndrome. Asymmetric association of the sixth and/or seventh cranial nerves is seen in acquired causes of floppy infant syndrome, namely poliomyelitis and diphtheritic polyneuropathy. Facial nerve involvement is symmetric in Guillaine–Barre syndrome. Deep tendon jerks are usually diminished in neuromuscular disorders but absent in SMA.

Contractures and arthrogryposis are common in congenital myotonic dystrophy and CMD. Nevertheless, Ullrich type of CMD is characterized by a peculiar combination of proximal contractures and distal laxity with congenital hip dislocation. Neonatal Schwartz–Jampel syndrome features pectus excavatum, camptodactyly, bowed lower limbs, and talipes.

Systemic Disorders

Apart from disorders of CNS and diseases of the motor unit, certain systemic disorders can present as floppy infant syndrome, as detailed in *Table 368.4*.

Table 368.4
Systemic disorders that may manifest floppy infant syndrome

Endocrine disorders
Hypothyroidism, hyperparathyroidism
Nutritional disorders
Primary: Severe childhood undernutrition (protein-energy malnutrition), rickets
Secondary: Malabsorption syndromes (celiac disease and cystic fibrosis), AIDS, cardiac disease, renal disease, pulmonary disease (tuberculosis)
Electrolyte disorders: Renal tubular acidosis, marble bone-marble brain disease (type III osteopetrosis)
Connective tissue disorders: Congenital laxity of ligaments, osteogenesis imperfecta, Ehlers–Danlos syndrome, Marfan syndrome, arachnodactyly.

Investigations

These investigations should be guided by the clinical presentation, symptoms, and the elicited physical signs. During the neonatal period, especially when there are features of encephalopathy or recurrent vomiting, investigations for inborn errors of metabolism should receive priority. Most inborn errors of metabolism, when presenting in the neonatal period, are lethal if specific treatment is not initiated immediately.

Measurement of serum concentrations of ammonia, bicarbonate, and pH should be done first. Many inborn errors of metabolism cause a metabolic acidosis due to excessive production of ketoacids, lactic acid, and/or other organic anions. Elevation of blood ammonia is usually caused by urea cycle defects. Such infants have normal serum pH and bicarbonate values. Determination of anion gap ($[Na^+] - [Cl] - [HCO_3]$) is the next pertinent step. High anion gap associated with serum ammonia is found in organic acidemias, whereas normal anion gap and normal serum ammonia are found in aminoacidopathies and galactosemia. Lactic acidosis unrelated to an enzymatic defect occurs in hypoxemia. When lactic acidosis results from an enzymatic defect in gluconeogenesis or pyruvate dehydrogenase complex, both lactate and pyruvate are increased and the ratio is normal. In hypoxemia and in mitochondrial diseases due to defects in the respiratory chain, the serum pyruvate concentration may remain normal with an increased lactate:pyruvate ratio. Elevation of lactic dehydrogenase (LDH), serum glutamate-oxaloacetate transaminase (SGOT), and serum glutamate-pyruvate transaminase (SGPT) indicates hepatic involvement in galactosemia, urea cycle defects, aminoacidurias, and organic acidurias. Other blood tests that should be done routinely include complete blood count (for neutropenia and thrombocytopenia seen in organic acidurias), glucose, urea, electrolytes (Na, K, and Cl), creatinine, blood gases, and thyroid function tests.

Biochemical neonatal screening is now available in many countries using tandem mass spectrometry (MS/MS); the diseases being screened emphasize differences in their incidence and prevalence among different populations. In addition to the tandem mass spectrometry, blood spots obtained from a newborn on Guthrie card can also be used to screen for hypothyroidism, biotinidase deficiency, congenital adrenal hyperplasia, and galactosemia, using high throughput fluorometric assays. In suspected cases of nonketotic hyperglycinemia, the diagnosis is highly significative by the demonstration of elevated plasma and cerebrospinal (CSF) glycine levels, with a high glycine CSF/plasma ratio, and confirmed by glycine cleavage enzyme assay on liver biopsy. In organic acidurias, findings in tandem mass spectrometry can be further confirmed by gas chromatography/mass spectrometry analysis of the urine organic acid profile.

In countries where a comprehensive neonatal screening program is not available, simple urine screening tests can be used. These tests include the ferric chloride test (phenylketonuria [PKU], tyrosinosis), the dinitrophenylhydrazine test (PKU, Maple syrup urine disease), the sodium cyanide-nitroprusside test (homocystinuria), Benedict's reagent or Clinitest tablets test (galactosemia), ketones (organic acidurias), and cetyltrimethylammonium bromide (mucopolysaccharidoses). These tests can be used as a basis for initiation of therapy when the clinical manifestations suggest the diagnosis. Nevertheless, they should never be considered definitive.

Special investigations when suspecting a disease of the motor unit include creatine kinase.

In Duchenne and Becker MDs, the level is grossly elevated (up to 50 times the normal limit) in the early stages, whereas in SCARMD and congenital muscular dystrophy, it is 5–10 times normal. Other forms of dystrophy such as Emery–Dreifuss MD may have a more modest elevation. In congenital myopathies with structural muscle abnormalities, it is likely to be normal or only slightly elevated. The levels are usually normal in neurogenic diseases, like the spinal muscular atrophies. Mild degrees of elevation are also seen in some carriers of Duchenne MD and in subclinical malignant hyperthermia.

CK is moderately elevated in congenital muscular dystrophy (CMD) but can range from normal to marked elevation, depending on the underlying degree of muscle degeneration. It is also likely to be normal or only slightly elevated in several congenital myopathies with structural abnormality, such as central core disease or nemaline myopathy. In Salih myopathy, serum CK is mildly elevated in the first 4 years of life (four times the upper normal limit) and increases slightly more by 10 years (5.5 times the upper normal limit). In SMA types 1 and 2 and other neurogenic syndromes serum CK is usually normal. The transminases (alanine aminotransferase, ALT and aspartate aminotransferase, AST) are also elevated in muscular dystrophy. Finding an associated elevation of CK will spare an unnecessary liver biopsy.

Chest X-ray is helpful in congenital myotonic dystrophy and may show diaphragmatic elevation due to hypoplasia of the diaphragm. It may also show thin ribs, which points to the antenatal origin of the condition. Cardiomegaly in Pompe's disease (type II glycogenosis) can also show on chest X-ray, as well as the radiologic features of rickets and osteopetrosis in the ribs and spine, respectively. Vertebral anomalies can also be seen in mucopolysaccharidosis, although bone survey is more suited for that.

Electrocardiography (ECG) is very useful in SMA since it shows the characteristic tremor (minipolymyoclonus) of the baseline, particularly in the limb leads, probably reflecting the fasciculation of skeletal muscle. In type II glycogenosis (Pompe's disease), ECG reveals features of hypertrophic cardiomyopathy, which is better assessed by echocardiography (➋ *Fig. 368.3d, e*).

Bone marrow aspiration and biopsy helps to show the characteristic cells in type 2 Gaucher disease and the Nieman–Pick disease (NPD) types A and C (➋ *Fig. 368.3b*).

Neuroimaging

Cystic encephalomalacia, intraventricular hemorrhage, porencephaly, and hydranencepahly can be detected by cranial ultrasound. Cranial computed tomography (CT) is helpful in detecting any neonatal intracranial hemorrhage or brain edema secondary to hypoxic-ischemic encephalopathy (HIE), some of the inborn errors of metabolism (e.g., glutaric aciduria type 1), and the presence of lissencephaly. It is also more sensitive than MRI in identifying intracranial calcification, which is seen with congenital TORCH infections, isolated sulphite oxidase deficiency, and marble brain disease with renal tubular acidosis (➋ *Fig. 368.3f*).

Later in infancy, it will show the periventricular leukomalacia and bilateral thalamic calcification of HIE and also of isolated sulphite oxidase deficiency. It may also show the basal ganglia cavitations that characterize biotin-responsive basal ganglia disease.

On the other hand, magnetic resonance imaging (MRI) is superior to CT in showing the features of HIE but it is difficult to use in the perinatal period. Nevertheless, MRI is the most sensitive modality to characterize the brain malformations associated with some forms of congenital muscular dystrophy (CMD). It also delineates the characteristic white matter alterations found in merosin-negative CMD, and basal ganglia and brainstem lesions in Leigh's disease.

Neurophysiology

Nerve conduction velocity (NCV) is a relatively simple technique requiring only surface electrodes, which can identify cases of peripheral neuropathy and characterize whether they are primarily axonal or demyelinating. On the other hand, electromyography (EMG), which requires needle insertion, is more invasive and frightening for babies. It does not detect myotonia in congenital myotonic dystrophy. However, myotonia can be confirmed in the asymptomatic mother on EMG. In a young child with a febrile illness and weakness, EMG is contraindicated in countries where oral poliovirus (OPV) vaccine is used. Intramuscular injection is a known risk factor for the development of vaccine-associated paralytic poliomyelitis. This also applies to places where vaccination coverage is still inadequate. It has long been noted that intramuscular injections administered during the incubation period of wild-type poliovirus causes what is known as "provocation" poliomyelitis. The author has seen a young child with extensive paralysis following an EMG, done at the start of weakness, within a few days after receiving OPV.

Decremental response following repetitive nerve stimulation (RNS) is diagnostic of congenital myasthenic syndrome (CMS) and can be positive when edrophonium test is negative. This test can be life saving in COLQ-mutant CMS where most patients are severely disabled from an early age with respiratory difficulties and no effect, or even worsening, after administration of acetyl choline esterase (AChE) inhibitors.

Muscle Biopsy

The muscle biopsy provides the definitive diagnosis in congenital myopathies and dystrophies, with the exception of congenital myotonic dystrophy when it may lead to misdiagnosis of other pathologies. In congenital myopathies, the specific structural defect can be revealed by histochemistry of muscle. Accumulation of glycogen is seen in type II glycogenosis (Pompe's disease) and accumulation of lipid in lipid storage myopathy. The characteristic ragged-red fibers may be seen in mitochondrial myopathy associated with absence of COX staining (complex IV of the mitochondrial respiratory chain). Electron microscopy, although time consuming and not widely available, has high diagnostic yield in the congenital myopathies. Dystrophic features are seen in muscular dystrophies, and immunohistochemistry can delineate the missing glycoprotein such as in merosin-deficient CMD.

References

Aicardi J (2009) Diseases of the nervous system in childhood. Mac Keith Press, London

Birdi K, Prasad AN, Prasad C, Chodirker B, Chudley AE (2005) The floppy infant: retrospective analysis of clinical experience (1990–2000) in a tertiary care facility. J Child Neurol 20:803–808

Dubowitz V (1980) The floppy infant. (Clinics in Developmental Medicine, No. 76.) Blackwell/Lippincott/Oxford, Philadelphia

Dubowitz V (1992) Lesson for the month: genetic counseling. Neuromusc Disord 2:85–86

Dubowitz V (1995) Muscle disorders of childhood. WB Saunders, London

El-Gazali LI, Varghese M, Varady E, Al-Talabani J, Scorer J, Bakalinova D (1996) Neonatal Schwartz-Jampel syndrome: a common autosomal recessive syndrome in the United Arab Emirates. J Med Genet 33:203–211

Laugel V, Cosse'e M, Matis J et al (2008) Diagnostic approach to neonatal hypotonia: retrospective study of 144 neonates. Eur J Pediatr 167:517–523

MacKinnon JA, Perlman M, Korpolani H et al (1993) Spinal cord injury at birth: diagnostic and prognostic data in twenty-two patients. J Pediatr 122:431–437

Menticoglan SM, Perlman M, Manning FA (1995) High cervical cord injury in neonates delivered with forceps: report of 15 cases. Obstet Gynecol 86:589–594

Naim-Ur-Rahman, Salih MAM, Jamjoom AH, Jamjoom ZA (1999) Congenital intramedullary lipoma of the dorsocervical spinal cord with intracranial extension: case report. Neurosurgery 34:1081–1084

Paine RS (1963) The future of the "floppy infant": a follow-up study of 133 patients. Dev Med Child Neurol 5:115–124

Salih MAM (2010) Muscular dystrophies and myopathies in Arab Populations. In: Teebi AS (ed) Genetic disorders among Arab Populations. Springer, New York, pp 145–180

Torres CF, Forbes GB, Decancq GH (1986) Muscle weakness in infants with rickets: distribution, course and recovery. Pediatr Neurol 2:95–98

Vasta I, Kinali M, Messina S et al (2005) Can clinical signs identify newborns with neuromuscular disorders? J Pediatr 146:73–79

Vialle R, Pie'tin-Vialle C, Ilharreborde B, Dauger S, Vinchon M, Gloriori C (2007) Spinal cord injuries at birth: a multicenter review of nine cases. J Matern Fetal Neonatal Med 20:435–440 misdiagnosis of other pathologies. In [illegible] myopathies, the specific structural [illegible] can be [illegible] of muscle. [illegible] [illegible] [illegible] myopathy [illegible] [illegible] microscopy [illegible] [illegible] and [illegible] [illegible]

Dubowitz V (1995) Muscle disorders of childhood. W.B. Saunders, London.

[illegible] (1998) [illegible] oral recessive [illegible] [illegible] 211

[illegible] [illegible] hypotonia [illegible] [illegible] [illegible]

[illegible] [illegible] two patients [illegible]

Montenegro [illegible] (1996) High cervical cord injury [illegible] report of 15 cases. Childs Nerv Syst [illegible]

[illegible] (1999) [illegible] of the [illegible] [illegible]

[illegible]

369 Cranial Nerve Disorders

Mustafa A. M. Salih

Congenital Cranial Dysinnervation Disorders

Congenital cranial dysinnervation disorders (CCDDs) are a group of neuromuscular diseases characterized by motor unit abnormalities involving ocular motility, eyelid, and/or facial muscles. These disorders result from developmental errors of cranial nerve (CN) innervations. The group includes Duane syndrome, congenital fibrosis of the extraocular muscles (CFEOM), congenital ptosis, horizontal gaze palsy with progressive scoliosis (HGPPS), Bosley–Salih–Alorainy syndrome (BSAS), congenital facial palsy (CFP), and Moebius syndrome.

Duane Syndrome

Duane syndrome is characterized by congenital limitation of horizontal eye globe movement and some globe retraction on attempted adduction of the eye. It constitutes the most common of the CCDs with prevalence of 1:10000 (1–4% of strabismus cases), and 10% of cases are familial. The condition results from reduction or absence of the abducent nerve (CN VI) motor neurons associated with aberrant innervations of the lateral rectus by the oculomotor nerve (CN III). In type 1 Duane syndrome (which constitutes about 80% of cases), abduction is affected with normal or minimally defective adduction, associated with narrowing of the palpebral fissure of the adducting eye. Both abduction and adduction are limited in type 3 Duane syndrome, whereas in type 2 Duane syndrome, adduction is limited.

Congenital Fibrosis of the Extraocular Muscles (CFEOM)

Various forms of CFEOM result from primary dysinnervation of oculomotor (CN III) and/or trochlear (CN IV) innervated extraocular muscles. Individuals with CFEOM1 have congenital nonprogressive bilateral external ophthalmoplegia, and congenital bilateral ptosis; inability to raise either eye above the horizontal midline and an infraducted primary position of each eye. The condition is inherited as autosomal dominant and, in most families, results from heterozygous mutations in *KIF21A* gene. Rare probands of CFEOM1 harbor mutations in the *FEOM3* gene.

Individuals with CFEOM2 are born with bilateral ptosis, with their eyes primarily fixed in an exotropic position and severely limited horizontal and vertical eye movements. The condition results from primary developmental defect of both oculomotor (CN III) and trochlear (CN IV) nuclei, and the only normally functioning extraocular muscle is the abducens (CN VI) innervated lateral rectus that pulls each eye outward. The condition is inherited as autosomal recessive and results from *PHOX2A* gene mutations. In CFEOM3, at least one affected family member does not meet CFEOM1 criteria. The condition results from a variable defect of the oculomotor (CN III) nucleus development. Inheritance is autosomal dominant with incomplete penetrance. Mutations of the *KIF21A* gene were detected in a minority of families with CFEOM3. Recently, and in 17 unrelated families and 12 unrelated individuals, CFEOM3 was found to be caused by heterozygous mutations in the *TUBB3* gene. These lead to a common defect in axonal guidance during development, which can result in additional neurologic involvements other than those manifesting in the ocular muscles.

Horizontal Gaze Palsy with Progressive Scoliosis (HGPPS)

Individuals affected with HGPPS are born with absent horizontal gaze movements and develop severe progressive scoliosis, starting in infancy or childhood (➋ *Fig. 369.1a*). Horizontal gaze palsy, which is nonprogressive, results from hypoplasia of the abucens (CN VI) nucleus with interneuron dysinnervation (medial longitudinal fasciculus and pontine paramedian reticular formation). Unlike other CCDDs, the abducens (CN VI) nerve is present bilaterally and the extraocular muscles are normal. Inheritance is autosomal recessive and the

Abdelaziz Y. Elzouki (ed.), *Textbook of Clinical Pediatrics*, DOI 10.1007/978-3-642-02202-9_369,

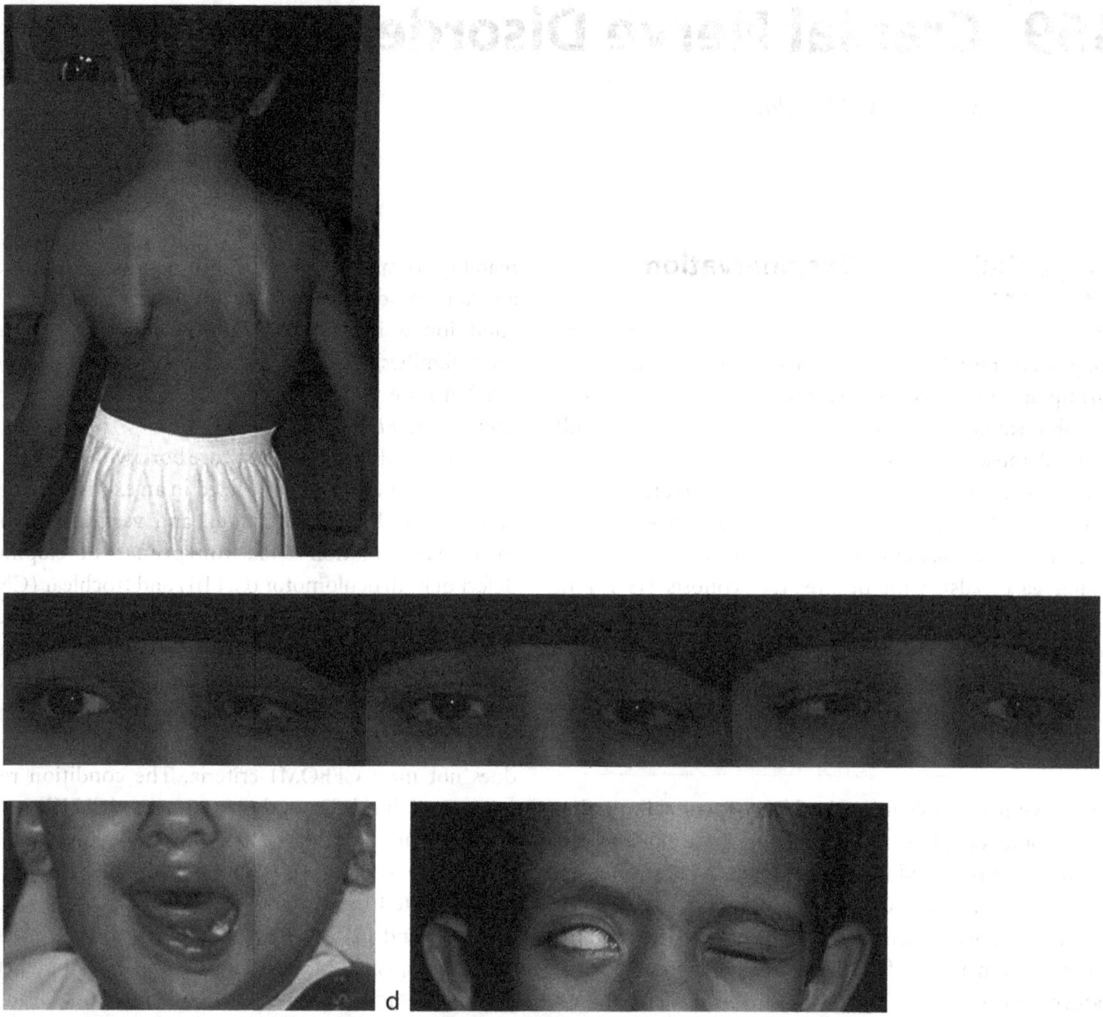

Figure 369.1

(a) Early scoliosis in a patient with horizontal gaze palsy with progressive scoliosis (HGPPS). (b) Bilateral Duane syndrome in an adolescent with Bosley-Salih-Alorainy syndrome (BSAS). There is limitation of horizontal eye globe movement with reduced abduction of both eyes associated with narrowing of the palpebral fissure of the adducting eye (Courtesy of Prof. Thomas M. Bosley). (c) Isolated weakness of the depressor angulae muscle. The right corner of the mouth fails to be lowered on crying. (d) Attempted closure of the eyes showing upward rolling of the right eye (Bell phenomenon) in a patient with right facial (VII cranial nerve) palsy

condition has been reported in consanguineous pedigrees of several different ethnicities. It results from homozygous or compound hererozygous mutations in *ROBO3*. The *ROBO3* gene encodes a transmembrane receptor required for hindbrain axon midline crossing. Electrophysiologic studies and tractography, using magnetic resonance imaging (MRI) diffusion tensor imaging, showed that affected individuals have ipsilateral corticospinal and dorsal column-medial lemniscus tract innervations.

Bosley–Salih–Alorainy (BSAS) and Athabascan Brainstem Dysgenesis Syndromes

Children with BSAS have bilateral Duane syndrome (*Fig. 369.1b*), associated in a subset of them with congenital sensorineural deafness secondary to bilateral absence of the cochlea, semicircular canals and vestibule, malformations of the internal carotid arteries and cardiac outflow tract, mental retardation and autism in some patients. The phenotype of BSAS overlaps with that of Athabascan brain dysgenesis syndrome (ABDS), which includes, in addition, central hypoventilation, facial weakness, and vocal cord paralysis. Both syndromes result from mutations in *HOXA1*, a homeobox gene essential to the development of head and neck structures, including hindbrain, ear, and occipital and hyoid bones. Homozygous mutations of *HOXA1* have been identified in BSAS consanguineous pedigrees in the Middle East (Saudi Arabia and Turkey) and as a sporadic trait in Native American (Athabascan) children from the American Southwest. In *Hoxa1*-knockout mice, the abducens nerve (CN VI) is absent, and it is likely that abducens (CN VI) development and consequent innervations of the lateral rectus muscle is aberrant in BSAS and ABDS patients.

Congenital Facial Palsy

Congenital nontraumatic facial weakness can occur in isolation or in association with abnormal ocular motility. Isolated congenital facial nerve (CN VII) weakness is thought to result from facial nuclei and/or nerve maldevelopment. The condition is unilateral or bilateral, often asymmetrical, and is inherited as autosomal dominant with variable penetrance. It can rarely be associated with congenital deafness.

Moebius Syndrome

Moebius syndrome is defined as facial weakness combined with an ocular abduction deficit. It is a rare sporadic disorder with an estimated prevalence of one case per 50,000 newborns in the USA and four cases per 189,000 newborns in the Netherlands. Necropsy studies in Moebuis patients have shown defects ranging from hypoplasia to agenesis of the respective cranial nuclei. Nevertheless, it has not been established yet whether nerve, brain stem, or muscle aplasia is the primary event leading to this phenotype. CNs IX (glossopharyngeal) and X (vagus) may be affected. The hypoglossal nerves (CN XII) are involved in a minority of cases, whereas the oculomotor (CN III) and trochlear (CN IV) can be involved on rare occasions.

Clinical Manifestations

The condition presents at birth with facial diplegia, incomplete eye closure during sleep, difficulty in sucking and drooling. Examination reveals masklike immobile facial appearance associated with various gaze palsies in about 80% of patients. Involvement of the hypoglossal (XII) nerve (in approximately 25% of cases) leads to atrophy and inability to protrude the tongue. Musculoskeletal abnormalities may be present in about a third of patients. These include talipes equinovarus, congenital amputations, arthrogryposis, syndactly, brachydactyly, and, occasionally (15% of patients), hypoplasia or absence of the pectoralis muscle and breast associated with ipsilateral hand malformation (also called Poland anomaly). Features of autism are known to be associated with some cases of Moebius syndrome.

Diagnosis and Differential Diagnosis

Most cases are recognized during infancy, but the diagnosis soon after birth may be difficult because of the rarity of the condition. Moebius syndrome can be confused with facial palsy secondary to birth trauma (especially with the use of forceps in breach deliveries), congenital myotonic dystrophy, congenital myopathies, or congenital muscular dystrophy.

On electromyography (EMG), no features of active denervation will be seen in the facial muscles, which are hypoplastic or aplastic. Conversely, in birth trauma, denervation potentials will be recorded 2–3 weeks (or more) after the facial nuclei or nerves are injured.

Cranial computed tomography (CT) may demonstrate bilateral calcifications in the region of the abducens (CN VI) nuclei. Bilateral calcifications of the basal ganglia have also been reported. MRI may show hypoplasia of the brain stem and exclude other associated cerebral malformations.

Treatment

This is generally supportive and symptomatic, depending on the severity of the patient's deficits. Attention should be given to check the development of corneal abrasion/ulceration, aspiration pneumonia, dysphagia, and poor nutrition. Physical and occupational therapies are useful for managing associated musculoskeletal problems. Speech therapy is also helpful, as well as psychiatric management when there is an associated autism. Symptomatic and cosmetic surgical care may be required such as tracheostomy, for supporting airway; gastrostomy, for feeding; and correction of foot deformities. Surgery for strabismus is usually delayed because the condition frequently improves with age, and plastic surgery may be required to counteract facial nerve paralysis.

Prognosis

Death may occur shortly after birth in 28% of patients, mainly due to bulbar or respiratory problems. Otherwise, Moebuis syndrome is a static neurologic defect with no mortality in its mild form.

Perinatal Factors and Other Causes of Congenital Facial Palsy (CFP)

Due to the relatively superficial course of the extracranial facial nerve (CN VII), it can be damaged during birth. This can follow instrumentation in assisted delivery, and intrapartum compression where the fetal head is compressed against the maternal bony prominences such as the ischeal spines, the pubic rami, and sacral prominence. Apart from Moebius syndrome and Poland sequence, other syndromes have CFP as part of their symptoms. These include Goldenhar syndrome, which is characterized by unilateral facial hypoplasia (occasionally associated with facial palsy), epibulbar dermoid, preauricular skin tags, and cervical vertebral defects. Cardiofacial syndrome can be confused with CFP. However, in this condition, there is isolated weakness of the depressor anguli oris and quadratus labii inferioris muscles, and the lower corner of the mouth on the involved side fails to move downward on crying (➋ *Fig. 369.1c*). On the same side, the lower lip may be slightly everted. In a minority of patients, the condition was found to be associated with congenital heart disease.

Acquired Facial Paralysis

Bell's Palsy

Definition/Classification

Bell's palsy is one of the most common neurologic disorders affecting the CNs and is characterized by abrupt unilateral peripheral facial paresis or paralysis with no detectable cause.

Epidemiology

The annual incidence of Bell's palsy is about 25 cases per 100,000 persons in the USA, similar to the rest of the world except for Japan, which has the highest incidence. The incidence of Bell's palsy is 2.7 per 100,000 in the first decade of life and 10.1 per 100,000 in the second decade. The palsy can occur bilaterally at a rate of less than 1%, and about 1.4% of patients have a family history of the disorder.

Etiology and Pathophysiology

Bell's palsy is thought to be caused by inflammation and swelling of the facial (VII) nerve resulting in its compression as it passes through the bony canal (a portion of the temporal bone commonly referred to as the facial canal). Nevertheless, the precise pathophysiology is still unclear, although it is assumed that herpes simplex virus (HSV) is the etiologic agent, being reactivated after remaining latent in the geniculate ganglion and causing, thereafter, local damage to the myelin of the facial nerve. The efferent component of the facial nerve stimulates the muscles of facial expression, with a small branch to the stapedius muscle in the middle ear. The afferent and smaller portion contains taste fibers to the anterior two-thirds of the tongue, some pain fibers and secretomotor fibers to the lacrimal and salivary glands.

Clinical Manifestations: Symptoms and Signs

Symptoms

The condition may manifest with posterior auricular pain, which precedes the paresis by 2–3 days in a quarter of patients. In the majority, it presents with acute onset of unilateral upper and lower facial paralysis over a period of 48 h. This might be associated with decreased tearing, taste disturbances, and hyperacusis due to paralysis of the stapedius muscle.

Signs

On the affected side, weakness and/or paralysis due to involvement of the facial (VII) nerve affects the entire upper and lower part of the face. When the child is asked to raise the eyebrows or look upward, without moving the head, the forehead with the palsy will remain flat. When asked to smile, the face lateralizes to the side opposite to the palsy. On attempted eye closure, Bell phenomenon is observed: the eye on the affected side rolls upward and outward (➋ *Fig. 369.1d*). This phenomenon is a normal response to eye closure. Although the disease can affect both sides, bilateral facial palsy should prompt workup for other causes besides Bell's palsy.

Diagnosis

Immediate imaging is not necessary if the history and physical examination lead to a diagnosis of Bell's palsy. Enhancement of the facial nerve, at or near the geniculate ganglion, may be detected on MRI. When the paralysis progresses over weeks, it is no longer Bell's palsy, and MRI brain is mandatory to exclude tumors compressing or involving CN VII, such as schwannoma, meningioma, hemangioma, pontine glioma, and rhabdomyosarcomas.

Differential Diagnosis

Otitis media and mastoiditis should always be considered as antibiotics and/or surgery may be requested. X-rays or CT of the temporal bone are indicated if the history and examination are suggestive. Hypertension is rarely associated with Bell's palsy and should systematically be looked for. Herpes zoster of the geniculate ganglion (Ramsay Hunt syndrome) is an uncommon cause of facial palsy in children. Other viruses that may cause facial weakness include mumps, chicken pox, and Epstein-Barr viruses.

Bacterial causes of facial palsy include Lyme disease (neuroborreliosis), in which it may be an early sign, brucellosis and diphtheria. Facial palsy may be associated with *Mycoplasma pneumoniae* infections, sometimes in the absence of respiratory symptoms. Traumatic paralysis of the facial nerve is revealed by history, and CT scan of the temporal bone may be required. Other causes include Guillain–Barré syndrome (bilateral facial palsy), sarcoidosis, and tumors of the brain stem or meninges.

Investigations

Laboratory studies should include serological tests for Lyme disease (IgG and IgM titres) and brucellosis (ELISA) in endemic areas. Serum titres for *Mycoplasma pneumoniae* (IgM) and for HSV may be obtained. Nerve conduction studies and EMG are useful in severe Bell's palsy. They are most informative when performed 3–10 days after the onset of paralysis. Comparison to the contralateral (unaffected) side has prognostic implications and helps to determine the extent of nerve injury.

Treatment

Impaired eye closure and abnormal tear flow require tear substitutes, lubricants, and eye protection with eye glasses or patches. Significant improvement in outcome was shown in two recent randomized controlled trials, when prednisolone was started within 72 h of symptom onset. The recommended pediatric dose is 1 mg/kg/day up to 60 mg/day for 7–10 days. Despite evidence to support HSV as a major cause of Bell's palsy, a recent trial showed no added benefit with the addition of acyclovir to prednisolone.

Prognosis

The majority of patients (85%) with Bell's palsy will achieve complete recovery, 10% have some persistent facial muscle asymmetry, and 5% have severe cosmotic sequelae. Patients showing complete paralysis during the acute phase are at a higher risk for severe sequelae. Bell's palsy recurs in 10–15% of patients, and recurrences are usually associated with a family history of recurrent Bell's palsy.

References

[Best Evidence] Sullivan FM, Swan IR, Donnan PT et al (2007) Early treatment with prednisolone or acyclovir in Bell's palsy. N Engl J Med 357:1598–1607

Baraitser M (1997) Genetics of Mobuis syndrome. J Med Genet 14:415–417

Bosley TM, Salih MA, Jen JC et al (2005) Neurologic features of horizontal gaze palsy and progressive scoliosis with mutations in ROBO3. Neurology 59:462–463

Bosley TM, Salih MA, Alorainy IA et al (2007) Clinical characterization of the HOXA1 syndrome BSAS variant. Neurology 69:1245–1253

Engle EC (2007) Genetic basis of congenital strabismus. Arch Ophthalmol 125:189–195

Engstrom M, Berg T, Stjernquist-Desatrik A et al (2008) Prednisolone and acyclovir in Bell's palsy: a randomized, double bind, placebo-controlled, multicentre trial. Lancet Neurol 7:993–1000

Gilden DH (2004) Clinical practice. Bell's Palsy. N Engl J Med 351:1323–1331

Guillberg C, Steffenburg S (1989) Autistic behavior in Moebuis syndrome. Acta Paediatr Scand 78:314–316

Katusic SK, Beard CM, Wiederholt WC, Bergstrach EJ, Kurland LT (1986) Incidence, clinical features, and prognosis in Bell's palsy, Rochester, Minnesota, 1968–1982. Ann Neurol 20:622–627

Kim YH, Choi IJ, Kim HM, Ban JH, Cho CH, Ahn JH (2008) Bilateral simultaneous facial nerve palsy: clinical paralysis in severe cases. Otol Neurotol 29:397–400

Lintas C, Persico AM (2008) Autistic phenotypes and genetic testing: state-of-the-art for the clinical geneticist. J Med Genet 46:1–8

Salih MA, Abdel-Gader AM, Al-Jarallah AA et al (2006) Infectious and inflammatory disorders of the circulatory system as a risk factor for stroke in Saudi children. Saudi Med J 27(Suppl 1):S42–S52

Salih MA, Suliman GI, Hassan HS (1981) Complications of diphtheria seen during the 1978 outbreak in Khartoum. Ann Trop Paediatr 1:97–101

Tischfield MA, Baris HN, Wu C et al (2010) Human TUBB3 mutations perturb microtubule dynamics, kinesin interactions, and axon guidance. Cell 140:74–87

Tischfield MA, Bosley TM, Salih MA et al (2005) Homozygous HOXA1 mutations disrupt human brain-stem, inner ear, cardiovascular and cognitive development. Nat Genet 37:1035–1037

370 Anterior Horn Cell Diseases

Mustafa A. M. Salih

Definition/Classification

Disorders of the anterior horn cell (AHC) can either be acquired or inherited. Acquired diseases are mainly of viral origin and most of these run an acute course. They include poliomyelitis and similar diseases due to enteroviruses other than poliovirus. Following the global control of poliomyelitis by widespread immunization, inherited degenerative diseases currently account for most cases of AHC disease.

Paralytic Poliomyelitis

The polioviruses belong to the Piccornaviridae family, in the genus *Entrovirus,* and include three antigenically distinct serotypes (types 1, 2, and 3). They spread by the fecal–oral route and humans are the only known reservoir. Polioviruses are known to be resistant and can retain infectivity for several days at room temperature.

Epidemiology

Paralytic poliomyelitis occurs in about 1/1,000 infections among infants to about 1/100 infections among adolescents. Prior to universal vaccination, epidemics of paralytic poliomyelitis occurred in developed countries primarily in adolescents, whereas in developing countries with poor sanitation, infections occurred early in life resulting in infantile paralysis. When the Expanded Program on Immunization (EPI) was established by the World Health Organization (WHO) in 1974, oral poliovirus (OPV) vaccine was introduced for developing countries to use exclusively. In the pre-EPI era, 600,000–800,000 cases of polio occurred annually, the vast majority in developing countries. Following the WHO program for global eradication of poliomyelitis (from 1988), paralytic poliomyelitis started to disappear. Nevertheless, due to occasional revertants (by nucleotide substitution) of these vaccine strains, a neuro-virulent phenotype leads to vaccine-associated paralytic poliomyelitis (VAPP). The annual incidence of VAPP was determined by the WHO to be 0.4–3.0/million vaccinated children with intercountry variations. The incidence of VAPP in India was estimated to be seven/million birth cohorts, one of the highest in the world. Cases of poliovirus following a circulating vaccine-derived poliovirus were documented in Egypt, the Dominican Republic and Haiti, Madagascar, the Philippines, and Romania.

Pathogenesis and Pathology

Polioviruses infect cells by adsorbing to poliovirus receptor and gain host entry via the gastrointestinal tract. Wild type poliovirus and neurovirulent revertant vaccine strains probably access the central nervous system (CNS) through the peripheral nerves. Infection by polioviruses is inapparent in 90–95% of cases or is associated with a mild nonspecific febrile illness in about 5% of patients (abortive) poliomyelitis. About 1% of patients infected with wild-type poliovirus develop lymphocytic meningitis (nonparalytic poliomyelitis), whereas paralytic poliomyelitis develops in about 0.1%. The pathological lesions primarily involve the motor neuron cells in the spinal cord (AHC) and the medulla oblongata (the cranial nerve nuclei). Involvement of the reticular formation compromises the vital centers controlling respiration and circulation. Hyperasthesia and myalgia, which are typical of acute poliomyelitis, are caused by the involvement of the intermediate and dorsal horn and dorsal root ganglia in the spinal cord. Other affected areas are the cerebellar vermis and, to a lesser extent, the thalamus and layers III and V of the motor cortex.

Clinical Manifestations

The clinical manifestations usually appear after an incubation period of 8–12 days (range 3–35 days). The initial symptoms comprise fever, malaise, and headache. There may also be sore throat, abdominal or muscle pain, and irregular vomiting. After an apparent recovery for 2–5 days, the previous symptoms recur associated with

Abdelaziz Y. Elzouki (ed.), *Textbook of Clinical Pediatrics,* DOI 10.1007/978-3-642-02202-9_370, fever, muscle pain, and sensory and motor phenomena (hyperesthesia, paraesthesia, spasms, and fasciculations). Paralysis appears within 2 days and is characterized by asymmetrical flaccid paralysis involving the legs, arms, and/or trunk with absent tendon reflexes. The proximal areas of the limbs tend to be involved to a greater extent than the distal areas. Sensation is intact and the presence of sensory disturbances suggests an alternative diagnosis. Urinary retention is present at onset in 20–30% of cases. In developing countries, history of intramuscular injections precedes paralytic poliomyelitis in 50–60% of patients (also termed provocation paralysis). Asymmetric involvement of the abdominal muscles results in bulging of the affected side (phantom hernia) (➋ *Fig. 370.1a*). Progression of the paralytic manifestation stops once the temperature returns to normal.

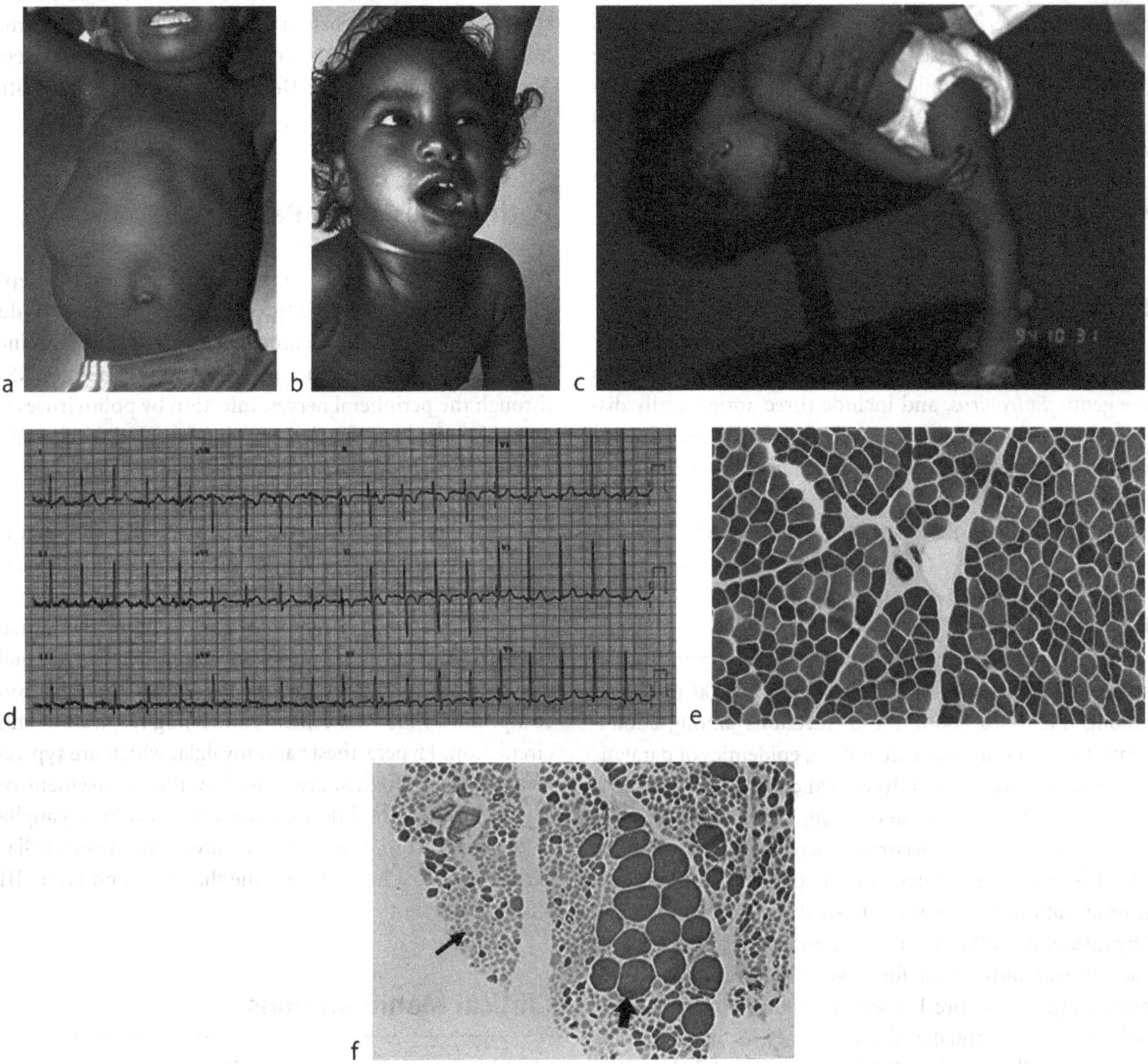

◘ Figure 370.1
(a) Asymmetric involvement of the abdominal muscles resulting in bulging of the right side (phantom hernia) following poliomyelitis. (b) Right lower motor facial nerve palsy in bulbar poliomyelitis. (c) Floppy infant syndrome due to spinal muscular atrophy (SMA) type 1. (d) Electrocardiography (ECG) showing baseline tremors in SMA type III. These are most prominent in leads II and III. (e) The checkerboard pattern in a normal muscle biopsy as compared to (f) which shows group atrophy (thin arrow) and compensatory hypertrophy (thick arrow) of muscle fibres

The bulbar form (bulbar poliomyelitis) is rarely isolated and the cervical cord is involved in at least 90% of cases. All cranially innervated muscles may be affected (➋ *Fig. 370.1b*). Involvement of vital centers in the medulla manifests as irregularities in rate, depth, and rhythm of respiration. It may also manifest as cardiovascular system alterations, including blood pressure changes, cardiac arrhythmias, and rapid changes in body temperature. A rare form of poliomyelitis is polioencephalitis in which higher centers of the brain are severely involved. Spastic paralysis with increased reflexes may be involved. Peripheral or bulbar paralysis may coexist with the condition or ensue during its course.

Diagnosis

Poliomyelitis should be suspected in any unimmunized or partially immunized child with paralytic disease. Paralytic disease occurring 7–14 days after receiving OPV is a major clue to the development of VAPP. In countries where wild-type poliovirus has been eradicated, VAPP can occur later if the OPV has been given to the child or contact.

Cerebrospinal fluid (CSF) examination shows a pleocytosis of 20–300 cells/mm^3. Initially, these cells are predominantly polymorphonuclear cells, followed after 5–7 days by a lymphatic pleocytosis. The cell count falls to near-normal values by the second week. Initially the CSF protein is normal or only slightly elevated but usually rises to 50–100 g/L by the second week. In polio encephalitis, the CSF may show minor changes or remain normal.

Poliovirus may be isolated from the stools of 80–90% of acutely ill patients and from <20% within 3–4 weeks after onset of paralysis. According to the WHO recommendations, two stool specimens should be collected 24–48 h apart, as soon as the diagnosis of poliomyelitis is suspected. Poliovirus isolates should be sent to either the Centre for Disease Control and Prevention in the USA or to one of the WHO-certified poliomyelitis laboratories, located in several regions of the world, where DNA sequence analysis can be performed. This investigation is performed to differentiate between wild poliovirus and neurovirulent revertant OPV strains.

Differential Diagnosis

Even in countries where the disease has been eradicated, the possibility of poliomyelitis should be considered in any case of acute flaccid paralysis. The diagnoses most often confused with polio are Guillaine–Barre syndrome, transverse myelitis, West Nile virus, and other enteroviruses. Guillaine–Barre syndrome differs in the mode of onset, the symmetrical distribution of weakness, and CSF characteristics (few cells but elevated protein level). Transverse myelitis is characterized by acute symmetric paralysis of the lower limbs associated with sensory level and bladder dysfunction. The CSF is usually normal. A syndrome closely resembling poliomyelitis (Hopkins syndrome) has been reported following acute attacks of asthma or status asthmaticus.

Injury of the spinal column, sometimes associated with periostitis or osteomyelitis, may present with a polio-like paralytic syndrome. Other rare causes include snakebite, spider bite, scorpion sting, tick bite, and schistomiasis involving the spinal cord. Chemical poisons that cause paralytic syndromes include arsenic, triorthocresyl phosphate, and organophosphorus insecticides.

Treatment

The management of paralytic poliomyelitis is supportive and there is no specific antiviral therapy. The objectives are to limit progression of the disease, prevent ensuing skeletal deformities, and provide psychological support for the child and family. Intramuscular injections, including insertion of an electromyography (EMG) needle, and surgical procedures are contraindicated since they precipitate provocation paralysis. This can happen particularly in the first week of illness.

The management of bulbar poliomyelitis consists of maintaining the airway, avoiding the risk of aspiration, observing for respiratory insufficiency, and circulatory disturbances. Tracheostomy and mechanical ventilation might be needed when there is vocal cord paralysis or constriction of the hypopharynx.

Prognosis

The mortality in spinal poliomyelitis, with or without less severe bulbar involvement, is about 5–10%. In severe bulbar poliomyelitis, the mortality rate may reach up to 60%. Following the paralytic phase of the illness, which takes 2–3 days, there is a period of stabilization followed by gradual return of muscle function. Recovery of affected muscles takes up to 6 months. Muscles still paralyzed thereafter, remain so indefinitely. Following an interval of 20–40 years, a progressive motor neuron disease (postpolio syndrome) may affect 30–40% of those who survived paralytic poliomyelitis in childhood.

Prevention

Vaccination is the only effective method that can prevent poliomyelitis. The live-attenuated OPV vaccine is more economic, easy to administer, and limits the replication of the wild poliovirus and its transmission by fecal spread. Nevertheless, it may undergo reversion to neurovirulence and cause VAPP. The more expensive to operate injectable inactivated poliovaccine (IPV) is equally immunizing and does not cause VAPP. In countries where the risk of VAPP is higher than the risk for transmission of poliomyelitis, IPV is being used routinely. Adoption of a policy of initial vaccination by the parenteral route (using IPV) followed by OPV has been shown to greatly reduce the risk of VAPP.

Spinal Muscular Atrophy

Definition/Classification

Spinal muscular atrophy (SMA) is an autosomal recessive inherited motor unit disease characterized by progressive muscle weakness resulting from degeneration and loss of the anterior horn cells in the spinal cord and the brain stem nuclei. The single gene responsible for SMA was mapped to chromosome 5q11.2–13.3 and identified as the survival motor neuron (SMN) gene. Classification of SMA, based on clinical criteria, was found to be useful for prognosis and management, although the phenotype of the disease-causing mutations of the SMN gene spans a continuum with no sharp distinction between the subtypes. These criteria include age of onset and maximum function attained. Spinal muscular atrophy type 1 (SMA I, Werdnig–Hoffman disease) is characterized by onset before 6 months of age, failure to achieve sitting without support and death by 2 years of age. Onset of SMA II (previously named chronic SMA) is between 6 months and 12 months, the patient ultimately attains independent sitting when placed and may live into adolescence or even longer. The onset of SMA III (juvenile SMA or Kugelberg–Welander disease) is after 12 months (usually after 18 months) and all patients walk independently at some stage of their life that extends into the sixth decade. Spinal muscular atrophy type IV is a disease of adults.

Epidemiology

In a world survey, the prevalence of SMA was estimated to be 12/million populations. The estimated prevalence among Norwegian children was $1.7/10^6$. Considerably higher prevalences of 133 and $172/10^6$ populations were found in Saudi Arabia and Tunisia, respectively, reflecting the high rate of consanguinity in these communities. Significantly higher carrier frequency of 5% was reported from Saudi Arabia, i.e., one carrier in each 20 persons compared to one in 50–80 in the USA and Europe.

Pathogenesis

The two genes associated with SMA are *SMN1* and *SMN2*. The *SMN1* gene is believed to be the primary disease-causing gene. Homozygous absence of exons 7 and 8 of *SMN1* is found in 95–98% of individuals with SMA. About 2–5% of patients are compound heterozygotes for absence of exons 7 and 8 of the *SMN1* and a point mutation in *SMN1*. On the other hand, there is a dose relationship between *SMN2* copies; most patients with the milder form (SMA II) have three *SMN2* copies, whereas most patients with the mildest form (SMA III) have three or four *SMN2* copies.

Pathology

Postmortem findings in SMA included decreased number of motor neurons and gliosis in the anterior horns of the spinal cord and motor cranial nerve nuclei V and VII–XII. This is reflected in the changes observed in muscle biopsy with features of acute and chronic denervation.

Clinical Manifestations

Onset of SMA I is from birth to 6 months. Sucking or swallowing problems may be noticed in the first few months of life, along with paradoxical or abdominal breathing. With inhalation, the chest caves in as the diaphragm contracts. There is poor muscle tone associated with muscle weakness manifesting as the "floppy infant syndrome" (➋ *Fig. 370.1c*). There is lack of motor development and the child never achieves ability to sit unsupported. Nevertheless, there is normal cerebral function and the baby has an alert appearance. Facial weakness is minimal or absent and fasciculations of the tongue are seen in most, but not all, affected children. Postural tremor of the fingers (minipolymyoclonus), due to fasciculations of intrinsic hand muscles, is seen occasionally. The distribution of muscle weakness is proximal and symmetrical, involving the upper and lower limbs. Contractures are mild, often at the knees and rarely at the elbows. Tendon reflexes are absent and there is no sensory loss. Survival is for about 2 years, although it can be extended with improved respiratory and nutrition care.

The usual onset of SMA II is after 6 months of age, but can be earlier. These patients achieve the ability to sit independently when placed in a sitting position, but will not be able to walk. They have decreased muscle tone, associated with symmetrical proximal muscle weakness and wasting, and may also present as "floppy infant syndrome." A postural tremor of the fingers is seen almost invariably and is a helpful diagnostic feature. Tendon reflexes are absent in 70% of affected children. Patients are cognitively normal with average intellectual skills during the formative years and above average by adolescence.

Onset of SMA III is after the age of 12 months (usually 18 months) and the patient will achieve the ability to walk. Weakness usually manifests between 2 years and 5 years with frequent falls or difficulty in walking up and down stairs. Symmetric proximal limb weakness and wasting ensues slowly with legs more severely affected than the arms. Examination shows a positive Gowers maneuver and absent knee jerks, with preservation of the ankle jerks and upper limb reflexes. Gait is waddling and calf hypertrophy may be present in some patients leading to an erroneous diagnosis of muscular dystrophy. Coarse tremor of the hands is shown by many patients. The disease progresses very slowly but the development of pes cavus is frequent.

Clinical Variants of SMA

A prenatal form of SMA with arthrogryposis associated with a deletion of *SMN* gene has been described. This form presents with weakness at birth with the face being minimally affected. Segmental SMA, with asymmetrical weakness and atrophy involving the distribution of several contiguous spinal roots, is a rare variant. Facial weakness and severe peripheral neuropathies have also been associated with a deletion of the SMA gene.

Diagnosis

Currently, the diagnosis of SMA is based on molecular genetic testing. Neurophysiological tests and muscle biopsy are done when the molecular genetic testing of the *SMN1* gene is normal.

The motor and sensory nerve conduction velocities are normal. Electromyography (EMG) reveals features of denervation and diminished motor action potential amplitude. Spontaneous motor unit activity is a unique feature of SMA and is most commonly seen in SMA I, occasionally in SMA II, but not in SMA III. Positive sharp waves and fibrillations are present in all individuals with SMA. This is reflected in the electrocardiogram (ECG), which shows tremor of ECG baseline even in SMA III (➋ *Fig. 370.1d*). Muscle biopsy shows signs of denervation in the form of group atrophy in type l and type ll muscle fibers as opposed to the normal checkerboard pattern (➋ *Fig. 370.1e* and *f*). Lipid deposits and glycogen are not seen, excluding lipid and glycogen storage disorders.

Differential Diagnosis

Arthrogryposis multiplex congenita (AMC) may be due to causes other than *SMN* mutations. For types I and II SMA, the differential diagnosis includes other causes of the floppy infant syndrome. A diagnosis of muscular dystrophy may be entertained in cases of SMA III with raised CK concentration. Congenital and metabolic myopathies may also present similarly.

Treatment

A recent consensus document has addressed the diagnosis and treatment of patients with SMA. This document included issues of respiratory and nutritional care in patients with SMA I, II, and III. Children with SMA I (Werdnig–Hoffman disease) can survive beyond 2 years of age on tracheostomy and noninvasive respiratory support. However, such an intervention raises ethical questions. Intermittent positive-pressure breathing was found to be effective in children with SMA, as well as other neuromuscular disorders, and leads to lung volume expansions and clearance of airway secretions. Nighttime use of continuous positive airway pressure prevents daytime fatigue caused by sleep apnea in SMA III patients.

About 50% of SMA patients develop scoliosis before age 10 years. Although orthosis allows the patient to be upright rather than bedridden, it does not prevent the development of scoliosis. Spinal surgery is required especially in those non-ambulatory patients who develop curvatures greater than 50°. Hip dislocation is common in SMA, but does not require surgical correction if it was asymptomatic. Clinic surveillance should be at least every 6 months and weaker children need more frequent visits. Clinical evaluations should include respiratory function, nutritional state, and orthopedic status.

While assessing respiratory function, note should be taken whether there is normal or abdominal breathing patterns. Children over the age of 4 years can accurately use the hand-held spirometer to measure the forced vital capacity (FVC). When FVC is above 40%, decompensation during respiratory infection is less likely. If abdominal breathing is noted and/or the FVC is less than 30%, options for management should be discussed with the family including "do not resuscitate" status.

During periods of intercurrent illness or fasting, children with SMA develop a poorly understood complication consisting of severe metabolic acidosis associated with dicarboxylic aciduria. Judicial administration of intravenous fluids prevents this condition.

Through the use of special education and electric wheelchairs, children with SMA type II can be integrated into normal schools. Parents and families with various types of SMA require active social and psychological support.

Specific medical treatment of SMA still does not exist. Nevertheless, several medications/chemicals that increase the activity of *SMN2* gene are under investigation. These include histone deacetylase (HDAC) inhibitors (aclarubicin), valproic acid, phenylbutyrate (a drug used in the treatment of urea cycle disorders), indoprofen (a nonsteroidal anti-inflammatory drug) and gabapentin. Clinical trials of Rilutek (Riluzole) in infants with SMA and hydroxyurea (a medication that enhances expression of human fetal hemoglobin gene and SMN protein levels) are underway.

Prognosis

Life expectancy reflects the type of SMA, although this has changed over the past few years with better respiratory and nutritional care. Recurrent pneumonia, scoliosis, and hip dislocation punctuate the progress of the disease.

Prevention

The optimal option for prevention is through family planning. In regions with high carrier rate, as in the Middle East, premarital screening is being introduced into the system. When faced with a married couple who are carriers of the disease, discussion of availability of prenatal testing should be made before pregnancy.

Prenatal testing is available for high-risk pregnancies. This can be achieved by analysis of fetal DNA obtained either through chorionic villous sampling (at 10–12 weeks of gestation) or through amniocentesis, usually at about 15–18 weeks of gestation. Samples will be analyzed for the known *SMN1* gene mutation or for the previously identified linked markers. Preimplantation genetic diagnosis (PIGD), available in centers with in vitro fertilization capability, can be done for parents in future pregnancies, when disease-causing mutations have been identified in an affected child.

References

Al Jumah M, Majumdar R, Al Rajeh S et al (2003) Molecular analysis of the spinal muscular atrophy and neuronal apoptosis inhibitory protein genes in Saudi patients with spinal muscular atrophy. Saudi Med J 24:1052–1054

Al Jumah M, Majumdar R, Rehana Z, Al Rajeh S, Eyaid W (2007) A pilot study of spinal muscular atrophy screening in Saudi Arabia. J Pediatr Neurol 5:221–224

Alexander LN, Seward JF, Santibanez TA et al (2004) Vaccine policy changes and epidemiology of poliomyelitis in the United States. JAMA 292:1696–1701

Bingham PM, Shen N, Renner H et al (1997) Arthrogryposis due to infantile neuronal degeneration associated with deletion of the SMNT gene. Neurology 49:848–851

Bosley AR, Speirs G, Markham NI (2003) Provocation poliomyelitis, vaccine associated paralytic poliomyelitis related to a rectal abscess in an infant. J Infect 47:82–84

Dawood AA, Moosa A (1983) Hand and ECG tremor in spinal muscular atrophy. Arch Dis Child 58:376–378

Emery AEH (1991) Population frequencies of inherited neuromuscular diseases – a world survey. Neuromuscul Disord 1:19–29

Gear JH (1984) Non-polio causes of polio-like paralytic syndromes. Rev Infect Dis 6(Suppl 2):S379–S384

Hergersberg M, Glatzel M, Capone A et al (2000) Deletions in spinal muscular atrophy gene repair in a newborn with neuropathy and extreme generalized muscular weakness. Eur J Paediatr Neurol 4:35–38

John TJ (2004) A developing country perspective on vaccine-associated paralytic poliomyelitis. Bull World Health Organ 82:53–58

Mizuno Y, Komori S, Shigetomo R, Kurihara E, Tamagawa K, Komiya K (1995) Poliomyelitis-like illness after acute asthma (Hopkins syndrome): a histological study of biopsied muscle in a case. Brain Dev 17(2):126–129

Strebel PM, Ion-Nedelcu N, Baughman AL, Sutter RW, Cochi SL (1995) Intramuscular injections within 30 days of immunization with oral poliovirus vaccine – a risk factor for vaccine-associated paralytic poliomyelitis. N Engl J Med 332:500–506

Summer CJ (2007) Molecular mechanisms of spinal muscular atrophy. J Child Neurol 22:979–989

Tangsrud S-E, Halvorsen S (1988) Child neuromuscular disease in Southern Norway. Prevalence, age and distribution of diagnosis with special reference to "non-Duchenne muscular dystrophy". Clin Genet 34:145–152

Wang CH, Finkel RS, Bertini ES et al (2007) Consensus statement for standard of care in spinal muscular atrophy. J Child Neurol 22:1027–1049

371 Plexopathies and Radiculopathies

Mustafa A. M. Salih

Several disorders of the brachial plexus and the lumbosacral plexus occur during childhood. These can either be traumatic or inflammatory disorders.

Brachial Plexus Palsy

Definition/Classification

The brachial plexus is composed of a group of nerves arising from the nerve roots of cervical segments 5 through thoracic segment (C5–T1). Injury to the upper plexus (C5 and C6 roots) leads to the Erb–Duchenne type of plexus paralysis. Involvement of the lower brachial plexus cervical 7, 8, and thoracic root 1 result in Klumpke paralysis.

Etiology

Brachial plexus injuries usually occur following shoulder dystocia in large-for-gestational-age newborns (macrosomic infants). This can result from forceful lateral deviation of the head from the shoulder during delivery due to impaction of fetal shoulders within maternal pelvis. Injury of the lower plexus results from traction on the trunk with breech delivery, or from traction on the adducted forearm during vertex delivery. Brachial plexus unassociated with shoulder dystocia or difficult delivery has been reported suggesting an intrauterine origin such as deformation from uterine constraint in cases of bicornuate uterus.

Pathogenesis and Pathology

Brachial plexus palsy has rarely been detected in babies delivered by cesarean section indicating that long-standing in utero stretching of the brachial plexus could lead to the development of palsy. In utero stretching could be due to constriction bands, uterine constraints from oligohydramnios or bicornuate uterus, intrauterine maladaptation or congenital aplasia of the roots of the brachial plexus. The most common and mildest form of brachial plexus injury is neuropraxia, which is due to edema following pressure on the nerve roots. Axonotmesis is more severe and is due to disruption of the axon of the nerve with an intact myelin sheath. Total disruption of the postganglionic nerve constitutes neurotmesis, whereas avulsion designates complete disruption of the ganglia from the spinal cord at both the anterior and posterior roots.

Clinical Manifestations

Paralysis is recognized from the first days of life in the majority of babies. In upper (Erb–Duchenne) palsy, the affected arm hangs limply adducted and internally rotated, with extended elbow, pronated forearm, and variably flexed wrist (➋ *Fig. 371.1a*). The Moro reflex is absent on the affected side (asymmetric Moro reflex), as well as the biceps and brachioradialis reflexes. Associated significant C7 involvement manifests as weakness of the triceps and extensors of forearm and digits. In lower brachial plexus (Klumpke) palsy (➋ *Fig. 371.1b*), intrinsic hand muscles are paralyzed, the grasp is absent and a Horner syndrome is frequently present. Horner syndrome manifests as meiosis, ptosis, and facial anhydrosis, and is caused by injury of the sympathetic fibers of the first thoracic root. The phrenic nerve, arising from C3, C4, and C5, can be involved in brachial plexus palsy resulting in ipsilateral diaphragmatic paralysis and produces symptoms of respiratory distress.

Diagnosis and Differential Diagnosis

Due to the unique physical findings of brachial plexus palsy, the diagnosis is readily apparent. Nevertheless, other possibilities that need to be considered are cerebral injury, cervical spine injury, fracture, dislocation or epiphyseal separation of the humerus, and fracture of the clavicle. Another brachial plexopathy that needs to be considered is brachial neuritis (neuralgic amyotrophy, Parsonage–Turner syndrome). Although pediatric cases are much rarer than in adults, this disease may occur from infancy.

Abdelaziz Y. Elzouki (ed.), *Textbook of Clinical Pediatrics*, DOI 10.1007/978-3-642-02202-9_371,

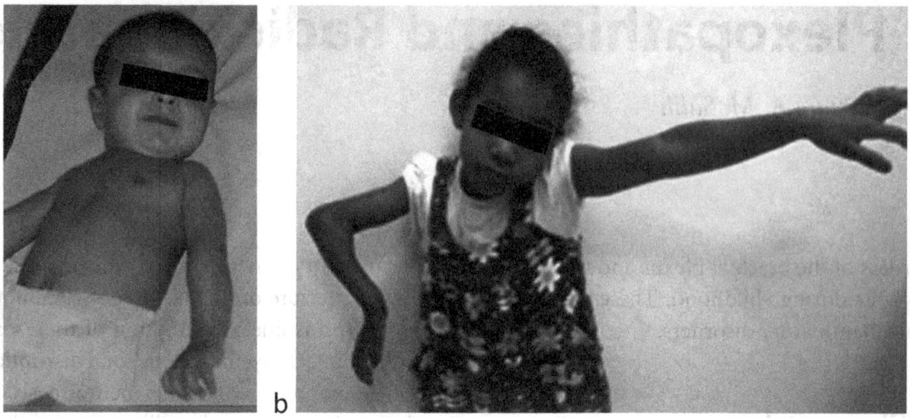

Fig. 371.1
(a) Erb-Duchenne palsy. The left arm is internally rotated, and the forearm is extended and pronated. (b) Lower brachial plexus (Klumpke) palsy of the right upper limb. The elbow is flexed and the hand is paralyzed and atrophic

Diagnostic work-up for brachial plexus palsy is best achieved by magnetic resonance imaging (MRI) of the spinal cord and roots. It has the advantage of avoiding the ionizing radiation of the computed tomography (CT). It also helps to detect the integrity of the brachial plexus, including root avulsion, and the presence of a pseudomeningocele. Electromyography (EMG) can be used to support the diagnosis of root lesions and is capable of detecting signs of denervation and reinnervation in recovery. Associated phrenic nerve injury leading to diaphragmatic involvement is assessed by plain radiography and real-time ultrasonography at the bedside.

Treatment

During the first 1 or 2 weeks, management consists of partial immobilization and appropriate positioning of the affected limb to prevent the development of contractures. Physiotherapy can be initiated after the first 10–14 days to allow delivery pain to subside. Immobilization should be intermittent, between feedings and while the infant is asleep, by abducting the arm to 90°, with external rotation at the shoulder, full supination of the forearm, slight extension at the wrist, and maintaining the palm turned toward the face. Splinting the wrist in the neutral position and placing a pad in the fist, is to be used in lower arm or hand paralysis. Range of motion exercises constitutes the required physical therapy to prevent ligament tightening and the discomfort following contractures. Monthly evaluations for range of motion, return of function, and development of contractures are required. Recovery of brachial plexus palsy occurs in about 70–80% of affected babies, with the remaining patients having residual deficits. Flaccid paralysis of the extremity, Horner syndrome, and diaphragmatic paralysis herald a poor outcome. Patients who do not show signs of recovery for 3–6 months require surgical intervention. Nevertheless, surgical intervention, which includes neurolysis, nerve grafting, and neurotization, requires the availability of microsurgical technique and intraoperative neurophysiologic recordings, and surgeons familiar with the techniques. For older children who did not improve, muscle release around the shoulder joint and tendon transfers may be required.

Prevention

Prompt recognition of shoulder dystocia and avoidance of excessive downward traction on the fetal head by the attending caregiver is the most important preventive step. Since this task requires skills and teamwork, conducting team training in shoulder dystocia as part of risk reduction strategy for improving perinatal outcome has been recommended.

Other Traumatic Plexopathies

After the neonatal period, brachial plexus injury affects principally adolescents, mainly due to motor vehicle (especially motorcycle) and sports accidents, and has guarded prognosis. Conversely, lumbosacral plexus injuries are rare, have been reported in neonates and children, and have favorable outcomes.

Inflammatory Plexopathies

Neuralgic Amyotrophy (Parsonage–Turner Syndrome, Brachial Plexus Neuritis)

Definition/Classification

Neuralgic amyotrophy is a syndrome characterized by episodes of neuropathic pain and rapid multifocal weakness and atrophy (amyotrophy) in the upper limbs. The syndrome has both an idiopathic and hereditary form with similar clinical symptoms but generally more episodes and an earlier age of onset in the hereditary form.

Etiology

An immune-mediated process is thought to underline the attacks, which may be triggered by viral or bacterial illnesses (influenza, Coxsackie-virus, parovirus B-19, Epstein-Barr virus, Q fever, human immunodeficiency virus (HIV) disease, mycoplasma pneumonia, bacterial pneumonia, typhoid, syphilis, and brucellosis). It can also follow immunizations such as tetanus toxoid, diphtheria, recombinant hepatitis B vaccination, swine flu, and immune sera. It may also be triggered by periods of physical or emotional stress. Hereditary neuralgic amyotrophy (HNA) is inherited as autosomal dominant. The proportion of HNA attributed to the mutations in the only known causative gene (*SEPT9*) is about 85%. Idiopathic neuralgic amyotrophy (INA) has a reported incidence of 2–3/100,000/year. The prevalence of hereditary neuralgic amyotrophy (HNA) is unknown and about 200 families are reported worldwide. Both disorders are likely to have higher prevalence because of underdiagnosis.

Pathogenesis and Pathology

Triggering factors are thought to render the brachial plexus more susceptible to an autoimmune damage. The limited nerve biopsies performed in this condition revealed focal decreases in myelinated fibers within individual nerves in the majority, and multiple perineural mononuclear infiltrates in three of four upper extremity nerve biopsies.

Clinical Manifestations

The disorder usually starts with intense pain localized to the shoulder or involving the whole upper limb. Weakness either develops simultaneously with the pain or follows it by days to few weeks. The mean age of onset of INA is about 40 years (range 10–80 years) with 3% of patients suffering the first attack in childhood (<16 years). The mean age of onset of HNA is significantly earlier at 28 years (range 3–56 years) with 23% having their first attack during childhood. Paralysis affects the upper part of the brachial plexus in the majority of patients (about 70%), the whole plexus in 14%, and involves predominantly the lower plexus in 3–8%. The mean time to onset of amyotrophy ranges between 8 days and 14 days after the initial pain. Sensory symptoms and signs are common during the attack affecting more than two third of patients in the form of large proximal hypoesthetic areas. Diaphragmatic paralysis (unilateral or bilateral) is present in about 7% of patients and may predominate in the clinical picture. Hereditary neuralgic amyotrophy affects a younger age group and is characterized by recurrent, often bilateral attacks. Dysmorphic features in the form of hypertelorism, long nasal bridge, and facial asymmetry can be present.

Diagnosis and Differential Diagnosis

Neuralgic amyotrophy needs to be differentiated from diseases that lead to pain or atrophic paralysis around the shoulder girdle and arm. Poliomyelitis can be distinguished by the absence of constitutional symptoms, cutaneous sensory symptoms and a normal CSF. Cervical disk disease and cervical root compression can be demonstrated by EMG and MRI or CT scan.

Routine laboratory studies are usually within the reference range. Complete blood count (CBC) and erythrocyte sedimentation rate (ESR) are helpful nonspecific indicators of systemic diseases presenting as neuralgic amyotrophy, such as systemic lupus erythematosis and lymphoma. Raised ESR may also point toward neurobrucellosis, sarcoidosis, and other granulomatous infiltrations of the brachial plexus. Human immunodeficiency virus (HIV) serology should be done in regions with high prevalence of childhood AIDS.

Imaging of the brachial plexus, using MRI, may reveal enlarged nerves with increased signal intensity on T2-weighted images. It may also help to rule out carcinomatous or granulomatous infiltration.

Electrodiagnostic tests (nerve conduction studies and EMG) are important for diagnostic and prognostic information. It is also important to rule out other conditions such as radiculopathy, neuropathy, and amyotrophic lateral sclerosis. Approximately 50% of unilateral clinical involvement demonstrates bilateral EMG abnormalities.

Features of denervation in affected muscles can be revealed by EMG 2–3 weeks after onset of disease.

Treatment

In the acute stage of the disease, pain management is the primary goal of therapy. Analgesics, using a nonsteroidal anti-inflammatory drug and opiates (if necessary) are required in the initial period. Immunosuppressive therapy, using steroids, do not alter the outcome of the disease. Intravenous immunoglobulin was reported to result in significant improvement in pain and to accelerate recovery of function. This should be followed by physical therapy in the form of passive and active range of motion exercises to avoid a frozen shoulder. Occupational therapy in the form of assistive devices and orthotics may be required when residual disabilities are established. A randomized placebo-controlled trial of oral prednisone is being conducted in the Netherlands.

Prognosis

Brachial neuritis has an overall good prognosis regarding functional recovery. About 80% of patients recover functionally within 2 years and 90% within 3 years. Patients with upper brachial plexus lesions improve earlier and bilateral disease has a less favorable outcome compared to unilateral disease. The recurrence rate of the idiopathic form is between 5% and 26%, and in the inherited form is approximately 75%.

Prevention

In hereditary neuralgic amyotrophy (HNA), at risk individuals younger than age 18 years are typically not offered genetic testing during childhood. This is because no preventive or ameliorating treatment is available for the disease. Since HNA does not affect intellectual or life span, prenatal testing for the condition is not required. However, preimplantation genetic diagnosis (PIGD) may be available for families in which the disease-causing mutation has been identified, although this technique is usually reserved for life-threatening hereditary diseases.

Lumbosacral Plexopathy

This is similar to neuralgic amyotrophy and constitutes its counterpart in the lower limb. The condition is rare but occasional cases are on record in adolescents and even in toddlers. It presents with pain located in a femoral or sciatic distribution, refusal to walk, or limping. The condition usually follows an intercurrent infection but has also been reported in association with schistosomiasis. Recovery is generally faster than neuralgic amyotrophy although mild residual weakness may persist.

References

Al Qattan MM, El Sayed AA, Al Kharfy TM (1996) Obstetrical brachial plexus injury in newborn babies delivered by caesarian section. J Hand Surg Br 21:263–265

Bahar AM (1996) Risk factors and fetal outcome in cases of shoulder dystocia compared with normal deliveries of a similar birthweight. Br J Obstet Gynaecol 103:868–872

Conway RR (2008) Neuralgic amyotrophy: uncommon but not rare. Mo Med 105:168–169

Foad SL, Mehlman CT, Ying J (2008) The epidemiology of neonatal brachial plexus palsy in the United States. J Bone Joint Surg Am 90:1258–1264

Hankin GD, Clark SM, Munn MB (2006) Cesarean section on request at 39 weeks: impact on shoulder dystocia, fetal trauma, neonatal encephalopathy, and intrauterine fetal demise. Semin Pernatol 30:276–287

Marra TA (1983) Recurrent lumbosacral and brachial plexopathy associated with schistosomiasis. Arch Neurol 40:586–588

Pondaag W, Malessy MJA, Gert van Dijk J, Thoameer RT (2004) Natural history of obstetric brachial plexus palsy: a systematic review. Dev Med Child Neurol 46:138–144

Thomson AJG (1993) Idiopathic lumbosacral plexus neuropathy in two children. Dev Med Child Neurol 35:258–261

van Alfen N, van Engelon BG (2006) The clinical spectrum of neuralgic amyotrophy in 246 cases. Brain 129:438–450

372 Peripheral Nerve Disorders

Mustafa A. M. Salih

Traumatic Mononeuropathy

The sciatic nerve can be injured as a result of injections into the nerve or its vicinity. This can follow intramuscular injections into the buttocks, or following injection of drugs into the umbilical artery leading to thrombosis of the inferior gluteal artery. Other causes include stretch injury following closed reduction of hip dislocation and rarely as a result of breech delivery. The resultant paralysis commonly affects the peroneal nerve but may affect the whole territory of the sciatic nerve. The condition frequently presents with foot drop and amyotrophy of the corresponding leg.

Radial nerve injury or paralysis may result from subcutaneous fat necrosis of the upper arm in the neonatal period or following constraint of the forearm for intravenous infusion. Injury of the median nerve may follow arterial stick at the wrist and attempted catheterization of the radial or humeral artery. Femoral nerve injury may follow attempted puncture of the femoral vein or, rarely, trauma to the nerve along the psoas muscle during herniorrhaphy or appendectomy. Peroneal nerve injury may follow casting and orthopedic appliance to the region.

Entrapment Neuropathy

Carpal tunnel syndrome is rare in childhood and usually presents with motor symptoms and wasting of the thenar muscles, rather than pain and paresthesia, which is more marked in adults. During childhood, it may be associated with mucopolysaccharidosis and hyporthyroidism.

Familial Pressure Neuropathy (Hereditary Neuropathy with Liability to Pressure Palsies)

This is a rare dominantly inherited condition due to a deletion at chromosome 17p11.2 locus that encodes peripheral myelin protein P22 (PMP22). Symptoms usually start after the first decade, but may be earlier. A single nerve trunk is usually involved, the most common being the popliteal nerve as a result of prolonged squatting or sitting cross-legged. The cubital nerve may also be involved secondary to pressure on the elbow and patients may develop a carpal tunnel syndrome of early onset. The diagnosis is made when the amount of trauma is out of proportion to the degree of paralysis and when there is a similar family history. Nerve conduction studies confirm the diagnosis by revealing delay in conduction velocities outside the affected territory. Recovery, which takes days to weeks, is usually complete.

Neuropathy of Infectious Diseases

Diphtheritic Neuropathy

Diphtheritic neuropathy is the most common severe complication of *Corynebacterium diphtheriae* infection. Following the introduction of childhood immunization, the disease became a rarity in the US and Western Europe. Nevertheless, the disease is endemic in countries of the Caribbean and Latin America. In the late 1970s, 1980s, and 1990s, outbreaks were reported in both industrialized (Germany, Sweden) and developing countries (Ecuador, China, Nepal, Sudan, Thailand). A large epidemic occurred from 1990 to 1995 throughout the States of the former Soviet Union. Outbreaks also occurred in Ecuador, Algeria, and Central Asia. Historically, diphtheria infected children less than 12 years and declined following childhood immunization with diphtheritic toxoid. Recently, due to incomplete immunization, or lack of it, the disease shifted to the adult population.

Pathogenesis and Pathology

C. diphtheria produces a 62-kd polypeptide exotoxin, which leads to demyelinating neuropathy because it

Abdelaziz Y. Elzouki (ed.), *Textbook of Clinical Pediatrics*, DOI 10.1007/978-3-642-02202-9_372,

inhibits the synthesis of myelin proteolipid and other basic proteins. The exotoxin also causes local tissue necrosis and cardiomyopathy.

Clinical Manifestations

Diphtheria neuropathy follows respiratory or cutaneous diphtheritic infection. Respiratory diphtheria usually involves the tonsils, pharynx, and larynx with a characteristic membranous exudate. The latency in development of diphtheritic polyneuropathy ranges between 5 and 70 (mean = 37) days. Bulbar disturbance appears first with nasal speech, nasal regurgitation, diplopia, and dysphoria. Palatal palsy is the commonest, affecting 72% of patients and is the first to appear at a mean of 22 (range 5–41) days after onset of diphtheria. Generalized peripheral neuropathy usually appears between the 5th and 6th week and may be associated with, or shortly followed by, pharyngeal paralysis, abducens (CN VI) palsy, and weakness of neck muscles (➲ *Fig. 372.1a*). Bilateral facial nerve (CN VII) palsy manifest between the 6th and 10th week (mean = 54 days). Patients have sensory disturbances of all modalities in the distal extremities, tendon reflexes are absent or depressed, and plantar responses are flexor. Autonomic instability is common in diphtheritic polyneuropathy and may be difficult to differentiate from myocarditis. Paralysis of the diaphragm and respiratory muscles may occur and require mechanical ventilation. Clinical recovery of the neurological complications of diphtheria follow the same pattern except for pharyngeal paralysis and peripheral weakness, which take longer to resolve (6–7 weeks), and facial weakness, which resolves more rapidly (about 4 weeks).

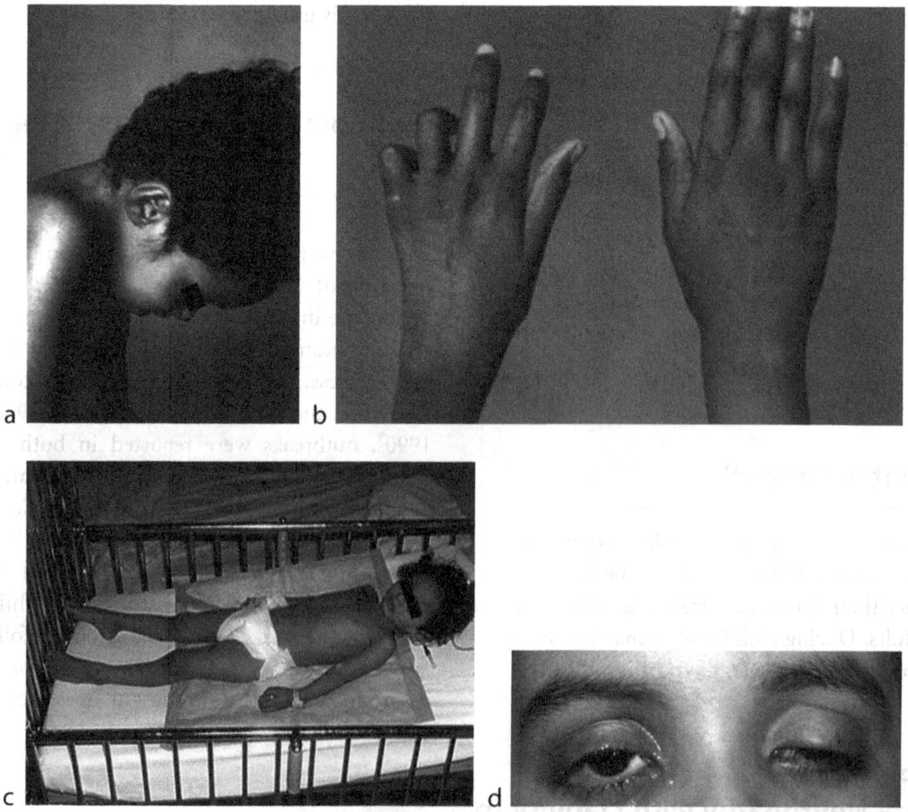

◘ Figure 372.1
(a) Weakness of neck extensors in a patient with diphtheritic polyneuropathy. (b) Left hand clawing following ulnar nerve mononeuritis in an adolescent with leprosy. Note the atrophy of the small muscles of the left hand and the hypothenar muscles. (c) Guillain-Barre syndrome (GBS). Nasogastric tube feeding was needed due to swallowing difficulties, and there is bilateral foot drop. (d) Bilateral ptosis of eyelids in Miller Fischer variant of GBS. The patient also had ophthalmoplegia

Diagnosis

Nose and throat swabs should be obtained from suspected cases and their close contacts, and cultured to isolate *C. diphtheriae*, determine the biotype (gravis, mitis, or intermedius), and whether the isolate produces toxin (toxigenicity test). Cultures are usually negative if the patient had received antibiotics before reporting to hospital. Nonviable *C. diphtheriae* organism can be detected by polymerase chain reaction (PCR) test from specimens taken after antibiotic therapy has been initiated. It can also confirm infection with toxigenic strains. Toxigenicity tests are not available in many laboratories and isolates need to be sent to a reference laboratory.

Neurophysiology studies show prolongation of distal motor latency, slowing of conduction velocity, and delayed F-wave latency. Because pathological changes appear later in the peripheral nerve segment than in the ganglia and root, the nerve conduction abnormalities might be mild even when the limb weakness is severe. Brainstem auditory evoked potentials (BAEP) may reveal auditory (VIII) nerve impairment, and autonomic tests may show impaired R-R variation on valsava testing.

Treatment

Diphtheritic polyneuropathy has no specific treatment. Attention should be paid to the airway and impending respiratory failure, which needs mechanical ventilation. Autonomic disturbances and circulatory collapse require prompt management.

Prognosis

The overall mortality of diphtheria is about 20% and is mainly due to mechanical airway obstruction or cardiac involvement. Mortality increases with severity of local disease and delay of administration of antitoxin. Gravis strain of *C. diphtheriae* accounts for the most severe and virulent disease. Other prognostic factors include the age and immunization status of the patient.

Prevention

The disease is preventable through routine childhood immunization programs and booster doses of diphtheria vaccine.

Leprosy

Leprosy is a systemic chronic granulomatous disease caused by infection with *Mycobacterium leprae*, and has a marked predilection for nerves and skin. The worldwide incidence of the disease is 2 cases per 10,000 populations and the disease is endemic in Africa and Asia, particularly in the Indian subcontinent. In northern Brazil, 10% of cases develop in children younger than 15 years.

Intimate person to person contact and vertical transmission have been considered the most likely routes of transmission. Hosts with high resistance to the organism develop paucibacillary (tuberculoid) leprosy, and those with low resistance develop multibacillary (lepromatous) leprosy. Borderline leprosy is characterized by the presence of single or multiple skin lesions with a raised central area.

The incubation period is long, averaging 5 years. The disease presents with hypopigmented lesions mostly observed in the cool areas of the body (earlobes, nose, dorsal surface of the hands, and feet). In multibacillary (lepromatous) leprosy, pure sensory polyneuritis develops in a glove and stocking distribution, with loss of touch, pain, and temperature sensation. Deep sensitivity is preserved. Pure mononeuritis is rare and enlargement of the peripheral nerves (such as the posterior auricular and ulnar nerves) may be present (➋ *Fig. 372.1b*). Nerve biopsy is useful for diagnosis and detection of persistent infection. To prevent antimicrobial resistance, treatment uses multidrug therapy including rifampin, dapsone, clofazimine, ofloxacin, minocycline, and clarithromycin. A single dose of bacilli Calmette-Guerin (BCG) vaccine was reported to be 50% protective in preventing leprosy.

Lyme Neuroborreliosis

Lyme disease is a multisystem infectious disease caused by a spirochete, *Borrelia burgdorferi* and affects, most commonly, the skin, nervous system, joints, and heart. It is transmitted from animals (deer) to man by the *Ixodes* tick. The disease is endemic in the US, with incidence averaging 9.1 cases per 100,000 persons. It is also prevalent throughout temperate Europe and Asia, and the estimated incidence was as high as 206 cases per 100,000 populations in Slovenia. Although few studies demonstrated multifocal perivascular inflammation in nerves, the pathophysiology of peripheral nerve and brain involvement remain to be clarified.

Clinical Manifestations

The first stage of the disease is characterized by an erythematous, macular, usually painless rash (erythema migrans), located in the area of the tick bite (the target sign). This is seen in 90% of infected patients and is associated with minor constitutional symptoms. The second stage of disseminated infection can involve the nervous system in approximately 15% of patients. This consists of part or all of the triad of lymphocytic meningitis, cranial neuropathy, and painful radiculitis. The facial nerve (CN VII) is the most commonly involved and may manifest as bilateral facial palsy. Other cranial nerves can be involved. The painful radiculitis may present as brachial plexopathy or lumbosacral plexopathy. A plexopathy resembling Guillain-Barre syndrome may also be seen. The third stage of persistent infection may be observed in untreated infection from one to several years. Its clinical features include chronic arthritis, chronic encephalomyelitis or a mild peripheral neuropathy, and focal mononeuropathy multiplex or polyradiculopathy.

Diagnosis and Differential Diagnosis

The diagnosis of Lyme disease rests on history of exposure in an endemic area, a clinical picture compatible with early Lyme disease (erythema migrans, constitutional flu-like symptoms) and laboratory demonstration of *Borrelia* infection. In suspected cases of neuroborreliosis, lumbar puncture is essential to evaluate the presence of specific antibodies to *B. burgdorferi*. Analysis of cerebrospinal fluid (CSF) will show significant pleocytosis, helping to differentiate the disease from Guillain-Barre syndrome, particularly when there is associated facial diplegia. In patients presenting with peripheral neuropathy, neurophysiologic studies are often consistent with axonal degeneration. Approximately 15–20% of patients with neurologic manifestations of Lyme disease show MRI abnormalities, usually in the form of punctuate lesions of the periventricular white matter.

Treatment

Treatment of neurologic Lyme disease is effectively accomplished with a 2-week course of parenteral penicillin, ceftriaxone or cefotaxime, or oral doxycycline. Approximately 90–95% of patients will be cured when receiving appropriate antimicrobial therapy early. A minority of patients, who had early treatment, develop late sequelae, but this rarely occurs in children.

Prevention

This is achieved by avoiding *Ixodes* tick bites through avoidance of infested areas, wearing appropriate clothing and using tick repellent with lower concentrations to avoid potential neurotoxicity in children.

Neurobrucellosis

On rare occasions, the nervous system is involved in systemic brucellosis. The clinical presentation of neurobrucellosis is diverse and reported neurological presentations in childhood range from acute to chronic forms. The former includes meningitis and meningoencephalitis, whereas the latter includes behavioral disturbance, brain abscess, stroke, myelitis, cerebellar ataxia (with or without cranial nerve involvement), radiculopathy, and peripheral neuropathy. Neurobrucellosis can present as Guillain-Barre syndrome, and bacteriological and serological tests should be part of the work-up for Guillain-Barre syndrome in endemic areas for brucellosis.

Toxic Neuropathies

Many toxins can induce polyneuropathy in children (➋ *Table 372.1*). Antimicrobial drugs that may cause neuropathy include nitrofurantoin, mainly in children with renal insufficiency. Isoniazid interferes with the metabolism of pyridoxine, which should be supplemented in patients treated with tuberculosis. Phenytoin neuropathy

Table 372.1
Exogenous toxins that cause polyneuropathy

Agent group	Name
Antimicrobial	Nitrofurantoin, isoniazid, ethambutol, ethionamide, metronidazole, amphotericin
Chemotherapy	Vincristine, cisplatin, chlorambucil, adenine arabinoside, cytosine arabinoside
Miscellaneous drugs	Phenytoin, lithium, thalidomide, amitriptyline, amiodarone, pyridoxine abuse
Metals	Lead, mercury, thallium, arsenic
Organic chemicals	Organophosphates, N-hexane, triorthocresyl phosphate, carbon monoxide, cyanate, hydroxyquinolines
Biological toxins	Tick bites, serum sickness, immunizations, cassava plant ingestion

is usually subclinical and most drug induced neuropathies are reversible following discontinuation of the causative drug. Lead poisoning rarely presents with peripheral neuropathy in children. Toxicity with other metals and organophosphates is associated with accidental ingestion of insecticides, usually in rural communities. Neuropathy from N-hexane results from glue sniffing, an addictive habit among adolescents. Cassava consumption causes tropical neuropathy because of its high cyanide content, whereas tick paralysis is seen in the US and Australia.

Guillain-Barre Syndrome

Definition/Classification

Guillain-Barre syndrome (GBS), or acute inflammatory demyelinating polyradiculoneuropathy (AIDP), is an inflammatory disease of the peripheral nervous system characterized by progressive motor weakness and areflexia. It can be divided into several forms based on the involved nerve fibers (motor, sensory and motor, cranial), and the predominant mode of fiber injury (demyelinating versus axonal). Autonomic and brainstem involvements are also common.

Epidemiology

Following virtual global eradication of poliomyelitis, GBS is the most common cause of acute paralysis in children. The overall incidence ranges from 0.6 to 2.4 cases per 100,000 population per year, whereas the incidence in individuals younger than 18 years ranges from 0.5 to 1.5 per 100,000. The disease has no racial predilection and males seem to be more susceptible to develop GBS, with a male to female ratio of 1.26:1. Seasonal predilections were observed in some countries with *Campylobacter*-related GBS (China, northern India, Bangladesh, northwestern Iran, Egypt, Mexico) occurring in the summer, and upper respiratory tract illness-related GBS occurring in winter. In children, the average age of onset ranges from 4 to 8 years, but can involve younger children.

Pathology and Pathophysiology

The mechanism of the disease is thought to involve an abnormal T-cell response triggered by a preceding infection. About two-thirds of cases of GBS follow an infection, usually viral (including cytomegalovirus, Epstein-Barr virus, HIV, hepatitis B or C, and smallpox-vaccinia), but sometimes mycoplasmal or bacterial (*Campylobacter jejuni*). An immune-mediated injury to the peripheral nerve occurs including cytotoxic T cell-mediated lyses and membrane damage from cytokines and free radicals. This is thought to be due to the molecular mimicry of the triggering pathogens, which resemble antigens on peripheral nerves including myelin P-2, ganglioside GQ1b, GM1, and GT1a. High titers of IgG anti-GM1, GM1b, or GD1a antibodies are more common in the acute motor axonal neuropathy (AMAN) than in the demyelinating forms of GBS. Acute motor axonal neuropathy is associated with infection by *C. jejuni*, the polysaccharide of which has a GM1 ganglioside-like structure. Other antecedent events associated with GBS include vaccination and surgery.

Clinical Manifestations

Symptoms

Onset of symptoms occurs within 2–4 weeks of illness or immunization. The preceding illness involves upper respiratory tract infection, fever, and muscle pains. History of vomiting is found in the demyelinating form of GBS and diarrhea is more likely to precede AMAN. The chief complaints include weakness and/or ataxia, associated with pain (in about half of affected children), dysesthesia, and urinary retention (in 10–15% of cases).

Signs

Weakness typically starts in the legs and ascends to the upper extremities, involving both sides of the body and evolving over a period of several days (➲ *Fig. 372.1c*). Evolution is complete after 2 weeks in half of the cases, after 3 weeks in over 80%, and after 4 weeks in over 90%. Weakness can be mild or severe leading to total paralysis and death from respiratory failure. Signs of autonomic dysfunction are common and include sinus tachycardia (in >50% of severe cases), bradycardia, orthostatic hypotension, and fluctuating hypertension and hypotension. Later in the disease course, objective sensory loss can be demonstrated in 75% of cases. Deep tendon jerks are usually absent or markedly diminished.

Other Variants of Guillain-Barre Syndrome

A small group of patients develop primary axonal degeneration associated with severe fulminant paralysis, sensory loss, and incomplete recovery. This variant is now termed *acute motor and sensory axonal neuropathy* (AMSAN). Conversely, the other variant of GBS (*acute motor axonal neuropathy* [AMAN]), usually follows antecedent *C. jejuni* infection and has a more rapid progression than the demyelinating form of GBS. Some patients with AMAN recover rapidly. The *Miller Fischer* variant of GBS is characterized by ophthalmoplegia, ataxia, areflexia, and relatively little weakness (➔ *Fig. 372.1d*). Some patients present with *polyneuritis cranialis* variant characterized by facial and ocular motor nerves involvement but infrequent limb weakness. The *pharyngeal-cervical-brachial* form of GBS is characterized by acute oropharyngeal, neck, and shoulder weakness, with sparring of the limb muscles. Another form is termed *acute sensory neuropathy of childhood* that presents as acute sensory loss but no weakness, although nerve conduction studies show features of demyelination. *Acute dysautonomia* variant, with no concomitant motor or sensory deficit, is rare. In this form of GBS, dysautonomia involves both the sympathetic and parasympathetic systems and may manifest with orthostatic hypotension, hypertension, sinus tachycardia, sweating abnormalities, and pupillary dysfunction.

Diagnosis

Support for the clinical diagnosis of GBS is provided by cerebrospinal (CSF) examination, neurophysiologic studies, and occasionally MRI findings. The CSF is acellular in all but 10% of patients; most of these have fewer than 10 cells/mm^3 and mild pleocytosis (10–50 cells/mm^3) may occasionally be seen. The finding of more than 50 cells/mm^3 on CSF examination suggests an alternative diagnosis. The CSF protein level rises about 1 week after the onset of symptoms, is usually elevated by 10 days, and reaches a peak in 3–4 weeks.

Nerve conduction studies (NCS) are frequently normal early. The most sensitive parameter of NCS is the F-wave. Within the first week of symptom onset, absent, impersistent, dispersed, or prolonged F response is seen in 88% of cases. This is compared to the finding, during this period, of increased distal latencies in 75%, conduction block in 58%, and reduced motor and sensory nerves conduction velocity in 50%. Electrodiagnostic criteria of the axonal forms of GBS are severe reduction in compound muscle action potential (CMAP) amplitudes, and minimal features of demyelination, with or without abnormalities in sensory nerves. F-wave latencies and blink response latencies are usually abnormal in Miller Fisher syndrome, but slowing of conduction velocities in the limbs may be absent. Electromyography (EMG) is contraindicated in GBS since the child may be harboring poliomyelitis, and EMG will lead to provocation paralysis.

Lumbosacral MRI may show, about 2 weeks after presentation of symptoms, enhancement of the cauda equina nerve roots with gadolinium in 95% of typical cases. The sensitivity of this study is 83% in acute GBS.

Serological Tests

High titers of IgG anti-GM1, GM1b, GD1a, and GalNac-GD1a was reported in 64% of children who develop the acute motor axonal neuropathy form of GBS, and was associated with more prolonged recovery and residual symptoms. Conversely, anti-GQ1b was found to be associated with Miller Fisher syndrome and anti-GT1a with pharyngeal-cervical-brachial variant of GBS.

Differential Diagnosis

Acute anterior horn infections by poliovirus, Coxsackie virus, and West Nile virus can produce an acute motor syndrome, but in contradistinction to GBS, CSF usually shows pleocytosis. Acute motor paralysis, associated with hyporeflexia or areflexia, can also be seen at the onset of transverse myelitis and acute spinal cord compression. The finding of a sensory level, associated with early involvements of the bowel or bladder, is supportive of these two diagnoses. In particular, acute spinal cord compression should not be missed to prevent the occurrence of a permanent cord infarct. Myasthenic crises and botulism may be considered when ophthalmoplegia is present in GBS. A history of fatiguabilily and fluctuating ocular symptoms favors the diagnosis of myasthenia, in which repetitive nerve stimulation on NCS shows decrement response. The presence of dilated unreactive pupil and severe constipation are indicative of botulism. Other causes of acute neuropathies include organophosphate poisoning, lead and heavy metals poisoning, and chemotherapy with vincristine. In endemic areas, tick paralysis can cause an ascending paralysis that dramatically improves after removal of ticks.

Treatment

Supportive therapy should be instituted immediately. Blood pressure, heart rate, temperature, respiratory capacity, blood gasses (when necessary), and urine output should be maintained. Children with oropharyngeal weakness with inability to protect their airway, vital capacity below 15 mL/kg body weight, or arterial pressure of oxygen below 70 mmHg should be considered for elective endotracheal intubation. These children and others with autonomic instability should be monitored in the intensive care unit. Orthostatic hypotension and urinary retention need judicious management. Measures to prevent infection (e.g., pneumonia and urinary tract infection), deep venous thrombosis, decubitus ulcers, and contractures should be instituted. After the acute phase, activity with physical and/or occupational therapy should be encouraged.

In children, immunomodulation using intravenous immunoglobulins (IVIG) is the treatment of choice. It reduces the severity of the disease and the duration of symptoms, although the long-term outcome may not be affected. It has several advantages over plasmapheresis, which is equally effective. Plasmapheresis is limited to children weighing more than 10–15 kg, requires a central line vascular access (which indicates intensive care unit management), and has several potential serious complications. These include bleeding due to depletion of clotting factors, autonomic instability, and hypercalcemia. Also, plasmapheresis would only remove free-circulating antibodies whereas IVIG can displace antibodies bound to motor nerves and possibly prevent complement activation. This may particularly be effective in cases of acute motor axonal neuropathy associated with positive autoantibodies.

The recommended dose of IVIG, which is administered by peripheral intravenous route, is 0.4 g/kg given daily for 5 days. This can lead to improvements within 2–3 days after start of therapy. When there are signs of rapid deterioration, IVIG can either be given as a single dose of 2 g/kg, or over 2 days using a single dose of 1 g/kg each day. Adverse reactions and effects to IVIG can occur in about 10% of patients and they are usually minor. These include fever, chills, wheezing and urticaria, headache, and 10% increased risk of aseptic meningitis.

Prognosis

Children with GBS have more favorable outcome compared to adults. The mortality rate is estimated to be less than 5% and usually follows respiratory failure, cardiac arrhythmias, and dysautonomia. The mortality rate is higher in areas with insufficient medical facilities. Approximately 90–95% of patients have full recovery within 3–12 months, 5–10% significant permanent disability and 5% have recurrence of GBS. Affected children with cranial nerve involvement, quadriplegia, and need for ventillatory support usually have significant delay in motor recovery. Patients with acute motor axonal neuropathy have longer recovery time compared to those who have the demyelinating variant of GBS. About 12% of patients may have recurrence 2–3 weeks after IVIG. When that happens, the differential must include *chronic inflammatory demyelinating polyneuritis (CIDP)*, which has a relapsing-remitting course in childhood, and unlike GBS, responds to steroids.

Hereditary Neuropathies

Charcot-Marie-Tooth Disease

Definition/Classification

Charcot-Marie-Tooth (CMT) disease or hereditary motor and sensory neuropathy was first recognized independently by Charcot and Marie in France and by Tooth in England.

Based on neurophysiologic and neuropathologic studies, two major types of CMT have been distinguished. The demyelinating form (CMT1) shows moderately to severely decreased nerve conduction velocity (NCV) of the median nerve (<38 m/s), whereas the axonal type (CMT2) exhibits normal or mildly reduced MCV (>38 m/s). Both CM1 and CMT2 are clinically indistinguishable and are usually inherited (in Europe and North America) as autosomal dominant disorders. A third form is autosomal dominant intermediate CMT, which is characterized by NCV overlapping those observed in CMT1 and CMT2, ranging between 25 and 50 m/s. The clinical, neurophysiological, and neuropathological phenotype of the X-linked forms of CMT is also intermediate between CMT1 and CMT2. The group of progressive motor and sensory axonal or demyelinating neuropathies with autosomal recessive inheritance is known as CMT4. Complex forms of CMT, in which the peripheral neuropathy is associated with other symptoms (ataxia, mental retardation, optic atrophy, pigmentary retinal degeneration) have also been recognized, and their pattern of inheritance and genes involved are being discovered. The autosomal dominantly inherited hereditary neuropathy with liability to pressure palsies (HNPP) is also included in the CMT group, and is clinically characterized by recurrent episodes of peripheral nerve palsies due to mechanical trauma.

Etiology

The disease is an inherited degenerative disorder of the peripheral nervous system with the primary pathological process affecting the axons of motor or sensory cells or both, or other myelin sheath and associated Schwann cells.

Epidemiology

Estimates of the frequency of CMT vary widely, yet the disease is one of the most common heritable neurologic disorders. A world survey estimated a prevalence of 10 cases per 100,000. The prevalence was reported to be 36 per 100,000 in Norway and 20 cases per 100,000 population in Finland. The incidence in Japan was estimated to be 10.8 per 100,000 population. The demyelinating autosomal dominant form (CMT1) accounts for about 50% of cases, the axonal autosomal dominant (CMT2) for 20–40%, whereas the X-linked inherited form constitutes 10–20% of cases. In contrast, in communities with a high percentage of consanguineous marriages (such as in North Africa and the Middle East), autosomal recessive CMT is likely to account for 30–50% of all CMT cases. In childhood, CMT constitutes approximately 40% of chronic neuropathies.

Pathogenesis

Charcot-Marie-Tooth (CMT) disease is inherited as autosomal dominant, X-linked or autosomal recessive. The inheritance pattern and molecular genetics constitutes the basis of classification of the various types of CMT. Nevertheless, mutations in a single gene are occasionally associated with both autosomal dominant and autosomal recessive inheritance, and/or both axonal, or demyelinating neuropathy. Tables ➋ *372.2–372.4* detail, respectively, the currently known molecular genetics of dominant, X-linked, and autosomal recessive forms of CMT. Demyelinating CMT is caused by diseases of the Schwann cell and the myelin, and the lesions are either diffuse or segmental (i.e., limited to the internode, which is formed by the part of the nerve depending on one Schwann cell). Diffuse demyelination leads to slowing of NCV, whereas segmental demyelination manifests as conduction block in some fibers and temporal dispersion as recorded on nerve conduction studies (NCS). Axonal CMT is characterized primarily by involvement of the axon and manifests with normal or only slightly slowed NCV.

The term *Dejerine–Sottas syndrome (DSS or CMT3)* was described as a hypertrophic polyneuropathy with onset in infancy or early childhood. It was first assumed to be inherited as autosomal recessive. Nevertheless, during the molecular biology era, patients with DSS were found to be heterozygous for point mutations in genes associated with CMT1 including *PMP22* (CMT1A), *MPZ* (CMT1B), and *EGR* (CMT1D). The entity designated as *congenital hypomyelination neuropathy (CHN)* is usually considered as a form of DSS, and can present as floppy infant syndrome. It is also associated with point mutations in *PMP22*, *MPZ*, and *EGR*. *Hereditary neuropathy with liability to pressure palsies* (HNPP) is a dominantly inherited disease characterized by acute onset of recurrent, painless, focal motor, and sensory neuropathy in a single nerve due to deletion or point mutations of *PMP22* gene.

Pathology

The pathology of CMT has mainly been studied by muscle or nerve biopsy. The rare postmortem examinations in CMT1 showed degeneration of the posterior columns, some loss of the anterior hom cells, and degeneration of the anterior and posterior spinal roots. Sural nerve biopsy shows reduced number of myelinated fibers, mainly those of large caliber with preservation of unmyelinated fibers. On electron microscopy, the classical onion bulbs are seen. These are thought to result from repeated demyelination and remyelination of Schwann cell wrappings around individual axons. In CMT2, the disease process is presumed to occur in the axon or cytoplasm of the anterior hom cell, and anterior hor cell loss has been found in two autopsies. Large-caliber fibers are reduced in number and the internodes are shortened and of irregular length. Three of the autosomal recessive forms of CMT (CMT4B1, CMT4B2, and CMT4H) are characterized by the presence, on sural nerve biopsy, of irregular redundant loops of focally folded myelin sheaths (➋ *Fig. 372.2a*). Onion bulbs are seen in CMT4A, CMT4C, CMT4D, CMT4F, and CMT4H. The onion bulbs in CMT4A are characteristically composed of basal laminae (➋ *Fig. 372.2b*).

Clinical Manifestations

Symptoms and Signs

The age of onset of CMT1 ranges from infancy (resulting in delayed walking) to the fourth or later decades but patients usually become symptomatic between age 5 and 25 years. The cardinal symptoms in children are difficulty in running or walking, or foot deformity. Gait disturbance includes clumsy walking, frequent falls, and high steppage gait. Foot deformity is characterized by pes cavus, often

Table 372.2

Genes and proteins involved in autosomal dominant demyelinating. (CMT1) and axonal (CMT2) forms of CMT

Type of CMT	Chromosomal locus of the gene	Gene symbol	Protein product
CMT1: Dominant; Demyelinating			
CMT1A	17p11	*PMP22*	Peripheral myelin protein 22
CMT1B	1q22	*MPZ*	Myelin P0 protein
CMT1C	16p13	*LITAF*	Lipopolysaccharide-induced tumor necrosis factor-alpha factor
CMT1D	10q21	*EGR2*	Early growth response protein 2
CMT2: Dominant; Axonal			
CMT2A1	1p36	*KIF1B*	Kinesin-like protein KIF1B
CMT2A2	1p36	*MFN2*	Mitofusin-2
CMT2B	3q13	*RAB7A*	Ras-related protein Rab-7a
CMT2B1	1q21	*LMNA*	Lamin A/C
CMT2B2	19q13.3	Unknown	Unknown
CMT2C	12q23–q24	*TRPV4*	Transient receptor potential cation channel subfamily V member 4
CMT2D	7p15	*GARS*	Glycyl-tRNA synthase
CMT2E*	8p21	*NEFL*	Neurofilament light polypeptide
CMT2F	7q11	*HSPB1*	Heat-shock protein beta-1
CMT2G	12q12–q13.3	Unknown	Unknown
CMT2L	12q24	*HSPB8*	Heat-shock protein beta-8

*Some individuals with mutations in NEFL, which typically cause CMT2E, have features of demyelination manifesting as slow nerve conduction velocities. This entity is referred to as CMT1F

Table 372.3

Genes and proteins involved in X-linked forms of CMT

Type of CMT	Chromosomal locus of the gene	Gene symbol	Protein product
CMTX1	Xq13	*GJB1*	Gap junction beta-1 protein (connexin 32)
CMTX2	Xp22.2	Unknown	Unknown
CMTX3	Xq26	Unknown	Unknown
CMTX4 (Cowchock syndrome)	Xq24–q26.1	Unknown	Unknown
CMTX5	Xq21.3–q24	*PRPS1*	Ribose-phosphate pyrophosphokinase 1

associated with hammer toes, but pes planus and valgus deviation of the feet may be present in some children. Symptoms are usually insidious and most patients are seen only after several years.

Difficulty in heel-walking is an early manifestation of the disease. Clinical examination reveals symmetrical peroneal muscle atrophy, later involving the calf muscles and eventually the lower third of the thigh, leading to stork leg appearance (*Fig. 372.2c*). Atrophy of the small muscles of the hands (including the thenar and hypothenar muscles) is usually late. When advanced, this leads to claw hands (*Fig. 372.2d*).

Loss of deep tendon reflexes (especially the ankle jerks) is a frequent early manifestation, and can be used to assess at risk children who have affected relatives. Sensory abnormalities are mild, and usually manifest after the age of 5 years. They are limited to subtle deficits in deep sensation, while pain and touch sensation are not impaired. Nerve enlargement is frequent whereas scoliosis, lordosis, and calf muscle hypertrophy may occur.

Table 372.4

Genes and proteins involved in autosomal recessive forms of CMT

Type of CMT	Chromosomal locus of the gene	Gene symbol	Protein product
CMT4A	8q13	*GDAP1*	Ganglioside-induced differentiation-associated protein 1
CMT4B1	11q22	*MTMR2*	Myotubularin-related protein 2
CMT4B2	11p15	*SBF2*	Myotubularin-related protein 13
CMT4C	5q32	*SH3TC2 (KIAA1985)*	SH3 domain and tetratricopeptide repeats containing protein 2
CMT4D (Lom)	8q24	*NDRG1*	Protein NDRG1
CMT4E	10q21	*EGR2*	Early growth response protein 2
CMT4F	19q13	*PRX*	Periaxin
CMT4H	12p11.2	*FGD4*	FYVE, RhoGEF, and PH domain-containing protein 4
CMT4J	6q21	*FIG4*	Polyphosphoinositide phosphatase

The full clinical picture of CMT1 may not occur until the second decade of life, progression is slow over many years, and arrests are common and often prolonged.

The age of onset of hereditary neuropathy with liability to pressure palsies (HNPP) ranges from the first to the eighth decade of life (typically the third or fourth decade), but can present at birth. The recurrent acute mononeuropathy is often related to minor nerve compression, usually after resting on a limb in an awkward position, such as squatting or sitting cross-legged. Affected nerves at sites of anatomic vulnerability to compression include the peroneal nerve at the fibular neck, the ulnar nerve at the cubital tunnel, the radial nerve at the spiral groove of the humerus, and the median nerve at the carpal tunnel. The brachial plexus may also be involved. Examination between episodes of focal weakness may be normal or mildly abnormal.

The clinical features of CMT2 are similar to those of CMT1 but onset is usually later, during the second or third decade, and the course of the disease is slower. Phenotypic variation is common between and within affected families. Areflexia, pes cavus and hammer toes may be less common than in CMT1, but nerve hypertrophy is absent.

In males, symptoms of CMTX1 usually begin in childhood or adolescence. Females are often asymptomatic but may have late onset of mild symptoms because of predominant inactivation of the X chromosomes that bears the normal allele of the gene. Atrophy, particularly of intrinsic hand muscles, paresthesia, and sensory loss, may be more common in this form of CMT than other subtypes.

The onset of the autosomal recessive type of CMT (CMT4) is significantly earlier than either CMT1 or CMT2. In its severe form, it overlaps with Dejerine–Sottas syndrome and can present at birth with congenital hypotonia.

CMT4A was first identified in families in Tunisia. It starts in early infancy with delayed motor development, and distal muscle weakness and atrophy of feet that progress to involve the proximal muscles by the end of the first decade. Atrophy of the hand muscles may occur later and loss of ambulation is often by the age of 30 years. Scoliosis and skeletal deformities may occur. The disease is associated with *GDAP1* mutations, which cause both demyelinating and axonal phenotypes. The axonal form is linked to vocal cord and diaphragmatic paralysis with onset in midlife.

CMT4B1 was first described in an Italian family. Mutations in the causative gene (the first identified autosomal recessive CMT gene) were found in families of Italian and Saudi Arabian ancestory. Onset is usually before the age of 4 years with progressive distal and proximal weakness of the lower limbs. Pes cavus foot deformity is common, and facial, bulbar, and diaphragmatic weaknesses are known associations. Adults frequently require wheelchairs by age 20 years and death may occur as early as the end of the second decade, or in the fourth to fifth decade.

A summary of the salient clinical features of the subtypes of CMT4 is depicted in (➋ *Table 372.5*).

Investigations

Electrodiagnostic Studies

When carefully done, electrodiagnostic studies (including nerve conduction study [NCS] and electromyography [EMG]) are almost always abnormal in cases of CMT.

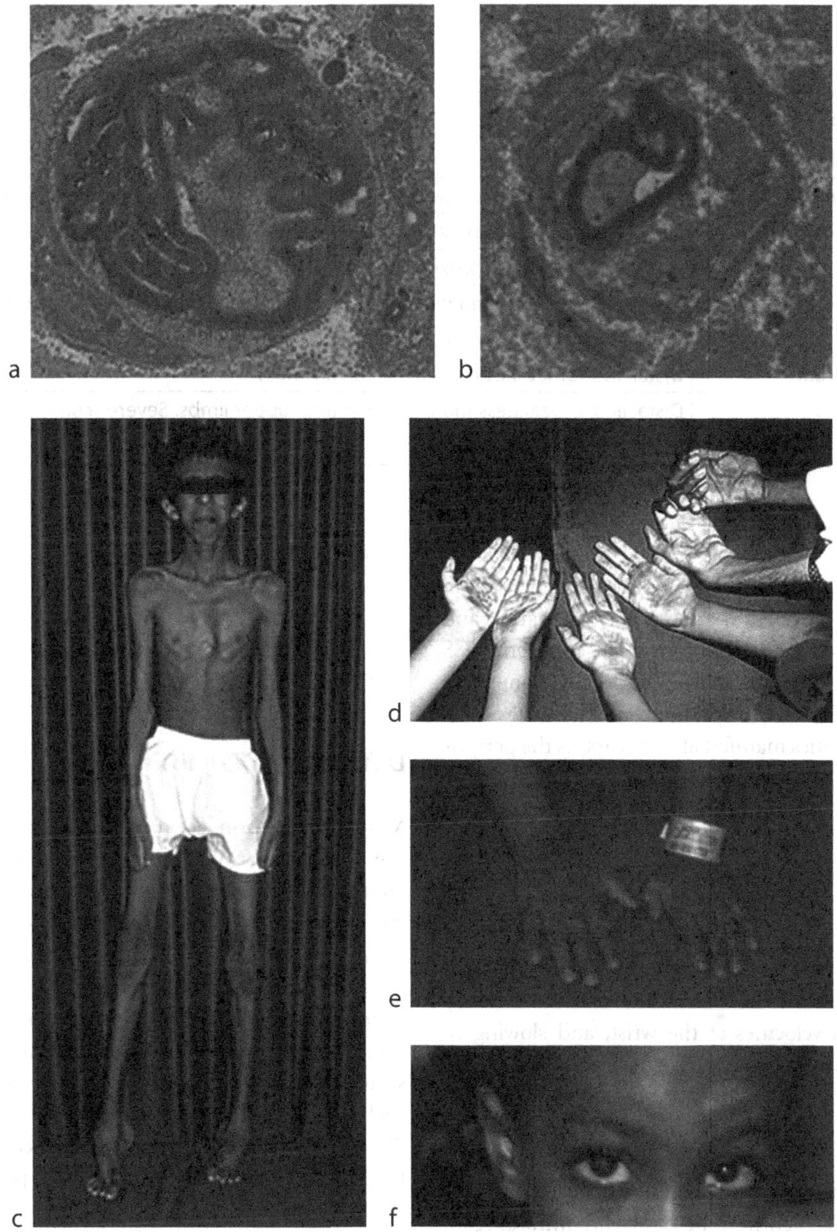

Figure 372.2

(a & b) Electron microscopic examinations of sural nerve biopsies showing (a) redundant loops of focally folded myelin sheaths, and (b) onion bulb formation. (c) Symmetrical distal muscle atrophy in Charcot-Marie-Tooth (CMT) disease. Note the stork leg appearance. (d) Progressive atrophy of the small muscles of the hands in two children and an adult from a family with CMT4B1. Note the development of claw hands in the elder patient to the right. (e) Healed traumatic hand injuries in a child with hereditary sensory and autonomic neuropathy. Note the resorption of the left thumb. (f) The patient had neuropathic keratitis leading to bilateral corneal opacities. Note the traumatic scar over the left eye-brow

Median motor nerve conduction velocity (NCV) is below 38 m/s in CMT1 and above in CMT2. Nerve conduction slowing is diffuse and uniform in CMT1 compared to acquired neuropathies where conduction block and temporal dispersion are common. F-wave responses are usually prolonged and EMG shows evidence of denervation. In CMT2, median NCV is typically above 38 m/s, and is associated with reduced compound muscle action

Table 372.5
Main clinical features of CMT4

Disease	Age at onset	Main clinical features
CMT4A	<3 years	Distal and proximal limb weakness, vocal cord, and diaphragmatic paralysis
CMT4B1	<4 years	Distal and proximal limb weakness. Facial, bulbar, and diaphragmatic weakness
CMT4B2	First decade	Distal and sometimes proximal limb weakness. Early-onset glaucoma
CMT4C	First or second decade	Distal and sometimes proximal limb weakness. Progressive, often severe, and early scoliosis
CMT4D	First decade	Distal and proximal limb weakness, sensorineural hearing loss, and tongue atrophy
CMT4E	Birth	Congenital hypotonia. Dejerine–Sottas syndrome-like presentation
CMT4F	First decade	Distal and sometimes proximal limb weakness
CMT4H	1–2 years	Distal limbs, weakness more in lower than upper limbs. Severe scoliosis
CMT4J	First decade	Severe childhood-onset demyelinating neuropathy

amplitude (CMAP) and reduced sensory nerve action potential (SNAP). Sural nerve sensory responses can be absent and EMG shows signs of chronic denervation. Nevertheless, the distinction between demyelinating and axonal CMT may not always be clear. In children, NCS shows normal results at birth, except for congenital hypomyelination neuropathy and Dejerine–Sottas syndrome. Abnormalities manifest at 2–4 years, as the peripheral nervous system matures, even in asymptomatic patients. The parents should always have NCS to ascertain asymptomatic neuropathy in either of them. In autosomal recessive forms (CMT4), both parents have normal findings on NCS.

Nerve conduction studies in hereditary neuropathy with liability to pressure palsies (HNPP) reveal bilaterally delayed median distal motor latency (DML), slowed median sensory nerve conduction velocities at the wrist, and slowing of peroneal nerve motor conduction velocity or DML.

Sural nerve biopsy is not routinely performed in children, but is occasionally helpful in establishing the diagnosis by showing relatively characteristic lesions in CMT1. It was found to be extremely helpful in autosomal recessive forms of CMT. Identification of myelin outfolding on sural nerve biopsy in two Saudi Arabian families lead to the recognition, and a later discovery in a joint research involving Italian families, of the gene for CMT4B1, which was the first identified gene for the recessive forms of CMT. The axonal form of CMT4A due to GDAP1 mutations is characterized by the presence of onion bulbs composed of basal laminae.

Imaging Studies

Enlarged nerves, both at the level of the spinal roots and also in the limbs, can be shown by magnetic resonance imaging (MRI), as well as subclinical central nervous abnormalities in several subtypes of CMT. Significant involvement of peroneal nerve-innervated muscles was seen in CMT1A patients, in contrast to fatty infiltration involving superficial posterior compartment in CMT2A cases.

Differential Diagnosis

Mental retardation, seizures, dementia, and blindness are not features of CMT and their presence should suggest another diagnosis. Acquired, especially treatable, causes of peripheral neuropathy should also be excluded such as vitamins B_1, B_6, B_{12}, folate, or E deficiencies. Vitamin E deficiency may be due to abetalipoproteinemia and biliary insufficiency that prevents normal emulsion of fat in the bowel lumen resulting in poor absorption associated with steatorrhea. Other diseases leading to fat malabsorption, such as cystic fibrosis and celiac disease, chronic liver disease (especially ductal hypoplasia) can lead to vitamin E deficiency. Other causes of acquired peripheral neuropathy include lead poisoning and heavy metal intoxication, leprosy, neurosyphilis, and immune-mediated neuropathies such as chronic inflammatory demyelinating polyneuropathy (CIDP).

Giant axonal neuropathy is a chronic polyneuropathy of childhood accompanied by characteristically kinky hair, curly eyelashes, and unique posture of legs. Sural nerve biopsy shows typical findings on electron microscopy, with the axons being distended by tightly woven neurofilaments. It is inherited as autosomal recessive and is caused by mutations encoding a protein named gigaxonin.

Hereditary neuropathies may constitute part of more complex neurological diseases involving the central nervous system (CNS). The autosomal recessively inherited

Friedreich's ataxia may present with sensory loss, depressed tendon reflexes, high-arched feet, and hammer toe. Some of the other degenerative disorders are either treatable or deserve accurate diagnosis to anticipate associated complications outside the CNS. These are briefly mentioned in (➋ *Table 372.6*).

Treatment

Treatment of CMT is symptomatic and therapy should focus on the management and prevention of the development of the physical disability related to CMT. Affected children are better evaluated by a multidisciplinary team

Table 372.6
Complex hereditary neurological diseases associated with neuropathies

Disorder	Brief clinical features	Suggestive diagnostic investigations
Mitochondrial disorders		
NARP	Neuropathy, ataxia, retinitis, pigmentosa	Muscle biopsy for biochemical, morphological, and mitochondrial DNA abnormalities
MNGIE	Mitochondrial neurogastrointestinal encephalomyopathy	Muscle biopsy for biochemical, morphological, and mitochondrial DNA abnormalities
Peroxisomal disorders		
Refsum disease	Ataxia, areflexia, atypical retinitis pigmentosa, deafness, ichthyosis, disorders of cardiac function	Very-long-chain fatty acids and phytanic acid
Juvenile adrenoleukodystrophy	Dementia, personality disorder, sensory ataxia, areflexia	Very-long-chain fatty acids
Leukodystrophies		
Krabbe	Floppiness, loss of milestones, seizures, ocular movement abnormalities	Galactocerebrosidase
Metachromatic	Progressive spastic diplegia, optic atrophy	Arylsulphatase A assay
Sialidosis type 1	Action and intension myoclonus, retinal cherry red spot, no dysmorphism, normal intelligence	Sialidase (α-neuraminidase) assay
Pelizaeus–Merzbacher disease	Rotary nystagmus, hypotonia, dystonia, pyramidal and cerebellar signs, optic atrophy	Intense signal from white matter on T2-weighted MRI sequence and absence of myelin signal on T1-weighted MRI sequence
DNA Processing(damage/repair) disorders		
Xeroderma pigmentosum	Photosensitivity, poikiloderma, skin cancer, hearing loss, cognitive impairment, microcephaly, neurodegeneration	BAEP
Cockayne syndrome	Photosensitivity, growth retardation, hearing loss, cognitive impairment, progeria, microcephaly, neurodegeneraion	Cerebellar atrophy on MRI
Ataxia telangiectasia	Ataxia, oculomotor apraxia, recurrent sinubronchial infections, immune defects, neurodegeneration, choreoathetosis, malignancy	Elevated levels of AFP and CEA, immunoglobulins profile (dysgammaglobulinemia)
Ataxia telangiectasia-like disease	Ataxia, oculomotor aprxia, neurodegeneration. Choreoathelosis	Normal levels of AFP, cerebellar atrophy on MRI
Spinocerebellar ataxia with neuropathy type 1 (SCAN1)	Ataxia, epilepsy (some cases)	Cerebellar atrophy on MRI
Ataxia and oculomotor apraxia type 2 (AOA2)	Ataxia, oculomotor apraxia, neurodegeneration	Normal levels of AFP, cerebellar atrophy on MRI

Abbreviations: AFP: alpha-fetoprotein; CEA: carcinoembryonic antigen; MRI: magnetic resonance imaging that includes pediatric neurologists, orthopedic surgeons, and physical and occupational therapists. Orthotics and ankle-foot orthosis (AFO) frequently enable patients to continue performing their daily activities while preventing falls that might result in injuries. Special shoes, including those with good ankle support can delay the need for ankle braces. Orthopedic surgery to correct severe pes cavus deformity and scoliosis might be needed at a certain stage. Exercise is encouraged within the child's capacity, daily heel cord stretching exercises are helpful in preventing Achilles tendon stretching, and obesity should be avoided because it makes walking more difficult. Medical conditions, situations, and interventions which can lead to systemic or focal neuropathies should be avoided or early managed. These include diseases such as diabetes mellitus and hypothyroidism, prolonged immobilization of limbs during surgery, vitamin deficiencies, carpal tunnel syndrome, and neurotoxic drugs. Symptoms of sleep apnea, vocal cord, and bulbar paralysis should be detected early and managed promptly.

Maladjustment and depression, especially in teenagers, should also be detected and managed. The importance of investing in education should be emphasized since CMT does not usually affect intellect, life span, or independent living.

Treatment with steroids (prednisone) or intravenous immunoglobulin has been reported to improve a few individuals with CMT1 who develop sudden worsening of their peripheral neuropathy. Other therapies under investigation include the effects of neurotrophin-3 on CMT1A patients. Ascorbic acid reduced PMP22 over expression and ameliorated the phenotype in a transgenic CMT1A mouse model, whereas a progesterone antagonist improved neuropathy in a transgenic rat model of CMT1A. A clinical trial is underway to address the possible role of high doses of ascorbic acid in CMT1A patients.

Prognosis

With the exception of CMT4, Dejerine–Sottas syndrome (DSS) and congenital hypomyelination neuropathy (CHN), life expectancy is normal in most patients with CMT. Nevertheless, the degree of disability varies according to the CMT subtype, and between and within families. Patients with CMT4A and CMT4B1 often require wheelchairs by the end of the second or third decade; and those with CMT4B1 may die by the third to fifth decade. Individuals with DSS are often disabled in early childhood and CHN may lead to early death. Approximately 10% of patients with HNPP have incomplete recovery from the acute nerve palsies, and cases of respiratory failure have been reported.

Prevention

Since CMT does not usually affect intellect, independent living, or life span, most affected parents choose to have children. Prenatal diagnosis for pregnancies at increased risk for some types of CMT4 is possible by chorionic villous sampling (at 10–12 weeks of gestation) and by amniocentesis (by about 15–18 weeks). Preimplantation genetic diagnosis may be available for families in which the disease-causing mutations have been identified.

Hereditary Sensory and Autonomic Neuropathy

Definition/Classification/Etiology

Hereditary sensory and autonomic neuropathy (HSAN) forms part of the inherited peripheral neuropathies where sensory dysfunction prevails and autonomic nervous system is involved to a varying degree. They are clinically and genetically heterogeneous with controversy over terminology. Based on clinical presentations, the distinct populations of affected nerve fibers, associated genes, and inheritance pattern, five types of HSAN have been defined (➋ *Table 372.7*). With the exception of HSAN type I, which is transmitted as autosomal dominant, the other types are transmitted as autosomal recessive traits.

Epidemiology

Type I variant of HSAN is the most frequent and has been described in Portuguese, Belgian, Australian, and English families. HSAN III (Riley–Day syndrome) is most prevalent among individuals of Eastern European Jewish extraction, with incidence of 1 per 3,600 live births. HSAN IV, also known as congenital insensitivity to pain and anhidrosis (CIPA), has been described in most ethnic groups but seems to have high prevalence in Bedouin Arabs living in Israel. Types II and V are rare autosomal recessively inherited forms of HSAN.

Table 372.7
Genes and loci associated with various types of hereditary sensory and autonomic neuropathy (HSAN)

HMSN type	Inheritance	Locus	Gene
HSAN I	Autosomal dominant	9q22.2	*SPTLC1*
HSAN II	Autosomal recessive	12p13.3	*HSN2*
HSAN III (Riley–Day syndrome, familial dysautonomia)	Autosomal recessive	9q31	*IKBKAP*
HSAN IV (Congenital insensitivity to pain and antidrosis [CIPA])	Autosomal recessive	1q21–22	*NTRK1*
HSAN V	Autosomal recessive	1p13.1	*NGFB*

Pathogenesis/Pathology

Mutations in the genes associated with HSAN are thought to lead to malfunction in vesicular transport along the axons. In humans, sensory axons can extend for one or more meters and most proteins must be transported along the axon to reach their destination at the cell bodies of nociceptive neurons. A founder mutation (C133N mutation) estimated to have originated 900–1,600 years ago, was found in British families with the dominantly inherited HSAN1. Pathological examination of this type showed degeneration of the dorsal root ganglia and the spinal dorsal roots supplying the lower limbs. Histopathological findings in HSAN III include loss of neurons in the posterior root, dorsolateral tract (Lissauer tract), and intermediolateral gray columns. The Lissauer tract and dorsal spinal roots are also affected in HSAN IV.

Clinical Manifestations: Symptoms, Signs

Symptoms of HSAN1 appear in late childhood or adolescence with a progressive loss of sensation in the lower extremities leading to acromutilations following episodes of cellulitis and trophic ulcerations of the feet. Spontaneous stabbing (lancinating) pain may occur. Initially, there is predominant loss of pain and temperature sensation with preservation of tactile sensation. Later, all sensory modalities are lost and the distal upper limbs may become involved. Variable distal motor weakness and wasting is also a feature of the disease.

The onset of HSAN II is either congenital or during first to second decades. There is universal absence of pain sensation resulting in burns and mutilations of the lips, tongue, and fingertips. There are also painless fractures, especially of the metatarsals, a delayed development and lack of fungiform papillae on the tongue. Bladder sensation may be impaired leading to its distension, and hearing loss affects 30% of patients.

The clinical manifestations of HSAN III are mainly due to autonomic disturbances. Sucking difficulties, a poor cry, vomiting, and hypotonia are present from birth. Affected children also have pain and temperature sensory loss, alacrima (loss of overflow tears), excessive sweating, and unstable temperature and blood pressure. On examination, they have absence of fungiform papillae on the tongue, and diminished or absent deep tendon reflexes. Death, which occurs in infancy or childhood, is usually caused by bouts of apnea and pneumonia. Intelligence remains normal but the occurrence of kyphoscoliosis, esophageal dilation, and impaired gastric motility are frequent.

The onset of HSAN IV is congenital with markedly decreased or absent sweating leading to episodic unexplained fever and hyperpyrexia, often related to environmental temperature. Insensitivity to pain is universal and promotes repeated traumatic and thermal injuries, and severe mutilations of the hands and feet (➲ *Fig. 372.2e*). Tongue-biting and osteomyelitis, especially of the lower extremities are frequent. Despite normal lacrimation, affected children are prone to neuropathic keratitis, associated with absent corneal sensation and very poor corneal healing, and resulting in corneal ulceration and opacities (➲ *Fig. 372.2f*). Affected children usually have mild mental retardation, frequently associated with hyperactivity and emotional liability. Examination reveals sequelae of anhidrosis in the form of calloused appearance of the skin, lichenification of the palms, areas of hypotrichinosis on the scalp, and dystrophic nail changes. Muscle power and deep tendon reflexes are usually preserved.

The phenotype of HSAN V is similar to that of HSAN IV with the exception of the presence of less severe anhidrosis and lack of mental retardation in patients with HSAN V. Affected patients have severe loss of deep pain perception, which prevents them from recognizing pain from bone fractures and joint injuries resulting in destroyed joints in childhood.

Diagnosis

The congenital or early-onset forms of HSAN can be suspected when an infant shows insensitivity or indifference to pain inflicted by the first intramuscular routine immunization injection. Attention should also be drawn to the condition when there are bouts of recurrent unexplained fever.

Investigations

Neurophysiologic Tests

Neurophysiologic tests that can be used to assess the various types of HSAN include nerve conduction studies (NCS) and electromyography (EMG). Sympathetic skin responses (SSR), utilizing the routine EMG equipment, can also be used to identify indirect evidence of sweat production via measurement of changes in skin conductance on the palm/sole in response to an electrical stimulus. Another helpful test is quantitative sensory testing (QST), which permits comparison of sensory thresholds by using vibration and temperature perception to assess both large- and small-fiber modalities. However, QST needs cooperation of the patient, which is usually lacking in young children.

Because the involved fibers in HSAN are small myelinated and unmyelinated fibers, motor nerve conduction velocity (NCV) and EMG are usually normal. Nevertheless, sensory NCV is low or absent in all forms except in HSAN V, and EMG may show features of chronic axonal neuropathy in HSAN I. Sympathetic skin responses (SSR) were reported to be absent in HSAN IV and temperature threshold is increased in HSAN V.

The histamine test is also a valuable diagnostic tool. This is done by injecting 0.1 ml of histamine (in a concentration of 0.275 mg histamine phosphale/ml) intradermally using a fine needle tuberculin syringe. In normal individuals, there is a bright red histamine flare (due to capillary vasodilation) within 5 min. Dyautonomic reaction demonstrates only a narrow areola surrounding the wheel. This lack of axon flare is universal and consistent in patients with HSAN II, III, and IV.

Histologic Findings

Sural nerve biopsy can indicate the diagnosis in HSAN by revealing the selective loss of particular fiber types. In HSAN I, there is reduction in the number of small myelinated and unmyelinated fibers, associated with loss of large myelinated fibers. HSAN II is characterized by severe reduction in the number of myelinated axons but unmyelinated fibers are usually normal or slightly diminished. Loss of unmyelinated and myelinated fibers in peripheral nerves, associated with decreased number of large myelinated fibers, characterizes HSAN III. Histopathological findings are striking in HSAN IV by the visual absence of unmyelinated nerve fibers in the peripheral nerves. In HSAN V, there is selective decrease in small myelinated fibers and mild reduction in unmyelinated fibers. Skin biopsy is useful in HSAN IV (congenital insensitivity to pain with anhidrosis) and shows lack of nerve fibers in the epidermis and only a few hypotrophic and uninnervated sweat glands in the dermis.

Treatment

Management of HSAN is symptomatic and preventative. Ulcero-mutilating complications are the most serious and should follow the guidelines given for diabetic foot care. Removal of pressure to ulcers, eradication of infection, and specific protective footwear are of paramount importance to avoid further complications like amputations. Careful daily inspection for unrecognized injury is important. Significant feeding problems, especially when associated with gastroesophageal reflux are managed with gastrostomy and fundoplication. The risk of aspiration pneumonia should be minimized in HSAN III by attention to posture and by meticulous precautions during feeding. Blood pressure liability (postural hypotension and hypertension) should be managed promptly. Alacrema and corneal analgesia, which predispose to corneal ulcerations, require frequent administration of topical lubricants. Control of hyperthermia in HSAN IV is important using acetaminophen and/or ibuprofen or direct cooling in a bath. Smoothing of the teeth or extraction, to prevent self-mutation of the tongue and lips, might be needed in some children. Chlorpromazine has been found to be effective in controlling bouts of rages, hyperactivity, and irritability, as well as behavior modification. Families of affected children need considerable psychological support.

Prognosis

HSAN I is a slowly progressive disease and does not influence life expectancy. Prognosis for the other congenital types is improving with time and increasing numbers of patients are reaching adulthood. This followed improved diagnosis and appropriate interventions and treatments. Understanding the pathomechanism underlying HSAN by knowing specific gene actions will have an impact on definitive therapeutic interventions.

Prevention

Prenatal diagnosis can be done in families where the diseases causing mutation is known. Nevertheless, termination of pregnancy is challenged with ethical justification, especially in HSAN I. Preimplantation genetic diagnosis is also another reproductive option following identification of the disease-causing mutation in the specific family.

References

Axelrod FB, Gold-von Simon G (2007) Hereditary sensory and autonomic neuropathies: types II, III and IV. Orphanet J Rare Dis 2:29 (doc:10.1186/1750-1172-2-39)

Bolino A, Muglia M, Conforti FL et al (2000) Charcot-Marie-Tooth type 4B is caused by mutations in the gene encoding myotubulism-related protein 2. Nat Genet 25:17–19

Burns J, Ouvrier RA, Yiu EM et al (2009) Ascorbic acid for Charcot-Marie-Tooth disease type 1A in children: a randomized, double-blind, placebo-controlled, safety and efficacy trial. Lancet Neurol 8:537–544 [Best Evidence]

Elovaara I, Apostolski S, van Doom P et al (2008) EFN guidelines for the use of intravenous immunoglobulin in treatment of neurological diseases: EFNS task force on the use of intravenous immunoglobulin in treatment of neurological diseases. Eur J Neurol 15:893–908 [Guideline]

Imbiriba EB, Hurtado-Guerero JC, Garnelo L, Levino A, Cunha Mda G, Pedrosa V (2008) Epidemiological profile of leprosy in children under 15 in Manaus (Northern Brazil), 1998–2005. Rev Saúde Pública 42:1021–1026

Korinthenberg R, Schess J, Kirschner J (2007) Clinical presentation and course of childhood Guillain-Barre syndrome: a prospective multicentre study. Neuropediatrics 38:10–17

Martin JJ, Brice A, Van Broeckhoven C (1999) 4th Workshop of the European CMT-Consortium-62nd ENMC International Workshop. Rare forms of charcot-marie-tooth disease and related disorders. 16–18 October 1998, Soestduinen, The Netherlands. Neurolmuscl Disord 9:279–287

Salih MA, Suliman GI, Hassan HS (1981) Complications of diphtheria seen during the 1978 outbreak in Khartoum. Ann Trop Paediatr 1:97–101

Schroder JM (2006) Neuropathy of Charcot-Marie-Tooth and related disorders. Neuromuscular Med 8:23–42

Verhoeven K, Timmerman V, Mauko B, Pieber TR, De Jonghe P, Auer-Grumbach M (2006) Recent advances in hereditary sensory and autonomic neuropathies. Curr Opin Neurol 19:474–480

Walton C, Interthal H, Hirano R, Salih MAM, Takashima H, Boerkoel CF (2010) Spinocerebellar ataxia with axonal neuropathy. In: Ahmad SI (ed) Diseases of DNA repair. Springer, New York, pp. 75–83

Yuki N (2007) Ganglioside mimicry and peripheral nerve disease. Muscle Nerve 35:691–711

Online Resourses

genetests.org

9783642022012VOL05